Handbuch
der inneren Medizin

Begründet von L. Mohr und R. Staehelin

Herausgegeben von
H. Schwiegk

Dritter Band: Verdauungsorgane
Fünfte, völlig neu bearbeitete und erweiterte Auflage

Teil 1 Esophagus

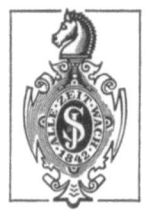

Springer-Verlag Berlin Heidelberg New York 1974

Diseases
of the Esophagus

By

G. Vantrappen and J. Hellemans

With Contributions of

C. Debray · W. Deloof · V. J. Desmet · D. A. W. Edwards · J. Fevery
G. Fransen · K. Geboes · J. De Groote · E. Hafter · A. Hancy
P. Heitmann · P. Housset · J. Janssens · A. Lacquet
H. P. Lazar · B. T. Le Roux · H. Monges · J. G. Pearson · W. Pelemans
E. Ponette · J. Pringot · J. A. Rinaldo · J. De Schryver
E. C. Texter · G. N. Tytgat · P. Valembois · F. Vilardell · B. S. Wolf

With 358 partly coloured Figures

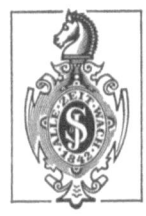

Springer-Verlag Berlin Heidelberg New York 1974

GASTON R. VANTRAPPEN, M.D., Agg. H.O. Professor of Medicine

JAN J. HELLEMANS, M.D., Agg. H.O. Professor of Medicine

Department of Medical Research and Department of Medicine,
Akademisch Ziekenhuis St. Rafaël, University of Leuven, B-3000 Leuven

ISBN-13: 978-3-642-65839-6   e-ISBN-13: 978-3-642-65837-2
DOI: 10.1007/978-3-642-65837-2

A special US edition is available under the title
G. VANTRAPPEN   J. HELLEMANS, Diseases of the Esophagus

Library of Congress Cataloging in Publication Data
Diseases of the Esophagus
(Verdauungsorgane, T. 1) (Handbuch der inneren Medizin, Bd. 3, T. 1)
Bibliography: p.
Esophagus—Diseases. II. VANTRAPPEN, G., ed. III. HELLEMANS, J., ed. IV. Series: Handbuch der inneren Medizin.
Bd. 3. T. 1.
RC41.H342 Bd. 3, T. 1 [RC815.7] 616'.026 74–13240

List of Contributors

DEBRAY, C., M.D., Professeur, Médecin des Hôpitaux, Chef du Service de Gastro-entérologie, Hôpital Bichat, Paris, France

DELOOF, W., M.D., Department of Medicine, Akademisch Ziekenhuis St. Rafaël, University of Leuven, 3000 Leuven, Belgium

DESMET, V. J., M.D., Professor of Pathology, Department of Medical Research and Department of Pathology, Akademisch Ziekenhuis St. Rafaël, University of Leuven, 3000 Leuven, Belgium

EDWARDS, D. A. W., M.D., F.R.C.P., MRC Department of Clinical Research, University College, Hospital Medical School, University Street London WC1E 6JJ, Great Britain

FEVERY, J., M.D., Associate Professor of Medicine, Department of Medical Research and Department of Medicine, Akademisch Ziekenhuis St. Rafaël, University of Leuven, 3000 Leuven, Belgium

FRANSEN, G., M.D., Department of Surgery, Akademisch Ziekenhuis St. Rafaël, University of Leuven, 3000 Leuven, Belgium

GEBOES, K., M.D., Department of Medical Research and Department of Medicine, Akademisch Ziekenhuis St. Rafaël, University of Leuven, 3000 Leuven, Belgium

GROOTE, De, J., M.D., Professor of Medicine, Department of Medical Research and Department of Medicine, Akademisch Ziekenhuis St. Rafaël, University of Leuven, 3000 Leuven, Belgium

HAFTER, E., M.D., Spezialarzt für innere Medizin F.M.H., Magen-Darmkrankheiten, Tödistrasse 36, CH-8002 Zürich, Switzerland

HANCY, A., M.D., 27, Bd. d'Athènes, F-1300 Marseille, France

HEITMANN, P., M. D., Krankenanstalten Düren, Abteilung für innere Krankheiten, 516 Düren, Germany

HELLEMANS, J., M.D. Agg. H.O., Professor of Medicine, Department of Medical Research, University of Leuven, Leuven, Belgium; Chief Geriatric Unit, Department of Medicine, Akademisch Ziekenhuis St. Rafaël, 3000 Leuven, Belgium

HOUSSET, P., M.D., Attaché de consultation à L'Hôpital Bichat, Membre de la Société Nationale Francaise de Gastro-Entérologie, Paris, France

JANSSENS, J., M.D., Aangesteld Navorser NFWO, Department of Medical Research and Department of Medicine, Akademisch Ziekenhuis St. Rafaël, University of Leuven, 3000 Leuven, Belgium

LACQUET, A., M.D., Professor of Surgery, Department of Surgery and Department of Surgical Pathology, Akademisch Ziekenhuis St. Rafaël, University of Leuven, 3000 Leuven, Belgium

LAZAR, H. P., M.D., 700 North Michigan, Chicago, Ill, 60611, USA

LE ROUX, B. T., Ch.M., F.R.C.S.E., Professor of Thoracic Surgery, Thoracic Unit, Department of Surgery, Wentworth Hospital, P. B. Jacobs, Durban, Natal, South Africa

MONGES, H., M.D., Professeur, Médecin des Hôpitaux, Clinique des maladies de l'appareil digestif et de la nutrition, Hôpital Nord, Marseille 15, France

PEARSON, J. G., M.D., Director of Radiotherapy, Provincial Cancer Hospitals Board, Dr. W. W. Cross Cancer Institute, 11560 University avenue, Edmonton, Alberta, T6G 1Z2, Canada

PELEMANS, W., M.D., Research Fellow, Department of Medical Research and Department of Medicine, Akademisch Ziekenhuis St. Rafaël, University of Leuven, 3000 Leuven, Belgium

PONETTE, E., M.D., Assistant Professor of Radiology, Department of Radiology, Akademisch Ziekenhuis St. Rafaël, University of Leuven, 3000 Leuven, Belgium

PRINGOT, J., M.D., Assistant Professor of Radiology, Department of Radiology, Cliniques Universitaires, U.C.L., 3000 Leuven, Belgium

RINALDO, J. A., Jr., M.D., Medical Director, Providence Hospital, 16001 W. Nine Mile Rd., Southfield, Michigan 48075, USA

SCHRYVER, DE, J., M.D., Wilhelmina Kinderziekenhuis, Nieuwe Gracht 137, Utrecht, The Netherlands

TEXTER, E. C., Jr., M.D., Professor of Medicine, Physiology and Biophysics, School of Medicine, Assistant Dean, School of Health, Related Professions, Associate Chief of Staff for Education, 300 E Roosevelt Rd., Little Rock, AR 72206, USA

TYTGAT, G. N., M.D., Lektor in Gastroenterologie, Akademisch Ziekenhuis bij de Universiteit van Amsterdam, Wilhelmina Gasthuis, Amsterdam, The Netherlands

VALEMBOIS, P., M.D., Aangesteld Navorser N.F.W.O., Consultant in Surgery, Department of Medical Research and Department of Surgery, Akademisch Ziekenhuis St. Rafaël, University of Leuven, 3000 Leuven, Belgium

VANTRAPPEN, G., M.D. Agg. H.O., Professor and Chairman, Department of Medical Research, University of Leuven, Leuven, Belgium; Chief Gastrointestinal Unit, Department of Medicine, Akademisch Ziekenhuis St. Rafaël, 3000 Leuven, Belgium

VILARDELL, F., M.D., D. Sc.Med., Director, School of Gastroenterology, Universidad Autonoma de Barcelona, Hospital Santa Cruz y San Pablo, Barcelona 13, Spain

WOLF, B. S., M.D., Chairman and Professor of Radiology, The Mount Sinai School of Medicine, 11 East 100th street, New York 10029, USA

Preface

This book aims to be a synthesis of our current knowledge about the normal and pathological esophagus. Although a number of excellent monographs on limited aspects of esophageal pathology are available, a recent handbook treating the whole of esophageal physiology and pathology is lacking. We attempted to present the collected material in such a way that even the neophyte in the field would not get lost in the wealth of data. For this reason we have included a number of illustrations such as classical radiological and endoscopic images, manometric tracings and uncomplicated graphs, which may seem superfluous for specialists but will be helpful to the reader who wants to be initiated in the subject. At the same time we tried to be fairly complete so as to make available to the esophageal specialist a book of references, to which he can readily turn when faced with rare diseases or unusual physiological or pathophysiological phenomena. In order to achieve both aims the authors often give their own point of view when faced with controversial topics, while classical as well as more recent features and concepts are mentioned and diverging opinions discussed.

Our knowledge about the structure and function of the normal and the pathological esophagus has increased considerably during the last few years. Our insight into the local and central innervation of the esophagus has improved; the behavior of the gastroesophageal sphincter has greatly been clarified and different types of esophageal motor responses have been recognized which, each in its own way, may be influenced pharmacologically. Therefore we thought it useful to thoroughly discuss the basic data, i.e. anatomy, histology, electron microscopy and physiology. Many diseases cause disturbances of esophageal mechanisms. The section on physiology was written to elucidate these mechanisms, starting from the normal motility. The examination of the esophagus has been improved by the refinement of the traditional methods, such as radiology, endoscopy and by the recent introduction of new techniques, such as electromyography, the acid infusion test and pH- and PD-measurements. Although the clinical and diagnostic value of these procedures has not yet been fully established, clinical correlations are discussed. In the chapter on diagnotic procedures, however, the stress is laid on procedures rather than on diagnosis, in order to minimize overlap with the chapters in which the diseases themselves are discussed.

There are many esophageal diseases in which the disorders or lesions of the esophagus are but a component of a more general condition. Motor disturbances may be found in collagen diseases, anatomical anomalies in various congenital malformations, mucosal lesions in several cutaneous diseases, esophageal varices in a series of extraesophageal conditions, etc. It is obviously unnecessary to give a detailed description of all these larger entities; for instance, we deemed it superfluous to elaborate on causes, symptoms and treatment of acute and chronic alcoholic intoxication because it may produce motility disturbances. Other conditions, such as systemic sclerosis, Chagas' disease and portal hypertension are discussed more thoroughly since their cause, evolution or treatment are important for the understanding of the esophageal component. In this discussion special prominence has been given to involvement of other parts of the gastrointestinal tract.

The necessity of subdividing the text in chapters and sections sometimes entails artificial classifications. For instance, hiatal hernia with gastroesophageal reflux, reflux esophagitis and peptic stenosis of the gullet are treated in three different sections, although they may be considered one coherent entity, which might equally well have been discussed under a single heading.

This book does not offer detailed descriptions of surgical interventions but surgery is treated to the extent that it may interest the non-surgeon.

We wish to express our gratitude to all those who have helped us so much in the preparation of this book. First of all we wish to mention the contributors, especially those not belonging to the Leuven group. Their competence and personal experience have greatly enhanced the value of this work. These, and the authors of our university, who have shown so much forbearance, will forgive us for the strict demands we imposed on them.

Our thanks are due also to our collegues of the Sint-Rafaël and Saint-Pierre University Hospitals, who have allowed us to draw on the work of their departments: at Sint-Rafaël Prof. J. Vandenbroucke, head of the department of internal medicine, Prof. A. Baert, head of the department of radiology, Prof. H. Degreef, head of the department of dermatology, and Dr. L. Broeckaert of the section of gastroenterology; at Saint-Pierre, Prof. P. Bodart, head of the department of radiology, Prof. P. J. Kestens, head of the department of surgery and Prof. C. Dive and Dr. R. Fiasse of the section of gastroenterology.

Dr. G. Tops (UFSIA) has ably assisted us in the translation of many texts into English.

Mr. Rummens carried out the photographic work on the pictures provided by the Leuven group. We also gratefully acknowledge the help of the Gevaert Company, Mortsel. We are particularly grateful for the secretarial assistance of Mrs. M. Vanderveken, R. Verbist and M. Rumbaut, who have done a great job in the preparation of the manuscript. And last but not least our thanks are due to the Springer Verlag. The spirit of cooperation and the courtesy of Mr. Bergstedt has been a great help throughout the preparation of this book.

Leuven, October 1974   G. Vantrappen
                                                     J. Hellemans

Contents

Chapter 1

Basic Data

Anatomy and Embryology. By G. FRANSEN and P. VALEMBOIS. With 6 Figures 1

1.	Anatomy	1
1.1.	Topographic Anatomy	1
1.1.1.	The Cervical Esophagus	1
1.1.2.	The Thoracic Esophagus	3
1.1.3.	The Abdominal Esophagus	3
1.2.	The Musculature of the Esophagus Proper	4
1.3.	The Pharyngoesophageal Junction	6
1.4.	The Esophagogastric Junction	6
1.4.1.	The Gastroesophageal Sphincter	6
1.4.2.	The Phrenoesophageal Membrane	7
1.4.3.	The Diaphragmatic Hiatus	7
1.5.	Arterial Blood Supply	9
1.6.	Venous Drainage	9
1.6.1.	Intrinsic Veins	10
1.6.2.	Extrinsic Veins	10
1.7.	Lymphatic Drainage	11
1.8.	Nerve Supply (Innervation)	12
1.8.1.	Parasympathetic Innervation	12
1.8.2.	Sympathetic Innervation	13
2.	Embryology	13
References	. . . .	15

Histology and Electron Microscopy. By V. J. DESMET and G. N. TYTGAT. With 8 Figures | 17

1.	Mucous Membrane (Tunica Mucosa)	17
1.1.	Epithelium	17
1.1.1.	Squamous Epithelium	17
1.1.1.1.	Histology	17
1.1.1.2.	Cell Kinetics	19
1.1.1.3.	Histochemistry	19
1.1.1.4.	Electron Microscopy	21
1.1.2.	Non-squamous Epithelial Structures, Cardia-type Glands	24
1.1.2.1.	Histology	24
1.1.2.2.	Electron Microscopy	27
1.2.	Lamina Propria	27
1.3.	Muscularis Mucosae	29
2.	Tunica Submucosa	29
3.	Tunica Muscularis	30
4.	Angio-architecture	35
5.	Innervation	35
6.	Adventitia, Elastic-muscular System, Serosa	37
References	. . . .	38

Physiology. By J. HELLEMANS and G. VANTRAPPEN. With 20 Figures . . . . | 40

1.	The Functions of the Esophagus	40
2.	The Esophagus at Rest	40
2.1.	The Pharyngoesophageal Sphincter	40
2.1.1.	Location	40
2.1.2.	The Pressure Profile of the Pharyngoesophageal Sphincter	41
2.1.3.	Manometric Measurements of the Resting Pressure in the Pharyngoesophageal Sphincter	42

2.1.4.	Respiratory Pressure Variations	43
2.1.5.	Elasticity or Tonic Contraction	43
2.2.	The Esophagus Proper	45
2.2.1.	The Resting Pressure	45
2.3.	The Lower Esophageal Sphincter (L.E.S.) (Gastroesophageal Sphincter)	45
2.3.1.	The Position of the Sphincter in Relation to the Squamocolumnar Junction	46
2.3.2.	The Pressure Profile of the Sphincter. The Pressure Inversion Point (P.I.P.)	46
2.3.3.	Manometric Measurements of the Resting Pressure in the Lower Esophageal Sphincter	48
2.3.4.	Other Measurements of Sphincter Strength	50
2.3.5.	Variations of the Sphincteric Pressure	51
2.3.5.1.	The Intrinsic Sphincteric Properties	51
2.3.5.2.	Hormonal Control of the Sphincter Strength	53
2.3.5.3.	The Response of the Lower Esophageal Sphincter to Increased Intragastric Pressure	56
2.3.5.4.	Nervous Control of the Lower Esophageal Sphincter Pressure	57
3.	Bolus Transport. Primary Peristalsis	59
3.1.	Mechanical Activity	59
3.1.1.	Oral Transport	59
3.1.2.	Pharyngeal Transport	62
3.1.3.	Electromyographic Studies of Deglutition	63
3.1.3.1.	Leading Complex	63
3.1.3.2.	Constrictor Musculature	64
3.1.3.3.	Variations in Ancillary Activity	65
3.1.4.	Esophageal Transport	65
3.1.4.1.	The Peristaltic Progression	65
3.1.4.2.	Longitudinal and Circular Musculature	65
3.1.4.3.	Striated and Smooth Muscles	67
3.1.5.	Transport through the Gastroesophageal Sphincter	68
3.2.	Intraluminal Pressure Variations	69
3.2.1.	The Deglutition Complex in the Pharynx and in the Pharyngoesophageal Sphincter	69
3.2.1.1.	Relaxion of the High Pressure Zone	69
3.2.1.2.	The e-(Elevation) Wave	71
3.2.1.3.	The t-(Tongue) Wave	71
3.2.1.4.	The p-(Peristaltic) Wave	71
3.2.2.	The Deglutition Complex in the Esophagus	71
3.2.2.1.	The Initial Negative Deflexion	72
3.2.2.2.	The First Positive Wave	72
3.2.2.3.	The Second Positive Wave	73
3.2.2.4.	The Peristaltic Contraction	73
3.2.3.	The Deglutition Complex in the Gastroesophageal Sphincter	74
3.3.	Innervation	75
3.3.1.	Innervation of Oropharyngeal Phase	75
3.3.1.1.	The Deglutition Center in the Rhombencephalon	75
3.3.1.1.1.	The Existence of a Deglutition Center	75
3.3.1.1.2.	Localization of the Deglutition Center	75
3.3.1.2.	The Peripheral Afferent System	76
3.3.1.3.	Elementary Reflexes Versus Swallowing	77
3.3.1.4.	The Central Afferent System	78
3.3.1.5.	The Cortical Control of the Deglutition Center	78
3.3.1.6.	Interference with Other Centers	80
3.3.1.7.	Efferent Pathways. Motoneurons	81
3.3.2.	Innervation of the Esophageal Phase	82
3.3.2.1.	Central Nervous Centers	82
3.3.2.2.	Afferent Pathways	82
3.3.2.3.	Efferent Pathways	84
3.3.2.4.	The Intramural Nervous System	85
3.3.2.4.1.	The Motor Neurons	85
3.3.2.4.2.	Local Nerve Fibers	85
4.	Reflex Responses of the Esophagus	86
4.1.	Secondary Peristalsis	86
4.2.	Esophageal Propulsive Force (E.P.F.)	87
4.3.	On- and off-Response; Duration Response	87
4.3.1.	The "On" Response (Circular Muscle)	87

4.3.2.   The "Off" Response (Circular Muscle) 88
4.3.3.   The Duration Response (Longitudinal Muscle) 89
4.4.   Inhibition 89
4.4.1.   Deglutitive Inhibition 89
4.4.2.   Inhibition by Distension 91
4.5.   Relaxion of the Gastroesophageal Sphincter 91
4.6.   Other Reflexes 91
5.   Retrograde Transport 92
5.1.   Rumination-Eructation 92
5.2.   Retching and Vomiting 92
5.3.   Belching 93
References 93

Chapter 2

Diagnostic Procedures

History and Symptoms of Esophageal Disease. By D. A. W. Edwards. With 5 Figures 103

1.   Symptoms and Syndromes 103
1.1.   Symptoms and their Significance 104
1.1.1.   The Sensation of Obstruction 104
1.1.1.1.   The Site of the Obstruction 104
1.1.1.2.   The Site of the Receptors 105
1.1.1.3.   The Sensation of "Choking" 105
1.1.2.   Regurgitation 105
1.1.2.1.   The Volume of Regurgitate 105
1.1.2.2.   The Taste 106
1.1.2.3.   The Content 106
1.1.2.4.   The Timing 106
1.1.2.5.   The Association with Position 106
1.1.3.   Pain 107
1.1.3.1.   The Distribution 107
1.1.3.2.   The Character 107
1.1.3.3.   The Timing 107
1.2.   Syndromes 108
1.2.1.   "Spill-Over" and "Spill-Into" Disease 108
1.2.2.   Obstruction Syndromes 109
1.2.2.1.   The Stricture Syndrome 109
1.2.2.2.   The Achalasia Syndrome 110
1.2.3.   The So-Called "Functional" Dysphagias 111
2.   History 112
2.1.   Pharyngeal Problems 113
2.1.1.   Pouch 113
2.1.2.   Stricture or Web 114
2.1.3.   Muscular and Neural 114
2.2.   Esophageal Problems 114

Radiological Examination of the Esophagus. By J. Pringot and E. Ponette. With 72 Figures 119

1.   The Radiological Technique 119
1.1.   Equipment 119
1.1.1.   The Standard Diagnostic X-Ray Unit 119
1.1.2.   The Image Intensifier 122
1.1.3.   Television Fluoroscopy 125
1.1.4.   Spot Filming 126
1.2.   The Recording Techniques Used with Image Intensifiers 127
1.2.1.   Photofluorography 127
1.2.2.   Cinefluorography 128
1.3.   Techniques of Recording the Television Images 131
1.3.1.   Cinefluorography 131
1.3.2.   Video Recording 131
2.   Contrast Materials 133
2.1.   Positive Contrast Materials 133
2.1.1.   Barium Sulfate 133
2.1.2.   Iodinated Contrast Materials 135

2.1.3.   Tantalum Powder 137
2.2.   Negative Contrast Materials 137
3.   The Radiological Examination 137
3.1.   General Principles 137
3.2.   Normal Radiological Anatomy and Physiology 138
3.2.1.   Hypopharynx and Cervical Esophagus 138
3.2.1.1.   Radiological Landmarks 138
3.2.1.2.   Hypopharynx and Cervical Esophagus during Swallowing 141
3.2.1.3.   Hypopharynx and Cervical Esophagus after Swallowing 146
3.2.1.4.   The Modified Valsalva Maneuver 147
3.2.2.   Thoracic Esophagus 147
3.2.2.1.   Normal Motor Activity 148
3.2.2.2.   Normal Esophagogram 150
3.2.3.   Esophagogastric Region 154
3.3.   Preparation of the Patient 156
3.4.   Radiological Examination without Contrast Material 157
3.4.1.   The Air Esophagogram 157
3.4.2.   Mediastinal Widening 159
3.4.3.   Mediastinal Calcifications 161
3.4.4.   Signs Related to Esophageal Perforation or Rupture 163
3.4.5.   Retention of Contrast Material 165
3.5.   Radiological Examination with Contrast Material 165
3.5.1.   Basic Technique of Examination 165
3.5.2.   Abnormal Images 166
3.5.2.1.   Filling Defects and Impressions 166
3.5.2.1.1. Malignant Tumors 166
3.5.2.1.2. Intraluminal Defects 171
3.5.2.1.3. Intramural Extramucosal Defects 173
3.5.2.1.4. Impressions 175
3.5.2.2.   Narrowings 178
3.5.2.2.1. Circular Tumors 178
3.5.2.2.2. Benign Strictures 179
3.5.2.2.3. Rings 180
3.5.2.3.   Changes in Mucosal Pattern 180
3.5.2.4.   Crater-like Images 180
3.5.2.5.   Diverticula, Perforations, Fistulas 184
3.6.   Special Procedures 184
3.6.1.   Examination of the Pharyngoesophageal Region 184
3.6.1.1.   Examination without Contrast Material 184
3.6.1.1.1. Technique of Examination 184
3.6.1.1.2. Abnormal Images 184
3.6.1.2.   Examination with Contrast Material 186
3.6.1.2.1. Single Films of the Swallowing Act 187
3.6.1.2.2. Single Films after Swallowing 187
3.6.1.2.3. Rapid Photofluorography of the Swallowing Act 187
3.6.1.2.4. Cinefluorography of the Swallowing Act 187
3.6.1.2.5. Contrast Laryngopharyngography 187
3.6.1.3.   Abnormal Images of the Opacified Pharyngoesophageal Region 190
3.6.1.3.1. Cricopharyngeal Indentation 190
3.6.1.3.2. Filling Defects 190
3.6.1.3.3. Extrinsic Compression 190
3.6.1.3.4. Narrowing 190
3.6.1.3.5. Obstruction 191
3.6.1.3.6. Dilatation of the Pharynx 191
3.6.1.3.7. Diverticula and Pouches 191
3.6.1.3.8. Motility Disorders of the Pharyngoesophageal Region 191
3.6.2.   The Demonstration of Esophageal Varices 192
3.6.3.   Pharmacoradiography 194
4.   The Radiological Examination of the Esophagus in Children 194
References 198

Esophagoscopy. By P. HOUSSET, A. SIMOENS and CH. DEBRAY. With 16 Figures . . . 204

1.   Introduction 204
2.   Common Recommendations for All Endoscopic Examinations 204
3.   Equipment and Techniques 204

3.1.   Rigid Esophagoscopy 205
3.1.1.   The Esophagoscope of Segal and Dubois de Montreynaud 205
3.1.2.   The Eder-Hufford Esophagoscope 206
3.1.3.   Results of Rigid Esophagoscopy 206
3.2.   Flexible Esophagoscopy 207
3.2.1.   Principle of the Fiberscopes 207
3.2.2.   Instruments 207
3.2.3.   Examination Technique 209
3.2.3.1.   Preparation and Positioning of the Patient 209
3.2.3.2.   Insertion of the Apparatus and Exploration 210
3.2.3.3.   Associate Maneuvers 213
3.2.3.4.   Advantages and Drawbacks 214
4.   Indications and Contraindications 215
5.   Accidents and Incidents 216
5.1.   Accidents 216
5.1.1.   Perforation 216
5.1.2.   Hemorrhage 216
5.2.   Incidents 216
5.2.1.   Failure to Pass Pharyngoesophageal Sphincter 216
5.2.2.   Respiratory Spasm 217
5.2.3.   Pain 217
5.2.4.   Bleeding 217
References 217

Exfoliative Cytology of the Esophagus. By F. VILARDELL. With 9 Figures 218
1.   Introduction 218
2.   Esophageal Cytological Techniques 218
2.1.   Techniques Combined with Esophagoscopy 218
2.2.   Abrasive Techniques 219
2.3.   Lavage Techniques 220
2.4.   Combined Techniques 220
3.   An Appraisal of Cytologic Techniques 221
4.   Normal Cytology of the Esophagus 221
5.   Criteria for Malignancy in Esophageal Cytology 221
6.   Cyto-Histological Correlations 225
7.   Indications of Esophageal Cytology 225
8.   Results of Esophageal Cytology 225
9.   Diagnostic Errors 226
10.   Cytology Compared with Other Diagnostic Techniques 228
11.   Fluorescent Techniques in Esophageal Cytology 228
12.   Cytology in Beningn Conditions of the Esophagus 229
13.   Effects of Roentgen Therapy on Esophageal Cells 230
14.   Cytology in the Early Diagnosis of Esophageal Cancer 231
References 232

The Manometric Examination of the Esophagus. By W. PELEMANS and E. C. TEXTER, JR.
With 6 Figures 235
1.   The Balloon-Kymographic Method 235
2.   Intraluminal Pressure Measurements 236
3.   Interpretation of Intraluminal Pressure Measurements 238
4.   The Perfused Catheter System 238
5.   The Technique of Intraluminal Pressure Measurements 243
References 243

pH Measurements. By W. PELEMANS and G. VANTRAPPEN. With 2 Figures 246
1.   pH Measurements in vitro 246
2.   pH Measurements in vivo 246
3.   The Pull-trough Technique 247
4.   Fixed Location of pH Electrode 248
5.   Interpretation of Results 249
6.   The Acid Clearing Test 250
7.   Protracted pH Measurements 251
References 251

PD Measurements. By J. Janssens and G. Vantrappen. With 1 Figure 253
1.   History 253
2.   The Origin of the Potential Difference 253
3.   Techniques of PD Measurements 255
4.   PD Measurements in the Esophagus 257
References 259

The Acid Infusion Test. By W. Pelemans and G. Vantrappen 262
1.   Procedure 262
2.   Hazards of the Test 263
3.   The Mechanism of Pain 263
References 265

Pharmacological Tests. By J. Janssens and J. Hellemans. With 2 Figures 266
References 269

Electromyography of the Esophagus. By J. Hellemans, G. Vantrappen and J. Janssens. With 14 Figures 270
1.   Introduction 270
2.   Registration Method 272
3.   The Electromyographic Tracings 273
3.1.   The Pharyngoesophageal Sphincter 273
3.2.   The Striated Muscle Segment of the Esophagus 274
3.3.   The Transitional Zone between Striated and Smooth Muscles 275
3.4.   The Smooth Muscle Segment of the Esophagus 276
3.5.   The Gastroesophageal Sphincter 279
4.   The Deglutitive Inhibition 280
5.   Electromyography in Esophageal Diseases 282
References 284

Chapter 3

Motility Disturbances of the Esophagus

Achalasia. By G. Vantrappen and J. Hellemans. With 27 Figures 287
1.   Definition 287
2.   Incidence 288
2.1.   Age Distribution 288
2.2.   Sex Distribution 288
2.3.   Geographical Distribution and Incidence 288
3.   Achalasia in Animals 289
4.   Etiology and Pathogenesis 289
4.1.   Genetic Factors 289
4.2.   Neuromuscular Abnormalities 290
4.2.1.   Anatomical Lesions 290
4.2.1.1.   The Nuclei of the Brainstem 290
4.2.1.2.   Vagal Nerve Fibres 290
4.2.1.3.   The Intramural Nerve Plexus 291
4.2.1.4.   Smooth Muscle 291
4.2.2.   Pharmacological Defects 292
5.   Clinical Features 293
5.1.   Symptoms and Signs 293
5.2.   Vigorous Achalasia 296
6.   Technical Examinations 297
6.1.   Radiology 297
6.1.1.   Plain Chest Film 297
6.1.2.   Radiological Examination with Contrast Medium 300
6.1.2.1.   Minimal Achalasia 300
6.1.2.2.   Mild Achalasia 301
6.1.2.3.   Moderate Achalasia 302
6.1.2.4.   Severe Achalasia 303
6.2.   Manometry 304
6.2.1.   Resting Pressures in the Gastroesophageal Sphincter 304
6.2.2.   Resting Pressure in the Esophagus 305

6.2.3.　　　The Deglutitive Response in the Gastroesophageal Sphincter 305
6.2.4.　　　Deglutitive Responses in the Esophagus 307
6.3.　　　　Mecholyl Test 308
6.4.　　　　Cytological Examination 308
6.5.　　　　Endoscopic Examination 308
7.　　　　　Differential Diagnosis 309
7.1.　　　　Other Causes of Megaesophagus 309
7.1.1.　　　Chagas' Disease 309
7.1.1.1.　　Acute Phase 309
7.1.1.2.　　Chronic Chagas' Syndrome 310
7.1.1.3.　　Megacolon 310
7.1.1.4.　　Megaesophagus 311
7.1.2.　　　Esophageal Cancer 312
7.1.3.　　　Rare Causes of Esophageal Dilatation 313
7.2.　　　　Other Causes of Aperistalsis 313
7.3.　　　　Achalasia-like Disorders 314
7.4.　　　　Diffuse Spasm 316
7.5.　　　　Post-Vagotomy Dysphagia 316
7.6.　　　　Differential Diagnosis in Children 316
8.　　　　　Complications and Associated Diseases 317
8.1.　　　　Carcinoma 317
8.1.1.　　　Incidence 317
8.1.2.　　　Age and Sex Distribution 318
8.1.3.　　　Pathology 318
8.1.4.　　　Pathogenesis 318
8.1.5.　　　Signs and Symptoms 318
8.1.6.　　　Treatment 318
8.2.　　　　Esophagitis 319
8.3.　　　　Bronchopulmonary Complications 319
8.4.　　　　Perforation 319
8.5.　　　　Associated Conditions 320
9.　　　　　Natural History 321
10.　　　　　Treatment 321
10.1.　　　　Medical and Psychiatric Therapy 321
10.2.　　　　Dilatations 321
10.2.1.　　　Types of Dilators 322
10.2.1.1.　　Mechanical System 322
10.2.1.2.　　Hydrostatic System 322
10.2.1.3.　　Pneumatic System 323
10.2.2.　　　Preventive Measures 324
10.2.3.　　　Results 325
10.2.3.1.　　Immediate Results 325
10.2.3.2.　　Immediate Complications 325
10.2.3.3.　　Late Results 327
10.3.　　　　Surgical Treatment 331
10.3.1.　　　Techniques 331
10.3.1.1.　　Operations Based on the Theory of "Idiopathic Dilatation" 331
10.3.1.2.　　Operations Based on the Theory of Disturbance in Esophageal Innervation 331
10.3.1.3.　　Operations Aimed at Decreasing the Resistance at the Cardia 332
10.3.1.4.　　Operations to Replace Part of the Esophagus by Intestine 333
10.3.2.　　　Results and Complications of Heller's Myotomy 334
10.3.2.1.　　Results 334
10.3.2.2.　　Complications 336
10.4.　　　　Sphincteric Pressures after Treatment 338
10.5.　　　　Myotomy or Forceful Dilatation ? 339
References 341

Diffuse Esophageal Spasm. By G. Vantrappen and J. Hellemans. With 3 Figures . . 355

1.　　　　　Definition 355
2.　　　　　Incidence 355
3.　　　　　Pathology 356
4.　　　　　Symptoms 356
5.　　　　　Technical Examinations 357
5.1.　　　　Radiology 357
5.2.　　　　Manometric Examinations 358

6.   Related Conditions 361
6.1.   Idiopathic Muscular Hypertrophy of Lower Esophagus 361
6.2.   The Hypertensive Sphincter 362
7.   Diagnosis 362
8.   Treatment 364
8.1.   Medical Treatment 364
8.2.   Dilatation 364
8.3.   Surgical Treatment 364
References 365

Post-Vagotomy Dysphagia. By D. A. W. EDWARDS. With 1 Figure 367
1.   Definition 367
2.   Incidence 367
3.   Symptoms 367
4.   Etiology and Pathogenesis 367
5.   Treatment 370
References 370

Presbyesophagus. By J. HELLEMANS and G. VANTRAPPEN. With 5 Figures 372
1.   Pharynx 372
2.   Esophagus 372
3.   Gastroesophageal Sphincter 375
4.   Nature of the Lesions 377
References 377

Esophageal Motility in Neonatal Infants. By J. DE SCHRYVER and J. HELLEMANS . . 379
1.   Introduction 379
2.   Normal Motility 379
2.1.   Mouth and Pharynx 379
2.2.   Esophagus 379
2.2.1.   The Esophagus at Rest 379
2.2.1.1.   Pharyngoesophageal Sphincter 379
2.2.1.2.   Esophageal Body 380
2.2.1.3.   Gastroesophageal Sphincter 380
2.2.2.   Deglutition 381
2.2.2.1.   Pharyngoesophageal Sphincter 381
2.2.2.2.   Esophageal Body 381
2.2.2.3.   Gastroesophageal Sphincter 381
References 381

Motor Disorders Due to Collagen Diseases. By J. HELLEMANS and G. VANTRAPPEN.
With 2 Figures 383
1.   Progressive Systemic Sclerosis 383
1.1.   Definition and General Data 383
1.2.   Esophageal Involvement in Progressive Systemic Sclerosis 385
1.2.1.   Incidence 385
1.2.2.   Pathology 386
1.2.3.   Radiological Examination 387
1.2.4.   Manometric Examination 387
1.2.5.   Differential Diagnosis 388
1.2.6.   Treatment 389
2.   Systemic Lupus Erythematosus 389
3.   Polymyositis-Dermatomyositis 389
4.   Related Syndromes 390
References 390

Motor Disorders Due to Muscle Disorders. By G. VANTRAPPEN and J. HELLEMANS. With
3 Figures 394
1.   Myotonic Dystrophy (Steinert's Disease) 394
1.1.   Definition and General Data 394
1.2.   Esophageal Involvement 394
2.   Ocular Myopathy and Oculopharyngeal Myopathy 397
2.1.   Definition and General Data 397

2.2.   Pharyngoesophageal Involvement 397
3.   Myasthenia Gravis 398
3.1.   Definition and General Data 398
3.2.   Pharyngoesophageal Involvement 398
4.   Endocrine Disorders of Muscle 399
References 400

Motor Disorders Due to Lesions of the Central Nervous System. By J. HELLEMANS and
G. VANTRAPPEN 402
1.   Brainstem Lesions 402
2.   Poliomyelitis 402
3.   Motor Neuron Disease 403
4.   Extrapyramidal Disturbances 404
5.   Stiff-man Syndrome 404
6.   Dysautonomia 404
References 404

Motor Disorders Due to Peripheral Nerve Lesions. By J. HELLEMANS and G. VANTRAPPEN 407
1.   Motor Disorders Associated with Diabetes 407
2.   Motor Disturbances Associated with Alcoholic Neuropathy 408
References 408

Emotional Disorders of the Esophagus. By H. MONGES and A. HANCY. With 6 Figures 409
1.   Globus Hystericus 409
1.1.   Definition and Generalities 409
1.2.   Clinical Findings 409
1.3.   Diagnosis 409
1.4.   Interpretation 410
1.5.   Treatment 410
2.   Esophageal Belching 410
2.1.   Definition 410
2.2.   Etiology 410
2.3.   Clinical Findings 410
2.4.   Pathophysiology 411
2.5.   Treatment 413
3.   Eructation or Belching 414
3.1.   Definition 414
3.2.   Mechanism of Eructation 414
3.3.   Treatment 415
4.   Merycism or Rumination 415
4.1.   Merycism in Infants 415
4.1.1.   Clinical Data 416
4.1.2.   Interpretation 416
4.1.3.   Treatment 417
4.2.   Merycism in Adults 417
4.2.1.   Clinical Data 417
4.2.2.   Mechanism 418
4.2.3.   Treatment 419
References 421

The Pathophysiological Basis of Gastroesophageal and Intestinoesophageal Reflux. By
P. HEITMANN 422
1.   The Gastroesophageal Closing Mechanism 422
2.   Conditions Associated with Gastroesophageal or Intestinoesophageal Reflux 424
2.1.   Sliding Hiatal Hernia 424
2.2.   Gastroesophageal Incompetence in the Absence of Demonstrable Hiatal
           Hernia 425
2.3.   Scleroderma with Esophageal Involvement and Related Conditions 425
2.4.   Following Myotomy for Achalasia of the Esophagus 425
2.5.   Vagotomy 425
2.6.   Pregnancy 426
2.7.   Gastric Operations 426
2.8.   Prolonged Gastric Intubation 426
References 427

Chapter 4
Tumors of the Esophagus

Benign Tumors and Cysts of the Esophagus. By G. VANTRAPPEN and J. PRINGOT. With
6 Figures 431
1.   Classification 431
2.   Incidence 432
3.   Intramural Tumors and Cysts 433
3.1.   Leiomyoma 433
3.1.1.   Age and Sex Incidence 433
3.1.2.   Pathology 433
3.1.3.   Symptoms 436
3.1.4.   Radiographic Signs 436
3.1.5.   Esophagoscopy 438
3.1.6.   Diagnosis 439
3.1.7.   Complications 441
3.1.8.   Treatment 441
3.2.   Cysts 441
4.   Intraluminal Tumors 443
4.1.   Fibrovascular Polyp 443
4.2.   Papillomas 444
4.3.   Adenomas 444
5.   Hemangiomas 444
References 445

Malignant Tumors of the Esophagus. By J. G. PEARSON and B. T. LE ROUX. With
20 Figures 447
1.   Esophageal Carcinoma 447
1.1.   Incidence and Etiology 447
1.2.   Pathology 448
1.2.1.   Squamous Cell Carcinoma 449
1.2.1.1.   Site 449
1.2.1.2.   Size 449
1.2.1.3.   Macroscopic Appearance 449
1.2.1.4.   Microscopic Appearance 449
1.2.1.5.   Direct Spread 451
1.2.1.6.   Lymphatic Metastases 454
1.2.1.7.   Blood-Borne Metastases 455
1.2.2.   Adenocarcinoma 456
1.2.3.   Mixed Squamous and Adenocarcinoma 458
1.3.   Clinical Features, Natural History, Symptoms and Signs 458
1.4.   Investigations 460
1.4.1.   Radiology 460
1.4.2.   Endoscopy 462
1.4.3.   Esophageal Cytology 463
1.4.4.   Cervical Lymph Node Biopsy 463
1.4.5.   Mediastinoscopy, Pneumomediastinography and Laparotomy 463
1.4.6.   Other Investigations 464
1.5.   Prognosis 464
1.5.1.   Factors Influencing Prognosis 464
1.5.1.1.   The Balance between the Aggressiveness of the Tumor and the Resistance of
            the Patient 464
1.5.1.2.   Treatment 465
1.5.1.3.   Sex 465
1.5.1.4.   Site 465
1.5.1.5.   Histology 466
1.5.1.6.   Condition of the Patient 466
1.5.1.7.   The Community in which the Patient Lives 466
1.6   Treatment 466
1.6.1.   Comparison of Surgery and Radiotherapy 467
1.6.2.   Anatomical Classification 470
1.6.3.   Radiation Therapy 470
1.6.3.1.   Squamous Carcinoma 470
1.6.3.2.   The Level of the Esophageal Cancer 477
1.6.3.3.   Adenocarcinoma 477

1.6.4.	Surgical Treatment	477
1.6.4.1.	Complications of Esophagogastrectomy	479
1.6.4.1.1.	Disruption or Leakage at the Site of the Anastomosis	479
1.6.1.1.2.	Hemorrhage from Aortic Erosion	479
1.6.4.1.3.	Death from Pulmonary Infection	480
1.6.4.1.4.	Pulmonary Embolism and Myocardial Infarction	480
1.6.4.1.5.	The Pleural Complications	480
1.6.5.	Preoperative and Postoperative Irradiation	480
1.6.6.	Intubation	481
1.6.7.	Cancer Chemotherapy	481
1.6.8.	Treatment of Esophagotracheal Fistula	482
1.6.9.	Results of Treatment	483
1.6.9.1.	Results of Surgical Management	483
1.6.9.2.	Results of Management of Squamous Esophageal Cancer by Irradiation	484
1.6.9.3.	Results of Management of Squamous Esophageal Cancer by Irradiation and Surgery	484
2.	Sarcoma	484
3.	Pseudosarcoma and Carcinosarcoma	485
4.	Malignant Melanoma	486
5.	Metastatic Tumors	486
6.	Other Rare Malignant Tumors of the Esophagus	486
6.1.	Carcinoid Tumor	486
6.2.	Paget's Disease	486
6.3.	Hodgkin's Disease	486
6.4.	Granular Cell Myoblastoma	487
6.5.	Verrucous Squamous Cell Carcinoma	487
Acknowledgements		487
References		487

Chapter 5

Inflammatory Lesions of the Esophagus

Reflux Esophagitis. By B. S. WOLF and H. P. LAZAR. With 12 Figures 493

1.	Introduction	493
2.	General Considerations	493
2.1.	Hiatal Hernia	494
2.2.	Esophagitis	497
2.3.	Reflux	499
2.4.	Heartburn	501
2.5.	Pathogenesis	502
3.	Clinical Features	504
4.	Roentgen Features	505
5.	Endoscopy	514
6.	Manometry	515
7.	Diagnosis and Differential Diagnosis	515
8.	Therapy	517
9.	Other Types of Reflux Esophagitis	519
References		521

Lower Esophagus Lined with Columnar Epithelium. By P. HEITMANN. With 12 Figures 525

1.	Historical Aspects, Definition, Incidence and Distribution	525
2.	Pathologic Anatomy	526
3.	Pathophysiology	529
4.	Symptomatology	531
5.	Diagnosis	532
6.	Differential Diagnosis	535
7.	Treatment	536
References		537

Caustic Lesions of the Esophagus. By W. PELEMANS and J. HELLEMANS. With 8 Figures 539

1.	Incidence	539
2.	Etiology	539
3.	Pathogenesis	539

4.   Pathology 541
4.1.   The Acute Necrotic Phase 541
4.2.   The Ulceration and Granulation Phase 541
4.3.   The Phase of Cicatrization and Stricture Formation 541
5.   Clinical Features 541
6.   Diagnosis 542
7.   Treatment 546
References 549

Acute Infectious Disease. By W. PELEMANS and G. VANTRAPPEN 551

1.   Suppurative Esophagitis 551
2.   Esophagitis Secondary to Infectious Disease 551
References 552

Tuberculosis of the Esophagus. By W. PELEMANS and J. HELLEMANS 553

1.   Incidence 553
2.   Pathogenesis 553
3.   Pathology 553
4.   Clinical Features 553
5.   Diagnosis 554
6.   Complications 554
7.   Prognosis 554
8.   Treatment 554
References 555

Syphilis of the Esophagus. By W. PELEMANS and G. VANTRAPPEN 556

1.   Incidence 556
2.   Pathology 556
3.   Clinical Features 556
4.   Technical Examination 556
5.   Diagnosis 557
6.   Complications 557
7.   Treatment 557
References 557

Esophageal Mycoses. By W. PELEMANS and G. VANTRAPPEN. With 2 Figures 558

1.   Monilial Esophagitis 558
1.1.   History 558
1.2.   Incidence 558
1.3.   Etiology 559
1.4.   Pathogenesis 559
1.5.   Clinical Features 560
1.6.   Technical Examination 561
1.7.   Diagnosis and Differential Diagnosis 563
1.8.   Complications 563
1.9.   Prognosis 564
1.10.   Treatment 564
2.   Other Mycotic Infections of the Esophagus 564
2.1.   Actinomycosis 565
2.2.   Mucormycosis 565
2.3.   Histoplasmosis 565
2.4.   Blastomycosis 565
References 566

Granulomatous Esophagitis. By W. PELEMANS and G. VANTRAPPEN 568

1.   Crohn's Disease of the Esophagus 568
2.   Sarcoidosis of the Esophagus 569
References 569

Chapter 6

Esophageal Webs and Rings. By J. A. RINALDO. With 5 Figures 571

1.   Introduction 571
2.   Upper Esophageal Web 572

2.1.   Definition 572
2.2.   Incidence 573
2.3.   Etiology and Pathogenesis 573
2.4.   Pathology 574
2.5.   Clinical Features 574
2.6.   Technical Features 575
2.7.   Diagnosis 576
2.8.   Differential Diagnosis 576
2.9.   Complications and Prognosis 577
2.10.   Treatment 577
3.   Middle Esophageal Web 577
3.1.   Incidence 577
3.2.   Etiology 578
3.3.   Clinical Features 578
3.4.   Technical Features 579
3.5.   Diagnosis 579
3.6.   Prognosis and Treatment 579
4.   Lower Esophageal Web 579
4.1.   Incidence and Etiology 579
4.2.   Clinical and Technical Features 580
4.3.   Diagnosis 581
4.4.   Comment 581
5.   Squamocolumnar Ring 581
5.1.   Definition 581
5.2.   Incidence 581
5.3.   Etiology and Pathogenesis 583
5.4.   Pathology 584
5.5.   Clinical Features 584
5.6.   Technical Features 584
5.7.   Diagnosis 586
5.8.   Differential Diagnosis 587
5.9.   Complications and Prognosis 587
5.10.   Treatment 587
5.11.   Comment 587
References 588

Chapter 7

Esophageal Diverticula. By G. VANTRAPPEN and W. DELOOF. With 12 Figures 591
1.   Lateral Pharyngeal Diverticula and Pouches 591
2.   The Hypopharyngeal Diverticulum (Zenker's Diverticulum) 593
2.1.   Incidence 593
2.2.   Pathophysiology and Pathogenesis 594
2.3.   Pathology 596
2.4.   Symptoms 596
2.5.   Diagnosis 597
2.6.   Complications of Untreated Diverticula 598
2.7.   Evolution and Prognosis 601
2.8.   Treatment 601
3.   Esophageal Diverticula 603
3.1.   Midesophageal Diverticula 605
3.1.1.   Pathogenesis and Pathology 605
3.1.2.   Symptoms 605
3.1.3.   Complications 606
3.1.4.   Diagnosis 606
3.1.5.   Treatment 606
3.2.   Epiphrenic Diverticula 606
3.2.1.   Incidence 606
3.2.2.   Pathology 607
3.2.3.   Etiology 607
3.2.4.   Symptoms 608
3.2.5.   Diagnosis 608
3.2.6.   Complications 609

3.2.7.   Treatment 610
3.3.   Subphrenic Diverticula 610
References 611

Chapter 8

Congenital Anomalies of the Esophagus

Esophageal Atresia. By G. FRANSEN and A. LACQUET. With 5 Figures 615
1.   History 615
2.   Incidence 615
3.   Embryology 616
4.   Pathological Anatomy 617
5.   Pathophysiology 619
5.1.   Hydramnios 619
5.2.   Prematurity 619
5.3.   Pneumonia 620
6.   Associated Anomalies 620
7.   Diagnostic Procedures 622
7.1.   Nasogastric Intubation 622
7.2.   Radiological Examinations 623
8.   Treatment 625
8.1.   Principles of Management 625
8.2.   Preoperative Management 626
8.3.   Operative Management 627
9.   Anastomotic Complications 629
9.1.   Leaks 629
9.2.   Strictures 630
9.3.   Recurrent Tracheoesophageal Fistula 631
9.4.   Neurogenic Dysfunction 631
10.   Trends in Survival 633
References 634

Isolated Tracheoesophageal Fistula. By A. LACQUET and G. FRANSEN 639
References 641

Bronchoesophageal Fistula. By G. FRANSEN and A. LACQUET 643
References 644

Cleft Larynx. Laryngotracheoesophageal Cleft. Persistent Esophagotrachea. By A. LACQUET
and G. FRANSEN 646
References 648

Vascular Rings. By G. FRANSEN and W. PELEMANS. With 7 Figures 649
Vascular Anomalies Causing Tracheoesophageal Symptoms 649
1.   Introduction 649
2.   Clinical Picture 649
2.1.   Respiratory Symptoms 649
2.2.   Feeding Problems 650
3.   Different Types of Anomalies 650
3.1.   Aberrant Right Subclavian Artery (A. lusoria) 650
3.2.   Double Aortic Arch 653
3.3.   Right-sided Aortic Arch 655
3.4.   Left-sided Aortic Arch with Right-sided Descending Aorta 657
3.5.   Cervical Aortic Arch 657
3.6.   Aberrant Left Pulmonary Artery 658
References 658

Chapter 9

Mechanical Lesions of the Esophagus

Traumatic Lesions of the Esophagus. By J. JANSSENS and P. VALEMBOIS 661
1.   Pathogenesis 661
1.1.   Blunt Trauma 661

1.2.   Penetrating Wounds 662
1.3.   Mechanical Agents Acting from Inside the Lumen 662
2.   Symptoms 662
3.   Diagnosis 663
4.   Treatment 663
References 663

Foreign Bodies in the Esophagus. By J. JANSSENS and P. VALEMBOIS 665

1.   Incidence 665
2.   Pathogenesis and Pathology 665
3.   Clinical Features 667
4.   Diagnosis 669
5.   Treatment 670
6.   Complications 672
7.   Esophageal Obstruction from Meat Impaction 672
References 673

Spontaneous Rupture of the Esophagus. (Boerhaave's Syndrome.) By J. JANSSENS and
P. VALEMBOIS. With 1 Figure 675

1.   Definition 675
2.   History and Incidence 675
3.   Pathogenesis 675
4.   Pathology 676
5.   Clinical Features 677
6.   Technical Examinations 678
7.   Diagnosis 679
8.   Prognosis 679
9.   Treatment 680
10.   Esophageal Rupture in Children 680
References 681

Iatrogenic Perforations of the Esophagus. By J. JANSSENS and G. VANTRAPPEN . . . 683

1.   Definition 683
2.   Incidence 683
3.   Etiology and Pathogenesis 684
4.   Symptoms and Diagnosis 685
5.   Treatment 686
References 687

Mallory-Weiss Syndrome. By J. JANSSENS and P. VALEMBOIS 689

1.   Definition 689
2.   History 689
3.   Incidence 689
4.   Pathogenesis 690
5.   Clinical Features 691
6.   Diagnosis 691
7.   Pathology 692
8.   Treatment 692
References 692

Intramural Rupture and Bleeding. J. JANSSENS and G. VANTRAPPEN 694

1.   Etiology 694
2.   Pathogenesis 694
3.   Symptoms 694
4.   Radiological Features and Diagnosis 695
5.   Treatment 695
References 696

Chapter 10

Esophageal Varices. By J. Fevery and J. De Groote. With 8 Figures 697

1.   Definition 697
2.   Anatomy and Histopathology 697
3.   Incidence 699
4.   Etiology and Pathogenesis 699
4.1.   Esophageal Varices Secondary to "Portal Hypertension" 699
4.1.1.   Presinusoidal Causes 699
4.1.1.1.   Prehepatic Pathology 699
4.1.1.1.1. Forward Flow Group 699
4.1.1.1.2. Portal Vein Thrombosis or Compression 701
4.1.1.1.3. Splenic Vein Thrombosis 702
4.1.1.2.   Presinusoidal Intrahepatic Disorders 702
4.1.1.2.1. Hepatic Schistosomiasis (Schistosoma Mansoni, Hematobium, Japonicum)
            (Mendes, 1965) 702
4.1.1.2.2. Myeloproliferative Disease, Myelofibrosis 703
4.1.1.2.3. Granulomatous Diseases 703
4.1.1.2.4. Congenital Hepatic Fibrosis (Fibroangioadenomatosis) 703
4.1.1.2.5. Polycystic Liver Disease 703
4.1.1.2.6. Liver Metastases 703
4.1.1.2.7. Wilson's Disease 704
4.1.1.2.8. Acute Hepatitis 704
4.1.2.   Sinusoidal Causes 704
4.1.2.1.   Acute Hepatitis 704
4.1.2.2.   Fatty Liver 704
4.1.2.3.   Early Stage of Chronic, Non-Suppurative, Destructive Cholangitis (Primary
            Biliary Cirrhosis) 704
4.1.2.4.   Kupffer Cell Hypertrophy with Perisinusoidal Fibrosis 704
4.1.3.   Postsinusoidal Portal Hypertension 705
4.1.3.1.   Postsinusoidal Intrahepatic Causes 705
4.1.3.1.1. Liver Cirrhosis 705
4.1.3.1.2. Liver Cirrhosis Associated with Metabolic Disorders 706
4.1.3.1.3. Alcoholic Hepatitis 708
4.1.3.1.4. Partial Nodular Transformation 708
4.1.3.1.5. Veno-Occlusive Disease 708
4.1.3.2.   Extrahepatic Postsinusoidal Portal Hypertension 708
4.1.3.2.1. Budd-Chiari Syndrome 708
4.1.3.2.2. Congestive Heart Failure 709
4.1.3.2.3. Obstruction of Inferior Vena Cava 709
4.2.   Esophageal Varices without Portal Hypertension 709
4.2.1.   Obstruction of Vena Cava Superior (Downhill Varices) 709
4.2.2.   Carcinoma at the Gastroesophageal Junction 709
4.2.3.   Idiopathic Esophageal Varices 709
4.2.4.   Esophageal Varices in Patients with Liver Disease, but Normal Portal Pressure 710
4.3.   Unclassified Miscellaneous Causes 710
5.   Clinical Features: Bleeding 711
5.1.   Incidence 711
5.2.   Pathogenesis of the Bleeding 711
5.3.   Clinical Symptoms 712
6.   Diagnosis 712
6.1.   Diagnosis of Esophageal Varices 712
6.1.1.   Barium Swallow 712
6.1.2.   Esophagoscopy 714
6.1.3.   Splenoportography 715
6.1.4.   Umbilical Vein Portography 717
6.1.5.   Ammonia Tolerance; Indirect Test for Esophageal Varices 718
6.1.6.   Evaluation of the Different Techniques Used 719
6.2.   Diagnosis of Bleeding from Esophageal Varices 719
7.   Therapy 720
7.1.   Medical Management of Bleeding Varices 720
7.1.1.   Blood Transfusion 720
7.1.2.   Prevention of Hepatic Encephalopathy (in Cirrhotics) 720
7.1.3.   Arrest of Further Bleeding 720
7.1.3.1.   Drugs 720

Contents

7.1.3.2.	Gastric Cooling	721
7.1.3.3.	Balloon Tamponade	721
7.1.3.4.	Intraarterial Infusion	721
7.2.	Surgical Management of Bleeding Esophageal Varices	722
7.2.1.	Emergency Surgical Treatment	722
7.2.2.	Elective Surgical Treatment in Liver Cirrhosis with Bleeding Varices	727
7.2.3.	Prophylactic Shunt Operations in Liver Cirrhosis	727
7.2.4.	Prophylactic Operations in Extrahepatic Block	727
7.3.	Thoracic Duct Drainage	728
7.4.	Transumbilical Portal Decompression	728
7.5.	Sclerosing Injections for Esophageal Varices	728
References		728

Chapter 11

Hiatus Hernia. By E. HAFTER. With 28 Figures		741
1.	Definition and Classification	741
2.	Incidence	742
3.	Anatomical Basis, Etiology and Pathogenesis	743
4.	Pathological Anatomy	746
5.	Clinical Features	747
5.1.	Symptoms	747
5.2.	Hiatus Hernia in Infants	749
5.3.	Hiatus Hernia during Pregnancy	749
5.4.	Postoperative Hernias	750
5.5.	Traumatic Hiatus Hernias	750
5.6.	Signs	750
6.	Technical Features	751
6.1.	Radiological Examination	751
6.1.1.	Technique of X-ray Examination	751
6.1.2.	Radiological Demonstration of Reflux	754
6.1.3.	Interpretation of X-ray Findings	757
6.1.4.	Paraesophageal Hernia	763
6.1.5.	Mixed Hernias	764
6.1.6.	Invagination	765
6.1.7.	Note on Terminology	765
6.2.	Endoscopy	765
6.2.1.	Esophagoscopy	766
6.2.2.	Gastroscopy	768
6.2.3.	Peritoneoscopy	768
6.3.	Manometry	768
6.4.	pH Measurements	769
6.5.	Acid Infusion Test	769
7.	Diagnosis	769
8.	Complications	771
9.	Associated Diseases	773
10.	Evolution and Prognosis	774
11.	Therapy	775
11.1.	Medical Treatment	775
11.2.	Surgical Treatment	776
References		779

Chapter 12

Resection and Reconstruction of the Esophagus. By P. VALEMBOIS and G. VANTRAPPEN. With 5 Figures		783
1.	Resection of the Esophagus	783
1.1.	Postoperative Complications	784
2.	Replacement of the Esophagus	784
2.1.	Mortality and Morbidity of the Esophageal Substitution	788
2.1.1.	Necrosis of the Esophageal Substitute	789
2.1.2.	Leakage at the Anastomosis	790
2.1.3.	Other Complications	791
2.2.	Functional Results	791
References		792

Chapter 13

Etiology and Non-Surgical Treatment of Organic Esophageal Stenosis. By G. VANTRAP-
PEN, J. HELLEMANS and K. GEBOES. With 7 Figures 795
1.   Etiology 795
2.   Techniques of Dilatation 797
3.   Indications for Dilatations 803
3.1.   Benign Strictures 803
3.2.   Malignant Stenoses 804
References 805

Chapter 14

Acquired Esophageal Fistula. By K. GEBOES and P. VALEMBOIS. With 3 Figures . . . 807
1.   Esophagorespiratory Fistula 807
1.1.   Etiology 807
1.1.1.   Malignant Esophageal Fistula 807
1.1.2.   Esophagorespiratory Fistula of Benign Origin 807
1.1.2.1. Traumatic Fistula 807
1.1.2.2. Fistula Secondary to Esophageal Diverticulum 809
1.1.2.3. Infectious Fistula 809
1.1.2.4. Esophageal Fistula and Bronchopulmonary Sequestration 810
1.2.   Location of the Fistula 811
1.3.   Symptoms 811
1.4.   Diagnosis 812
1.5.   Treatment 813
2.   Aortoesophageal Fistula 814
2.1.   Benign Aortoesophageal Fistula 814
2.2.   Malignant Aortoesophageal Fistula 814
2.3.   Other Fistulas between the Esophagus and the Cardiovascular System . . 815
2.3.1.   Fistula between the Esophagus and the Pericardial Cavity 815
2.3.2.   Kommerell's Diverticulum 815
2.3.3.   Esophagocardiac Fistula 816
2.3.4.   Fistula between Larger Veins and Esophagus 816
3.   Esophagocavitary Fistulas 816
3.1.   Etiology and Pathogenesis 816
3.2.   Localization 817
3.3.   Symptoms 817
3.4.   Diagnosis 818
3.5.   Treatment 818
4.   External Esophageal Fistula 818
References 819

Chapter 15

The Esophagus in Cutaneous Diseases. By K. GEBOES and J. JANSSENS. With 2 Figures 823
1.   Bullous Dermatoses 823
1.1.   Pemphigus 823
1.2.   Bullous Pemphigoid (Parapemphigus) 823
1.3.   Benign Mucosal Pemphigoid (Cicatricial Pemphigoid) 824
1.4.   Epidermolysis Bullosa Dystrophica 824
1.5.   Toxic Epidermal Necrolysis (Lyell's Disease, Ritter's Disease) 826
1.6.   The Stevens-Johnson Syndrome 827
1.7.   Recurrent Aphtae 827
1.8.   Esophagitis Superficialis Dissecans. Benign or Idiopathic Esophageal Casts 827
2.   Disorders of Keratinization 828
2.1.   Keratosis Follicularis, Darier's Disease 828
2.2.   Keratoderma 829
2.3.   Acanthosis Nigricans 829
3.   Hypertrophic Osteoarthropathy 830
4.   Dermatomyositis 830
5.   Leukoplakia and Other Yellow-White Spots on the Esophageal Mucosa . . 830
References 831

Chapter 16

Miscellaneous and Rare Diseases. By K. GEBOES and W. PELEMANS. With 2 Figures   . 835
1.   Idiopathic Retroperitoneal Fibrosis 835
2.   Amyloidosis 835
3.   Lupus Erythematosus Disseminatus   835
4.   Intramural Diverticulosis 836
5.   Pneumatosis Cystoides 837
6.   Eosinophilic Granuloma 838
7.   Extensive Necrosis of the Esophagus 838
8.   Esophagogastric Invagination. Transmigration of the Esophageal Mucosa . 838
9.   Cervical Osteophytes. External Compression 838
10.   Ulcerative Colitis 839
11.   Pancreatitis 839
12.   Amebic Abcess 839
13.   Worms   839
13.1.   Hydatid Cyst 839
13.2.   Spirocerca Lupus 839
14.   Ectopic Tissues   839
14.1.   Primary Melanosis of the Esophagus 839
14.2.   Sebaceous Glands   840
14.3.   Liver Tissue 840
14.4.   Pancreatic Tissue 840
14.5.   Heterotopic Gastric Mucosa 840
14.6.   Tracheobronchial Remnants 840
14.7.   Aberrant Origin of Right Main Bronchus 841
14.8.   Thyroid Tissue 841
References 841

Subject Index   845

Chapter 1

Basic Data

Anatomy and Embryology

G. Fransen and P. Valembois

With 6 Figures

1. Anatomy

1.1. Topographic Anatomy

(Fig. 1)

The esophagus is a tube closed at both ends by sphincter mechanisms. Starting at the lower edge of the cricoid cartilage it forms the continuation of the pharynx, runs through the posterior mediastinum and the esophageal hiatus of the diaphragm, and ends in the cardiac orifice of the stomach at the level of T 11.

In adults the lower edge of the cricopharyngeal muscle is located 18 cm distal from the upper incisors and the cardia 40 cm; thus the overall length of the esophagus is about 22 cm. Small individual variations are possible, depending on the length of the thorax. In neonates the distance between incisors and cardia averages 18 cm, in 3-year-olds 22 cm, and in 10-year-olds 27 cm.

1.1.1. The Cervical Esophagus

The cervical part of the esophagus extends to the suprasternal notch (at the level of transition T 2–T 3) and runs between the trachea and the spinal column. At the ventral side it is separated from the posterior wall of the trachea by loose fibrous tissue; in some persons it is strongly connected to the membraneous posterior wall of the trachea by elastic tissue. The few tracheo-esophageal muscle fibers that have been described are insignificant. Dorsally the esophagus is connected to the prevertebral portion of the deep cervical fascia by loose connective tissue.

The recurrent nerves run bilaterally in the groove between the trachea and the esophagus. As the cervical esophagus deviates slightly to the left, and as the right recurrent nerve bends around the subclavian artery, the left recurrent nerve runs somewhat closer to the gullet than the right one. The lateral aspect of the lobes of the thyroid and the parathyroids rest on the esophagus. To the left and the right of the gullet run the carotid sheaths with the structures they contain. Because of its slight left deviation, the esophagus is somewhat closer to the left carotid artery.

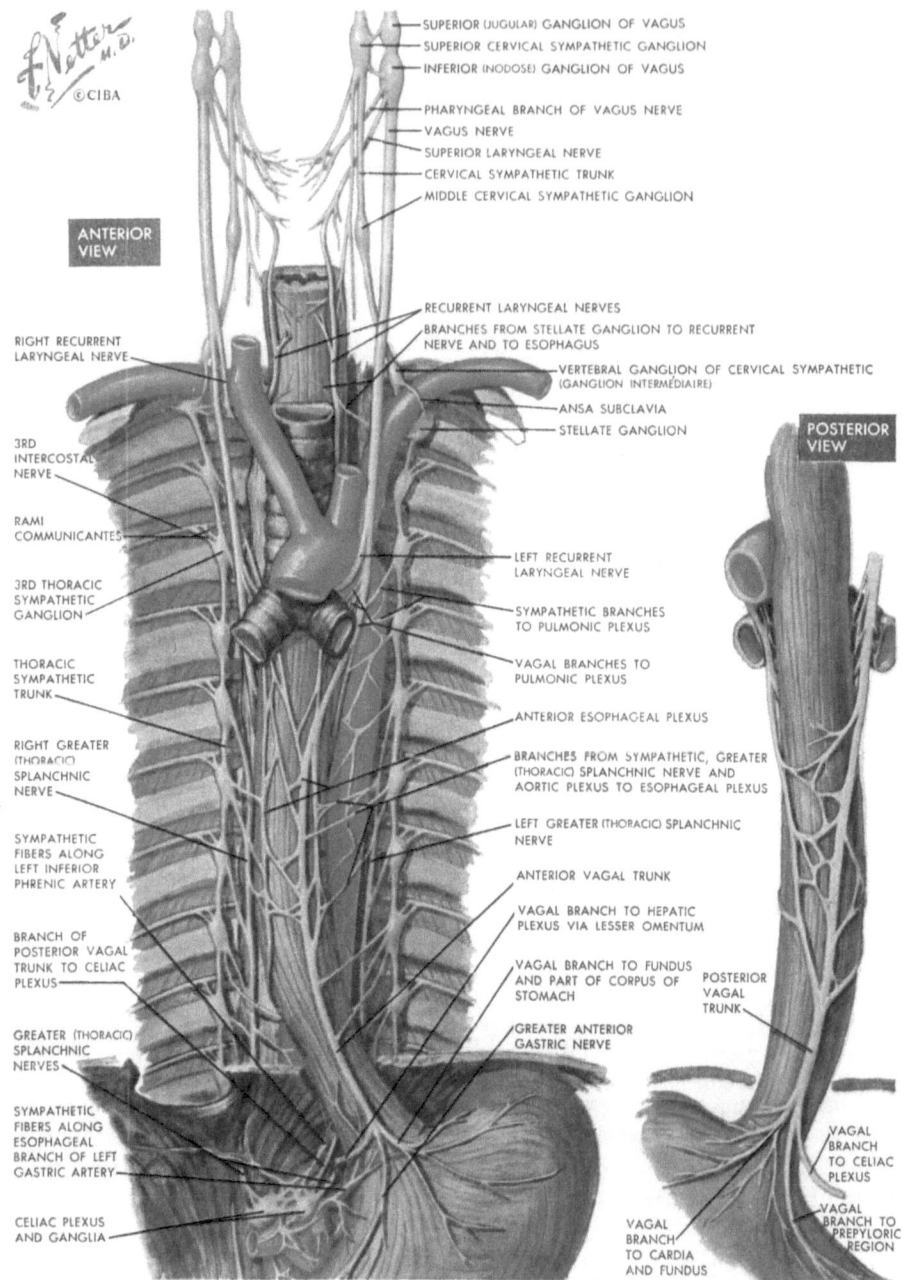

Fig. 1. Topographic relationship and innervation of the esophagus. (From Netter, F. H.: The Ciba collection of medical illustrations, vol. 3: Digestive system, part I: Upper digestive tract, 1959, p. 44)

1.1.2. The Thoracic Esophagus

In its thoracic part the esophagus remains in intimate relationship with the posterior wall of the trachea and with the prevertebral fascia. As a result of the slight deviation of the esophagus to the left, and of the terminal part of the trachea to the right, part of the gullet appears behind the trachea as the bed of a groove in which runs the left recurrent nerve. Farther down, the esophagus passes to the right of the aortic arch from which it receives a radiologically observable notch. Immediately below this notch the esophagus crosses the bifurcation of the trachea and the left main bronchus. From there on it runs along the pericardium of the left atrium. In this portion the course of the esophagus is slightly convex to the right of the midline. The right aspect of the gullet is completely covered by the parietal pleura except at the level of T4, where the azygos vein turns to the ventral side. On its left, the upper part of the thoracic esophagus is covered anterolaterally by the left subclavian artery and posterolaterally by the parietal pleura. Distally from the aortic arch (T4), the esophagus is located to the right of the descending aorta. From T8 onward the aorta disappears behind the gullet, and the left esophageal wall comes into closer contact with the mediastinal pleura. From the bifurcation of the trachea onward, both vagal nerves and the esophageal nerve plexus lie in close contact with the esophagus. In the postero-anterior plane the esophagus follows the curvature of the spine; dorsally it remains in close contact with the vertebral bodies through the prevertebral fascia. From T8 onward it runs a more ventral course, away from the spine, and after passing through the esophageal hiatus of the diaphragm, lies in front of the aorta. Dorsally the esophagus is crossed by the first five intercostal arteries and the hemiazygos vein. The thoracic duct, which passes through the aortic hiatus of the diaphragm, at first runs a course dorsal to the esophagus, between the azygos vein on the right and the aorta on the left. From the level of T5 onward it gradually moves to the left and then continues upward between the left side of the esophagus and the parietal pleura, dorsally to the aortic arch and the thoracic part of the subclavian artery. In the neck it turns away from the esophagus and ends in the junction of the subclavian and the internal jugular veins.

1.1.3. The Abdominal Esophagus

The abdominal part of the esophagus is short; in dorsal decubitus, when the stomach sags to the right of the spinal column, it is 2 to 3 cm long. The cardiac orifice may ascend as high as the esophageal hiatus of the diaphragm; when the abdominal part is severed, the esophagus usually disappears into the thorax.

The anterior part and to some extent the right side of the abdominal esophagus lie in a small hollow in the posterior aspect of the left liver lobe. The dorsal aspect of the esophagus rests on the crura of the diaphragm, and on the left the gullet may come in close contact with the spleen.

The esophageal lumen can be narrowed in several locations, four of which are fairly constant: (1) the narrowing at the entrance of the esophagus caused by the cricopharyngeal muscle and the cricoid cartilage; (2) the small indentation in the left esophageal wall caused by the crossing of the aortic arch—at this point aortic pulsations may be observed during esophagoscopy; (3) an indentation on the left anterior aspect caused by the left main bronchus; (4) the narrowing caused by the esophagogastric sphincter mechanism at or slightly above the passage through the diaphragm.

1.2. The Musculature of the Esophagus Proper
(Fig. 2)

Schematically the musculature of the esophagus can be divided into an exterior longitudinal and an interior circular muscle layer, but this representation is a simplification of a structure that is actually much more complex (KAUF-MANN et al., 1968).

The upper 2 to 6 cm contain only striated muscle. From there on, smooth muscle fibers gradually become more abundant, so that at a distance of 4 to 8 cm from the superior end the smooth musculature constitutes 50% of the esophageal tunica muscularis. The junction of striated and smooth muscle in the inner "circular" layer is located at a higher level than in the outer "longitudinal" layer.

Most muscle fibers of the longitudinal layer originate from a strong tendon in the center of the dorsal upper edge of the cricoid. Two bundles of muscles emanate from this tendon; their fibers diverge distally and form a fan around the esophagus. Both diverging bundles meet on the dorsal midline at about 3 cm below the cricoid. From this point on, the entire circumference of the esophagus is covered by a layer of longitudinal fibers. On both sides two additional smaller muscle bundles participate in the formation of this layer; ipsilaterally they originate from the posterolateral part of the cricoid and contralaterally from the cricopharyngeal muscle. Thus the configuration of the longitudinal muscle fibers around the most proximal part of the esophagus leaves a V-shaped defect in the posterior wall, called the triangle of Laimer. The upper edge of this V-shaped area is formed by the lower edge of the cricopharyngeal muscle; its floor by the fibers of the inner circular layer. Only a few fibers originating at the lower edge of the cricopharyngeal muscle, and the rare fibers that leave both longitudinal bundles are scattered over this defect.

In the upper third of the esophagus the longitudinal layer is clearly thicker at the lateral aspects than at the ventral and dorsal sides; more distally, the layering around the esophagus becomes more uniform. Also, the overall thickness seems to decrease a little distally.

The longitudinal muscle fibers do not follow the axis of the esophagus quite closely; it is as though the end of the esophageal tube were turned to the left through 90° in relation to the pharyngoesophageal junction; in other words, the course of the fibers is that of an elongated spiral, turning round one quarter of the esophageal circumference (KAUFMANN et al., 1968).

Offshoots of the longitudinal muscle layer may veer off into the inner coat; these offshoots are spread irregularly over the circumference of the esophagus. A few fibroelastic and muscle fibers connect the anterior esophageal wall with the posterior wall of the trachea. Occasionally smooth muscle fibers emanate from the membraneous part of the left main bronchus and from the left pleura (bronchoesophageal and pleuroesophageal muscle).

In contrast with the musculature elsewhere in the gastrointestinal tract, the inner, so-called circular muscle layer of the esophagus is thicker than the outer, longitudinal layer. It is as yet uncertain whether or not the circular layer receives fibers from the cricopharyngeal muscle. At any rate, the caudal horizontal fibers of this muscle surround the upper fibers of the esophagus and a tight connection certainly exists. The fibers of the so-called circular layer run horizontally only in the isolated and retracted esophagus. In the esophagus in situ their course is elliptical and their inclination varies according to the level of the esophagus: in the cervical part, the highest points of the ellipses are located dorsally; in the upper thoracic part, right laterally; behind the heart, ventrally; and in the abdominal part, left laterally (KAUFMANN et al., 1968). Moreover,

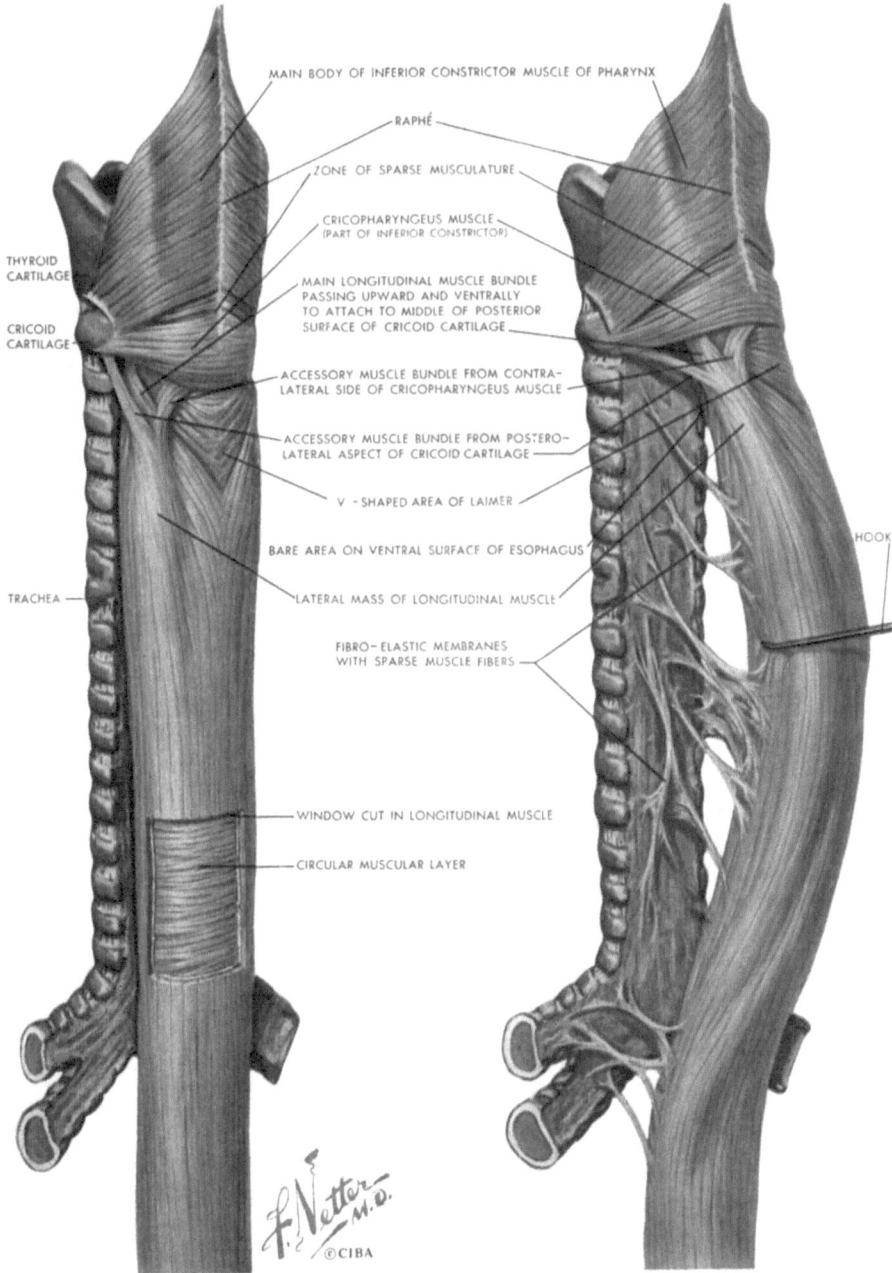

Fig. 2. Musculature of the esophagus. (From NETTER, F. H.: The Ciba collection of medical illustrations, vol. 3: Digestive system, part I: Upper digestive tract, 1959, p. 36)

completely parallel and uniform courses of the circular fibers do not seem to occur at any level of the esophagus; everywhere there are fibers that leave their expected course and join higher or lower bundles.

1.3. The Pharyngoesophageal Junction
(Fig. 2)

The cricopharyngeal muscle, in other words, the cricopharyngeal part of the lower constrictor of the pharynx, originates on both posterolateral sides of the cricoid cartilage and covers the dorsal aspect of the pharyngoesophageal junction. It has no median raphe and some of its lower muscle bundles diverge into the esophageal wall itself, so that its upper boundary can usually be recognized more easily than its transition to the esophageal wall proper (Zaino et al., 1970).

Although, anatomically speaking, this muscle belongs to the pharyngeal wall, it is of the utmost importance for the normal functioning of the esophagus because it constitutes the upper esophageal sphincter. It is still not certain whether the closing mechanism of this sphincter in its resting state is due to a tonic contraction or to stretching of the cricopharyngeal muscle fibers. The relaxation and the contraction of this sphincter constitute an integral part of normal deglutition and initiate the primary peristaltic wave of the esophagus. Most hypopharyngeal diverticula find their origin in the weak muscle wall of the upper part of the cricopharyngeus.

1.4. The Esophagogastric Junction
1.4.1. The Gastroesophageal Sphincter

The consensus of opinion is that the circular and longitudinal muscle layers of the esophagus become continuous with those of the stomach. The longitudinal muscle layer diverges distally from the cardia over the gastric body as the outer longitudinal muscle coat; the inner muscle layer of the esophagus continues into the stomach, on the one hand into the middle muscle layer, whose fibers run more or less horizontally, and on the other hand into the inner muscle layer, whose fibers are turned in a sling-like manner across the cardiac incisura. To the latter muscular arrangement some authors ascribe a certain role in the antireflux mechanism. Other factors to which a role in the closing mechanism of the cardia has been ascribed are the sharp angle between the lower esophagus and the right side of the gastric fundus (angle of His), the rosette-like configuration of the gastric mucosa around the cardiac orifice, the lower esophageal sphincter, the intraabdominal part of the esophagus, the phrenoesophageal membrane and the configuration of the esophageal hiatus of the diaphragm. None of these structures, however, can be termed an anatomical sphincter. In the most distal segment

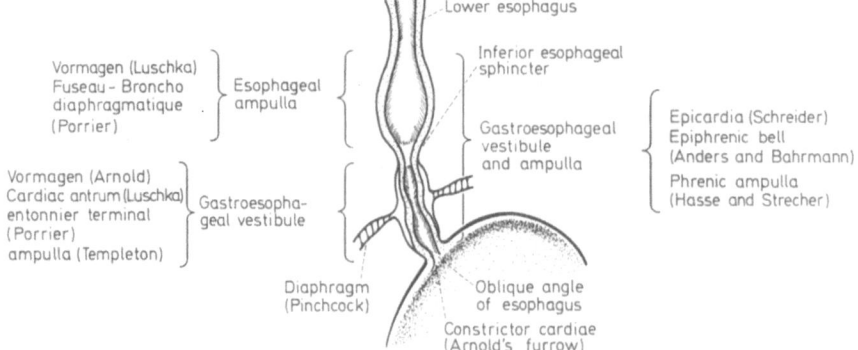

Fig. 3. Schematic diagram of the anatomy of the gastroesophageal junction. [From Van-trappen et al.: Amer. J. Med. 28, 564 (1960)]

of the esophagus (from about 2 cm above the diaphragm to the cardiac orifice) the muscular wall is slightly thicker because of the increased thickness of the inner circular musculature and because of the presence of extra muscle bundles immediately below the submucosa (ZAINO et al., 1960). This zone has been called the esophagogastric vestibule. The upper border of the vestibule has been described by LERCHE (1950) as the lower esophageal sphincter (Fig. 3) and can be visualized radiologically as a contractile ring, the A-ring of WOLF (1970) (Fig. 25). This structure has also been observed in 4% of the cadavers as a ring-like muscular narrowing (GOYAL et al., 1970, 1971). The lower end of the vestibule has been described as the constrictor cardiae (LERCHE, 1950). Manometric studies indicate that the vestibule functions as a unit. In the resting state it is closed and its intraluminal pressure is high (high-pressure zone). Upon deglutition or other stimuli, it opens (relaxation). Although the vestibule cannot be considered an anatomical sphincter, it has been termed a physiological sphincter, because of its functional characteristics (FYKE et al., 1956; VANTRAPPEN et al., 1960).

1.4.2. The Phrenoesophageal Membrane

The vestibular complex is surrounded by the phrenoesophageal membrane, a fibroelastic ligament arising from the subdiaphragmatic fascia. This phrenoesophageal membrane divides at the lower margin of the esophageal hiatus into a thin, elongated ascending leaf, which surrounds the terminal segment of the esophagus in a tent-like fashion, and into a shorter and thicker descending leaf, which merges with the peritoneal covering of the stomach. The upper division of the membrane attaches itself in a circumferential fashion around the esophageal segment, about 2 to 3 cm above the level of the esophageal hiatus (CAREY and HOLLINSHEAD, 1955; ZAINO et al., 1960; BOMBECK et al., 1966). Between the lower division of the membrane and the cardia there is a ring of fairly solid fatty tissue, which in certain places may be somewhat more fibrous and contributes to the fixation of the esophagus (BOUTELIER and LEFORT, 1970). The vagus nerves and blood vessels pierce the upper and lower divisions of the membrane and run along the esophagus to the stomach.

1.4.3. The Diaphragmatic Hiatus
(Fig. 4)

The anatomy of the esophageal hiatus of the diaphragm is certainly not uniform, though usually its many variants can readily be derived from the standard type found in 46% of the individuals (COLLIS et al., 1954). The tendinous sheets of the diaphragmatic crura originate from the anterolateral aspect of the first four lumbar vertebrae and their intervertebral disks; both crura are separated from each other by the celiac trunk. During its ventrally ascending course the right crus bifurcates into a more superficial muscle bundle, which bends to the right around the esophagus, and into a deeper bundle which bends to the left proximally to the celiac trunk, and forms the left margin of the diaphragmatic hiatus. Ventrally their sinewy insertions cross each other in the central tendon of the diaphragm. The entire circumference of the hiatus is therefore formed by muscle bundles of the right crus. The left crus, which runs in a postero-anterior direction, meets those muscle bundles of the right crus that run to the left of the esophagus, but does not itself take part in the formation of the esophageal hiatus. The most common anatomical variants of this standard type show what is called the shift to the left. A shift to the left can be of first, second or third degree, depending on the extent to which the margins of the hiatus are formed

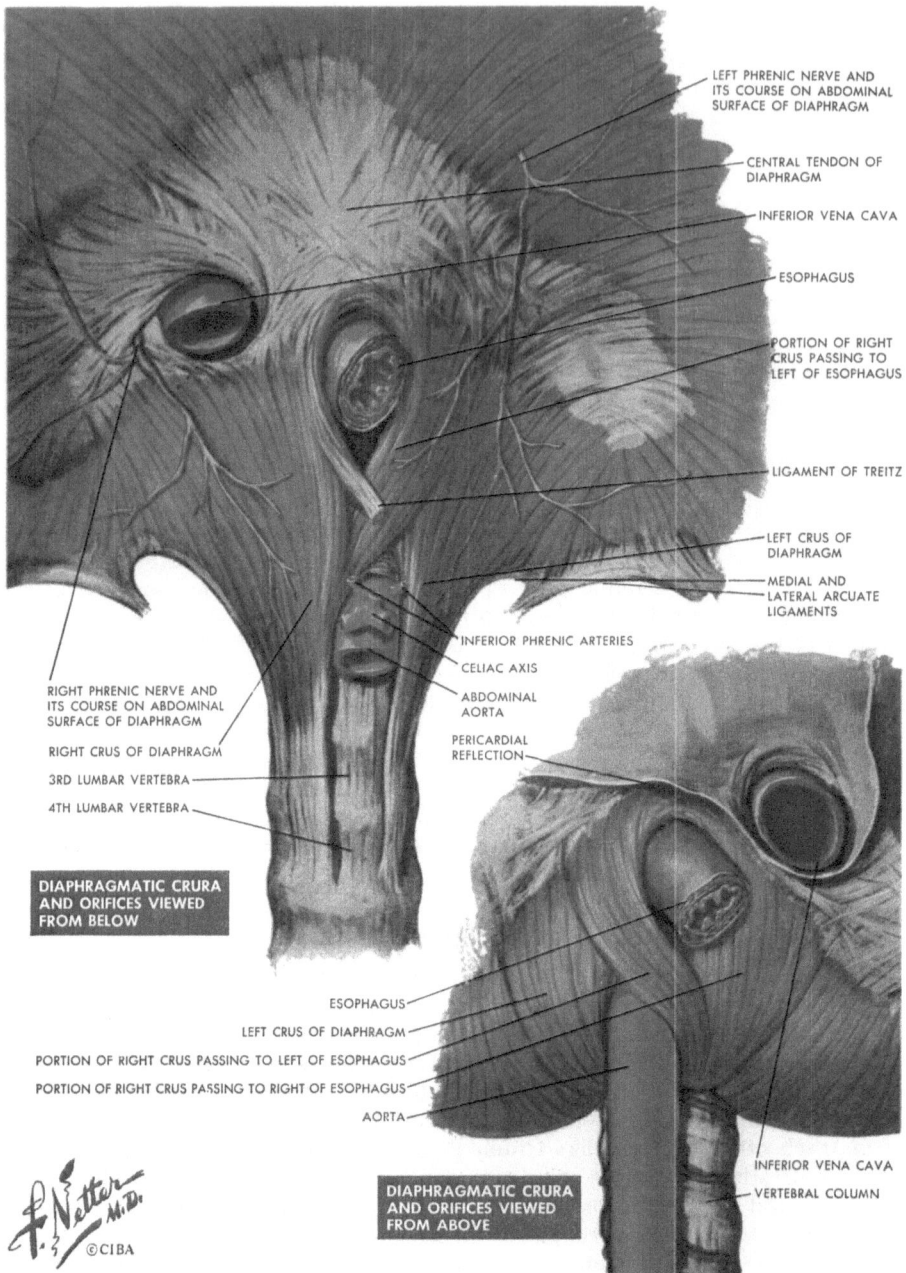

Fig. 4. Anatomy of the esophageal hiatus. (From Netter, F. H.: The Ciba collection of medical illustrations, vol. 3: Digestive system, part I: Upper digestive tract, 1959, p. 39)

by muscle bundles of the left crus (Collis et al., 1954). A number of other bands and muscles have been described; among them the muscle of Low, types I and II, the transverse intertendinous muscle, and the ligament of Treitz.

1.5. Arterial Blood Supply

The cervical part of the esophagus receives its blood supply mainly from the lower thyroid artery, a branch of the truncus thyreocervicalis. The blood is supplied both directly, via the final branches of these arteries, and indirectly via the rami esophagei, which arise from them. The branches which originate from the ascending part of the lower thyroid artery are mostly larger and extend more distally than those originating from the distal part of the artery. Although the right lower thyroid artery usually has more branches than the left, the blood supply to both sides of the esophagus is of the same order. Very often the ascending part of the right thyroid artery has an important tracheoesophageal branch, which follows the course of the recurrent laryngeal nerve, supplies the trachea, the hilar nodes and the posterolateral side of the esophagus, and finally anastomoses with branches of the bronchial arteries. An additional, individually very variable blood supply is provided by small, direct branches of various arteries, such as the a. subclavia, a. carotis communis, a. vertebralis, a. thyroidea superior, a. cervicalis superficialis and the truncus costocervicalis.

The thoracic part of the esophagus receives its blood supply from the branches of the aorta, the bronchial arteries and the right intercostal arteries. At the level of the bifurcation of the trachea the main supply comes from branches of the bronchial arteries, which descend on the ventral side of the esophagus. Fifty percent of all individuals also have accessory esophageal branches which originate directly from the aortic arch and the aorta as well as from the a. mammaria interna, the a. carotis communis and the upper aa. intercostales. Below the bifurcation of the trachea the thoracic esophagus receives its blood supply from two esophageal branches that arise directly from the right ventral side of the aorta. The upper branch is usually the smaller of the two (3–4 cm) and originates at the level of T6–T7; the lower is longer (6–7 cm) and originates at the level of T8–T9. Both arteries run to the dorsal side of the esophagus, where they split into a right and a left branch. These in turn split into ascending and descending branches which anastomose between themselves, with the descending branches of the lower thyroid artery, and with the ascending branches of the left gastric artery and the left lower phrenic artery.

The abdominal part of the esophagus is supplied mainly from the esophageal branches of the left gastric artery and of the left lower phrenic artery. These esophageal branches run mainly alongside the right anterolateral and dorsal aspect of the esophagus and anastomose with the lower two rami esophagei, which originate directly from the thoracic aorta. An additional blood supply may be provided by branches of the aorta, the splenic artery, the celiac trunk and an aberrant left hepatic artery.

In general the arterial blood supply of the human esophagus can be considered as segmental. A periesophageal dissection during surgery can therefore easily lead to devascularization and ischemic necrosis, in spite of the existence of anastomoses with neighbouring vessels.

1.6. Venous Drainage

The arrangement of the venous drainage, in both fetuses and adults has been clearly outlined by the work of BUTLER (1951). The esophageal veins may conveniently be classified as intrinsic veins and extrinsic veins.

1.6.1. Intrinsic Veins

The subepithelial venous plexus lies in the lamina propria, close to the epithelium, and extends over the whole length of the esophagus as a coarse polygonal meshwork, slightly elongated in the line of the long axis of the esophagus. The average diameter of these veins varies from 30 μm in the fully developed fetus to 170 μm in adults. There are no valves in this plexus. Numerous small veins perforate the muscularis mucosae to join the submucosal plexus.

At the cardia, where the veins follow a more longitudinal direction, the plexus joins the denser subglandular venous plexus of the stomach; at the lower margin of the cricoid the veins are also more longitudinally arranged and join the irregular subepithelial plexus of the pharynx.

The submucosal venous plexus lies midway between the muscularis mucosae and the circular muscle coat and consists of 10 to 15 longitudinal veins, evenly distributed around the circumference of the esophagus and connected by numerous cross-anastomoses. The diameter varies from 50 μm in the fully developed fetus to 1 mm in adults.

At the distal end of the esophagus the veins increase in number but decrease in diameter; at the cardia they become aggregated in the longitudinal folds of the mucosa and are markedly tortuous. They join the submucosal veins of the stomach. Valves to direct the blood flow to the stomach may be found at this level, but are not always present.

At the level of the vestibule the intrinsic venous drainage is chiefly subepithelial; in the rest of the esophagus it runs chiefly in the submucosal layer. In the upper esophagus the veins become tortuous with fusiform and globular dilatations which give them a varicose appearance; they increase in diameter (up to 4 mm) but their number is reduced to about eight, arranged in a ventral and a dorsal group; they drain into the pharyngolaryngeal venous plexus.

The perforating veins arise from the longitudinal submucosal plexus and at frequent intervals perforate the muscle layers, which are also drained by them. Most of these veins reach the outer surface along the lateral border of the esophagus; at the point of exit from the muscle coat, valves direct the blood outwards.

1.6.2. Extrinsic Veins

The perforating veins run for a short distance on the surface of the esophagus before uniting in the greater periesophageal veins. Two of these run longitudinally on the outer esophageal surface in close proximity to the vagus nerves and pursue their spiral course around the esophagus; they are called venae comitantes nervi vagi and connect the left gastric vein to the azygos or hemiazygos veins, either directly or via the posterior bronchial veins. The periesophageal veins of the cervical gullet drain into the inferior thyroid vein, the venous plexus on the lower pole of the thyroid gland, the vertebral and deep cervical veins and the peritracheal venous plexus. Valves, when present, direct the blood away from the esophagus. Most of the intrathoracic periesophageal veins drain on the right into the azygos vein and on the left into the hemiazygos vein. The number of periesophageal veins is always smaller on the left than on the right, especially if the hemiazygos system is poorly developed. When the hemiazygos is absent, the esophageal veins join the intercostal veins. Above the level of the arch of the azygos vein the esophageal veins drain into the superior intercostal veins. At the cardia several small esophageal veins join the superior and inferior phrenic veins. In the abdomen the esophageal veins join mainly the left gastric vein, but smaller veins may reach the vena phrenica inferior, vena gastroepiploica sinistra, or vena splenica.

1.7. Lymphatic Drainage

Both in the mucosa and in the submucosa there is a dense network of lymph vessels, which are so closely interconnected as to constitute a single plexus. Indeed there are more lymph vessels than blood capillaries in the submucosa. The flow in the submucosal plexus runs chiefly in the longitudinal direction and, on injection of contrast medium, the longitudinal spread of the medium is seen to be about six times that of the transverse spread. In the upper two thirds of the esophagus the flow is mostly cranially directed; in the lower third, mostly distally. Especially in the thoracic part of the esophagus the submucosal lymph vessels run over a long distance in a longitudinal direction before penetrating through the muscle layer into the adventitia. Some lymph vessels of the submucosal plexus, however, penetrate directly through the muscular wall into the adventitia.

There are fewer lymph vessels in the muscle layers. It is still uncertain whether or not connections exist between the submucosal plexus and the lymph chain in the muscle layers; beyond the esophageal wall the lymph vessels of the submucosa and musculosa are no longer separate. The short course of the lymph vessels on the outside of the esophagus is also mainly longitudinal, although much more irregular than in the submucosal plexus.

Except for the lymph vessels in the most proximal part of the esophagus, which flow directly into the deep cervical chain, all lymph vessels drain into the nearest lymph nodes after reaching the adventitia, i.e., into the internal jugular, the tracheal, the tracheobronchial, the posterior mediastinal or the paracardial nodes. The internal jugular chain, which belongs to the deep cervical nodes, follows the course of the internal jugular vein from the parotid gland until the clavicle and ends in the thoracic duct or the right lymph duct. The tracheal nodes, which are located in the groove between esophagus and trachea, and the tracheobronchial nodes, located in the angles formed by the bifurcation of the trachea, drain proximally via the bronchomediastinal trunk into the thoracic duct. Anastomoses with the internal mammary chain and the lower lymph nodes of the internal jugular chain may occur, as well as direct connections with the surrounding veins.

The posterior mediastinal lymph nodes form a chain located against the dorsal side of the esophagus and in front of the aorta; they drain chiefly into the tracheal and tracheobronchial nodes. The diaphragmatic nodes, located just above the diaphragm at the dorsal aspect of both esophagus and aorta, drain the most distal part of the gullet.

In 25% of all individuals, one or two lymph nodes are found ventrally to the esophagus in the phrenopericardial angle, and retrocardially; but these drain cranially, into the tracheal and tracheobronchial nodes. The pericardial lymph nodes are located below the diaphragm; they are part of the upper left gastric group and provide the lymph drainage of the abdominal esophagus. Some lymph vessels, however, ascend through the hiatus and join other local lymph vessels. Thus the arrangement of the lymph drainage of the esophageal wall is not segmental. This explains why lymph node invasion can occur at a site remote from the primary esophageal lesion.

1.8. Nerve Supply (Innervation)
(Fig. 1)

1.8.1. Parasympathetic Innervation

The complete parasympathetic innervation of the esophagus is provided by the vagal nerves; the visceral afferent and efferent cell bodies are located in the nucleus dorsalis; the fibers that innervate the striated muscles of the pharynx and of the upper segment of the esophagus originate in the nucleus ambiguus. The vagus branches also receive fibers emanating from the paravertebral sympathetic chains; this makes their composition from the neck onward a mixture of both sympathetic and parasympathetic fibers (Youmans, 1968). The pharyngo-esophageal junction is innervated by the pharyngeal plexus, which is located on the middle constrictor of the pharynx and is formed by the pharyngeal branches of the vagal nerves. Smaller branches coming from the ninth and eleventh cranial nerves also arrive via the vagal nerves. While a single nerve derived from the vagus supplies the cricopharyngeal muscle in the dog, no such nerve can be demonstrated in man (Lund, 1965).

The cervical part of the esophagus is innervated by the recurrent laryngeal nerves. These originate on the vagal nerves: the right recurrent nerve at the lower margin of the subclavian artery, the left one at the lower margin of the aortic arch. They are slung dorsally around these vessels and ascend in the groove between esophagus and trachea, to which the esophageal and tracheal nerves branch off.

The upper thoracic esophagus is innervated by branches of the left recurrent laryngeal nerve and by smaller branches, split off directly from the vagal nerves. After their passage through the carotid sheaths, the vagal nerves descend into the posterior mediastinum, pass behind the lunghili and bend medially until they reach the esophageal wall. There they join with fibers of the sympathetic chain to form the esophageal plexus. According to Peden et al. (1950), the left vagus splits before the esophageal plexus forms two main branches; the first branch runs through the ventral part of the esophageal plexus and constitutes the main element of the anterior abdominal vagus trunk; the second branch runs around the left esophageal wall, joins the dorsal part of the eso-phageal plexus and contributes to the formation of the dorsal trunk of the abdominal vagus. According to the same authors, a large branch of the right vagus constitutes the main element of the dorsal part of the esophageal plexus and of the dorsal trunk of the abdominal vagus, whereas several lesser branches participate in the formation of the neutral esophageal plexus. As a result of the intertwining of the left and right vagus in the esophageal plexus, both the anterior and the posterior vagus trunk contain fibers of the left and of the right vagus when they differentiate out of the esophageal plexus. The level at which the ventral and dorsal vagal trunk are formed out of the esophageal plexus varies from immediately to 6 cm above the diaphragm (Chamberlin and Winship, 1947); the average distance above the diaphragm at which the anterior trunk becomes single is 5.13 cm; for the posterior trunk it is 3.7 cm (Jackson, 1949). However, sometimes several anterior and/or posterior vagal trunks are found (Jackson, 1949; Peden et al., 1950), or a single anterior and/or posterior vagal trunk may already have split once more before its passage through the esophageal hiatus (Jackson, 1949). According to Chamberlin and Winship (1947) these anatomical variants are much more frequent (40% of all cases) than the study of Dragstedt et al. (1947) suggests.

The anterior vagal trunk splits in the abdomen into two branches; the hepatic branch courses in the smaller omentum and its smaller branches innervate the porta hepatis, the arteria hepatica, the duodenum and the arteria gastroduodenalis; the anterior gastric branches (usually four, but the number can vary from one to nine) form the gastric plexus on the anterior aspect of the stomach. The dorsal vagus gives rise to about six smaller gastric nerves, which intertwine into the gastric plexus on the posterior aspect of the stomach; a larger branch of the dorsal vagus follows alongside the left gastric artery to the celiac plexus. In some cases the dorsal vagal trunk is bent just below the diaphragm and proceeds directly, alongside the aorta, to the celiac plexus (JACKSON, 1949); in that case, the posterior wall of the stomach is innervated by small branches, veering off the dorsal vagal trunk at different levels.

1.8.2. Sympathetic Innervation

The cell bodies of the centroganglionary connectors lie in the spinal marrow at the level of the segments T4–T5–T6 on the lateral side of the columna grisea anterior et posterior. The preganglionary fibers of these cell bodies leave the spine via the ventral roots and reach the sympathetic chain via the rami communicantes albi. Here they make synapses with the excitatory neuron of the corresponding ganglion, or they turn to a higher or lower ganglion. The postganglionary fibers reach the esophagus via nerve branches that veer off from the sympathetic chain; some reach the esophageal wall directly, others join the vagus trunk. Thus the vagal nerves always contain a number of postganglionary sympathetic fibers from their entrance into the neck (YOUMANS, 1968).

The pharyngeal plexus, which innervates the pharyngoesophageal junction, receives from the rami pharyngei of the vagal nerves, sympathetic fibers which arrive directly from the superior cervical ganglion and fibers which are supplied by the arteriae pharyngeae. Further distally other fibers leave the ganglion cervicale medium, the ganglion stellatum and the ansa subclavia for the esophagus. The esophageal plexus, formed by the intertwining of the vagal nerves, in addition receives sympathetic fibers emanating directly from the thoracic aortic plexus, the sympathetic chain, and the major splanchnic nerve. The latter originates on the sixth to the ninth thoracic sympathetic ganglia as independent bundles that run medially and caudally and combine to form one trunk near the diaphragm.

The distal esophageal segment also receives direct sympathetic fibers coming from the celiac ganglion. These fibers reach the esophagus via the periarterial plexuses around the left gastric artery and the lower phrenic artery.

2. Embryology

The elements of the esophageal wall derive from: (1) an internal tube of entoderm, which is the primary tissue that eventually becomes the epithelial lining, including its glandular ingrowths; (2) an investing layer of splanchnic mesoderm, which differentiates into lamina propria, submucosa and muscularis mucosa; (3) nervous elements deriving from the neural crest.

The esophagus develops from the foregut. Its cranial part, between the buccopharyngeal membrane and the pulmonary buds, dilates and eventually becomes the pharynx (Fig. 5). At the end of the third week the buccopharyngeal membrane disappears without leaving any trace in the later stages (LANGMAN, 1963). The esophagus develops from that part of the foregut which extends from the respiratory diverticulum to the fusiform dilatation that develops into the stomach.

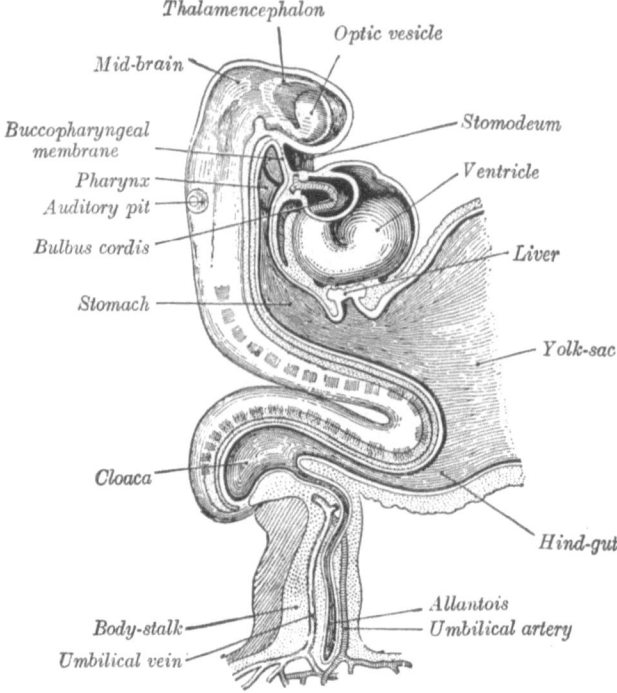

Fig. 5. Human embryo, about 15 days old. Brain and heart represented from the right side. Digestive tube and yolk sac in median sections. (From Gray, H.: Anatomy of the human body. 28th edition by C. M. Goss. Philadelphia: Lea & Febiger 1966, p. 1162)

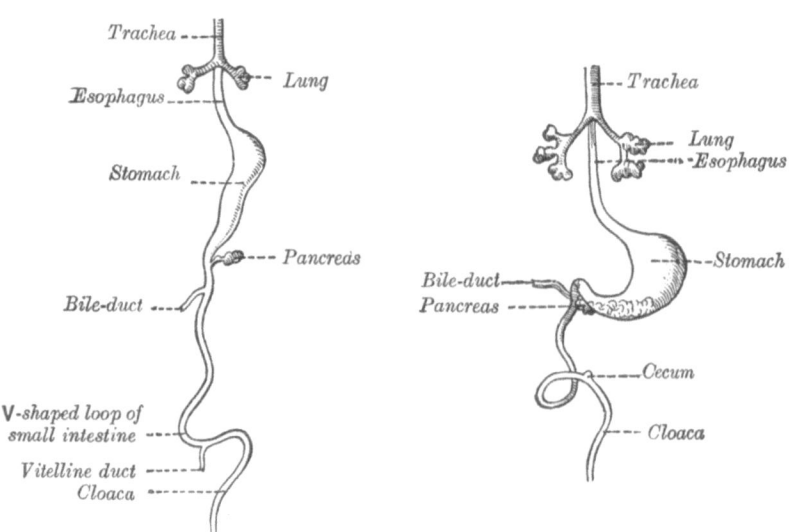

Fig. 6. Embryonic development of the esophagus. At about the fourth week a fusiform dilatation of the primitive gut appears and above this the tubular esophagus can be recognized. The latter soon elongates. (From Gray, H.: Anatomy of the human body. 28th edition by C. M. Goss. Philadelphia: Lea & Febiger 1966, p. 1164)

A tubular esophagus becomes recognizable around the third week (BOTHA, 1963). At four weeks it is still a short tube extending from the pharynx to the fusiform dilatation of the foregut (Fig. 6), but it elongates rapidly, keeping pace with the differentiating neck and the growing heart and lungs alongside.

Concentric depositions of mesodermal elements are found around the esophagus. These elements differentiate into muscle and connective tissue. The inner circular layer of muscle differentiates at the 10–40 mm stage (6th week) and the outer longitudinal layer at the 20–75 mm stage (8th week) (BOTHA, 1963). The muscularis mucosae differentiates even later and becomes apparent at the 30–90 mm stage (10th week) (BOTHA, 1963).

Neuroblasts reach the embryonic esophagus along the vagi before the 10 mm stage, and form a complete circlet outside the circular muscle before the longitudinal muscle begins to develop (SMITH and TAYLOR, 1972). Groups of large neuroblasts are visible within the vagi of the 10 mm embryo.

Migration of neuroblasts along the vagi continues, so that these cells increase in number as development proceeds. In fetuses of 65 mm or less, the myenteric plexus is visible throughout the whole length of the esophagus. As growth proceeds, the cells from the upper quarter apparently migrate lower down the esophagus so that a myenteric plexus is not found in the upper part after the 80 mm stage. With cholinesterase methods, both the periesophageal and myenteric plexuses are visible in the 35 mm fetus. At the 65 mm stage the myenteric plexus stains more darkly. In the 90 mm fetus, most ganglia show enzyme activity (SMITH and TAYLOR, 1972). It seems that the ganglion cells continue to develop after birth (LORENZ, 1962). The epithelium becomes two-layered between the 23 mm and the 34 mm stage; it subsequently changes to a multilayered sheath. It begins to acquire cilia after the 70 mm stage. The ciliated epithelium first appears as islands which then grow together. This change begins in the middle part of the esophagus and extends upwards and downwards (JOHNS, 1952). It is not until the fifth month that a stratified squamous epithelium starts to replace it. This change also begins in the middle reach of the esophagus and extends upwards and downwards. At birth the epithelium numbers 10 layers but may still include some ciliated patches. Superficial glands develop during the fifth month, whereas the deep glands form mostly after birth (AREY, 1965).

References

AREY, L. B.: Developmental anatomy. A textbook and laboratory manual of embryology. Philadelphia-London: W. B. Saunders Co. 1965.

BOMBECK, C. T., DILLARD, D. H., NYHUS, L. M.: Muscular anatomy of the gastroesophageal junction and role of phreno-esophageal ligament: autopsy study of sphincter mechanism. Ann. Surg. 164, 643–654 (1966).

BOTHA, G. S. M.: Gastro-oesophageal junction: clinical applications to oesophageal and gastric surgery. Boston: Little, Brown & Co. 1963.

BOUTELIER, P., LEFORT, R.: Etude anatomique du "meso-œsophage abdominal". J. Chir. (Paris) 100, 371–384 (1970).

BUTLER, H.: The veins of the oesophagus. Thorax 6, 267–296 (1951).

CAREY, J. M., HOLLINSHEAD, W. H.: An anatomic study of the esophageal hiatus. Surg. Gynec. Obstet. 100, 196–200 (1955).

CHAMBERLIN, J. A., WINSHIP, T.: Anatomic variations of the vagus nerves. Their significance in vagus neurectomy. Surgery 22, 1–19 (1947).

COLLIS, J. L., KELLY, T. D., WILEY, A. M.: Anatomy of the crura of the diaphragm and the surgery of hiatus hernia. Thorax 9, 175–189 (1954).

DRAGSTEDT, L. R., FOURNIER, H. J., WOODWARD, E. R., TOVEE, E. B., HARPER, P. V.: Transabdominal gastric vagotomy. A study of the anatomy and surgery of the vagus nerves at the lower portion of the esophagus. Surg. Gynec. Obstet. 85, 461–466 (1947).

Fyke, F. E., Code, C. F., Schlegel, J. F.: The gastroesophageal sphincter in healthy human beings. Gastroenterologia (Basel) **86**, 135–150 (1956).

Goyal, R. K., Bauer, J. L., Spiro, H. M.: The nature and location of the lower esophageal ring. New Engl. J. Med. **284**, 1175–1180 (1971).

Goyal, R. K., Glancy, J. J., Spiro, H. M.: Lower esophageal ring. New Engl. J. Med. **282**, 1298–1305, 1355–1361 (1970).

Jackson, R. G.: Anatomy of the vagus nerves in the region of the lower esophagus and the stomach. Anat. Rec. **103**, 1–18 (1949).

Johns, B. A. F.: Developmental changes in the oesophageal epithelium in man. J. Anat. (Lond.) **86**, 431–442 (1952).

Kaufmann, P., Lierse, W., Stark, J., Stelzner, F.: Die Muskelanordnung in der Speise-röhre (Mensch, Rhesusaffe, Kaninchen, Maus, Ratte, Seehund). Ergebn. Anat. Entwickl.-Gesch. **40**, 3–33 (1968).

Langman, J.: Medical embryology: human development—normal and abnormal. Baltimore: Williams & Wilkins Co. 1963.

Lerche, W.: Esophagus and pharynx in action: a study of structure in relation to function. Springfield (Ill.): Charles C. Thomas, Publisher 1950.

Lorenz, J.: Observations comparatives sur l'innervation intramurale du cardia, du pylore et de la valvule iléo-coecale chez l'homme normal au cours de l'âge. Z. mikr.-anat. Forsch. **68**, 540–563 (1962).

Lund, W. S.: A study of the cricopharyngeal sphincter in man and in the dog. Ann. Roy. coll. Surg. Engl. **37**, 225–246 (1965).

Netter, F. H.: Anatomy of the esophagus. The Ciba collection of medical illustrations, vol. 3: Digestive system, part I: Upper digestive tract (1959).

Peden, J. K., Schneider, C. F., Bickel, R. D.: Anatomic relations of the vagus nerves to the esophagus. Amer. J. Surg. **80**, 32–34 (1950).

Smith, R. B., Taylor, I. M.: Observations of the intrinsic innervation of the human foetal oesophagus between the 10-mm and 140 mm crown-rump length stages. Acta anat. (Basel) **81**, 127–138 (1972).

Vantrappen, G., Texter, E. C., Barborka, C. J., Vandenbroucke, J.: The closing mecha-nism at the gastroesophageal junction. Amer. J. Med. **28**, 564–577 (1960).

Wolf, B. S.: The inferior esophageal sphincter. Anatomic, roentgenologic and manometric correlation, contradiction, and terminology. Amer. J. Roentgenol. **110**, 260–277 (1970).

Youmans, W. B.: Innervation of the gastrointestinal tract. In: Handbook of physiology, section 6: Alimentary canal, by C. F. Code, p. 1655–1663. Baltimore: Williams & Wilkins 1968.

Zaino, C., Jacobson, H. G., Lepow, H., Ozturk, C. H.: Pharyngoesophageal sphincter. Springfield (Ill.): Charles C. Thomas, Publisher 1970.

Zaino, C., Poppel, M. H., Jacobson, H. G., Lepow, H., Ozturk, C. H.: The lower eso-phageal vestibular complex. An anatomic-roentgen study. Amer. J. Roentgenol. **84**, 1045–1055 (1960).

Histology and Electron Microscopy

V. J. Desmet and G. N. Tytgat

With 8 Figures

The esophagus is a relatively straight but deformable muscular tube extending from the pharynx to the stomach, and subject to longitudinal tension (Kaufmann et al., 1968). Its wall is composed of the four typical layers which characterize the tubular digestive system: the mucous membrane (tunica mucosa), the submucosa (tunica submucosa), the muscularis externa (tunica muscularis), and adventitia (tunica adventitia).

1. Mucous Membrane (Tunica Mucosa)

In cross-section the lumen of the empty esophagus has a collapsed stellate appearance, brought about by the presence of seven to ten longitudinal folds of the mucous membrane. During passage of a food bolus these longitudinal folds are more or less "ironed out" by esophageal dilatation, but reappear at the same site afterwards (Bargmann, 1967).

The mucosal surface of the esophagus is moistened and lubricated by saliva and mucous secretions of the pharyngeal and esophageal glands. Like any "tunica mucosa" of the tubular digestive tract, the mucous membrane of the esophagus is composed of an epithelial membrane, and supported by a layer of connective tissue (the lamina propria) and a third thin outer layer of smooth muscle (the muscularis mucosae). The total thickness of these three layers may reach 500 to 800 μ (Bargmann, 1967).

1.1. Epithelium
1.1.1. Squamous Epithelium
1.1.1.1. Histology

The normal esophagus is lined over its full length by a tough non-keratinizing stratified squamous epithelium (Fig. 7A) except for a short segment of columnar epithelium at the gastro-esophageal junction.

In animals which consume fibrous food, like ruminants or rodents, the esophageal epithelium undergoes complete cornification, similar to the mammalian epidermis, with a well developed granular and horny layer.

The lower border of the epithelium is irregular, due to the presence of transitory folds of the lamina propria and more particularly due to the presence of large numbers of high conical papillae (Fig. 7B). The latter are arranged in linear rows running parallel with the longitudinal axis of the esophagus and resembling in their general arrangement those found in the skin of the palmar surfaces (Goetsch, 1910). Besides conical papillae, elongated ridges of the lamina propria also occur; they run in a direction parallel with the long axis of the esophagus and are connected with one another by oblique ridges (Goetsch, 1910).

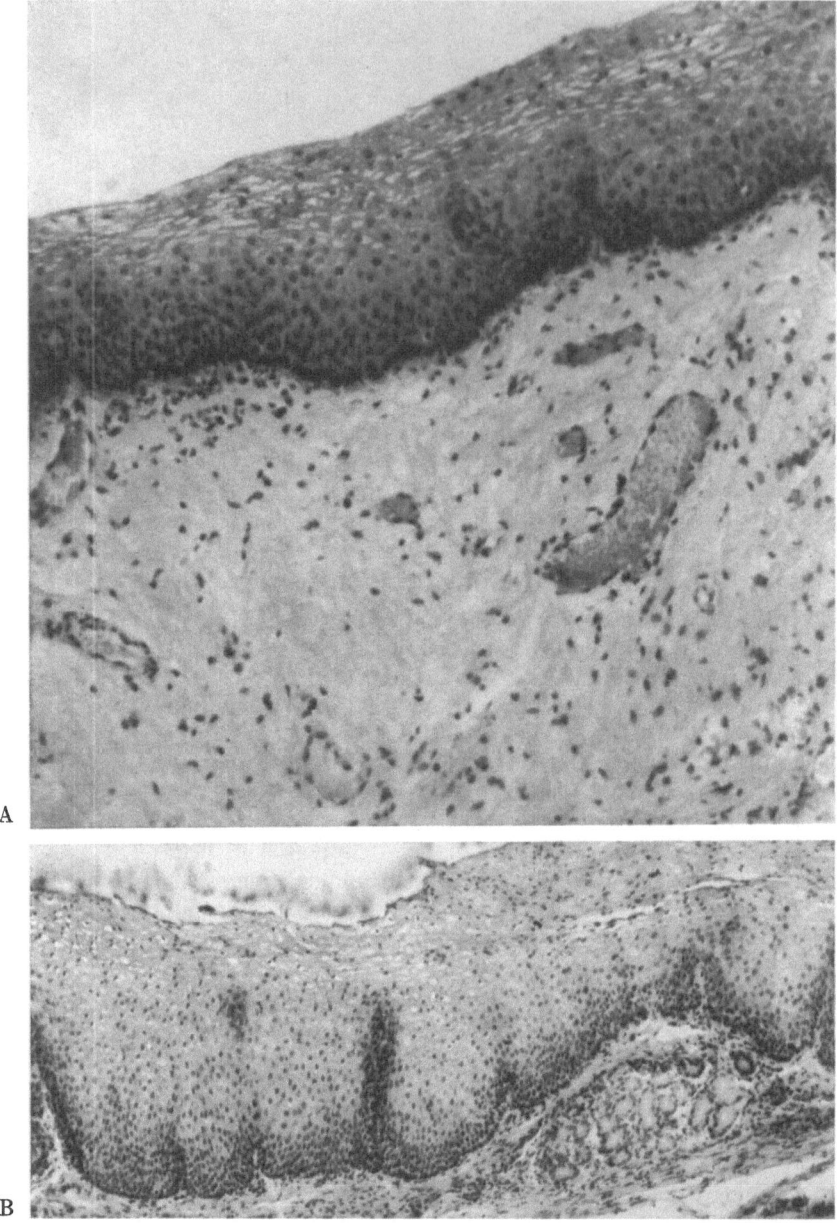

Fig. 7. A Esophageal mucosa, covered by non-keratinizing squamous epithelium. The lamina propria consists of loose areolar connective tissue. H.E. ×160. B Cardia-type glands in esophageal mucosa, located between squamous epithelium and muscularis mucosae. H.E. ×64

This stratified squamous epithelium comprises different layers of cells. The basal or germinative layer is made up of cylindrical, basophilic cells and is covered by several intermediate layers of polyhedral cells. The layers show a progressive flattening of the cells, which, however, retain their nucleus. Although no true cornification occurs, some cells in the surface layers occasionally contain some keratohyalin granules (PARAKKAL, 1967; LEESON and LEESON, 1970). The surface cells desquamate as single cells or in small groups. The esophageal epithelium has a remarkable regenerative capacity, as exemplified in a recent report of pathological sloughing of the whole epithelial coat along the entire esophagus (FOROOZAN et al., 1967).

Foci of epithelial hyperplasia with intracellular accumulation of glycogen ("glycogenic acanthosis") are a common finding in the lower third of the esophagus in older people (RYWLIN and ORTEGA, 1970).

1.1.1.2. Cell Kinetics

The squamous esophageal epithelium, like other epithelia, is a dynamic cell population which is renewed continuously. The production of new cells in the deeper layers is balanced by the loss of cells from the surface (LEBLOND and WALKER, 1965). Part of the daughter cells formed in the basal layers migrate upward and differentiate into intermediate, and ultimately superficial squamous cells. The time required for the migration of cells from the basal layers to the luminal surface in man is not known; the average migration time in rats is 8.8 days in the upper esophagus and 10.6 days in the lower esophagus (BERTALANFFY, 1960). In rats, virtually every cell of the basal layer becomes labeled after repeated injections of tritiated thymidine, which indicates that all basal cells are capable of desoxyribonucleic acid (DNA) synthesis and presumably of cell proliferation (LEBLOND et al., 1964). This renewal system is not caused by "differential mitoses" in which one daughter cell remains in the deeper layers to divide again, and the other daughter cell migrates towards the surface to differentiate, and is sloughed off eventually. In fact, the mitoses are "equivalent" (MARQUES-PEREIRA and LEBLOND, 1965), yielding identical daughter cells with similar potentialities. One, or both, or neither of the two daughter cells of any mitosis can be transferred to the upper, differentiating layers, whereas any cell remaining in the basal layer will divide again. This is consistent with the concept that transfer of basal cells to the spinous layers occurs randomly except during DNA synthesis and mitosis.

1.1.1.3. Histochemistry

Histochemical studies on esophageal epithelium have been conducted mainly in rats (MAEIR and ANGRIST, 1962; CABRINI and CARRANZA, 1958) and chickens (HINSCH, 1966, 1968). In chickens, ribonucleic acid is concentrated in the cytoplasm of the basal cells of the epithelium; the presence of triglycerides or neutral fats cannot be demonstrated. Acid phosphatase and non-specific esterase are confined to the deeper layers; adenosine triphosphatase, 5'-nucleotidase, nonspecific glycerophosphatase, thiamine pyrophosphatase and glucose-6-phosphatase reactions are negative in the epithelium (HINSCH, 1966). Oxidative enzymes (succinic dehydrogenase, NADP diaphorase, NAD diaphorase, alpha-glycerophosphate dehydrogenase, glutamic and lactic dehydrogenase) can be demonstrated in fully developed esophageal epithelium of the chicken; most enzymes show a higher concentration in the basal layers, correlating with a higher number of mitochondria in these cells. Choline-oxidase and d-aminoacid oxidase are reported to be located mainly in the luminal region of the epithelium, where they may play a role in the aging of these cells (HINSCH, 1968).

In rats (MAEIR and ANGRIST, 1962), acid phosphatase is found mainly in the stratum granulosum, whereas alkaline phosphatase activity is almost absent.

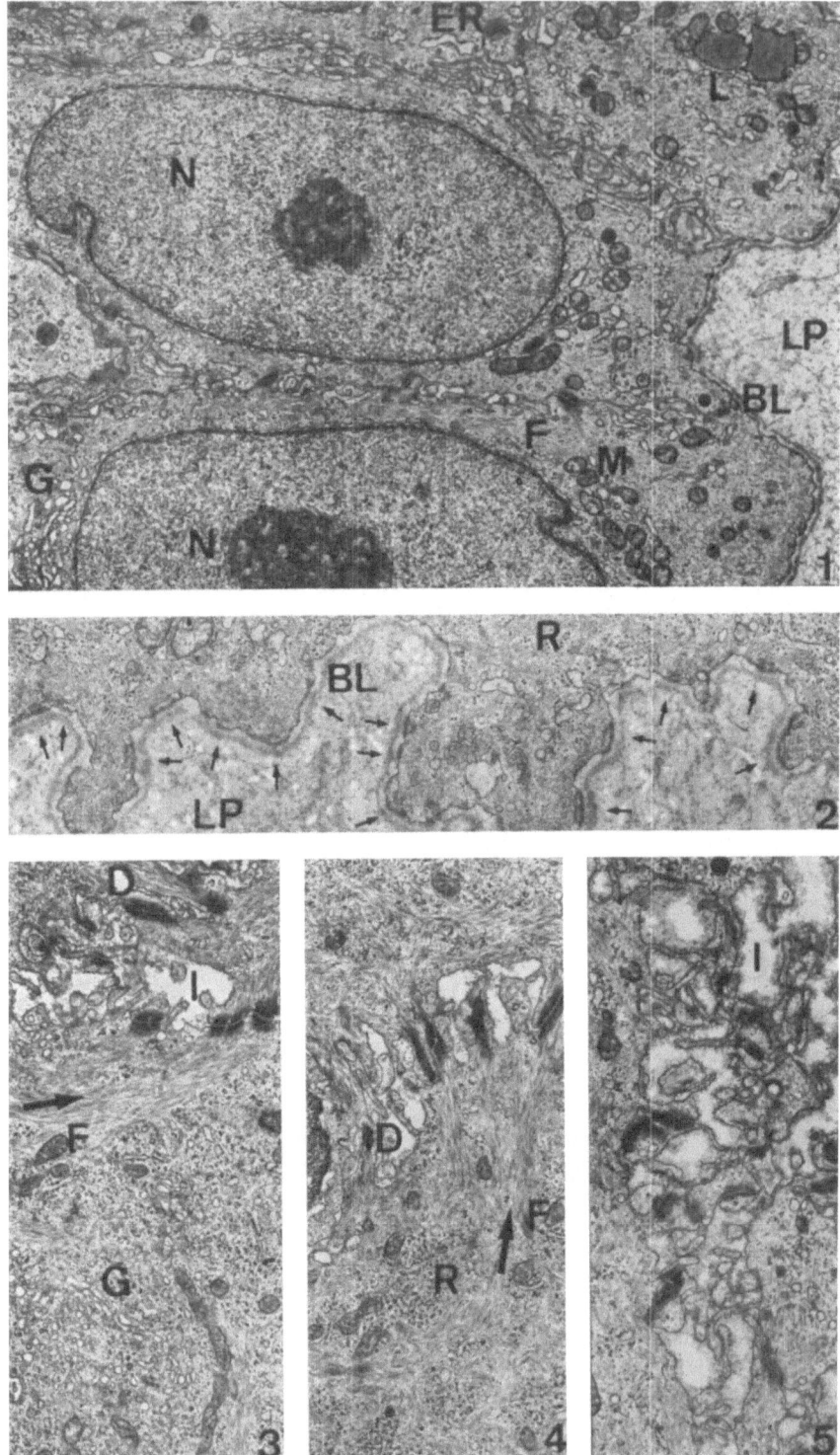

Fig. 8

Adenosine triphosphatase is found in the cell membranes of the basal layer, which also stains positively for NAD diaphorase. This zone shows focal areas of positive adenosine monophosphatase. The beta-glucuronidase activity in the basal layers is thought to be related to the proliferation of the cells of this layer (CABRINI and CARRANZA, 1958).

MAEIR and ANGRIST (1962) demonstrated that quantitative and qualitative variations exist within the stratified squamous epithelia of different organs in the same animal (e.g. skin, vagina, esophagus and cervix in rats). Conclusions concerning a tissue in one species do not necessarily hold true for this tissue in another species, even when they are morphologically identical by ordinary staining methods. For this reason, no valid histochemical conclusions can be drawn from these reports concerning the human esophageal epithelium.

1.1.1.4. Electron Microscopy

The germinative or basal cell layer rests upon a distinct moderately dense basal lamina (BL) (Fig. 8[1, 2]), approximately 400–600 Å thick and separated from the inferior epithelial cell border by a space approximately 400–500 Å wide. The cell border adjacent to the basal lamina has an irregular course and reveals numerous fingerlike extensions, protruding into the underlying connective tissue of the lamina propria (LP) (Fig. 8[2]). Occasionally small invaginations and vesicles, reminiscent of pinocytotic vacuoles are present along the inferior cell border. Thickened areas are observed with irregular intervals along the cytoplasmic membrane, facing the basal lamina (Fig. 8[2], arrows). These structures have been compared to hemidesmosomes, which are thought to attach the epithelial cells to the underlying basal lamina. No cell junctions seem to be present between adjacent basal cells at the level of the basal lamina but more proximally the irregularly interdigitated lateral cell membranes are interconnected through a few typical desmosomes (Fig. 8[1]). Desmosomes consist of two dense attachment plaques, each approximately 150 Å thick, separated by an interval of approximately 350 Å. Within this space there is a dense, 40 Å dick, intercellular contact layer in the center, separated by an interval of approximately 65 Å from an intermediate layer on either side. A 50 Å light layer, apparently continuous with the light middle layer of the trilaminar cell membrane, separates the intermediate layers from the attachment plaques. The shape of the basal cells is roughly columnar or fusiform, particularly when seen in longitudinal sections (Fig. 8[1]). The cytoplasm of the basal cells contains the usual set of cell organelles in relatively small quantities: a few mainly infranuclear mitochondria (M), a relatively rudimentary supranuclear Golgi Apparatus (G) and discrete rough-surfaced endoplasmic reticulum (ER). Large numbers of free ribosomes (R) are inter-

Fig. 8. Details of squamous epithelium in esophageal biopsies from healthy volunteers; tissue fixed in collidin or bicarbonate-buffered osmium tetroxide and stained with uranyl acetate and lead citrate. 1 Basal cells, resting upon basal lamina (BL). Lamina propria (LP), nucleus (N), mitochondria (M), rough endoplasmic reticulum (ER), Golgi apparatus (G), lipid inclusions (L), tonofilaments (F). Mag. ×8300. 2 Hemidesmosomes (arrows) along the basal plasma membrane, which closely follows the basal lamina (BL) within a distance of approximately 400 Å. Note the occasional small (pinocytotic) vesicles along the basal plasma membrane. Lamina propria (LP), scattered free ribosomes (R). Mag. ×13500. 3—5 Cells in basal and middle portion of stratum spinosum. More elaborate Golgi complex (G), large number of desmosomes (D), bundles of cytoplasmic filaments (F) oriented towards (arrows) and apparently attached to desmosome plaques, clusters of free ribosomes (R) numerous fingerlike projections of the cytoplasm into the intercellular space (I), resulting in a complex desmosome-studded intercellular cytoplasmic network. Mag. ×8300

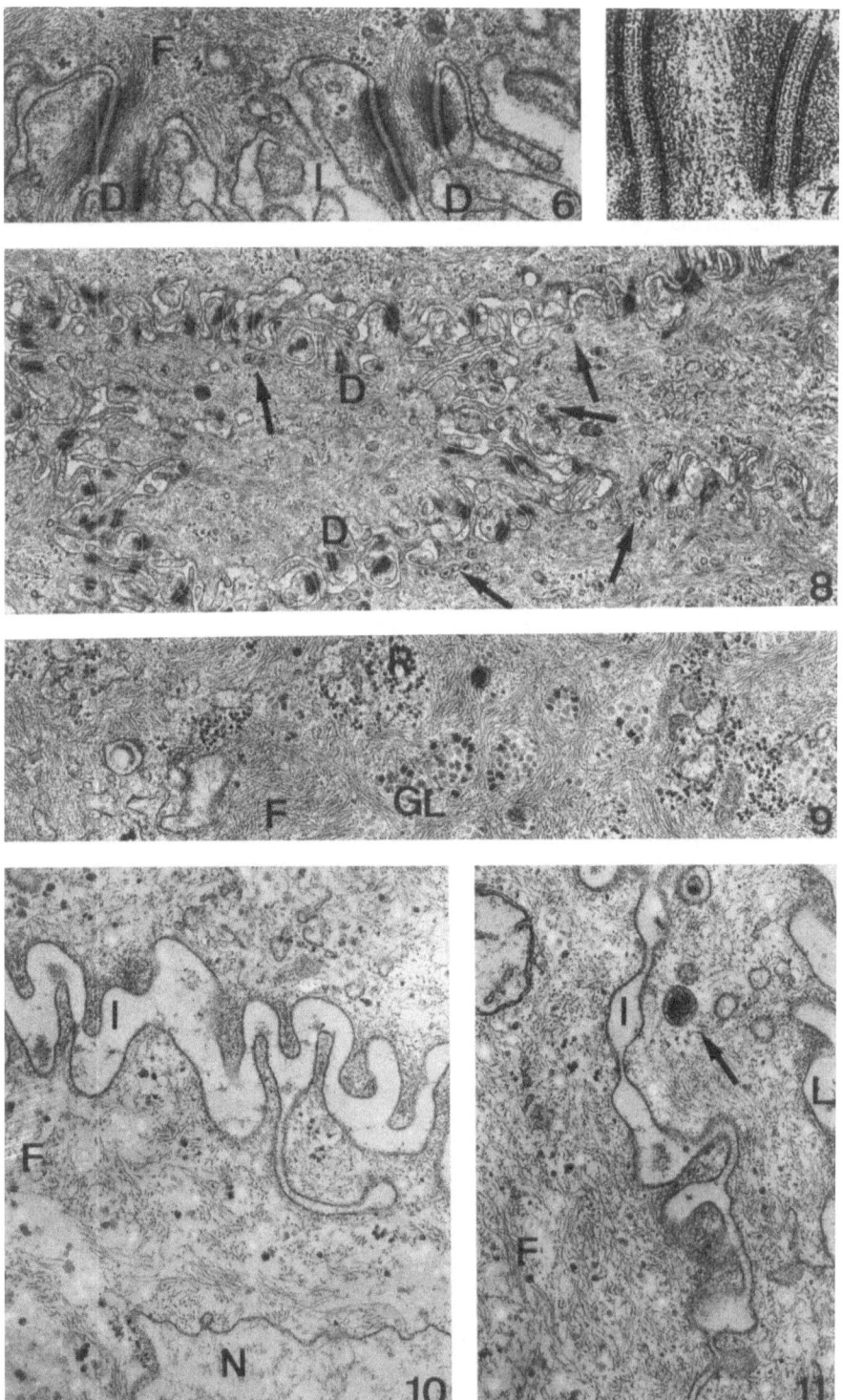

Fig. 9

spersed between loosely woven bundles of tonofilaments (F) (Fig. 8[1, 2]). These tonofilaments (circa 60 Å in diameter) are a characteristic structure in basal cells and run mainly in their long axis, making contact with the attachment plaques of the desmosomes. Tonofilaments are almost absent from an area at the inferior pole of the nucleus where mitochondria are more abundant. Lipid inclusions (L) are occasionally seen near the inferior pole of the nucleus of some basal cells (Fig. 8[1]).

The basal cell nucleus (N) is elongated, may contain an infolding, and is enclosed by a somewhat undulent nuclear membrane. Often one or more nucleoli are visible (Fig. 8[1]).

As the cells differentiate and move from the germinal layer out into the stratum spinosum, they flatten and their bundles of cytoplasmic filaments become more abundant and more tightly packed (Fig. 8[3, 4]). The polyhedral cells from the basal portion of the stratum spinosum are structurally similar to the basal cells, except for their location away from the basal lamina. The plasma membrane of these cells, in contrast to that of the basal cells, is richly supplied with well developed desmosomes (D) (Fig. 8[3, 5]). Fingerlike projections of the cytoplasm into the intercellular space become prevalent and result in a complex desmosome-studded intercellular cytoplasmic network (Fig. 8[3, 4]). The desmosomes are composed of multiple layers arranged parallel to each other (Fig. 9[6, 7]). Where junctional structures exist, the cell surfaces of adjacent cells are in proximity; elsewhere they tend to be separated, enclosing the intercellular space (I) (Figs. 8[3], 9[6]). The cell surface in these areas may have a finely fibrillar extracellular coating (Fig. 8[5]). The cytoplasm reveals the same set of organelles in a distribution similar to that described for basal cells. The Golgi complex (G) is somewhat more elaborate (Fig. 8[3]) and clusters of free ribosomes (R) are more voluminous (Fig. 8[4]). In addition, the cytoplasm of these cells appears to contain more tonofilaments (F) than the cytoplasm of the basal cells. In the cell periphery thick bundles of tonofilaments (each bundle representing a tonofibril) become oriented perpendicular to the cell surface and appear to anchor in the attachment plaques of the desmosomes (Fig. 8[3, 4] arrows).

Indentations of the nuclei become more frequent and deeper as the cells migrate towards the surface.

In the luminal portion of the stratum spinosum, the cells gradually become flattened, appear shrunken and primarily composed of densely packed tonofilaments (Fig. 9[8, 9]). Cytoplasmic organelles, when present, are not easily recognized.

Fig. 9. Details of squamous epithelium in esophageal biopsies from healthy volunteers; tissue fixed in collidin- or bicarbonate-buffered osmium tetroxide and stained with uranyl acetate and lead citrate. 6—7 Detail of desmosomal structures. The intercellular space is occupied by a disc of dense material, the intercellular contact layer. The lateral dense lines, the intermediate layers, appear to be continuous with the outermost leaflet of the unit membrane. The attachment plaques are closely applied to, and seemingly continuous with, the innermost leaflet of the unit membrane. Bundles of cytoplasmic filaments emerge on the inner aspect of each plaque. Mag. respectively ×27000 and ×70000. 8—9 Cells of the luminal portions of the stratum spinosum. Note the progressive flattening of the cells and the concentration of tonofilaments (F) in the peripheral cytoplasm. Membrane-enclosed dense granules (arrows) accumulate along the plasma membrane. Separate or clustered granules, probably representing glycogen (GL), are easily distinguished from ribosomes (R). Mag. respectively ×8300 and ×27000. 10—11 Topmost squamous cells, facing the lumen (L). The markedly flattened cells appear to separate from the underlying cells. Note the disappearance of desmosomes. Moderate swelling of cytoplasm brings out its filamentous (F) nature. Intercellular space (I), remnants of nuclear envelope (N). Mag. ×27000

Small dense granules, bound by a limiting membrane, can be observed, especially in the peripheral cytoplasm (Fig. 9[8, 11] arrows). Separate or clustered granules, different in size from ribosomes (R) and probably representing glycogen (GL), appear occasionally in cells of the upper stratum spinosum (Fig. 9[9]). Keratohyaline granules are virtually absent from these cells. Towards the surface the nuclei appear shrunken and more or less deeply indented. Occasionally desintegration of the nucleus (N) occurs, leaving only remnants of the nuclear envelope (Fig. 9[10]).

The topmost cell, facing the lumen (L) appears markedly flattened (Fig. 9[11]). Cells from this superficial layer seem to separate from the underlying cells by rupture of the desmosomes (Fig. 9[10, 11]). This absence of desmosomal structures is in striking contrast with their abundance in the deeper layers of the stratum spinosum. The entire cytoplasm is essentially occupied by fine filaments with a few interspersed ribosomes and glycogen particles, whereas the other cell organelles have disappeared to a large extent.

1.1.2. Non-squamous Epithelial Structures, Cardia-type Glands
1.1.2.1. Histology

Taste buds may occasionally be found in the upper third of the esophagus (BARGMANN, 1967).

Persistence of embryonic, ciliated epithelium has been recorded in premature and newborn infants (RECTOR and CONNERLY, 1941; HEALY, 1920; JOHNS, 1952) and even in an adult woman (RAEBURN, 1951). This is not surprising in view of the complex changes that occur in the types of epithelium lining the esophagus during its development.

More complex is the fact that the esophagus may be lined by gastric mucosa. This seems to be related to the caudal descent of the stomach before the seventh week of fetal life, when a few nests of cells, destined to become gastric mucosa, remain in the esophageal portion of the gut and become islets of typical gastric mucosa (ABRAMS and HEATH, 1965). This "anomaly" seems to be very common. SCHRIDDE (1904) found patches of ectopic gastric mucosa up to 2 cm in diameter in the postcricoid region of the esophagus in 70% of his necropsied cases. This high incidence is probably the reason why classical textbooks on histology (BARGMANN, 1967; BLOOM and FAWCETT, 1962; BÜCHER, 1948; LEESON and LEESON, 1970; CHÈVREMONT, 1966) usually mention the possible occurrence of islands of ectopic gastric mucosa in the esophagus.

In these islands, the tunica propria contains small groups of glandular acini composed of clear, mucoid cells, resembling very much those of the cardia of the stomach (Fig. 7B). These cardia-type glands are usually described as occurring at both the upper and lower extremities of the esophagus. They are commonly associated with a chronic type of inflammatory cell infiltration. The glands found at the level of the cricoid cartilage and first tracheal rings are sometimes referred to as the glands of SCHAFFER and RÜDINGER (CHÈVREMONT, 1966; GOETSCH, 1910). These glands as well as those in the distal esophagus are of the mucoid type and secrete non-metachromatic mucus (CHÈVREMONT, 1966).

The description by BARRETT (1950) of the syndrome which bears his name arose new interest in the nature (congenital or acquired) of these areas of ectopic gastric mucosa. As stated by ADLER (1963), remarkably little is known about the cardiac glands of the esophagus. They vary widely among mammals and their function is unknown. In a study of esophageal mucosae from over 250 routine autopsies, in which special care was taken to examine the entire esophageal mucosa, cardiac glands were found scattered diffusely throughout the length of some esophagi, and not only at either end of the tube as stated in classical descriptions (ADLER, 1963). In a subsequent study, covering 500 esophagi (DE LA PAVA et al., 1964), the incidence of ectopic gastric mucosa was reported to be at least 12%. The anomalous glandular epithelium was frequently superficial and replaced the lining squamous epithelium; in other esophagi the glands were entirely subepithelial. These gastric glands were seen most frequently in the lower part of the organ, adjacent to the cardia, and were thought to be congenital anomalies, representing rests of gastric mucosa from faulty descent during embryologic development.

Islands of ectopic gastric mucosa may be the cause of the "lower esophagus lined by columnar epithelium": when ulceration of the squamous epithelium occurs in an area in which there are ectopic glands in the lamina propria, the defect may not heal from regeneration of the squamous epithelium, but by surfacing of the ectopic glands. It has been suggested also that these glands may pierce the squamous epithelium, eventually reach the surface, and replace the lining squamous epithelium without ulceration.

The heterotopic mucosa is not always of the gastric cardia type. The presence of parietal (or oxyntic) cells, suggesting a more fundic type of mucosa, was reported by several authors (HEWLETT, 1900; BENSLEY, 1902; GOETSCH, 1910; JOHNSON, 1910; TAYLOR, 1927; IRELAND, 1933; RECTOR and CONNERLY, 1941; WILLIS, 1958; ABRAMS and HEATH, 1965; CORRIN et al., 1970). More rarely the heterotopic mucosa is of the intestinal type.

Recently TRIER (1970) reported 5 cases with midesophageal peptic strictures in which the distal esophagus was lined by a distinctive columnar epithelium which could readily be distinguished by optical and electron microscopy from the epithelia lining the normal gastric fundus, the gastroesophageal junction, and the small intestinal villi.

It is not clear at the present time whether the columnar epithelium in the esophagus is congenital or acquired. It has not been established whether it has its origin from upward migrating junctional epithelium (HAYWARD, 1961; BREMNER et al., 1970), from heterotopic embryonic remnants of gastric-like columnar cells, or from metaplasia.

Most of these reports are concerned with esophageal pathology such as peptic strictures and reflux esophagitis and are therefore not directly applicable in normal histological descriptions. It must be stressed in this chapter on histology that more knowledge is needed about the variations in normal epithelial covering of the esophageal mucosa in order to solve the pathogenesis and histogenesis of the above mentioned pathological states.

The squamous epithelial lining of the esophagus and the cylindrical epithelium of the stomach join each other right at the transition from the tube to the "sac" or a couple of centimeters higher up in the gullet (Fig. 10). This problem is discussed also in Chapter 6.

The squamo-columnar junction is macroscopically visible from the luminal surface as a dentate line (BARGMANN, 1967). According to some (DE LA PAVA et al., 1964), the lack of a clear-cut demarcation between the esophagus and the stomach results from the surfacing of the subepithelial inclusions of ectopic gastric epithelium which occur quite commonly in this area. Recently, experimental evidence was obtained on the squamocolumnar junction of the rat stomach (TRUDINGER and WILHELM, 1969) and on the esophagogastric junction in the dog (BREMNER et al., 1970). It showed that squamous epithelium cannot

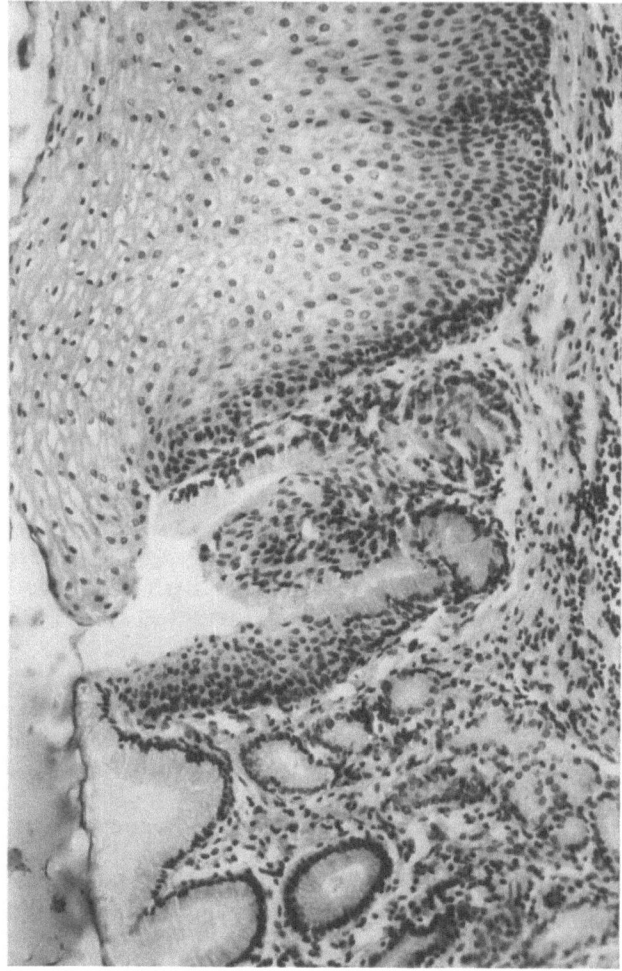

Fig. 10. Junction of squamous epithelium of the esophagus and cylindrical epithelium of the stomach. H.E. ×400

regenerate as well as columnar gastric epithelium in an acid-pepsin environment. These experiments favor the concept that "the lower esophagus lined by columnar epithelium" is an acquired condition. They may also explain the variable location of the squamocolumnar junction in the esophagogastric transition zone. Further studies on the redistribution of squamous and columnar epithelium after gastric mucosal wounds in the rat (WONG and FINCKH, 1970) have stressed the importance of the subepithelial mesenchyme; there seems to be a specific effect of the superficial subepithelial mesenchyme upon the selection of cells that cover some anatomical areas of the body after superficial trauma. This action may help to ensure that regeneration is provided by the appropriate type of cells, and may well account for the persistence throughout life of an abrupt transition in epithelial cell types at the esophagogastric junction, anorectal junction, and cervix uteri (WONG and FINCKH, 1970).

1.1.2.2. Electron Microscopy

The mucosa along the luminal (L) border and in the crypt-like glands at the gastroesophageal junction is lined by columnar epithelial cells which resemble the gastric epithelial cells that line the surface of other parts of the stomach (Fig. 11). Intestinal-type goblet cells, intestinal absorptive cells, and enterochromaffin cells are absent from this junctional epithelial layer. The apical surface of junctional epithelial cells is characterized by the presence of only a few rudimentary microvilli (MV), the fine structure of which resembles that of other alimentary epithelial cells (Fig. 11[14]). They are enclosed by a trilaminar apical plasma membrane. A well developed filamentous glycoprotein surface coat (SC) lies directly against the outer leaflet of this apical plasma membrane (Fig. 11[14]). The cores of the microvilli contain fine filaments which occasionally penetrate into the apical cytoplasm just beneath the microvillous border. The terminal web area is virtually non-existent (Fig. 11[12, 14]). Peculiar small spherical bodies of unknown nature, which consist of a moderately dense core, enclosed by a trilaminar membrane of the same dimensions as the apical plasma membrane, are occasionally seen within vesicles located in the apical cytoplasm (Fig. 11[15], arrows).

Frequent infoldings due to interdigitation of cytoplasmic processes of adjacent epithelial cells are regularly observed in sections of adjacent lateral plasma membrane (Fig. 11[12]). Although the lateral plasma membranes are closely adjacent to each other, intercellular spaces of significant size are not uncommon. Specialized attachment zones between adjacent cells include tight junctions at the apical aspects (T), intermediate junctions just beneath the tight junctions and various numbers of desmosomes (D) (Fig. 11[12, 14]). The basal plasma membrane is close to a continuous basal lamina, which separates the epithelium from the connective tissue in the lamina propria.

Secretory mucous granules (MG) are abundantly present in the apical cytoplasm (Fig. 11[12, 15]). These spherical granules are enclosed by a trilaminar membrane (Fig. 11[14, 15]). The majority of the secretory granules contain material of various electron densities, which causes their stippled heterogeneous appearance (Fig. 11[12]). In some sections there is morphological evidence suggesting secretion of these granules into the esophageal lumen. The membrane enclosing the secretory granules appears to fuse with the apical plasma membrane; this suggests that it probably delivers the content of the granule into the esophageal lumen by merocrine secretion.

Typical spherical or rod-shaped mitochondria (M) are distributed throughout the cytoplasm of the lower half of the epithelial cells.

A well developed accumulation of Golgi material (G) is seen regularly in the supranuclear cytoplasm (Fig. 11[12, 13]). Formed secretory granules are frequently seen close to the Golgi complex. A prominent rough-surfaced endoplasmic reticulum (ER), indicative of high protein synthetic activity, is present in the supra- and infranuclear cytoplasm (Fig. 11[12, 13]).

1.2. Lamina Propria

This lamina is a loose areolar connective tissue, containing a network of collagenous and elastic fibers and very few cells (Fig. 7A). It projects with high, vascularized papillae and ridges between the pegs of the basal layer of the overlaying epithelium (Fig. 7B). It contains scattered lymphocytes, mainly in the immediate subepithelial zone, and solitary lymph follicles which are located preferentially along the excretory ducts of the esophageal submucosal glands.

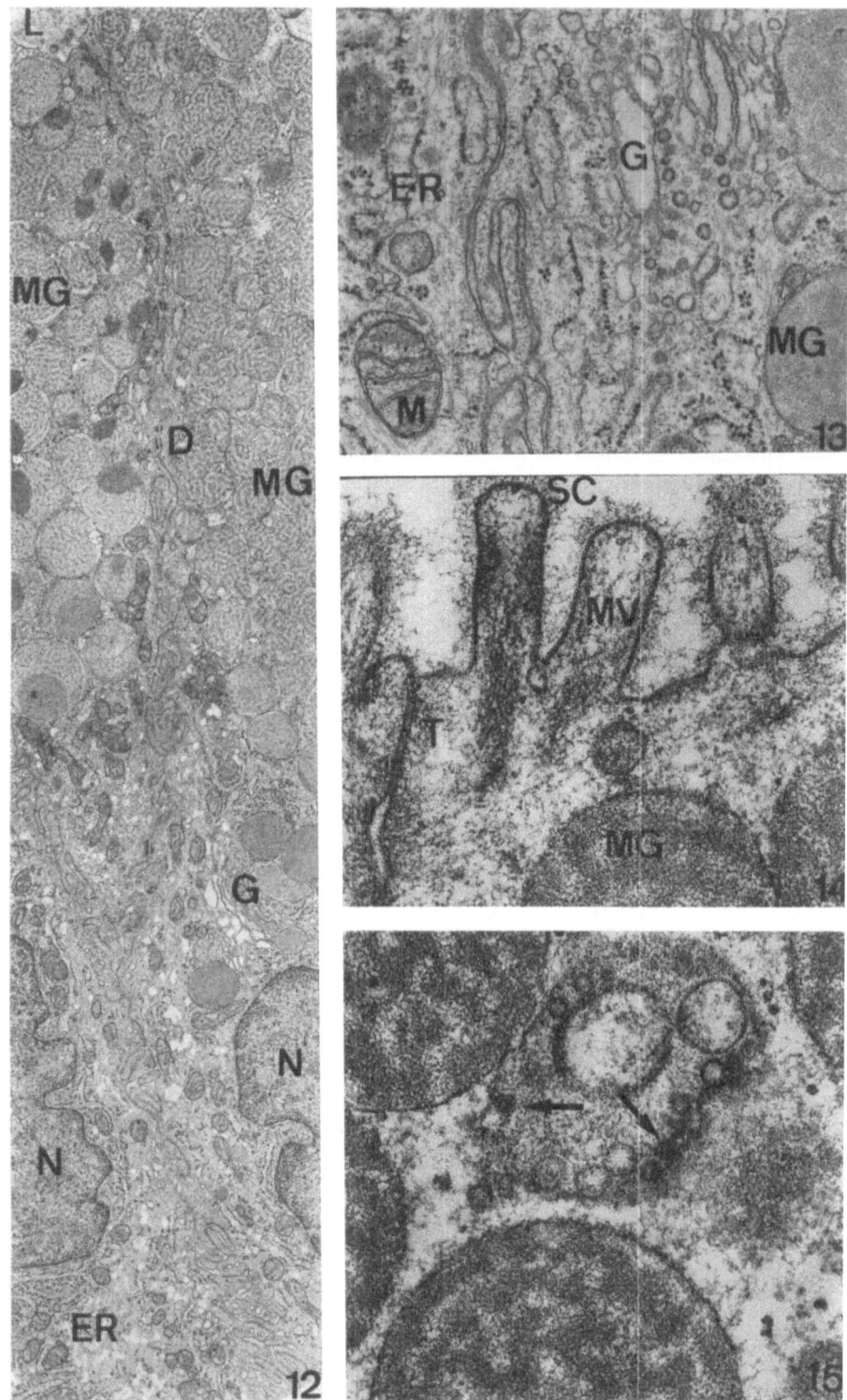

Fig. 11

The mucoid glands of the cardia type in the esophagus are also located in this lamina (Fig. 7 B). The elastic fiber network of the lamina propria represents the continuation of elastic "tendons" of the muscle fibers of the muscularis mucosae (NAGEL, 1938; BARGMANN, 1967).

1.3. Muscularis Mucosae

This layer forms the boundary between the lamina propria and the submucosa, and follows the mucosal longitudinal folds. It is composed of smooth muscle fibers, oriented in longitudinal direction, and with spiral disposition at the proximal and distal ends of the esophagus (PANNESE, 1954). The muscle bundles are frequently interrupted by intercalated elastic tendons (NAGEL, 1938; BARG-MANN, 1967). The thickness of the muscularis mucosae increases towards the distal part of the organ, reaching up to 300 μ at the level of the cardia (PANNESE, 1954). The muscularis mucosae at the level of the cricoid cartilage is continuous with the elastic layer of the pharynx.

2. Tunica Submucosa

The tunica submucosa, a thick layer of dense fibroconnective tissue, constitutes a shifting layer between the mucous membrane and the muscular coat of the esophageal tube. When the esophagus is empty, it is pulled up into the longitudinally arranged folds of the mucosa.

It contains large blood vessels and has a rich elastic meshwork which is part of the elastic-muscular system (NAGEL, 1938).

The typical esophageal glands are located in the submucosa (Fig. 12); they occur mainly on the ventral side in the upper and lower segments of the esophagus (BARGMANN, 1967) but are quite variable in number, size, and distribution. A comparative study of esophageal glands in different species was made by GOETSCH (1910). The body of the glands is composed of a number of acini, built up exclusively of mucous cells. Their mucus stains metachromatically (CHÈVREMONT, 1966).

They resemble the glands of the bucco-pharyngeal cavity; short ducts connect them with a main duct, which passes through the muscularis mucosae and ends with a narrow lumen between the epithelial ridges of the mucosa. The main duct is covered by a cuboidal epithelium, which becomes a stratified epithelium with superficial columnar cells in its terminal part. Sometimes the squamous epithelium of the mucosa covers the terminal part of the duct. Before their passage through the muscularis mucosae the ducts show an ampullary dilatation. They are frequently surrounded by a lymphocytic infiltration. From time to time the esophageal glands may form cysts.

According to GOETSCH (1910), the great variation in number of the esophageal glands, the constant presence of cyst formation, stasis of secretions,

Fig. 11. Details of columnar esophagogastric epithelium in biopsies from healthy volunteers; tissue fixed in collidin- or bicarbonate-buffered osmium tetroxide and stained with uranyl acetate and lead citrate. The columnar epithelial cells contain only sparse rudimentary microvilli (MV), bearing an obvious glycoprotein surface coat (SC). The supranuclear cytoplasm is filled with mucous granules (MG). Arrows point towards peculiar spherical structures within vesicles in the apical cytoplasm. Elaborate Golgi (G), elaborate rough endoplasmic reticulum (ER), mitochondria (M), tight junction (T), desmosome (D), lumen (L), nucleus (N). Mag. respectively ×8300, ×13500, ×38500 and ×38500

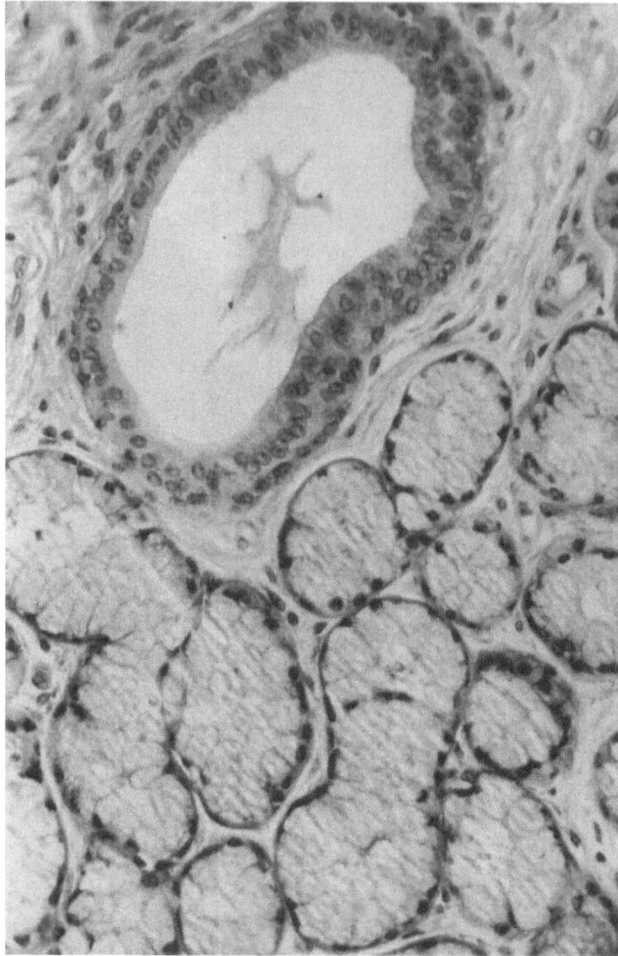

Fig. 12. Detail of submucosal esophageal gland, composed of several mucoid acini. The main duct is covered by a cuboidal to cylindrical epithelial lining; its lumen is somewhat dilated and contains some precipitated mucoid secretory material. H.E. ×400

and atrophy of the glandular cells might be taken as an indication that these glands represent a disappearing structure in man.

3. Tunica Muscularis

In textbooks the tunica muscularis of the esophagus is classically described as composed of an inner circular and an outer longitudinal layer. However, there seems to be no real separation into two different layers. The most recent, and at the same time the most original study of the esophageal musculature is that of Kaufmann et al. (1968).

In principle, three types of muscle arrangement can be distinguished:

1. A *spiral* arrangement, characterized by muscle fibers, which run in a horizontal plane, while their distance from the lumen decreases with each turn.

2. A *winding* arrangement, which can be considered as a muscle bundle around a cylinder, arranged in such a way that the beginning and the end of the bundle are at a different vertical level, whereas the distance from the lumen remains the same.

3. A *screw*, which can be considered as a muscle bundle arranged around a cone: the distance from the lumen is decreasing, while the beginning and the end of the bundle are located at different vertical levels.

This last type of muscle arrangement (screw) has been observed in the human esophagus. In a screw-like construction, four different types can be distinguished according to the course and direction of the muscle fibres. All four screw systems begin at the outside (adventitia) and end at the inside (submucous layer). When fibers run from the outside to the inside and from proximal to distal, the screw is said to be descending. Screwfibers may follow a clock-wise or an anti-clock-wise direction along the vertical cranio-caudal axis of the esophagus.

A system containing only ascending or only descending screws, is called a polar system. When a system is composed of both ascending and descending screws, running both clockwise and anti-clockwise, it is called an apolar system. The tunica muscularis of the esophagus corresponds to an apolar screw construction; the more steeply descending and ascending parts of the screws form the classical "outer longitudinal" layer, whereas the more horizontally running end-parts of the screws from the classical "inner circular" layer. The muscle arrangement of the human esophagus is even more complicated than a simple apolar screw system. One has to consider the esophageal tube as twisted to the left, over 90° at its lower end, whereas its attachment to the pharynx remains as a "punctum fixum".

This explains why the longitudinal fibers do not run parallel to the longitudinal axis of the tube, but are arranged as steep, left-turning windings, running around $1/_4$ of the circumference. At the same time the arrangement of the more horizontal end-parts of the screw is changed in the so-called circular layer: the bundles turning to the left (anti-clockwise) run in an even more horizontal plane, while those turning to the right (clockwise) follow a slightly steeper course. Furthermore, the "ring fibers" (i.e. the more horizontal end-parts of the screws) lie in planes which make an angle of 10 to 20° with the horizontal plane. The highest points of these oblique planes occupy different positions in the esophageal circumference, describing a left turn over 315°: they are located dorsally in the cervical esophagus, at the right lateral side in the upper thoracic part, ventrally in the retrocardiac part, and at the left lateral side in the abdominal part of the esophagus. This arrangement causes an undulated appearance of the "circular" fibers when viewed through the longitudinally opened esophagus, at least when care is taken to avoid shortening of the organ.

The transitions of the "longitudinal" towards the "circular" musculature are unevenly distributed around the esophageal circumference. The transition maxima of the descending screws lie opposite those of the ascending ones; the transition maxima of the descending screws coincide with the highest points of the oblique planes; the transition maxima of the ascending muscle bundles coincide mostly with the lowest points of the oblique planes. The number of ascending screws is always higher than that of descending ones, especially in the cervical part of the esophagus.

The thickness ratio of the "longitudinal" versus the "circular" layer corresponds to 1:2 in the cervical part, to 2:2 in the thoracic part and to 3:2 in the abdominal part of the esophagus. These figures express at the same time the increase in thickness of the tunica muscularis towards the caudal part of the esophagus. In addition there are longitudinal muscle bundles, lying outside the screw system without intercalated connective tissue sheet. They begin at the lateral side of the cricoid cartilage and form two elevated ridges, which irradiate fan-wise in caudal direction. Only in the cervical part of the esophagus is this longitudinal layer composed of separate longitudinal bundles apart from the screw system. In the thoracic segment of the esophagus they are composed of very steep outer parts of the screw system and run parallel to the longitudinal axis of the organ. No such outside longitudinal ridges are observed in the abdominal part of the esophagus.

In the pharyngo-esophageal and gastro-esophageal junctional segment, the muscle arrangement is somewhat different from the rest of the organ; so-called "sphincters" are formed. In the cervical segment of the esophagus, up to 3 to 4 cm from the cricoid cartilage, the ascending (screw) bundles, winding upwards in the circular layer, run at a rising angle of about 45°. Higher up the bundles lie in a more horizontal plane, so that over a distance of 1–1.5 cm below the cricoid cartilage the bundles form almost horizontal spirals. In the upper 2–4 cm of the esophagus only very few or no outer longitudinal bundles are found. In this segment the last ascending screws have already bent inwards to the "circular" almost horizontal layer. Over this stretch, only two bundles of the already mentioned separate longitudinal musculature reach up to the cricoid cartilage. Between these longitudinal muscle ridges, a free area is delineated at the dorsal side: it forms a triangle with upper base and lower top of about 4 cm height, the so-called Trigonum Laimeri, which is a predilection site for pulsion diverticulum of Zenker.

Although the layer of circular bundles at the esophageal entrance is thicker than in the rest of the esophageal tube, there is no anatomically isolated "upper esophageal sphincter". These horizontal and circular bundles may function as a sphincter, but they do not correspond to the anatomical definition of a sphincter, since the circular bundles are continuous with longitudinal fibres. Indeed, inside "the upper esophageal sphincter", at the dorsal side, a few longitudinal fibers are found, which run as ascending screws upwards into the pharyngeal wall. They were described already in 1898 by Birmingham as "musculus pharyngo-esophagus" (Kaufmann et al., 1968).

In the lower end of the esophagus, a similar sort of "sphincter" is found. Two centimeters above the entrance of the "esophageal tube" into the gastric sac the terminal ends of the muscle screws assume an almost horizontal layering. Again there is no real anatomical sphincter, since these circular muscle segments are continuations of the outer longitudinal bundles which end higher up, or lower down. In other words, "longitudinal" fibers coming from the stomach and from the thoracic segment of the esophagus end into this "lower esophageal sphincter". This "sphincter" is better developed than its cervical counterpart. Since neither the upper nor the lower "sphincter" correspond to a real anatomical sphincter, it has been proposed to call these muscular structures "closing segments" (Kaufmann et al., 1968).

Another factor complicating the structure of the esophageal tunica muscularis is the occurrence of smooth and striated muscle in the same organ. Different authors described different proportions of smooth and skeletal muscle, with different proportions even in the "circular" and the "longitudinal" layers (Kaufmann et al., 1968).

In man, Kaufmann et al. (1968) found striated skeletal muscle in the cervical part and often also in the upper thoracic part of the esophagus (pars retro-

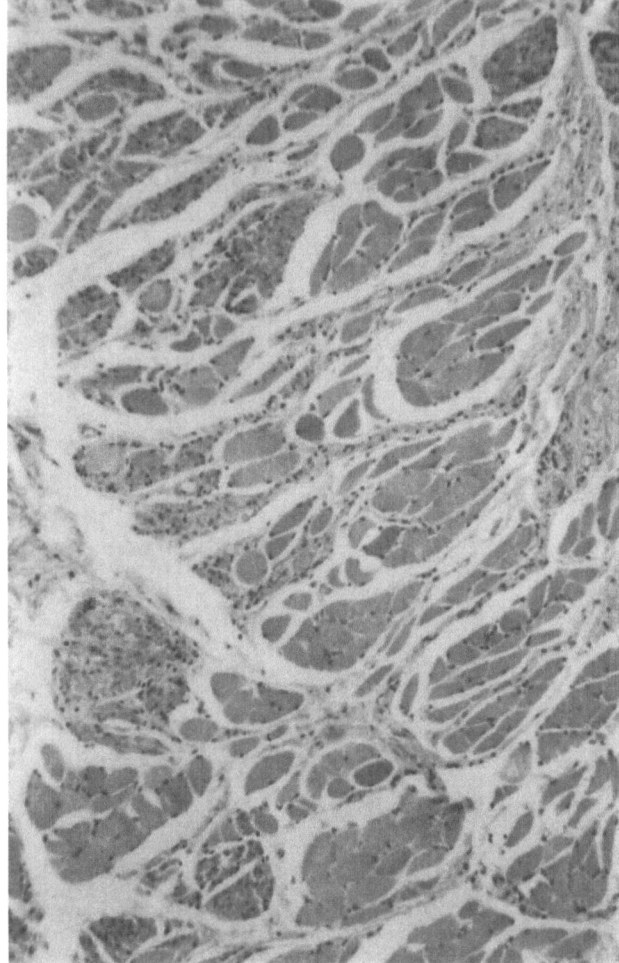

Fig. 13. Longitudinal section of esophagus at ± 8 cm from the pharyngoesophageal sphincter. The picture shows a detail of the cross-sectioned "circular layer" of the tunica muscularis, composed of striated muscle fibres, intermingled with several smooth muscle bundles. H.E. ×160

trachealis). The upper two to six centimeters contain only striated muscle. From there smooth muscle fibers gradually become more abundant (Fig. 13), so that at a distance of 4 to 8 cm from the superior end the smooth musculature constitutes 50% of the esophageal tunica muscularis.

The retrocardiac segment of the esophagus has no striated muscle fibers: they may occasionally be found in the abdominal part and seem to be continuations of the muscle bundles of the diaphragm. The smooth muscle cells in the circular layer lie closer to the lumen than the striated fibres. Smooth and striated muscle cells are arranged together in such a way that they run a similar course

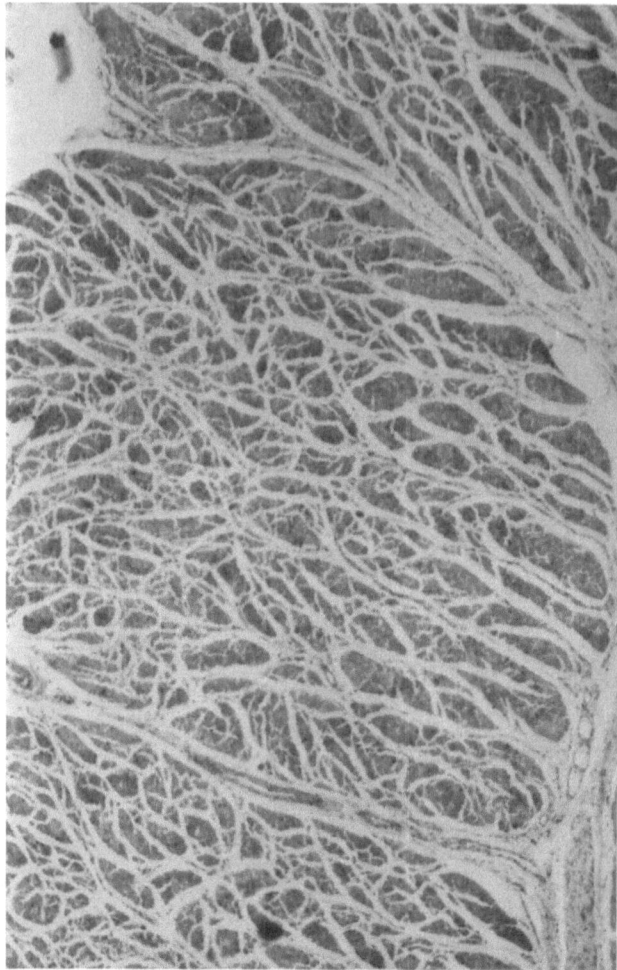

Fig. 14. Longitudinal section of distal esophagus. The picture shows a detail of the cross-sectioned "circular layer" of the tunica muscularis, composed exclusively of smooth muscle cells and subdivided by oblique connective tissue septa. H.E. ×64

and belong to the same construction system. In the "circular" layer the bundles of smooth or striated muscle fibers may be subdivided by connective tissue septa; on longitudinal sections of the esophagus these septa appear as oblique lines, running in caudal direction from the outside to the inside, so that the "circular" layer is divided in blocks piled up like roofing tiles (Fig. 14).

Most important for a good understanding of the structure and function of the esophageal musculature is the fact that the esophagus is subject to longitudinal tension (Kaufmann et al., 1968). On the basis of their observations, Kaufmann et al. (1968) propose a possible explanation for the function of the esophageal musculature in deglutition and peristaltic contraction as well as in closing and opening the lower esophageal sphincter.

4. Angio-architecture

According to recent studies (DE CARVALHO, 1966; GÜNTHER and LIERSE, 1968) there is a general parallelism between the muscle architecture and the course of the blood vessels in the esophageal wall. Generally, the longitudinal arteries do not run along the full length of the esophagus. Two arteries begin at the proximal end as branches of the truncus thyreocervicalis; they receive new arterial branches from the descending aorta as they pass down the esophagus. The blood supply of the caudal part of the esophagus is secured by ascending branches of the left gastric artery. Longitudinal arteries of the first order, lying in the adventitia, give off ring arteries which accompany the muscle fibers of the muscular coat. Longitudinal arteries of the second order located in the submucosa are branches of these ring arteries.

The venous system of the esophagus constitutes an anastomosis between the cranial drainage area, leading towards the superior vena cava, and the caudal drainage area, leading towards the portal system. The venous angio-architecture of the transition zone between esophagus and stomach in man was studied by DE CARVALHO (1966). He divides the junctional segment into 4 zones: "gastric" zones 1 and 2 (the latter including the epithelial squamo-columnar junction or "Z" line) and the "esophageal" zones 3 and 4.

Zone 1 shows a dense irregular venous network in the submucosa. It is situated from 0.5 to 1.0 cm below the squamo-columnar junction line to 0.5 to 1.0 cm more distally. In zone 2 there are five groups of veins, arranged longitudinally in the submucosa. This zone is about 1 cm high and is intersected by the epithelial "Z" line. The veins of zone 3 are located mainly in the mucosa, and not in the submucosa as they are in the more distal zones 1 and 2. These vessels are arranged longitudinally and form palisades of parallel veins of quite regular outline. Zone 3 extends from 1.5 to 3.5 cm at the proximal side of the epithelial junction line. The most cranial zone (zone 4) is characterized by a return of the longitudinal subepithelial vessels towards the submucosa. These veins are small and are not arranged in palisades, but form a fine irregular network. The veins of the esophago-gastric junctional segment pass twice through the muscularis mucosae. In the segment that extends from 1.5 to 3.5 cm proximally from the squamo-columnar mucosal junction the main venous plexus is located in the mucosa, right underneath the epithelial layer. This arrangement suggests that the muscularis mucosae plays an important role in the venous drainage of esophagus and stomach. The thickening of the muscularis mucosae in the lower part of the esophagus (PANNESE, 1954) as well as its elastic tendons at the site of vascular penetration (NAGEL, 1938) may be important in this respect.

This special venous arrangement is thought to play a physiological role in the so-called "angio-muscular wring-closure system" of the terminal esophagus (GÜNTHER and LIERSE, 1968; STELZNER and LIERSE, 1967; KAUFMANN et al., 1968). It may also be important in pathological conditions, such as portal hypertension and esophageal varices (DE CARVALHO, 1966).

5. Innervation

The autonomic innervation of the esophagus originates from branches of both vagal and sympathetic nerves. The nerve fibers form a series of plexuses in the adventitial, muscular and submucosal layers, recently studied in the rabbit (CECIO and CALIFANO, 1967).

The vagal and sympathetic branches in the adventitial layer form a relatively abundant plexus of interlacing fibers (Rash and Thomas, 1962) which is more evident in the lower third of the organ (Cecio and Califano, 1967).

Branches from this adventitial or extramural plexus and branches of the rami esophagi of the vagal nerve (Gruber, 1968) run across the outer muscular layer and reach the myenteric plexus of Auerbach.

In man, the first ganglia of Auerbach's plexus are found 1 to 2 cm distally from the proximal end of the esophagus (Treacy et al., 1963). This plexus contains groups of ganglion cells at the crossing points of the nervous network. The highest number of ganglion cells is found in the distal part of the esophagus (Cecio and Califano, 1967). Thin terminal branches of the myenteric plexus end at the motor endplates of striated muscle fibers. In silver preparations each muscle fiber is usually found to be innervated by a single motor endplate, although some muscle cells have two endplates innervated by two branches of the same axon (ultraterminal or ultraexpansional endplates) (Cecio and Califano, 1967). In histochemical acetyl cholinesterase preparations of a rat esophagus, no such ultraterminal endplates could be detected (Gruber, 1968).

Branches of the myenteric and adventitial plexus form the delicate network of the submucosal plexus. The meshes of the submucosal plexus of Meissner lie in different levels of the submucosa and contain groups of ganglion cells. A thinner web of fibers occupies the lamina propria of the mucosa; some delicate fibers arising from it terminate between the basal cells of the squamous epithelium.

The sensory innervation of the rabbit esophagus is largely limited to the submucosal connective tissue (Cecio and Califano, 1967). It is composed of Ruffini's corpuscules which are small and non-encapsulated.

In recent years several histochemical studies have been performed on the innervation of the esophagus, using techniques for specific and non-specific cholinesterase for cholinergic fibers, and formaldehyde-induced fluorescence on freeze-dried specimens for adrenergic fibers.

It has been shown that the vagal trunk and its ramifications into the lower esophagus and cardia also contain adrenergic nerve fibers, of which only a small portion correspond to vasomotor sympathetic nerves (Baumgarten and Lange, 1969). Therefore the vagus serves as a conducting structure for adrenergic fibers from the sympathetic chain to certain parts of the esophageal musculature; this observation is important for electrophysiological and pharmacological studies. The adrenergic innervation of the esophagus was studied recently in the cat, the rhesus monkey (Baumgarten and Lange, 1969), and the dog (Jacobowitz and Nemir, 1969).

It has been shown that the mammalian esophagus receives sympathetic adrenergic fibers which supply blood vessels and the muscularis mucosae but innervate mainly ganglia of the myenteric plexus. A small percentage of the adrenergic neurons contact nerve cells of the submucosal plexus in rhesus monkeys. Only a few fibers are confined to the tunica muscularis. The outer "longitudinal" layer receives more terminal ramifications than the inner "circular" layer. The liberation of endogeneous noradrenaline is supposed to affect the following structures which control the motor activity of the esophagus: (1) smooth muscle cell of the tunica muscularis (direct influence of the transmitter); (2) smooth muscle cells of the muscularis mucosae (direct influence); (3) nerve cells of the myenteric and submucosal ganglia (indirectly influencing the smooth muscle layer). Since it is not known at the present time whether the adrenergic endings contact inhibitory or excitatory cholinergic neurons of the myenteric plexus, it is difficult to make a definite statement concerning the physiological role of noradrenaline release in esophageal ganglia. Regional differences in the adrenergic innervation of sphincteric and nonsphincteric parts of the esophagus have not been observed. The question is still open whether or not the lower esophageal segment really represents a nervously controlled sphincteric division of the alimentary canal. As far as the adrenergic innervation is concerned, no structure corresponding to a sphincteric mechanism has been detected. The circularly arranged smooth musculature of the lower esophageal segment does not have a specialized adrenergic innervation comparable to that of the sphincter ani internus, which would account for a tonic and permanent closure (BAUMGARTEN and LANGE, 1969). These authors also describe adrenergic fibers around the mucous glands.

Cholinergic fibers (JACOBOWITZ and NEMIR, 1969) were described in the dog esophagus primarily in the regions of smooth muscles, both the muscularis mucosae and the tunica muscularis. The circular layer of the esophagus is richly innervated with cholinergic nerves. Such fibers also innervate blood vessels and mucous glands.

Ganglion cells of Auerbach's plexus stain densely for acetyl-cholinesterase in histochemical preparations. Pseudo-cholinesterase, the function of which is unknown, was demonstrated histochemically in smooth muscle cells and in the myenteric plexus, but not in striated muscle of the esophagus.

In the rat esophagus, GRUBER (1968) found about 10% of the ganglion cells of the myenteric plexus to be positive for acetyl-cholinesterase. However, the cholinesterase positive ganglion cells were not always larger than the less positive or negative ones, as was the case in the observations of GUNN (1968) in her study of the myenteric plexus of the stomach and the gut.

6. Adventitia, Elastic-muscular System, Serosa

The outermost layer of the esophageal wall, the tunica adventitia, is a connective tissue sheath whose fibers are the continuation of the connective tissue of the tunica muscularis. The adventitia not only contains vascular and nervous plexuses but also an important network of elastic fibers. This elastic fiber system is continuous with the elastic networks of the inner esophageal layers and the elastic tendons in the muscular coats, creating a real elastic-muscular system (NAGEL, 1938). It extends without interruption from the elastic networks of the adventitial layer up to the elastic fiber-sheath at the border of epithelium and tunica propria of the mucosa. By means of elastic tendons between the muscle fibers, the smooth musculature of the esophagus can regulate the continuous tension of the elastic components of the esophageal wall. This tension helps the esophagus to reassume its original form, size, and shape following each deglutition. The elastic tendons intercalated between the smooth muscle bundles of the muscularis mucosae and the tunica muscularis also serve to protect the blood vessels from being ripped off when shifting of the different layers of the esophageal wall occurs. Furthermore, the branching points of the vessels are protected by a network of loosely arranged elastic fibers, tending to return the displaced vessel into its original bed.

The adventitial layer also connects the esophagus with the surrounding mediastinal tissues.

Only small areas of the thoracic segment and the short abdominal segment are covered with a serosal coat (BÜCHER, 1948).

References

ABRAMS, L., HEATH, D.: Lower esophagus lined with intestinal and gastric epithelia. Thorax **20**, 66–72 (1965).

ADLER, R. H.: The lower esophagus lined by columnar epithelium. Its association with hiatal hernia, ulcer, structure and tumor. J. thorac. cardiovasc. Surg. **45**, 13–34 (1963).

BARGMANN, W.: Histologie und mikroskopische Anatomie des Menschen, 6. Aufl. Stuttgart: Thieme 1967.

BARRETT, N. R.: Chronic peptic ulcer of the oesophagus and oesophagitis. Brit. J. Surg. **38**, 175–182 (1950).

BAUMGARTEN, H. G., LANGE, W.: Adrenergic innervation of the oesophagus in the cat (Felis domestica) and rhesus monkey (Macacus rhesus). Z. Zellforsch. **25**, 529–545 (1969).

BENSLEY, R. R.: The cardiac glands of mammals. Amer. J. Anat. **2**, 105 (1902–1903).

BERTALANFFY, F. D.: Mitotic rates and renewal times of the digestive tract epithelia in the rat. Acta anat. (Basel) **40**, 130–148 (1960).

BLOOM, W., FAWCETT, D. W.: A textbook of histology. Philadelphia-London: W. B. Saunders Co. 1962.

BREMNER, C. G., LYNCH, V. P., ELLIS, F. H.: Barrett's esophagus: congenital or acquired? An experimental study of esophageal mucosal regeneration in the dog. Surgery **68**, 209–216 (1970).

BUCHER, O.: Histologie. Bern: Hans Huber 1948.

CABRINI, R. L., CARRANZA, F. A.: Histochemical localization of β-glucuronidase in stratified squamous epithelia. Naturwissenschaften **45**, 553 (1958).

CECIO, A., CALIFANO, G.: Neurohistological observation on the oesophageal innervation of rabbit. Z. Zellforsch. **83**, 30–39 (1967).

CHÈVREMONT, M.: Notions de cytologie et histologie, vol. II, 2º édition. Liège: Editions Desoer 1966.

CORRIN, B., HARRISON, G. K., JOHNSON, H. R. M.: High oesophageal stricture with hiatal hernia and a lower oesophagus lined by columnar epithelium. Thorax **25**, 89–91 (1970).

DE CARVALHO, C. A. F.: Sur l'angio-architecture veineuse de la zone de transition œsophago-gastrique et son interprétation fonctionnelle. Acta anat. (Basel) **64**, 125–162 (1966).

DE LA PAVA, S., PICKREN, J. W., ADLER, R. H.: Ectopic gastric mucosa of the esophagus. A study on histogenesis. N.Y. J. Med. **64**, 1831–1835 (1964).

FOROOZAN, P., ENTA, T., WINSHIP, D., TRIER, J.: Loss and regeneration of the esophageal mucosa in pemphigoid. Gastroenterology **52**, 548–558 (1967).

GOETSCH, E.: The structure of the mammalian oesophagus. Amer. J. Anat. **10**, 1–40 (1910).

GRUBER, H.: Über Struktur und Innervation der quergestreiften Muskulatur des Oesophagus der Ratte. Z. Zellforsch. **91**, 236–247 (1968).

GÜNTHER, S., LIERSE, W.: Die Angioarchitektur im Oesophagus des Kaninchens, der Ratte und der Maus. Ergebn. Anat. Entwickl.-Gesch. **40**, H. 4 (1968).

GUNN, M.: Histological and histochemical observations on the myenteric and submucous plexuses of mammals. J. Anat. (Lond.) **102**, 223–239 (1968).

HAYWARD, J.: The lower end of the oesophagus. Thorax **16**, 36 (1961).

HEALEY, F. H.: Note on the occurrence of ciliated epithelium in the esophagus of a 7-month human fetus. J. Anat. (Lond.) **54**, 180 (1920).

HEWLETT, A. W.: The superficial glands of the oesophagus. J. exp. Med. **5**, 319 (1900).

HIMSCH, G. W.: Histochemistry of the chick esophagus and trachea. II. Enzymes, nucleic acids, proteins, carbohydrates and fats. J. Morph. **119**, 327–340 (1966).

HINSCH, G. W.: Oxidative enzyme histochemistry of the chick esophagus and proventriculus. J. Morph. **125**, 403–418 (1968).

IRELAND, P. E.: Glands of esophagus. Laryngoscope (St. Louis) **43**, 351 (1933).

JACOBOWITZ, D., NEMIR, P.: The autonomic innervation of the oesophagus of the dog. J. thorac. cardiovasc. Surg. **58**, 678–684 (1969).

JOHNS, B. A. E.: Developmental changes in the oesophageal epithelium in man. J. Anat. (Lond.) **86**, 431–442 (1952).

JOHNSON, F. P.: The development of the mucous membrane of the esophagus, stomach and small intestine in the human embryo. Amer. J. Anat. **10**, 521 (1910).

KAUFMANN, P., LIERSE, W., STARK, J., STELZNER, F.: Die Muskelanordnung in der Speiseröhre. Ergebn. Anat. Entwickl.-Gesch. **40**, H. 3 (1968).

LEBLOND, C. P., GREULICH, R., MARQVES-PEREIRA, J. P.: Relationship of cell formation and cell migration in the stratified squamous epithelia. Advances in biology of skin, vol. 5, p. 39–67. Dorking, England: Edward Adlard and Son Ltd. 1964.

LEBLOND, C. P., WALKER, B. E.: Renewal of cell populations. Physiol. Rev. **36**, 255–275 (1956).

LEESON, T. S., LEESON, C. R.: Histology, 2nd ed. Philadelphia-London-Toronto: W. B. Saunders Co. 1970.

MAEIR, D. M., ANGRIST, A. A.: Comparative enzymatic histochemistry of various stratified squamous epithelia. Lab. Invest. 11, 440–451 (1962).

MARQVES-PEREIRA, J. P., LEBLOND, C. P.: Mitosis and differentiation in the stratified squamous epithelium of the rat esophagus. Amer. J. Anat. 117, 73–90 (1965).

NAGEL, A.: Das Bindegewebegerüst des menschlichen Oesophagus. Gegenbaurs morph. Jb. 81, 449–492 (1938).

PANNESE, E.: Sulla muscolaris mucosae dell'esofago umano. Monit. zool. ital. 62, 146–153 (1954).

PARAKKAL, P.: An electron microscopic study of esophageal epithelium in the newborn and adult mouse. Amer. J. Anat. 121, 175–196 (1967).

RAEBURN, C.: Columnar ciliated epithelium in the adult oesophagus. J. Path. Bact. 63, 157–158 (1951).

RASH, R. M., THOMAS, M. D.: The intrinsic innervation of the gastro-oesophageal and pyloro-duodenal junctions. J. Anat. (Lond.) 96, 389–396 (1962).

RECTOR, L. W., CONNERLEY, M. L.: Aberrant mucosa in the esophagus in infants and children. Arch. Path. 31, 285–294 (1941).

RYWLIN, A. M., ORTEGA, R.: Glycogenic acanthosis of the esophagus. Arch. Path. 90, 439–443 (1970).

SCHRIDDE, H.: Über Magenschleimhautinseln vom Bau der Cardialdrüsenzone und Fundus-drüsenregion und den unteren, oesophagealen Cardialdrüsen gleichende Drüsen im obersten Oesophagusabschnitt. Virchows Arch. path. Anat. 175, 1–16 (1904).

STELZNER, F., LIERSE, W.: Über das Verschlußsystem der terminalen Speiseröhre. Thorax-chirurgie 15, 676–679 (1967).

TAYLOR, A. L.: The epithelial heterotopias of the alimentary tract. J. Path. Bact. 30, 415–449 (1927).

TREACY, W. L., BAGGENSTOSS, A. H., SLOCUMB, C. H., CODE, C. F.: Scleroderma of the esophagus. A correlation of histologic and physiologic findings. Ann. intern. Med. 59, 351–356 (1963).

TRIER, J. S.: Morphology of the epithelium of the distal esophagus in patients with mid-esophageal peptic strictures. Gastroenterology 58, 444–461 (1970).

TRUDINGER, B. J., WILHELM, D. L.: Regeneration of gastric mucosa at the squamo-columnar junction in the rat. J. Path. 27, 127–135 (1969).

WILLIS, R. A.: The borderland of embryology and pathology. London: Butterworth 1958.

WONG, J., FINCKH, E. S.: Redistribution of squamous and columnar epithelium after gastric mucosal wounds in the rat. Pathology 2, 147–159 (1970).

Physiology

J. Hellemans and G. Vantrappen

With 20 Figures

1. The Functions of the Esophagus

The main function of the esophagus is the active transport of food and drink from the pharynx into the stomach. Above and below, the esophagus is closed by a sphincter. The upper sphincter prevents the undesirable passage of air from the pharynx into the esophagus as well as the reflux of fluid from the gullet into the pharynx. The lower esophageal sphincter is important to prevent gastroesophageal reflux. Under certain circumstances, e.g. vomiting or belching, the transport through the esophagus takes place in the retrograde direction. Little is known about the secretory function of the normal esophageal mucosa. No absorption takes place in the gullet.

2. The Esophagus at Rest
2.1. The Pharyngoesophageal Sphincter
2.1.1. Location

The upper end of the esophagus is closed by the so-called pharyngoesophageal sphincter over a distance of 2.5 to 4.5 cm. It has been known for a long time that this segment remains closed while the esophagus is at rest. This closure can be observed by direct inspection and on introduction of instruments a resistance is felt at this level (INGELFINGER, 1958). At the time of the rigid esophagoscopes this constantly closed gate leading into the esophagus was called the Gate of Tears of the inexperienced esophagoscopist (JACKSON and JACKSON, 1950). The musculature of this region is fairly complex (Fig. 2); moreover it shows considerable individual variations (PERROT, 1962). The sphincter has been described by anatomists for many years as being formed by the cricopharyngeal muscle, which arises from the lower side of the cricoid cartilage, the fibers spreading backwards and medially. A dorsal median raphe, similar to that of the pharynx, is lacking from this level onward. LUND (1965a, b) has shown that in dogs the whole sphincter contracts after unilateral electrical stimulation of the vagal branch to the cricopharyngeal muscle, i.e. the whole sphincter behaves as one unit in contrast with the pharyngeal muscles above. In humans also the pharyngoesophageal sphincter behaves as one unit, but no special vagal branch is found; instead vagal fibers arrive via the pharyngeal plexus (LUND, 1968). The anterior wall of the sphincter is rigid as it consists of the lamina of the cricoid cartilage (LUND, 1965a, b, 1968). The boundary with the thyropharyngeal muscle above it is variable (PERROT, 1962).

Most radiologists locate the sphincter at the level of the transition between C5 and C6. On the basis of an anatomico-roentgen study, ZAINO et al. (1967) questioned the identity of the cricopharyngeal muscle with the pharyngo-esophageal sphincter in man. They found that the cricopharyngeal muscle had considerable anatomical variability and that there were no consistently present transverse fibers that could act as a sphincter. The fibers spread out in a fan-shaped manner from one edge of the cricoid to the other, but chiefly spread upwards. According to these authors the sphincter consists mostly of the rather thick circular muscle bundles of the esophagus itself. In their radiological studies they demonstrated a narrowed area between the sixth and seventh cervical vertebra, which they interpreted as a sphincter. This is lower than the normal anatomical location of the cricopharyngeal muscle (C5–C6). Their designation of this segment as a "sphincter" is not based on the observation of physio-logical properties normally to be expected in a sphincter. Especially vague are the grounds on which they decided that the circular esophageal muscles, earlier already described as the post-cricoid sphincter of the esophagus (PERROT, 1962), can be considered as a sphincter and the cricopharyngeal and thyropharyngeal muscles cannot. Several studies, using simultaneous manometric and radiological techniques, suggest that the high pressure zone is located at the lower border of the cricoid cartilage (see 2.1.2.).

2.1.2. The Pressure Profile of the Pharyngoesophageal Sphincter

Pressure measurements have been correlated with radiologic observations by SOKOL et al. (1966). In the resting state, the sphincter may be seen dividing a column of air in the pharynx and in the upper part of the esophagus. Pressures higher than the atmospheric pressure begin immediately below the air column

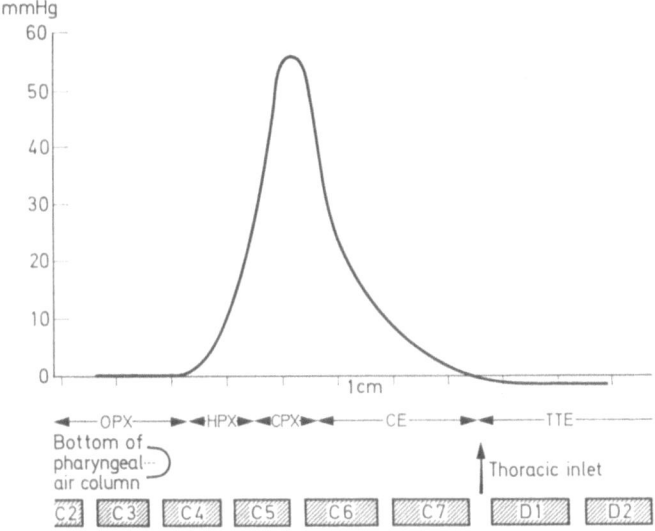

Fig. 15. Resting pressure profile of the pharyngoesophageal region, related to radiological and anatomical landmarks. *OPX* oropharynx; *HPX* hypopharynx; *CPX* cricopharynx; *CE* cervical esophagus; *TTE* thoracic-tubular esophagus. The vertebral bodies are as labeled. [From SOKOL, E. M. et al.: Gastroenterology 51, 960 (1966)]

in the hypopharynx and continue to increase distally until a peak is reached near the lower border of the cricoid cartilage (C5–C6) (Fig. 15). More distally, within the cervical esophagus, resting pressures decline until slightly subatmospheric pressures are recorded at the thoracic inlet or at the C7–T1 intervertebral level (Cohen and Wolf, 1968). The high pressure zone extends over a length of 2.5 to 4.5 cm. The highest pressure is noted at the level of the cricopharyngeal muscle. This muscle has a width of only 1 to 2 cm, but the pharyngeal muscle just above (the m. thyropharyngeus) and the circular muscles of the esophagus just below, also contribute to the build-up of a fairly wide high pressure zone. Atkinson et al. (1957a), Lund (1965a) and Fyke and Code (1955) also locate the peak of the high pressure zone at the level of the cricopharyngeal muscle.

2.1.3. Manometric Measurements of the Resting Pressure in the Pharyngoesophageal Sphincter

Most measurements of the resting pressure at the level of the cricopharyngeal muscle were done with non-perfused catheters. This technique mostly underevaluates the sphincter pressure. In one study (Atkinson et al., 1957a) the maximal elevation of pressure varied between 10 and 60 mm Hg above atmospheric pressure with a mean of 35 mm Hg. Using a tiny (3 mm) cylindrical pressure transducer Fyke et al. (1956) found the mean sphincteric pressure to be 39 cm of water above the esophageal pressure; individual values varied between 20 and 60 cm of water. By means of a perfusion technique pressures up to 75 mm Hg above the esophageal pressure can be recorded at the level of the cricopharyngeal muscle. It seems, however, that the recorded pressure depends on the spatial orientation of the perfused side holes (see p. 239—240) and on the speed of perfusion (Rinaldo and Levey, 1968). Using perfused catheters (0.078 ml/min) Goyal et al. (1970) found an end-expiratory pressure of 26.2 mm Hg and an end-inspiratory pressure of 32.7 mm Hg above the atmospheric pressure, while Dodds et al. (1972), perfusing at a rate of 1.6 ml/min, found 65 ± 20 mm Hg. With an intraluminal strain gauge system (Honeywell Probe) a pressure of 66 ± 23 mm Hg was recorded (Dodds et al., 1972).

The sphincter can probably resist pressures of at least 5 to 15 cm of H_2O, whether applied from above or below, before it opens (Ingelfinger, 1958). On occasion it can resist even higher pressures. A certain control over the sphincter can be acquired, e.g. by laryngectomized patients with esophageal speech.

Certain stimuli such as an increase in the cervical esophageal pressure (Car and Roman, 1970a) or an increase in intragastric pressure (Rosenberg and Harris, 1971a) also increase the sphincter tonus. Sphincter closure tension appears to be more than two times as high in patients with reflux esophagitis (32 mm Hg above the esophageal pressure), as in normals (14.6 mm Hg). This high resting pressure decreases again after repair of the hernia or after the appearance of a distal stricture and loss of heartburn (Hunt et al., 1970; Smiley et al., 1970). The resting pressure in the upper esophageal sphincter of patients with a Zenker's diverticulum has been reported to be high (Hunt et al., 1970), normal (Kodicek and Creamer, 1961) or low (Ellis et al., 1969). These studies were all done with a non-perfused catheter system. Data on the effect of hormones on the upper esophageal sphincter are lacking. But in the course of a few minutes substantially different resting pressures can be measured in the same subject.

The resting pressure also depends upon the species. It is lower in monkeys than in dogs and lower in dogs than in humans (Code and Schlegel, 1968).

2.1.4. Respiratory Pressure Variations

In man inspiration is associated with a fall in pressure in the cervical esophagus from $+0.9$ to -3.4 mm Hg. In the pharynx inspiration causes a drop in the intraluminal pressure from $+1.4$ to -0.2 mm Hg. In the high pressure zone between the pharynx and the cervical esophagus, however, the pressure rises on inspiration. The end-inspiratory pressure rise is maximal at the level of the peak of the high pressure zone (from 26.2 to 32.7 mm Hg, GOYAL et al., 1970). The inspiratory increase in sphincteric pressure is probably an active phenomenon. In sheep (CAR and ROMAN, 1970a), in dogs (KAWASAKI et al., 1964; LEVITT et al., 1965; HELLEMANS and VANTRAPPEN, 1971), in rats (ANDREW 1956b, c) and even in humans (HELLEMANS and VANTRAPPEN, 1971) inspiration is frequently, though not always, associated with spiking activity (Fig. 16). This inspiratory contraction of the upper esophageal sphincter probably helps to prevent the entry of air into the esophagus during inspiration.

2.1.5. Elasticity or Tonic Contraction

The mechanism of the high resting pressure in the upper esophageal sphincter is still controversial. DOTY (1968) ascribes the high resting pressure and the sphincteric properties of this zone to the narrowness of the junction and the elasticity of the tissue composing it. "Relaxation" of the sphincter is then considered as a passive opening by hyoid and larynx displacements. DOTY (1968) argues that there is no electromyographic evidence of tonic contraction in the resting state. Moreover a pale striated muscle, such as the cricopharyngeal muscle (BIRMINGHAM, 1899), appears to be particularly appropriate for fast contractions of short duration but not for tonic contractions. KAWASAKI et al. (1964) and LEVITT et al. (1965) did not find an electromyographic equivalent of a tonic contraction in the pharyngoesophageal sphincter in dogs. However, CAR and ROMAN (1970a), using thin wire electrodes chronically implanted in sheep did find continuous spiking of the cricopharyngeal muscle. A continuous spiking activity can also be recorded in the upper esophageal sphincter of humans by means of an intraluminal suction capsule containing needle electrodes which penetrate the wall from the mucosal side (HELLEMANS, 1970). But this does not prove that the sphincter contracts at rest because the presence of the suction capsule can cause distension and, by reflex means, contraction. The experiments of LUND (1965a, b) are hardly to be reconciled with the idea of a sphincter that is merely elastic. He demonstrated that in dogs the cricopharyngeal muscle, when isolated from the larynx, keeps its resting tone if the innervation is intact and looses it partially if the muscle is denervated. ANDREW (1956a, b) found a certain resting activity in the cricopharyngeal muscle of slightly anesthetized rats. Some motor units discharged continuously throughout the respiratory cycle, with a maximal frequency during inspiration. In the efferent nervous fibers to the cervical esophagus one or two fibers discharged at low frequencies. At its lowest detectable level, the activity consisted of a few impulses during inspiration only. At higher levels of respiratory activity there was a continuous discharge with a maximal frequency during inspiration.

The interpretation of these observations is difficult due to the fact that the cricopharyngeal muscle is a very reactive muscle. Implantation of an electrode and introduction of an intraluminal catheter or of an electromyographic capsule already provoke an active contraction. The surgical isolation of the sphincter from the surrounding structures in the experiments of LUND (1965a, b) may also induce reflex spasm (DOTY, 1968). Indeed, in laryngectomized patients the

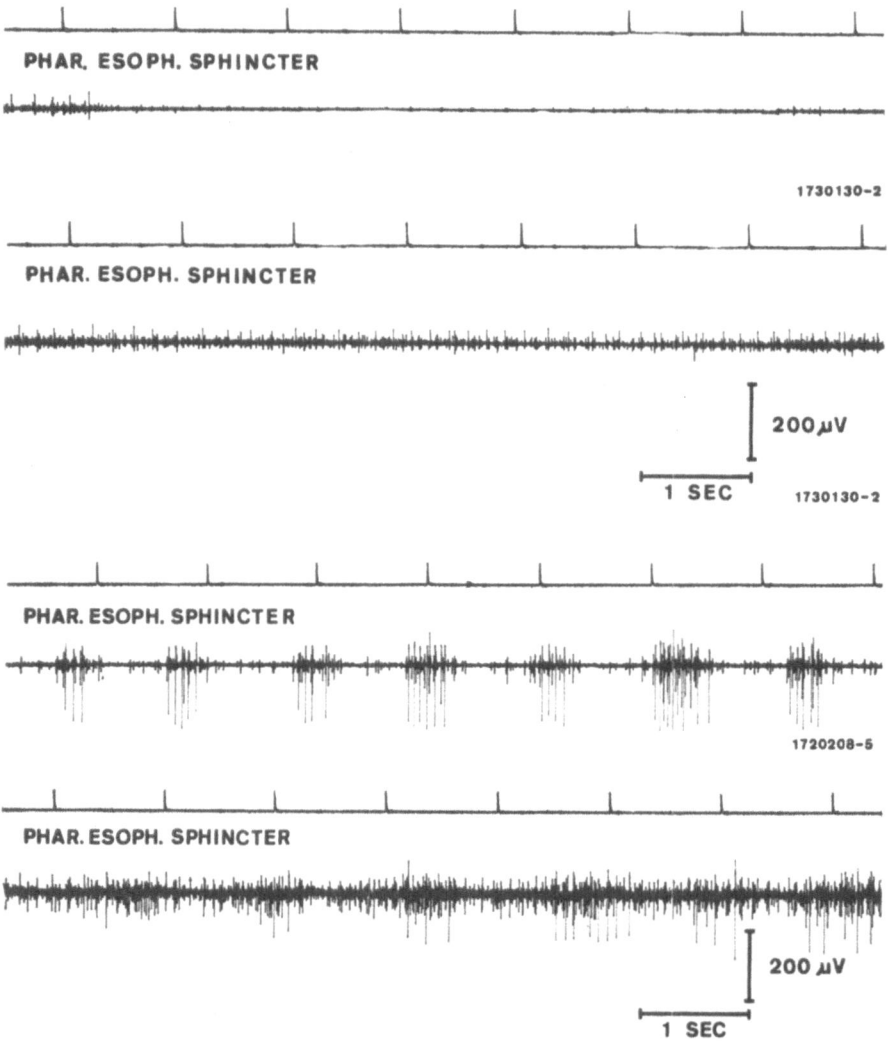

Fig. 16. Different electromyographic tracings from the pharyngoesophageal sphincter at rest. The tracings were obtained in dogs by means of a chronically implanted bipolar electrode. The upper two tracings were registered during the same experiment. When the animal is very quiet, spontaneous activity is minimal (upper tracing). However, the slightest excitation gives rise to a continuous spiking activity (second tracing). Often spiking activity increases synchronously with inspiration, whether the sphincter is nearly silent (third tracing) or rather active (fourth tracing) in the intervals between the inspirations

cricopharyngeal muscle becomes prominent on radiographies and dysphagia occurs (Schobinger, 1958). In our experiments on non-premedicated dogs with chronically implanted electrodes, periods of electromyographic inactivity during expiration occurred when the animal was very quiet. The slightest excitation resulted in the appearance of a continuous spiking activity (Fig. 16) which was modulated by respiration and became richer on each inspiration. These observations suggest that the "spontaneous" activity could be ascribed to the irritation by the electrode, no matter how minimal it may be.

2.2. The Esophagus Proper

In contrast to the other parts of the gastrointestinal tract the normal esophagus does not contract spontaneously. In the resting state, i.e. when no deglutition or no distension has taken place, the musculature of the esophagus is relaxed. No muscular activity can be shown either mechanically or electromyographically. Spontaneous activity is always clearly pathological. The normal esophagus empties in a few seconds after food or drink has been swallowed. Although small quantities of liquid or air can remain in the gullet, stasis of considerable amounts of material is always pathological.

2.2.1. The Resting Pressure

The resting pressure in the esophagus correlates with the intrathoracic pressure. Simultaneous measurements of intrapleural and intraesophageal pressures in dogs without thoracotomy have indicated that intraesophageal pressures are higher than intrapleural pressures recorded at the same levels in the thorax (RUTISHAUSER et al., 1966).

The pressure varies with respiration. On inspiration the intrathoracic and, therefore, the intraesophageal pressure decreases. On quiet inspiration in dorsal decubitus the intraluminal pressure drops to -12 to -15 cm H_2O. On expiration it again increases to -2 to -1 cm H_2O (CODE and SCHLEGEL, 1968). In the proximal few centimeters, close to the pharyngoesophageal sphincter, the respiratory pressure changes are less pronounced (GOYAL et al., 1970). In the abdominal cavity on the other hand the average resting pressure is higher than the atmospheric pressure and it increases on inspiration. Coughing results in changes in esophageal pressure of -65 cm H_2O to $+150$ cm H_2O (HIGHTOWER, 1955).

In dorsal decubitus the resting pressures are about the same over the total length of the esophagus. In the upright position the resting pressures are lower. A pressure gradient is found of about 1.0 cm H_2O per cm below the superior heart border. Above this border a small or no gradient exists. These differences in intraesophageal pressures at different heights in the thorax are ascribed to the weight of the thoracic contents (BANCHERO et al., 1967).

Smaller variations in pressure are caused by the pulsations of the heart and the large blood vessels. Their exact morphology and amplitude depend on the level of registration in the esophagus. Four types of cardiovascular artifacts are described by TROP et al. (1970): (1) the ventricular esophageal pulse, recorded at the level of the ventricle; (2) the pure auricular pulse, recorded at the level of the left atrium; (3) the auricular pulse with arterial impact, registered at the upper part of the left atrium and (4) the aortic pulse, registered at the level of the aortic arch.

The auricular pulse is positive and is ascribed to the filling of the left auricle. The other three are mainly negative and are related to the direct action of the ventricular contraction pulling on the esophagus.

2.3. The Lower Esophageal Sphincter (L.E.S.) (Gastroesophageal Sphincter)

Manometric evidence for the existence of a lower esophageal sphincter mechanism in man was first offered by FYKE et al. (1956). They showed the presence in the lower 2 to 4 cm of the esophagus of a high pressure zone, in which the resting pressure is higher than in the esophagus proper or in the gastric fundus. This elevated pressure can be observed even in patients with a sliding hiatal hernia and therefore is caused by intrinsic esophageal mechanisms (Vantrappen et al., 1958; Cohen and Harris, 1972). In the resting state this segment is closed, but it relaxes soon after swallowing or distension of the esophagus. This segment thus seems to have the typical physiological characteristics of a sphincter. In the new-born human (Gryboski et al., 1963; Gryboski, 1965) and in the adult macaca mulatta (Winship et al., 1965) this high pressure zone is less marked.

2.3.1. The Position of the Sphincter in Relation to the Squamocolumnar Junction

The location of the squamocolumnar epithelial junction in relation to that of the sphincter is variable. The junction bears little relationship to the structure and function of the underlying muscle (Ingelfinger, 1958). Mostly the squamocolumnar mucosal junction lies in the upper portion of the abdominal esophagus (Wolf, 1970), but the columnar mucosa can extend upward as high as 4 cm above the incisura cardiae (Botha, 1962).

2.3.2. The Pressure Profile of the Sphincter. The Pressure Inversion Point (P.I.P.)

The high pressure zone is located partially below and partially above the diaphragm (Fig. 140). Below the diaphragm the pressure increases on inspiration: above the diaphragm a short drop in pressure is observed during inspiration and a longer lasting period of relatively high pressure during expiration. About in the middle of the sphincter a zone of 0.5 cm is found in which the inspiratory pressure increase of the intraabdominal portion of the sphincter suddenly changes into an inspiratory drop in pressure and where sometimes biphasic pressure changes occur during inspiration. The point where this respiratory pressure swing changes from inspiratory positive to inspiratory negative has been called the pressure inversion point (P.I.P.). The maximal end-inspiratory pressure is found just below this P.I.P., the maximal end-expiratory pressure just above it (Fig. 17 A).

Whether this respiratory pressure reversal is registered at the very level of the diaphragmatic hiatus is doubtful. Most investigators agree that in health the P.I.P. corresponds to the diaphragmatic narrowing (Code and Schlegel, 1968; Heitmann et al., 1966). According to Winans and Harris (1967), however, the P.I.P. in the tracing from an uninfused open-tip catheter occurs in the distal end of the high pressure zone, shortly after the recording tip enters it. When a perfused catheter system is used, the P.I.P. is seen at the proximal end of the high pressure zone. Winans and Harris (1967) explain the difference by offering the hypothesis that the orifice of an uninfused system is sealed as it enters the lower sphincter; the entire length of tube lying within the chest would then act as a long narrow balloon and respond to intrathoracic respiratory pressure fluctuations (Harris and Pope, 1966).

Simultaneous pressure measurements by several catheters indicate that the P.I.P. is not always found at the same distance from the incisors, whether a non-perfused or perfused catheter system is used (Harris and Pope, 1966; Kaye and Showalter, 1971). The latter authors used three perfused catheters (0.5 ml/min) with lateral orifices located at the same level. The P.I.P. was registered at different levels by different catheters and in quite a few normal subjects a double P.I.P. was found in one or more catheters. They ascribed

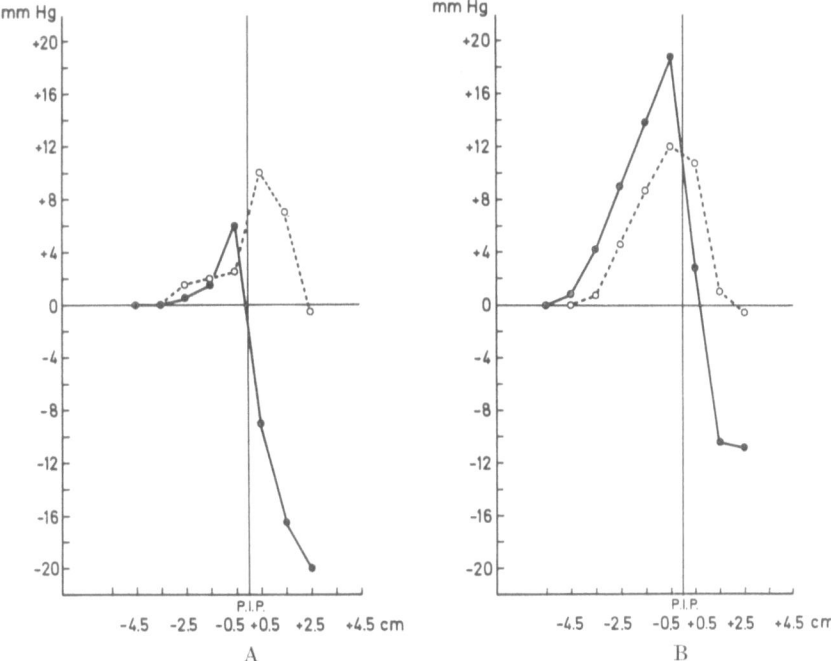

Fig. 17 A and B. Pressure prolife of the gastroesophageal sphincter at rest. A Measured with non-perfused open tip catheters. (From VANTRAPPEN, G.: Slokdarmmotiliteit, p. 52. Brussel: Arscia 1961.) B Measured with perfused (1.2 ml/min) catheters with lateral orifices. In these conditions, higher pressures are measured and the P.I.P. is found more proximally in the high pressure zone. Solid lines: end-inspiratory pressures. Broken lines: end-expiratory pressures. P.I.P.: pressure inversion point. On the horizontal axis: distance in centimeters above (+) or below (−) the P.I.P. On the vertical axis: pressure in mm Hg above (+) or below (−) the fundic pressure

these findings to the spatial orientation of the recording system, but this orientation was not always checked in the course of the experiments. WINANS (1972b) demonstrated that the highest pressures are recorded with lateral openings directed towards the left dorsal aspect of the sphincter. This is possibly due to the lateral margin of the diaphragmatic hiatus.

The high pressure zone lies deeper during held inspiration than during held expiration (KAYE and SHOWALTER, 1971). On quiet inspiration it lies about 1 to 3 cm more distally than on expiration (WINANS, 1970, 1972a). When abdominal compression is applied the pressure inversion point shifts proximally (HENDERSON and RODNEY, 1971).

Is the P.I.P. determined by the diaphragm, which separates the thoracic from the abdominal cavity or by the lower esophageal sphincter, which separates the gastric cavity from the esophageal lumen? Probably both the diaphragmatic hiatus and the sphincter can play a role. Indeed, in patients with large hernias CODE et al. (1962) found a double P.I.P., one at the level of the diaphragm and one at the level of the sphincter. Maybe the P.I.P. at the level of the diaphragm is determined by the sealing of the orifice when the catheter passes from the stomach into the herniated sac. In patients with a sliding hernia, the P.I.P. is frequently above the diaphragmatic narrowing, seen on roentgen examination (Rinaldo and Clark, 1964). Harris and Pope (1966) also demonstrated that the P.I.P. is produced not by the diaphragm but by the lower esophageal sphincter, whether it was in a normal position or displaced as a result of hiatal hernia. They also quote results of Mann et al. (1964) demonstrating that after transplantation of the lower esophageal sphincter into the abdomen, the P.I.P. is transplanted together with the sphincter. Actually the illustrations of Mann et al. (1964) show a double P.I.P., one at the level of the sphincter and one at the level of the surgically displaced hiatus.

2.3.3. Manometric Measurements of the Resting Pressure in the Lower Esophageal Sphincter

The resting pressure in the lower esophageal sphincter is usually defined as the difference between the intrasphincteric and fundic pressure. If non-perfused catheters are used, rather low resting pressures are measured. Some authors (Fyke et al., 1956; Vantrappen, 1961) find the maximal end-expiratory pressure to be somewhat higher than the maximal end-inspiratory resting pressure, but

Table 1. Yield pressures in the lower esophageal sphincter

Authors	Subjects without reflux		Number of subjects	Subjects with reflux	
	Yield pressures			Yield pressures	
	Range mm Hg	Mean mm Hg		Range mm Hg	Mean mm Hg
Pope 1967	10–43	24.8 ± 9.3 (SD)	15 N	3–20	11.6 ± 4.8 (SD)
	11–38	26.1 ± 9.3 (SD)	9 N	6–17	10.9 ± 4.3 (SD)
Winans and Harris, 1967	15–31		14 N	1–10	
Rinaldo and Levey, 1968		18.3 ± 1.5 (SE) (dist. cath.)	10		
		14.6 ± 2.1 (SE) (midd. cath.)			
Castell and Harris, 1970		15.0 ± 1.7 (SE)	18 N		
Cohen and Harris, 1970	8–36		25 N		
Haddad, 1970	6–20	13.2 ± 4.7 (SD)	10 N	3.2–14	6.9 ± 3.4 (SD)
				0 –10.7	3.4 ± 2.6 (SD)
Castell and Levin, 1971		17.6 ± 2.6 (SE)	14 N	3 – 9	5.5 ± 1.0 (SE)
		16.4 ± 2.6 (SE)	9 N		
		16.0 ± 2.1 (SE)	6 N		
Cohen and Harris, 1971	13–20	20.4 ± 2.1 (2SE)	25 N	0 – 6	3.8 ± 1.2 (2SE)
	12–30	19.6 ± 1.2 (2SE)	25 HH	1 – 6	3.0 ± 1.3 (2SE)
Cohen et al., 1971		19.4 ± 1.3 (SE)	20 N		
Moran et al., 1971				3 –17	9 ± 4 (SD)

N = normal subjects; HH = patients with hiatus hernia; OD = outer diameter; ID =

others observed the reverse (KELLEY et al., 1960; RINALDO and LEVEY, 1968). The maximal end-inspiratory pressure is found just below and the maximal end-expiratory pressure above or at the P.I.P. (Fig. 17 A). FYKE et al. (1956) found an end-expiratory pressure of about 8 to 12 cm H_2O and an end-inspiratory resting pressure which was lower, 2 to 5 cm H_2O. In our own experiments we found an end-inspiratory pressure of 5.8 mm Hg and an end-expiratory pressure of 10.3 mm Hg in one series of patients (VANTRAPPEN, 1961). In other series of subjects of different ages end-expiratory pressure values of 8.2 to 11.2 mm Hg were found (HELLEMANS, 1970). If balloons are used higher values are found, which depend on the diameter of the balloons.

In recent years the necessity of perfusing the catheters continuously has been stressed. Non-perfused catheters are said to seal on penetrating into the sphincter and to indicate mainly the already existing pressure (HARRIS et al., 1966). It is argued that a pressure is a force per unit of surface. Theoretically, therefore, no pressure can be measured in a closed sphincter which has no surface. Continuous perfusion gives a measure of the resistance of the sphincter to distension by a force acting from within its lumen (WINANS and HARRIS, 1967). The

of subjects without and with gastroesophageal reflux

	Technical data			Pressure measured	Criteria for gastroesophageal reflux
Number of subjects	Rate of perfusion ml/min	Diameter of tube mm			
10 6	0.18 (0.048–0.84)	2.5 OD		Mean	Presence of heartburn (10) Posit. Tuttle-test (intraesophageal pH probe) (6)
7	0.36–0.48	1.4 ID		Mean	Free gastroesophageal reflux of barium
	0.3	1.77 ID		EI	
	0.2	1.4 ID		Mean	
	1.2	1.4 ID		Mean	
14 26	0.6	1.4 ID		EE	Reflux of barium by straining (14) Free reflux of barium (26)
6	0.4	1.4 ID		Mean	Abnormally low pressure (incompetent sphincter)
13 12 HH	1.2	1.4 ID		Mean	Subject sympt. of gastroesophageal reflux as a major reason for seeking medical advice
		1.4 ID		Mean	
16	0.2	1.4 ID		Mean	Preoperative before Belsey and Nissen-operation, which was performed only after strict medical therapy had failed to control the symptoms and complications of prolonged and persistent reflux

inner diameter; EE = end-expiratory pressure; EI = end-inspiratory pressure.

fluid infusion causes the pressure within the recording system to increase to the level necessary to displace the sphincter tissues sealing the recording orifice ("yield pressure"). Pressures measured with perfusion are higher than pressures measured without perfusion (Fig. 17B). Mean L.E.S. pressures measured with catheters with lateral orifices perfused at a rate of 1.2 ml/min are 20.4 ± 2.1 mm Hg (mean ± 2 SE) above the gastric pressure (Cohen and Harris, 1971). Other published values are shown in Table 1. Pressures measured with perfusion are said to be better reproducible in the same individual. In the experiments of Pope (1967) yield pressures had an average coefficient of variation of 39%, whereas the resting pressures measured without perfusion had a coefficient of 53%.

The strong argument in favour of perfusion is the good correlation of the determined yield pressure with the presence or absence of gastroesophageal reflux. Pressures measured with non-perfused catheters, on the other hand, do not correlate very well with reflux (MacLaurin, 1963; Winans and Harris, 1967; Pope, 1967). No good correlation is found with miniature balloons either (MacLaurin, 1963).

The yield pressures in hernia patients without reflux are similar to those in normal subjects without reflux, but they are considerably lower in patients with reflux, whether they have or do not have a hiatus hernia (Pope, 1967; Cohen and Harris, 1971). The question can be asked whether an incompetent sphincter is incompetent at each and every moment. If not, a certain amount of overlap between normals and patients with reflux seems unavoidable. Indeed Haddad (1970) found that sometimes intraesophageal pH-measurements did not show reflux in patients with peptic esophagitis and a positive acid infusion test. These patients had both normal resting pressures at manometry and a negative Tuttle test. From the data of Cohen and Harris (1971) it can be presumed that in their series no such patients were present: all 25 patients with serious symptoms of gastroespohageal reflux as a major reason for seeking medical advice had a low resting pressure, not higher than 6 mm of Hg. Pope (1967) and Bennett (1973), however, did find a certain overlap between patients with and without heartburn, as well as between patients with negative and positive Tuttle test; but the overlap was much higher if non-perfused catheters were used (Pope, 1967). Skinner and Booth (1970) studied patients with and without reflux. If a non-perfused catheter system was used, the sphincteric pressures in the refluxing patients were not significantly different from those in the non-refluxing patients; with a perfused system significant differences were observed but there was a considerable overlap. Benz et al. (1972) also studied patients with and without symptoms of gastroesophageal reflux. They found that the resting lower esophageal sphincter pressures, measured with a perfused catheter system, overlapped partially, 17% of the symptomatic group having normal pressures and 19% of the asymptomatic group having low pressures. A better correlation with symptoms was obtained by means of the acid perfusion test or pH probe measurement of acid reflux.

2.3.4. Other Measurements of Sphincter Strength

Another means to assess accurately the strength of the lower esophageal sphincter is the measuring of the force required to pull a 12 mm Teflon ball from the stomach through the sphincter (Cohen and Harris, 1970). Comparison of this value with L.E.S. pressures shows a good correlation in normal subjects, resting in the supine position or during increased abdominal pressure. The contribution of the diaphragm to the values obtained by these measurements is minor because the test correlated fairly faithfully with the measured pressures even in patients with a hiatus hernia without reflux.

2.3.5. Variations of the Sphincteric Pressure

2.3.5.1. The Intrinsic Sphincteric Properties

In order to be competent the gastroesophageal sphincter must be able to prevent gastroesophageal reflux. The problem then arises: to what extent is the sphincter competence dependent on the surrounding structures or an intrinsic property of the sphincter itself? Two important observations have often thrown doubt upon the intrinsic value of the sphincter to prevent reflux (EDWARDS, 1967). (1) The sphincter is often incompetent in cases of hiatus hernia but the symptoms provoked by reflux diminish (in varying degrees) after repair of the hernia. (2) The measured resting pressures amount to only 10 mm Hg, whereas the abdomino thoracic pressure gradient can be much higher. Therefore the competence of the gastroesophageal junction has been ascribed, in part or completely, to factors outside of the sphincter itself, e.g. a pinchcock mechanism of the diaphragmatic slings (JACKSON, 1922; ALLISON, 1951; PETERS, 1955; EARLAM et al., 1967); the oblique muscle fibers of the stomach (loop of Willis) (SMIDDY and ATKINSON, 1960; GAHAGAN, 1962; WILLIAMS and INGRAM, 1964; KARAS et al., 1966; DEMOS et al., 1967); the acute angle of entry of the esophagus in the stomach or the angle of HIS (BARRETT, 1954; NAUTA, 1956; GOLDBERG, 1960; STERN et al., 1964; KARAS et al., 1966; BOMBECK et al., 1967); a flutter valve mechanism (EDWARDS, 1967; TOCORNAL et al., 1968); the existence of an intraabdominal sphincter segment which keeps the sphincter pressure always slightly above the abdominal pressure (BRAASCH and ELLIS, 1956; MACLAURIN, 1963; SICULAR et al., 1967); the insertion, at the proper location, of the phrenicoesophageal ligament (DILLARD, 1964; MICHELSON and SIEGEL, 1964; DILLARD and ANDERSON, 1966; BOMBECK et al., 1966, 1967; ANDERSON et al., 1967); the mucosal seal of the mouth of the esophagus (BOTHA, 1958).

To determine the relative importance of all these factors experiments have been carried out on the sphincter outside of its natural surroundings. In experiments with the isolated esophagus of both guinea pigs and kittens a sphincteric function could be demonstrated in the lower esophagus even when the gullet was lying free in a water bath (MANN et al., 1968a, b). In the guinea pig the sphincter had a tonus of its own and relaxed in response to distension of the lower part of the esophagus. The observation of MEI and SALDUCCI (1971) that continuous afferent vagal impulses from the lower esophageal sphincter can be recorded in the nodose ganglion of cats, indicates that an intrinsic sphincteric mechanism exists. ARIMORI et al. (1970) and THOMAS and EARLAM (1972) recorded in the resting gastroesophageal sphincter of dogs rhythmic electrical activity, disappearing on swallowing or distension of the esophagus; they consider this activity to be related to the tone of the sphincter. Dogs were subjected to a whole series of procedures designed to cause or eliminate reflux. The results of these experiments are often conflicting. The gastroesophageal sphincter was brought into the abdominal cavity (MANN et al., 1964) by reattaching the diaphragm to the esophagus 6 cm above the gastroesophageal junction. This sphincter remained competent although the resting pressure was clearly lower and the amplitude of the sphincter relaxation and contraction was reduced. Perhaps the sphincters of these dogs had their innervation disturbed. Indeed, three dogs in which the hiatus was mobilized but not displaced also had a lowered sphincter pressure. The same authors reported on a series of experiments in dogs in which the lower esophageal sphincter was placed into the thorax by creating a large hiatus hernia. The resting pressures in these sphincters were lowered by the procedure, they were much less competent and reflux occurred (Greenwood et al., 1965). Lind et al. (1969) also transposed the gastroesophageal junction of dogs into the thorax. In their experiments this procedure did not cause reflux but following vagotomy reflux did occur. Studies in the macaque (Karas et al., 1966) confirm that the intrinsic properties of the sphincter play the most important role and not the diaphragm, nor the phrenoesophageal ligament, nor the loop of Willis. The angle of His did seem to be important; if it was widened by lowering the gastric fundus reflux took place, although the sphincter kept its tonus. The question can be asked, however, whether such procedures do not interfere with the vagus-mediated increases in tone of this sphincter which must protect the esophagus from reflux (see below).

Vandertoll et al. (1966) showed that in dogs complete removal of the musculature of the proximal stomach or implantation of the esophagogastric junction into the fundus of the stomach did not impair gastroesophageal competence. They consider the role of the oblique fibers of the stomach and the angle of His in maintaining the competence of the gastroesophageal junction insignificant. For humans also it is generally accepted that many patients with a hernia have a competent sphincter.

One cannot escape the impression that the sphincter itself is not the only factor preventing reflux. The sphincter behaves best in its normal position, being less effective when transposed either into the chest or into the abdomen (Ellis, 1971). As contributory factors the mucosal folds (Botha, 1958) and the intraabdominal segment of the sphincter acting as a flutter valve (Edwards, 1967) may be important. The exact mechanism which allows the sphincteric pressure to increase again after hernia repair (Lind et al., 1965; Skinner and Booth, 1970; Moran et al., 1971; Csendes and Larrain, 1972; Hill, 1972) is not yet understood completely. Moran et al. (1971) found a mean preoperative sphincteric pressure of 9 mm Hg in 16 patients and a mean postoperative pressure of 15.6 mm of Hg in 22 patients after a Belsey repair or a Nissen fundoplication, but they did not find a correlation between the postoperative L.E.S. pressure and the relief from symptoms. Csendes and Larrain (1972) evaluated the long term effects of a posterior gastropexy (Hill repair) for hiatal hernia in 29 patients. Mean resting pressures in the gastroesophageal sphincter increased from 3.5 mm Hg preoperatively to 12.5 mm Hg 2 months after operation. The individual data suggest a correlation with the clinical result. In a second test 16 months after operation, no change was observed when compared with the results obtained 2 months after operation. The sphincter response to abdominal compression (see 2.3.5.3.) became normal in 21 of these subjects, a fact already observed by Lind et al. (1965).

It is a fairly constant finding that damage to the sphincter leads to the development of gastroesophageal reflux. The intrinsically incompetent sphincter, regardless of its location, will permit reflux. Many authors also confirm that in humans the yield pressure of the sphincter correlates fairly well with the presence or absence of reflux whether there is a hernia or not. Consequently it is safe to assume that the gastroesophageal sphincter is the main barrier preventing gastroesophageal reflux. In most publications reporting experiments which manipulated the sphincter or its surroundings, no data are found about the reactions of the sphincter to hormonal or nervous stimuli after these procedures. This might explain some contradictory conclusions drawn by different investigators. In addition peptic esophagitis and gastroesophageal reflux should not be equated. The occurrence of gastroesophageal reflux is only one factor in the pathogenesis of peptic esophagitis (BOYD, 1971). Other factors, e.g. acid clearing, are also important and are not always evaluated (BOOTH et al., 1968; SKINNER and BOOTH, 1970).

2.3.5.2. Hormonal Control of the Sphincter Strength

In vitro, BENNETT et al. (1967) have shown that the human esophageal smooth muscle responds to physiological doses of gastrin and that the response to pentagastrin is less marked. GILES et al. (1969 a) have shown that hog gastrin or pentagastrin, slowly administered intravenously, stimulate the cardiac sphincter to increase its tone. The motor effects of pentagastrin on the cardiac sphincter are less obvious than those seen after injection of gastrin, which provokes a marked response in a rather low dose of 0.005 units/kg. Secretion of endogenous gastrin, provoked by the introduction of meat extract, has a similar effect, independent of its secretory stimulus (GILES et al., 1969 a).

Endogenous as well as exogenous gastrin therefore increases the lower esophageal sphincteric pressure. CASTELL and HARRIS (1969, 1970) and CASTELL and LEVINE (1971) showed that acidification of the antrum, which inhibits the gastrin production, lowers the sphincteric pressure and that alkalinization of the antrum increases this pressure. However, when the gastric aspect of the sphincter mucosa is perfused with acid (pH 3) the intraluminal sphincter pressure increases. Atropine abolishes this reflex (GILES et al., 1969 b).

The effect on the sphincter of an I.V. injection of gastrin I reaches its maximum after 3 min (Fig. 18). The sphincteric pressure increases to 460% of the initial value after an optimal dosis of 0.7 µg/kg of gastrin (COHEN and LIPSHUTZ, 1971).

The peak sphincter responses at increasing doses of gastrin permit to calculate a dose-response curve. The log dose-response curve is sigmoid shaped. At doses higher than 0.7 µg/kg, the sphincter response declines below the maximal response (Fig. 19). Gastrin antiserum markedly reduces the resting pressure of the sphincter and diminishes its response to endogenous or exogenous gastrin (LIPSHUTZ et al., 1972).

Incompetent sphincters can also increase their tonus under the influence of alkalinization of the antrum. This has practical consequences for the therapy of reflux (CASTELL and LEVINE, 1971). The absolute change in sphincter pressure is directly related to the initial sphincter pressure (COHEN and LIPSHUTZ, 1971). ROSENBERG and HARRIS (1971 b) proposed the hypothesis that an incompetent lower esophageal sphincter is not a primary defect of the sphincter muscle itself but is secondary to decreased stimulation by endogenous gastrin. They made dose-response curves with pentagastrin in normal and incompetent sphincters and found the shape and the percentage increase of the curve to be the same in both groups but at least twice as much pentagastrin was required for peak response in patients with an incompetent sphincter. The gastric acid dose-response curve also had the same shape in both groups but in patients with incompetent sphincters the acid output was only half normal at each dose. These findings indicate that the function of the parietal cell mass of patients with lower esophageal sphincter incompetence is reduced to approximately 50% normal.

In patients with achalasia, however, there is a parallel shift of the dose-response curve toward lower doses (Fig. 20); their serum gastrin levels were found to be normal so that an oversensitivity of the sphincter to gastrin was postulated (COHEN et al., 1971).

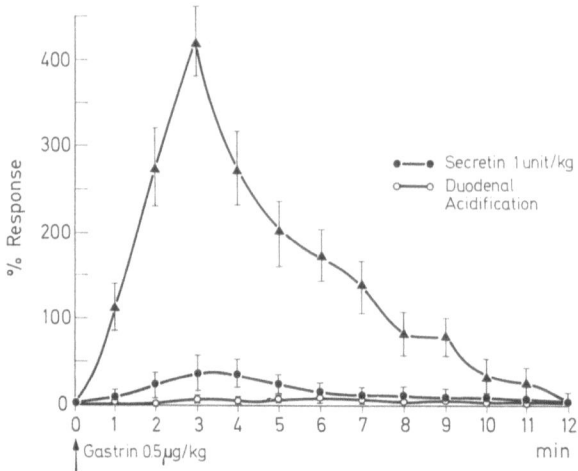

Fig. 18. Increase (in %) of the yield pressure in the lower esophageal sphincter after the injection of gastrin I 0.5 µg/kg (△———△). This gastrin effect can be inhibited by exogenous secretin (●———●) or by endogenous secretin, released by duodenal acidification (○———○). [From COHEN, S., LIPSHUTZ, W.: J. clin. Invest. **50**, 449 (1971)]

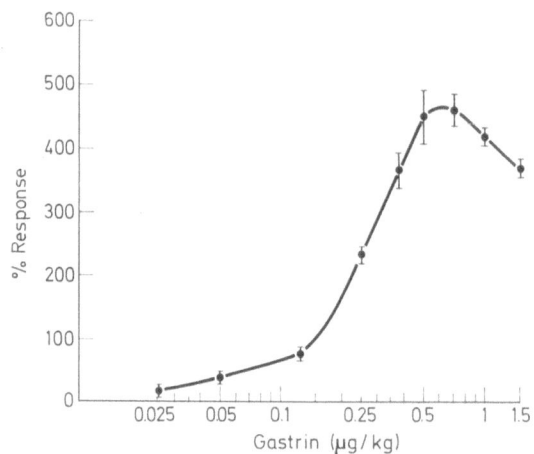

Fig. 19. Dose-response curve of the effect of gastrin on the lower esophageal sphincter. The response of the sphincter is expressed as the per cent increase of the yield pressure above its initial value. [From COHEN, S., LIPSHUTZ, W.: J. clin. Invest. **50**, 449 (1971)]

More reflux is said to occur in persons with a partial gastrectomy, which eliminates the antrum as a source of gastrin (BIRMINGHAM, 1958; COX, 1961; WINDSOR, 1964). Strangely enough some rise in pressure occurs after administration of alkali to these patients too (CASTELL and HARRIS, 1970), but this could be due to gastrin producing cells in the duodenum. It is also hard to understand why patients with pernicious anemia, who have a high serum gastrin level do not have an increased L.E.S. pressure (HARRIS, 1970). COHEN et al. (1971) found normal or low normal pressures in patients with Zollinger-Ellison syndrome;

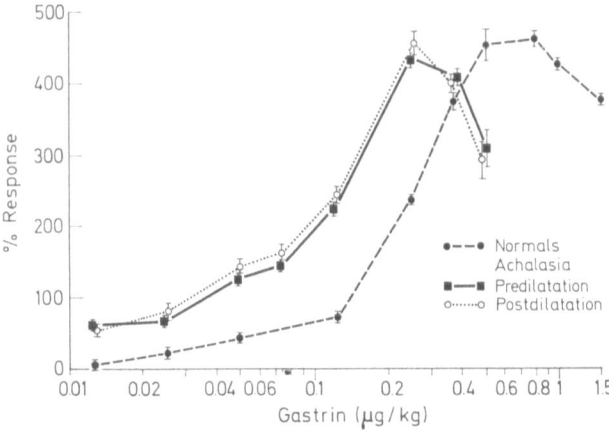

Fig. 20. Dose-response curves of the effect of gastrin on the lower esophageal sphincter in normals and in achalasia patients. The response of the sphincter is expressed as a per cent increase of the initial resting pressure. The L.E.S. in patients with achalasia is more sensitive to lower doses of gastrin, but not capable of a greater per cent response. [From COHEN, S. et al.: J. clin. Invest. 50, 1241 (1971)]

others (ISENBERG et al., 1971) measured values which were significantly higher in 6 patients than in normals (27.2 ± 2.1 mm Hg versus 12.4 ± 1.6 mm Hg). However, the responsiveness of the L.E.S. to exogenous gastrin is distinctly diminished in these patients. The L.E.S. of patients with Zollinger-Ellison syndrome seem less responsive to both endogenous and exogenous gastrin than are the L.E.S. of normal subjects (COHEN and HARRIS, 1972). Secretin interferes with the action of gastrin on the lower esophageal sphincter by a selective and competitive type of antagonism.

Exogenous and endogenous secretin counteract the effect of gastrin (COHEN and LIPSHUTZ, 1970a, 1971) (Fig. 18). However, secretin has considerably less effect in lowering the normal level of the resting sphincteric pressure (COHEN and LIPSHUTZ, 1970a, 1971). Ingestion of a corn oil meal results in a striking decrease in L.E.S. pressure. Even greater decreases occur when corn oil is instilled directly into the duodenum. This effect is more pronounced than the decrease in pressure noted after the intravenous injection of secretin (CASTELL and NEBEL, 1971). After protein ingestion the L.E.S. pressure increases. The inhibition of this increase by acidification of the antrum suggests a mechanism through antral gastrin release (CASTELL and NEBEL, 1971). Secretin interferes with the action of gastrin on the lower esophageal sphuncter by a selective and competitive type of antagonism.

Caerulein in low doses (20 ng per kg) decreases the sphincter pressure in dogs and man; at higher dose levels (200 ng per kg) it causes an increase of sphincter pressure. As a continuous infusion of caerulein results in a shift to the left of the pentagastrin dose-response curve, a competitive mechanism may be postulated (JENNEWEIN et al., 1972). The octapeptide of cholecystokinin causes a slight decrease in L.E.S. pressure in man (RESIN et al., 1972). Prostaglandins E_1 and E_2 cause a potent inhibition of the L.E.S. and it has been suggested that they have a physiological role in the sphincteric relaxation. This actions seems to be a direct action on the muscle (GOYAL et al., 1973).

Insulin-induced hypoglycemia decreases the L.E.S. pressure as a result of the stimulation of acid secretion in the stomach. If the gastric acid is neutralized with antacids the pressure increases during the hypoglycemia. This effect is also observed in patients who underwent vagotomy and who therefore no longer react to hypoglycemia with an increased acid secretion. In patients with antrectomy insulin does not increase the lower esophageal sphincter pressure (CASTELL, 1971). This author attributed the decrease in lower esophageal sphincter pressure during hypoglycemia to the suppression of gastrin release by the acid secreted in the stomach. Actual measurements of serum gastrin levels in normals, however, have shown a 247% increase in serum gastrin during insulin-induced hypoglycemia (HANSKY et al., 1971). These observations suggest that other factors (secretin ?, vagal influences ?) interfere with the hypoglycemia-induced changes in sphincteric pressure.

Glucagon markedly reduces the lower esophageal sphincter pressure and inhibits the normal response of the sphincter to pentagastrin by a non-competitive mechanism. This effect is not due to the concomitant hyperglycemia (JENNE-WEIN et al., 1972). Calcitonin does not directly affect the sphincter pressure, but lowers the pentagastrin response, without causing a shift of the dose-response curve of the pentapeptide, i.e. it acts by a non-competitive mechanism. Carminatives such as essence of peppermint decrease the intrasphincteric pressure and favor belching (SIGMUND and McNALLY, 1969).

The site of action of gastrin was thoroughly studied on smooth muscle strips of the opossum (LIPSHUTZ et al., 1971). In the circular smooth muscle of the lower esophageal sphincter as well as in the gastric antrum, gastrin I stimulates the postganglionic cholinergic nerves to release acetylcholine. Gastrin is antagonized by atropine, hyoscin, tetrodotoxin, and hemicholinium, but not by ganglionic blocking agents. In the guinea pig ileum BENNETT (1965) found the same site of action for gastrin II. The same author (BENNETT et al., 1967) found a direct action of gastrin on the human esophageal smooth muscle. It is not clear whether or how gastrin acts on striated muscle sphincters of certain species. In vitro the circular muscle of the L.E.S. is more sensitive to gastrin than the circular muscle of the esophagus or of the antrum (LIPSHUTZ and COHEN, 1971). In vivo the L.E.S. of achalasia patients is said to be more sensitive to gastrin than that of normals (COHEN et al., 1971).

2.3.5.3. The Response of the Lower Esophageal Sphincter to Increased Intragastric Pressure

When the sphincter is challenged by an increase of pressure in the abdomen, the pressure within the whole length of the sphincter increases by intrinsic muscular contraction (WANKLING et al., 1965). The intraluminal pressure in a tubular esophagus proximal to a competent gastroesophageal sphincter does not change during abdominal compression. But if the sphincter is incompetent the esophageal pressure does increase (VAN DERSTAPPEN and TEXTER, 1964; LIND et al., 1966; BUTTERFIELD et al., 1970, 1972). An increase of the intraabdominal and intragastric pressures due to straight-leg raising or inflation of an abdominal binder or a Valsalva maneuver causes a greater increase in intrasphincteric pressure than in intragastric pressure (Fig. 21), regardless of the presence or absence of a hernia (LIND et al., 1966; COHEN and HARRIS, 1971). The greater increase is found especially below the P.I.P. (NAGLER and SPIRO, 1961; BUTTERFIELD et al., 1970). LIND et al. (1966) found that, although the pressure increased both above and below the P.I.P., an increase higher than the intragastric pressure increase was observed only below the P.I.P.

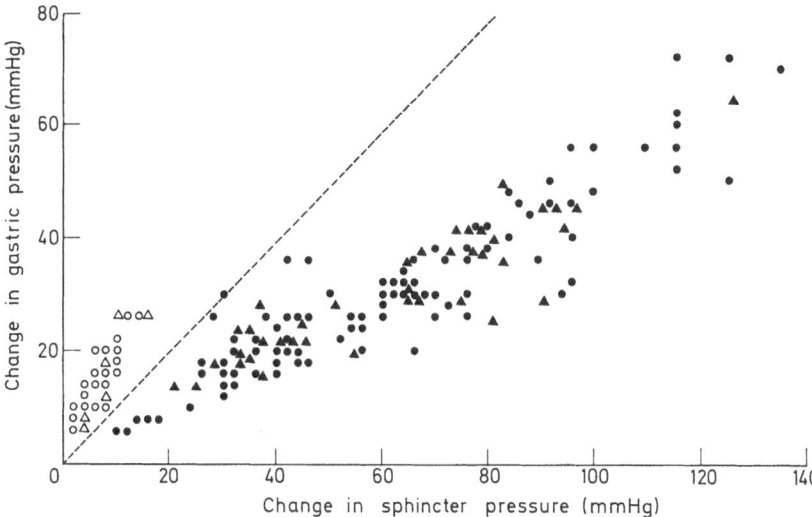

Fig. 21. Increase in lower esophageal sphincter pressure related to the increase in intragastric pressure caused by a Valsalva maneuver (△ and ▲), or by either inflation of an abdominal binder or lifting of the legs while the patient was supine (○ and ●). In asymptomatic hernia patients (black symbols), the increase in sphincter pressure is greater than the rise in intragastric pressure. In symptomatic hernia patients (open symbols) the sphincteric pressure increase is less than the rise in intraabdominal pressure. [From COHEN, S., HARRIS, L. D.: New Engl. J. Med. **284**, 1053 (1971)]

In patients with symptomatic reflux, on the other hand, the increase in L.E.S. pressure is always exceeded by the increase in gastric pressure (Fig. 21) (COHEN and HARRIS, 1971). An excellent correlation was found between the yield pressure in the lower esophageal sphincter and the degree to which sphincteric pressure increased together with gastric pressure (COHEN and HARRIS, 1969). The response of the lower esophageal sphincter to an increase in intraabdominal pressure is probably due to a reflex mediated by the vagal nerve, because it is inhibited by vagotomy (CRISPIN et al., 1967) and after the administration of atropine (LIND et al., 1968; COHEN and LIPSHUTZ, 1970b). Even more pronounced than the increase of the L.E.S. pressure caused by an increase in intraabdominal pressure, is the response of the lower esophageal sphincter when the pressure in the gastric fundus increases as a result of gastric contractions. In that case the sphincter pressure increases 8 times as much as the pressure in the fundus (DIAMANT and AKIN, 1970, 1972). CLARK and VANE (1961) found that in cats the lower esophageal sphincter tonus increased when the gastric pressure increased moderately but that it decreased when the stomach was distended further. These effects were abolished by bilateral vagotomy.

2.3.5.4. Nervous Control of the Lower Esophageal Sphincter Pressure

Extensive sympathectomy does not affect the resting pressure profile of the gastroesophageal sphincter in dogs (GREENWOOD et al., 1962). On the contrary, section of the vagal nerves at different levels decreases the lower esophageal sphincter pressure but does not abolish the high pressure zone completely. After a variable period of time the sphincter may even regain its normal strength

(Higgs and Ellis, 1965). Electrolysis of the motor centers of the vagus (Higgs et al., 1965), bilateral supranodosal vagotomy (Higgs and Ellis, 1965), left cervical vagotomy combined with a high right thoracic vagotomy (Carveth et al., 1962), bilateral hilar vagotomy (Carveth et al., 1962) and even trans-abdominal supradiaphragmatic vagotomy (Elebute et al., 1966) decrease the sphincteric pressures in dogs and, except for the latter procedure, impair sphinc-teric relaxation. Cervical vagotomy causes a decrease in the sphincteric pressure of monkeys as well (Binder et al., 1968). Denervation of the feline esophagus seems to provoke sphincteric disturbances different from those recorded in the denervated dog and monkey esophagus. After bilateral cervical vagotomy, the resting sphincteric pressure was unchanged for 6 months and deglutitive relaxa-tions were rare. But later on the incidence of relaxations gradually returned to normal and resting pressures increased definitely. After sympathectomy, deglutitive relaxations were normal and the resting sphincteric pressure was unchanged for the first month. The resting pressures at 2 and 3 months, however, were very low (Burgess et al., 1972). These results are difficult to reconcile with previous observations in dogs. However, the late appearance of these changes points to some indirect effect. Secondary degeneration of Auerbach's plexus was looked for, but not found. Maybe the centrally regulated equilibrium of the sympathetic and parasympathetic system had changed in the post-operative period? Examination of other parameters of sympathetic and parasympathetic activity could have answered this question. Precisely the L.E.S. pressure is one of the elements that have always hampered the experimental reproduction of achalasia: following vagotomy the pressure decreases in experimental animals, but in patients with achalasia it is normal (Vantrappen et al., 1963) or even more than double (Cohen et al., 1971). This difference is ascribed to the fact that vagotomy eliminates all vagal fibers and achalasia only some of them (Higgs et al., 1965).

The result of high vagotomy in man is unknown. Transabdominal vagotomy did not affect the mean lower esophageal sphincter pressure of 10 ulcer patients (Blackman et al., 1971) or had only a slight effect (Mann and Hardcastle, 1968). In some patients vagotomy causes a decrease in sphincteric pressures (Williams and Woodward, 1967; Blackman et al., 1971), but this may be due to variations in the vagal innervation or to marginal lesions of the esophageal wall. The normal response of the sphincter to abdominal compression, however, is altered by vagotomy (Crispin et al., 1967).

Both the resting tone of the sphincter (Skinner and Camp, 1968) and its normal response to abdominal compression are diminished by atropine (Crispin et al., 1967). Moreover, Cohen and Lipshutz (1970b) have demonstrated that atropine blocks the sphincteric effects of both endogenous and exogenous gastrin. Certainly the competence of the sphincter is not improved by the administration of atropine. Smoking 1 or 2 cigarettes is sufficient to cause a fall in lower esoph-ageal sphincter pressure (Dennish and Castell, 1971), probably because the inhaled nicotine blocks the cholinergic control mechanisms as it does in vitro (Bennett, 1972). Beta adrenergic stimulation has been reported to cause inhibi-tion of the circular muscle of the lower esophagus including the sphincteric zone (Christensen and Daniel, 1968; Misiewicz et al., 1969).

In dogs transection and reanastomosis of the esophagus does not cause dis-turbances in the sphincter (Carveth et al., 1962). In children whose esophagus was partially replaced by a colon transplant but who kept the distal 3 to 4 cm of the esophagus, manometric measurements at the level of the sphincter were also normal (Sieber and Sieber, 1968).

3. Bolus Transport. Primary Peristalsis

Normally, swallowing elicits a contraction which starts high up in the pharynx and continues throughout the whole esophagus until it reaches the cardia. This contraction is called "primary peristalsis". It pushes a solid bolus down the esophagus into the stomach. Fluids taken in the upright position reach the cardia under influence of gravity several seconds before the peristaltic contraction. Taken in horizontal decubitus or in the head down position they are propelled by the peristaltic contraction, if necessary against the force of gravity. Studies of swallowing incidence over 24-hour periods in normal young subjects show a mean deglutition frequency of 585 per day (range 203–1008) (LEAR et al., 1965). Secondary peristalsis is elicited by distension of the esophageal wall. A bolus which for some reason was held up in the esophagus after swallowing can be propelled into the stomach by secondary peristalsis. Tertiary contractions are defined as contractions which occur simultaneously at different levels of the esophagus.

The transport from mouth to stomach can be divided in three phases, which follow each other very closely.

a) The *oral phase* during which voluntary movements take food and drink into the pharynx.

b) The *pharyngeal phase* during which the bolus is transported through the pharynx into the esophagus. This phase requires the complex cooperation of different groups of muscles and nerves because the pharynx is part of the respiratory system as well. This phase is not voluntary but it is brought about by reflexes caused by stimuli from the first phase of deglutition.

c) The *esophageal phase* including the transport through the gastroesophageal sphincter.

The mechanical activities, the intraluminal pressure changes and the nervous impulses belonging to each phase will be discussed separately.

3.1. Mechanical Activity

3.1.1. Oral Transport

The movements in the oral and pharyngeal cavities during swallowing were studied mainly by radiocinematography (RAMSEY et al., 1955; CHRISTRUP, 1964; FARRIAUX and MILBLED, 1965; SOKOL et al., 1966; COHEN and WOLF, 1968) and by means of electromyography (DOTY and BOSMA, 1956; DOTY, 1968). The previous literature on this subject has been thoroughly discussed by BOSMA (1957) and INGELFINGER (1958). This complex phenomenon has been beautifully illustrated by NETTER (1959).

After food has been masticated and mixed with the necessary quantity of saliva a bolus of appropriate size and consistency is separated and transported to a groove in the middle of the tongue. The base of the tongue is displaced a little backward, narrowing the lumen of the oral pharynx. Once the decision to swallow has been made the forepart of the tongue is pressed firmly against the anterior part of the palate (Fig. 22 A). A rolling movement brings an ever increasing part of the tongue against the palate (Fig. 22 B, C). The posterior part of the tongue makes a rather brusk forward movement to form a grooved chute down (Fig. 22 B). This projects the bolus through the isthmus into the pharynx. In the mean time the nasopharynx is being cut of from the oropharynx. To achieve this the soft palate is brought up (Fig. 22 A), the relaxed posterior pillars approximate one another and a bulge begins to form in the upper part of the

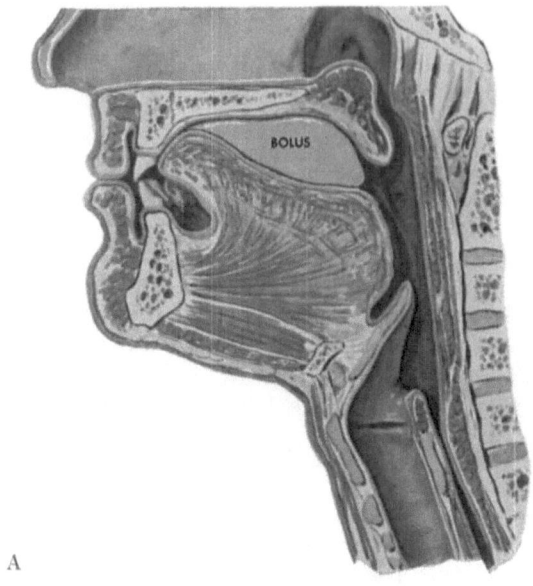

A

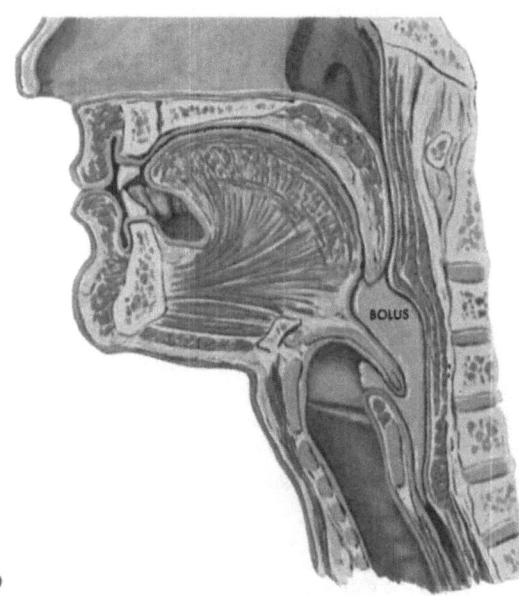

D

Fig. 22 A—F. Schematic representation of the successive phases of the deglutition act. (From
Netter, F. H.: Ciba collection of medical illustrations, Digestive system, part I, 1959,
p. 74–75.) A Tip of tongue in contact with anterior part of palate bolus is pushed backward
in groove between tongue and palate. Soft palate is being drawn upward. Bulge has begun
to form in upper part of posterior pharyngeal wall (Passavant's ridge) and approaches rising
soft palate. B Gradually pressing more of its dorsal surface against hard palate, tongue
pushes bolus backward into oral pharynx. Soft palate is drawn upward to make contact
with Passavant's ridge, closing off nasopharynx. Receptive space in oral pharynx forms
by slight forward movement of root of tongue. Contraction of stylopharyngeus and upper
pharyngeal constrictor muscles draws pharyngeal wall upward over bolus. C Bolus has
reached valleculae. Hyoid bone and larynx move upward and forward. Epiglottis is tipped

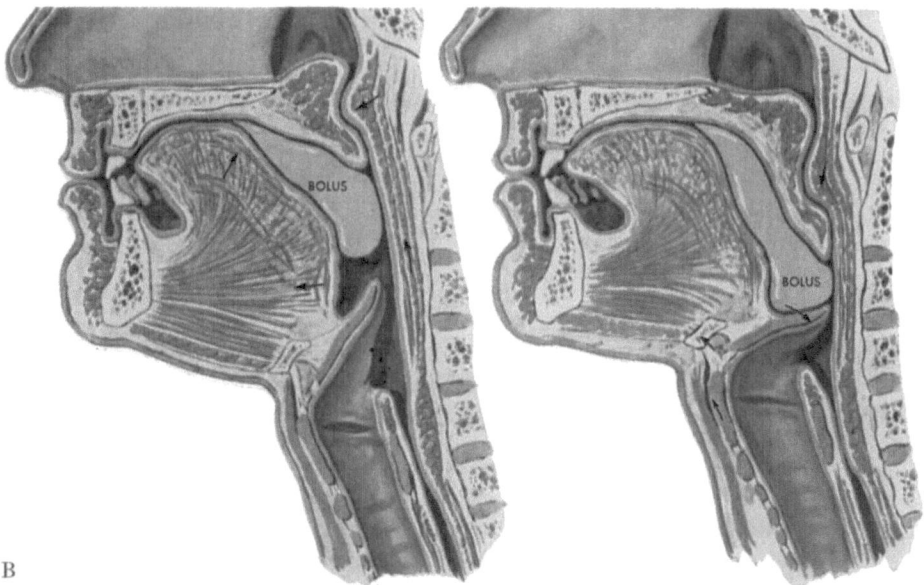

B C

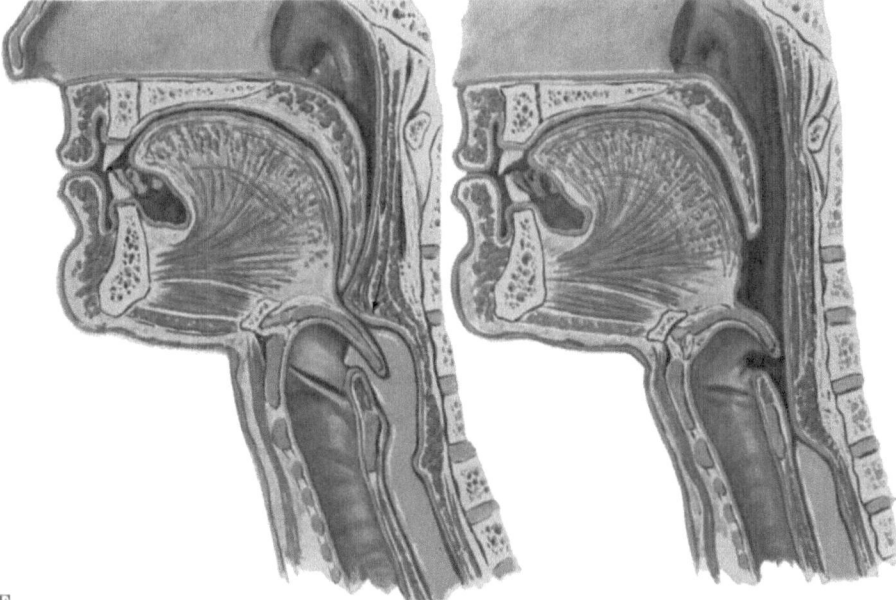

E F

downward. "Stripping wave" on posterior pharyngeal wall moves downward. D Soft palate
has been pulled down and approximated to root of tongue by contraction of pharyngo-
palatine muscles (posterior pillars), and by pressure of descending "stripping wave"; oropharyngeal cavity closed by contraction of upper pharyngeal constrictors. Cricopharyngeus
muscle is relaxing to permit entry of bolus into esophagus. Trickle of food entres also laryngeal
aditus but is prevented from going farther by closure of ventricular folds. E "Stripping
wave" has reached vallecula and is pressing out last of bolus therefrom. Cricopharyngeus
muscle has relaxed and bolus has largely passed into esophagus. F "Stripping wave" has
passed pharynx. Epiglottis is beginning to turn up again as hyoid bone and larynx descend.
Communication with nasopharynx has been re-established

posterior pharyngeal wall (Passevant's ridge) and comes into contact with the weak palate (Fig. 22B). This manoeuvre prevents the penetration of food and drink into the nasopharynx; if the soft palate is paralyzed, this penetration does take place. Coincident with the elevation of the soft palate the posterior pharyngeal wall begins to make an upward excursion (Fig. 22B). The soft palate is then pulled down again by contraction of the pharyngo-palatinus muscles situated in the posterior faucial pillars (Fig. 22C). It descends onto the back of the bolus and, after this has passed, lies on the dorsum of the tongue, while it maintains its contact with the posterior pharyngeal wall (Fig. 22D).

3.1.2. Pharyngeal Transport

The bolus stimulates tactile receptors in the mouth and the pharyngeal cavity and elicits a complex series of reflex muscle activities, which are so meticulously coordinated that they succeed in pushing the bolus down in the right direction. As already mentioned the pharynx is pulled up by contraction of the stylo-pharyngeal muscle and by the pharyngeal muscles themselves (Fig. 22B). Immediately prior to the act of swallowing the hyoid bone is brought in a position of moderate elevation; the mylohyoid muscle is the first to contract. Just before the bolus reaches the valleculae the hyoid and the larynx move abruptly upward and forward (Fig. 22C). The degree of the forward movement depends on the properties of the bolus.

Respiration is momentarily inhibited and the airways are closed off. Some of the air trapped in the laryngopharynx ahead of the bolus vanishes through the still open glottis. Then the larynx is closed by the false and the true vocal cords. The epiglottis is tipped down over the laryngeal aditus because the thyroid cartilage approaches the hyoid bone (Fig. 22C, D); thus the larynx climbs faster then the hyoid and hides partially under the base of the tongue. A solid bolus will itself push the tip of the epiglottis backward over the aditus of the larynx (Fig. 22D). A fluid bolus is split by the epiglottis into two parts which run at both sides of the epiglottis toward the piriform fossae. They reunite behind the cricoid at the level of the upper esophageal sphincter, which on their arrival is already relaxed in order to allow the bolus to pass through (Fig. 22D). When fluids are passing, the superior aperture of the larynx and the lumen of the vestibule are reduced to a narrow channel; however, when a solid bolus is swallowed the lumen of the vestibule may be relatively wide open (Staple and Ogura, 1966). Although the epiglottis protects the larynx, this closing mechanism is not perfect. Some swallowed fluid may penetrate into the larynx (Fig. 22D), where it is stopped by the glottis which closes quickly when fluids are swallowed. These small quantities of fluid are pushed up again by a sort of stripping wave of the laryngeal sphincters occurring just before pharyngeal peristalsis (Fig. 22E). As a matter of fact the epiglottis mechanism is not even necessary. A beer guzzler can drink a whole glass with the epiglottis in an upright position. Patients who underwent a supraglottic subtotal laryngectomy, by which epiglottis, aryepiglottic folds, false vocal cords and the upper third of the thyroid cartilage were removed, can avoid false passage by means of the remaining structures. The mechanisms they may call upon are the closing of the true vocal cords and the movements of the tongue. Exhalation at the end of swallowing clears the airway of any residual food (Staple and Ogura, 1966).

The tail of the bolus is followed by the stripping wave of the pharyngeal wall, moving downward (Fig. 22D). This contraction ring retains the contact with the soft palate and, together with the contraction of the palate and the tongue, it is the major force pushing the bolus on. Below the root of the tongue the anterior wall no longer plays an important part in the stripping wave (Fig. 22 E, F). The propulsion is much more important for the transport of the bolus than any sucking force which may be created by the foreward movements of the hyoid and the trachea, the airways being closed.

All these swallowing movements take place rather quickly. The bolus is tipped off the back of the tongue and through the pharynx at high speed (40 to 50 cm/sec). It slows down as it passes through the relaxed sphincter. The sphincter closes quickly behind the bolus but not before all of it has passed (Fig. 22 E). In patients with Zenker's diverticulum the sphincter is said to be uncoordinated with the pharyngeal contractions (ELLIS et al., 1969). On the average 200 msec elapse between the moment liquid starts to descend and the onset of the pharyngeal contraction. After 300 msec the bolus reaches the cricopharyngeal muscle; after 750 msec (330 to 1000 msec) the liquid bolus has passed the cricopharyngeal sphincter. This whole phase takes a second or less. These data are valid for humans and were obtained by cinefluorography (CHRISTRUP, 1964).

Variants of swallowing movements have been described in champion beer guzzling and in swallowing sticky material (RAMSEY et al., 1955; ATKINSON et al., 1957 a). The expert beer drinker eliminates a series of musculatory movements because he does not form a bolus. Before he starts the whole assembly of hyoid bone, larynx, pharynx and the base of the tongue are placed about one vertebral lower than normal. The epiglottis does not descend but the glottis remains closed the whole time. As soon as the mouth is filled the soft palate rises upward, the tongue comes foreward and the liquid runs down into the pharynx. The tongue, in cooperation with the soft palate forms a short stripping wave which empties the pharynx while the mouth is filled again. The tongue continuously makes pumping movements, about one per second. The pharyngoesophageal sphincter remains open throughout.

Another phenomenon is observed during quick successive swallows to get rid of a viscous paste: the pharynx contracts repeatedly while the hyoid bone is raised very high and the epiglottis closes the larynx.

3.1.3. Electromyographic Studies of Deglutition

The sequence in which the muscles contract during deglutition has been studies in several species by DOTY and BOSMA (DOTY and BOSMA, 1956; BOSMA, 1957; DOTY, 1968).

3.1.3.1. Leading Complex

Swallowing is initiated by an abrupt onset of activity in some intrinsic and supporting muscles of the oropharynx. The first noticeable movement is a contraction of the mylohyoid muscle (Fig. 23). In species in which the anterior digastric muscles and the internal pterygoid muscles are active during swallowing, they contract at the same moment. Just afterwards or at the same time the posterior part of the tongue, the upper constrictor pharyngis, the palatoglossus, the stylohyoideus and sometimes the geniohyoideus start contracting. Together these muscle contractions form the leading complex. Some variations according to species exist. In cats and dogs the palatopharyngeus starts contracting 40 msec later than the leading complex. In the monkey the palatopharyngeus and palatoglossus fire with the leading complex but they usually continue their action for 80 msec after other lead muscles are silent.

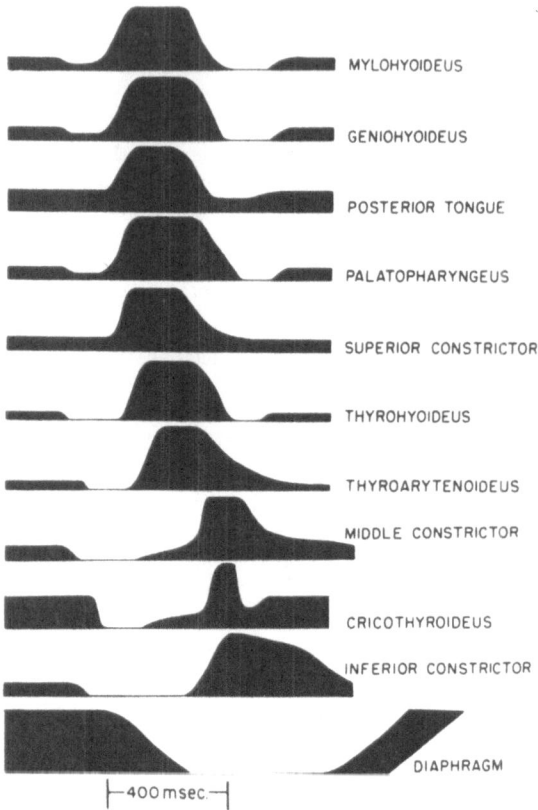

MYLOHYOIDEUS

GENIOHYOIDEUS

POSTERIOR TONGUE

PALATOPHARYNGEUS

SUPERIOR CONSTRICTOR

THYROHYOIDEUS

THYROARYTENOIDEUS

MIDDLE CONSTRICTOR

CRICOTHYROIDEUS

INFERIOR CONSTRICTOR

DIAPHRAGM

├─400 msec.─┤

Fig. 23. Schematic representation of the electromyographic activity in different muscles of the dog during swallowing. Height of line for each muscle indicates intensity of action observed, ranging from complete silence to maximum occurring after deglutition. [From Doty, R. W., Bosma, J. F.: J. Neurophysiol. **19**, 44 (1956)]

3.1.3.2. Constrictor Musculature

The constrictors of the pharynx fire in overlapping sequence. The muscles of the upper, middle and lower constrictor pharyngis form a continuous sheet of striated muscle. The middle constrictor is activated when about one third of the leading complex has elapsed. The inferior constrictor starts firing while the leading complex decreases. This E.M.G. activity is preceded and followed by a period of inhibition during which background or provoked activities are inhibited. The inferior constrictor is inhibited during almost the entire course of lead muscle activity.

Though the duration of each E.M.G. pattern is very dependent on the level of anesthesia or the prevailing level of medullary excitation, the temporal pattern of action among the different muscles is changed only slightly by these variations of overall duration. The total duration of the swallowing act can vary but the temporal organization of the different muscle groups remains quite constant.

3.1.3.3. Variations in Ancillary Activity

Several muscles of the face and neck contract during swallowing but their activity is of minor importance. Two types of activity can be observed in man. In the first type, considered normal beyond infancy, the teeth are together and the jaw muscles contract during swallowing, but the circumoral muscles do not participate. In the other, normal in infants but considered abnormal beyond this age, the teeth are apart, with the tongue often thrust against them; the circumoral muscles contract, but the activity in the masseter or temporalis muscles is minimal. The persistance of the last type of swallowing in adolescents is abnormal and is associated with malocclusion of the teeth (TULLEY, 1953; BARIL and MOYERS, 1960). It has not yet been established whether these variations in muscle activity during swallowing are due to a variable pattern of activity in higher nervous centers or to a variable organization of these centers in different individuals (DOTY, 1968). An individual variability can also be observed in decerebrated animals. Sometimes the geniohyoid muscle contracts together with the leading complex; more frequently the contraction is simultaneous with the activity of the middle pharyngeal constrictor. Exceptionally the pattern varies in the course of the experiment (DOTY et al., 1967).

3.1.4. Esophageal Transport

3.1.4.1. The Peristaltic Progression

The contraction of the upper pharyngeal constrictor coincides with the relaxation of the pharyngoesophageal sphincter, allowing the bolus to pass through the sphincter. Three forces propel the bolus: the buccopharyngeal pressure, squirting the bolus into the esophagus, gravity and the peristaltic wave. The latter follows immediately after the bolus and passes over the cricopharyngeal muscle into the esophagus. The speed of this peristaltic contraction is 3.44 ± 0.45 cm/sec in the upper part and 3.53 ± 0.44 cm/sec in the distal part of the esophageal body. In the most distal segment peristalsis slows down again. The speed of progression is markedly slower in a short segment 4–6 cm below the pharyngoesophageal sphincter, where it is only 1.87 ± 0.15 cm/sec. In older subjects this slower speed at 4–6 cm below the sphincter is less evident (2.56 ± 0.29 cm/sec) than in younger persons (Fig. 29) (HELLEMANS and VANTRAPPEN, 1971). In other species, different speeds of peristaltic progression are found: 35–40 cm/sec in the horse (MELTZER, 1899), 6.5 cm/sec in the dog (SCHLEGEL and CODE, 1958), 42 cm/sec in the cow (STEVENS and SELLERS, 1960) and 0.7 to 3.3 cm/sec in the monkey (WINSHIP et al., 1965).

It is difficult to measure the length of the contracting segment. Judging from the duration of the deglutitive pressure complex and the speed of the progression, it is estimated to be 4–6 cm in the upper part of the esophagus and 10–13 cm in the lower part (INGELFINGER, 1958).

Afferent impulses seem to influence the esophageal activity much more than the buccopharyngeal phase (see 3.3.2.2.).

3.1.4.2. Longitudinal and Circular Musculature

Studies in vivo have been done on the coordination of longitudinal and circular muscle coats. To study these movements DODDS et al. (1970) attached clips to the mucosa of the cat esophagus and X-rayed the animal during deglutition. Immediately following the onset of peristalsis all the clips went upwards. This confirms data of JOHNSON (1968) and CLARK et al. (1970). As the bolus

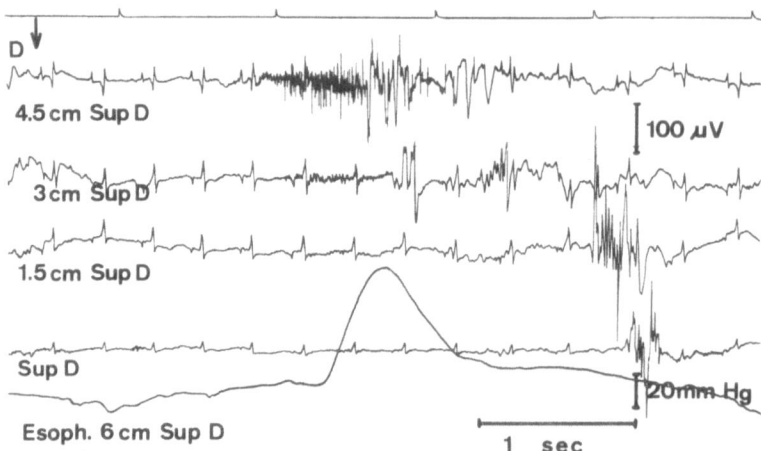

Fig. 24. E.M.G. simultaneously recorded at different levels of the esophagus in a monkey. *D* deglutition signal. At 4.5 cm above the diaphragm (Sup. D), the spike burst begins with striated muscle spikes. In the second half of the burst, smooth and striated muscle spikes are intermingled. At 3 cm sup. D, both types of spikes still occur. At 1.5 cm sup. D and at the diaphragmatic level, only smooth muscle spikes occur. The lower trace is a pressure recording

tail passed the marker sites, the opposing esophageal walls approximated one another and commenced aboral movements. Each marker reached its original initial resting position at the time the pressure peak of the peristaltic wave traversed the esophageal wall at the marker site. Afterwards the markers moved down about one cm. BERRIDGE et al. (1966) implanted radiopaque clips in the esophagus of humans. The passage of the stripping wave down the esophagus was attended by an oral movement of the markers, followed by a distal movement of the clips behind the swallowed semi-solid bolus. After swallowing the lower esophageal segment, the so-called "vestibulum", was first lengthened and then shortened. Electromyographic studies of the deglutitive response in the transition zone between the striated and the smooth musculature of monkeys suggest that the longitudinal muscle contracts first to be followed by a contraction of the circular muscle (HELLEMANS et al., 1968) (Fig. 24). Using force transducers sewn on the tubular esophagus of dogs, RINALDO et al. (1970) demonstrated that both the longitudinal and the circular muscles contract upon swallowing. In the gastroesophageal sphincter, on the other hand, both muscle coats relax and, judged from the published tracing, this relaxation is followed by a fairly long-lasting contraction. Different results were obtained by NAUTA (1956). He found that the movement of lead pellets implanted in the tubular esophagus and the gastroesophageal sphincter of dogs moved in similar patterns: as the bolus approached, the longitudinal coat was first lengthened and then shortened to 55% of its original length.

There is a general agreement that the longitudinal muscle coat contracts and, when the peristalsis has passed, relaxes again. It is less clear at which moment this contraction begins and how long the contracting segment of the longitudinal muscle coat is. Both BERRIDGE et al. (1966) and RINALDO et al. (1971) agree that the longitudinal coat of the sphincter zone relaxes prior to contraction.

In vitro studies of the distal 8 cm of the opossum esophagus indicate that the two muscle coats react differently to stimulation (LUND and CHRISTENSEN, 1969; CHRISTENSEN and LUND, 1969) (see 4.3.).

3.1.4.3. Striated and Smooth Muscles

In many animal species, such as dogs and sheep, the esophagus is composed entirely of striated muscle. In dogs only the inner muscle coat of the gastro-esophageal sphincter contains smooth muscle (BOTHA, 1962).

The distal part of the esophagus consists of smooth muscle in the human, the cat, the monkey (BOTHA, 1962) and the opossum (CHRISTENSEN and LUND, 1969; CHRISTENSEN, 1969). In the human the pharynx and the proximal 2–6 cm of the esophagus contain only striated muscle (TREACY et al., 1963). This striated muscle still shows a few primitive characteristics such as the muscle proprioceptors (see 3.3.1.2.), the arrangements of the motor endplates and the multiple innervation of individual muscle fibers (DOTY, 1968; FLOYD, 1971). The innervation ratio in humans is unknown. DUTTA and BASMAJIAN (1960) described it as low in the pharynx of the rabbit, both in the lower constrictor (4–6 muscle fibers per motoneuron) and in the upper and middle constrictor (2–4 muscle fibers per motoneuron). The primary peristaltic contraction of the striated muscle esophagus of dogs is fairly similar to that of humans, but its speed of progression is greater (6.5 cm/sec) and the duration of the contraction waves is shorter (1.5–1.8 sec) (SCHLEGEL and CODE, 1958).

The striated muscle of the canine esophagus reaches its maximal tetanic tension on electrical stimulation of the muscle at a rate of 35–40 per sec. With direct supramaximal stimulation of the muscle the time to reach the peak amplitude of the twitch contraction was 75 msec. Dog esophageal muscle is of the twitch type composed of a uniform population of muscle cells that are relatively slow mechanically (DIAMANT, 1971).

The electrical and mechanical properties of the smooth muscle of the esophagus are not very well known either. In vitro studies on smooth muscle strips of cat esophagus reveal no basic electrical rhythm in the resting state (CHRISTENSEN and DANIEL, 1966, 1968). Nor have spontaneous slow waves been found in isolated smooth muscle from the esophageal body of the opossum (CHRISTENSEN and LUND, 1969; CHRISTENSEN, 1970b). In vivo studies suggest that the smooth muscle of the esophagus is not spontaneously active. In the resting state no spike potentials and no slow waves are found (HELLEMANS, 1970), whereas spontaneous slow wave activity can easily be demonstrated in the longitudinal muscles of stomach and small intestine (DANIEL and CHAPMAN, 1963) and in circular muscles of the colon (CHRISTENSEN and HAUSER, 1961). In cats, however, spontaneous activity of the longitudinal smooth muscle was found after vagotomy (ROMAN et al., 1969; ROMAN and TIEFFENBACH, 1971). Occasional spontaneous contractions have been observed in longitudinal smooth muscle strips from the opossum esophagus (WEISBRODT and CHRISTENSEN, 1972).

No qualitative differences in pharmacological response of sphincteric and non-sphincteric circular muscles seem to exist, although more tension was developed by sphincteric than by non-sphincteric circular muscle at any given level of the drugs tested (acetylcholine, norepinephrine e.a.) (CHRISTENSEN and DONS, 1968; CHRISTENSEN, 1970a). From in vitro studies by LIPSHUTZ and COHEN (1971) it appears that the circular muscle of the lower esophageal sphincter is more sensitive to gastrin I than the circular muscle of the esophagus or the stomach.

3.1.5. Transport through the Gastroesophageal Sphincter

Deglutition results in a relaxation of the sphincter, followed by a contraction which is a continuation of the esophageal peristalsis. The relaxation begins a few seconds before the arrival of the peristaltic contraction, usually about 2 sec after the relaxation of the upper sphincter, though sometimes both sphincters relax simultaneously (CODE and SCHLEGEL, 1968). Radiocinematography reveals the sphincter to be open before the barium reaches the cardia under the influence of gravity. This fact greatly hampers the anatomo-radiological correlations.

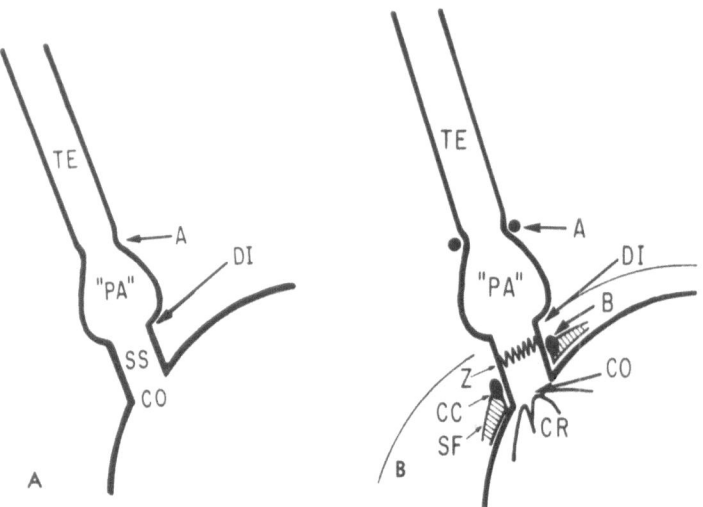

Fig. 25 A and B. Diagrammatic representation of the normal esophagogastric region. A Appearance of the lumen when filled with fluid barium. B Anatomic features added to the scheme. *TE* tubular esophagus; *PA* phrenic ampulla; *SS* submerged segment; *A* A-ring; *DI* diaphragmatic indentation; *B* B-ring; *CO* cardiac orifice; *Z* Z-line or squamocolumnar mucosal junction; *SF* sling fibers; *CC* constrictor cardiae; *CR* cardiac rosette. [From WOLF, B. S.: Amer. J. Roentgenol. **150**, 251 (1970)]

WOLF (WOLF et al., 1968; WOLF, 1970) proposed the following radiological points of reference (Fig. 25):

— *the A ring* corresponds to LERCHE's "inferior esophageal sphincter" and is a short functional contractile ring. It may become evident during the course of a pinchcock maneuver when barium refluxes back into the body of the esophagus; it may be seen fleetingly during filling; sometimes it persists as a shallow indentation at the end of the tubular esophagus.

— *The B ring* corresponds to TEMPLETON's circumferential web-like ring, and distends passively to a constant caliber. It cannot be seen when the sphincter is in its normal position but becomes visible as a static ring when the segment can be distended because of its supradiaphragmatic position. It is located approximately at the level of the squamocolumnar mucosal junction.

— *The cardiac orifice* is the entrance of the esophagus into the stomach. Under certain circumstances it may be incorporated into the body of the stomach.

The different segments in the region of the cardia have been defined by WOLF (1970); these definitions are shown in Table 2:

Table 2

Name	Technique	Proximal limit	Distal limit
High pressure zone Gastroesophageal sphincter	Manometry	A ring (approxim.)	Cardiac orifice
Vestibulum	Roentgen (hernia)	A ring	B ring event. Schatzki ring
Phrenic ampulla	Roentgen (normals)	A ring + "apical cap"	Diaphragmatic indentation
Submerged segment	Roentgen (normals)	Diaphragmatic indentation	Cardiac orifice

Though manometry indicates relaxations over the whole length of the high pressure zone, cineradiography does not show distension of the submerged segment after deglutition. The relative lack of distensibility of the submerged segment, however, is related to its location in and below the hiatus. When it is displaced above the hiatus it expands upon deglutition and a static indentation, the B ring, can be seen.

Both manometric and radiological studies indicate that the submerged segment relaxes but does not contract. Peristaltic contractile activity seems to occur down to but not beyond the level of the Schatzki ring (HEITMANN et al., 1966). Upon relaxation the supradiaphragmatic part of the sphincter expands more than the tubular esophagus. The oncoming peristaltic contraction distends this segment even more, particularly on deep inspiration, thus causing a phrenic ampulla. If the phrenic ampulla fails to empty due to continued deep inspiration, retrograde flow of barium into the tubular esophagus may occur through the relaxing A ring (MONGES and SALDUCCI, 1966).

Sphincter relaxations of considerable duration can be obtained by repeated swallows in rapid succession. The sphincter relaxes with the first and remains relaxed until the last swallow.

3.2. Intraluminal Pressure Variations

3.2.1. The Deglutition Complex in the Pharynx and in the Pharyngoesophageal Sphincter

The peristaltic contraction (p-wave) is preceded by a series of pressure changes which have been described and correlated with radiocinematographic images by SOKOL et al. (1966) and COHEN et al. (1968). In the pharynx the deglutition complex consists of a positive e-wave, a positive t-wave and a pressure plateau during the filling phase, which are followed by the peristaltic contraction (Fig. 26). In the high pressure zone, relaxation occurs just before or simultaneously with the e-wave; this relaxation lasts until the arrival of the peristaltic contraction. The duration of the sphincteric contraction is variable, but mostly quite long (Fig. 27).

3.2.1.1. Relaxation of the High Pressure Zone

Manometry shows that the relaxation of the pharyngoesophageal sphincter begins before the bolus leaves the mouth. This drop in pressure begins simultaneously over the whole length of the high pressure zone. The peak pressure in the upper pharynx occurs 0.3 sec after the drop in the pharyngoesophageal

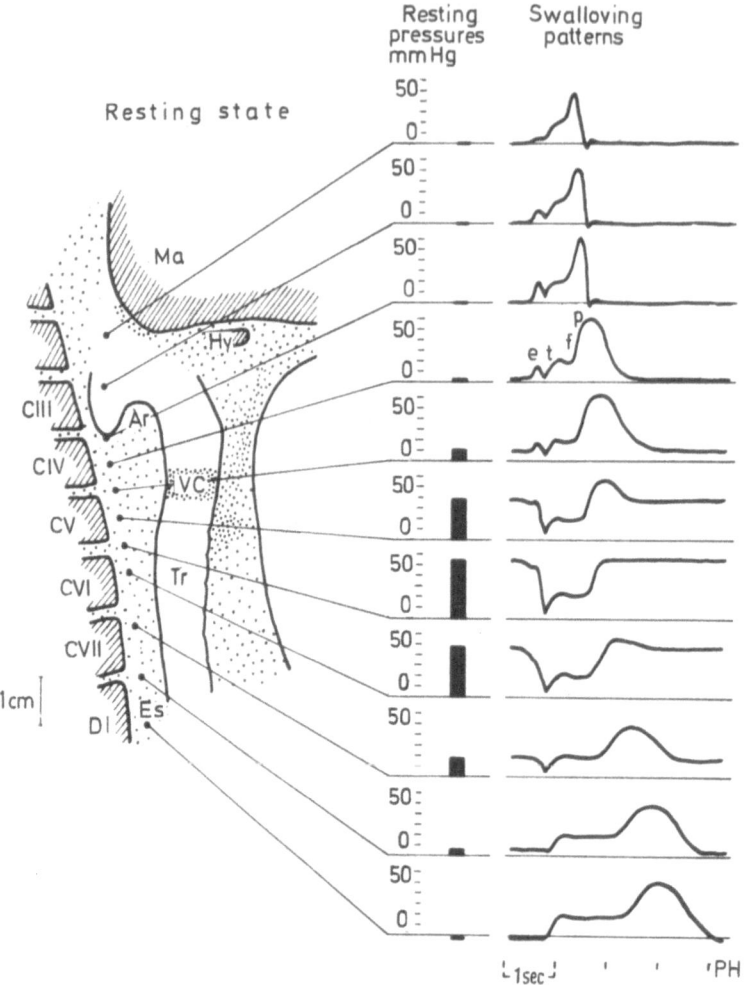

Fig. 26. Composite diagram of resting pressure and swallowing complexes obtained from oropharynx, hypopharynx and cervical esophagus. The vertebral bodies (C III through D I) are shown in relation to the pharyngeal air column, the arytenoids (*Ar*), the mandible (*Ma*) the hyoid bone (*Hy*), the vocal cords (*VC*), the trachea (*Tr*) and the proximal esophagus (*Es*). The resting pressures are indicated by vertical bars and are followed by swallowing pressure patterns. The c, t, and p waves and the flow period (f) are labeled on one of the curves. [From SOKOL, E. M. et al.: Gastroenterology 51, 960 (1966)]

sphincteric pressure (ATKINSON et al., 1957a). The relaxation of the sphincter lasts 0.5–1.2 seconds (INGELFINGER, 1958), i.e. until after the bolus has passed and the peristaltic contraction arrives (CODE and SCHLEGEL, 1968). The drop in pressure is most pronounced at the level of the cricopharyngeus where the resting pressure is highest. The pressure may fall below atmospheric level especially after dry swallows (SOKOL et al., 1966) though it never falls below the intraesophageal pressure (ATKINSON et al., 1957a). It remains unsettled whether this sphincter undergoes genuine relaxation or whether it is pulled open by the surrounding structures. Indeed the upward and forward lifting of the hyoid and larynx practically coincides with the onset of the sphincter opening.

3.2.1.2. The e-(Elevation) Wave

The e-(elevation) wave coincides with the elevation of the laryngopharynx or follows it by a short interval. Simultaneously, a barium bolus begins to enter the pharynx and the soft palate moves backward. This wave is most prominent in the distal oropharynx and the adjacent hypopharynx, it is minimal in the cricopharyngeal region and is no longer present in the cervical esophagus. If present, it begins shortly after or together with the onset of the relaxation of the sphincter. The e-wave occurs simultaneously in all places where it is visible. It is not greater than a few mm of Hg and quite short (0.2 sec). Perhaps there is an electromyographic equivalent for this e-wave. Occasionally a short increase of the spiking activity may be observed in sheep (CAR and ROMAN, 1970a) and in humans (HELLEMANS and VANTRAPPEN, 1971), just before the deglutitive inhibition of the pharyngoesophageal sphincter.

3.2.1.3. The t-(Tongue) Wave

When the back of the tongue moves forward barium begins to flow into the oropharynx. Just before that, the nasopharynx has been closed by the contraction of the weak palate and of the posterior wall of the pharynx (PASSE-VANT's ridge). At that moment a pressure peak can be registered in the velopharyngeal channel, which can be considered the onset of the perstaltic pressure wave. Backward movement of the posterior aspect of the tongue completes propulsion of the bolus into the pharynx. The backward movement of the tongue is a vigorous motion and is represented in pressure recordings by an abrupt positive "t" wave (tongue wave). In the upper pharynx this wave merges with the beginning peristaltic pressure wave. The t-wave is a simultaneously or a rapidly progressive wave. The time interval between the t-wave and the peristaltic contraction increases in the more distal segment. The t-wave is also visible distally from the high pressure zone, and in the esophagus it is called the first positive pressure wave. Dry swallows produce a rather small t-wave.

3.2.1.4. The p-(Peristaltic) Wave

The peristaltic wave originates in the upper part of the oropharynx at the same moment as the t-wave and almost immediately clears the swallowed barium from the proximal part of the oropharynx. As the p-wave proceeds through the pharynx at the rate of 5 to 10 cm/sec, the time interval between the simultaneous t-wave and the p-wave gradually increases. During this phase barium flows through the pharynx. This "flow" or f-phase corresponds to a manometric pressure plateau. Its duration depends on the size of the swallowed bolus and on the pharyngoesophageal level (ATKINSON et al., 1957a; COHEN and WOLF, 1968). In the horizontal position, the beginning of the p-wave coincides with the disappearance of barium from the segment. While the cricopharyngeal region is emptying the pharynx again descends to its resting position, and the oropharynx is again filled with air. The small negative pressure caused thereby is manometrically visible as a small dip, just after the p-wave in the oropharynx.

3.2.2. The Deglutition Complex in the Esophagus

Deglutition causes a series of intraesophageal pressure variations which together form the deglutition complex. This complex consists of an initial negative followed by three positive waves (BUTIN et al., 1953; CODE et al., 1958; VAN-TRAPPEN, 1961; VANTRAPPEN and HELLEMANS, 1967).

3.2.2.1. The Initial Negative Deflexion

The initial negative deflexion is a wave which begins 0.1 to 0.2 sec after deglutition, almost simultaneously with the pressure drop in the pharyngo-esophageal sphincter (Fig. 27). Its amplitude usually is 5 to 10 mm Hg but sometimes waves of 20 mm Hg have been observed. Its duration is 0.3 to 0.5 sec (VANTRAPPEN, 1961). It occurs with the same frequency in the upper, middle and lower third of the esophagus. Its incidence increases with age (HELLE-MANS, 1970).

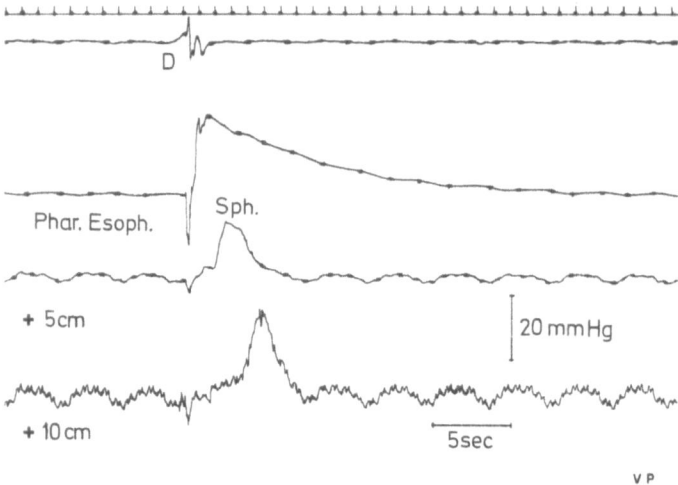

Fig. 27. Manometric recording of a deglutition complex in the pharyngoesophageal sphincter and in the proximal esophagus. *D* deglutition signal

Mostly this negative pressure wave is ascribed to the so-called "Schluck-atmung", a respiratory movement which was found in experimental animals to accompany deglutition. In humans the presence or absence of a pressure drop in the pleural cavity at deglutition correlates fairly well with the presence or absence of the initial negative deflexion (VANTRAPPEN, 1961).

3.2.2.2. The First Positive Wave

When a large bolus is swallowed the initial negative deflexion is followed by an increase in pressure which may continue into a plateau of positive pressure. This first positive wave has been ascribed to the transmission of the intrapharyngeal pressures into the esophagus through the open pharyngoesophageal sphincter, and to the sudden propulsion of a large non-compressible bolus into the lumen of the esophagus. So-called dry swallows only rarely cause this first positive pressure wave. The same wave has been described in the pharynx as the "t"-wave.

Usually this wave is found most clearly in the upper part of the esophagus. After the administration of high doses of anticholinergics it can become so large that it may be confused with the contraction wave proper (HELLEMANS, 1970). In the distal part of the esophagus it occurs somewhat later than in the proximal part (0.56 sec for a distance of 10 cm) and it is markedly weaker.

3.2.2.3. The Second Positive Wave

The second positive pressure wave originates simultaneously over the whole length of the esophagus at the time that the esophageal peristalsis runs through the upper third of the gullet. It is most marked in the lower part of the esophagus (Fig. 28) and is found in 25% of the deglutition complexes. Its incidence increases after the age of 50. This wave is probably caused by a compression of the lower esophageal compartment, between the gastroesophageal sphincter

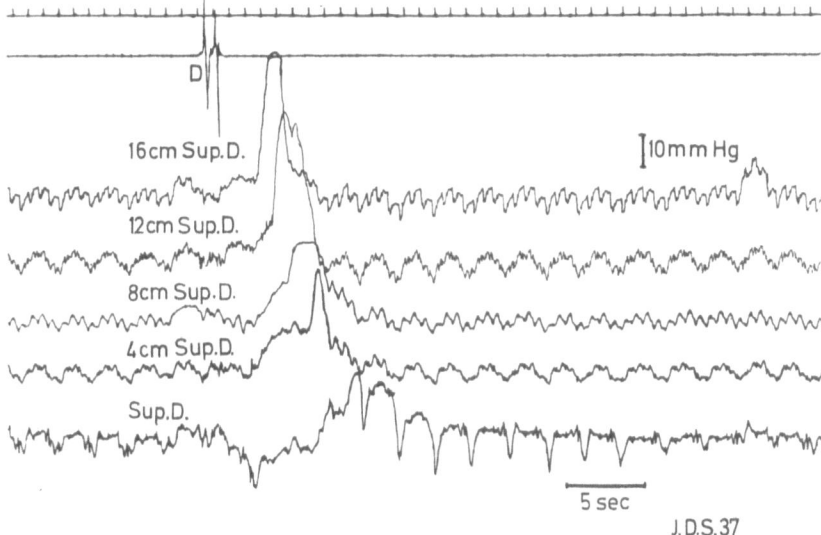

Fig. 28. Manometric recording of a deglutition complex in the gastroesophageal sphincter (Sup. D) and at different levels above the diaphragm (cm Sup. D). This is a normal peristaltic contraction, accompanied by sphincteric relaxation and contraction. At 12, 8 and 4 cm Sup. D, a "second positive wave" can be recognized. *D* deglutition signal

and the approaching peristaltic contraction. If the lumen of the gastroesophageal sphincter is obstructed artificially (e.g. by a gastric tube) the incidence of this wave is markedly increased (VANTRAPPEN and HELLEMANS, 1967). It also occurs more frequently with forceful than with weak peristaltic contractions.

3.2.2.4. The Peristaltic Contraction

The final positive wave is caused by the esophageal contraction itself. In man the speed of the peristaltic contraction depends on the level in the esophagus. In the pharyngoesophageal sphincter it is still rapid, but it slows down in the first few cm of the esophagus. The greatest slowing effect is observed in a zone 4 to 6 cm or, in other subjects, 6 to 8 cm below the pharyngoesophageal sphincter (Fig. 29). Simultaneous electromyographic and manometric studies show that the zone of slow progression of the pressure wave corresponds to the zone in which both striated and smooth muscle spikes are found on electromyography (HELLEMANS et al., 1971). In the distal part of the esophagus 4 to 5 cm above the diaphragm the speed of progression again slows down. The duration of the pressure wave is 2 to 4 sec in humans and 1 to 2 sec in dogs (CODE and SCHLEGEL, 1968). It increases towards the distal part of the esophagus.

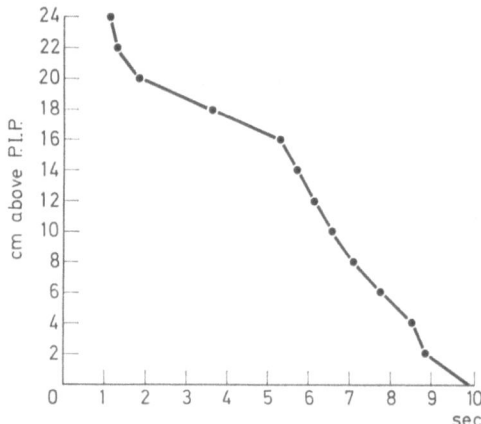

Fig. 29. Progression of the peristaltic contraction along the esophagus in a normal individual, in whom the slowing effect at 4–8 cm below the upper sphincter is rather marked. Each dot represents the mean of 25 deglutition complexes

The amplitude of the pressure wave depends, among other factors, on the nature (Roman, 1966) and on the temperature (Winship et al., 1970) of the swallowed bolus and on the time interval since the previous deglutition (see 4.4.1.). It also depends on the level of the esophagus; it reaches its lowest value at 6 cm below the pharyngoesophageal sphincter, increases more distally, but decreases again in the lowest segments, where the duration becomes much longer.

3.2.3. The Deglutition Complex in the Gastroesophageal Sphincter

The gastroesophageal sphincter, which is closed at rest, relaxes about 1.5 to 2.5 sec after deglutition and reaches its lowest pressure after 5 to 6 sec (Fyke et al., 1956). On manometric studies the relaxation is most frequently visible at 0.5 cm above the pressure inversion point. In the supradiaphragmatic part of the sphincter the relaxation manifests itself by a decrease of end-expiratory and often also of end-inspiratory pressure (Fig. 28). The relaxation lasts on the average 5.0 ± 0.9 sec and is followed by a sphincter contraction in peristaltic sequence with that of the esophagus. Measuring the pressures by means of a perfused catheter system in normal subjects, relaxations lasting 9 sec (Cohen, 1965) and about 8 sec (Kaye and Showalter, 1971) were found.

The sphincteric contraction is long lasting (9.8 ± 0.48 sec) (Vantrappen, 1961) (7 to 10 sec) (Code and Schlegel, 1968) and has a low amplitude (15.4 ± 1.46 mm Hg) (Vantrappen, 1961), (20 to 35 cm H_2O) (Code and Schlegel, 1968). In the part of the sphincter below the pressure inversion point deglutition causes only relaxation, which is followed by restoration of the resting tone, but no increase of pressure above it (Kelley et al., 1960). The onset of relaxation is simultaneous over the whole length of the sphincter (Vantrappen, 1961) or proceeds very rapidly (Kelley et al., 1960) but the contractions proceed in a caudal direction through the sphincter. EMG tracings in dogs and monkeys show spike potentials in the supradiaphragmatic part of the sphincter during the phase of the pressure increase caused by the contraction. During the slow decrease of the pressure no spikes can be detected. The mechanism of this latter part of the pressure wave is unknown. In the infradiaphragmatic part of the sphincter no deglutitive spikes are found (Hellemans and Vantrappen, 1967; Hellemans et al., 1968).

3.3. Innervation

3.3.1. Innervation of the Oropharyngeal Phase

3.3.1.1. The Deglutition Center in the Rhombencephalon (Fig. 30)

3.3.1.1.1. The Existence of a Deglutition Center

Once it has been initiated the act of deglutition and all its complex associated muscle activities follow a set pattern, regardless of the provoking stimulus. There is no feedback regulation (DOTY and BOSMA, 1956). Indeed, proprioceptive fibers or receptors are lacking in many of the muscles involved in deglutition. Even after curarization of the neuromuscular junction the nervous impulses of the deglutition act retain their normal sequence (SUMI, 1963, 1964; JEAN, 1972). Absence of muscle activities of the leading complex (see 3.1.3.1.), due to lesions of the hypoglossal nuclei or of the trigeminal motoneurons does not interfere with the deglutition (DOTY et al., 1967). Patients with poliomyelitis may lack the pharyngeal phase of the deglutition act, yet show a clear esophageal phase (SANCHEZ et al., 1953).

It thus seems unlikely that swallowing could be organized solely by sequential linkages between motor cells. On the contrary, most observations suggest the presence of a well-organized central nervous mechanism, i.e. the deglutition center, which determines the deglutition act in an almost always identical way. In addition the center must be able to exert a strong influence on other activities involving the musculature of the laryngopharynx such as respiration, vomiting, gagging, barking, whining, coughing, etc.

3.3.1.1.2. Localization of the Deglutition Center

Swallowing is abolished by destroying the brainstem rostral to the obex, which is situated at the distal end of the 4th ventricle. Serial surgical sections show that the swallowing center lies in the reticular substance rostrally from the obex at a level between the posterior pole of the facial nucleus and the rostral pole of the inferior olive of the medulla oblongata, 1 to 3 mm dorsal to these structures and about 1.5 mm off the midline (DOTY et al., 1967). The data presented by SUMI (1971) lend support to the assumption that apart from such a center there exists a rather dispersed reticular area which can exert a facilitating or an inhibiting influence upon chewing or swallowing evoked by cortical stimulation.

CAR and ROMAN (1970b) also found a somewhat wider dispersion and a somewhat differently located center in the medulla oblongata of sheep. The excitation of one end of the center can be propagated throughout the whole center without any afferent reinforcement (JEAN, 1972). The deglutition center consists of two half-centers. Stimuli of one superior laryngeal nerve reach both half-centers. Bilateral coordination of deglutition is brought about by connections between the two half-centers, rather than via projections from one center towards bilateral motor centers. Sometimes, under the artificial conditions of unilateral electrical stimulation of the superior laryngeal nerve, the activity of the contralateral middle and inferior constrictor laryngis and of the other participating ipsilateral muscles is more vigorous than that of the opposite side (DOTY et al., 1967). Normally, however, swallowing is a symmetrical phenomenon. Both half-centers inhibit each other; unilateral swallows are often more protracted than normal bilateral swallowing. The connecting fibers run partially at the level of the trapezoid body, partially posterior to the obex. Each center stimulates the ipsilateral deglutitive muscles except the middle and lower constrictor pharyngis

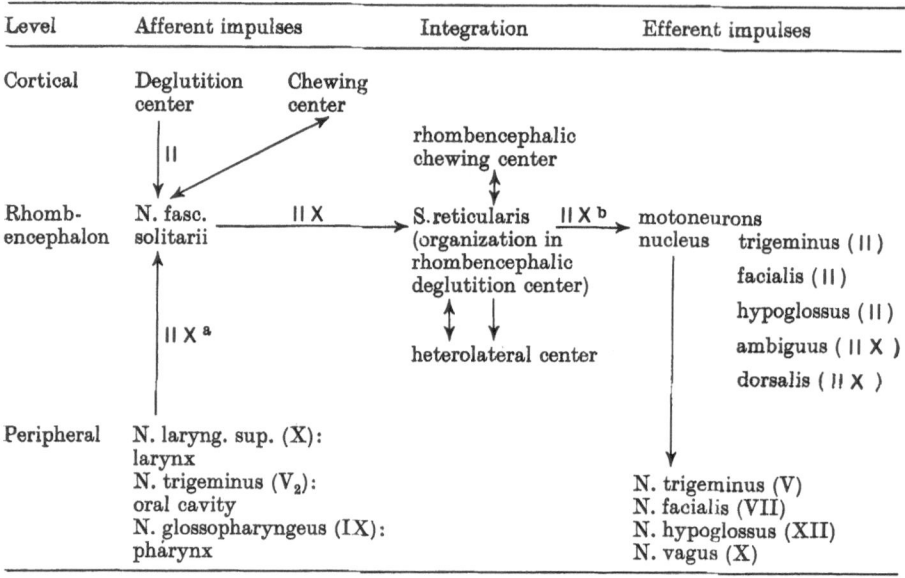

Level	Afferent impulses		Integration	Efferent impulses

→ Stimulation.

←→ Inhibition.

|| Homolateral connection.

X Heterolateral connection.

[a] Crossed in case of elementary reflexes.

[b] Crossed for inferior (and middle) constr. pharyngis in case of deglutition, not in case of respiration or inhibition.

in dogs and cats, and the lower constrictor in macaques, which are stimulated contralaterally. However, the fibers for the deglutitive inhibition of these constrictors and the connections from the rhombencephalon to these muscles for their participation in respiratory movements run ipsilaterally. Indeed, section on the midline posterior to the obex eliminates these constrictors for swallowing but leaves their participation in respiration, in elementary reflexes and in deglutitive inhibition intact (Doty et al., 1967). The motor nuclei regulating the deglutition are discussed below (see 3.3.1.7.).

3.3.1.2. The Peripheral Afferent System

Swallowing can be initiated voluntarily but is very difficult if there is no bolus to stimulate the pharynx or when the pharyngeal wall has been anesthetized. This points out the importance of tactile stimuli initiated by the contact of the bolus with the peripheral receptors. The base of the tongue, tonsils, anterior and posterior pillars of the fauces, soft palate, uvula and posterior pharyngeal wall are all sensitive areas which, when stimulated by tactile stimuli, will initiate the swallowing reflex. The receptor is thought to belong to the beaded type of free nerve endings, present throughout the epithelial surface of palate, pharynx, larynx and esophagus. The literature on this subject has recently been reviewed by Doty (1968). In the rabbit and the macaque the swallowing reflex seems to originate mainly in the palatal area, innervated by the maxillary branch of the trigeminal nerve; in the cat and the dog rather in the upper pharynx, innervated by the glossopharyngeal nerve (KAHN, 1903). The optimal sites for eliciting deglutition in man are the anterior pillars and, to a lesser degree, the posterior pillars and the posterior pharynx (POMMERENKE, 1928; BOSMA, 1957). The afferent stimuli which can elicit a deglutition movement run via the maxillary branch of the trigeminus, the glossopharyngeus and the superior laryngeal nerve. As can be expected from its innervation area (ANDREW, 1956b) the superior laryngeal nerve plays only a subordinate role in eliciting normal deglutition. However, electrical stimulation of this nerve is used frequently as a method to provoke deglutition movements in experimental animals (DOTY and BOSMA, 1956; ROMAN and CAR, 1970). Stimulation of the entire vagus can also provoke deglutition. These tactile and electrical stimuli will induce a deglutition movement even more easily if there is a facilitation at the level of the bulbus (ROMAN and CAR, 1970).

In addition to touch or chemical receptors in the mucosa of the tongue, larynx and pharynx, there are other types of endings that serve as proprioceptors in joints, tendons and muscles of this area. No true spindle afferent gamma system exists in the muscles of the tongue, larynx or palate of animals, although spiral nerve endings around ordinary muscle fibers can occasionally be discovered (BLOM, 1960; WILLIAMS and DIXON, 1963; SZENTAGOTHAI, 1948). In humans a number of true muscle spindles were found in the m. tensor veli palatini, but none in the mylohyoideus, levator veli palatini or posterior digastricus (WINCKLER, 1964). Their relevance to swallowing is questionable. The pattern of discharge must be centrally determined without feedback regulation by stimuli from the muscles themselves.

Gagging is thought to be elicited by stimulation of receptors in palate and pharynx that are also responsible for swallowing (DOTY, 1968). The length of the stimulation seems to be important; if a solid bolus is held up by means of a counterweight gagging occurs at swallowing (SCHREIBER, 1904). It is possible also that gagging is temporarily inhibited by the swallowing center. Anybody who has some experience of swallowing a tube knows that the difference between swallowing and gagging depends partially on voluntary factors and that swallowing may inhibit gagging for a very short time.

3.3.1.3. Elementary Reflexes Versus Swallowing

In the previous paragraphs it has been described how different stimuli can lead to a series of sequential events which are called swallowing. Less appropriate stimulations of the superior laryngeal nerve does not induce deglutition but provoke only isolated muscular contractions (elementary reflexes) (DOTY and BOSMA, 1956). They begin after a minimal latency period of 8 to 10 msec (ROMAN and CAR, 1970), which corresponds to a central delay of 4 to 7 msec (CAR and ROMAN, 1970b). This indicates a paucisynaptic reflex pathway. Elementary reflexes are seen most frequently in the geniohyoideus, palatopharyngeus, thyrohyoideus, cricohyoideus and thyrearytenoideus. It is also possible to elicit elementary reflexes in the esophagus (ROMAN and CAR, 1970). These reflexes are followed by a refractory period of 30–40 msec, which corresponds to a hyperpolarisation of the neuron after each action potential (PORTER, 1965). When the rate of stimulation exceeds 1 per second, facilitation develops progressively and ultimately leads to a deglutition reflex. After this deglutition reflex has occurred the elementary reflex is greatly reduced (ROMAN and CAR, 1970).

Electrical stimuli of the superior laryngeal nerve can elicit bilateral muscle contractions but the ipsilateral response is more pronounced (DOTY, 1968; ROMAN and CAR, 1970).

3.3.1.4. The Central Afferent System

The afferent impulses of the maxillary branch of the trigeminal nerve, the glossopharyngeal nerve and the vagal nerve seem to converge centrally into two systems (Fig. 30) (Ramon y Cajal, 1909). The first, the descending or spinal trigeminal system, receives fibers from the trigeminal, facial, glossopharyngeal and vagal nerves and conducts the pain sensations. The second system, consisting of the fasciculus solitarius and its nucleus, conduct the stimuli which induce deglutition (Doty, 1968; Car and Roman, 1970b). Fibers arrive in the solitary system via the descending trigeminal system, which receives stimuli from the mandibular and maxillary areas via the glossopharyngeal nerve and via the vagal nerve. Some of these fibers cross the midline and join the contralateral nucleus tracti solitarii. The neurons of the solitary system do not go directly to the motor neurons of the cranial nerves, but mainly toward the adjacent reticular formation (Car and Roman, 1970b).

Electrical stimulation of the fasciculus solitarius induces deglutition reflexes and causes antidromal potentials in the superior laryngeal nerve. Lesions of the rostral part of the fasciculus solitarius prevent deglutition reflexes elicited by stimulation of the ipsilateral superior laryngeal nerve, while leaving intact certain elementary reflexes from that superior laryngeal nerve, and preserving bilateral symmetry of swallowing in response to stimulation of the other superior laryngeal nerve (Doty et al., 1967).

In rats (Torvik, 1956), cats (Brodal et al., 1956), sheep (Car, 1969, 1970) and rabbits (Sumi, 1971) corticofugal fibers, predominantly from frontal areas, reach the solitary system in considerable numbers.

3.3.1.5. The Cortical Control of the Deglutition Center

Stimulation of the anterolateral area of the frontal cortex can produce swallowing movements alone or together with chewing. In rabbits a narrow cortical motor area for swallowing and a relatively wide area for chewing were found. Swallowing was shown to be more susceptible to depression by anesthetics than chewing (Sumi, 1969). In sheep Car and Roman (Car and Roman, 1968; Car, 1969, 1970) could provoke deglutition movements and sometimes esophageal peristalsis by means of stimulation of the cortex just in front of the gyrus orbitalis. In contrast to the impulses from the superior laryngeal nerve, the corticobulbar impulses follow a polysynaptic course via the capsula interna, the substantia nigra and the substantia reticularis of the mesencephalon and ultimately they reach the nucleus tracti solitarii and its surrounding substantia reticularis.

Cortical and laryngeal impulses thus converge on the same nerve elements of the bulbar centers. Impulses of both systems can therefore facilitate each other. Facilitation can also be obtained by previous tetanization of the contralateral cortex (Car, 1970). Splits on the midline in the lower midbrain or the upper pons do not abolish cortically evoked swallowing (Sumi, 1971).

Continuous stimulation of the cortical deglutition center results in a discontinuous discharge of the rhombencephalic center at a rate of about 1 per second. Initially these rhythmical deglutitions comprise only the buccopharyngeal phase, the esophageal peristalsis being inhibited. Later the rhythm of the deglutitions slows down gradually and peristaltic esophageal movements take place (Car and Roman, 1968). The same phenomenon occurs on prolonged faradization of the bulbus (Car and Roman, 1970b) and of the superior laryngeal nerve (Doty, 1968; Roman and Car, 1970).

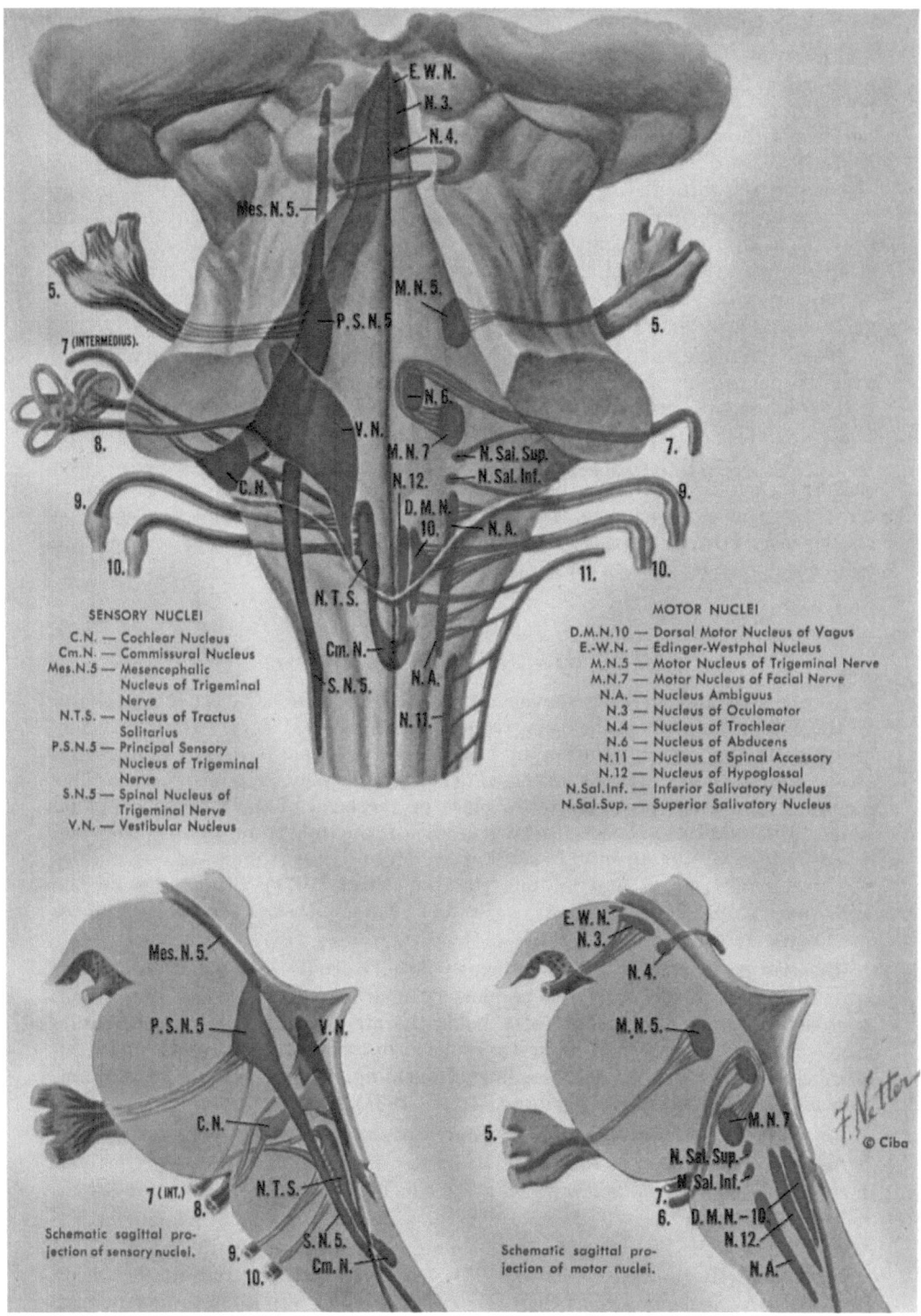

Fig. 30. Localization of the principal sensory (blue) and motor (red) nuclei in the rhomb-encephalon. (From NETTER, F. H.: Ciba collection of medical illustrations, vol. I, Nervous system, 4th printing, p. 47. New York 1958)

The cortical center is not necessary for normal deglutition. Decerebrated animals and anencephalic fetal monsters can swallow. The centers that are absolutely necessary for swallowing are located completely within the rhombencephalon. These centers receive stimuli from the cortex or from the peripheral deglutition organs. However, a voluntary (cortical) deglutition is difficult to perform without a bolus to provide afferent stimuli from the periphery to the deglutition center. Subjects whose oropharyngeal mucosa has been anesthetized also experience difficulty in swallowing. The peripheral afferent stimuli therefore seem to be more important than the cortical ones to activate the deglutition center. The rhythmical deglutitions elicited at a rate of 1 per second by continuous stimulation of the cortical center weaken very quickly if the peripheral afferent stimuli are eliminated by section of both superior laryngeal nerves or of the glossopharyngeal nerves (Car, 1970).

There is some evidence that under certain circumstances a voluntary control over the pharyngoesophageal sphincter can be established. For instance, patients with poliomyelitis can swallow air and keep the sphincter closed, so that the swallowed air is forced into the airways (glossopharyngeal respiration) (Dail et al., 1955). Esophageal speech in patients who have undergone laryngectomy presupposes such control over the sphincter. "Charging" of esophageal air is a critical step in esophageal speech and is accomplished by maneuvers other than swallowing. Lower pressures in the upper esophageal sphincter facilitate esophageal speech (Reichbach and Winans, 1970).

3.3.1.6. Interference with Other Centers

Swallowing and chewing movements seem to inhibit each other on several levels. Stimulation of the chewing center in the frontal cortex inhibits reflex deglutitions due to stimulation of the superior laryngeal nerve. Conversely, strong stimuli of the superior laryngeal nerve can stop chewing movements. This reciprocal inhibition probably takes place at the level of the rhombencephalon (Car, 1970). On stimulation certain areas of the midbrain induce chewing, others reduce it, but all inhibit swallowing. More distal stimulation can induce swallowing movements and inhibits chewing (Sumi, 1971). Stimulation of the upper pons stops chewing, results in closing of the mouth and eventually induces swallowing movements.

Swallowing inhibits respiration during 0.5 to 3.5 sec (Clark, 1920), by inhibiting the spiking activity of the respiratory neurons (Jean, 1972). The reason is obvious: during the passage of a bolus the airways must be closed. Adults mostly swallow during the expiratory phase of respiration (Clark, 1920). In infants there is a one to one coupling of suckling, swallowing and respiration, with swallowing setting the rhythm (Peiper, 1961).

Just before swallowing there is a short abrupt inspiratory movement, 20 to 30 msec after the onset of the mylohyoideus contraction. This can be registered in the neurons of the medulla, which spike synchronously with respiration (Sumi, 1963).

The heart rate also changes at the moment of deglutition by inhibition of tonic vagal activity (Okada et al., 1961). Another series of reflexes has been described, among them vasomotoric reflexes. The tonic activity in the splanchnic, hypogastric and renal nerve branches is increased by pouring water in the pharynx and is inhibited by swallowing (Okada et al., 1961).

3.3.1.7. Efferent Pathways. Motoneurons

The most important motor nuclei of the brainstem involved in deglutition are the nucleus of the trigeminal nerve, the facial nucleus, the hypoglossal nucleus and the nucleus ambiguus (Fig. 30). The trigeminal motor nucleus and the facial nucleus are less important for deglutition. The trigeminus is involved mainly in chewing. A small part of the facial nucleus participates in normal deglutition. The percentage of participating neurons in the hypoglossal nerve must be much higher. All neurons of the nucleus ambiguus presumably participate in swallowing, but not all parts of the nucleus are equally important (DOTY, 1968). Lesions in the rostral part (Fig. 31) mainly cause dysphagia (BAKER et al., 1950). Lesions in the caudal part mainly cause dysartria. The palatal, pharyngeal and striated esophageal muscles project into the compact, rostral part of the nucleus ambiguus; the laryngeal musculature into the scattered magnocellular elements of the caudal two thirds of this nucleus (LAWN, 1964, 1966; CAR and ROMAN, 1970b).

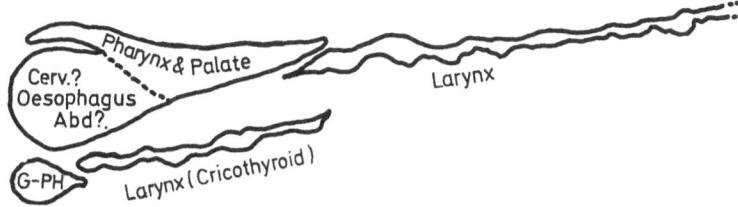

Fig. 31. Muscle representation in the nucleus ambiguus of the rabbit. The medial cell column [glossopharyngeal (G-PH) and cricothyroid] of the nucleus has been shown below the principal cell column to avoid confusion. *G-PH* glossopharyngeal neurons; *Cerv.* and *Abd.* cervical and abdominal portions of the esophagus with motoneurons to the cervical portion, probably occupying a dorsal position. [From LAWN, A. M.: J. comp. Neurol. **127**, 293 (1966)]

Vagal fibers reach the pharynx via the pharyngeal plexus. Contrary to what has been found in dogs the human cricopharyngeus does not seem to receive a special branch (LUND, 1965a).

The motor end fibers serving the cervical esophagus emerge from the vagus either above or below the nodose ganglion, depending on the species (HWANG et al., 1948). The cervical esophagus of dogs, cats and rabbits receives its vagal innervation from the pharyngoesophageal nerves; monkeys, guinea pigs and rats receive their vagal innervation from the external branch of the superior laryngeal nerve. In humans there is still uncertainty about this innervation.

Disturbance of the pharyngeal innervation may sometimes result in dysfunction of the cervical esophagus (HWANG and GROSSMAN, 1953; LUND, 1965a). In addition there is an overlap of the pharyngeal plexus with the zone innervated by the recurrent laryngeal nerve (ANDREW, 1956c). This overlap also exists in humans. In dogs electrical stimulation of the branch that innervates the cricopharyngeus results in contraction of the sphincter but not in relaxation (LUND, 1965a). This sphincter continues to function normally after unilateral section of this branch but the relaxations disappear when the sphincter is separated from the pharynx. According to LUND (1965a) these observations suggest that afferent impulses via the pharyngeal innervation are necessary for a normal reflex activity.

The nerve fibers reach the striated muscles without passing by the myenteric plexus. In the striated esophageal muscles the neuromuscular junction is formed by a neuro-muscular endplate, sensitive to curare but not to atropine.

3.3.2. Innervation of the Esophageal Phase

3.3.2.1. Central Nervous Centers

Two motor nuclei of the vagus control the motor activity of the esophagus below the upper sphincter. The ambiguus innervates the striated musculature. The motoneurons are located in the rostral part of the caudal nucleus. The nucleus dorsalis innervates the smooth esophageal muscles in species with a mixed esophageal musculature. Some authors, however, hold that the vagal motoneurons of the smooth muscles are not located in the dorsal nucleus but in the area between the nucleus ambiguus and the trigeminal spinal nucleus (KERR, 1967, 1969). Destruction of the nucleus ambiguus in dogs and of the nucleus ambiguus and nucleus dorsalis in cats causes a state of "achalasia" characterized by, among other things, loss of the peristaltic progression (HIGGS et al., 1965).

Yet the central nervous system does not seem to be absolutely required to initiate esophageal peristalsis in smooth muscles. Peristaltic contractions can sometimes be induced by mechanical or electrical stimulation of the isolated esophagus of the opossum (CHRISTENSEN and LUND, 1969). As the peristaltic contractions of this preparation are abolished by tetrodotoxin, it may be assumed that they are brought about by a local neural mechanism, probably the intramural nerve plexus (CHRISTENSEN, 1970b). In the distal esophagus of monkeys peristalsis can be induced by stimulation of the distal cut end of the vagus after bilateral vagotomy (VANTRAPPEN and HELLEMANS, 1970). In cats peristalsis in the lower esophageal segment reappears 8–9 months after vagotomy (BURGESS et al., 1972). It has been claimed that the central organization of the peristaltic mechanism is so strong that esophageal peristalsis, once initiated, cannot be interrupted by a second swallow. This is true for the thoracic esophagus of the dog, but in the human esophagus the progression of peristalsis can be interrupted at any level of the smooth muscles by a second deglutition (HELLEMANS, 1970).

3.3.2.2. Afferent Pathways

During the passage of peristalsis afferent vagal impulses from the striated (HWANG, 1954; ANDREW, 1956a) as well as from the smooth esophageal muscles (MEI, 1965a) can be registered. In his studies on the smooth esophageal musculature of cats, MEI (1965a) found slowly and rapidly adapting receptors whose afferent impulses could be registered at the level of the nodose ganglion. The conduction velocity of these impulses is 1 to 14 m/sec (mean 7 m/sec) (IGGO, 1957; MEI, 1965a, b).

Afferent impulses, emanating from the esophageal wall, clearly influence the progression of a peristaltic contraction in the esophagus proper (ROMAN, 1967). Esophageal peristalsis stops at the level of a forceful distention (see 4.2.). The nature (ROMAN, 1966) and the temperature (WINSHIP et al., 1970) of a bolus influence the speed of progression. The vagal output destined to the esophagus of sheep was recorded in the m. trapezius by ROMAN (1966) who connected the vagus to the nervus accessorius. He found that the pattern of discharge in various efferent esophageal units was strongly affected by afferent feedback. These vagal afferent impulses have a bilateral effect. The importance of these afferent impulses is confirmed by the experiments of BURGESS et al. (1969) and LONGHI and JORDAN (1971). Surgical separation of the mucosa and the muscle coats around the complete circumference of the esophagus interferes with normal peristalsis and gives rise to simultaneous repetitive contractions after swallowing. This

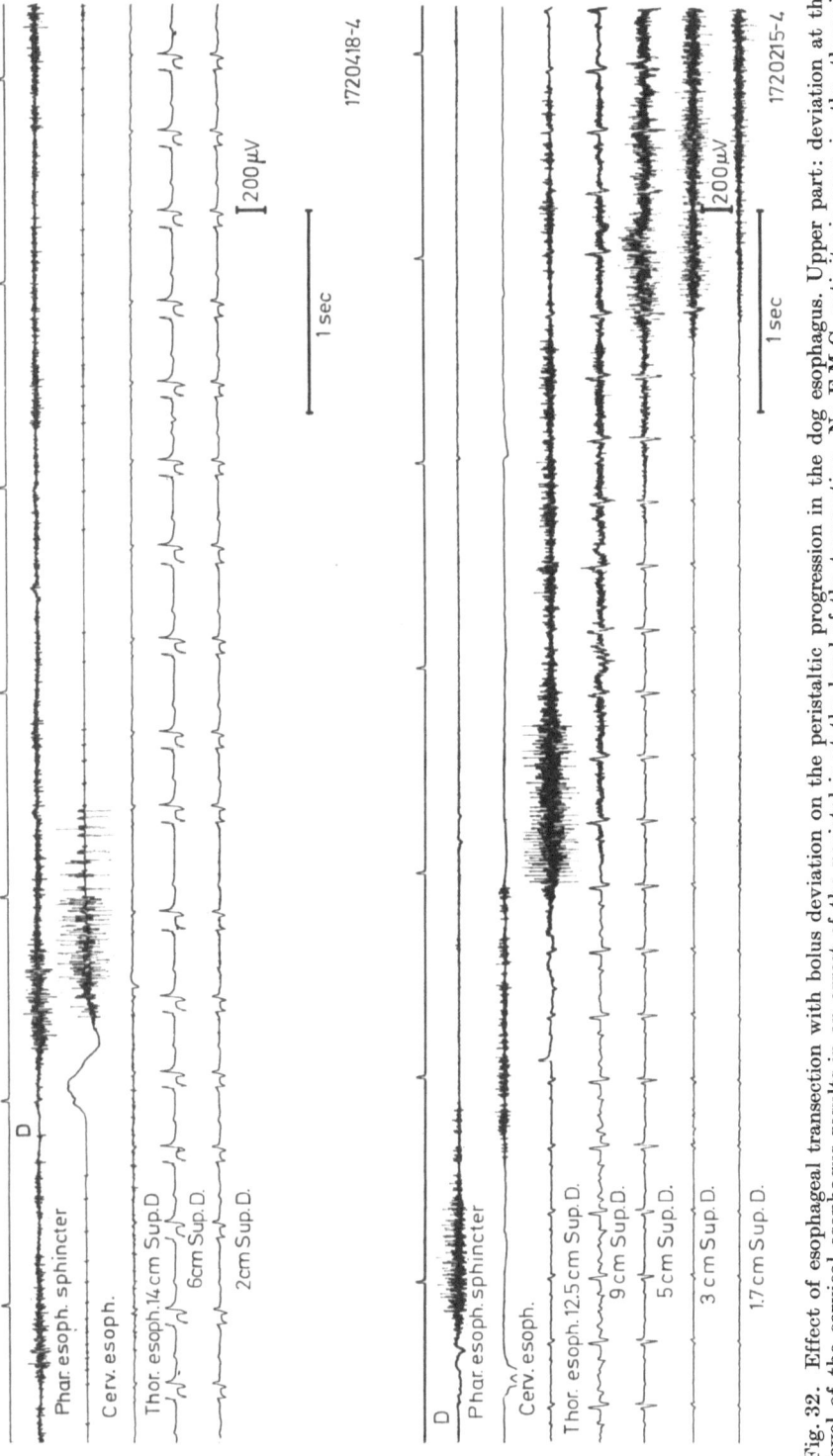

Fig. 32. Effect of esophageal transection with bolus deviation on the peristaltic progression in the dog esophagus. Upper part: deviation at the level of the cervical esophagus results in an arrest of the peristalsis at the level of the transection. No E.M.G. activity is seen in the thoracic esophagus. Lower part: after bolus deviation at a level between 9 and 5 cm above the diaphragm (Sup. D), the peristaltic contraction continues its course across the transection

effect lasts for no longer than 3 weeks. The sphincteric function of the gastro-esophageal region remains normal. The sphincter still relaxes in response to distention of the esophagus, which implies the intervention of receptors deeper in the wall (Burgess et al., 1969). Longhi and Jordan (1971) found that the dog esophagus can no longer contract in a peristaltic way if the bolus is deviated in the cervical esophagus. However, once the contraction has reached the thoracic esophagus it can progress in a normal peristaltic way even without an intra-luminal bolus (Fig. 32) (Janssens et al., 1972). At least two mechanisms seem to be involved in the production and progression of a normal peristaltic contraction in dogs: the central mechanism in the medulla oblongata and afferent impulses from the esophagus. The latter are a prerequisite for peristalsis in the cervical, but not in the thoracic esophagus. If present, however, these afferent impulses greatly improve the peristaltic performance of the thoracic part of the gullet.

3.3.2.3. Efferent Pathways

The role the sympathetic system plays in the esophageal transport is not clear but seems to be of minor importance (Greenwood et al., 1962; Burgess et al., 1972).

The main efferent impulses arrive via the vagal nerve. The cervical esoph-agus is innervated by pharyngeal branches, whereas the recurrent nerve inner-vates the lower part of the cervical esophagus and the upper part of the thoracic esophagus. The innervation of the more distal part of the esophagus is supplied by the vagal branches (Hwang, 1954; Roman and Car, 1967; Andrew, 1956a, b, c). In sheep the conduction velocity of the impulses to the cervical esophagus is 15 to 30 m/sec, to the thoracic esophagus 50 to 60 m/sec. This difference in conduction velocity is due to a difference in diameter of the nerve fibers (Car and Roman, 1965).

Electrical stimulation of the vagus causes the esophagus to contract, the gastroesophageal junction first to relax and subsequently to contract. Vagotomy in dogs abolishes peristalsis in the body of the esophagus and gives rise to the appearance of weak simultaneous contractions. In addition, vagotomy decreases the incidence of deglutitive relaxations of the gastroesophageal sphincter. These observations have repeatedly been confirmed in several animal species (see 2.3.5.4.) but they do not allow to distinguish clearly between the roles of afferent and efferent pathways.

The effects of vagotomy on the smooth esophageal musculature are not permanent (Jurica et al., 1926; Burgess et al., 1972). In cats, peristalsis is regained after 8 months in the lower part of the esophagus (Burgess et al., 1972); local reflexes can take over part of the peristaltic mechanism (Christensen, 1970b). After vagotomy peristaltic contractions can be observed upon inflation of a balloon in the esophagus and spontaneous activity occurs in the longitudinal muscle coat (Roman et al., 1969, 1971). Such peristaltic contractions, occurring without the intervention of the central nervous system, have been called "tertiary peristaltic contractions".

In the esophageal striated musculature of sheep, two distinct types of motor nerve endings are found: motor endplates and small multiple endings (Floyd, 1971). Muscle fibers innervated by small multiple endings occur more frequently near the cardia and have smaller diameters ($4–19\ \mu$) than fibers with motor endplates ($18–43\ \mu$). The vagal fibers to the smooth muscles do not run directly into the muscle coat, but form synapses in Auerbach's plexus.

3.3.2.4. The Intramural Nervous System

In the esophagus both nerve cells and nerve fibers are found.

3.3.2.4.1. The Motor Neurons

The motor neurons are located mainly in Auerbach's plexus. On the basis of their affinity for silver, the myenteric neurons can be divided into an argyrophil and an argyrophobe type (SMITH, 1970). Argyrophil cells have dendrites that end on argyrophobe cells in the same ganglion and two or three axons that lead to other ganglia. These axons do not leave the myenteric plexus. On the basis of these observations, SMITH (1970) suggested that the argyrophil cells stimulate the argyrophobe cells, which produce the acetylcholine stimulating the muscle fiber.

Little is known about the role of the various types of these neurons. The study of their action potentials has only recently been started (WOOD, 1970). For instance, the role of Auerbach's plexus in the striated esophageal musculature is still obscure.

Some adrenergic nerves terminate in an apparently synaptic relation with neurons in the intramural plexus, which are called secondary parasympathetic ganglion cells. This has been demonstrated in rabbits (NISHIMURA and TAKASU, 1969), in dogs (JACOBOWITZ and NEMIR, 1969), in cats and in monkeys (BAUMGARTEN and LANGE, 1969).

3.3.2.4.2. Local Nerve Fibers

Several varieties of motor nerve fibers have been found in the smooth muscles of the esophagus (1) Cholinergic excitatory fibers whose activity is eliminated by atropine. (2) Adrenergic fibers which can activate either α-receptors and thus cause contraction or β-receptors and thus cause relaxation (MISIEWICZ et al., 1969). (3) Non-cholinergic, non-adrenergic inhibitory fibers for which ATP or a related nucleotide has been proposed as transmitter (BURNSTOCK et al., 1970). (4) Non-cholinergic excitatory fibers which trigger contraction of the circular muscle coat at the end of a period of distention or electrical stimulation (the off-response) (CHRISTENSEN, 1969; LUND and CHRISTENSEN, 1969).

Striated esophageal muscles cannot contract in a peristaltic way without impulses from the central nervous system. Interruption of the local nerve system by transection and reanastomosis of the esophageal wall does not interrupt the peristaltic progression (Fig. 32).

Smooth esophageal muscles are capable of an occasional peristaltic contraction after they have been separated from the central nervous system (VANTRAPPEN and HELLEMANS, 1970; CHRISTENSEN, 1971; BURGESS et al., 1972). Local nerve impulses are necessary to produce this peristalsis, as is shown by the fact that tetrodotoxin eliminates them (CHRISTENSEN, 1971). Few studies have been done on the effects of transection and reanastomosis of the smooth muscle esophagus (VANTRAPPEN, 1970). In children who underwent anastomosis because of esophageal atresia, the motor activity in the distal part of the esophagus is disordered (SHEPARD et al., 1966). Several years after surgical repair of an atresia an aperistaltic segment is found above and below the suture, while normal peristalsis persists above and below this aperistaltic segment (BURGESS et al., 1968). It is difficult to determine whether lesions of the local innervation, of the muscles, or of the extrinsic innervation cause these disturbances.

4. Reflex Responses of the Esophagus

4.1. Secondary Peristalsis

According to MELTZER's definition (1899, 1907) primary peristalsis is initiated by swallowing and secondary peristalsis is the response to a local stimulus of the esophageal wall. Such a local stimulus can be provided by a bolus of food that remains stuck in the gullet. Because this bolus itself elicits secondary peristaltic contractions, it is pushed further down. Rapid inflation and deflation of a balloon also can evoke secondary peristalsis. Actually the secondary peristaltic contraction follows the deflation of the balloon (CREAMER and SCHLEGEL, 1957; FLESHLER et al., 1959). Distension of the esophageal wall by means of inflation results in an increase in pressure proximally of the balloon and a decrease in pressure in the gastroesophageal sphincter (CREAMER and SCHLEGEL, 1957) (see 4.2.). HWANG (1954) demonstrated that in dogs the degree of distension necessary to provoke secondary peristaltic contractions is higher in the cervical than in the thoracic esophagus. This difference did not show up in sheep (ROMAN, 1966). In humans the upper third of the esophagus seems to be the most sensitive area to elicit secondary peristalsis (CREAMER and SCHLEGEL, 1957). The threshold for secondary peristalsis is increased after unilateral vagotomy (ROMAN, 1966). JORDAN and LONGHI (1971) demonstrated in dogs with a transection of the cervical esophagus that swallowing reduces the threshold stimulus required for esophageal secondary peristalsis.

Secondary peristaltic contractions start proximally of the site of stimulation, and run distally at the same progression velocity as those after swallowing (SIEGEL and HENDRIX, 1961). The exact level at which peristaltic contractions start seems to depend on the location and the nature of the provoking stimulus, among other factors. Inflation of a balloon or rapid injection of water in the esophagus increases the upper esophageal sphincter pressure, especially if the inflation is done in the cervical esophagus (CREAMER and SCHLEGEL, 1957). Others (SIEGEL and HENDRIX, 1961) found that the pharyngoesophageal sphincter relaxed upon inflation and deflation of a balloon and that esophageal peristalsis occurred subsequently. If the secondary peristalsis is elicited fairly high in the canine esophagus, the pharyngoesophageal sphincter contracts but does not relax (JANSSENS et al., 1972). If it is provoked distally of a transection of the canine esophagus, a contraction also occurs in the segment immediately above the transection (VALEMBOIS et al., 1972).

MELTZER (1899, 1907) considered the propagating mechanism of secondary peristaltic contractions to be different from that of primary peristalsis. He thought that the latter was determined centrally and that, once initiated, it was independent of local reflexes. Secondary peristaltic contractions he considered mediated by local reflexes with continuous afferent stimuli, released from the esophageal wall as it is sequentially stimulated by a moving bolus. It is now generally accepted that the same mechanism ensures the coordinated progression of both primary and secondary peristaltic contractions. On the one hand, primary peristaltic contractions are not totally independent of afferent impulses from the esophageal wall (see 3.3.2.2.). On the other hand, the propulsion of a secondary peristaltic contraction is less dependent on afferent impulses than was originally thought. It may move past transections (SIEGEL and HENDRIX, 1961) or past a zone whose mucosa has been cocainized (HWANG, 1954). Secondary peristaltic contractions do not appear to be bolus-dependent in the thoracic esophagus, just as primary contractions. If a thoracic esophageal transection with bolus deviation is performed in dogs, a secondary peristaltic contraction elicited just proximally of the transection can continue its normal peristaltic course in the esophageal segment distal of the transection (VALEMBOIS et al., 1972). HWANG (1954) and FLESHLER et al. (1959) found that both the propagation velocity and the contraction force were identical in primary and secondary peristalsis. In an experiment necessitating a unilateral vagotomy, however, ROMAN (1966) found some differences.

4.2. Esophageal Propulsive Force (E.P.F.)

Transient distension of the esophagus for 5 sec or less with small volumes (5 ml or less) often evokes a secondary peristaltic wave in the esophagus. When this distension is due to an inflated fixed intraluminal balloon, the secondary peristalsis seems to begin upon deflation of the balloon rather than at the distension proper (FLESHLER et al., 1959). The latter causes a contraction above the point of stretch and an inhibition distally of the balloon (CREAMER and SCHLEGEL, 1957).

WINSHIP and ZBORALSKE (1967) have investigated the mechanical effects of a large fixed obstructing bolus in the human esophagus. Distension of the esophagus by a thick-walled balloon elicits an "esophageal propulsive force" exerted upon the obstructing bolus and oriented to propel it aborally into the stomach. The E.P.F. occurs promptly, and, once initiated, is sustained until deflation of the balloon. Its force varies from 4 to 200 g and is variable in the same individual. In the dog the maximal force of propulsion was measured with similar techniques in the middle third of the esophagus, and was found to be between 240–400 g (HWANG, 1954). The E.P.F. is inhibited upon deglutition, but arrival of the primary peristaltic wave at the bolus results in an increase of the force. No associated motor phenomena are recorded from the body of the esophagus proximal or distal to the balloon.

When the obstructing balloon is freed from its attachment the persistent stationary force is converted to a propagating one, which propels the balloon before it. If the balloon is arrested before entering the stomach, the moving contraction is also arrested. The velocity of the moving contraction wave is determined to a great extent by the resistance offered by the bolus.

The esophageal response to intraluminal distention is thus determined by the nature of the distending bolus. Transient distension by a mobile or collapsible bolus elicits a propagated secondary peristaltic wave. An obstructing bolus, on the other hand, evokes a persistent, often rather powerful muscular contraction, presumably localized at the proximal margin of the bolus and oriented to propel it. This reflex probably plays a physiological role when large lumps of food become stuck.

4.3. On- and Off-Response; Duration Response

The data on E.P.F. are in accordance with experiments performed on the smooth musculature of the opossum esophagus, both in vivo and in vitro.

CHRISTENSEN (1970b) studied the response to stretch and to electrical stimulation in the distal 12 cm of the isolated opossum esophagus by means of electromyographic recordings and observed three types of responses.

4.3.1. The "On" Response (Circular Muscle)

Rostral to the point of stretch by an inflated balloon a burst of action potentials is registered, with a delay of 0.29 to 0.36 sec. It usually occurs just above the point of stretch. This "on" response can also be elicited by direct electrical stimulation. If a 2 to 10 sec train of square waves (30 V, 1 msec, 10 to 20 cycles/ sec) is applied, strips of circular muscle contract briefly at the beginning of the stimulus.

The "on" response is not affected by drugs and should be considered as a direct response of the circular muscle to stimulation. Tetrodotoxin does not suppress it. However, this does not constitute absolute proof that nervous pathways are not involved (Carter, 1969). The "on" response seems to be related to the E.P.F. in humans, elicited by an obstructing balloon.

4.3.2. The "Off" Response (Circular Muscle)

After deflation of the balloon, a brief burst of action potentials occurs caudal to the point of stretch with a delay of 0.96 to 1.08 sec. The burst of action potentials usually begins well below the point of stretch and involves a long segment of distal esophagus. It is commonly propagated caudally, but sometimes it is simultaneous throughout the distal segment. The "off" response may also be recorded at the end of a train of electrical stimuli.

The "off" response is abolished by tetrodotoxin, but not by phenoxybenzamine, tolazoline, hexamethonium, atropine or methysergide. Hence the nervous

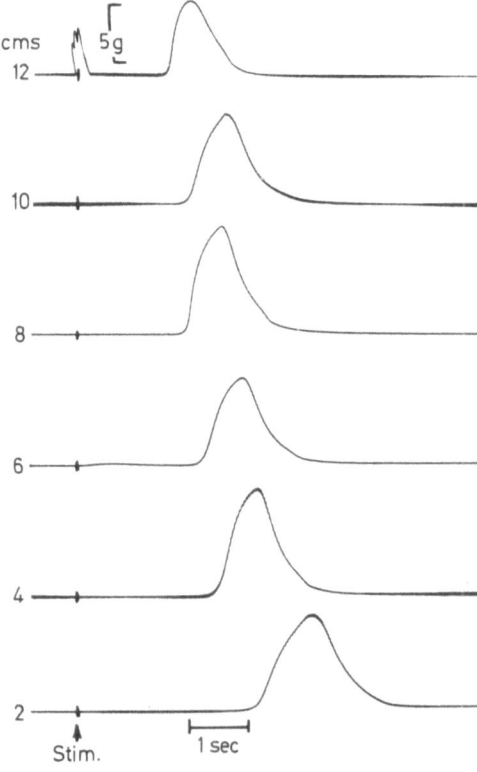

Fig. 33. Response of isolated strips of circular smooth muscle from different levels of the opossum esophagus. Arrow indicates time of electrical stimulation. Distance is in centimeters from gastroesophageal junction. The delay between the end of the transmural stimulation and the contraction (off-response) of the circular muscle strip gradually increases along the esophagus. [From Weisbrodt, N. W., Christensen, J.: Gastroenterology **62**, 1159 (1972)]

pathway must be a non-cholinergic excitatory nerve, as yet insufficiently known (CHRISTENSEN, 1970b), or the "off" response is an after-contraction elicited by excitation of nonadrenergic inhibitory nerves (WEISBRODT and CHRISTENSEN, 1972). This "off" response resembles a secondary peristaltic contraction quite well. Thus it seems that, at least in smooth muscle, the secondary peristaltic contraction does not require intervention from the central nervous system, though it may be influenced by it.

The time interval between the end of the electrical transmural stimulation of circular smooth muscle strips and the beginning of the "off"response progressively increases in progressively more distal segments of the esophagus (Fig. 33). This gradient may partially account for the segmental nature of the peristaltic contraction (WEISBRODT and CHRISTENSEN, 1972).

4.3.3. The Duration Response (Longitudinal Muscle)

The reflex responses of the esophagus involve not only the circular muscle layer, but the longitudinal and mucosal muscles can react as well. The latter contract throughout an electrical or mechanical stimulus. This response contains both atropine-sensitive and atropine-insensitive components, but it is nerve-mediated, as it is completely abolished by tetrodotoxin.

4.4. Inhibition

4.4.1. Deglutitive Inhibition

In humans a series of deglutitions taken in rapid succession elicits only one esophageal contraction, starting after the last deglutition. The gastroesophageal sphincter relaxes from the first deglutition onward and remains relaxed during the whole series. This observation indicates that every deglutition is accompanied by an inhibition of esophageal peristalsis. From manometric, electromyographic and radiocinematographic evidence the following picture of deglutitive inhibition in humans can be constructed (HELLEMANS, 1970).

If a second deglutition occurs when the peristaltic contraction elicited by the first deglutition is still in the striated part of the esophagus, this contraction stops immediately. The pressure peak drops, and the spike burst on the EMG is cut off. The progress of the barium bolus is halted. If the first contraction has already reached the smooth musculature of the esophagus at the time of the second deglutition, the spike burst is not immediately interrupted, though it is shortened. A pressure wave that had already begun can rise to a nearly normal amplitude and a barium bolus does not stop at once. The distal progression of the EMG and of the pressure waves, however, are inhibited, so that the peristaltic wave dies out.

The contraction which follows the second deglutition is often abnormal itself. The deglutition that follows another swallow at an interval of four to six seconds elicits a contraction which progresses in the upper part of the esophagus at a very high speed. It is as though the second contraction catches up with the first, after which both continue together (Fig. 34). This high speed of the second contraction was also noted by ROMAN (1966). Even if the interval between two deglutitions is as long as 10 to 12 sec, the pressure complex of the second contraction is often abnormal in its amplitude and its peristaltic progression (VANTRAPPEN, 1971).

In other species different types of deglutitive inhibitions can be observed. In the canine thoracic esophagus a second deglutition causes an immediate

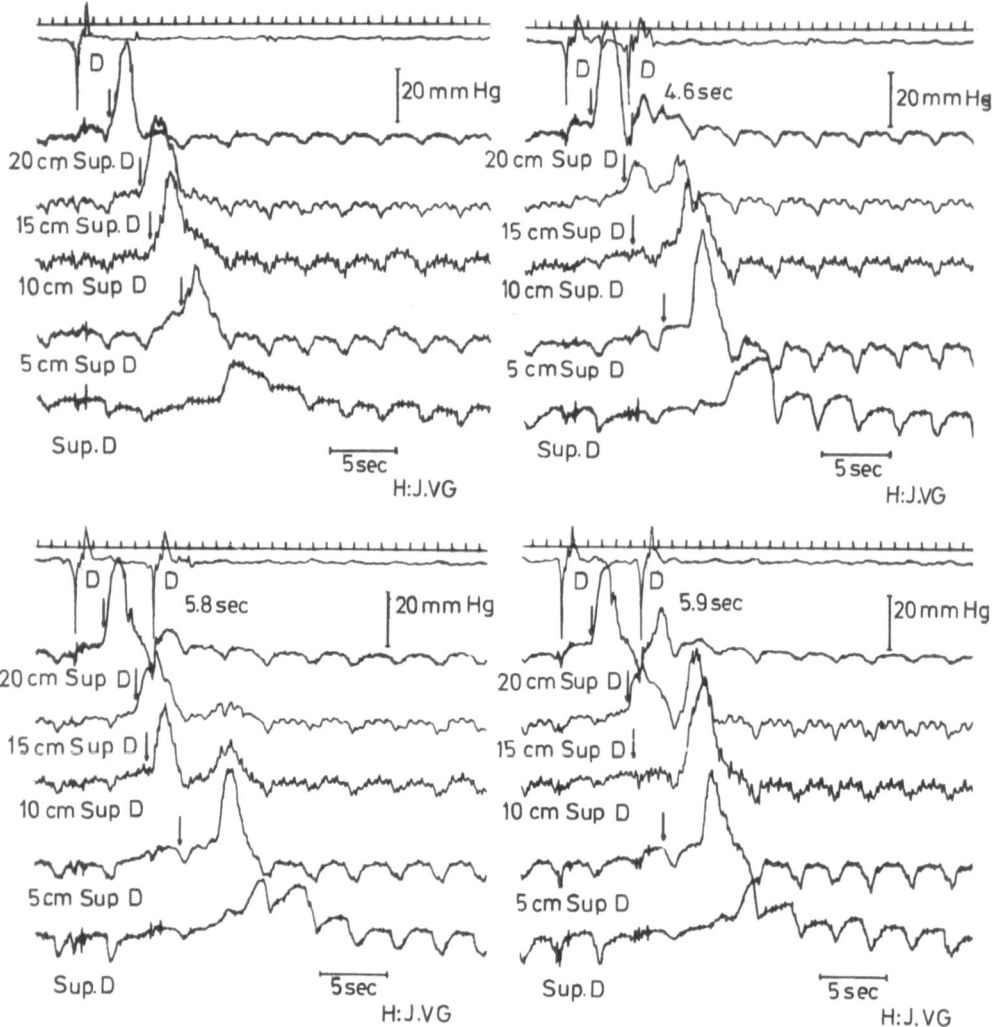

Fig. 34. Deglutitive inhibition in man. The first deglutition complex does not appear in the distal part of the esophagus if a second swallow takes place 4–6 sec after the first swallow. cm Sup. D: centimeters above the pressure inversion point. D deglutition signal

but brief (0.1 to 0.2 sec) interruption of the burst of muscle spikes, which then continues normally. High in the esophagus the spike burst is cut off, as it is in humans (HELLEMANS and VANTRAPPEN, 1967). In monkeys the deglutitive spike burst stops at the moment of a second deglutition even if the contraction had reached the smooth musculature (HELLEMANS et al., 1968). In the thoracic esophagus of sheep a spike burst is blocked if a contraction of the cervical esophagus is elicited by stimulation of the afferent vagal fibers (ROMAN and CAR, 1970). Secondary peristalsis (ROMAN, 1966) and a stationary contractile ring proximal of a distending balloon (WINSHIP and ZBORALSKE, 1967) are also inhibited by a deglutition.

The deglutitive inhibition originates in the swallowing center and is not caused by stimuli from the esophagus. In dogs it occurs almost immediately upon swallowing, is nearly simultaneous over the entire length of the esophagus, and persists even after esophageal transection (HELLEMANS and VANTRAPPEN, 1967). ROMAN (1967) demonstrated that in sheep also, secondary peristalsis is abruptly inhibited, even before the appearance of buccopharyngeal activity.

4.4.2. Inhibition by Distension

Experiments of HWANG (1954) demonstrate that balloon distension of the cervical portion of the esophagus inhibits the thoracic gullet. This inhibition lasts as long as the activity in the proximal part of the esophagus. During distension of the cervical esophagus, a contraction of the supradiaphragmatic segment of the esophagus, caused by electrical stimulation of the thoracic vagus, is suppressed or diminished (ROMAN and CAR, 1970). This can be considered as an instance of the more general law of BAYLISS and STARLING.

4.5. Relaxation of the Gastroesophageal Sphincter

Deglutition or distension of the esophagus cause the gastroesophageal sphincter to relax. The mechanism of this relaxation is poorly understood. It is certain that the relaxation of the sphincter can occur independently of a peristaltic contraction. Several deglutitions in quick succession cause the sphincter to relax, though a peristaltic contraction follows only upon the last deglutition (see 4.4.1.). If an inflated balloon is kept at a fixed location in the esophagus, the sphincter relaxes though no contractions can be recorded distally of the balloon (see 4.2.). After dissection of the mucosa in the thoracic esophagus, distension still causes relaxation of the sphincter,' but no longer peristaltic contractions (BURGESS et al., 1969). Simultaneous contractions can be accompanied by sphincter relaxations.

Electrical stimulation of the vagus causes the sphincter to relax and vagotomy or administration of anticholinergics clearly disturb the sphincter relaxation. However, after its dissociation from the central nervous system the sphincter still relaxes on distension of the esophagus and on the introduction of acid into the sphincter (TITCHEN and WHEELER, 1971). THOMAS and EARLAM (1972), using an isolated preparation of the guinea pig esophagus, found that the sphincter possesses an intrinsic tone and relaxes in response to distension of the lower part of the esophagus. The mechanism controlling relaxation was shown to be associated with the muscle coat. The role of the sympathetic innervation in the sphincter relaxation is probably minimal, though the muscle contains β-adrenergic receptors which cause relaxation when they are stimulated. The α-adrenergic receptors, however, cause contraction (CHRISTENSEN and DANIEL, 1968).

Electrical stimulation of the non-adrenergic inhibitory nerves produces an inhibition of the acetylcholine stimulated circular muscle of the L.E.S. of the opossum. This inhibition is maximal at the level of the L.E.S., less pronounced 2 cm above and zero 4 cm above the L.E.S. (TUCH and COHEN, 1973).

4.6. Other Reflexes

Swallowing (CANNON and LIEB, 1911, 1912) or distension of different parts of the esophagus (VEACH, 1926; LIND et al., 1961) cause prompt and pronounced relaxation of the stomach, particularly of the gastric fundus. The gastric relaxation is mediated by a vago-vagal reflex, which disappears after cervical vagotomy.

This reflex is not blocked by atropine or guanethidine (ABRAHAMSSON and JANSSON, 1969). Hence the neurotransmitter of these vagal relaxatory fibers must be a non-adrenergic inhibitory substance, which has not yet been identified with certainty (serotonin ?).

5. Retrograde Transport

5.1. Rumination-Eructation

Rumination is a complex act, typical of cud-chewers which transport food from the stomach back to the mouth, where it is chewed again and subsequently swallowed once more. The sequence of events during rumination has been studied manometrically (STEVENS and SELLERS, 1960) and electromyographically (ROUS-SEAU, 1970). The cycle begins with a contraction of the reticulum followed by a forceful inspiration against a closed nasopharynx, which causes an intrapleural and intraesophageal pressure drop; this on its turn causes an increased gastro-esophageal pressure gradient and expels the contents of the stomach into the esophagus. Following this, a strong positive pressure wave proceeds orally along the esophagus. The progression velocity of this antiperistaltic rumination pressure wave is twice that of an aboral peristaltic contraction.

The motility tracing of the eructation of ruminants shows 2 pressure peaks (STEVENS and SELLERS, 1960). The first component can be accounted for on the basis of filling with gas from the rumen sac; in this phase the pharyngoesophageal sphincter relaxes. The second component is an antiperistaltic "clearing contraction", traveling orally at a very high speed. Such types of orally oriented transport are not found in man.

5.2. Retching and Vomiting

During vomiting the role of the esophagus is rather passive (SMITH and BRIZZEE, 1961; LUMSDEN and HOLDEN, 1969). On the basis of radiocinematographic studies in cats, SMITH and BRIZZEE (1961) describe four phases in each retching movement: esophageal dilatation, expulsion of gastric contents, return into the stomach and esophageal collapse. Apparently external pressures provide the forces for expelling vomitus from the stomach.

The initial action is a contraction of the thoracic cage, while the glottis remains closed, and the diaphragm moves downward. The esophagus rapidly dilates, so that the line of demarcation between esophagus and stomach is obscured (Phase I). After 0.07 to 0.53 sec, the abdominal wall forcefully contracts and the thoracic walls move outward. The barium is propelled through the gastro-esophageal junction as a rapidly moving jet (Phase II). Before it opens, the cardia is raised so that the abdominal esophagus is non-existing at that moment, and the high abdominal pressure no longer prevents the gastroesophageal transport (TORRANCE, 1958; JOHNSON and LAWS, 1966; LUMSDEN and HOLDEN, 1969). The opening of the cardia can be at least partially explained as a reflex elicited by the high intragastric pressure (TITCHEN and WHEELER, 1971). The role of the gastric antrum in this phase does not seem to be entirely passive (LUMSDEN and HOLDEN, 1969). Indeed, the contents of the stomach accumulate in the gastric fundus while the antrum contracts. When the abdominal contraction ceases, the oral movement of the vomitus stops, and the esophageal contents return to the stomach (Phase III), after which the esophagus again assumes its normal shape (Phase IV). The whole cycle is repeated for the following retching movement.

5.3. Belching

If the human stomach is distended with air, either simple gastroesophageal reflux or reflux with belching can occur. This reflux usually occurs during inspiration.

During simple reflux, the gastroesophageal barrier opens and a common gastroesophageal cavity is established after 2 sec to 2 min (usually 6–10 sec). The esophagus is emptied of air by a secondary peristalsis. On manometry the gastroesophageal sphincter is seen to relax, the intraesophageal pressure rises and the respiratory pressure changes in the esophagus assume an intraabdominal pattern. No sensation is experienced during this reflux of air. Gaseous reflux with belching differs from simple reflux in that air is expelled from the common gastroesophageal cavity into the mouth. This action requires contraction of somatic muscles (McNALLY et al., 1964). Some people swallow air or can easily force it into the esophagus. Belching of this air can be accomplished at will by an increase in intrathoracic pressure and a relaxation of the pharyngoesophageal sphincter (CODE and SCHLEGEL, 1968).

References

ABRAHAMSSON, H., JANSSON, G.: Elicitation of reflex vagal relaxation of the stomach from pharynx and esophagus in the cat. Acta physiol. scand. **77**, 172–178 (1969).

ALLISON, P. R.: Reflux esophagitis, sliding hiatal hernia, and the anatomy of repair. Surg. Gynec. Obstet. **92**, 419–431 (1951).

ANDERSON, H. N., MAY, K. J., STEINMETZ, G. P., OFSTUN, M., HARRISON, H. G., LEYSE, R. M. DILLARD, D. H.: The lower esophageal intrinsic sphincter and the mechanism of reflux: experimental observations supporting a new concept. Ann. Surg. **166**, 102–108 (1967).

ANDREW, B. L.: The extrinsic neural control of the oesophagus during swallowing. J. Physiol. (Lond.) **132**, 13 P (1956a).

ANDREW, B. L.: A functional analysis of the myelinated fibres of the superior laryngeal nerve of the rat. J. Physiol. (Lond.) **133**, 420–432 (1956b).

ANDREW, B. L.: The nervous control of the cervical oesophagus of the rat during swallowing. J. Physiol. (Lond.) **134**, 729–740 (1956c).

ARIMORI, M., CODE, C. F., SCHLEGEL, J. F., STURM, R. E.: Electrical activity of the canine esophagus and gastroesophageal sphincter: its relation to intraluminal pressure and movement of material. Amer. J. dig. Dis. **15**, 191–208 (1970).

ATKINSON, M., EDWARDS, D. A. W., HONOUR, A. J., ROWLANDS, E. N.: The oesophagogastric sphincter in hiatus hernia. Lancet **1957 II**, 1138–1142.

ATKINSON, M., KRAMER, P., WYMAN, S. M., INGELFINGER, F. J.: The dynamics of swallowing. I. Normal pharyngeal mechanisms. J. clin. Invest. **36**, 581–588 (1957a).

BAKER, A. B., MATZKE, H. A., BROWN, J. R.: Poliomyelitis. III. Bulbar poliomyelitis; a study of medullary function. Arch. Neurol. Psychiat. (Chic.) **63**, 257–281 (1950).

BANCHERO, N., SCHWARTZ, P. E., WOOD, E. H.: Intraesophageal pressure gradient in man. J. appl. Physiol. **22**, 1066–1074 (1967).

BARIL, C., MOYERS, R. E.: An electromyographic analysis of the temporalis muscles and certain facial muscles in thumb- and finger-suckling patients. J. dent. Res. **39**, 536–553 (1960).

BARRETT, N. R.: Hiatus hernia: a review of some controversial points. Brit. J. Surg. **42**, 231–243 (1954).

BAUMGARTEN, H. G., LANGE, W.: Adrenergic innervation of the oesophagus in the cat (Felix domestica) and rhesus monkey (Macacus rhesus). Z. Zellforsch. **95**, 529–545 (1969).

BENNETT, A.: Effect of gastrin on isolated smooth muscle preparations. Nature (Lond.) **208**, 170–173 (1965).

BENNETT, A., MISIEWICZ, J. J., WALLER, S. L.: Analysis of the motor effects of gastrin and pentagastrin on the human alimentary tract in vitro. Gut 8, 470–474 (1967).

BENNETT, J. R.: Smoking and the gastrointestinal tract. Gut **13**, 658–665 (1972).

BENNETT, J. R.: Section 5 in: Symposium on gastroesophageal reflux and its complications. Gut **14**, 246–249 (1973).

Benz, L. J., Hootkin, L. A., Margulies, S., Donner, M. W., Cauthorne, R. T., Hendricks, T. R.: A comparison of clinical measurements of gastro-esophageal reflux. Gastroenterology **62**, 1–5 (1972).

Berridge, F. R., Friedland, G. W., Tagart, R. E. B.: Radiological landmarks at the oesophago-gastric junction. Thorax **21**, 499–510 (1966).

Binder, H. J., Bloom, D. L., Stern, H., Solitare, G. B., Thayer, W. R., Spiro, H. M.: The effect of cervical vagectomy on esophageal function in the monkey. Surgery **64**, 1075–1083 (1968).

Birmingham, A.: A study of the arrangement of the muscular fibres at the upper end of the esophagus. J. Anat. Physiol. **33**, 10–21 (1899).

Birmingham, J. A. W.: Oesophageal stricture after gastric surgery and nasogastric intubation. Brit. med. J. **1958** II, 817–819.

Blackman, A. H., Rakatansky, H., Nasrulla, H. M., Thayer, W. R.: Transabdominal vagectomy and lower esophageal function. Arch. Surg. **102**, 6–8 (1971).

Blom, S.: Afferent influences on tongue muscle activity. A morphological and physiological study in the cat. Acta physiol. scand. **49**, Suppl. 170, 97 P (1960).

Bombeck, C. T., Aoki, T., Nyhus, L. M.: Anatomic etiology and operative treatment of peptic esophagitis: an experimental study. Ann. Surg. **165**, 752–764 (1967).

Bombeck, C. T., Dillard, D. H., Nyhus, L. M.: Muscular anatomy of the gastroesophageal junction and role of phrenoesophageal ligament. Autopsy study of sphincter mechanism. Ann. Surg. **164**, 643–654 (1966).

Booth, D. J., Kemmerer, W. K., Skinner, D. B.: Acid clearing from the distal esophagus. Arch. Surg. **96**, 731–734 (1968).

Bosma, J. F.: Deglutition: pharyngeal stage. Physiol. Rev. **37**, 275–300 (1957).

Botha, G. S. M.: Mucosal folds at the cardia as a component of the gastro-oesophageal closing mechanism. Brit. J. Surg. **45**, 569–580 (1958).

Botha, G. S. M.: Gastro-oesophageal junction: clinical applications to oesophageal and gastric surgery. Boston: Little, Brown & Co. 1962.

Boyd, D. P.: Transabdominal repair of hiatal hernia. Surg. Clin. N. Amer. **51**, 597–606 (1971).

Braasch, J. W., Ellis, F. H., Jr.: The gastroesophageal sphincter mechanism, an experimental study. Surgery **39**, 901–905 (1956).

Brodal, A., Szabo, T., Torvik, A.: Corticofugal fibers to sensory trigeminal nuclei and nucleus of the solitary tract: an experimental study in the cat. J. comp. Neurol. **106**, 527–555 (1956).

Burgess, J. N., Carlson, H. C., Ellis, F. H.: Esophageal function after successful repair of esophageal atresia and tracheoesophageal fistula. J. thorac. cardiovasc. Surg. **56**, 667–673 (1968).

Burgess, J. N., Kelly, K. A., Schlegel, J. F., Ellis, F. H.: Effect of esophageal mucosal denervation on the motility of the canine esophagus. J. surg. Res. **9**, 605–610 (1969).

Burgess, J. N., Schlegel, J. F., Ellis, F. H.: The effect of denervation on feline esophageal function and morphology. J. surg. Res. **12**, 24–33 (1972).

Burnstock, G., Campbell, G., Satchell, D.: Evidence that adenosine triphosphate or a related nucleotide is the transmitter substance released by non-adrenergic inhibitory nerves of the gut. Brit. J. Pharmacol. **40**, 668–688 (1970).

Butin, J. W., Olsen, A. M., Moersch, H. J., Code, C. F.: A study of esophageal pressures in normal persons and patients with cardiospasm. Gastroenterology **23**, 278–291 (1953).

Butterfield, D. G., Struthers, J. E., Showalter, J. P.: A test of gastroesophageal sphincter competence: the common cavity test. Gastroenterology (Abstract) **58**, 932 (1970).

Butterfield, D. G., Struthers, J. E., Showalter, J. P.: A test of gastroesophageal sphincter competence. The common cavity test. Amer. J. dig. Dis. **17**, 415–421 (1972).

Cannon, W. B., Lieb, C. W.: The receptive relaxation of the stomach. Amer. J. Physiol. **29**, 267–273 (1911–1912).

Car, A.: La commande corticale du centre déglutiteur bulbaire; sa voie d'expression. J. Physiol. (Paris) **61**, Suppl. 2, 239 (1969).

Car, A.: La commande corticale du centre déglutiteur bulbaire. J. Physiol. (Paris) **62**, 361–386 (1970).

Car, A., Roman, C.: Etude des vitesses de conduction des fibres nerveuses motrices de l'œsophage. C. R. Soc. Biol. (Paris) **159**, 1767–1770 (1965).

Car, A., Roman, C.: Déglutitions produites par la stimulation du cortex frontal chez le mouton. C. R. Soc. Biol. (Paris) **162**, 740–743 (1968).

Car, A., Roman, C.: L'activité spontanée du sphincter œsophagien chez le mouton. Ses variations au cours de la déglutition et de la rumination. J. Physiol. (Paris) **62**, 505–511 (1970a).

Car, A., Roman, C.: Déglutitions et contractions œsophagiennes réflexes produites par la stimulation du bulbe rachidien. Exp. Brain Res. **11**, 75–92 (1970b).

CARTER, R. H.: Resistance to tetrodotoxin in toad sympathetic nerves. J. Pharm. Pharmacol. 21, 394–395 (1969).

CARVETH, S. W., SCHLEGEL, J. F., CODE, C. F., ELLIS, F. H.: Esophageal motility after vagotomy, phrenicotomy, myotomy and myomectomy in dogs. Surg. Gynec. Obstet. 114, 31–42 (1962).

CASTELL, D. O.: Changes in lower esophageal sphincter pressure during insulin-induced hypoglycemia. Gastroenterology 61, 10–15 (1971).

CASTELL, D. O., HARRIS, L. D.: The link between control of gastric acid secretion and control of lower esophageal sphincter strength. Gastroenterology (Abstract) 56, 1249 (1969).

CASTELL, D. O., HARRIS, L. D.: Hormonal control of gastroesophageal sphincter strength. New Engl. J. Med. 282, 886–889 (1970).

CASTELL, D. O., LEVINE, S. M.: Lower esophageal sphincter response to gastric alkalinization. Ann. intern. Med. 74, 223–227 (1971).

CASTELL, D. O., NEBEL, O. T.: Physiologic controls of lower esophageal sphincter competence. Rendic. Gastroenterol. 3, 140–141 (1971).

CHRISTENSEN, J.: Responses of the smooth muscle portion of the esophagus to distension and to electrical stimulation. Rendiconti Rom. Gastro-enterol. 1 (Suppl. 2), 127 (1969).

CHRISTENSEN, J.: Pharmacologic identification of the lower esophageal sphincter. J. clin. Invest. 49, 681–691 (1970a).

CHRISTENSEN, J.: Patterns and origin of some esophageal responses to stretch and electrical stimulation. Gastroenterology 59, 909–916 (1970b).

CHRISTENSEN, J.: The controls of gastrointestinal movements: some old and new views. New Engl. J. Med. 285, 85–98 (1971).

CHRISTENSEN, J., DANIEL, E. E.: Electric and motor effects of autonomic drugs on longitudinal esophageal smooth muscle. Amer. J. Physiol. 211, 387–394 (1966).

CHRISTENSEN, J., DANIEL, E. E.: Effects of some autonomic drugs on circular esophageal smooth muscle. J. Pharmacol. exp. Ther. 159, 243–249 (1968).

CHRISTENSEN, J., DONS, R. F.: Regional variations in response of cat esophageal muscle to stimulation with drugs. J. Pharmacol. exp. Ther. 161, 55–58 (1968).

CHRISTENSEN, J., HAUSER, R. L.: Circumferential coupling of electric slow waves in circular muscle of the cat colon. Amer. J. Physiol. 221, 1033–1037 (1971).

CHRISTENSEN, J., LUND, G. F.: Esophageal responses to distension and electrical stimulation. J. clin. Invest. 48, 408–419 (1969).

CHRISTRUP, J.: Normal swallowing of foodstuffs of pasty consistence. A cinefluorographic investigation of a normal material. Dan. med. Bull. 11, 79–91 (1964).

CLARK, C. G., VANE, J. R.: The cardiac sphincter in the cat. Gut 2, 252–262 (1961).

CLARK, G. A.: Deglutition apnoea. J. Physiol. (Lond.) 54, LIX (1920).

CLARK, M. D., RINALDO, J. A., EYLER, W. R.: Correlation of manometric and radiologic data from the esophagogastric area. Radiology 94, 261–270 (1970).

CODE, C. F., CREAMER, B., SCHLEGEL, J. F., OLSEN, A. M., DONOGHUE, F. E., ANDERSON, H. A.: An atlas of esophageal motility in health and disease. Springfield (Ill.): Charles C. Thomas 1958.

CODE, C. F., KELLEY, M. L., Jr., SCHLEGEL, J. F., OLSEN, A. M.: Detection of hiatal hernia during esophageal motility tests. Gastroenterology 43, 521–531 (1962).

CODE, C. F., SCHLEGEL, J. F.: Motor action of the esophagus and its sphincters. In: Handbook of physiology, section 6, Alimentary canal, vol. IV, Motility, p. 1821–1839. Washington, D.C.: Amer. Physiol. Soc. 1968.

COHEN, B. R.: "Cardiospasm" in achalasia: demonstration of an abnormally elevated esophagogastric sphincter pressure with partial relaxation on swallowing. Gastroenterology (Abstract) 48, 864 (1965).

COHEN, B. R., WOLF, B. S.: Cineradiographic and intraluminal pressure correlations in the pharynx and esophagus. In: Handbook of physiology, section 6, Alimentary canal, vol. IV, Motility, p. 1841–1860. Washington, D.C.: Amer. Physiol. Soc. 1968.

COHEN, S., HARRIS, L. D.: The adaptive response of the lower esophageal sphincter. Clin. Res. (Abstract), 17, 300 (1969).

COHEN, S., HARRIS, L. D.: Lower esophageal sphincter pressure as an index of lower esophageal sphincter strength. Gastroenterology 58, 157–162 (1970).

COHEN, S., HARRIS, L. D.: Does hiatus hernia affect competence of the gastroesophageal sphincter? New Engl. J. Med. 284, 1053–1056 (1971).

COHEN, S., HARRIS, L. D.: The lower esophageal sphincter. Gastroenterology 63, 1066–1073 (1972).

COHEN, S., LIPSHUTZ, W.: Hormonal control of lower sphincter competence: interaction of gastrin and secretin. Gastroenterology (Abstract) 58, 937 (1970a).

COHEN, S., LIPSHUTZ, W.: Anticholinergic therapy: a triple threat to lower esophageal sphincter competence. Ann. intern. Med. 72, 792 (1970b).

Cohen, S., Lipshutz, W.: Hormonal regulation of human lower esophageal sphincter competence: interaction of gastrin and secretin. J. clin. Invest. 50, 449–454 (1971).

Cohen, S., Lipshutz, W., Hughes, W.: Role of gastrin supersensitivity in the pathogenesis of lower esophageal sphincter hypertension in achalasia. J. clin. Invest. 50, 1241–1247 (1971).

Creamer, B., Schlegel, J. F.: Motor responses of the oesophagus to distension. J. appl. Physiol. 10, 498–504 (1957).

Crispin, I. S., McIver, D. K., Lind, I. F.: Manometric study of the effect of vagotomy on the gastroesophageal sphincter. Canad. J. Surg. 10, 299–303 (1967).

Csendes, A., Larrain, A.: Effect of posterior gastropexy on gastroesophageal sphincter pressure and symptomatic reflux in patients with hiatal hernia. Gastroenterology 63, 19–24 (1972).

Dail, C. W., Affeldt, J. E., Collier, C. R.: Clinical aspects of glossopharyngeal breathing. Report of use by 100 post-poliomyelitis patients. J. Amer. med. Ass. 158, 445–449 (1955).

Daniel, E. E., Chapman, K. M.: Electrical activity of the gastrointestinal tract as an indication of mechanical activity. Amer. J. dig. Dis. 8, 54–102 (1963).

Demos, N. J., Timmes, J. J., Di Bianco, J.: Experimental study of a new operation for the treatment of reflux oesophagitis. J. thorac. cardiovasc. Surg. 54, 832–838 (1967).

Dennish, G. W., Castell, D. O.: Inhibitory effect of smoking on the lower esophageal sphincter. New Engl. J. Med. 284, 1136–1137 (1971).

Derstappen, G. Van, Texter, E. C., Jr.: Response of the physiologic gastroesophageal sphincter to increased intraabdominal pressure. J. clin. Invest. 43, 1856–1868 (1964).

Diamant, N. E.: In vitro characteristics of dog esophageal striated muscle. Rendiconti Rom. Gastro-enterol. 3, 138 (1971).

Diamant, N. E., Akin, A. N.: Response of the lower esophageal sphincter to gastric contractile activity. Gastroenterology (Abstract) 58, 940 (1970).

Diamant, N. E., Akin, A. N.: Effect of gastric contractions on the lower esophageal sphincter. Gastroenterology 63, 38–44 (1972).

Dillard, D. H.: Esophageal sphincter and reflux. Surg. Clin. N. Amer. 44, 1201–1209 (1964).

Dillard, D. H., Anderson, H. N.: A new concept of the mechanism of sphincter failure in sliding esophageal hiatal hernia. Surg. Gynec. Obstet. 122, 1030–1038 (1966).

Dodds, W. J., Hogan, D. P., Reid, E. T., Stewart, E. T., Stef, J. J., Arndorfer, R. C.: Evaluation of pharyngeal peristalsis using a strain sensitive recording system. Gastroenterology (Abstract) 62, 743 (1972).

Dodds, W. J., Stewart, E., Hodges, D., Zboralske, F. F.: Esophageal motion associated with peristalsis. Gastroenterology (Abstract) 58, 942 (1970).

Doty, R. W.: Neural organization of deglutition. In: Handbook of physiology, section 6, Alimentary canal, vol. IV, Motility, p. 1861–1902. Washington, D. C.: Amer. Physiol. Soc. 1968.

Doty, R. W., Bosma, J. F.: An electromyographic analysis of reflex deglutition. J. Neurophysiol. 19, 44–60 (1956).

Doty, R. W., Richmond, W. H., Storey, A. T.: Effect of medullary lesions on coordination of deglutition. Exp. Neurol. 17, 91–106 (1967).

Dutta, C. R., Rasmajian, J. V.: Gross and histological structure of the pharyngeal constrictors in the rabbit. Anat. Rec. 137, 127–134 (1960).

Earlam, R. J., Schlegel, J. F., Ellis, F. H., Jr.: Effect of ischemia of lower esophagus and esophagogastric junction on canine esophageal motor function. J. thorac. cardiovasc. Surg. 54, 822–831 (1967).

Edwards, D. A. W.: Sphincter mechanisms in the gastrointestinal tract. Amer. J. dig. Dis. 12, 267–276 (1967).

Elebute, E., Kelly, M. L., Jr., Schwartz, S. I.: Pressure effects of transabdominal supradiaphragmatic vagotomy on the inferior esophageal sphincter of dogs. Surg. Gynec. Obstet. 123, 326–332 (1966).

Ellis, F. H.: Gastroesophageal reflux. Indications for fundoplication. Surg. Clin. N. Amer. 51, 575–588 (1971).

Ellis, F. H., Jr., Schlegel, J. F., Lynch, V. P., Payne, W. S.: Cricopharyngeal myotomy for pharyngo-esophageal diverticulum. Ann. Surg. 170, 340–349 (1969).

Farriaux, J. P., Milbled, G.: Physiologie de la déglutition. 1. Etude physiologique de la déglutition. Bol semi-liquide, bol liquide. Presse méd. 73, 343–350 (1965).

Fleshler, B., Hendrix, T. R., Kramer, P., Ingelfinger, F. J.: The characteristics and similarity of primary and secondary peristalsis in the esophagus. J. clin. Invest. 38, 110–116 (1959).

Floyd, K.: Small multiple nerve endings in sheep oesophageal muscle. Proc. Physiol. Soc. 216, 37P–38P (1971).

FYKE, F. E., Jr., CODE, C. F.: Resting and deglutition pressures in the pharyngo-esophageal region. Gastroenterology **29**, 24–34 (1955).

FYKE, F. E., Jr., CODE, C. F., SCHLEGEL, J. F.: The gastroesophageal sphincter in healthy human beings. Gastroenterologia (Basel) **86**, 135–150 (1956).

GAHAGAN, T.: The function of the musculature of the esophagus and stomach in the esophagogastric sphincter mechanism. Surg. Gynec. Obstet. **114**, 293–303 (1962).

GILES, G. R., HUMPHRIES, C., MASON, M. C., CLARK, C. G.: Effect of pH changes on the cardiac sphincter. Gut **10**, 852–856 (1969 b).

GILES, G. R., MASON, M. C., HUMPHRIES, C., CLARK, C. G.: Action of gastrin on the lower oesophageal sphincter in man. Gut **10**, 730–734 (1969 a).

GOLDBERG, H. M.: Role of the fundus in the prevention of gastroesophageal regurgitation. Lancet **1960 I**, 613–615.

GOYAL, R. K., RATTAN, S., HERSCH, T.: Comparison of the effects of prostaglandins E_1, E_2, and A_2, and of hypovolemic hypotension on the lower esophageal sphincter. Gastroenterology **68**, 608–612 (1973).

GOYAL, R. K., SANGREE, M. H., HERSCH, T., SPIRO, H. M.: Pressure inversion point at the upper high pressure zone and its genesis. Gastroenterology **59**, 754–759 (1970).

GREENWOOD, R. K., SCHLEGEL, J. F., CODE, C. F., ELLIS, F. H., Jr.: The effect of sympathectomy, vagotomy, and oesophageal interruption on the canine gastro-oesophageal sphincter. Thorax **17**, 310–319 (1962).

GREENWOOD, R. K., SCHLEGEL, J. F., HELM, W. J., CODE, C. F.: Pressure and potential difference characteristics of surgically created canine hiatal hernia. Gastroenterology **48**, 602–611 (1965).

GROSSMAN, M. I.: How does insulin stimulate the lower esophageal sphincter? Gastroenterology **61**, 119–120 (1971).

GRYBOSKI, J. D.: The swallowing mechanism of the neonate. I. Esophageal and gastric motility. Pediatrics **35**, 445–452 (1965).

GRYBOSKI, J. D., THAYER, W. R., Jr., SPIRO, H. M.: Esophageal motility in infants and children. Pediatrics **31**, 382–395 (1963).

HADDAD, J. K.: Relation of gastroesophageal reflux to yield sphincter pressures. Gastroenterology **58**, 175–184 (1970).

HANSKY, J., KORMAN, M. G., COWLEY, D. J., BARON, J. H.: Serum gastrin in duodenal ulcer. Part II. Effect of insulin hypoglycemia. Gut **12**, 959–962 (1971).

HARRIS, L. D.: Letter to the editor. New Engl. J. Med. **282**, 1375 (1970).

HARRIS, L. D., POPE, C. E., II: The pressure inversion point: its genesis and reliability. Gastroenterology **51**, 641–648 (1966).

HARRIS, L. D., WINANS, C. S., POPE, C. E., II: Determination of yield pressures; a method for measuring anal sphincter competence. Gastroenterology **50**, 754–760 (1966).

HEITMANN, P., WOLF, B. S., SOKOL, E. M., COHEN, B. R.: Simultaneous radiocineradiographic-manometric study of the distal esophagus: small hiatal hernias and rings. Gastroenterology **50**, 737–753 (1966).

HELLEMANS, J.: Invloed van de leeftijd op de motorische funktie van de slokdarm. Thesis. Tielt: Uitg. Lannoo 1970.

HELLEMANS, J., VANTRAPPEN, G.: Electromyographic studies on canine esophageal motility. Amer. J. dig. Dis. **12**, 1240–1255 (1967).

HELLEMANS, J., VANTRAPPEN, G.: Unpublished data (1971).

HELLEMANS, J., VANTRAPPEN, G., JANSSENS, J., PELEMANS, W., VALEMBOIS, P.: Electromyographic and manometric studies of the transitional zone between striated and smooth esophageal muscle. Rendiconti Rom. Gastro-enterol. **3**, 138–139 (1971).

HELLEMANS, J., VANTRAPPEN, G., VALEMBOIS, P., JANSSENS, J., VANDENBROUCKE, J.: Electrical activity of striated and smooth muscle of the esophagus. Amer. J. dig. Dis. **13**, 320–334 (1968).

HENDERSON, R. D., RODNEY, K.: Tone of the gastroesophageal junction: its response to abdominal compression and to swallowing. Canad. J. Surg. **14**, 328–334 (1971).

HIGGS, B., ELLIS, F. H.: The effect of bilateral supranodosal vagotomy on canine esophageal function. Surgery **58**, 828–834 (1965).

HIGGS, B., KERR, F. W. L., ELLIS, F. H., Jr.: The experimental production of esophageal achalasia by electrolytic lesions in the medulla. J. thorac. cardiovasc. Surg. **50**, 613–625 (1965).

HIGHTOWER, N. C., Jr.: Esophageal motility in health and disease. Dis. Chest **28**, 150–169 (1955).

HILL, L. D.: Surgery and gastroesophageal reflux. Gastroenterology **63**, 183–185 (1972).

HUNT, P. S., CONNELL, A. M., SMILEY. T. B.: The cricopharyngeal sphincter in gastric reflux. Gut **11**, 303–306 (1970).

HWANG, K.: Mechanism of transportation of the content of the esophagus. J. appl. Physiol. 6, 781–796 (1954).

HWANG, K., GROSSMAN, M. I.: A note on the innervation of the cervical portion of the human esophagus. Gastroenterology 25, 375–377 (1953).

HWANG, K., GROSSMAN, M. I., IVY, A. C.: Nervous control of the cervical portion of the esophagus. Amer. J. Physiol. 154, 343 (1948).

IGGO, A.: Gastrointestinal tension receptors with unmyelinated afferent fibers in the vagus of the cat. Quart. J. exp. Physiol. 42, 130–143 (1957).

INGELFINGER, F. J.: Espohageal motility. Physiol. Rev. 38, 533–584 (1958).

ISENBERG, J., CSENDES, A., WALSH, J. H.: Resting and pentagastrin-stimulated gastro-esophageal sphincter pressure in patients with Zollinger-Ellison syndrome. Gastroenterology 61, 655–658 (1971).

JACKSON, C.: The diaphragmatic pinchcock in so-called "cardiospasm". Laryngoscope (St. Louis) 32, 139 (1922).

JACKSON, C., JACKSON, C. L.: Bronchoesophagology, p. 226–230. Philadelphia: W. B. Saunders Co. 1950.

JACOBOWITZ, D., NEMIR, P., Jr.: The autonomic innervation of the esophagus of the dog. J. thorac. cardiovasc. Surg. 58, 678–684 (1969).

JANSSENS, J., VALEMBOIS, P., PELEMANS, W., HELLEMANS, J., VANTRAPPEN, G.: Is the primary peristaltic contraction of the canine oesophagus bolus dependent? Europ. symposium on the function of the oesophagus. Odense, October 1972.

JEAN, A.: Localisation et activité des neurones déglutiteurs bulbaires. J. Physiol. (Paris) 64, 227–268 (1972).

JENNEWEIN, H. M., WALDECK, F., SIEWERT, R., WEISER, F.: The action of gastro-intestinal hormones and drugs on the lower oesophageal sphincter in man and dog. Europ. symp. on the function of the oesophagus. Odense, October 1972.

JOHNSON, H. D.: The cardia and hiatus hernia. Springfield (Ill.): C. C. Thomas 1968.

JOHNSON, H. D., LAWS, J. W.: The cardia in swallowing, eructation, and vomiting. Lancet 1966 II, 1268–1273.

JORDAN, P. H., LONGHI, E. H.: Relationship between size of bolus and the act of swallowing on esophageal peristalsis in dogs. Proc. Soc. exp. Biol. and Med. (N.Y.) 137, 868–871 (1971).

JURICA, E. J.: Studies on the motility of the denervated mammalian esophagus. Amer. J. Physiol. 77, 371–384 (1926).

KAHN, R. H.: Studien über den Schluckreflex. 1. Die sensible Innervation. Arch. Physiol., Suppl. 27, 386–426 (1903).

KARAS, L. M., STERN, H., BLOOM, D., BINDER, H. J., POINDEXTER, B. S., THAYER, W. SPIRO, H. M.: The gastroesophageal junction in the monkey and its relation to reflux. J. surg. Res. 6, 469–477 (1966).

KAWASAKI, M., OGURA, J. H., TAKENOUCHI, S.: Neurophysiologic observations of normal deglutition. I. Its relationship to the respiratory cycle. Laryngoscope (St. Louis) 74, 1747–1765 (1964).

KAYE, M. D., SHOWALTER, J. P.: Manometric configuration of the lower esophageal sphincter in normal human subjects. Gastroenterology 61, 213–223 (1971).

KELLEY, M. L., WILBUR, D. L., SCHLEGEL, J. F., CODE, C. F.: Deglutitive responses in the gastroesophageal sphincter of healthy human beings. J. appl. Physiol. 15, 483–488 (1960).

KERR, F. W. L.: Function of the dorsal motor nucleus of the vagus. Science 157, 451–452 (1967).

KERR, F. W. L.: Preserved vagal visceromotor function following destruction of the dorsal motor nucleus. J. Physiol. (Lond.) 202, 755–789 (1969).

KODICEK, J., CREAMER, B.: A study of pharyngeal pouches. J. Laryng. 75, 406–411 (1961).

LAWN, A. M.: The localization, by means of electrical stimulation, of the origin and path in the medulla oblongata of the motor nerve fibers of the rabbit oesophagus. J. Physiol. (Lond.) 174, 232–244 (1964).

LAWN, A. M.: The localization, in the nucleus ambiguus of the rabbit, of the cells of origin of motor nerve fibers in the glossopharyngeal nerve and various branches of the vagus nerve by means of retrograde degeneration. J. comp. Neurol. 127, 293–306 (1966).

LEAR, C. S. C., FLANAGAN, J. B., MORREES, C. F. A.: The frequency of deglutition in man. Arch. oral Biol. 10, 83–99 (1965).

LEVITT, M. N., DEDO, H. H., OGURA, J. H.: The cricopharyngeus muscle, an electromyographic study in the dog. Laryngoscope (St. Louis) 75, 122–136 (1965).

LIND, J. F., BURNS, C. M., MACDOUGALL, J. T.: "Physiological" repair for hiatus hernia—manometric study. Arch. Surg. 91, 233–237 (1965).

LIND, J. F., COTTON, D. J., BLANCHARD, R., CRISPIN, J. S., DIMOPOLOS, G. E.: Effect of thoracic displacement and vagotomy on the canine gastroesophageal junctional zone. Gastroenterology 56, 1078–1085 (1969).

LIND, J. F., CRISPIN, J. S., MCIVES, D. K.: The effect of atropine on the gastroesophageal sphincter. Canad. J. Physiol. Pharmacol. 46, 233–238 (1968).

LIND, J. F., DUTHIE, H. L., SCHLEGEL, J. F., CODE, C. F.: Motility of the gastric fundus. Amer. J. Physiol. 201, 197–202 (1961).

LIND, J. F., WARRIAN, W. G., WANKLING, W. J.: Responses of the gastroesophageal junctional zone to increases in abdominal pressure. Canad. J. Surg. 9, 32–38 (1966).

LIPSHUTZ, W., COHEN, S.: Physiological determinants of lower esophageal sphincter function. Gastroenterology 61, 16–24 (1971).

LIPSHUTZ, W., HUGHES, W., COHEN, S.: The genesis of lower esophageal sphincter pressure: its identification through the use of gastrin antiserum. J. clin. Invest. 51, 522–529 (1972).

LIPSHUTZ, W., TUCH, A. F., COHEN, S.: A comparison of the site of action of gastrin I on lower esophageal sphincter and antral circular smooth muscle. Gastroenterology 61, 454–460 (1971).

LONGHI, E. H., JORDAN, P. H., Jr.: Necessity of a bolus for propagation of primary peristalsis in the canine esophagus. Amer. J. Physiol. 220, 609–612 (1971).

LUMSDEN, K., HOLDEN, W. S.: The act of vomiting in man. Gut 10, 173–179 (1969).

LUND, G. F., CHRISTENSEN, J.: Electrical stimulation of esophageal smooth muscle and effect of antagonists. Amer. J. Physiol. 217, 1369–1374 (1969).

LUND, W. S.: A study of the cricopharyngeal sphincter in man and in the dog. Ann. roy. Coll. Surg. Engl. 37, 225–246 (1965 a).

LUND, W. S.: The function of the cricopharyngeal sphincter during swallowing. Acta otolaryng. (Stockh.) 59, 497–510 (1965 b).

LUND, W. S.: The cricopharyngeal sphincter: its relationship to the relief of pharyngeal paralysis and the surgical treatment of the early pharyngeal pouch. J. Laryng. 82, 353–367 (1968).

MacLAURIN, C.: The intrinsic sphincter in the prevention of gastro-oesophageal reflux. Lancet 1963 II, 801–805.

MANN, C. V., CODE, C. F., SCHLEGEL, J. F., ELLIS, F. H.: Intrinsic mechanisms controlling the mammalian gastro-oesophageal sphincter deprived of extrinsic nerve supply. Thorax 23, 634–639 (1968 a).

MANN, C. V., ELLIS, F. H., Jr., SCHLEGEL, J. F., CODE, C. F.: Abdominal displacement of the canine gastroesophageal sphincter. Surg. Gynec. Obstet. 118, 1009–1018 (1964).

MANN, C. V., HARDCASTLE, J. D.: The effect of vagotomy on the human gastroesophageal sphincter. Gut 9, 688–695 (1968).

MANN, C. V., SCHLEGEL, J. F., ELLIS, F. H., CODE, C. F.: Studies of the isolated gastroesophageal sphincter. Surg. Forum 13, 248–250 (1968 b).

McNALLY, E. F., KELLY, J. E., Jr., INGELFINGER, F. J.: Mechanism of belching: effects of gastric distension with air. Gastroenterology 46, 254–259 (1964).

MEI, N.: Etude électrophysiologique des récepteurs sensibles de l'œsophage thoracique du chat. C. R. Acad. Sci. (Paris) 260, 302–305 (1965 a).

MEI, N.: Etude de la vitesse de conduction et du cycle d'excitabilité des fibres vagales afférentes appartenant aux groupes A, B, et C. C. R. Soc. Biol. (Paris) 159, 1373–1377 (1965 b).

MEI, N., SALDUCCI, J.: Afferent vagal impulses from the lower oesophageal sphincter. Rendiconti Rom. Gastro-enterol. 3, 139 (1971).

MELTZER, S. J.: On the causes of the orderly progress of the peristaltic movements in the esophagus. Amer. J. Physiol. 2, 266–272 (1899).

MELTZER, S. J.: Deglutition through an esophagus partly deprived of its muscularis, with demonstration. Proc. Soc. exp. Biol. (N.Y.) 4, 40–43 (1907).

MICHELSON, E., SIEGEL, C. I.: The role of the phrenico-esophageal ligament in the lower esophageal sphincter. Surg. Gynec. Obstet. 118, 1291–1294 (1964).

MISIEWICZ, J. J., WALLER, S. C., ANTHONY, P. P., GUMMER, J. W. P.: Achalasia of the cardia: pharmacology and histopathology of isolated cardiac sphincteric muscle with and without achalasia. Quart. J. Med. 38, 17–30 (1969).

MONGES, H., SALDUCCI, J.: Etude physiologique de l'ampoule épiphrénique de l'œsophage par la méthode manométrique et la radiocinématographie combinées. Arch. Mal. Appar. dig. 55, 871–882 (1966).

MORAN, J. M., PIHL, C. O., NORTON, R. A., RHEINLANDER, H. F.: The hiatal hernia-reflux complex. Current approaches to correction and evaluation of results. Amer. J. Surg. 121, 403–411 (1971).

NAGLER, R., SPIRO, H. M.: Segmental response of the inferior esophageal sphincter to elevated intragastric pressure. Gastroenterology 40, 405–407 (1961).

NAUTA, J.: The closing mechanism between the oesophagus and the stomach. Gastroenterologia (Basel) 86, 219–232 (1956).

NETTER, F. H.: Ciba collection of medical illustrations. Digestive system, part I: Upper digestive tract, ed. E. OPPENHEIMER. New York 1959.

Nishimura, T., Takasu, T.: The adrenergic innervation in the esophagus and respiratory tract of the rabbit. Acta oto-laryng. scand. 67, 444–452 (1969).

Okada, H., Okamoto, K., Nisida, I.: The activity of the cardioregulatory and abdominal sympathetic nerves during swallowing. Jap. J. Physiol. 11, 44–53 (1961).

Peiper, A.: Die Eigenart der kindlichen Hirntätigkeit. Leipzig: Thieme 1961.

Perrot, J. W.: Anatomical aspects of hypopharyngeal diverticula. Aust. N.Z. J. Surg. 31, 307–317 (1962).

Peters, P. M.: Closure mechanism of the cardia with special reference to the diaphragmatico-esophageal elastic ligament. Thorax 10, 27–36 (1955).

Pommerenke, W. T.: A study of the sensory areas eliciting the swallowing reflex. Amer. J. Physiol. 84, 36–41 (1928).

Pope, C. E., II: A dynamic test of sphincter strength: its application to the lower esophageal sphincter. Gastroenterology 52, 779–786 (1967).

Porter, R.: Synaptic potentials in hypoglossal motoneurones. J. Physiol. (Lond.) 180, 209–224 (1965).

Ramon y Cajal, S.: Histologie du système nerveux de l'homme et des vertébrés. Tome I, translated by L. Azoulay, Madrid: Consejo Sup. Invest. Cient. (1909), p. 669–959 (1952).

Ramsey, G. H., Watson, J. S., Gramiak, R., Weinberg, S. A.: Cinefluorographic analysis of the mechanism of swallowing. Radiology 64, 498–518 (1955).

Reichbach, E. J., Winans, C. S.: Esophageal manometrics in the postlaryngectomy patient. Gastroenterology (Abstract) 58, 987 (1970).

Resin, H., Stern, D. H., Sturdevant, R. A., Isenberg, J. I.: Effect of octapeptide of cholecystokinin on lower esophageal sphincter pressure in man. Gastroenterology (Abstract) 62, 797 (1972).

Rinaldo, J. A., Clark, M. D.: Simultaneous cineradiographic and manometric analysis of the gastroesophageal junction. Gastroenterology (Abstract) 46, 757 (1964).

Rinaldo, J. A., Levey, J. F.: Correlation of several methods for recording esophageal sphincteral pressures. Amer. J. dig. Dis. 13, 882–890 (1968).

Rinaldo, J. A., Levey, J. F., Smathers, H. M., Gardner, L. W., McGinnis, K. D.: An integrated anatomic, physiologic and cineradiologic study of the canine gastroesophageal sphincter. Amer. J. dig. Dis. 16, 556–565 (1971).

Roman, C.: Contrôle nerveux du péristaltisme œsophagien. J. Physiol. (Paris) 58, 79–108 (1966).

Roman, C.: La commande de la motricité œsophagienne et sa régulation. Thèse Doctorat ès Sciences, Marseille, 181 p. (1967).

Roman, C., Car, A.: Contractions œsophagiennes produites par la stimulation du vague ou du bulbe rachidien. J. Physiol. (Paris) 59, 377–398 (1967).

Roman, C., Car, A.: Déglutitions et contractions œsophagiennes réflexes obtenues par la stimulation des nerfs vague et laryngé supérieur. Exp. Brain Res. 11, 48–74 (1970).

Roman, C., Orengo, M., Tieffenbach, L.: Etude électromyographique du muscle lisse œsophagien chez le chat. J. Physiol. (Paris) 61, Suppl. 2, 390–391 (1969).

Roman, C., Tieffenbach, L.: Motricité de l'œsophage à musculature lisse après bivagotomie. Etude électromyographique (EMG). J. Physiol. (Paris) 63, 733–762 (1971).

Rosenberg, S. J., Harris, L. D.: A single physiologic mechanism for changing strength of both esophageal sphincters. Gastroenterology (Abstract) 60, 798 (1971a).

Rosenberg, S. J., Harris, L. D.: Heartburn and hormones: the mechanism of gastro-esophageal sphincter incompetence. Gastroenterology (Abstract) 60, 711 (1971b).

Rousseau, J. P.: Contribution à l'étude de la rumination et de l'éructation. Thèse Doctorat ès Sciences, Marseille, 156 p. (1970).

Rutishauser, W. J., Banchero, N., Tsakiris, A. G., Edmundowicz, A. C., Wood, E. H.: Pleural pressures at dorsal and ventral sites in supine and prone body positions. J. appl. Physiol. 21, 1500–1510 (1966).

Sanchez, G. C., Kramer, P., Ingelfinger, F. J.: Motor mechanisms of the esophagus, particularly of its distal portion. Gastroenterology 25, 321–332 (1953).

Schlegel, J. F., Code, C. F.: Pressure characteristics of the esophagus and its sphincters in dogs. Amer. J. Physiol. 193, 9–14 (1958).

Schobinger, R.: Spasm of cricopharyngeal muscle as cause of dysphagia after total laryngectomy. Arch. Otolaryng. 67, 271–275 (1958).

Schreiber, J.: Ueber den Schluckmechanismus. 91 S. Berlin: A. Hirschwald 1904.

Shepard, R., Fenn, S., Sieber, W. K.: Evaluation of esophageal function in postoperative esophageal atresia and tracheoespohageal fistula. Surgery 59, 608–617 (1966).

Sicular, A., Cohen, B., Zimmerman, A., Kark, A. E.: The significance of an intra-abdominal segment of canine esophagus as a competent antireflux mechanism. Surgery 61, 784–790 (1967).

Sieber, A. M., Sieber, W. K.: Colon transplants as esophageal replacement; cineradiographic and manometric evaluation in children. Ann. Surg. **168**, 116–122 (1968).

Siegel, C. I., Hendrix, T. R.: Evidence for the central mediation of secondary peristalsis in the esophagus. Bull. Johns Hopk. Hosp. **108**, 297–307 (1961).

Sigmund, C. J., McNally, E. F.: The action of a carminative on the lower esophageal sphincter. Gastroenterology **56**, 13–18 (1969).

Skinner, D. B., Booth, D. J.: Assessment of distal esophageal function in patients with hiatal hernia and/or gastroesophageal reflux. Ann. Surg. **172**, 627–637 (1970).

Skinner, D. B., Camp, T. F.: Relation of esophageal reflux to lower esophageal sphincter pressures decreased by atropine. Gastroenterology **54**, 543–551 (1968).

Smiddy, F. G., Atkinson, M.: Mechanisms preventing gastroesophageal reflux in dogs. Brit. J. Surg. **47**, 680–687 (1960).

Smiley, T. B., Caves, P. K., Porter, D. C.: Relationship between posterior laryngeal pouch and hiatus hernia. Thorax **25**, 725–731 (1970).

Smith, B.: The neurological lesion in achalasia of the cardia. Gut **11**, 388–391 (1970).

Smith, C. C., Brizzee, K. R.: Cineradiographic analysis of vomiting in the cat. Gastroenterology **40**, 654–664 (1961).

Sokol, E. M., Heitmann, P., Wolf, B. S., Cohen, B. R.: Simultaneous cineradiographic and manometric study of the pharynx, hypopharynx, and cervical esophagus. Gastroenterology **51**, 960–974 (1966).

Staple, T. W., Ogura, J. H.: Cineradiography of the swallowing mechanism following supraglottic subtotal laryngectomy. Radiology **87**, 226–230 (1966).

Stern, H., Karas, L. M., Bloom, D. L., Winship, D. H., Melnick, G. S., Thayer, W. R., Spiro, H. M.: Evaluation of factors involved in gastroesophageal reflux. J. thorac. cardiovasc. Surg. **48**, 906–911 (1964).

Stevens, C. E., Sellers, A. F.: Pressure events in bovine esophagus and reticulorumen associated with eructation, deglutition and regurgitation. Amer. J. Physiol. **199**, 598–602 (1960).

Sumi, T.: The activity of brain-stem respiratory neurons and spinal respiratory motoneurons during swallowing. J. Neurophysiol. **26**, 466–477 (1963).

Sumi, T.: Neuronal mechanisms in swallowing. Pflügers Arch. ges. Physiol. **278**, 467–477 (1963–1964).

Sumi, T.: Some properties of cortically evoked swallowing and chewing in rabbits. Brain Res. **15**, 107–120 (1969).

Sumi, T.: Modification of cortically evoked rhythmic chewing and swallowing from midbrain and pons. Jap. J. Physiol. **21**, 489–506 (1971).

Szentágothai, J.: Anatomical considerations of monosynaptic reflex arcs. J. Neurophysiol. **11**, 445–454 (1948).

Thomas, P. A., Earlam, R. J.: Electrical activity of the isolated perfused canine gastroesophageal junction. Gastroenterology (Abstract) **62**, 821 (1972).

Titchen, D. A., Wheeler, J. S.: Contraction of the caudal region of the oesophagus of the cat. J. Physiol. (Lond.) **215**, 119–137 (1971).

Tocornal, J. A., Snow, H. D., Fonkalsrud, E. W.: A mucosal flap valve mechanism to prevent gastroesophageal reflux and esophagitis. Surgery **64**, 519–523 (1968).

Torrance, H. B.: Studies on the mechanism of gastro-oesophageal regurgitation. J. roy. Coll. Surg. Edinb. **4**, 54–62 (1958).

Torvik, A.: Afferent connections to the sensory trigeminal nuclei, the nucleus of the solitary tract and adjacent structures—an experimental study in the rat. J. comp. Neurol. **106**, 51–141 (1956).

Treacy, W. L., Baggenstoss, A. H., Slocumb, C. H., Code, C. F.: Scleroderma of the esophagus. A correlation of histologic and physiologic findings. Ann. intern. Med. **59**, 351–356 (1963).

Trop, D., Peeters, R., Van de Woestijne, K. P.: Localization of recording site in the esophagus by means of cardiac artefacts. J. appl. Physiol. **29**, 283–287 (1970).

Tuch, A., Cohen, S.: Lower esophageal sphincter relaxation: studies on the neurogenic inhibitory mechanism. J. clin. Invest. **52**, 14–20 (1973).

Tulley, W. J.: Methods of recording patterns of behaviour of the oro-facial muscles using the electromyography. Dent. Rec. **73**, 741–748 (1953).

Valembois, P., Janssens, J., Pelemans, W., Hellemans, J., Vantrappen, G.: Central or peripheral regulation of secondary peristalsis in the canine oesophagus. Europ. symposium on the function of the oesophagus. Odense, October 1972.

Vandertoll, D. J., Ellis, F. H., Schlegel, J. F., Code, C. F.: An experimental study of the role of gastric and esophageal muscle in gastroesophageal competence. Surg. Gynec. Obstet. **122**, 579–586 (1966).

Vantrappen, G.: Slokdarmmotiliteit. Brussel: Arscia Uitgaven 1961.

Vantrappen, G.: Measurement of electrical activity. American Gastroenterological Association, Postgraduate Course "The Esophagus". Bal Harbour, Florida, May (1971), p. 26.

Vantrappen, G., Goidsenhoven, G. E. van, Verbeke, S., Vandenberghe, G., Vandenbroucke, J.: Manometric studies in achalasia of the cardia before and after pneumatic dilatations. Gastroenterology 45, 317–325 (1963).

Vantrappen, G., Hellemans, J.: Studies on the normal deglutition complex. Amer. J. dig. Dis. 12, 255–266 (1967).

Vantrappen, G., Hellemans, J.: Esophageal motility. Rendiconti Rom. Gastro-enterol. 2, 7–19 (1970).

Vantrappen, G., Liemer, M. D., Ikeya, J., Texter, E. C., Jr., Barborka, C. J.: Simultaneous fluorocinematography and intraluminal pressure measurements in the study of esophageal motility. Gastroenterology 35, 592–602 (1958).

Veach, H. O.: Studies on the innervation of smooth muscle. IV. Functional relations between the lower end of the esophagus and stomach of the cat. Amer. J. Physiol. 76, 532–537 (1926).

Wankling, W. J., Warrian, W. G., Lind, J. F.: The gastroesophageal sphincter in hiatus hernia. Canad. J. Surg. 8, 61–67 (1965).

Weisbrodt, N. W., Christensen, J.: Gradients of contractions in the opossum esophagus. Gastroenterology 62, 1159–1166 (1972).

Williams, G. S., Ingram, P. R.: A comparative intraluminal oncometric study of the experimentally reconstructed esophagogastric junction. Surg. Gynec. Obstet. 118, 1205–1216 (1964).

Williams, J. A., Woodward, D. A. K.: The effect of subdiaphragmatic vagotomy on the function of the gastroesophageal sphincter. Surg. Clin. N. Amer. 47, 1341–1344 (1967).

Williams, T. H., Dixon, A. D.: The intrinsic innervation of the soft palate. J. Anat. (Lond.) 97, 259–267 (1963).

Winans, C. S.: Axial movements of the human esophageal high pressure zone with respiration and swallowing. Gastroenterology (Abstract) 58, 1008 (1970).

Winans, C. S.: Alteration of lower esophageal sphincter characteristics with respiration and proximal esophageal balloon distension. Gastroenterology 62, 380–388 (1972a).

Winans, C. S.: Manometric asymmetry of the lower esophageal high pressure zone. Gastroenterology 62, 830 (1972b).

Winans, C. S., Harris, L. D.: Quantitation of lower esophageal sphincter competence. Gastroenterology (Abstract) 52, 773–778 (1967).

Winckler, G.: L'équipement nerveux du muscle tenseur du voile du palais. Arch. Anat. (Strasbourg) 47, 313–316 (1964).

Windsor, C. W. O.: Gastro-esoophageal reflux after partial gastrectomy. Brit. med. J. 1964 II, 1233-1234.

Winship, D. H., de Andrade, S. R., Zboralske, F. F.: Influence of bolus temperature on human esophageal motor function. J. clin. Invest. 40, 243–250 (1970).

Winship, D. H., Poindexter, R. E., Thayer, W. R., Jr., Spiro, H. M.: Esophageal motility in the monkey. Gastroenterology 48, 231–236 (1965).

Winship, D. H., Zboralske, F. F.: The esophageal propulsive force: esophageal response to acute obstruction. J. clin. Invest. 46, 1391–1401 (1967).

Wolf, B. S.: The inferior esophageal sphincter. — Anatomic, roentgenologic and manometric correlation, contradictions, and terminology. Amer. J. Roentgenol. 110, 260–277 (1970).

Wolf, B. S., Heitmann, P., Cohen, B. R.: The inferior esophageal sphincter, the manometric high pressure zone and hiatal incompetence. Amer. J. Roentgenol. 103, 251–276 (1968).

Wood, J. W.: Electrical activity from single neurons in Auerbach's plexus. Amer. J. Physiol. 219, 159–169 (1970).

Zaino, C., Jacobson, H. G., Lepow, H., Ozturk, C.: The pharyngoesophageal sphincter. Radiology 89, 639–645 (1967).

Chapter 2

Diagnostic Procedures

History and Symptoms of Esophageal Disease

D. A. W. EDWARDS

With 5 Figures

1. Symptoms and Syndromes

In this chapter the author is confronted with a conflict between two approaches to the use of clinical information. When learning and trying to understand, or describing in a text book, the manifestations of a disease process, the more information one is given the better, provided that it does not cause confusion. A picture of what is happening and what may (but does not always) happen is built up. An unusual symptom or sign may then be more easily recognized as a manifestation of the disease, and so anxiety about its meaning is relieved. It is for this reason, because the doctor is anxious about missing a clue to a disease and because he does not know or understand that it may not be necessary to use that clue, that there is a demand for a detailed list of all the possible symptoms and signs which may arise from the disease process in text book descriptions.

When taking a history or questioning a patient, the contrasting need is for economy of effort and thinking when making a diagnosis. Symptoms or signs which are common to many conditions are not helpful in making a distinction between conditions; they merely alert the doctor to the possibilities. Many diseases can be characterized by a small number of features which should be sought for in the most economical sequence. If the defining features are present, the diagnosis is established and any further information is redundant unless it is used to determine management or prognosis. In the same way, however, it is more economical of time, manpower, and money, and intellectually more stimulating, to decide what information will influence action, and what will not, and to confine one's search for information that will influence action. All information which is not *necessary* for making a decision is redundant.

The next problem is the definition of "necessary". Clearly, some doctors seem to require more information before they will act than others. Information may also be unnecessary for a decision about diagnosis, but necessary for a decision about management. One doctor may be influenced by the number or age of a patient's children and to him this information is necessary in deciding whether to operate, whereas another doctor may consider it to be unnecessary or redundant. Information may also be necessary to one doctor because he is not intellectually satisfied until he has filled in all the details of the clinical picture, although only a few of the details are necessary to identify the disease.

For these reasons the information in this chapter is presented in the following way. The common symptoms associated with dysphagia are described and an attempt is made to explain how they are produced and how they should be produced.

Many symptoms are common to many conditions and are merely *indicative* of disease; for example "I get a pain in my chest" gives very little useful information and does not distinguish between the possible lesions. More detailed information such as a description of the position or character of the pain adds to the picture by its *descriptive* nature, but does not necessarily provide *discriminative* information; for example "The pain starts in the middle of the chest and radiates to the neck, jaw and shoulders". Discriminative information may be offered by the patient or sought by direct questioning and the information "The pain comes on when I bend or turn on to my right side in bed" makes the diagnosis of gastroesophageal reflux. These common symptoms which discriminate between diseases will be described, so that the diagnostic features of the disease are emphasized, but rare symptoms will not be included unless they are characteristic and discriminate clearly between diseases or unless they are specific indicators upon which the diagnosis can be made forthwith.

Part 2 describes how this discriminative information may be built into a logical decision tree for making a diagnosis on the basis of symptoms only.

1.1. Symptoms and their Significance

The main symptoms which characterize esophageal causes of dysphagia are (1) a sensation of obstruction, (2) regurgitation, and (3) pain.

1.1.1. The Sensation of Obstruction

The patient commonly complains of a sensation of obstruction but this symptom is often misleading. The patient says that food sticks, or that he cannot swallow, or that there is something that he cannot swallow away and points to a site at which he feels something is happening. If the sensation occurs or is worsened at the time of, or within 20 sec of swallowing, it is a true dysphagia. If the sensation is not present when eating or drinking it is a pseudo-dysphagia, either functional or a referred sensation from another lesion.

1.1.1.1. The Site of the Obstruction

The site at which the obstruction is localized by the subject is so frequently incorrect that no importance can be attached to it. Table 3 illustrates the sites

Table 3. Site at which an obstruction is localized by the patient in various conditions

Site at which subject localizes block	Actual site of upper level of lesion (stricture may be benign or malignant)					
	Achalasia	Lower esoph. strict.	Fundal cancer	Mid. esoph. strict.	Upper esoph. strict.	Total
Above thyroid cartilage	0	5	0	2	0	7
At thyroid cartilage	28	6	1	3	6	44
Sternal notch	27	23	4	8	10	72
Upper sternal	42	25	5	11	2	85
Lower sternal and xiphoid	69	50	19	13	2	153
Epigastric	7	10	3	2	0	22
Total	173	119	32	39	20	383

of localization in various conditions. If the subject points to the neck or sternal notch region, the likelihood that the lesion is in that area is very small. If the subject points to the xiphoid or lower sternal area, the likelihood that the lesion is at the lower end of the esophagus is greater, but two subjects with an obstructing stricture (web) at the pharyngoesophageal junction pointed to the xiphoid as the site of the block.

1.1.1.2. The Site of the Receptors

The site of the receptors which are stimulated and the pathways of transmission of the sensory impulses are not defined. The sense of impaction or pain seems likely to be produced by pressure upon mucosal receptors and unlikely to be produced by stimulation of muscle "receptors" or "spasm". "Spasm" as a cause of pain is a confused and nebulous concept which has no proven meaning unless it relates to the compression of mucosal receptors by a solid bolus impacting on an area of increased resistance to stretch. In the early stages of dysphagia from carcinoma of the esophagus the impaction of food commonly causes pain similar to that produced by the impaction of food on a peptic structure, but it is not unusual for the pain to be less severe as the carcinoma progresses. If this symptom pattern is present the likelihood of carcinoma is very high.

1.1.1.3. The Sensation of "Choking"

The sensation of "choking" or compression of the lungs or trachea which follows swallowing against an obstruction is difficult to explain unless it is a paresthesia. Indeed, distension of the upper esophagus and local pressure on the tracheobronchial tree is commonly seen during the radiological examination of a subject tilted head-down, yet symptoms do not occur. Sometimes this sensation of "choking" occurs when the subject attempts to swallow a bolus when the esophagus is full and will accept no more, so that spill-over into the larynx occurs.

1.1.2. Regurgitation

The volume, taste, contents, timing, and associations of regurgitation give valuable clues about the lesion. Regurgitation must first be differentiated from vomiting. Patients usually only know one word, "vomiting", for food or liquid coming back into the mouth, but can, when asked, distinguish readily between the powered projection of retching and vomiting with contraction of abdominal muscles and proceeding nausea, and the effortless efflux of regurgitation, in which material flows up out of the chest as if of its own accord or by deliberate provocation by the subject. Regurgitation refers to the flow of material from the esophagus into the pharynx or mouth; reflux is confined to the flow from stomach to esophagus. The regurgitated material may come from the stomach, as for example when the rate of flow and volume of reflux is enough to flood the esophagus and broach the cricopharyngeal closing mechanism. Alternatively, it may come only from the esophagus which has failed to empty into the stomach because of obstruction. Regurgitation may induce nausea and subsequent vomiting so that both may occur in the same subject, but if they do, a narrow rigid obstruction is unlikely.

1.1.2.1. The Volume of Regurgitate

The volume of regurgitate in the presence of obstruction depends partly upon the capacity of the esophagus. Short peptic strictures are rarely associated with a dilated proximal esophagus except in systemic sclerosis. A long tight post-intubation stricture, a carcinomatous stricture of the lower esophagus, an esophagus that has been obstructed for many hours by impaction of solid material, a severe post-vagotomy constriction, and most, but not all, untreated achalasias have a degree of dilatation of the esophagus that will accommodate 100 ml or more. A patient may be able to drink this volume at normal speed before feeling full, and then wait many minutes to allow the esophagus to empty. Their capacity to take fluid in this way may cause misunderstandings of the severity or the obstruction. When these subjects regurgitate, the volume returned has been estimated as usually 30 ml or more, whereas the amount regurgitated when the esophagus is not dilated is less than 30 ml, and usually the volume just swallowed.

1.1.2.2. The Taste

The taste provides some information. If the regurgitate clearly tastes of vomit or gastric contents or is very bitter or burns, then it must have been in the stomach. Moreover, there cannot be a completely closed obstruction and the gastroesophageal closing mechanism must be ineffective. The taste of gastric contents must and can usually be distinguished from the taste of decomposing residues in a pharyngeal pouch or in the esophagus obstructed by carcinoma or achalasia. Regurgitation of tasteless mucus or of undigested food or fluid with its own natural taste suggests obstruction, although in those who ruminate shortly after a meal the regurgitated material may come from the proximal part of the stomach apparently unmixed with the gastric juices.

1.1.2.3. The Content

The content of the regurtitate may be helpful. If bile is present, the material must have come from the stomach. Large quantities of clear mucus suggests achalasia or total obstruction with much salivation.

1.1.2.4. The Timing

The timing of regurgitation after swallowing gives some indication of the nature of the lesion. If food impacts on a peptic or early carcinomatous stricture and an attempt is made to push it on by drinking, regurgitation may follow within 15 to 30 sec. If the interval is 30 to 90 sec carcinoma or achalasia are more likely, and if the interval is longer than 90 sec or apparently unrelated to swallowing, then hiatus hernia reflux, rumination or pouch is more likely.

1.1.2.5. The Association with Position

The association of regurgitation with position may distinguish a stricture from other causes. A peptic or early carcinomatous stricture allows liquids to pass easily. On the other hand, solids either pass, or impact and regurgitation follows within a few seconds. There is no residue in the esophagus, so that if the subjects bends over or lies down the only regurgitation possible is of gastric contents. Some patients with a greatly dilated achalasic esophagus will regurgitate if they bend over or lie down, but this is unusual because bending or lying does not increase the volume of the contents of the esophagus. When there is severe obstruction the continual swallowing of saliva during sleep may result in regurgitation during the night. Regurgitation occurring on bending or lying and especially after a meal is most likely to result from severe gastroesophageal reflux.

1.1.3. Pain

Pain in esophageal disorders may characterize the lesion.

1.1.3.1. The Distribution

The distribution of the pain is unhelpful because it is similar in all esophageal disorders. Heartburn from gastroesophageal reflux and the pain of food impaction are commonly felt retrosternally, but when severe they may radiate to one or both sides of the neck, the floor of the mouth, the lower jaw, up to the ear, to the shoulders, and into the arms, mimicking the pain of myocardial ischemia. Radiation to the teeth and gums of the lower jaw has resulted in the erroneous removal of teeth. There is probably a rough correlation between severity of pain and the extent of radiation. The spontaneous pain of achalasia may be very severe and commonly radiates to the neck and shoulders.

1.1.3.2. The Character

The character of the pain is equally unhelpful and may be misleading. Many "pains" in the chest are interpreted by the patient as "indigestion" which is not considered by them to be a pain, but might be described as "heartburn". When questioned they can distinguish between the discomfort of bolus obstruction, the sensation of reflux when bending, and the effect of drinking hot fluids or alcohol, although all may be described as "burning". Similarly, the patient with achalasia may recognize four different discomforts: that of food held up at the sphincter, that of "pressure" or "bursting" when drinking or eating too quickly, that of gastroesophageal reflux if it occurs, and that of the spontaneous pain characteristic of achalasia.

1.1.3.3. The Timing

The timing of the pain or discomfort is the most discriminating feature. Pain which (a) occurs only after swallowing solids, (b) is always within 10 sec of swallowing, (c) is associated with a sensation that food is not moving on, and continues until the sense of obstruction is relieved either by the regurgitation of the obstructed bolus, or its passage through the obstruction, means stricture, either benign or malignant. Two other syndromes overlap and may be confused with stricture, namely obstruction due to an extrinsic mass and the "tender" esophagus. The extrinsic mass may be a benign or malignant tumor which displaces the esophagus but does not invade the wall, or may be a grossly enlarged heart chamber, usually the left atrium. The difference between these syndromes and stricture is that although there is a painful sensation of food moving on slowly, the food bolus will always move on. The "tender" esophagus may be various degrees of esophagitis or the nonspecific variety described in detail later under functional dysphagia. In all examples the pain begins within a few seconds of swallowing the bolus.

Retrosternal discomfort or pain which is present all the time, but which is worsened by swallowing solids or hot liquids or alcohol or fruit juices indicates esophagal ulceration, almost always consequent upon severe peptic esophagitis. Occasionally it develops in carcinoma of the esophagus.

Retrosternal pain provoked by swallowing solids or hot or cold liquids, developing abruptly with or without previous symptoms of gastroesophageal reflux and lasting days or weeks, is likely to be acute monilial esophagitis or occasionally the "tender" esophagus syndrome.

Pain of esophageal distribution, which comes on at any time of day or night, without relationship to posture or movement or to eating or drinking, which is often very severe, and lasts for a few seconds to many minutes, is almost pathognomonic of achalasia. It is often thought to be more frequent at night because it wakes the subject, is usually attributed to "indigestion" or duodenal ulcer (3 of 180 patients with achalasia mistakenly had vagotomy or partial gastrectomy for this pain), and is often treated, unsuccessfully, with alkalis and antisecretory or "antispasmodic" drugs. The pain is commonly stopped by one or two swallows of cold water. It's cause is unknown although it has been called "spasm". During repeated fluoroscopy of 200 subjects with achalasia the author has watched a total of many hours of vigorous abnormal esophageal motility that was painless, and on the one occasion when pain developed at the time of screening, the amount and type of movement was not obviously different. The pain often precedes the development of dysphagia and regurgitation by many months, is almost always reduced in severity and frequency by a cardio-myotomy, but may continue for many years after cardiomyotomy when it is again often mistaken for reflux.

Pain of esophageal distribution which may occur apparently spontaneously an hour or more after meals, but is consistently provoked by bending, or lying flat, or turning on to one side, particularly the right, in bed, or by sobbing or breathing deeply, or by certain types of exertion, involving contraction of the abdominal wall muscles, and is relieved within 1 min by an adequate dose of a potent antacid, is characteristic of gastroesophageal reflux. Confirmation of the sensitivity of the esophageal mucosa is provided if hyperesthesia to heat exists; that is, the subjects finds that hot drinks are unexpectedly and unbearably hot. The mucosa is also unduly sensitive to alcoholic drinks and fruit juices. The sensation of heartburn or pain may occur in subjects whose esophagus is not abnormally sensitive to heat, or alcohol, or infused N/10 HCl.

A not uncommon syndrome of undetermined etiology, which causes much anxiety to patient and physician alike, consists of attacks of severe retrosternal pain which may radiate to the epigastrium or right hypochondrium or over the chest to the neck, occur commonly at night when the subject is asleep, and are shortly followed by vomiting which does not relieve the pain. Both pain and vomiting continue for up to several hours, abating slowly, and usually are un-affected by alkali. The electrocardiogram, pyelogram and cholecystogram are normal and the barium meal reveals nothing abnormal except a minor degree of hiatal herniation in the head-down position. The attacks are usually many months apart and the subject is otherwise well, with few if any symptoms of gastroespohageal reflux. Some episodes have been called "esophageal spasm" but there is no contraction that obstructs the flow of food or liquid, and drinking large volumes of cold water may sometimes induce relief.

1.2. Syndromes

1.2.1. "Spill-Over" and "Spill-Into" Disease

When swallowing is rapidly followed by coughing the laryngeal or tracheo-bronchial mucosa is being stimulated. Simple distension of the upper esophagus adjacent to the trachea does not seem to provoke coughing, but occasionally a subject with a large pharyngeal pouch feels a "compression" which induces a dry cough which does not seem to be due to "spill over".

Coughing is more likely to follow the swallowing of fluid than the swallowing of solid or dry food and the faster the drinking, the greater the likelihood. Saliva swallowed unconsciously in a small amount is often tolerated well. If coughing starts immediately after the pharyngeal swallow movement the lesion is causing failure of the epiglottic closure of the larynx or there is a fistula between the upper few cm of the esophagus and the trachea. Failure of the pharyngeal mechanism for closing off the larynx is almost always from either (a) upper or lower motor neuron lesions, so that there is associated dysarthria, and sometimes pharyngonasal regurgitation because the posterior nares are not closed, or (b) from muscle disease such as polymyositis, dermatomyositis, or myasthenia gravis with associated difficulty in carrying through the swallow movement and often dysarthria.

If there is delay of 1 to 10 or more seconds there are three possible causes. (a) In the early stages of a fistulous track between the esophagus and the tracheobronchial tree, fluid does not flow along the tract unless there is an adequate force behind it and an adequate quantity. There is also a finite time interval between the movement of the pharyngeal phase of swallowing and the moment when the fluid reaches a sensitive area of tracheobronchial mucosa. This fistula is nearly always the result of carcinoma of bronchus or trachea, or radiation-necrosis. (b) When there is an almost total block to solids and fluids there may be dilatation of the esophagus which will accommodate several tens of milliliters, so that the subject swallows several mouthfuls with ease and then suddenly finds that the esophagus is full to overflowing and some spill-over to the larynx is likely to occur. This may follow carcinoma of the esophagus or fundus or a severe and long post-intubation stricture. The subject is aware of the sequence and can distinguish it from the sequence of events due to fistula. Spill-over with delayed cough response is most likely to result from neoplastic involvement of the recurrent laryngeal nerve and is then associated with dysphonia. When the subject swallows a radiopaque liquid during fluoroscopy, some of the liquid is seen to enter the larynx and descend the trachea, often for several centimeters and taking several seconds to do so, before the cough reflux is elicited. The likely explanation is that the sensitivity of the laryngeal and adjacent tracheal mucosa is reduced and the "spill-over" is not appreciated until sensitive mucosa is reached, when coughing becomes severe. All examples examined by the author have had primary or secondary neoplastic involvement of the recurrent laryngeal nerve in the paratracheal area. The distinguishing feature of this cause is the coincident dysphonia.

1.2.2. Obstruction Syndromes

There are two main obstruction syndromes which can be characterized, the "stricture" syndrome and the "achalasia" syndrome.

1.2.2.1. The Stricture Syndrome

The stricture syndrome is that of a rigid or semi-rigid narrowing which is open and therefore allows liquid to pass through easily but obstructs solids. The rate of flow of liquid through a tube of circular cross section is approximately determined by Poiseuille's equation:

$$\text{rate} = \frac{\pi \times \text{pressure} \times \text{radius}^4}{8 \times \text{length} \times \text{coefficient of viscosity}}$$

This relationship is not difficult to apply to a short peptic stricture, and it is most unusual for these to become less than 4 mm diameter. At this bore most subjects are able to drink at a normal speed. Long post-intubation strictures and carcinomatous strictures may so reduce the rate of flow, that the rate of drinking is slowed. Because the flow is proportional to the 4th power of the radius, when the lumen is only a few mm in diameter, small reductions have a considerable effect, so that as a carcinoma grows into the lumen, drinking remains easy until, over a period of a week or two, it becomes rapidly progressively slower and then stops.

Solids become impacted at the narrowed rigid zone in proportion to their viscosity, the size of the bolus, and the diameter of the constriction. The distinction between benign and malignant stricture can frequently be made on the rate of change of the symptoms. The benign stricture begins as a circumferential increase in resistance to stretch, at the junction of squamous and columnar epithelium, which slowly and intermittently increases over months or years. The length is 2 to 10 mm and the bore is circular. There is an early awareness of the resistance to stretch by a large bolus, so that obstruction occurs only occasionally and the rate of change is slow. The bolus is usually forced through for months or years and fluids flow normally for an indefinite period.

By contrast the malignant lesion starts from a point source and grows round the lumen and up and down. The remaining flexible wall stretches to allow the bolus to pass until about two thirds of the circumference are infiltrated. Once bolus obstruction has occurred it is likely to re-occur with increasing ease as the growth extends around and along the lumen. From the time of the first episode of bolus obstruction there is a rapid progression in the difficulty with food. Often the subject will say that the food stuck at one meal and at every meal thereafter unless he was progressively more careful to cut up or chew his food, and that within two weeks he had given up solid food. Within a few weeks liquids pass more slowly, and from the time that he is aware that he cannot drink at a normal speed, it is only a matter of a few weeks before he can hardly drink at all. The length of the malignant stricture is 20 to 100 mm, the bore is irregular and cauliflower-like on section. A fundal carcinoma obstructing the esophagogastric junction tends to produce symptoms abruptly, but they progress much more slowly. They are more severe than those of benign stricture and there may be some slowing of the speed of drinking, but, in contrast to esophageal carcinoma, many months may elapse before there is severe obstruction to fluids.

Peptic stricture is commonly associated with sensitivity to hot drinks and alcohol, whereas carcinoma is rarely so. Pain is usual when food impacts on a peptic structure. It is common in the early stages of cancer, but often becomes less as the lesion progresses, perhaps because the mucosal receptors are destroyed and perhaps because the power of the peristaltic wave to drive the bolus into the stricture is impaired.

1.2.2.2. The Achalasia Syndrome

The achalasia syndrome is characterized by the properties of a tube closed by an elastic process, that is, the closure is not rigid and may be forced open by intraesophageal pressure high enough to let liquids and solids through slowly. Both liquids and solids are difficult from the beginning. When the patient presents with this pattern the distinction between achalasia and carcinoma can again be made with considerable accuracy from the pattern of symptoms. Achalasia usually causes difficulty with liquids and solids from the beginning, whereas carcinoma causes difficulty with solids for a few weeks before there is any awareness of difficulty with liquids. Achalasia is frequently associated with the characteristic spontaneous pain (see above), whereas in carcinoma the pain is clearly associated with bolus obstruction. The patient with achalasia frequently has a history of many months' duration before he presents to the doctor, and is still in good general health. The patient with carcinoma usually has a history of only a few weeks.

1.2.3. The So-Called "Functional" Dysphagias

This group includes difficulties in swallowing for which no demonstrable pathological cause is found and a presumptive diagnosis of "psychogenic" is made. There are undoubtedly examples of hysterical dysphagia and there is a syndrome of a sensation of a "lump in the throat", or "tightness in the throat", or "dryness in the throat" which comes on when a person is frightened. The syndrome is intermittent and clearly related to stress.

There are several syndromes, however, which are superficially similar but have a definable organic cause if examined in detail. Errors in diagnosis most commonly arise because the nature, timing and associations of the sensations complained of are not determined accurately, because radiology is very limited in its usefulness, and because the thyroid cartilage and suprasternal notch area are points of reference for sensation provoked by stimulation of distant receptors (see above).

Pain, or tenderness, or discomfort, which is present all the time and *worsened* by swallowing movements should be considered organic and probably inflamma- tory, possibly neoplastic. Pain or tenderness or discomfort which is not present when the subject is not swallowing, but occurs with each swallow movement should be considered to be organic. Inflamed lymph glands, an inflamed or tender oral or pharyngeal mucosa, sometimes associated with impaired secretion of saliva or a low serum iron or low serum vitamin B_{12} are common causes. An uncommon cause is a viral thyroiditis associated with measles, mumps, or influenza. In addition to pain, there is local tenderness over the thyroid gland.

The painless sensation of a "crumb" in the throat that cannot be swallowed away, which is continually present but unnoticed during eating and drinking, is commonly caused by lumps of debris in mucosal crypts overlying lymphatic tissue, e.g., the tonsil. Careful examination of the pharyngeal mucosa is necessary to exclude evidence of carcinoma. Considerable enlargement of the tonsil, or neoplastic tissue will be appreciated during swallowing.

The sensation of "a lump" or "something to swallow away", or "food sticking in the back of the throat" or other description, which is *not* present while eating or drinking, but develops 10 min to 2 hours *after* eating and then persists for 30 min or more is almost characteristic of the hiatus hernia-reflux syndrome. The essential question to ask is whether the sensation comes on some- time *after* eating and is absent at the time of eating and drinking. Usually other symptoms of gastroesophageal reflux occur. The radiological demonstration of hiatal herniation or reflux may require special maneuvers such as swallowing barium when tilted 10° head-down, or toe-touching, because the symptoms may occur when only minor degrees of herniation or reflux are demonstrable. It seems likely that the sensation in the throat is a referred sensation or a paresthesia arising from stimulation of the lower esophageal mucosa.

The sensation that food is sticking in the neck may be an incorrect localization of a site of obstruction (see above) and a radiological or endoscopic examination which does not include the whole pharynx, esophagus and upper part of stomach cannot be relied upon to exclude an obstructing or sensitive lesion which produces symptoms located in the neck or "throat".

Inability to swallow, or difficulty in initiating a swallow may be the result of neural or muscular damage so that initiation, power, or coordination of the swallowing sequence is disturbed, or the result of cortical inhibition because of loss of appetite, distaste for food, fear of the consequences of eating, depression, or an hysterical aversion. The food is chewed, and rolled round in the mouth but the subject declares that he "just can't seem to swallow it" and will often eventually spit it out. There is no dysarthria, chewing movements are normal, saliva is usually swallowed unconsciously without any difficulty, and often drinking occurs normally. The initiation, motor, and coordination processes of swallowing are, therefore, intact.

Some subjects complain of a sensation of being choked, or that the windpipe is being compressed when they lie down or turn on to one side, or when they eat or drink fast. When associated with posture the symptom is highly suggestive of gastroesophageal reflux; when associated with drinking or eating it is highly suggestive of an obstructive lesion such as achalasia or carcinoma of the body of the stomach, in which no clear sense of impaction of food occurs. Barium swallow and esophagoscopy may be normal when this is "gastric" dysphagia.

The "tender esophagus" syndrome is a source of anxiety and frustration for the physician and much distress to the patient. The main complaint is that all solids cause pain or discomfort as they pass through the esophagus as though passing over a raw or inflamed area. There is no real obstruction to their passage and no sense of impaction. Drinking will speed the transit but increase the pain. Drinking slowly in the absence of solids does not provoke pain, but drinking quickly may do so. Commonly, but not always, hot liquids feel excessively hot. Sometimes there is an abrupt outset of pain 3 to 4 sec after swallowing the bolus. Pain persists until the bolus is felt to pass the sensitive area, and sometimes a soreness perists for minutes or hours. There may or may not be symptoms provoked by bending or lying. Esophagoscopy is repeatedly normal with no sense of a constricting process and a normal looking mucosa. Fluoroscopy with liquid barium fails to reveal any lesion of the peristaltic wave, the mucosa, or the size and shape of the lumen. Screening with a radiopaque solid bolus, however, shows that pain develops consistently when the bolus reaches a particular point, and stops when the bolus moves on. The commonest sites at which pain develops are just proximal to the arch of the aorta and the lowest few cm of the esophagus. Because all routine methods of investigation do not reveal any abnormality and the patient has no other signs, his symptoms are frequently called hysterical or functional. Most examples that the author has seen have been unhappy, but their mental state may be the consequence of lack of effective treatment and sympathy together with continuing discomfort and anxiety. The condition may continue for months or years.

2. History

In the preceding paragraphs the discriminating symptoms and their patterns have been described for a variety of causes of dysphagia. Because the patterns are characteristic, it is possible to make an accurate diagnosis of the cause of the symptoms from an accurate history in almost all cases. Because of the limitations of esophagoscopy and radiology, and the incompleteness of some radiological examinations, the history is often more accurate and informative than radiology or esophagoscopy. Esophagoscopy may be reported as normal in early or mild achalasia, and in many examples of ring stricture, early peptic stricture and almost always in "tender esophagus". The correlation between esophagoscopic "esophagitis" and the patient's symptoms is poor. Radiography of the esophagus in the erect position will not infrequently miss mild or early achalasia, ring stricture, "tender esophagus", hiatus hernia, mid and low peptic strictures and fundal carcinoma. The patient is correct more often than the physician who can be correct more often than the radiologist who can be correct more often than the esophagoscopist. Radiology and esophagoscopy should always include special techniques aimed at explaining the details of a patient's symptoms, which must therefore be clearly defined before the special examination.

The following scheme summarizes a sequence of questioning which in most instances will make the diagnosis at the first interview so that confirmatory questions and investigations may be applied.

2.1. Pharyngeal Problems

These can be grouped as pouch, stricture or web, neuromuscular and fistula (see Fig. 35).

2.1.1. Pouch

The characteristics are that sometimes *both food and liquid* are swallowed out of the mouth beyond awareness, but some returns *immediately*, that is, without a definable interval, or they return *minutes or hours later* unchanged, particularly if the patient lies down or turns the head to one side or bends the head over to the left.

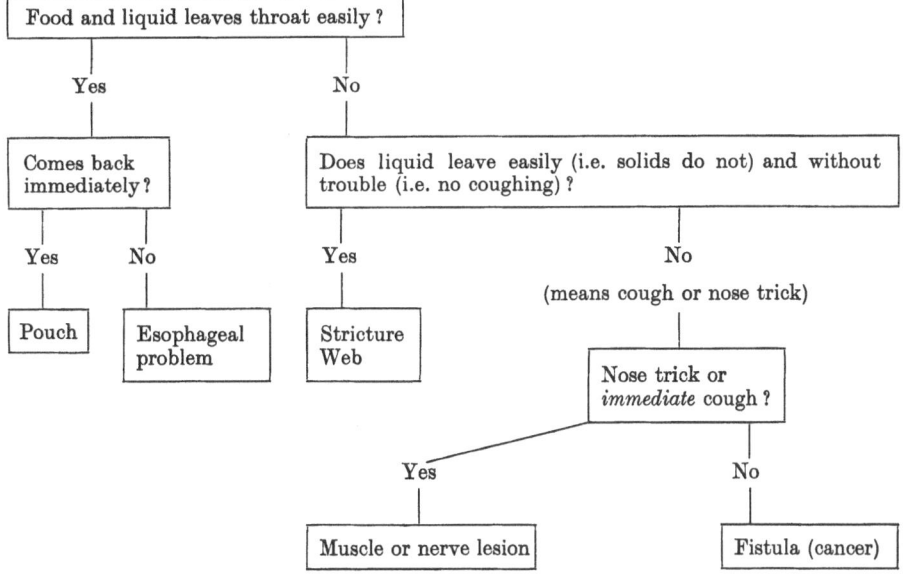

Pharyngeal problems

Lesions include pouch, stricture or web, neuro-muscular lesion and fistula

Pouch: Food and liquid leave mouth and return immediately

Stricture
Web   } Liquid flows easily; solids impact or are rejected within 1 sec of swallow

Muscular   } Fail to close nose from pharynx = "nose trick"; fail to close larynx from
Neurological } pharynx = cough (cough caused also by fistula)

Fig. 35

2.1.2. Stricture or Web

Whether benign or malignant an obstruction in the pharynx allows fluids to pass (at least for many months) without returning. Solids are held up partially or completely and rejected within 1 sec of swallowing; commonly the solid cannot be swallowed out of the pharynx beyond the area of awareness.

2.1.3. Muscular and Neural

The symptoms are of lack of power to project the bolus into the esophagus and of failure to close the pharynx from the nose or larynx. There is no sense of obstruction to solid or liquid and no return from the esophagus. In both primary muscle disease and neural disorder there is usually associated dysarthria, and other symptoms and signs in addition to dysphagia will be present. Coughing *immediately* upon swallowing, that is, without a detectable interval, means spill-over because of failure to close the larynx. Regurgitation through the nose means neural or muscular failure except when widespread destruction prevents proper sealing. Cough which begins several seconds after drinking means fistula or recurrent laryngeal nerve damage (see above).

2.2. Esophageal Problems
(Fig. 36)

If, therefore, food and drink leave the mouth without difficulty and do not return for at least 2 sec, the problem is esophageal (except for pouch; see above).

Esophageal problems

Stricture = Open tube narrowed by *rigid* process; liquids flow through easily; solids impact with pain; no pain except when solids stuck.

Achalasia or "diffuse spasm" = Closed by elastic contraction of sphincter but can be opened by pressure; both liquids and solids slow to move on; no impact sensation or pain; commonly spontaneous pain.

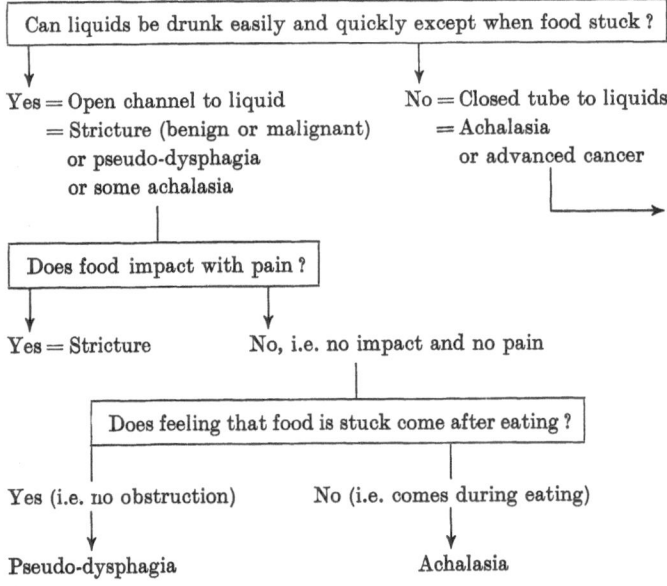

Fig. 36

Cancer and achalasia

In both, the tube is partially or completely closed to liquids.
Achalasia = Slow progression in months; liquids and solids always equally difficult; no
impact pain at beginning; commonly spontaneous pain; rarely period when liquids easy and
solids stick.

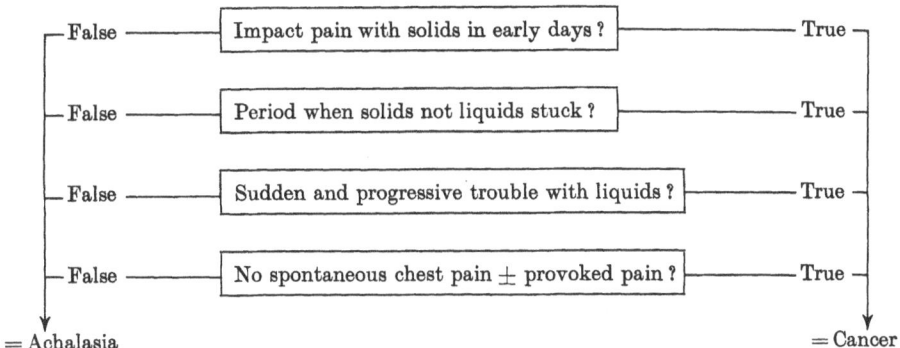

Fig. 37

Esophageal problems are grouped into (1) the *stricture* type characterized by the open tube narrowed by a rigid process through which fluids flow easily (at least in the earlier stages), solids impact with an abrupt sensation of pain or discomfort, 2nd there is no pain except when solids stick, unless there is an additional lesion; at) the *achalasia* type (which includes diffuse spasm, hypertensive sphincter, severe post-vagotomy and post hernial repair dysphagia), characterized by a tube which is closed to both liquids and solids, but the closure is elastic and can be opened by increasing intraesophageal pressure. Both liquids and solids are therefore slow to move on, there is no impact sensation with pain, but there is spontaneous pain; (3) the *advanced cancer* type characterized by a tube closed by a rigid material which obstructs the flow of liquid and solid and cannot be opened by building up intraesophageal pressure.

The distinction between (1) and (2 and 3) is made by the question "Can liquids be drunk as easily as normal except when food is stuck?". The answer "yes" means an open channel to liquid, that is, a stricture (benign or malignant) or pseudo-dysphagia or some examples of achalasia in which habit or the volume of the esophagus allows drinking to occur rapidly. These are distinguished by the question "Does food impact with pain?" The answer "yes" means stricture and the distinction must then be made between benign or malignant (see below). The answer "no", that is, there is no impact pain, is followed by the question "Does the feeling that food is stuck come some time after eating?" The answer "yes" to this means there is no true obstruction and the patient has one of the "pseudo-dysphagias". The answer "yes", that is, the sense of obstruction occurs during eating, means achalasia.

The answer "no" to the question "Can liquids be drunk easily?" means the tube is partially or completely closed to liquids, that is, the problem is either achalasia or advanced cancer. These two may be distinguished by four questions designed to bring out the differences in the natural history of the two conditions (Fig. 37). No question will give an absolutely reliable answer but the answer "yes" in each case gives a likelihood in favor of cancer and "no" in favor of achalasia.

Benign and malignant stricture

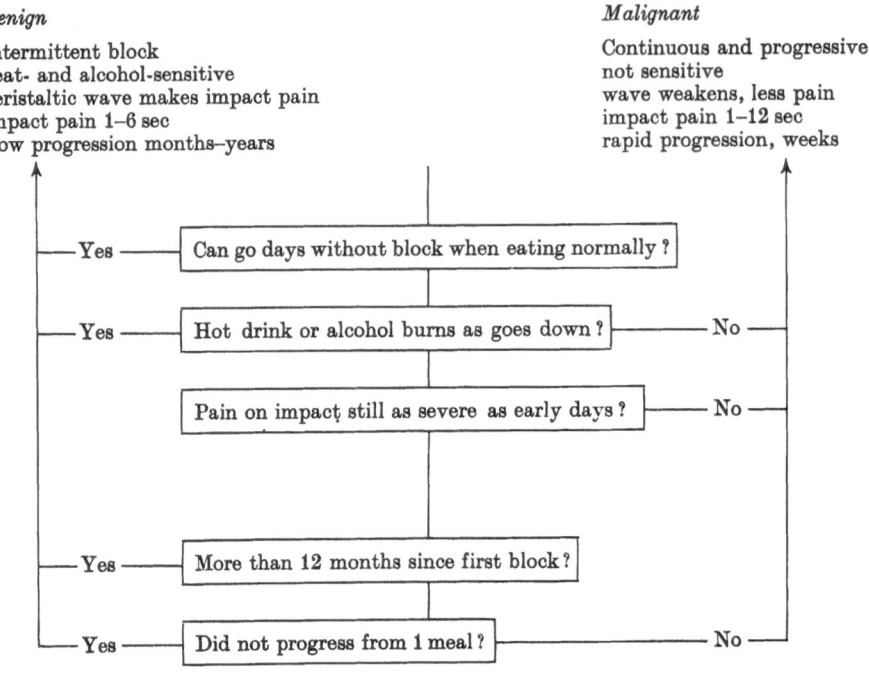

Benign

Intermittent block
heat- and alcohol-sensitive
peristaltic wave makes impact pain
impact pain 1–6 sec
slow progression months–years

Malignant

Continuous and progressive
not sensitive
wave weakens, less pain
impact pain 1–12 sec
rapid progression, weeks

—Yes —— | Can go days without block when eating normally ? |

—Yes —— | Hot drink or alcohol burns as goes down ? |—— No —

| Pain on impact still as severe as early days ? |—— No —

—Yes —— | More than 12 months since first block? |

└—Yes —— | Did not progress from 1 meal? |—— No —

Fig. 38

"Was there impact pain in the early days of the trouble?" asks whether there was a sensation of impact which caused pain or discomfort, and either still occurs or the pain or discomfort is now less or absent. This sequence is strongly in favour of cancer. If there has never been any clear-cut impact sensation even at the beginning the diagnosis is almost certainly achalasia.

"Was there a period when solids stuck or impacted but liquids were as easy as normal?" asks whether there was a time when solids obstructed in a rigid narrowing but the tube was open and liquids flowed easily but now there is slowing of the flow of liquids. This sequence is strongly in favor of cancer. If the awareness of difficulty for both solids and liquids came on about the same time, achalasia is a much more likely cause than cancer.

The question "Has there been a sudden and progressive trouble with liquids in the last few weeks?" is not entirely independent of the last question but enquires whether the difficulty with liquids developed progressively to a severe degree over a period of only a few weeks and had not been previously noticed. This sequence is almost characteristic of cancer, either in the lumen or around it. It is rare for dysphagia for liquids to become steadily and progressively more severe in only a few weeks in achalasia.

The question "No spontaneous chest pain . . ." enquires about the existence of *spontaneous* pain. Spontaneous pain is common in achalasia and rare in carcinoma. There may or may not be associated pain or discomfort which is provoked by bending or drinking or eating solids, but this *provoked* pain may occur in a variety of conditions and does not discriminate. Hence the importance of ascer-

Scheme of questions to diagnose the cause of dysphagia

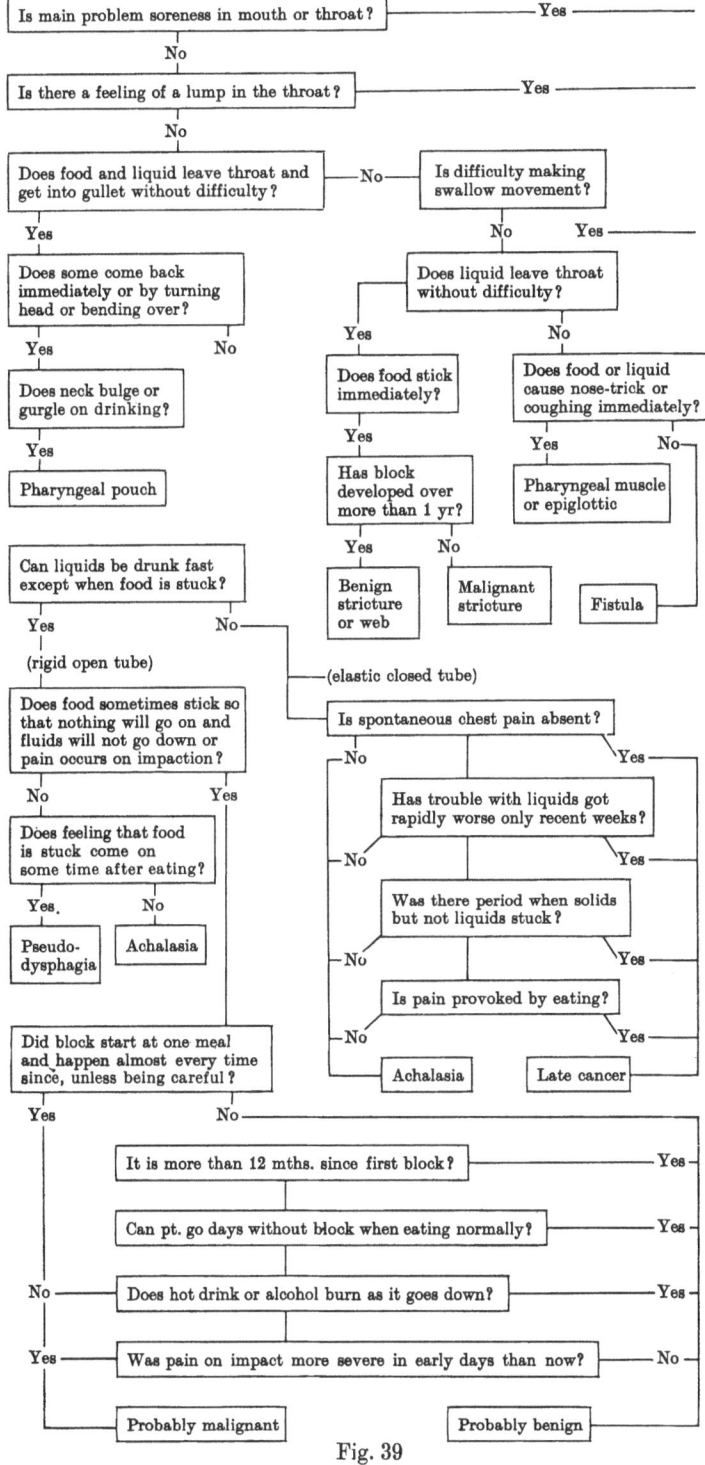

Fig. 39

taining whether it is spontaneous, and the arrangement of the question so that false means achalasia.

The distinction between *benign* and *malignant* stricture again depends on a group of questions (Fig. 38). "Can you go for days without a block when eating normally?" enquires about the severity of the block. The benign ring stricture or lower esophageal web is characterized by its wide bore and infrequency of bolus obstruction so that a long history of intermittent block is much in favor of a mild degree of benign stricturing. The answer "no" is not very helpful because both benign and malignant strictures may cause block to solid food at every meal.

"Does a hot drink or alcohol burn as it goes down?" enquires whether esophagitis or mucosal inflammatory ulceration is present. The answer "yes" is strongly in favor of a benign stricture and the answer "no" is strongly in favor of a cancer, but occasionally a cancerous stricture is sensitive, and sometimes an old benign stricture with healed overlying mucosa is insensitive.

"Is pain on impact still as severe as in early days?" relates to the reduction in pain on impact which sometimes develops in cancer, perhaps because of the loss of the peristaltic wave force above the cancer, or due to the destruction of mucosal endings. Care must be taken that this reduction in pain is not simply a consequence of being more careful about what is eaten. If pain on impact is as severe as in earlier days the answer is unhelpful since both benign or malignant lesions may be present.

"Is it more than 12 months since the first sensation of block?" relates to the rapid progression of dysphagia due to cancer. The answer "yes" means a benign lesion except in an occasional example of fundal carcinoma where no other evidence may be available for as long as 18 months. If less than 12 months have elapsed since the first block the lesion may be benign or malignant.

"Did not progress from 1 meal?" again refers to the rapid rate of progression in the annular variety of cancer. (Plaques developing in a dilated or atonic presbyesophagus may not cause dysphagia because they do not cause obstruction.) One of the characteristics of annular carcinoma is that once obstruction to food has occurred there is a rapid worsening almost from meal to meal, whereas the benign stricture may be painful from almost one meal but the degree of obstruction increases much more slowly. If dysphagia did start at one meal and progress from that meal, cancer is very likely, whereas if the dysphagia has been present for more than 4 weeks and is not progressing, a benign stricture is more likely, although dysphagia from cancer of the fundus may not progress for many months, until there is a sudden and rapid increase so that dysphagia for liquids may be present within a few weeks.

Such a scheme of questions can be run together in the form of Fig. 39, which provides a diagnostic tree for most causes of dysphagia. Careful attention to the details of the symptomatology will not infrequently provide the correct answer when radiology or esophagoscopy fail to do so. In the author's experience the symptom pattern has been especially useful in the diagnosis of early achalasia, of carcinoma of the fundus, of ring stricture, and "tender esophagus", and has made a precise diagnosis when routine radiology and esophagoscopy have been reported as normal.

Radiological Examination of the Esophagus

J. Pringot and E. Ponette

With 72 Figures

If the radiological examination of the esophagus has been improved in recent years and has led to a more accurate diagnosis of esophageal diseases, this progress is due mainly to the use of improved equipment, i.e. the image intensifier and related techniques. Another important factor in this progress has been the correlation of radiological, manometric, endoscopic and anatomical observations, which has resulted in a better understanding of the functional phenomena and a more accurate interpretation of new and old X-ray images. Recent advances in diagnostic radiology of the esophagus have been reviewed by several authors (Wolf and Khilnani, 1966; Kramer, 1968; Kaufmann, 1969; Wolf, 1969; Pope, 1970).

The pharynx is anatomically distinct from the esophagus; however, the functions of esophagus and pharynx are so well integrated that the technique of radiological examination of the pharynx will be included in this chapter.

1. The Radiological Technique

1.1. Equipment

1.1.1. The Standard Diagnostic X-Ray Unit

A diagnostic X-ray unit should offer optimal technical conditions for the examination. Therefore, the equipment of a standard X-ray unit should comprise (1) a tilt table which permits to examine the patient in vertical, horizontal and head-down position of 15°; (2) a fluoroscopic filming device designed for both fluoroscopy and spot filming under fluoroscopic control; (3) an image intensifier which permits special fluoroscopic and television techniques; (4) a powerful generator for high voltage radiography at short exposure time and (5) an automatic exposure control system.

Two types of tilt table are used for gastrointestinal examinations (Figs. 40, 41). Both have advantages and drawbacks. The conventional table supports the X-ray tube under, and the fluoroscopic filming device in front of the table top. The main advantages of this system are the direct contact with the patient, the possibility of performing compression in prone position and of palpating with the hand under fluoroscopic control. The spot film device, equipped with an image intensifier, however, is heavier and less handy than the simple fluoroscopic screen. The main disadvantage of the conventional system is that a second tube is needed for Bucky work on the same table and that filming with the additional overhead tube must be performed without fluoroscopic control. The second, more recent type of table supports the spot film device under and the X-ray tube on top of the table and requires a closed circuit television chain for fluoroscopy. It was originally designed for remote control and remote fluoroscopy

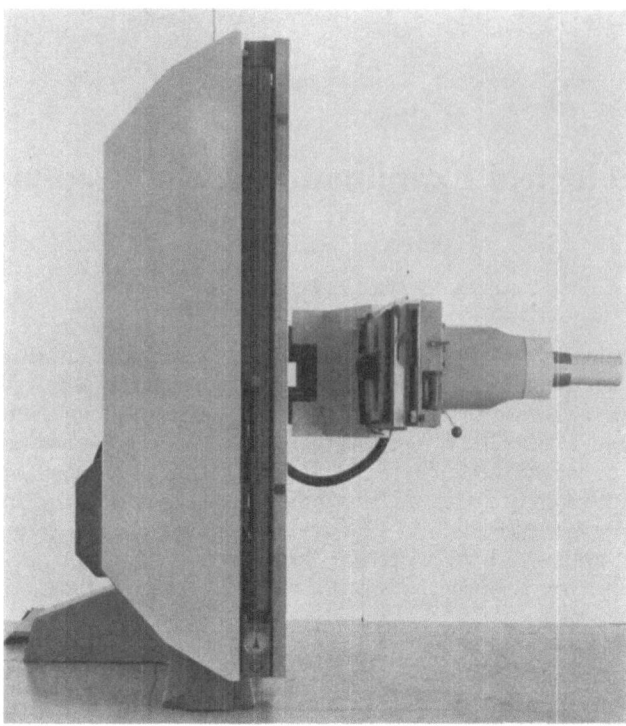

Fig. 40. So-called conventional type of tilt table; the X-ray tube is attached below and the fluoroscopic filming device in front of the table top

in order to reduce the radiation hazard for the radiologist (Jutras and Duckett, 1958). The main advantages of this system are that Bucky films can be taken under fluoroscopic control and that the X-ray tube can be angulated. When the patient is in prone, right anterior oblique position, a caudal angulation of the tube offers a better fluoroscopic approach to the esophagogastric junction because overlapping of the terminal esophagus by the stomach is avoided (Berridge, 1971). However, as a consequence of the remote control, compression can be done only in a rectilinear direction and with the patient in supine position. The distance between tube focus and film is greater than with the conventional system and therefore the exposure under otherwise identical conditions has to be longer. The main disadvantage of this newer type of table is the relative inaccessibility of the patient during fluoroscopy, due to the radiation hazard. It means a delay in positioning of patients particularly when they are severely ill or helpless, an increased duration of fluoroscopy and a diminished possibility of examination under compression and palpation. Obviously these drawbacks apply mainly to the examination of the abdominal portion of the gastrointestinal tract. Pharynx and esophagus can be examined quite satisfactorily. This type of table is well suited for combined radiological and manometric or esophagoscopic techniques.

The modern spot film device is automatized and allows an easy selection of the proper film size. Serial films can be taken under fluoroscopic control and even long esophageal segments can be filmed in successive phases of filling

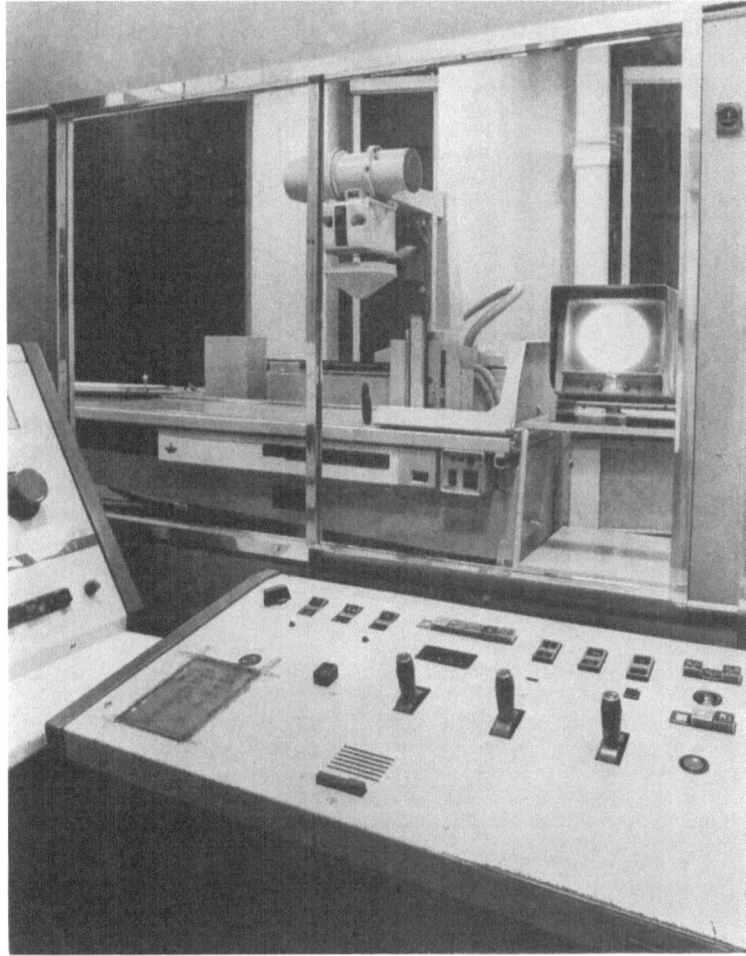

Fig. 41. X-ray table with spot filming device under, and X-ray tube in front of the table top

and contraction. The system, however, remains too slow to record fast changes. If the spot film device is designed for films not larger than 24×30 cm, the Bucky technique must be used for films of greater size, which are often wanted by surgeons and radiotherapists for localization of esophageal lesions.

Fluoroscopy of the gastrointestinal tract is almost always performed by means of an X-ray image intensifier (WOLF and KHILNANI, 1966). The four major reasons for using this system are (1) the ability to observe details with greater precision and to recognize patterns more rapidly by utilizing high resolution cone vision; (2) the convenience of being able to conduct fluoroscopic examination without adaptation to the dark; (3) the reduced amount of radiation to the patient and (4) the possibility of utilizing the techniques derived from the image intensifier. These changes in the technique of fluoroscopy have markedly increased the diagnostic accuracy of the radiological examination and have made it possible to supplement or change the conventional methods of spot filming.

1.1.2. The Image Intensifier

Intensification of the X-ray image can be obtained by two different systems. The fluoroscopic screen can be replaced by an image intensifier tube sensitive to X-rays (Fig. 42). In this conventional X-ray intensifier the fluoroscopic screen

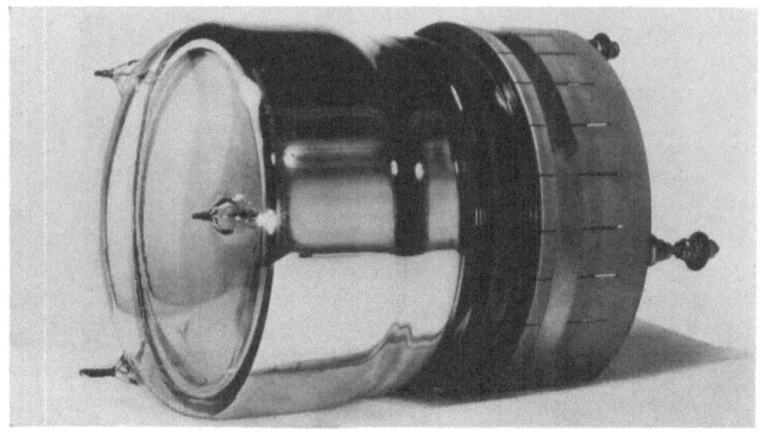

A

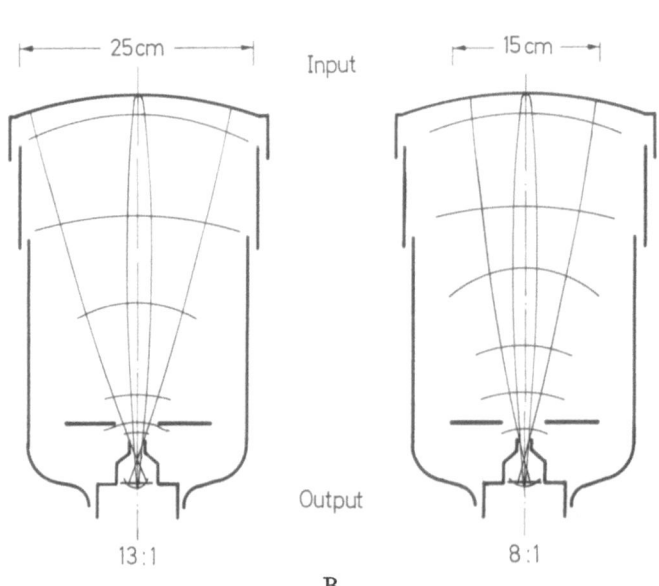

B

Fig. 42. A Outside view of X-ray image intensifier. B Scheme illustrating the principle of a dual-mode X-ray image intensifier

is incorporated in the tube. The fluoroscopic screen can also be coupled optically with a light amplifier tube. This second system is called Cinelix-Delcalix (Fig. 43). In both systems the method of X-ray image intensification is identical; the X-ray image is converted into a light image by a fluorescent screen and the light image is intensified by the same type of light amplifier (TER-POGOSSIAN, 1967).

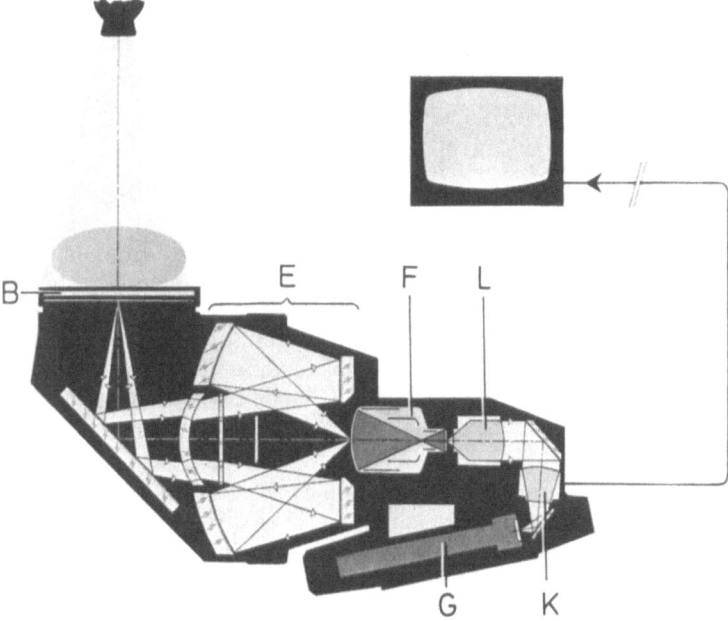

Fig. 43. Schematic representation of the electron-optical image intensifier system of Delcalix. The light image delivered by the fluorescent screen (B) is projected by means of a Brouwer's concentric mirror system (E) on the photocathode of the light image intensifier (F) and is then intensified and displayed on the screen of a TV monitor (L, K, G)

An X-ray image intensifier system can be characterized by (1) the luminance gain it produces, (2) the diameter of the input fluorescent screen, (3) the possibility of electron-optical magnification, (4) the diameter of the output screen and (5) the quality of the delivered image, i.e. the resolution in lines pairs per cm (lp/cm).

The luminance gain of an X-ray intensifier is about 5000 to 15000 times greater than that of a conventional fluorescent screen at the same exposure rate, so that this is no longer a limiting factor in an image intensifier system. The most important property of the image intensifier is the effective absorption of the input radiation which reduces the quantum noise to a minimum and results in pictures of high contrast and high resolution.

The diameter of the input fluorescent screen determines the diameter of the X-ray field. The gain of an intensifier is inversely proportional to the diameter of the input fluorescent screen. The diameter of the input screen in the commonly used X-ray image intensifier is 6 or 7 in. and 9 or 10 in. This corresponds to a fluoroscopic field of 15 or 17 cm for the small intensifier and a field of 22 or 25 cm for the larger intensifier.

The 9 or 10 in. dual-mode intensifier permits electron-optical magnification by a factor of approximately 1.7 (HELLEKAMP and ENDLICH, 1965), thus resulting in a reduction of field to a diameter of 5 and 6 in. resp. When an electron-optical magnification system is used, the brightness of the output screen is reduced by a factor of 3.3 (KUEHL and VAN OVERHAGEN, 1965). This has to be compensated either by increasing the sensitivity of the optical system, or by changing the gain of the video amplifier or by increasing the exposure rate.

The highest resolution achieved by conventional X-ray intensifiers in the center of the image is about 20 pairs of lines per cm, which was about half that of the universal intensifying screens used in radiography (Boijsen et al., 1969). The luminance gain to a level which permits high resolution cone vision is the main reason why the perceptibility of details is increased. Other characteristics of these conventional image intensifiers are a decrease in brightness gain at the periphery of the image (the so-called vignetting) and a decrease in resolution of the peripheral parts of the image due to the geometrical lay-out of the electron-optical system. This non-uniform resolution and vignetting are reduced by electron-optical magnification. The advantages of intensifiers with an input screen of small diameter are the compactness and the better performance owing to the higher resolving power. The main disadvantage is the limited field which in Europe is considered to be inadequate for general gastrointestinal examinations. The disadvantage of the dual-mode intensifier is that the electron-optical magnification and the resulting gain in resolution necessitate an increase of the input exposure rate.

The Delcalix system has a fluorescent screen with a diameter of 12.5 in., which corresponds to a fluoroscopic field of 32 cm. With electron-optical magnification this field is reduced to 20 cm. The Delcalix system has several advantages over conventional X-ray image intensifiers. The fluoroscopic screen is larger, plane and can be changed at will. The light amplifier tube of small diameter can be replaced at a low cost. This system has also some disadvantages: the apparatus is not easy to use on a conventional table, it does not offer the possibility of fluorography and the large screen results in a loss of brightness (Ter-Pogossian, 1967).

The quality and specific characteristics of the image produced by an intensifier are determined not only by its contrast and resolution and by the signal to noise ratio. Contrast and resolution can be defined by the so-called modulation transfer function (M.T.F.), which permits to represent graphically the relation between contrast and resolution (Dutreix, 1965; Hendee, 1970). The signal to noise ratio, which depends upon the effective X-ray absorption of the input screen, allows to calculate the average input exposure necessary to obtain a certain contrast. M.T.F. and signal to noise ratio are reliable criteria for the evaluation of imaging systems (Feddema et al., 1969).

Recently a new generation of image intensifiers has been introduced into clinical radiology (Kühl, 1969; Fuchs and Hofmann, 1971). The improved quality of the image delivered by these intensifiers is due to the introduction of caesium iodide fluorescent screens, which has resulted in increased resolution and increased absorption, to newly calculated electron optics and to the application of improved technology for the construction of the output screen. The resolution of the small screen image intensifier is increased from about 2 periods per mm to about 4 periods per mm and vignetting has been reduced by a factor of 3 (Kühl, 1969; Hofmann, 1972). The resolution thus approaches that of the universal film screens. The resolution at the center of the large screen dual-mode intensifier is increased to about 3 periods per mm. With the use of electron-optical magnification it is further increased up to about 4 periods per mm, which is equal to the resolution of fast film screens. Other advantages of these new image intensifiers are the better modulation transfer function over the entire frequency range, less quantum noise at lower exposure rate and a better imaging quality at high kilovoltage. Consequently the quality of the cine-, photo-fluorographic and fluoroscopic images is greatly improved (Fig. 44).

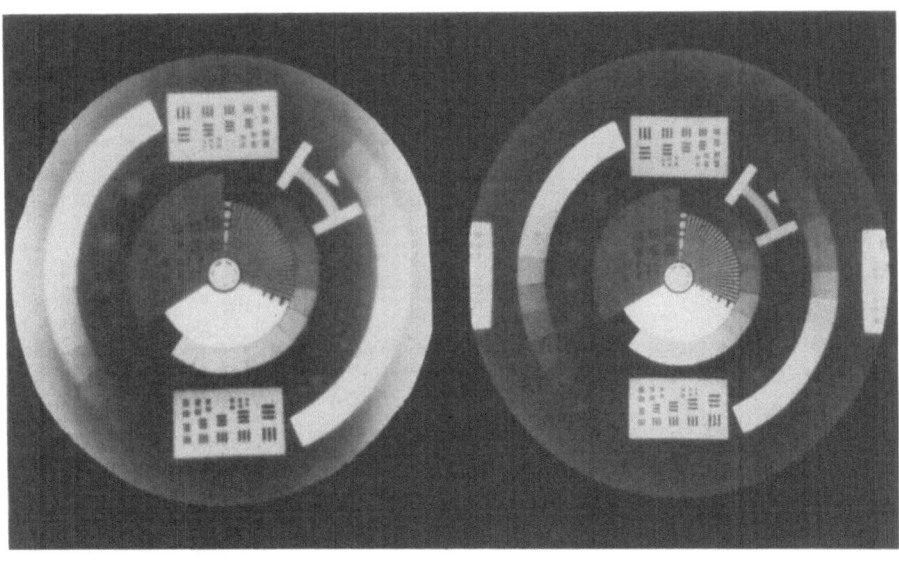

Fig. 44 A and B. Comparative test pictures made with the former (A) and with the new (B)
X-ray image intensifier

1.1.3. Television Fluoroscopy

The image produced by the intensifier can be observed either on a mirror
viewer or on the screen of a television monitor (Fig. 45). Television fluoroscopy
is preferred because it offers many advantages; the detail perceptibility of the
image displayed on the TV screen is increased; the brightness and contrast
of the image can be controlled electronically; the image is sufficiently large for
direct observation; remote monitors can be used simultaneously; finally, video-
and kinescopic recording can be performed.

A television chain consists of an electronic circuitry used in connection with
a TV camera (TER-POGOSSIAN, 1967; GEBAUER et al., 1967). The function of
the camera is to convert an optical image into a modulated electrical signal

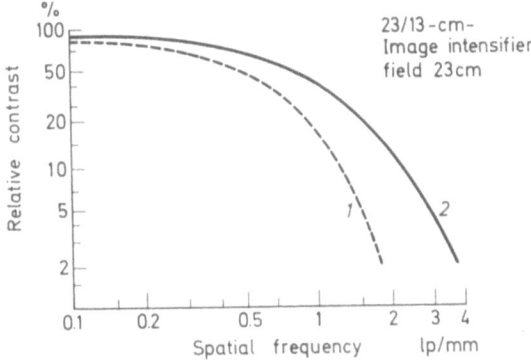

Fig. 45. Comparative modulation transfer function (M.T.F.) with the former (1) and with
the new (2) 23 cm image intensifier

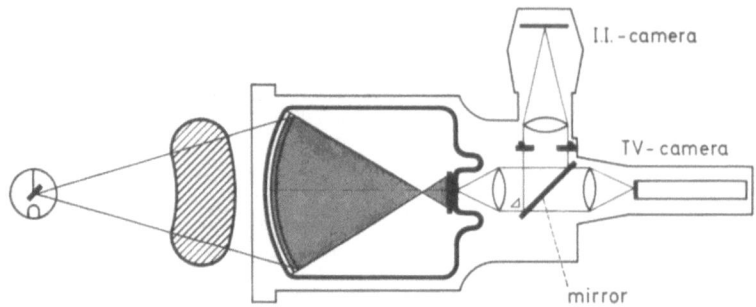

Fig. 46. Scheme of optical coupling between X-ray image intensifier, image-intensifier camera and television camera tube by means of tandem optics which permit the use of a folding mirror

—the video signal—by means of a pick-up tube. Two types of pick-up tube with different characteristics are commonly used in TV camera's, the Vidicon-Plumbicon tubes, and the super Orthicon-Isocon tubes. The tubes of the first type have a relatively simple construction and a small size, are durable and relatively inexpensive. This is the reason why they are commonly used with conventional X-ray intensifiers. In comparison to the Plumbicon tube, the Vidicon tube has a higher remanence, which results in pictures with increased movement unsharpness and a reduced noise. The Orthicon-Isocon tubes are rather cumbersome, fragile and more expensive. The Isocon tube which is used, e.g., in the Delcalix system, has a high sensitivity and a wide dynamic range enabling it to display within the same fluoroscopic field satisfactory images of both highly absorbing and more transparent parts of the body (Bouwers, 1971).

The maximal resolution which can be achieved by a television system is theoretically limited by two related factors, the number of horizontal lines scanned and the bandwidth of frequencies transmitted by the electronic circuitry. In practice television fluoroscopy, when performed with a bandwith of 5 to 6 megahertz and approximately 625 scanning lines, will not limit the performance of a modern fluoroscopic system. The real limitations are still the image intensifier, the camera pick-up tube and the monitor display tube.

Usually the TV camera is coupled to the output screen of the intensifier by means of tandem optics (Fig. 46). This type of coupling results in a slight loss of quality at the periphery of the image due to vignetting and marginal loss in the response of the optics. This drawback can be overcome by integrated coupling of output screen and TV camera by means of two fiber optic plates (Botden et al., 1969). The main advantage of the tandem optical system is the possibility of mounting 3 camera's on the intensifier: TV, cine and photospot.

1.1.4. Spot Filming

The amount of information which can be obtained in diagnostic radiography is related to detail perceptibility, which depends on the contrast and sharpness of the image. The image unsharpness is the main limiting factor in gastrointestinal films and results from motion unsharpness and geometrical unsharpness. In esophageal radiography motion unsharpness is the predominant factor and must be reduced before improvement in geometric sharpness can play a significant role.

It is generally considered useless to try to increase the image sharpness by reducing the focus size of the X-ray tube to a diameter of less than 1 mm, unless the exposure time is shorter than 0.03 sec (ELMER, 1967). Furthermore, high speed screens yield better resolution than detail screens (RAO, 1971).

In conclusion, to obtain films of satisfactory sharpness, fast screens, an exposure time of less than 0.06 sec and a focal spot size of less than 1.5 mm should be used. This requires a high capacity X-ray tube energized by a powerful 3-phase generator.

At present the exposure of the films is usually controlled by an automatic exposure timer.

1.2. The Recording Techniques Used with Image Intensifiers

There are two methods of recording the fluoroscopic images supplied by the image intensifier. (1) Photofluorography. (2) Cinefluorography.

1.2.1. Photofluorography

The fluoroscopic images are photographed by means of a still camera, either of the 70 mm or of the 100 mm format (Fig. 47). The 70 mm camera takes single and serial pictures on roll films at a frequency varying from 1 to 6 frames per second (f.p.s.). With the 100 mm camera single and serial pictures can be taken on sheet films at a frequency of 1 f.p.s. A 105 mm camera which would permit serial filming at a rate of 0.5 to 12 f.p.s. on perforated roll film has been announced.

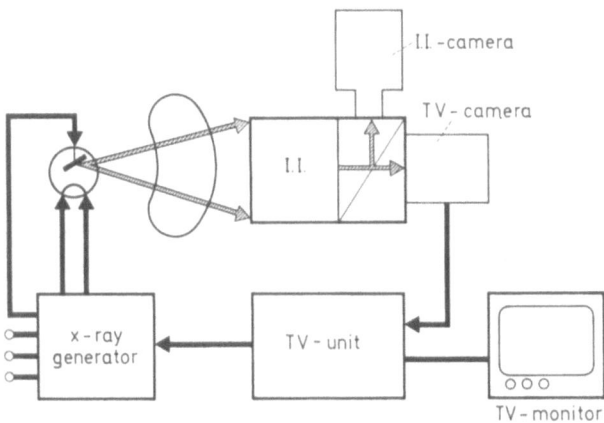

Fig. 47. Scheme of arrangement of image-intensifier fluoroscopy with an X-ray television chain

Fluorography is used in diagnostic radiology of the gastrointestinal tract for several reasons. The quality of the image is adequate to record the diagnostic information delivered by the intensifier; this technique represents a convenient technical means for spot filming and allows serial spot filming; the exposure rate per frame is reduced and hence the radiation to the patient can be reduced. Finally, small size films are easy to handle. To obtain films of good quality, optimal X-ray factors and high-definition, high-contrast films should be used. The optimal X-ray factors for the examination of the esophagus include a focus size not exceeding 1.0 or 1.2 mm, the highest milliamperage and the lowest kilovoltage which allow an exposure time of approximately 0.03 sec and excellent collimation (WOLF and KHILNANI, 1966; BODART and PRINGOT, 1968; ELMER,

1971). The presently available high-contrast films can be developed to a gamma of about 3 and yield images with a good detail perceptibility (Elmer, 1971). Detail rendering on small films can be enhanced by reducing the recorded anatomical field, using either an intensifier with an input screen of small diameter (6 or 7 cm), or an intensifier with a larger input screen and geometric or electronic magnification (Feddema, 1962; Bodart and Pringot, 1968).

It appears clearly from M.T.F. calculations and from phantom studies (Boijsen et al., 1969) that photofluorographic films of static objects cannot deliver the same amount of information as do full-size films. In practice, however, when moving organs are examined, the total amount of diagnostic information obtained by small films is at least equal to the amount of information obtained by conventional films (Wolf and Khilnani, 1966; Kaude, 1967; Bodart and Pringot, 1968).

However, the image quality of photofluorography has been remarkably improved by the new generation of intensifiers which yield an amount of information comparable to that of the presently available cassette screens (Kühl, 1969; Fuchs and Hofmann, 1971). The dose of radiation to which the patient must be exposed is at least 5 times less than with the conventional spot film technique when measured under the technical conditions (Beranbaum and Lignon, 1964; Samuel and Summerling, 1964; Bodart and Pringot, 1968; Carlsson and Kaude, 1968). However, when electron-optical magnification is used, the factor of reduction is only about 3. With the modern image intensifier the exposure rate can be reduced to 50% as compared with the former type, thanks to the increased X-ray absorption. As radiologists seem to have a natural tendency to increase the number of photofluorographic exposures, photofluorography does not necessarily lead to a considerable reduction of the irradiation of the patient. The disadvantages of photofluorography include the limitation of the field to the area covered by the intensifier, the delay in the opportunity to check the processed radiograph, and the increased care and time requested for handling the pictures (Townsend, 1969). In conclusion, photofluorography is a valuable method of spot filming, particularly useful for the examination of pharynx and esophagus, when the area to be examined is of limited size.

1.2.2. Cinefluorography

In this technique the fluoroscopic images of an image intensifier are recorded cinematographically, i.e. at frame rates corresponding to the usual standards for cinematography (Chesney and Chesney, 1971) (Fig. 47). The framing speed should be adapted to the speed of the phenomenon to be analyzed and if sharp pictures are to be obtained exposures should be short. Cinefluorography can be carried out with a standard diagnostic X-ray unit. Additional equipment, particularly useful for cinefluorography of the esophagus, is the exposure control system.

Cinefluorography can be carried out using either a non-synchronized cinefluorographic system, which generates X-rays continuously, or a synchronized system in which X-rays are produced only during the time the shutter of the cinecamera is open (Hendee, 1970).

Cinefluorography with a non-synchronized generator exposes the patient needlessly to X-rays during the time the camera shutter is closed (Fig. 48A). The heat storage capacity of the X-ray tube is rapidly exceeded, which limits each cinematographic sequence to a short run. If the voltage applied to the X-ray tube is non-uniform, due to the use of a single phase generator, the frame

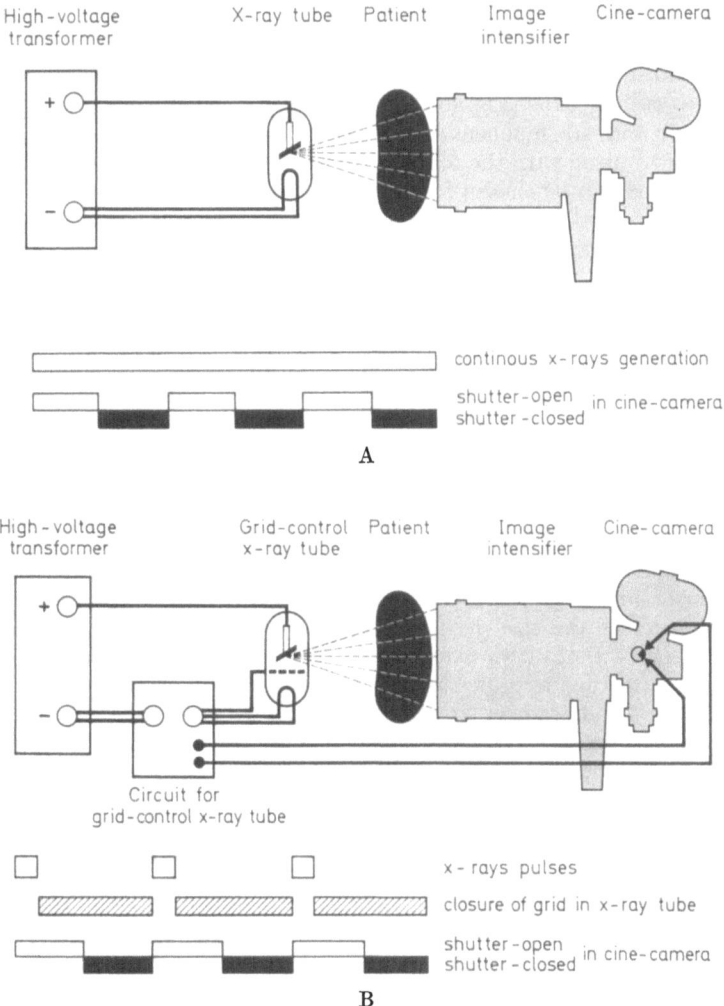

Fig. 48 A and B. Scheme illustrating the difference in radiation to the patient. A X-rays generated continuously by means of a non-synchronized cinefluorographic system. B X-rays generated in pulses by means of a grid control X-ray tube in a synchronized cinefluorographic system

rate is limited to 25 f.p.s. At this rate unequal exposure of different frames represents a serious drawback. This difficulty can be overcome by using a camera with shutter-open and shutter-closed times of equal duration, powered by a synchronous motor. The filming speed of such a camera is fixed to the frequency of the alternating current or its submultiples, i.e. with a.c. of 50 Hz the filming speed is limited to 50, 25, 12.5 and 6.25 f.p.s. Synchronitazion between the X-ray production and the opening of the shutter in the cinecamera can be achieved in two different ways. The technique of primary pulsing uses two switching tubes in the primary circuit of the generator which are controlled by an electrical signal provided by the synchronous motor powering the cinecamera. With this technique, the filming speed is limited to the frequency of the alternating current or its submultiples and the exposure time depends on the number of frames per second used. Most radiologists prefer the technique of pulsing in the high-voltage circuit of the generator by means of a grid control tube or a grid-controlled switching tube (Fig. 48 B). With this method the X-ray exposures can be kept short and are independent of the framing speed used. As the timing circuit is synchronized with the mechanism supplying the film to the cinecamera, the filming speed can be chosen freely.

The cameras used in cinefluorography are derived from those used in conventional cinematography. A typical camera permits adaptation of the filming speed to the motion. The standard filming speed is 24 frames per second, which corresponds to the standard projection speed of sound cineprojectors. Lower projection speeds may be used; 16 frames per second, however, is the minimum speed which will give a smooth appearance of movement. The cinefluorographic image is usually recorded on 16 mm or 35 mm film. The 35 mm film provides images with higher detail rendering because the area of each frame is five times larger and thus allows lower minification of the image being recorded on the film. This can be turned to full advantage if the cinefluoroscopic system is composed of an intensifier with an input screen of 9 or 10 in. and if a system with high resolving power is used (Feddema et al., 1969; Ter-Pogossian, 1967). A new cinefluorographic system, called system 180, uses a 16 mm film which is exposed with the long side of its frames running in the direction of the pellicule. This permits to increase the size of the exposed area of the film 2.5 times without overframing and 4 times with overframing. The quality of the image is improved and, with overframing, approaches that of the 35 mm films. The optical coupling system of the 16 mm camera is nearly four times faster than that of a 35mm camera, and the number of frames per meter is 2.5 times greater. The advantages of the 16 mm film, however, are obviated by the currently available faster 35 mm film and by the possibility of reading 35 mm film directly through a Tago-Arno viewer. For teaching purposes 35 mm films may be copied on 16 mm films. Cinefluorography is usually carried out with negative films to obtain images comparable to a radiograph. Reversal films are also used; after a negative-type processing they provide high-contrast images. High-speed, high-contrast emulsions with reduced grain size are now available in both 16 and 35 mm films.

Cine films should be viewed with equipment which permits to observe the films at normal, fast or reduced cinespeeds, as frame-by-frame and as stationary frames. The method of viewing the film in frame-by-frame motion should never be omitted and is particularly useful to observe low contrast details more easily (Ardran, 1964).

The viewing distance should be $^1/_2$ to 2 times the projection distance, and the image should be projected on a white mat screen to avoid enhancement of the grain by the beads of the screen. The size should correspond to the input diameter of the image intensifier to avoid loss of luminosity (Lichtenberg and Dutreix, 1969). Owing to their special processing needs the cinefilms cannot usually be viewed immediately after fluoroscopy. For this reason either full-size or 70 mm films or, better still, a simultaneous video-tape recording should be obtained for demonstration or interpretation purposes. Cinefluorography is employed mainly for studying the motor activity of pharynx and esophagus (Ardran, 1964; Seaman, 1969; Mandelstam and Lieber, 1970); it is useful for studying the esophagogastric junction, demonstrating gastroespohageal reflux, esophageal varices and fistulas. Some authors feel that even small morphologic changes can adequately be evaluated with this technique (Berridge and McGregg, 1958; Stilson, 1965; Jorgens, 1969). For diagnostic purposes it should be considered as a technique to supplement conventional roentgen examinaton and not as an exclusive method of examination (STAPLE and MARGULIS, 1964). In spite of the availability of videotape recording, cinefluorography remains indicated in clinical radiology when high image quality is required, or when images are changing so rapidly that they cannot be observed readily on a fluorescent screen, e.g., during the process of swallowing (ARDRAN, 1964; STIEVE, 1969). A further application of cinefluorography is the simultaneous recording of roentgen configurations and measured parameters, such as intraluminal pressures (VAN-TRAPPEN et al., 1958; HEITMANN et al., 1966).

1.3. Techniques of Recording the Television Images

The fluoroscopic images supplied by a television chain can be recorded by two main techniques, cinefluorography and video recording.

1.3.1. Cinefluorography

In this technique, the fluoroscopic images on a television monitor are photographed either as motion pictures by means of a cinescope recorder, or as single-shot photography by means of a still camera operating at $1/30$ sec (CHESNEY and CHESNEY, 1971). Cinescopy can be performed by synchronizing the framing frequency of the cinecamera with the scanning frequency of the television chain (Fig. 49). The pictures can be taken during fluoroscopy or during the display of the video record. It is the only way to record cinematographically the fluoroscopic images supplied by the television system composed of a Delcalix image intensifier and an Isocon pick-up tube (BOUWERS, 1971). The best results are obtained with reversal films. The image quality of the film is similar to that of the fluoroscopic image supplied by the television monitor (JANSEN, 1969).

The main advantage of this technique of cinerecording is the reduction of the radiation dose to the level required for fluoroscopy. Cinescope recording is limited to frame rates equal to or a submultiple of the scanning frequency of the T.V. chain. The quality of the photographic images is poorer than that of cinefluorography (BOUWERS and KREBS, 1968).

However, with equipment of good quality, cinescope recording may be a valuable substitute for cinefluorography, particularly when the information to be recorded is displayed clearly on the T.V. monitor.

1.3.2. Video Recording

The fluoroscopic images are converted in the television camera to a video signal and recorded on video tape or on video disk (GEBAUER et al., 1967).

The video tape recorder has proved to be very useful in diagnostic radiology (Fig. 50). In most cases it is an acceptable substitute for cineradiology if it has a double scanning head which permits slow motion playback and improves the quality of the still picture. The still picture delivered by the playback of a video tape record represents only half of the television picture (one of the two interlaced scans). The still and slow motion pictures delivered by the video disc recorder correspond in quality to the pictures displayed by a moving type recorder because they represent the whole television picture. Moreover, the disc recorder system with its electronic signal processing allows discontinuous updating of information, subtraction techniques and video enhancement. Its application in clinical radiology, however, is still limited due to the high cost of the apparatus and the limited storage capacity of the magnetic disk. At present video tape

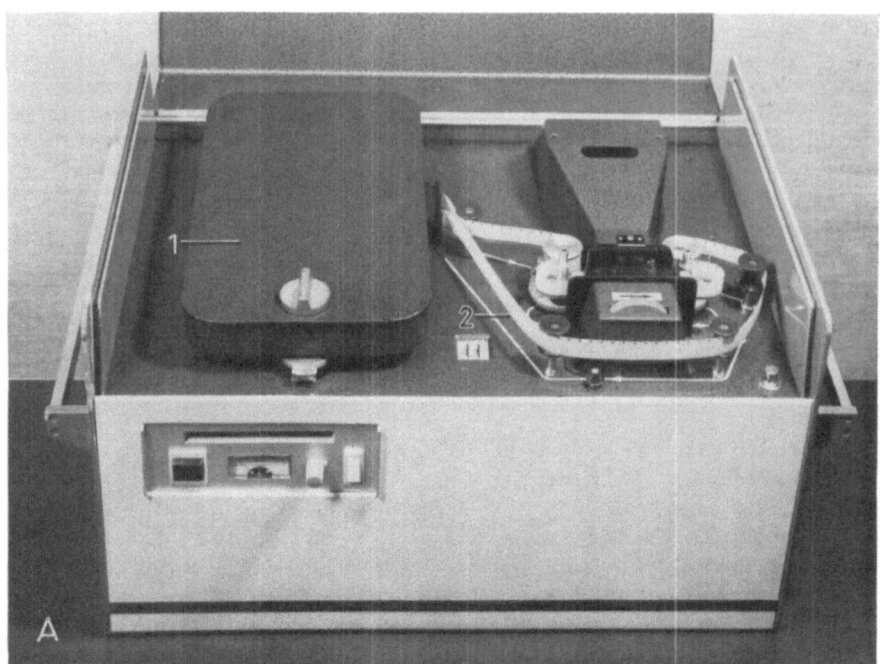

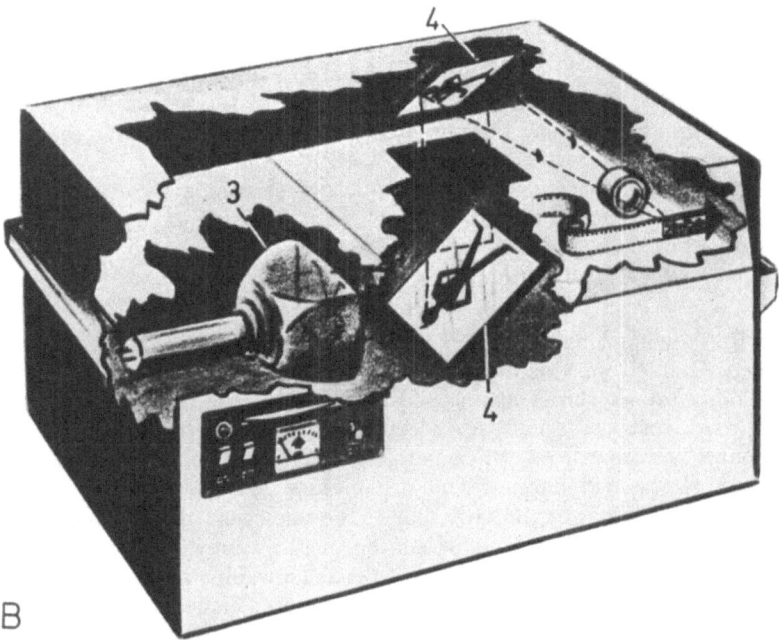

Fig. 49. A Outside view of kinescope "Old Delft" with film container (*1*) and 16 mm film disposed for recording (*2*). B Inside scheme showing the small TV monitor (*3*) with flat screen, the mirrors (*4*) and the light beam path to the film

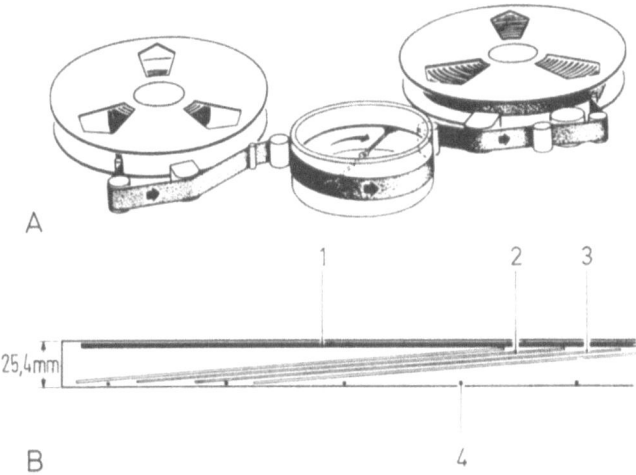

Fig. 50 A and B. Scheme of video tape recorder of the helically scanning type. A Magnetic tape moves on the double scanning head. B Principles of recording. 1 Sound track; 2 half picture track of odd lines; 3 half picture track of even lines; 4 synchronisation pulse (distances between pulses are not to scale)

replaces cinefilms in dynamic gastrointestinal radiology. It has the great advantage that it can be used as a monitor of fluoroscopy and that the tape can be displayed for interpretation immediately after completion of the recording. If a permanent record is not needed, it can be erased and used again. Video tape is easier to use when it is equipped with remote control and, particularly with a conventional table, when the record can be started from the spot filming device. If the bandwidth approaches 4 megahertz, the quality of the image is nearly equal to that of the original television image. Still and slow motion replay, however, results in a considerable loss of quality. In addition slow motion display is associated with jerkiness due to the limited recording speed. Consequently video tape is a less satisfactory technique than cinefluorography for the recording of rapid movement. Another disadvantage is the poor interchangeability of tape recordings between machines from different manufacturers.

2. Contrast Materials

Different contrast materials can be used in diagnostic radiology of the esophagus. The positive contrast substances include (1) barium sulfate, (2) iodinated contrast media in aqueous solution (Gastrografin, Hypaque), in aqueous suspension (Dionosil, Hytrast), in oil suspension (Dionosil) or as Lipiodol and (3) tantalum powder. The negative contrast material is air or gas.

2.1. Positive Contrast Materials
2.1.1. Barium Sulfate

This is the contrast material of choice, because it is non-toxic, non-absorbable and gives an adequate mucosal coating. The quality of the barium powder and of the thick barium suspensions has recently been improved. The particle size has been decreased to about 1 μ and additives have enhanced the stability of the colloidal suspension (Embring and Mattson, 1968; James and Goddard, 1971). It is now possible to prepare suspensions of low aggregation tendency and of considerably greater density without increase in viscosity (Micropaque and Mixobar, etc.) (Embring and Mattson, 1968; James and Goddard, 1971). Micropaque and Mixobar are commercially prepared thick suspensions which can be used directly or after adequate dilution. Two different systems are used to indicate the amount of barium contained in the commercially available preparations: the weight/weight (w/w) and the weight/volume percentage systems (w/v). One system can be converted into the other, as 100% w/v equals 60% w/w. The weight/weight system is used for dry powder and barium paste, the weight/volume system for barium suspensions. When a barium suspension has to be freshly prepared either from dry powder or from a commercially available suspension both barium and water are usually measured by volume (Miller, 1965) (the volume/volume system).

Barium is commonly used at three different degrees of concentration: as a creamy paste (barium 70% w/w), as a highly opaque liquid suspension (commercial preparations of barium 100% w/v or 60% w/w or freshly prepared barium suspensions 50% v/v) and as a moderately opaque liquid suspension (commercial preparation of barium diluted to 50% or freshly prepared barium 40% v/v) (Templeton, 1964). Barium paste is used for the study of the mucosal folds or to outline the whole esophagus. The paste should have a creamy consistency (Prevot and Lassrich, 1959; Templeton, 1964). Too thick a paste has a high degree of thixotrophy, is difficult to swallow, travels through the esophagus as a compact bolus and, therefore, results in poor mucosal coating (Miller, 1965). A highly opaque liquid suspension is the contrast medium of choice for studies of the mucosal pattern and the motor activity of the esophagus and is frequently used for double contrast pictures. This type of contrast material is too opaque to study the filled esophagus and not sufficiently fluid to be recommended for the examination of the gastroesophageal junction or the demonstration of gastroesophageal reflux (Wolf, 1967; Sandmark, 1963). Moderately opaque suspensions are better suited for these purposes. The formation of foam or air bubbles may produce disturbing artifacts and can be very inconvenient, particularly if one is looking for varices. Water containing more than 50 mg of sodium or potassium salts per liter is likely to cause foaming (Miller, 1965). Bubble formation can be reduced by decreasing the hardness of the water used in the preparation of the barium mixture, and by avoiding overstirring and agitating just before ingestion. Foaming can also be avoided by adding 1–2 ml of silicone (dimethylpolysiloxane) to the barium cup (Doi, 1971). This agent, however, decreases the adhesive properties of a barium suspension, a drawback which is particularly evident in some commercial preparations. Barium may also be used as compressed tablets 1.25 cm in diameter (Wolf, 1967), as barium-filled gelatine capsules (Schatzki and Gary, 1956) or as barium marshmallows (Kelly, 1961) to demonstrate an esophageal stenosis. An acid barium suspension of pH 1.7 has been advocated as a screening test for acid-induced esophageal pain (Donner et al., 1966). The test demonstrates the reactivity of the esophagus to acid and is said to identify those patients whose symptoms are likely to be due to reflux fo gastric contents into the lower esophagus (Donner et al., 1961). An acid barium of pH 1.7 is prepared by mixing 100 ml of standard barium sulfate suspension and 0.5 ml of concentrated hydrochloric acid (37%). The patients are examined in the horizontal position and the esophageal response to acid barium is compared with the response to standard barium. The esophageal motility of normal subjects, as observed on X-ray, does not change when acid barium is given. In most patients with reflux symptoms the normal peristaltic activity after a standard barium swallow is replaced by segmental non-peristaltic contractions when acid barium is swallowed.

The use of barium sulfate as a contrast medium is contraindicated in all perforations of the gastrointestinal tract and in obstructions of the distal half of the colon.

Most authors consider barium sulfate to be contraindicated in patients who are likely to aspirate it into the airways because of neuromuscular disturbances, lesions of the central nervous system and pharyngeal or upper esophageal obstructions (JACOBSON et al., 1958; LESSMAN and LILIENFELD, 1959; NELSON et al., 1963).

Accidental aspiration of barium sulfate is thought to expose the patient to mechanical obstruction of the airways, necrotizing bronchopneumonia or granulomatous lesions (LESSMAN and LILIENFELD, 1959) and may even cause death (SAUVEGRAIN, 1969). Experimental studies, however, have failed to produce acute pulmonary distress, abscesses, scarring or granulomatous lesions in animals after the introduction of barium into their bronchial tree (WILLSON et al., 1959; FRECH et al., 1970).

Clinical experience has confirmed that barium sulfate is a safe contrast material for bronchography (DI RENZO and PEREIRA-DUARTA, 1957; NELSON et al., 1964). Mechanical obstruction can be avoided by using highly viscous barium which is less readily aspirated (STAPLE and OGURA, 1966) and, if aspirated, remains in the main bronchi for a longer period of time so that it can more easily be eliminated by coughing. This is the main reason why some authors still use small amounts of highly viscous barium sulfate in patients who are predisposed to aspiration into the airways (SAUVEGRAIN, 1969).

2.1.2. Iodinated Contrast Materials

Water-soluble iodinated contrast media can be used to visualize the upper gastrointestinal tract (JACOBSON et al., 1958; SHEHADI, 1960). These contrast materials are considered safer than barium sulfate in patients with esophageal perforation or communication between esophagus and airways and when there is a risk of aspiration into the bronchi. They are also used for the examination of the esophagus in the early postoperative period following esophageal surgery or correction of a hiatal hernia. The demonstration of a leak is a contraindication for the withdrawal of the postoperative gastric tube (MATHESON and DUDLEY, 1963).

The most commonly used iodinated water-soluble contrast media are Gastrografin and Hypaque (JACOBSON et al., 1958; LESSMAN and LILIENFELD, 1959; SHEHADI, 1960; WÜRDINGER, 1962). Gastrografin is a 76% meglumine diatrizoate solution to which flavoring agents are added. It is a ready-for-use preparation. Hypaque, sodium diatrizoate, is available as a powder containing a flavoring agent and must be diluted before use. Animal studies and clinical experience indicate that these preparations have no direct toxicity (SHEHADI, 1960). Effusion of contrast material into the mediastinum, peritoneal cavity or retroperitoneal tissues appears to be well tolerated and harmless (MEYERS and JACOBSON, 1964). In normal intestinal conditions only a small amount of these contrast materials is absorbed by the intestine and secreted by the kidneys (JACOBSON et al., 1958; TOSCH, 1961). Larger amounts may be absorbed when intestinal obstruction or intestinal mucosal lesions are present (TOSCH, 1961; MORI and BARRETT, 1962) and when there is effusion of contrast material into the pleural or abdominal

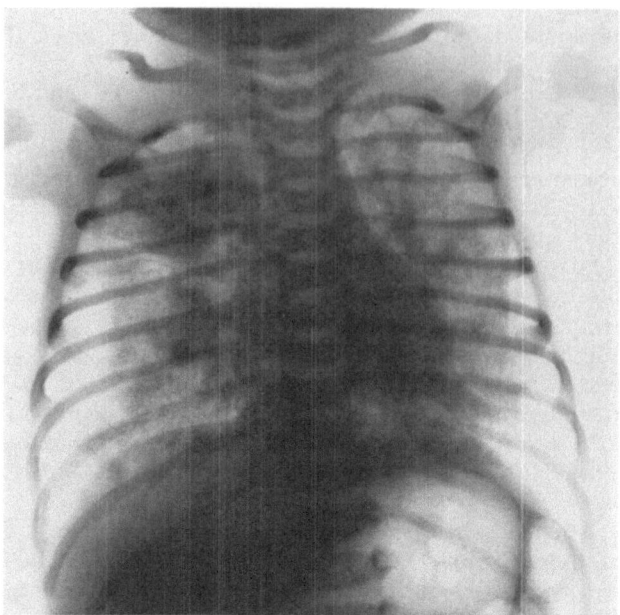

Fig. 51. This newborn with a laryngo-tracheo-esophageal cleft was admitted for acute respiratory distress, following a radiological examination with gastrografin. The contrast medium had been massively aspirated in the lungs

cavity (MEYERS and JACOBSON, 1964). These contrast media may produce dramatic side effects on the intestinal tract and the lungs because of their hypertonicity (the osmolarity of gastrografin is 6 times that of blood serum). Their cathartic effect on the intestinal tract is usually well tolerated in the absence of dehydration. However, it may be dangerous and cause death in dehydrated children (HARRIS et al., 1964). This complication can be prevented by correction of the dehydration before the contrast material is given and by the parenteral administration of fluid to compensate the induced hypovolemia. The side effects of these contrast media on the lungs have recently been emphasized (Fig. 51). Following the report of REICH (1969) on the death of an adult patient with cor pulmonale after aspiration into the airways of a mouthful of Gastrografin, the effect of water-soluble contrast materials on the lungs after its introduction into the tracheobronchial tree, has been studied experimentally (REICH, 1969; FRECH et al., 1970). Gastrografin, Hypaque or Renografin introduced into the tracheobronchial tree of anesthetized cats caused acute respiratory distress and death of the animals. This dramatic effect is due to pulmonary edema, caused by the hyperosmolarity of these materials after their alveolarization. When the same amount of contrast medium was administered to unanesthetized animals, pulmonary edema developed but cleared within hours, and no death was observed.

These studies suggest that the acute respiratory distress caused by these hypertonic contrast media will resolve in patients with normal pulmonary function but may be dramatic and even fatal in patients with poor pulmonary function or reduced coughing reflex. The aqueous suspensions of iodinated material used for bronchography, Dionosil and Hytrast, are less dangerous when they happen to be aspirated (GRAINGER et al., 1970). Introduced into the airways of anesthetized animals, Dionosil causes only very slight pulmonary edema (REICH, 1969). Hytrast has a higher viscosity and a higher iodine content and is well tolerated clinically if it is used without dilution (GRAINGER et al., 1970). Lower viscosities may be dangerous and even lethal. It must be stressed that all pulmonary contrast materials interfere with lung function by obstructing the bronchi and that large amounts of any contrast material in the airways can be fatal (CHRISTOFORIDIS et al., 1962).

Hytrast and Dionosil in oil suspension are used as contrast media for laryngo-pharyngography (POWERS et al., 1957; COLLARD, 1964).

Lipiodol is not recommended as a substitute of barium sulfate for gastro-intestinal examinations because of the irregular mucosal coating it produces (BACHMAN, 1963; SAUVEGRAIN, 1969).

2.1.3. Tantalum Powder

Tantalum powder may visualize the esophageal lumen fairly well when sprayed on the esophageal mucosa (NADEL et al., 1969) or when swallowed as a paste (DODDS et al., 1972). The principal advantage of this method is that mucosal coating lasts for a long period of time, at least 10 min. It can be a useful research tool but has not yet found wide application in clinical radiology.

2.2. Negative Contrast Materials

In newborn infants suspected of having esophageal atresia, air may be in-sufflated through an esophageal tube in order to determine the level of the stenosis. Air is also used as a contrast medium in the double contrast technique of examination.

3. The Radiological Examination

3.1. General Principles

The radiological examination is an essential step in the clinical exploration of the esophagus. In many cases it allows the correct diagnosis; in some conditions such as wide rings, intramural diverticulosis, extramural tumors and esophago-tracheal fistulas, it is the most reliable diagnostic method (SCHATZKI and HARVES, 1942; SCHATZKI and GARY, 1956; SOM et al., 1960; GWINN, 1969; CREELY and TRAIL, 1970). It is the easiest and sometimes the only way to obtain a morpho-logical analysis of a narrow stricture. Usually it precedes endoscopy and other investigative procedures. Radiological examination of the esophagus is indicated when esophageal disorders are suspected on clinical grounds, and when it is necessary to know whether or not the esophagus is involved in diseases such as portal hypertension, mediastinal tumors, bronchial carcinoma, systemic diseases and cardiovascular anomalies. The esophagus should also be examined rapidly at every X-ray examination of the upper gastrointestinal tract. In this way unsuspected abnormalities or lesions, such as diverticula, arterial impressions, small tumors or varices may be detected. Sometimes it may even lead to the discovery of symptomless large malignant tumors (Fig. 52).

As the localization of the lesions by the patient is frequently incorrect, the whole length of the esophagus should be examined. A complete X-ray examina-tion of the esophagus must include a study of the swallowing act and of the pharyngoesophageal region as well as a careful examination of the esophago-gastric junction with a search for gastroesophageal reflux. The presence of esoph-

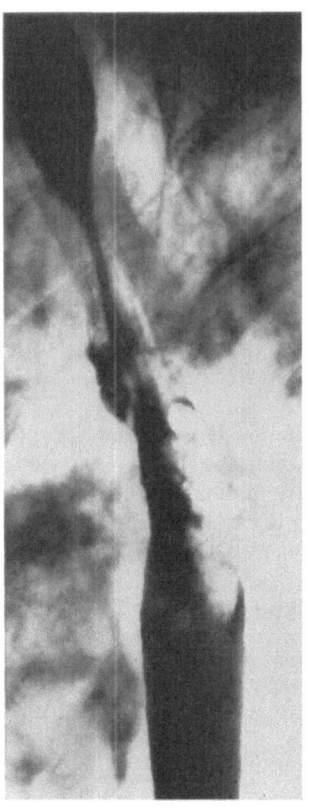

Fig. 52. Ulcerated carcinoma in the middle third of the esophagus detected by systematic screening of the esophagus during an X-ray examination of stomach and duodenum. This examination was requested because of an epigastric mass in a patient who had no dysphagia. The epigastric mass turned out to be a hepatic metastasis

ageal varices calls for an examination of stomach and duodenum in order to detect associated gastric or duodenal varices, and, in cases of gastrointestinal hemorrhage, to detect gastric or duodenal causes of bleeding (Dagradi et al., 1955). Narrowing of the distal esophagus also calls for further examination, because this lesion may be tumoral and due to a carcinoma originating in the upper part of the stomach (Dodge, 1961) or it may be peptic and be associated with an active gastric or duodenal ulcer (Cruze et al., 1959; Skinner et al., 1966); it may even be secondary to duodenal stenosis (Johnston and Stevenson, 1966).

Since X-ray image intensifiers have become available for routine fluoroscopy, it is unusual for even small lesions to be missed by an experienced examiner during fluoroscopy. Consequently, fluoroscopy has become the most important part of the gastrointestinal radiological examination. The fluoroscopic findings should be documented by spot films. X-ray pictures of the entire esophagus on large films should also be made in order to show the localization of a lesion or to document a negative fluoroscopy. These large films must be checked immediately after processing. Any abnormality which cannot be explained by the preceding fluoroscopic observation is an indication to repeat the fluoroscopy. The technique of fluoroscopic examination must be standardized to avoid omissions and to give the radiologist the experience to decide what he should record and which technique of recording is the most valuable for the diagnosis (Templeton, 1964). As other examinations of the gastrointestinal tract, the X-ray examination of the esophagus is more than a passive watching in different positions of the barium passing through the gullet. Good diagnostic results depend on a precise knowledge of what one is looking for and requires intensive thinking and effort (Schatzki, 1966).

3.2. Normal Radiological Anatomy and Physiology

3.2.1. Hypopharynx and Cervical Esophagus

3.2.1.1. Radiological Landmarks

The hypopharynx extends from the level of the hyoid bone to the lower border of the cricoid cartilage, at the level of C6–C7 (Bachman, 1963) (Figs. 53, 60) The hypopharynx may be further divided into three main parts: the pyriform

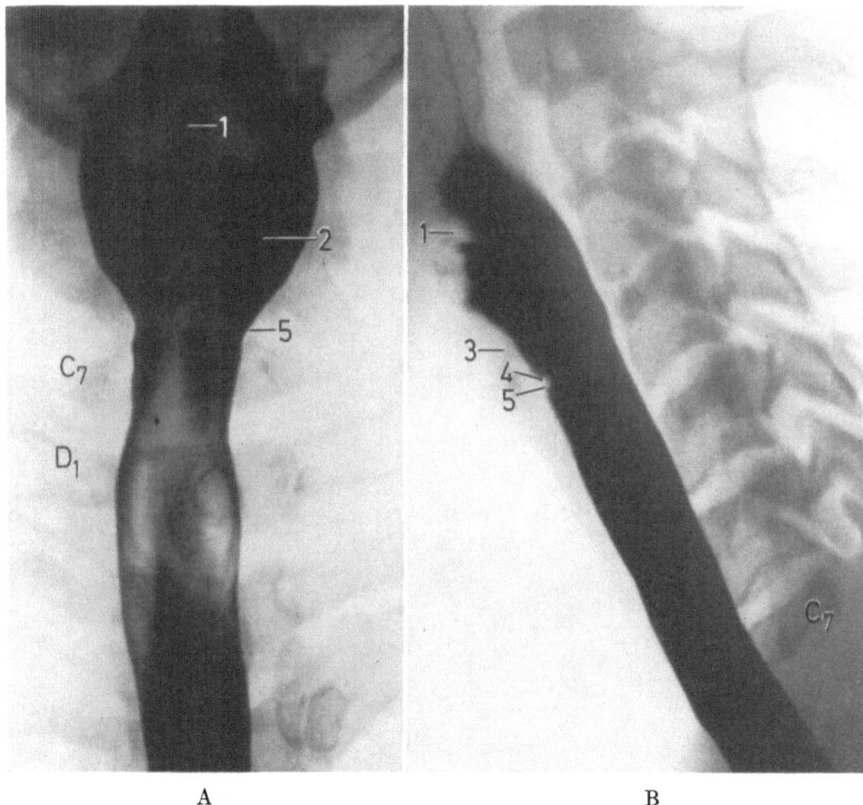

A   B

Fig. 53 A and B. Frontal (A) and lateral (B) view of hypopharynx during swallowing ot
show epiglottis (1), lower lateral food channels or pyriform sinuses (2), postcricoid area (3),
postcricoid venous plexus (4) and pharyngoesophageal junction (5)

sinuses, the posterolateral walls and the postcricoid area (SEAMAN, 1967 b).
The cervical portion of the esophagus extends downwards to the level of the
thoracic inlet, corresponding to T1–T2. The pharyngoepiglottic folds or valleculae and the tip of the epiglottis mark the upper limit of the opacified hypopharynx. The distal limit is marked by the lower margin of the cricoid cartilage
impression and by the level of the postcricoid venous impression. On lateral views,
the indentation of the cricopharyngeal muscle, and on frontal views, the level
at which the converging lateral walls of the hypopharynx begin to run parallel
may also indicate this distal limit. The term "pharyngoesophageal junction" refers
to the sphincter area at the proximal end of the esophagus, which may be marked
by the cricopharyngeal indentation (SEAMAN, 1969; ZBORALSKE and DODDS,
1969). On plain films the lower part of the hypopharynx is only visible when
distended by air, e.g. by the modified Valsalva maneuver. The soft tissue density
of the collapsed hypopharynx and cervical esophagus is indistinguishable from
that of the prevertebral space (Fig. 54 A). Air can be seen in the proximal 2 to
3 cm of the esophagus during a dry swallow (CIMMINO, 1969) and sometimes
even at rest (ZAINO et al., 1970) (Fig. 54 B). The anterior border of the prevertebral soft tissue shadow runs parallel to the cervical spine. The thickness

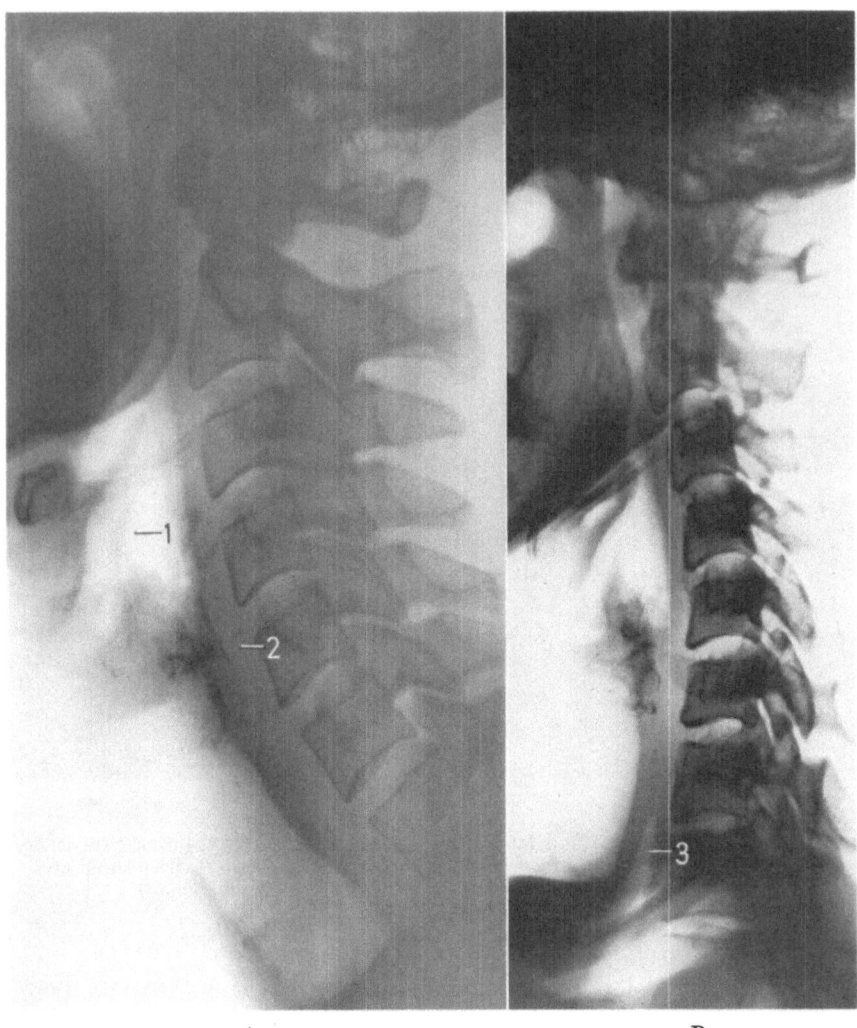

Fig. 54. A Plain film of neck in profile showing the air-contrasted upper part of the hypopharynx (*1*) and the collapsed lower part, obscured by the soft tissue shadow of the prevertebral space (*2*). The posterior wall of the hypopharynx appears straight. B In another patient, a small amount of air (*3*) was incidentally seen in cervical esophagus

of this soft tissue layer is less than the diameter of the adjacent vertebral body (Brenner, 1964) or, when measured at the level of the tip of the lower horn of the thyroid cartilage, less than the diameter of the adjacent tracheal shadow (Woods and Chance, 1965). In adults the thickness of the prevertebral layer at the retrolaryngeal level ranges from 3 to 5 cm (Zaino et al., 1970); it decreases during inspiration and increases during expiration and phonation. At the end of a deep expiration it may bulge into the pharynx, particularly in children (Fig. 55).

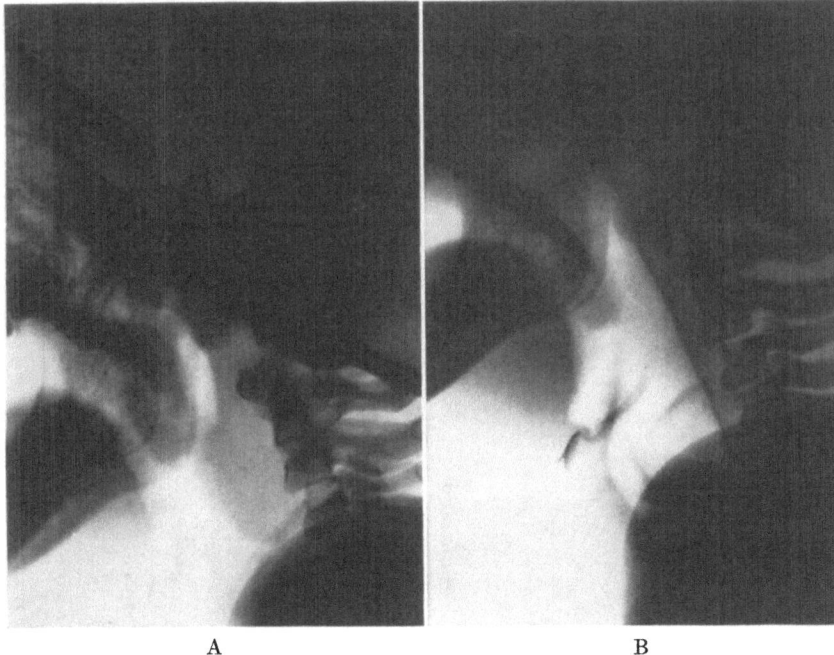

A   B

Fig. 55 A and B. In children expiration may result in marked bulging of the posterior wall
of the hypopharynx (A), disappearing on inspiration (B)

3.2.1.2. Hypopharynx and Cervical Esophagus during Swallowing

The appearance of the opacified hypopharynx and cervical esophagus depends
upon the phase of swallowing at the time of the exposure. The act of swallowing
has been described in detail in the section "Physiology". The most important
radiological aspects can be summarized as follows (Fig. 56).

At the onset of swallowing, the bolus of contrast material is thrown against
the posterior wall of the oropharynx by the backward and upward movement
of the tongue and deflected by the epiglottis into the pyriform sinuses on either
side. During the pharyngeal phase of deglutition, the larynx is raised towards
the hyoid bone, the lower part of the pyriform sinuses opens and the cricopharyngeus relaxes, allowing the bolus to fill the hypopharynx and to enter
the esophagus. Turning the head to one side closes the lateral part of the hypopharynx on that side, and results in barium going down on the opposite side.
By the action of the peristaltic contraction, the bolus is pushed downwards
from the pharynx into the esophagus like toothpaste out of a tube. As the tail
of the bolus leaves the pharynx, the cricopharyngeus contracts and the peristaltic
wave moves down the esophagus. When the peristaltic contraction has passed
the level of the clavicles, the larynx descends again. Successive swallows inhibit
the progression of the peristaltic wave down the esophagus as well as the descent
of the larynx. The whole pharyngeal phase of swallowing takes one second or less.

On lateral view, the hypopharynx is distended with contrast medium during
swallowing and appears as a barium column in continuity with the cervical
esophagus (Figs. 53–57). The posterior wall runs parallel to the anterior border

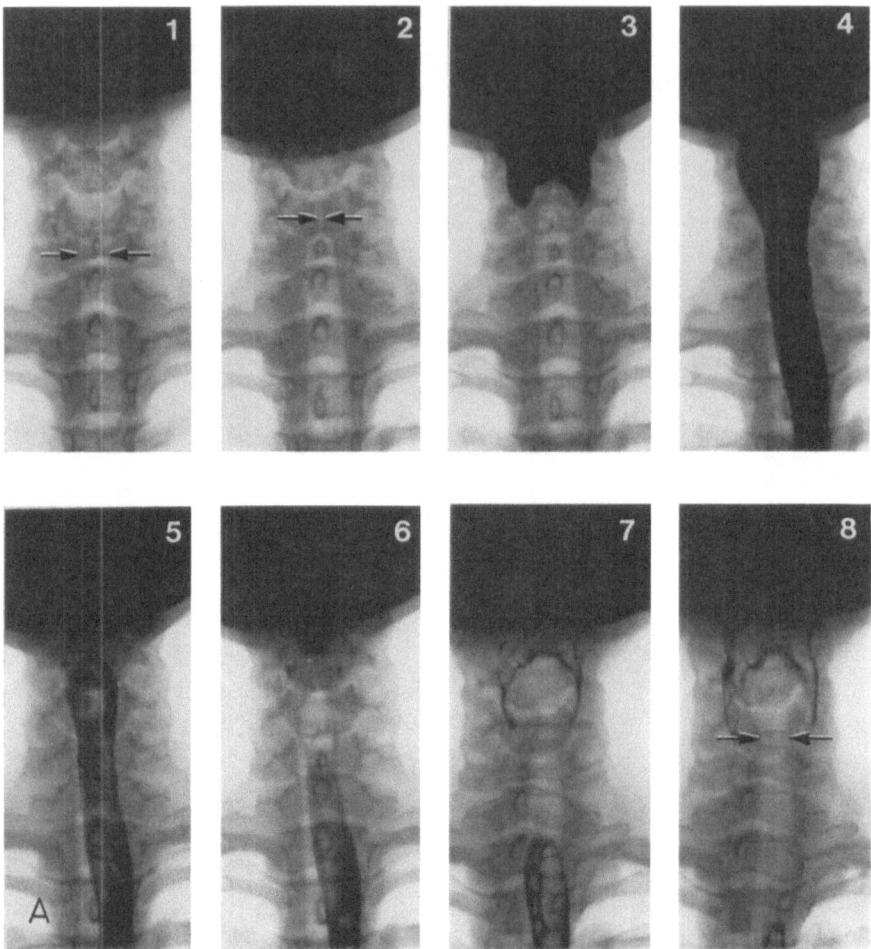

Fig. 56A and B. Serial filming of the swallowing act (70 mm film taken at a rate of 6 f.p.s.) in anteroposterior (A) and lateral (B) projections. Pictures *1* and *2* show upward movement and closure of larynx; *3* and *4* filling of hypopharynx and upper esophagus; *5* peristaltic contraction of hypopharynx; *6* closure of pharyngoesophageal junction and onset of primary esophageal peristalsis; and *7* and *8* downward movement and reopening of larynx

of the cervical spine at a distance of only 2 mm. Osteophytes and other lesions of the cervical spine may produce impressions on the posterior pharyngeal wall (Fig. 277). The pharyngoesophageal junction is normally not discernible. A posterior indentation due to the cricopharyngeal muscle is seen in 5% of the barium swallows and may be considered as a variant of normal swallowing (Seaman, 1966) (Fig. 103). The anterior wall has an irregular outline at the level of the valleculae, the epiglottis and the laryngeal vestibule (Bachman, 1959). A shallow curved indentation is sometimes apparent at the level of C5–C6, and is caused by the posterior lamina of the cricoid cartilage. At or immediately below the inferior margin of the cricoid cartilage the postcricoid venous impression is seen (Pitman and Fraser, 1965). It is produced by mucosal prolaps over the anterior

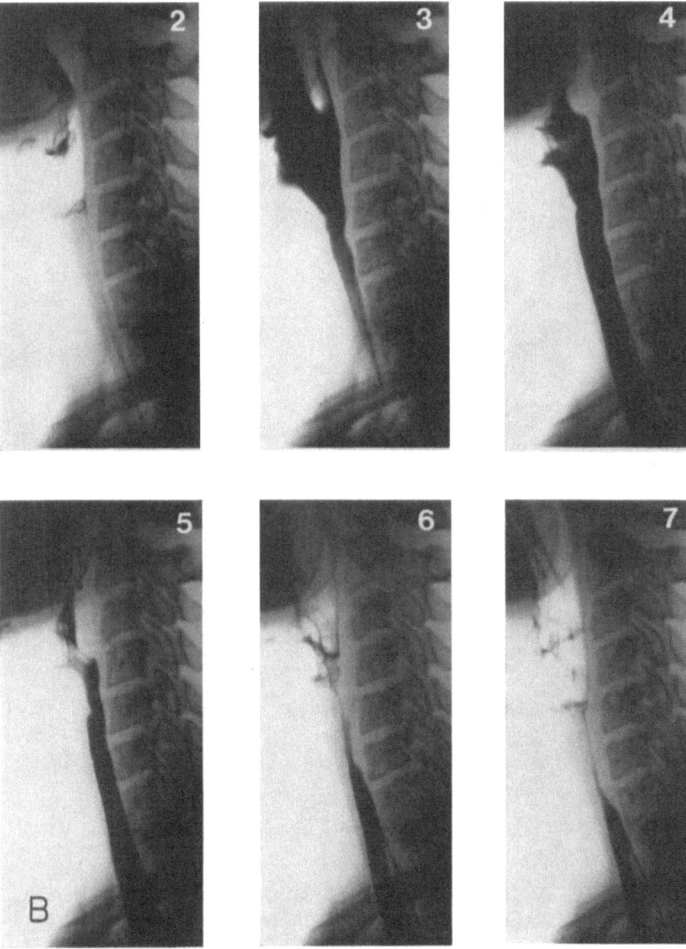

Abb. 56 B

submucosal venous plexus and may cause a curved impression, or a filling defect, or it may even mimic a web. Characteristically the appearance of this venous plexus is quite variable during the course of a single deglutition as well as on consecutive swallows (Fig. 58). A web-like post-cricoid venous impression can be distinguished from a true web by the gap between the two halves of the venous plexus visible on the midline. The walls of the barium-filled esophagus follow a smooth course behind the radiolucent trachea. The normal thyroid does not cause any anterior impression on the cervical esophagus (KREEL et al., 1965). On a frontal view the lateral walls of hypopharynx and cervical esophagus have a regular outline, but they may bulge more or less between the hyoid bone and the upper edge of the thyroid cartilage (BACHMAN et al., 1968) (Figs. 53–57). The central area of the hypopharynx is less opacified than the lateral parts as a result of laryngeal compression. The lumen of the hypopharynx narrows toward the proximal end of the esophagus where it becomes tubular. When the

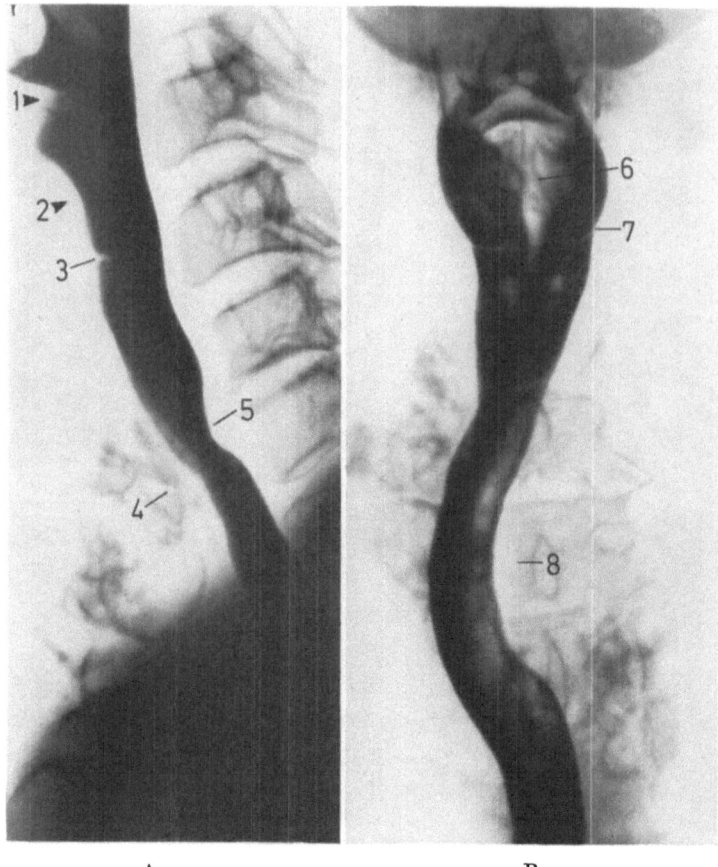

A   B

Fig. 57 A and B. Pharyngoesophageal region. The lateral view (A) shows the irregular outline of this region at the level of the laryngeal vestibule (1), the impression by the cricoid cartilage (2), a web-like venous plexus (3), the impression by a calcified goiter (4) and an impression by cervical osteophytes (5). The frontal views (B) shows the radiolucent central area of the hypopharynx (6) and a web-like venous plexus with a typical gap at the midline (7). The cervical esophagus is deviated to the right by a goiter (8)

esophagus is distended, the pharyngoesophageal junction sometimes appears as a slightly narrowed ring (Templeton, 1964). Lateral notching and horizontal mucosal folds may be seen in the lower portion of the pyriform sinuses (Zaino et al., 1970). When the lower part of the hypopharynx is not fully distended, the arched mucosal folds behind the laryngeal impression may cause a seal-like pattern (Brombart, 1961). Below the pharyngoesophageal junction the lateral lobes of the thyroid frequently cause slight symmetrical impressions (Kreel et al., 1965). At the level of the thoracic inlet, where the esophagus curves slightly to the left, a right-sided impression caused by the trachea is often noted. In subjects with a narrow thoracic inlet this impression may be very prominent, extending from C6–T7 and having a lobulated medial contour (Fig. 59). Typically it decreases in size or disappears by binding the neck or turning the head to the left (Kendall et al., 1962).

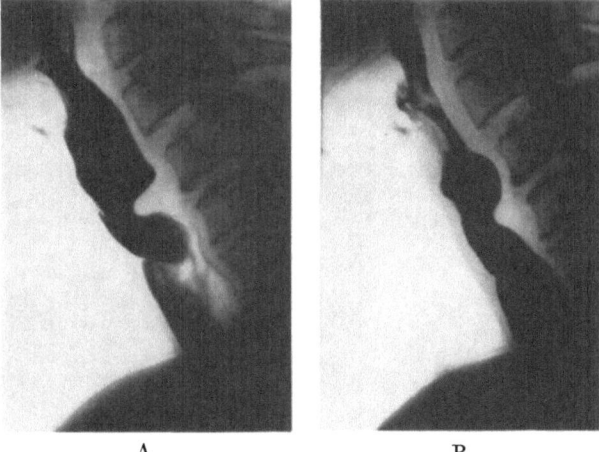

Fig. 58 A and B. The appearance of the venous plexus changes from one swallow to an other. A Web-like appearance. B Arc-like indentation (see further on Fig. 103)

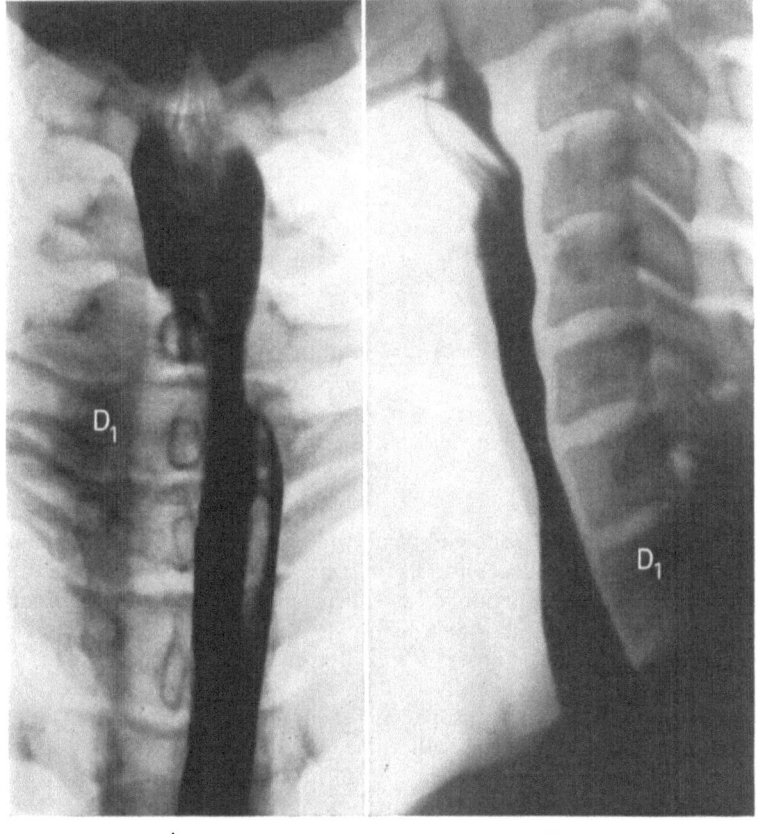

Fig. 59 A and B. Impression on the cervical esophagus by the trachea. As can be seen on the frontal view (A) the impression is right-sided. On the lateral view (B), there is overlapping of esophageal and tracheal outlines below the site of the impression

3.2.1.3. Hypopharynx and Cervical Esophagus after Swallowing

If a subject swallows only once, a small amount of contrast medium is retained in the valleculae and in the pyriform sinuses and some mucosal coating remains so that hypopharynx and esophagus are outlined (Fig. 60). On lateral views the

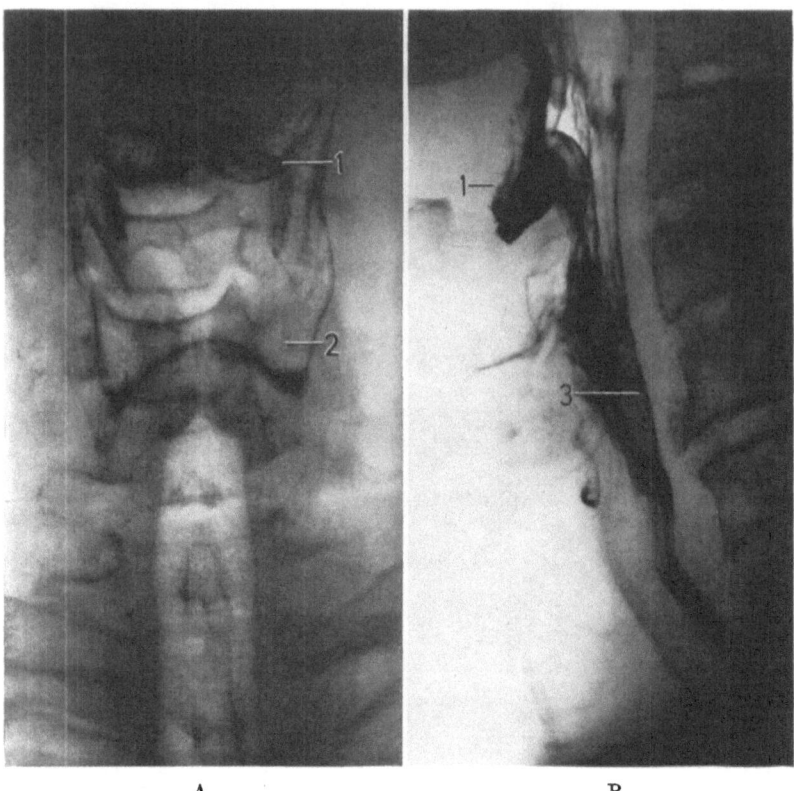

A   B

Fig. 60A and B. Normal hypopharyngogram after swallowing, in frontal (A) and lateral (B) view. The pharyngoepiglottic folds or valleculae (1), the upper part of the pyriform sinuses (2) and the posterolateral walls (3) are outlined

epiglottis is raised after swallowing and the upper part of the hypopharynx gapes slightly. The valleculae and the pyriform sinuses are super-imposed one on the other. The lower portion of pyriform sinuses and pharyngoesophageal junction are contracted and appear empty. The cricopharyngeal indentation cannot usually be identified, unless a Valsalva maneuver is performed. A small amount of barium may occasionally be held up at the upper margin of the cricopharyngeal muscle and must not be mistaken for a diverticulum (Fig. 103A). In an anteroposterior view, the valleculae are outlined with barium on each side of the glossoepiglottic fold. The pyriform sinuses appear as two inverted pyramids separated by a central area with arched mucosal folds. In the resting state, the lower portion of the pyriform sinuses is frequently not obliterated and may contain barium residues (ARDRAN and KEMP, 1961). The pharyngoesophageal orifice is collapsed and not distinguishable from the collapsed esophageal lumen.

3.2.1.4. The Modified Valsalva Maneuver

This maneuver consists of blowing against closed lips and nose and distends the hypopharynx. When the mucosa is coated with contrast medium, the contours of the distended air-filled hypopharynx become clearly outlined (Fig. 61). In

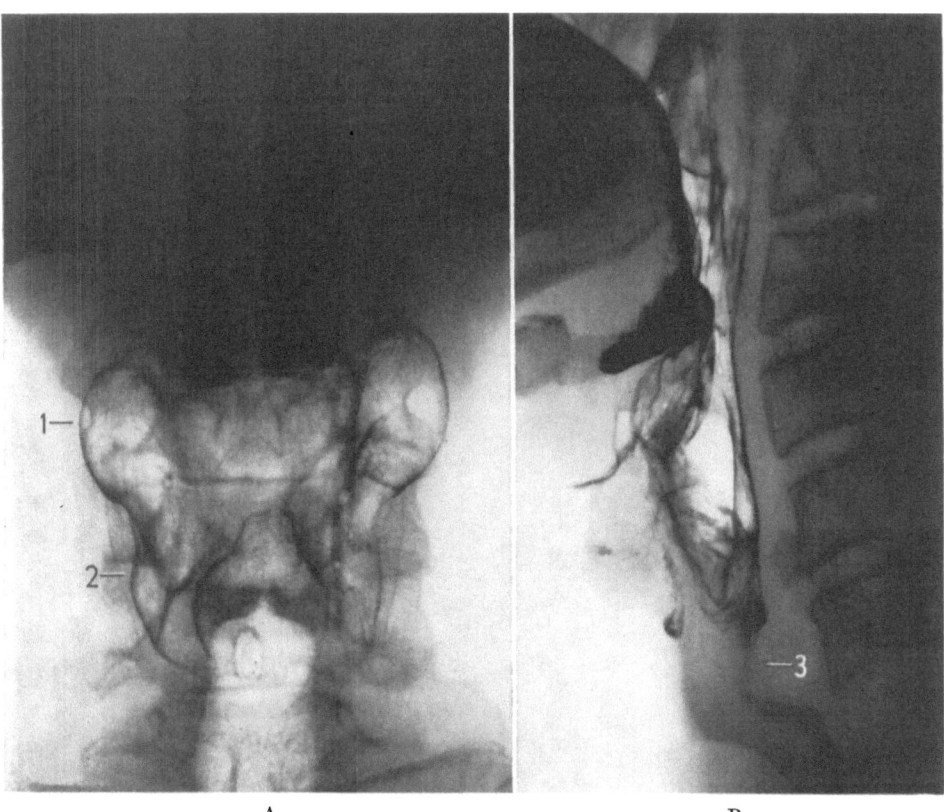

A   B

Fig. 61. Normal hypopharyngogram during a modified Valsalva maneuver. The lower part of the pyriform sinuses (2) and the cricopharyngeal indentation (3) are outlined. The frontal view shows slight outbulging (1) of the upper part of the hypopharynx

lateral projection, the distended lower part of the hypopharynx reaches down to the upper border of the cricopharyngeal muscle, which becomes apparent as an indentation on the posterior border of the pharyngoesophageal junction. In the anteroposterior projection, the pyriform sinuses balloon out and protrude laterally between the hyoid bone and the upper edge of the thyroid cartilage. They are sometimes very prominent, particularly in older people and are called pharyngeal pouches or lateral pharyngeal pseudo-diverticula (BACHMAN et al., 1968).

3.2.2. Thoracic Esophagus

The thoracic esophagus begins at the thoracic inlet at level T2–T3, runs between the mediastinal aspect of the lungs and extends down to the esophageal hiatus (CIMMINO, 1969). The terminal few centimeters of the esophagus form a physiologically and radiologically separate entity which is called the vestibule. The esophagovestibular junction is located at a short distance above the esophageal hiatus and is often defined by a short contractile ring (Berridge et al., 1966; Friedland et al., 1966; Wolf, 1970). A strictly topographic definition of the thoracic esophagus would include the supradiaphragmatic portion of the vestibule as well as the tubular esophagus. The radiologic features of the vestibule will not be discussed in this section.

3.2.2.1. Normal Motor Activity

Following deglutition, the contrast medium is squirted into the relaxed esophagus, and gives it the appearance of a continuous radiopaque column. A peristaltic wave soon follows and empties the esophagus (Fig. 62). If a subject takes several swallows in rapid succession, the peristaltic contraction is delayed until after the last deglutition. In the upright position liquid falls down the esophagus and is completely evacuated into the stomach before the peristaltic wave is

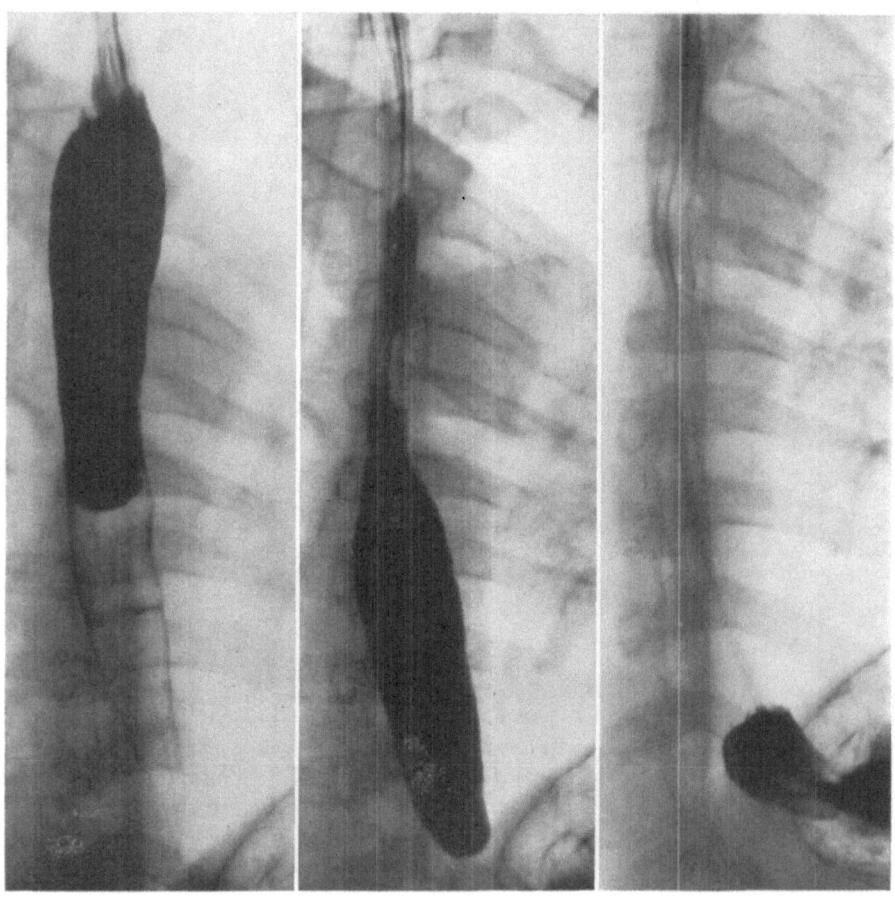

A   B   C

Fig. 62 A–C. Normal esophagogram in right anterior oblique position, taken at three different intervals after swallowing. Immediately after deglutition (A) the filled esophagus appears as a continuous radiopaque column; B shows the peristaltic wave trailing the barium column and obliterating the esophageal lumen. In C only a small amount of barium coating the mucosal folds is left

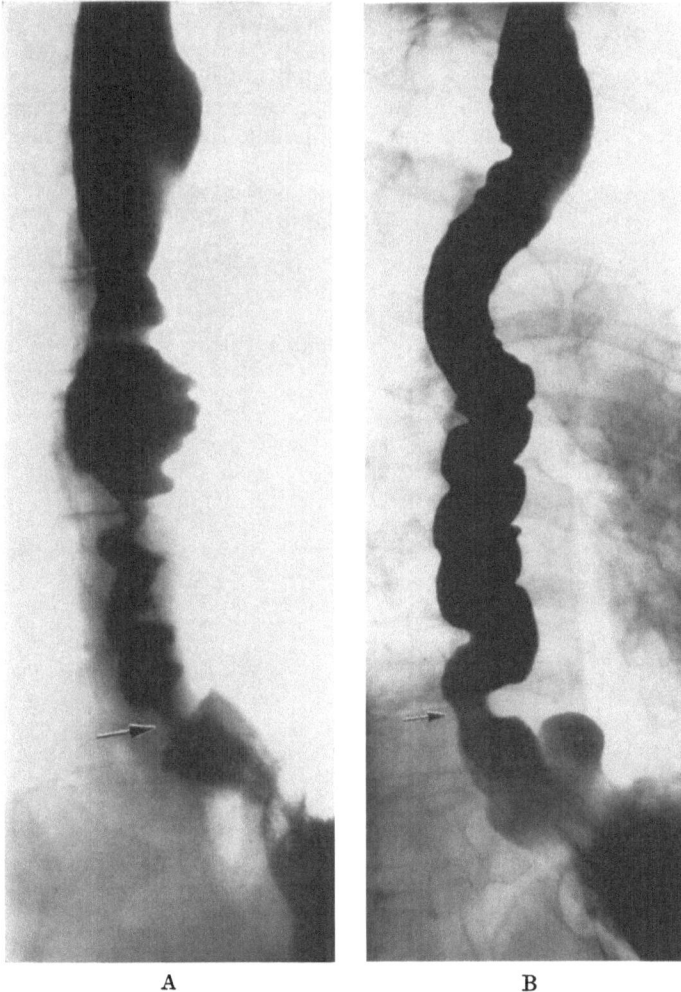

A   B

Fig. 63. Tertiary contractions in two different patients (Curling). An A-ring is shown in
the two patients (→). A small hiatus is demonstrated in patient B

completed. In the horizontal position also, liquid moves along the esophagus
faster than the peristaltic wave, apparently as a result of the propulsive force
of the pharyngeal contraction. The propulsion of pasty contrast medium, however, depends on the peristaltic wave. Esophageal peristalsis is visualized radiologically as a lumen-obliterating contraction which sweeps down the esophagus
in a coordinated progressive fashion and seems to stop at the upper margin
of the vestibule. In front of the peristaltic contraction, the tail of the barium
column assumes an inverted V configuration (ZBORALSKE and DODDS, 1969).
Non-peristaltic contractions in response to swallowing appear roentgenologically
as annular or segmental narrowings of the radiopaque column, which displace
barium both orally and aborally. These contractions may be single or repetitive
and uncoordinated and may also occur independently of swallowing. They are
commonly designated as tertiary contractions (Fig. 63).

At rest the tubular esophagus is relaxed and collapsed so that the mucosal folds are visible.

3.2.2.2. Normal Esophagogram

For descriptive purposes the thoracic esophagus is divided into upper, middle and lower third. The junction of upper and middle third is located near the level

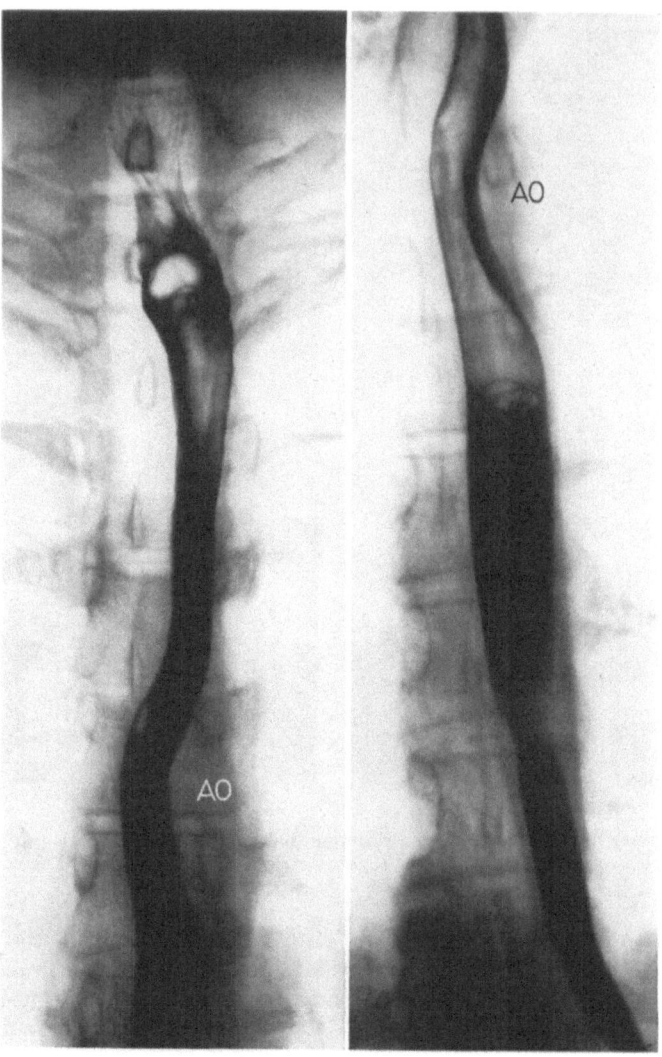

Fig. 64. Normal esophagogram in frontal view. Above and below the aortic knob (AO) the esophagus lies to the left of the midline

of the aortic arch. The aortic arch and the left main bronchus cause impresssions on the left esophageal border. The esophagopulmonary interphase produces a right paraesophageal line. When filled, the normal esophagus has a diameter of up to 3 cm (Frik, 1965). On anteroposterior films the upper third of the

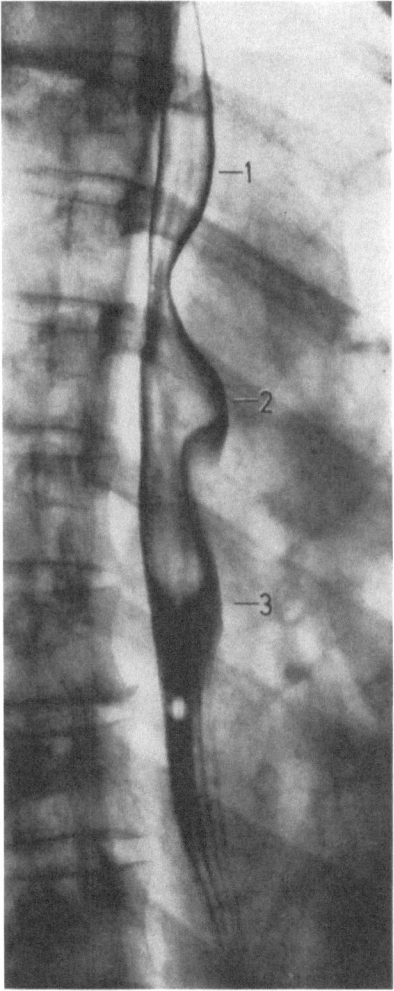

Fig. 65. Normal esophagogram in frontal view showing the bulge of the left esophageal border above the aortic knob (*1*), the bulge between the impressions caused by the aortic knob and the left main bronchus (*2*) and the bulge between the bronchial indentation and the cardiac impression (*3*)

normal esophagus curves gently to the left of the midline. At the level of the aortic arch, the curve is inverted and directed to the right to accommodate the aortic knob (Fig. 64). Below the level of the tracheobroncheal bifurcation, the course of the esophagus is more variable, because it may be displaced by the heart and the descending aorta. It lies always to the left of the midline, even in subjects with a right-sided aorta, except if the right-sided aorta is elongated and tortuous (KLINKHAMER, 1969). The deviation to the left of this part of the esophagus is more apparent in old people, in whom the esophagus follows the aorta, and in subjects with pulmonary emphysema. The left border of the barium-filled esophagus balloons out between the impression of the aortic knob and that of the left main bronchus, and may give rise to two or three successive

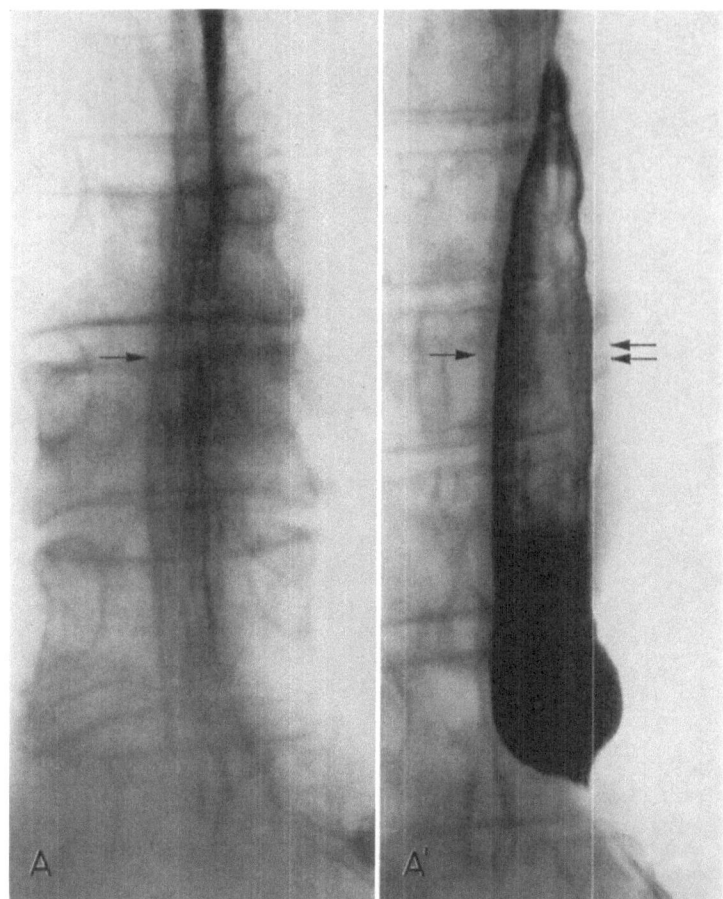

Fig. 66. AA′ The right pleuroesopahgeal line (single arrow) can be seen on both the collapsed (A) and the distended (A′) esophagus. On A′ the left pleuroesophageal line is also visible (double arrow). BB′ Laminograms before (B) and after (B′) a barium swallow demonstrate the posterior mediastinal line (between arrows)

bulges: a bulge above the aortic arch indentation, a bulge between the aortic arch and the tracheobronchial impression, and a bulge between the tracheobronchial bifurcation and the cardiac impression (Fig. 65). The bulge of the aortic arch is of great radiological significance for the evaluation of mediastinal masses (BERNE et al., 1969). The lateral walls of the thoracic esophagus are separated from the lungs only by some adventitial tissue and by the mediastinal pleura. If the interphase between the air-containing lung and the paraesophageal mediastinal pleura is X-rayed tangentially, it is indicated roentgenologically by a line, the paraesophageal line or pleuraesophageal stripe (BERNE et al., 1969; CIMMINO, 1969; ORMOND et al., 1963) (Fig. 66A). This line is clearly seen on the right side below the level of the right main bronchus. At the left side it is not always visualized because of the orientation of this interphase and the interposition, between esophagus and left lung, of the subclavian artery and the descending aorta. The right paraesophageal line follows the course of the esophagus

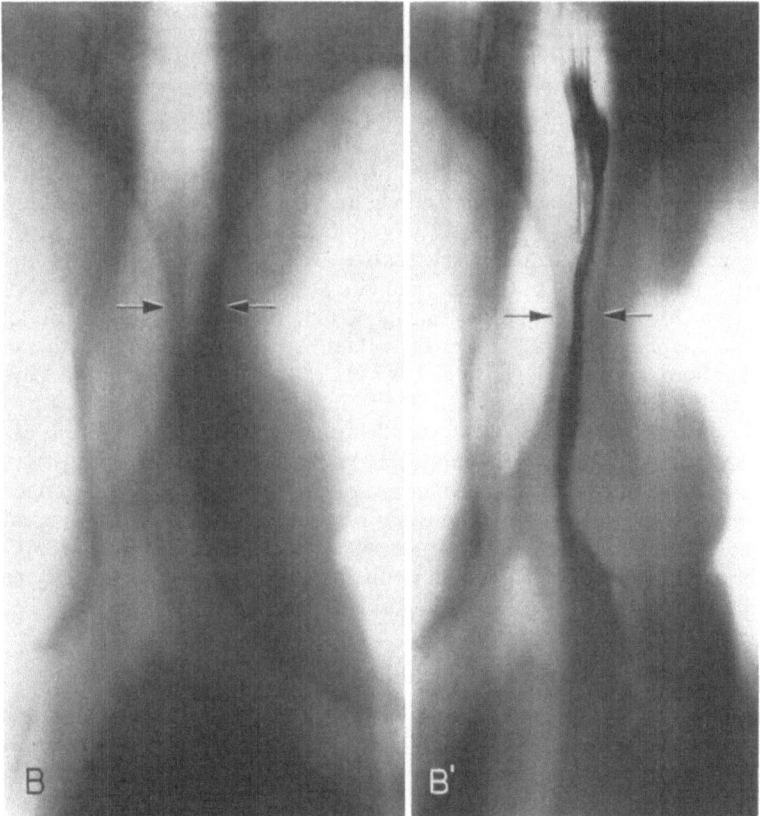

Fig. 66 B

and has a typical aspect which permits to distinguish it from other mediastinal lines. Sometimes, however, this distinction is possible only after opacification of the esophageal lumen. The posterior mediastinal line or posterior junction line is another mediastinal line which may be modified by abnormalities of the esophagus. It is produced by the junction of the right and left pleural layers in the space between the esophagus and the dorsal spine. The posterior junction line is visible in the posterior mediastinum behind the trachea as a fine vertical line extending cranially above the clavicles (Fig. 66B). The soft tissue shadow between the paraesophageal line and the esophageal lumen, outlined by air or barium, is an index of the thickness of the esophageal wall (ORMOND et al., 1963), although it depends on the thickness of the pleural layers and the adventitial tissue with its vessels as well as on the thickness of the esophageal wall. The thickness of this line tends to be uniform and varies with the degree of esophageal filling. It usually measures 2 to 3 mm, with a maximum of 5 mm when the esophagus is distended by barium. In the collapsed phase it measures 4 to 5 mm but may be as thick as 8 mm.

The right paraesophageal line is interrupted at the level of the azygos vein. It may also be obscured by prominent right pulmonary veins, an enlarged left atrium, interposition of the descending aorta or pleural effusion. Visualization of normal paraesophageal and posterior junction lines establishes the lack of esophageal distension (Figley, 1969).

On lateral views, the esophagus courses straight behind the trachea and curves gently forwards as it descends through the retrocardiac space. The soft tissue shadow between the air-filled trachea and the barium-filled esophagus corresponds to the joined tracheal and esophageal walls. In normal conditions it has a uniform thickness. Sometimes the left main bronchus causes an indentation on the anterior border of the esophagus. In longilineal subjects a longitudinal impression may be seen on the posterior wall of the lower esophagus caused by the aorta. The esophageal indentations by the aortic arch, by the left main bronchus and by the left auricle as well as the corresponding esophageal bulges are best visualized in the right anterior oblique position (Fig. 62). In the left anterior oblique position, the esophagus appears almost straight with only an indentation on its posterior border at the level of T5–T6, related to the descending part of the aortic arch. The mucosal pattern, best apparent in the resting state after a deep inspiration, shows vertical parallel mucosal folds (Jutras et al., 1949). These are also apparent in the contracted esophagus but are completely obliterated in the barium-filled gullet. The radiologic appearance of the mucosal folds is an unreliable indicator of the type of epithelium (squamous or columnar) covering it (Allison and Johnstone, 1953; Friedland et al., 1966). In only a minority of the cases is it possible to diagnose an "esophagus lined by columnar epithelium" on the basis of the mucosal pattern (Wright, 1965).

3.2.3. The Esophagogastric Region

The terminology of the radiological landmarks at the espohagogastric junction is rather confusing (Vantrappen et al., 1960). Recent concepts and terms based on anatomic, roentgenologic and manometric correlations have brought simplification and some clarity (Berridge et al., 1966; Wolf, 1970). There is, however, no uniformity in the definition of some important terms such as esophagogastric junction and vestibule, due to the fact that either the mucosal or the muscular junction is used to denote the end of the terminal esophagus. From a radiological standpoint this discordance is of limited importance because there is general agreement about the existence and the roentgenological characteristics of a morphologic and functional unit in the esophagogastric region, the vestibule.

In normal conditions the esophagogastric region lies partly within and partly below the diaphragmatic hiatus. Unlike in specimens in vitro, the normal vestibule does not appear in vivo as a single distensible segment and a distal ring or notch is not visible in it. X-ray pictures of the distended vestibule show that it is limited at its proximal end by a contractile A-ring and that it comprises an ampullary supradiaphragmatic portion and a tubular infradiaphragmatic submerged segment (Fig. 67). The submerged segment has longitudinal mucosal folds and it stretches on deep inspiration. Its identification permits to locate radiologically the position of the hiatus. As studies with radiopaque markers have shown (Botha, 1957; Berridge et al., 1966; Monges, 1956) the hiatus is located slightly above the level of the diaphragmatic shadow, and moves forward and downward on inspiration. The mucosal folds of the submerged segment are larger and more numerous than those of the esophagus above it, and in the absence of a B-ring or notches the esophagogastric mucosal junction is usually not recognized radiologically (Fig. 68). The esophagogastric region has specific functional characteristics different from those of the esophagus proper. It fills as a unit and distends to a greater degree than the esophagus. It contracts

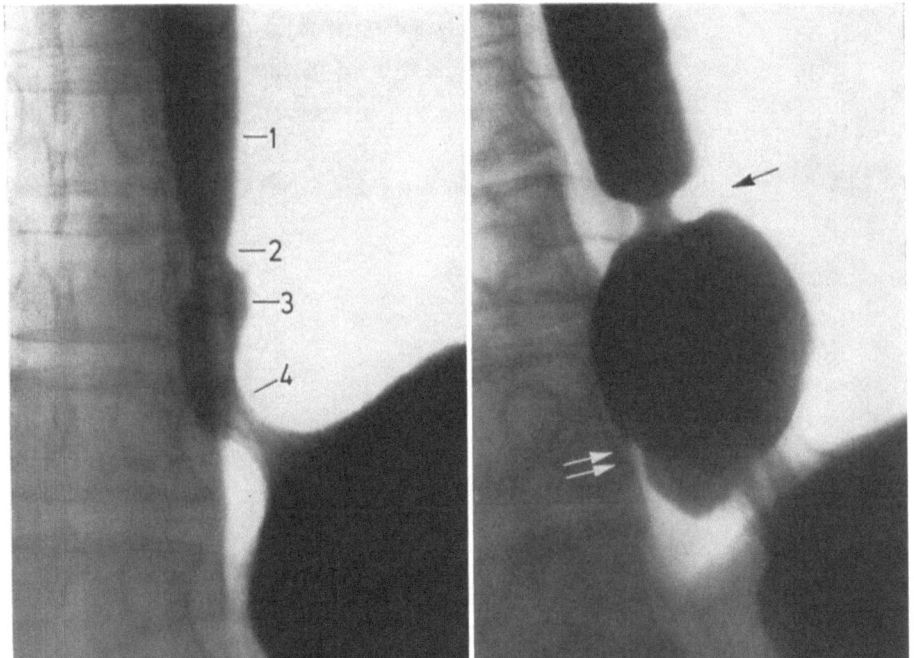

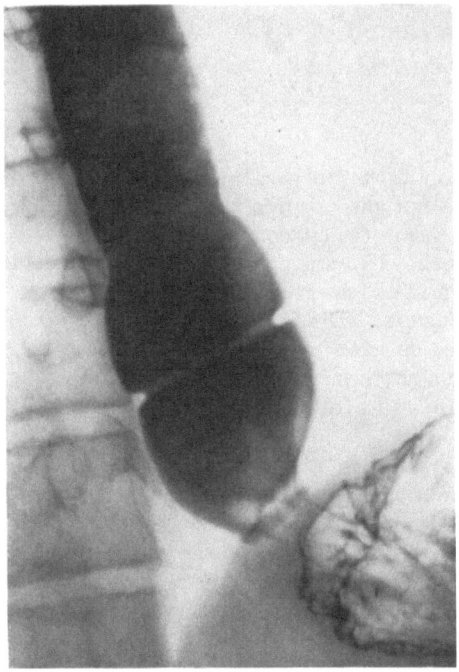

Fig. 67 A–C. Different aspects of the esophagogastric region. A Radiological appearance of the normal esophagogastric region: (1) tubular esophagus, (2) A-ring, (3) supradiaphragmatic ampullary part and (4) submerged segment. B Prominent A-ring (→) and notch (⇉).
C Non-stenotic B-ring

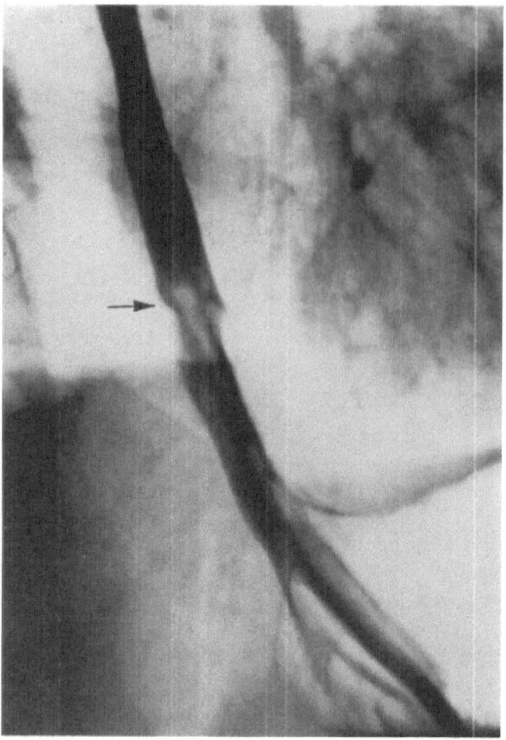

Fig. 68. Radiological demonstration of the level where the mucosal folds of esophageal and
gastric aspect join (→)

in a sequential fashion with the peristaltic wave in the esophagus. A barium
swallow taken in the upright position may be held up for a short while if it
reaches the vestibule before the latter is relaxed (Wolf, 1970). If the subject takes
a deep breath the pinch-cock action of the diaphragm and the increased gastroesophageal pressure gradient may delay the passage of the barium at the level
of the hiatus (Templeton, 1964). During continuous drinking the esophagogastric junction closes on each inspiration so that the passage of barium into
the stomach occurs in a rhythmical way. On relaxation of the vestibule the proximal ring moves upwards and the submerged segment shortens (Berridge et al.,
1966).

The term "phrenic ampulla" refers to the characteristic roentgen appearance
of the supradiaphragmatic portion of the gullet, which assumes a variable inverted
pear-shaped configuration when barium is trapped by the pinch-cock action
of the diaphragm between the hiatus and the progressing peristaltic wave (Templeton, 1964). It does not refer to a specific anatomic structure. In patients
with a small hernia, the hernia may also contribute to the ampullary configuration (Wolf, 1970).

3.3. Preparation of the Patient

In principle the patient must be fasting in order to permit, if necessary,
the examination of stomach and duodenum. When the esophageal lumen is

dilated, as a result of functional or organic obstruction, any residue should be removed to avoid misleading or poor results (WYCHULIS et al., 1971). Before beginning the examination the radiologist should have a clear idea about the patient's symptomatology, about the type of operation which has been performed (if any), and he should have checked the previous X-ray pictures which are available.

3.4. Radiological Examination without Contrast Material

Plain films of neck and chest may give important clues for the diagnosis of some pathologic conditions in pharynx and esophagus. They are particularly indicated when a foreign body is suspected (see Foreign bodies). Special procedures for plain film examination of the pharyngoesophageal region are discussed in 3.6.1.1. In this section only those features will be discussed which are detectable on routine plain films of the chest.

3.4.1. The Air Esophagogram

Accumulation of air in the esophagus without dilatation is a normal finding in children (CAFFEY, 1967). In adults it occurs in numerous abnormal conditions which prevent the esophagus to collapse, such as systemic sclerosis (Fig. 69),

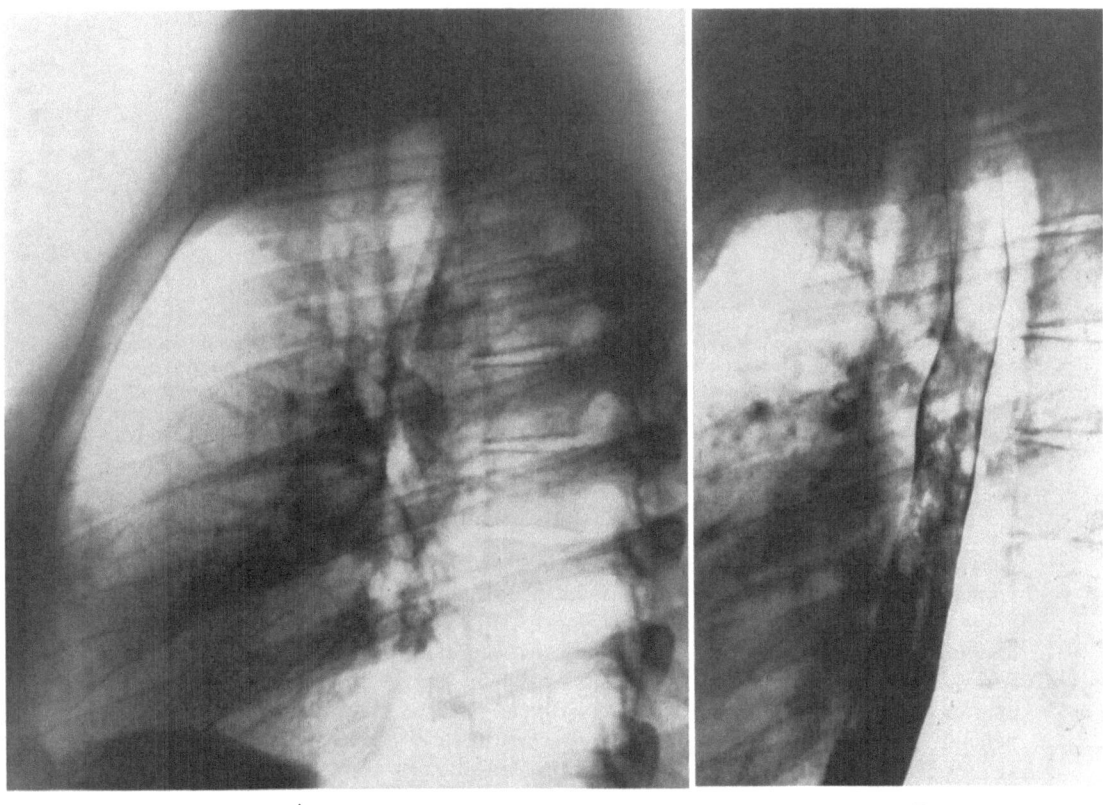

A   B

Fig. 69A and B. Air esophagogram in systemic sclerosis. A Lateral chest film shows the characteristic radiolucent band in the retrotracheal area. B Same view with barium outlining the slightly dilated gullet

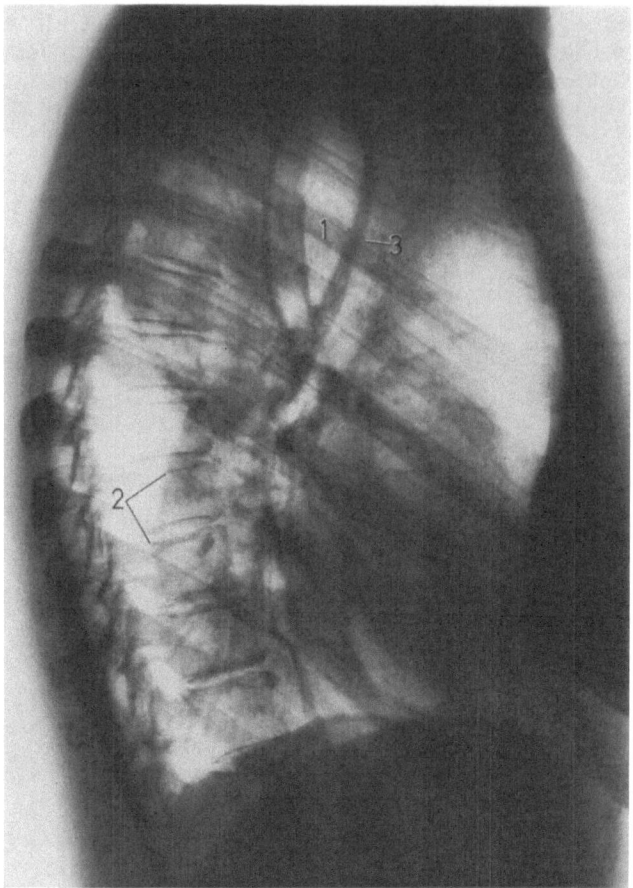

Fig. 70A and B. Plain chest films in untreated achalasia. A Lateral chest film shows air esophagogram (*1*) in retrotracheal area and a strongly outlined dilated esophagus (*2*) projecting on the lower part of the dorsal spine. Note that the retrotracheal line (*3*) appears thickened because the density of the esophageal wall fuses with that of the posterior tracheal wall. B Same view of the opacified gullet. The lower esophagus is displaced posteriorly and to the right of the dorsal spine

achalasia (Fig. 70), inflammatory mediastinal processes (Fig. 71), myotonic dystrophy (KRAMER, 1968), severe caustic esophagitis (MARTEL, 1972), intraluminal benign or malignant tumors (POWELL et al., 1971; McCORT, 1972) and primary circular carcinoma (WOLF et al., 1967). It also occurs in patients with esophageal speech after laryngectomy and in patients who have undergone a pneumonectomy. In old people it may occasionally be observed secondary to a massive belch (CIMMINO, 1969), or spontaneously. We have also observed an air esophagogram above an esophageal narrowing caused by metastatic mediastinal lymph nodes.

The air-filled esophagus is best visualized on lateral films and appears as a band-like accumulation of air behind the trachea (DINSMORE et al., 1966); the posterior wall of the trachea becomes clearly apparent and looks thicker

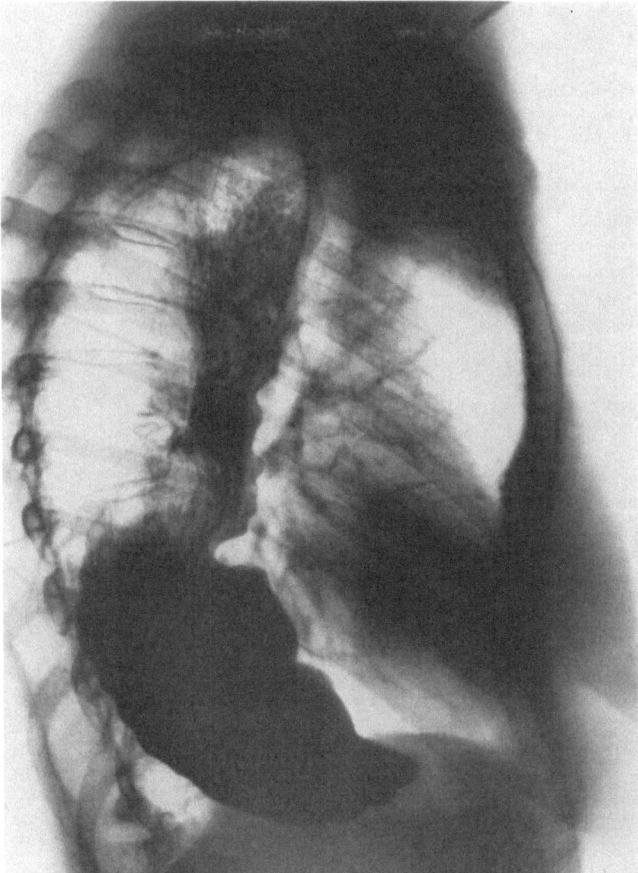

Fig. 70 B

than expected (FIGLEY, 1969) (Fig. 70). On anteroposterior films air in the esophagus results in a separation of the right and left paraesophageal lines in the retrotracheal area. The air esophagogram, when associated with typical lung changes, is highly suggestive of systemic sclerosis. In myotonic dystrophy an air esophagogram may be found in association with megacolon (GOLDBERG and SHEFT, 1972). In non-treated achalasia the esophagus may be markedly dilated and show an air-fluid level (Fig. 72).

3.4.2. Mediastinal Widening

Mediastinal widening due to diffuse esophageal dilatation appears as a displacement to the right of the right paraesophageal line over its entire length but particularly in its upper portion (Fig. 165). On anteroposterior films this results in a double contour on the right border of the heart shadow or in an obvious displacement of the right border of the mediastinum (Figs. 166, 167). On lateral films the trachea is displaced anteriorly and, if esophageal dilatation is marked, the lateral and posterior aspect of the mediastinum may be displaced

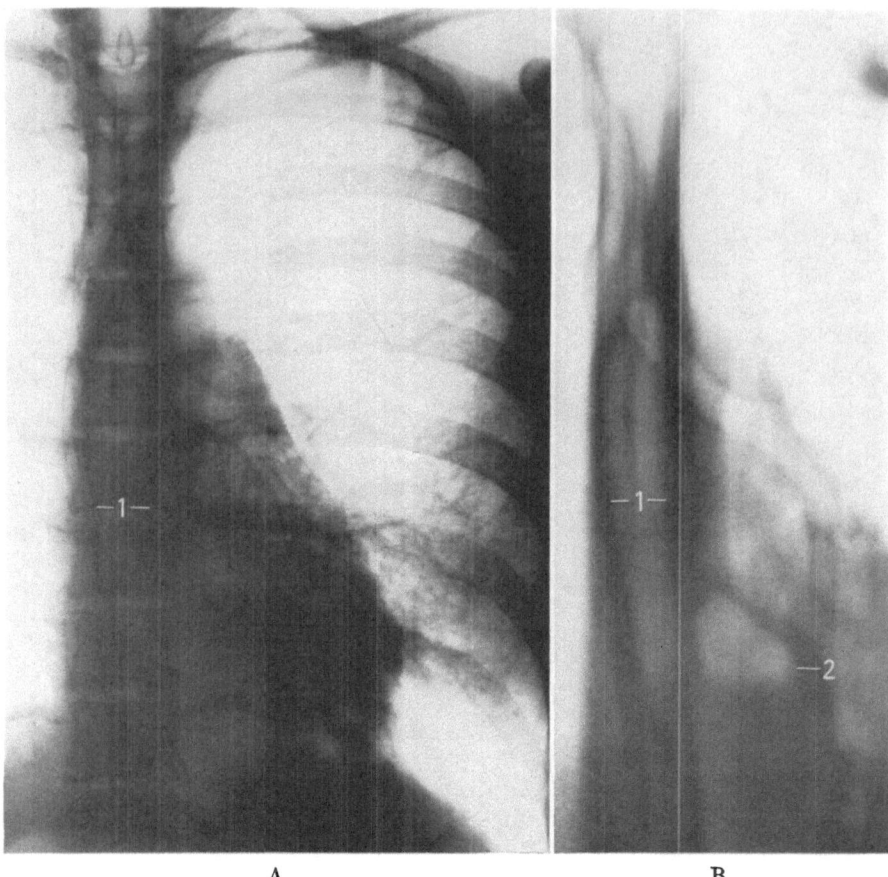

A   B

Fig. 71 A and B. Mediastinitis due to esophageal perforation during dilatation of caustic stenosis. The frontal chest film (A) shows in middle and lower esophagus an air esophagogram (1) which is more clearly demonstrated by laminography (B). Note also the fluid level in a mediastinal collection (2)

to such an extent that it becomes apparent and looks like an unrolled dilated aorta (Fig. 70).

Segmental widening of the proximal portion of the thoracic esophagus is first seen on lateral films as an anterior displacement of the trachea with anterior bulging of the retrotracheal space. On frontal films it appears as a displacement to the right of the right paraesophageal line in the retrotracheal area and results in the absence of the posterior junction line (FIGLEY, 1969). Later the corresponding right mediastinal border is further displaced to the right, and the trachea to the left (Fig. 181). When the esophagus is almost completely filled with liquid the resulting density will obscure the posterior wall of the trachea (FIGLEY, 1969) (Fig. 72).

Circumscribed widening of the middle mediastinum may be caused by large esophageal tumors, epiphrenic diverticula, hiatus hernia, esophageal duplication and venous dilatation. An air fluid level may be observed not only if there is

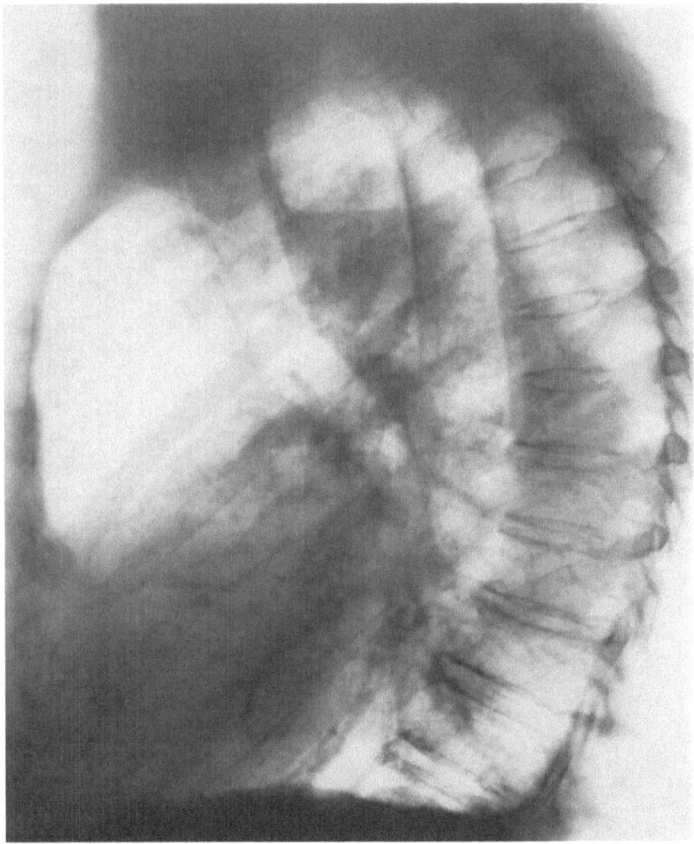

Fig. 72. Lateral chest film showing fluid level in the retrotracheal area in a case of non-treated achalasia. The retrotracheal line is obscured below the fluid level due to the lack of air-soft tissue interphase

retention of fluid and air in the esophagus but also in cases of diverticula, hiatus hernia and communicating duplication (Fig. 73). An extraluminally developed leiomyoma often appears as a round opacity in the middle mediastinum behind the trachea or the heart (LEIGH and WEENS, 1969; KAVLIE and WHITE, 1972). Dilatation of the hemiazygos vein or huge esophageal varices may appear on chest films as a retrocardiac mediastinal shadow which changes in size with changes in posture and respiration (JONSSON and RIAN, 1970).

3.4.3. Mediastinal Calcifications

Stippled calcifications within an esophageal leiomyoma have been observed on chest films but are considered to be rare (Fig. 210) (WEYLMAN and SIMON, 1961; GUTMAN, 1972; HUDDY and GRIFFITHS, 1972). When looked for specifically with laminography we found it in 2 out of 5 cases of leiomyoma. Calcified mediastinal lymph nodes frequently indent or displace the anterior wall of the middle third of the esophagus.

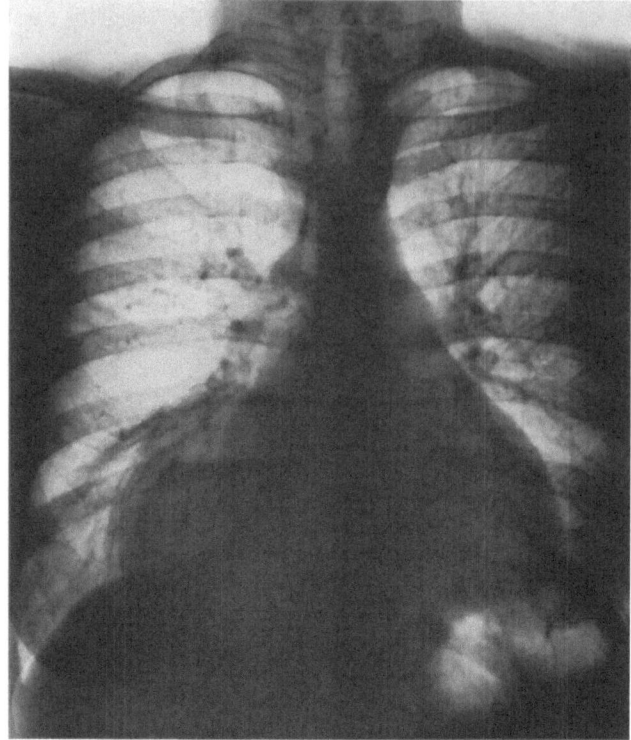

A

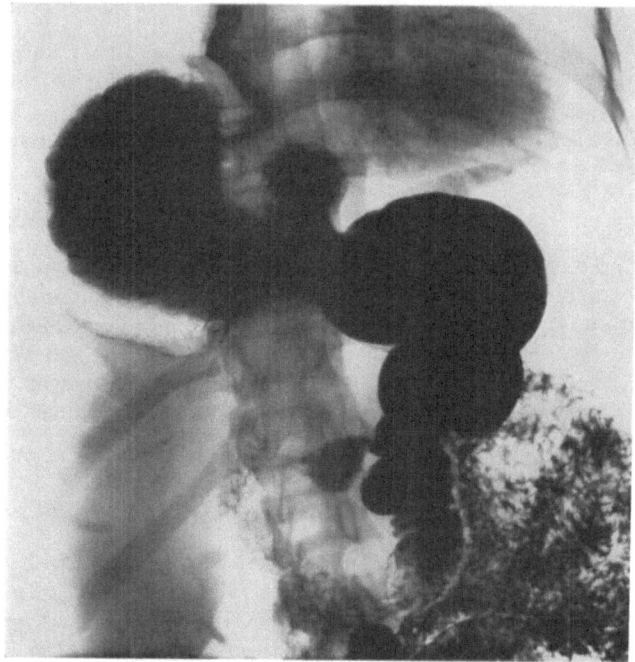

B

Fig. 73. A Frontal chest film showing a density with a fluid level in the right retrocardiac area. B Barium examination demonstrates that it is due to a hiatus hernia

3.4.4. Signs Related to Esophageal Perforation or Rupture

Perforation of the thoracic esophagus results in extravasation of air into the mediastinum with mediastinal, and later cervical, supraclavicular and wide-spread subcutaneous emphysema. Mediastinal emphysema appears on a chest X-ray as radiolucent streaks of air along aorta, heart and diaphragmatic dome

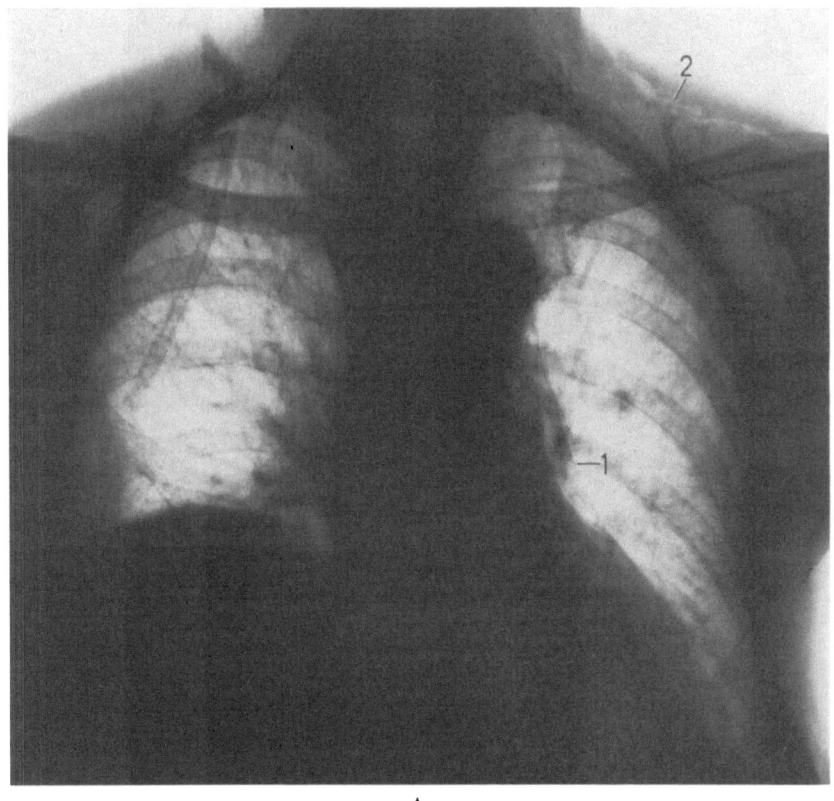

A

Fig. 74 A and B. Esophageal perforation after esophagoscopy in a 72-year old patient. Frontal chest film (A) shows mediastinal (1) and subcutaneous (2) emphysema. The lateral chest film (B) shows a streak of air (3) along the posterior and inferior contour of the heart

(Fig. 74). The isolated finding of paracardiac air may represent pneumomediastinum but may also be due to pneumopericardium or pneumothorax. To differentiate these conditions the patient should be placed in the horizontal position; air in the pericardial or pleural space moves while mediastinal air remains in the same place (TOLEDO et al., 1972). Occasionally air diffuses into the subdiaphragmatic retroperitoneal space. Free gas in the peritoneal cavity or in the subdiaphragmatic retroperitoneal space has been observed exceptionally after forceful dilatation for achalasia (WOLF and KHILNANI, 1966). Later, mediastinitis will cause mediastinal and paraspinal widening, pulmonary densities and pleural effusion and, when the pleura has finally ruptured, pneumothorax. The most valuable clues for the diagnosis of esophageal perforation are provided by chest

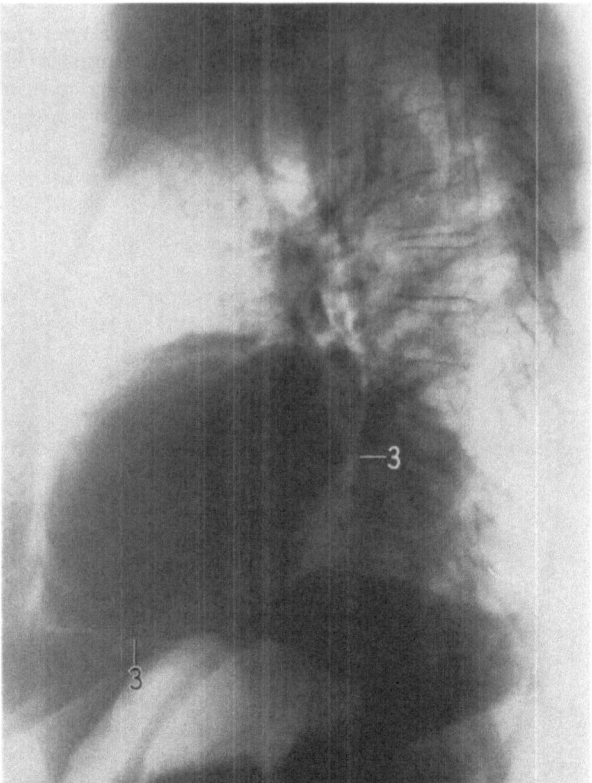

Fig. 74 B

films and esophagograms (Wychulis et al., 1969a). The standard chest film is likely to show evidence of mediastinal and subcutaneous, unilateral or bilateral pleural effusion with or without pneumothorax. Hydropneumothorax without detectable pneumomediastinum may be the initial finding when the esophagus perforates directly into the pleural space (Fleischli, 1966). Penetrated chest films of the recumbent patient will usually reveal paraspinal widening (Fleichli, 1966; Panaro and Leslie, 1965), and films taken with a horizontal beam may reveal a mediastinal collection appearing as a fusiform opacity with a fluid level (Fig. 71). Radiological examination with water-soluble contrast medium will usually demonstrate the site of perforation by showing extravasation of contrast material into mediastinum or pleura (Fig. 183). False negative results have been reported so that the examination must be repeated if a perforation is strongly suspected (Abbott et al., 1970).

In Boerhaave's syndrome (Fig. 303) the perforation is usually located in the left lateral aspect of the lower third of the esophagus, just above the diaphragm. The initial signs consist of localized mediastinal emphysema, pleural effusion and patchy densification in the lung on the side of the esophageal rupture (Panaro and Leslie, 1965; Rogers et al., 1972). Mediastinal widening with a fluid level near the site of rupture is best detected on penetrated chest films (O'Connell, 1967). The "V sign" of Nacleiro refers to the radiolucent streaks of air visible

Fig. 75. Frontal view of dorsal spine. Contrast material, given for cholecystography, was retained in the lower esophagus above a malignant lesion, which was demonstrated by a subsequent X-ray examination of the esophagus

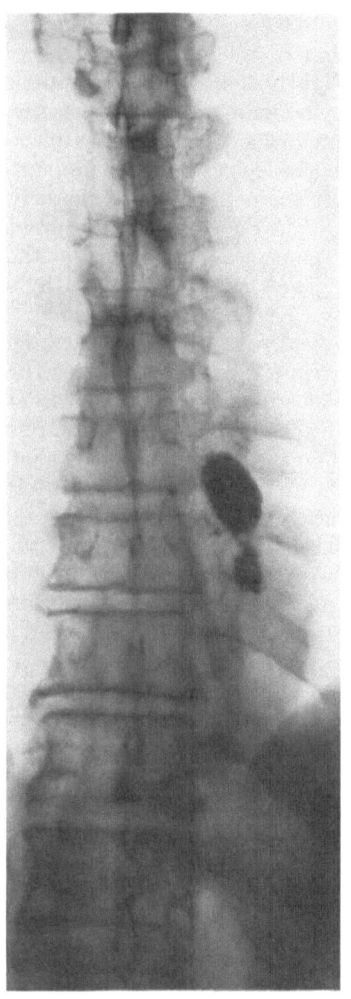

along the left border of the descending thoracic aorta and under the diaphragmatic pleura. It is typical of Boerhaave's syndrome but is rarely seen in its complete form (ROGERS et al., 1972). Usually the mediastinal air is best visible along the aortic arch in the superior mediastinum. The diagnosis is often missed until unilateral or bilateral pleural effusion and hydropneumothorax have developed (WYCHULIS et al., 1969; ABBOTT et al., 1970; KEIGHLEY et al., 1972). Displacement of the esophagus by a mediastinal fluid collection may be the only sign of a rupture when contrast material fails to extravasate.

3.4.5. Retention of Contrast Material

Retention of contrast material in the esophagus late after its ingestion may reveal an asymptomatic pharyngeal or esophageal diverticulum, a hiatus hernia, achalasia or an esophageal narrowing (Fig. 75). It may be observed without anatomical obstruction in old people (EDELL, 1972), in severe esophagitis (MARTEL, 1972), in scleroderma and in cases of intramural dissection of the esophagus (LOWMAN et al., 1969; MARTEL, 1972).

3.5. Radiological Examination with Contrast Material

3.5.1. Basic Technique of Examination

Before giving contrast material a brief fluoroscopy of the chest and abdomen, particularly of the mediastinum and gastric fundus, should be performed. There are three main methods of examination: the classical follow-through, the study of the filled esophagus and the double-contrast technique. In the follow-through study both the motility and the morphology of the esophagus are evaluated. A few swallows of semiliquid barium are watched to evaluate first the pharyngeal phase of deglutition and thereafter the passage through the esophagus. Next, the patient is asked to drink liquid barium and the expanded esophagus is examined at least in two positions. The radiological features of the normal pharyngeal and esophageal motility are discussed in 3.2.1.2. and 3.2.2.1. Any abnormality of the esophageal contractions should be noted. Although tertiary contractions frequently have no pathological significance, a stenotic or inflammatory lesion should be looked for if they are found.

An essential step in the morphological study of the esophagus is the examination of the fully expanded gullet, because this is the only way to visualize a slightly stenosing lesion radiologically. Drinking in the upright position produces a moderate dilatation of the esophageal lumen. To obtain a more complete expansion the patient is placed in the prone horizontal position with a bolster in the epigastrium and pictures are made while he is taking a deep breath or performing a Valsalva maneuver.

The double-contrast method is another means of obtaining good esophageal expansion and is the best method to visualize the mucosal surface. Double-contrast pictures may be obtained by swallowing air during the injection of barium and by various maneuvers, such as taking a small amount of effervescent powder (equal parts of sodium bicarbonate and tartric acid) (Templeton, 1964), injecting barium into the esophagus through a nasogastric tube followed by air injection, and administering anticholinergics. If the stomach is filled with air beforehand, anticholinergics will allow reflux of air into the gullet at each deglutition and then result in double contrast (Suzuki et al., 1972).

Fluoroscopy is the most important part of the radiological examination of the esophagus. X-ray pictures should be taken mainly to document the fluoroscopic observations. The position in which the patient should be placed to take the X-ray picture is determined by fluoroscopy. Both pictures of the entire gullet and spot films of the suspected region should be taken. The problem has been raised whether the radiological examination of the esophagus should be performed in the upright or in the recumbent position (Brombart, 1961; Templeton, 1964; Wolf, 1967; Donner and Margulies, 1972). If the examination is carried out as part of a routine upper gastrointestinal study on a patient who has no esophageal symptoms it can be done only in the upright position. However, if the patient presents with esophageal symptoms or if esophageal lesions are strongly suspected, an examination in the recumbent position is indicated. In some instances it may be necessary to use special procedures, such as those described in 3.6. and in the chapter on hiatus hernia and reflux esophagitis.

3.5.2. Abnormal Images

3.5.2.1. Filling Defects and Impressions

The radiological characteristics of a mass involving the esophageal wall depend in part on whether the lesion is intrinsic or extrinsic (Schatzki and Harves, 1942). An intrinsic mass appears as a sharply outlined filling defect. The abrupt margin of the lesion, where the tumor meets the normal esophageal wall, is best visible on lateral views. If an extraluminal soft tissue density is noticeable, it corresponds in size and shape to the intraluminal defect and does not interrupt the bulging pleuroesophageal line. An extrinsic lesion indenting the esophageal contour produces a gently sloping impression with ill-defined margins, particularly on a frontal view. If an extraluminal soft tissue density is seen it may exceed largely the size of the luminal projection and may interrupt the adjacent pleuroesophageal line. However, if an extrinsic lesion is adherent to, or invades the wall of the esophagus it may mimic closely a primary intrinsic lesion.

3.5.2.1.1. Malignant Tumors

A primary carcinoma may appear as a filling defect, an ulcerated lesion or a rigid infiltrating process (Chiari and Wanke, 1971). A sharp, angulated

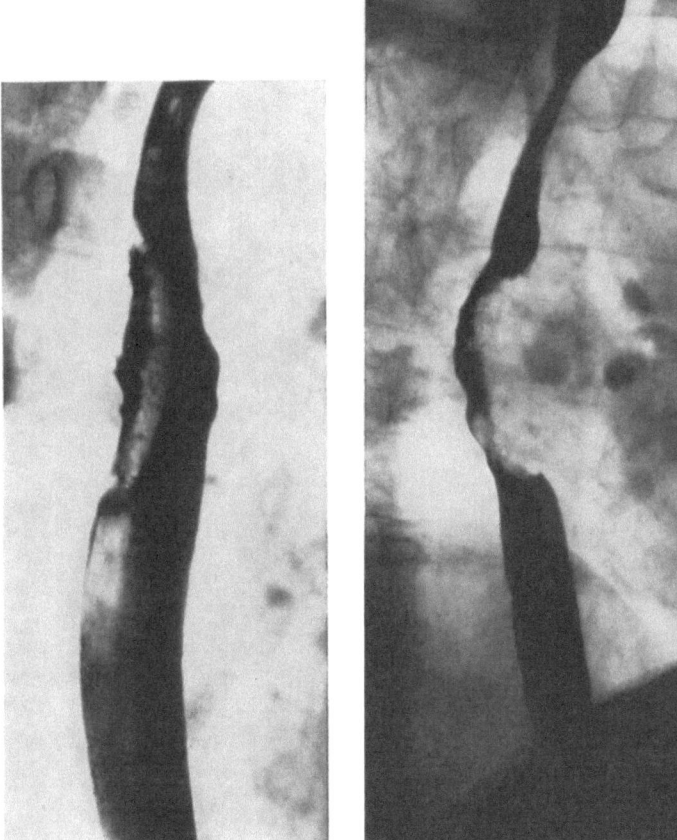

Fig. 76   Fig. 77

Fig. 76. Typical meniscus sign due to ulcerated carcinoma in the middle third of the esophagus

Fig. 77. Lobulated filling defect in non-ulcerated carcinoma

margin is present in the two former types, but may fail in the latter one. The ulcerated type is most frequently seen in the middle third of the esophagus. When the pictures are made with the ulcer in lateral projection while the esophagus is distended by barium, it produces a typical meniscus sign (Fig. 76). Malignant filling defects usually have a broad base and an irregular fungating outline (Fig. 77); a more smoothly outlined filling defect of malignant nature often shows a superficial ulceration (Fig. 78). Sometimes the filling defect is plateau-like and then has a sharply outlined appearance on frontal view (Fig. 79). As a rule, malignant lesions have a linear extension of at least 1.5 to 3 cm along the longitudinal axis of the esophagus (NABEYA, 1970; ENDO et al., 1971). A small carcinoma appears radiologically as a marginal circumscribed zone of irregularity (Fig. 80) or, more often, as true filling defects (Fig. 81). As the lesion advances it extends circumferentially and transmurally. Carcinomas of the ulcerating type have a tendency to encircle the entire circumference and to produce a circular narrowing, limited at its two extremities by rolled and irregu-

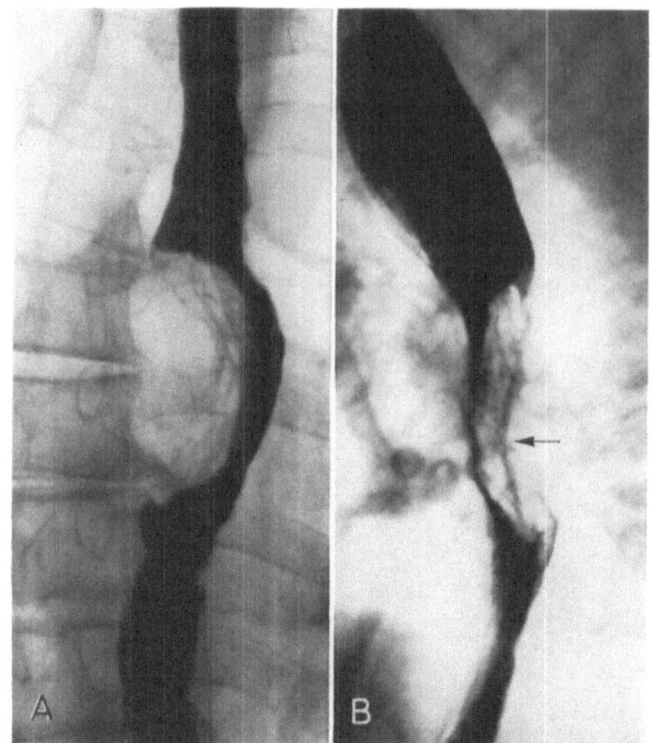

Fig. 78 A and B

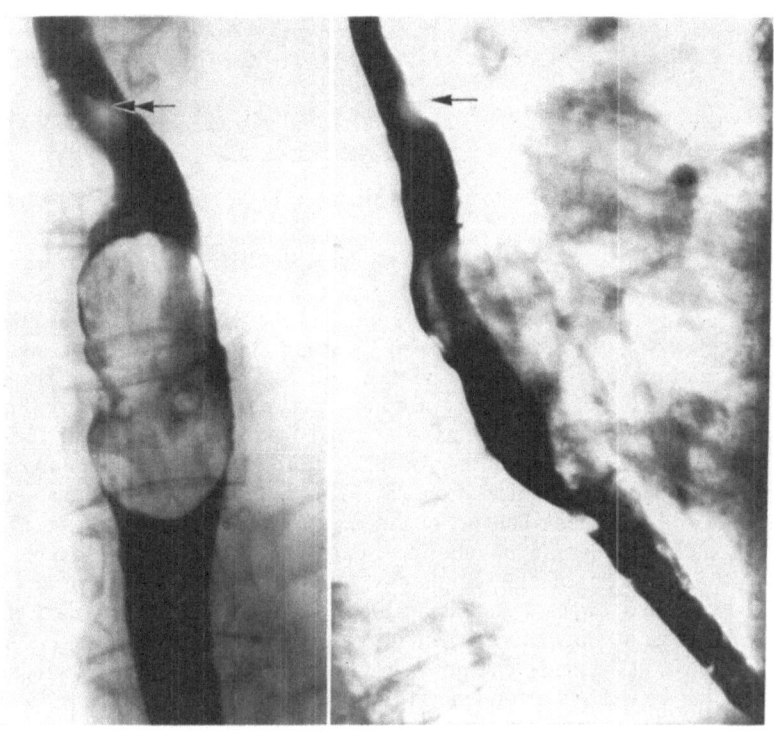

A   Fig. 79   B

Fig. 78 A and B. Squamous cell carcinoma. The profile view (A) suggests a tumor of extramucosal origin, but the superficial ulceration (←), a feature visible on the oblique view (B), is a feature commonly observed in malignant tumors of epithelial origin

Fig. 79. Esophageal carcinoma producing a plateau-like filling defect. Satellite filling defect (←) corresponding to a submucosal metastasis

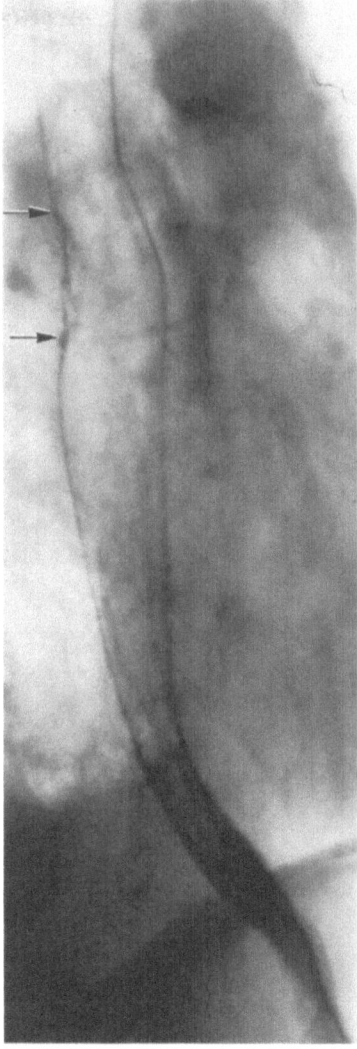

Fig. 80. Small squamous cell carcinoma of middle third, appearing in double contrast as a short segmental irregularity of the posterolateral border (between arrows)

larly outlined margins (Fig. 92). X-ray signs of transmural extension are fixity, paraesophageal soft tissue density and fistula formation with the tracheo-bronchial tract. A paraesophageal mass is usually observed only when the luminal signs of the carcinoma are evident (MARSHAK, 1956).

The infiltrating type of carcinoma occurs more often in the lower esophagus, sometimes in association with a hiatus hernia. It has no sharp line of demarcation and is rapidly stenotic, so that it may simulate a benign stricture or achalasia. Signs of diagnostic value are an irregular outline, mural rigidity, an eccentric lumen and an asymmetric margin (Fig. 82). However, these signs may be discrete and only perceptible by a careful examination of the junction between the stricture and the normal esophagus. Metastatic tumors developing in the submucosa of the esophagus often appear as small, multiple and ulcerated filling defects (Fig. 83); secondary carcinomas invading the esophagus from adjacent

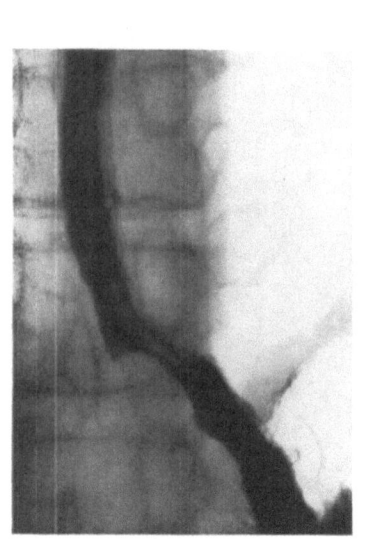

Fig. 81

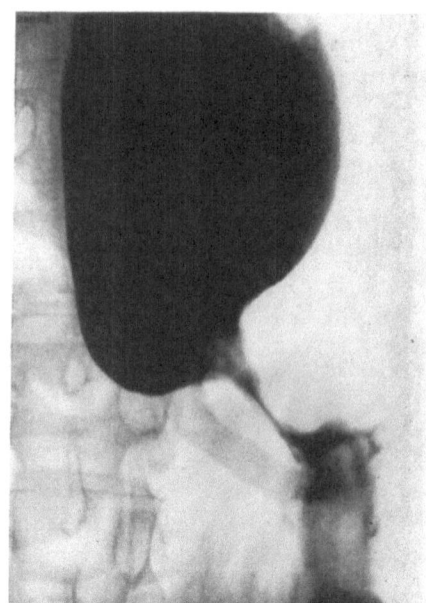

Fig. 82

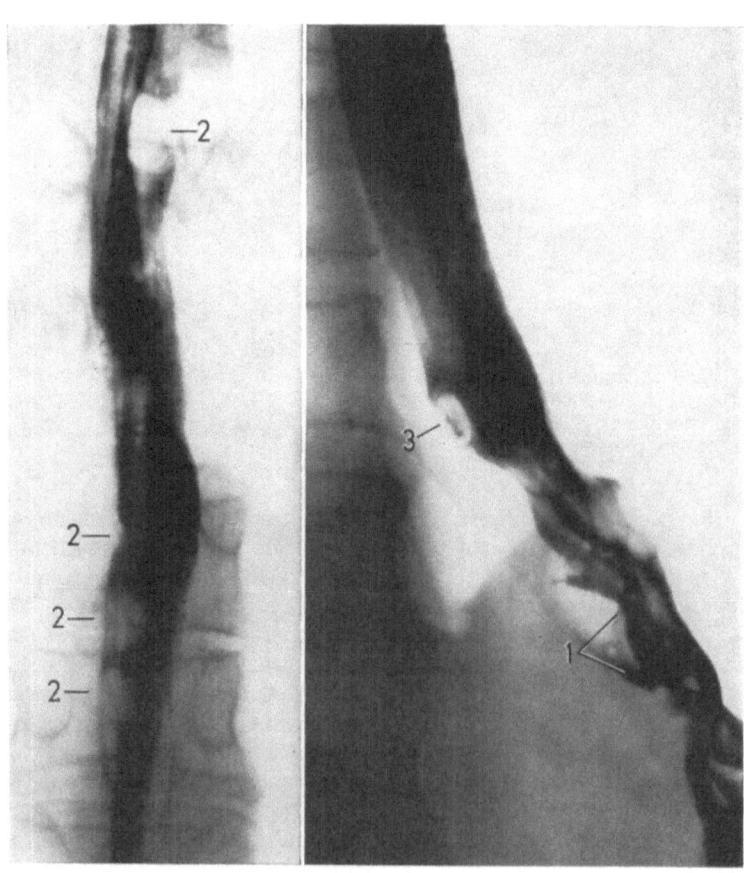

A   Fig. 83   B

structures appear as broad defects which may excavate and then simulate a primary carcinoma (Fig. 95), or as infiltrating extramucosal strictures with signs of a tumor in mediastinum or gastric fundus.

3.5.2.1.2. Intraluminal Defects

Intraluminal defects may be produced by polypoid tumors, which are sessile and then generally malignant, or pedunculated and most often benign. Pedunculated polyps appear as radiolucent defects completely surrounded by contrast

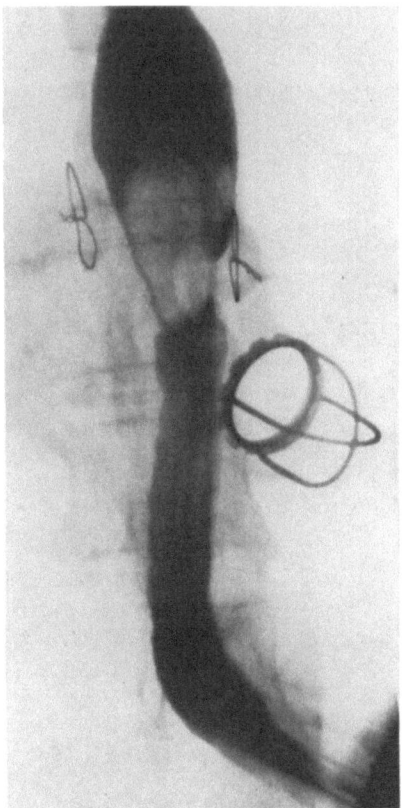

Fig. 84. Intraluminal filling defect caused by radiolucent foreign body

medium, except for the stalk which, however, is often difficult to see. Small polyps are masked when the esophagus is filled with too much contrast medium. Large polyps may distend the esophageal lumen and fork the barium column (NAHUM et al., 1972). In the rare eventuality of malignancy the defect shows

Fig. 81. Small carcinoma of the lower esophagus appearing as a 20 mm smooth filling defect

Fig. 82. Infiltrating carcinoma of the lower esophagus with esophageal dilatation above it. The margins of the narrowed segment are asymmetrical

Fig. 83A and B. Ulcerated adenocarcinoma of the esophagogastric junction (1) with multiple submucosal metastases (2) in middle (A) and lower (B) esophagus; one of them is ulcerated (3)

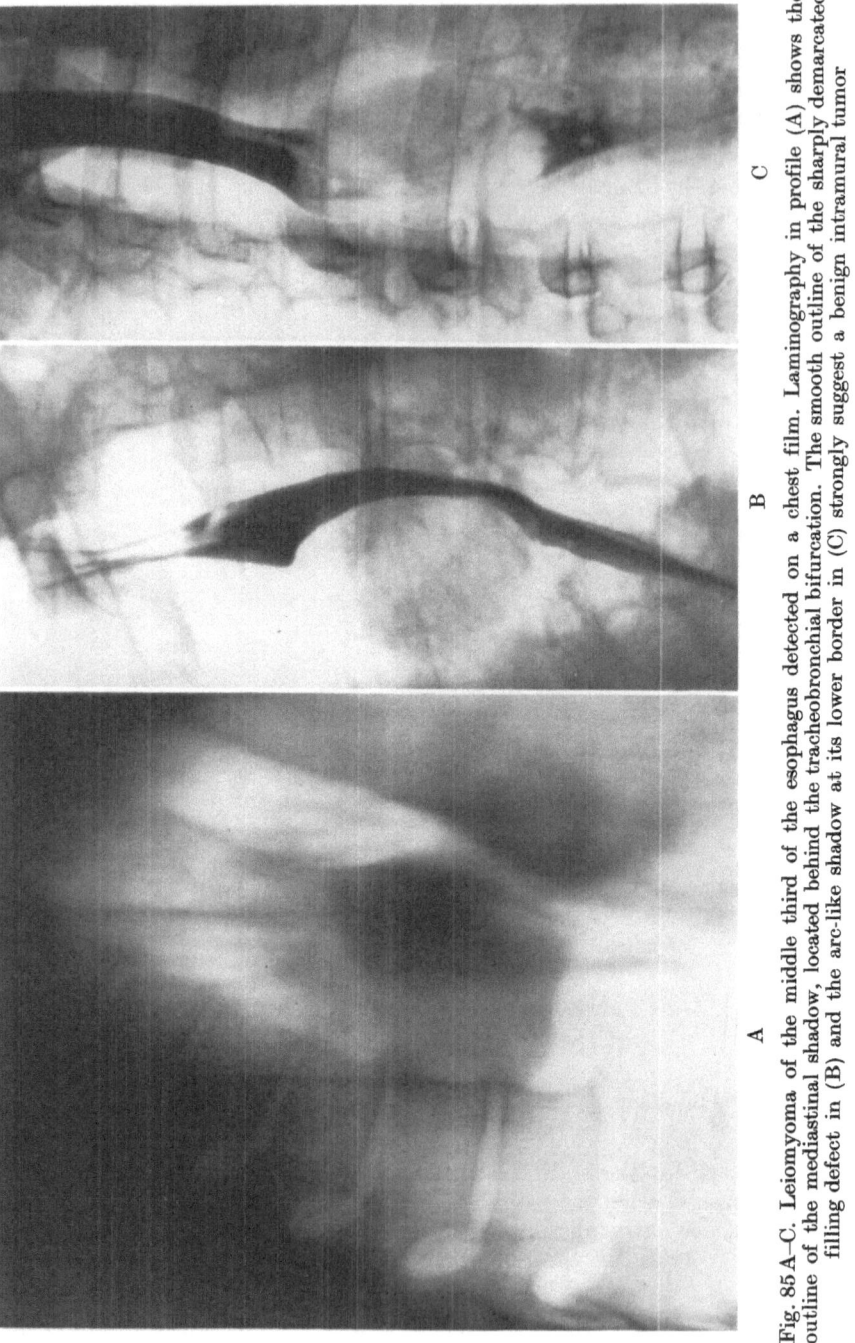

Fig. 85 A–C. Leiomyoma of the middle third of the esophagus detected on a chest film. Laminography in profile (A) shows the outline of the mediastinal shadow, located behind the tracheobronchial bifurcation. The smooth outline of the sharply demarcated filling defect in (B) and the arc-like shadow at its lower border in (C) strongly suggest a benign intramural tumor

irregular outlines, a broad-based pedicle and there are associated signs of wall infiltration; these malignant tumors are often carcinosarcoma and pseudo-sarcoma (CALENOFF, 1962; McCORT, 1972). Impacted non-opaque foreign bodies may give a similar image (Fig. 84). The differentiation is made possible by the clinical

Fig. 86. Bronchial carcinoma with mediastinal metastases causing polycyclic compression and rigidity of the esophageal wall

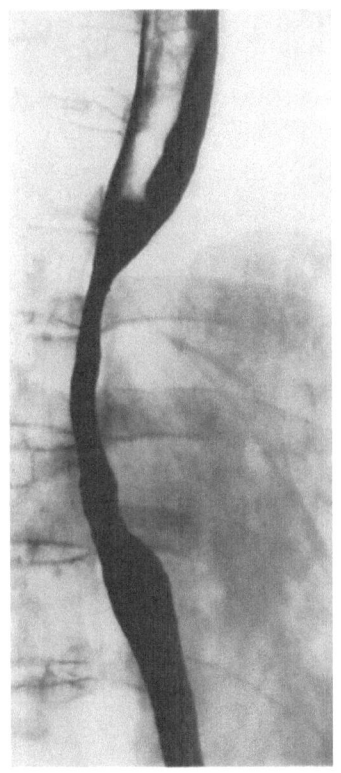

history, the fact that the site of impaction is related to a physiological narrowing or to an organic structure and by the particular shape of the foreign body.

Polypoid hyperplasia of gastric mucosa at the esophagogastric region may produce a markedly protruding intraluminal defect (FAGAN and PALMER, 1963). Mucosal cast is a rare cause of an intraluminal defect (Fig. 356).

3.5.2.1.3. Intramural Extramucosal Defects

Filling defects of these nature are all characterized by their smooth outline.

3.5.2.1.3.1. Benign Tumors and Cysts. A smooth oval or crescent-shaped and sharply outlined defect, normal wall flexibility and a neatly delineated paraesophageal soft tissue density are the characteristic features of benign tumors and cysts (SCHATZKI and HARVES, 1942) (Fig. 85). The lower border of the mass is often more sharply demarcated than the upper one and shows an arc-like shadow (HARPER and TISCENCO, 1945). There is no retention of barium above the lesion, even if it reduces the diameter of the esophagus. Leiomyomas are the most frequent benign tumors and may present additional particular features, such as multiple localization (GODARD and McCRANIE, 1973), calcifications (GUTMAN, 1972; HUDDY and GRIFFITHS, 1972), and an encircling development (BÖTTGER, 1970) with sometimes a pouch-like dilatation of the esophageal lumen, particularly in the lower esophagus (Fig. 210) (BOZORGI et al., 1973).

3.5.2.1.3.2. Malignant Tumors. In primary carcinomas, careful study of an apparently smooth extramucosal defect will usually demonstrate rigidity of the wall and a superficial ulceration (Fig. 78). Non-ulcerated filling defects due to secondary carcinoma may show a confusing appearance; however, the polycyclic appearance of the outline and the mural rigidity in general permit to make the differentiation with benign lesions (Fig. 86).

3.5.2.1.3.3. Varices. An individual varix may become so prominent as to appear as a distinct filling defect (Fig. 310). As a single finding, it is exceptional, though it sometimes occurs as a residuum after a portocaval shunt. Usually, however, varices appear as a cluster of nodular images or as a worm-like dilated submucosal vein (Fig. 309). The particular features of varices are the variable shape in relation to peristalsis and the fact that they cannot often be visualized in the terminal portion of the esophagus. This permits to distinguish them from he hypertrophic gastric folds, which are seen at the esophagogastric region int association with hiatus hernia (DAGRADI et al., 1971).

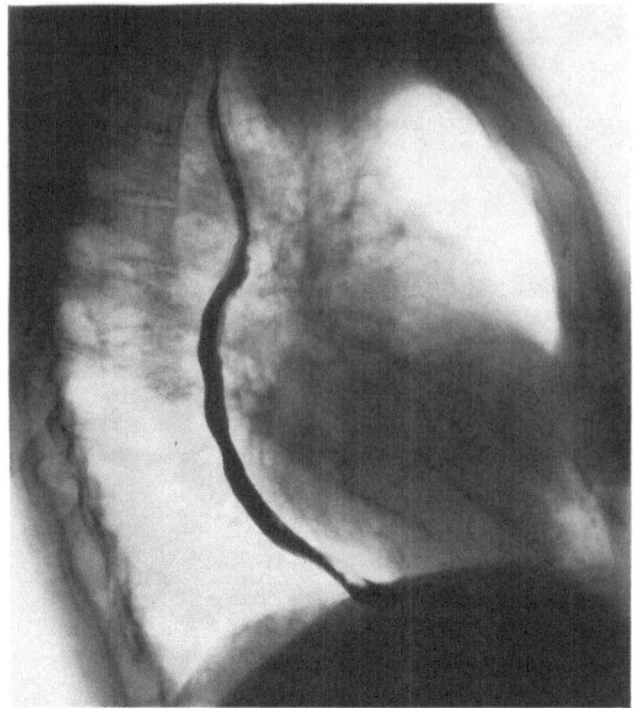

Fig. 87. Impression on the lower esophagus due to enlarged left atrium

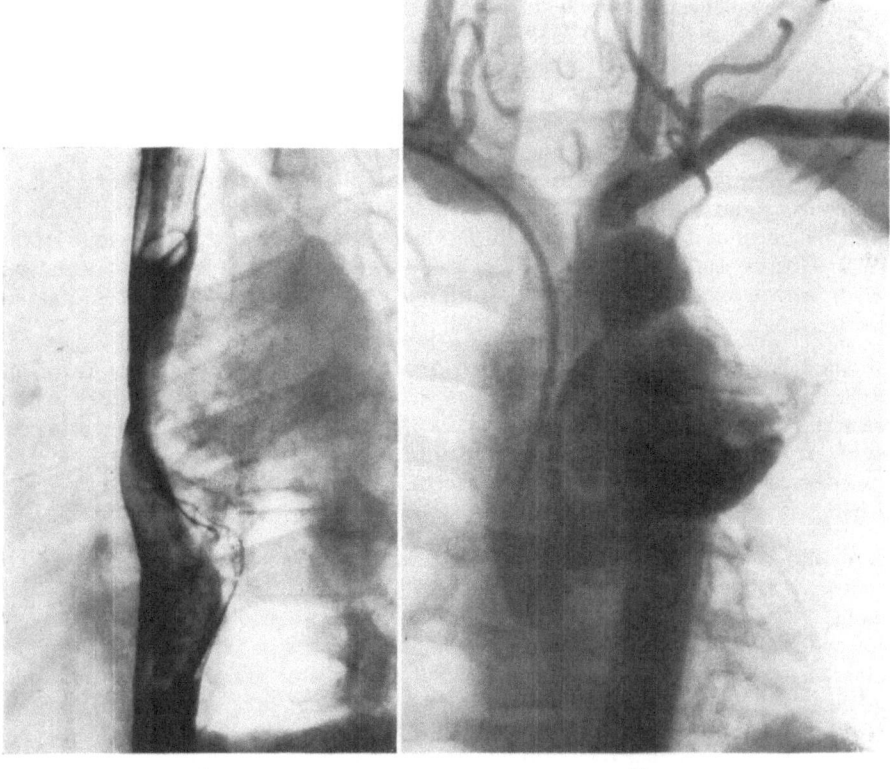

A   B

Fig. 88 A and B. Posttraumatic aneurysm of the aorta (A) causing a smooth impression
on the posterior aspect of the middle esophagus (B)

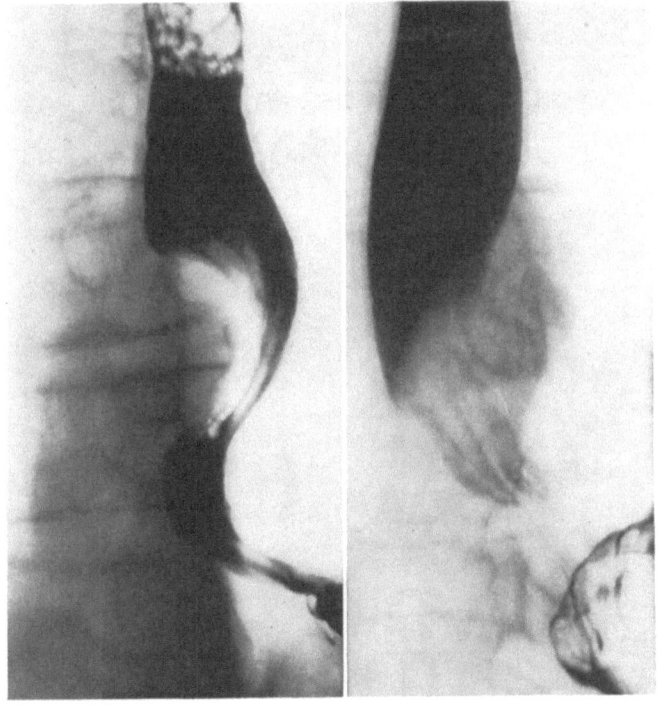

Fig. 89 A and B. The right oblique anterior view of the lower esophagus (A) shows an indentation on the posterior wall. On the frontal view (B) an oblique band-like impression appears, typical of a tortuous descending aorta

3.5.2.1.4. Impressions

3.5.2.1.4.1. Cardiovascular Abnormalities. A large arc-like impression and, in severe cases, displacement of the esophagus occur if the left atrium is enlarged (Fig. 87) (SWISCHUK, 1970) and if there is an aneurysm of the aortic arch (Fig. 88) (COOLEY and SCHREIBER, 1967; WILLIAMS and BONTE, 1961), or of the descending aorta (SAKIYALAK, et al. 1972). Correlation of measured left atrial volume with readings on cardiac X-ray series has shown that the enlargement of the left atrium must be at least 2.5 times to be detectable on esophagograms (LEVIN et al., 1972). Indentations produced by anomalous vessels may occur on the posterior wall of the esophagus at the level of the aortic arch in cases of vascular rings related to an aberrant right subclavian artery (Fig. 292), a right aortic arch (Fig. 295) or a double aortic arch (KLINKHAMER ,1969; VIDNE et al., 1972); on the anterior wall of the esophagus they are found in cases of a vascular sling due to an aberrant left pulmonary artery. Indentation of the anterior wall of the lower esophagus at the level of the left atrium may be produced by an anomalous left pulmonary vein (JACOBS et al., 1972); an indentation immediately above the diaphragmatic shadow may be due to an anomalous pulmonary venous connection below the diaphragm (EISEN and ELLIOT, 1968). In the elderly an indentation on the posterior contour may be due to tortuosity of the descending aorta (Fig. 89); the esophagus passing the aorta undergoes a very typical deviation to the left anterior side; sometimes the esophagus slips from one side of the aorta to the other. In general, indentations caused by vascular anomalies appear on frontal views as bands of radiolucency and on lateral views as notch-like indentations.

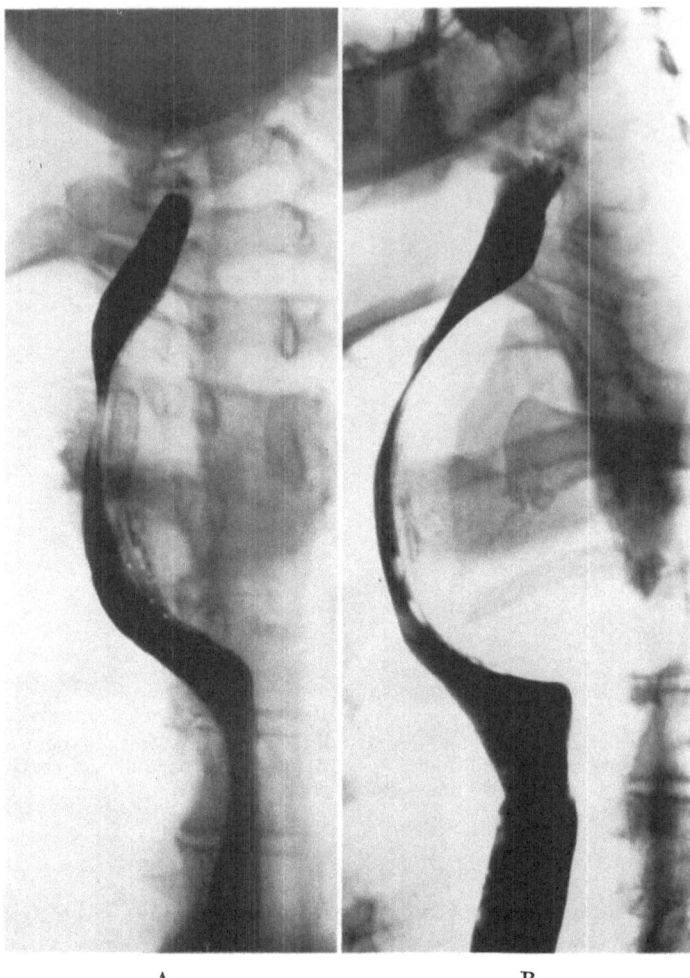

A   B

Fig. 90A and B. Posttraumatic hematoma in the left thyroid lobe resulting in an upper
mediastinal mass. Thyroid scanning failed to show accumulation of iodine in the mass.
On the frontal view (A) the upper esophagus is displaced to the right. The left oblique anterior
view reveals a large impression with a sharp lower margin (B). At operation, the mass was
found to adhere to the esophageal wall

3.5.2.1.4.2. Mediastinal Tumors and Cysts. Space-occupying processes in the
posterior mediastinum first impress the esophageal contour, and as they continue
to develop, displace and compress the esophagus against solid structures. If the
impression occurs on the upper third of the esophagus it may be caused by an
intrathoracic goiter which has extended posteriorly in the upper mediastinum
(Fig. 90), more often on the right than the left side (Shin et al., 1972). In this
case the esophagus and the trachea are displaced to the mid and to the front,
and the paraesophageal soft tissue density which corresponds to the goiter
extends upwards above the level of the clavicles and is in continuity with the
density of the soft tissues of the neck. Thyroid scanning may fail to show any

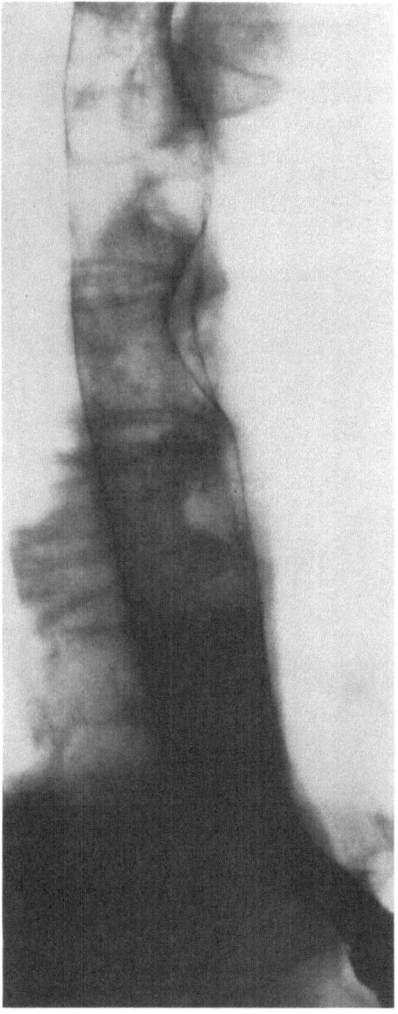

Fig. 91. Double contrast picture of the esophagus showing a smooth impression which was the first sign of a bronchial carcinoma

accumulation of iodine in the region of the mass and is not entirely reliable for the diagnosis (Fig. 90). Impressions on the middle third are often caused by enlarged lymph nodes such as metastatic adenopathies, particularly in cases of bronchial carcinoma (Figs. 86, 91) and lymphomatous or tuberculous adenopathies. These adenopathies commonly indent the anterior or lateral wall of the esophagus at the level of the carina. Typically the indentations have ill-defined margins on frontal as well as on lateral views, except if the adenopathy invades the wall of the gullet (STEPHAN, 1970). Calcifications are frequently observed in tuberculous adenopathies (CHRISTIEN et al., 1972) but may also be observed in Hodgkin's disease after radiation therapy (FISHER et al., 1962).

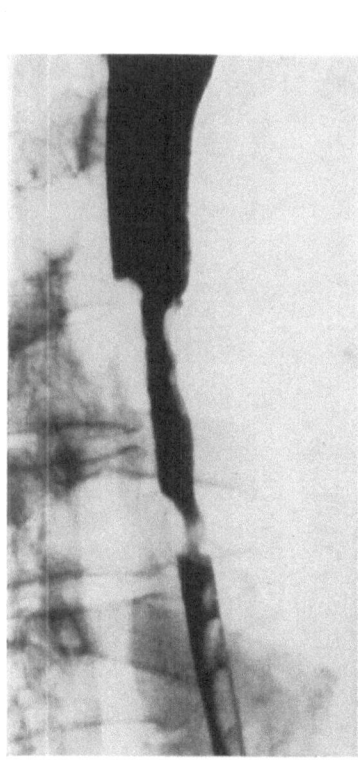 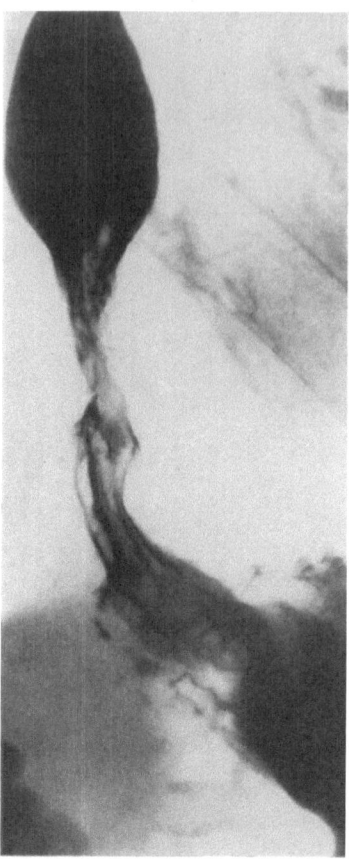

Fig. 92   Fig. 93

Fig. 92. Circular carcinoma in the middle third of the esophagus producing a narrowing
with typical rolled margins

Fig. 93. Tapered narrowing of the terminal esophagus due to carcinoma in a patient with
hiatus hernia. The differentiation between reflux esophagitis and infiltrating carcinoma
in this case is difficult. The asymmetry of the left border was the only sign which suggested
a malignant lesion

3.5.2.2. Narrowings

3.5.2.2.1. Circular Tumors

A narrowing due to primary carcinoma is rigid, irregularly outlined, often
asymmetric and in typical cases bordered by rolled margins (Fig. 92). The lesion
is rapidly obstructing, produces retention even if there is but a slight degree
of distension and may result in fistula formation with the tracheobronchial
tract. Such lesions occur most often in the middle third of esophagus. They
may be simulated by invasive bronchial or mediastinal carcinoma at a late
stage of development. An extramucosal infiltrating carcinoma produces smoothly
outlined narrowings with sometimes tapered borders.

When it is associated with a hiatus hernia, the narrowing must be distinguished
from reflux esophagitis (Fig. 93). A localized rigidity and asymmetrical flattening

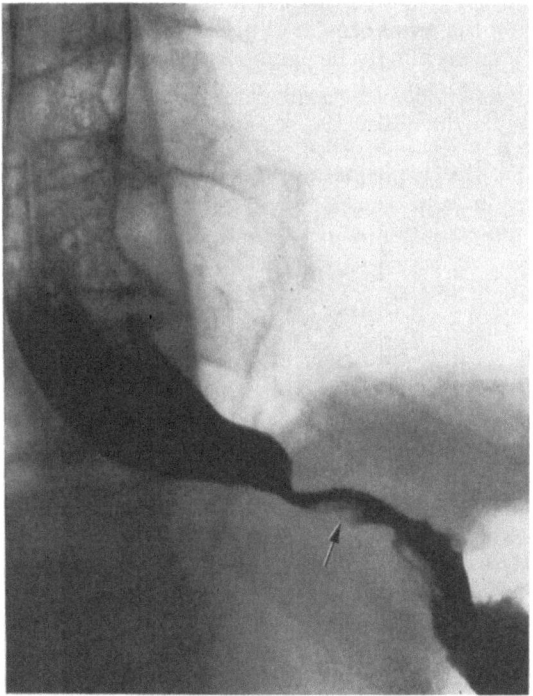

Fig. 94. Tapered narrowing of the terminal esophagus with slight dilatation and aperistalsis. The elongated esophagogastric junction and the filling defect (↑) suggest the correct diagnosis (carcinoma)

of the esophageal wall suggest that the narrowing is due to submucosal extension of a carcinomatous infiltration above rather than to esophagitis. When esophageal dilatation and aperistalsis are present it may be difficult to distinguish carcinomatous infiltration from achalasia (Fig. 94). In this case mucosal irregularity, eccentricity of the lumen, slight flattening of one wall of the esophagus, depression and elongation of the esophagogastric junction are helpful signs which all suggest malignancy. Rarely a smooth narrowing may be due to a benign intramural tumor encircling the esophagus, e.g. leiomyoma of the lower esophagus. The absence of rigidity, a normal mucosal pattern, and the presence of an extraluminal mass, which may be calcified, permit the correct diagnosis.

3.5.2.2.2. Benign Strictures

Benign strictures are characterized by the tapered aspect of the narrowing and by the absence of rigidity. Their distensibility is limited during filling but during emptying the area contracts in a segmental fashion. A peristaltic wave can travel through the narrowing but this sign is not an absolute proof of benignity (TEMPLETON, 1964). The narrowings may be single or multiple. Depending upon the length of the stricture they appear annular, fusiform or tubular. The overlying mucosal pattern is normal in lesions of extramucosal or extrinsic nature, such as atresia and mediastinal fibrosis. If the mucosa is involved by the pathologic process, due to scar formation or to an associated active chronic inflammation, the mucosal pattern is abnormal. A non-obstructing benign stricture may be overlooked unless the esophagus is carefully examined in horizontal position and in full distension. Seemingly benign strictures associated with hiatus hernia do not exclude the possibility of carcinoma. In active inflammations the degree of narrowing may be increased by spasm. Reflux esophagitis usually causes short strictures of 1 to 2 cm near the esophagogastric junction. Long strictures in the middle third of the esophagus are frequently a sequel of caustic esophagitis. Ring-like strictures may be caused by scar formation due to an ulcer at the squamocolumnar mucosal junction and may be indistinguishable from a non-inflammatory ring.

3.5.2.2.3. Rings

The contractile A-ring often seen at the tubulovestibular junction appears as a functional collar-like indentation (Fig. 67B). A particularly prominent A-ring may be an isolated finding, or an associated abnormality in early achalasia, diffuse spasm, epiphrenic diverticulum or hiatal hernia (Fig. 63). The mucosal B-ring is a static, fine and sharply demarcated diaphragm-like constriction of constant diameter. It may be symmetrical but often it is deeper on one side of its circumference. Depending on its diameter, it may be stenotic or not (Figs. 67C, 348). It is located at the squamo-columnar mucosal junction. Sometimes it may be difficult to distinguish a B-ring from an A-ring, except if it can be demonstrated that the ring one is trying to identify is not located at the end of the tubular esophagus or if an A-ring is visible at the same time. Congenital rings and webs are located higher in the tubular esophagus.

3.5.2.3. Changes in Mucosal Pattern

Hypertrophy or absence of folds yield abnormal fold patterns; hazy, coarse or cobblestone appearances on frontal views and serrated contours on lateral views are abnormal mucosal patterns. Fold abnormalities can best be demonstrated in semi-repletion whereas mucosal abnormalities are more clearly visualized in double contrast. These abnormalities are the common feature of active esophagitis and are associated in various degrees with lack of distensibility, stricture or atony (Fig. 96). A cobblestone appearance is a typical feature of esophageal moniliasis (Fig. 267).

3.5.2.4. Crater-like Images

Crater-like images may be due either to malignant or to benign lesions. An ulceration of a mass in the esophagus is diagnostic of malignancy, either primary or secondary and results in typical (Fig. 95) images such as a niche in a filling defect or a crater surrounded by rigid and irregularly elevated margins. Benign ulcerations occur in the course of severe ulcerative esophagitis, caused, for instance, by reflux or by moniliasis (Figs. 96, 268). Sometimes a distinct esophageal ulcer appearing as a niche is the predominant X-ray feature. A benign ulcer niche appears on lateral views as a barium projection outside the esophageal contour with an ulcer collar (Fig. 97) and on frontal views as a barium fleck with punched-out borders, which is round or elongated along the longitudinal axis of the esophagus. The niche may have a length up to 3 cm and may be single or multiple (Fig. 98). It may occur as a marginal ulcer located at the squamocolumnar mucosal junction (Fig. 98C), or as an ulcer in the body of the esophagus, either in the esophageal mucosa above the esophagogastric junction (Fig. 97), or beneath this junction in an esophagus lined with columnar

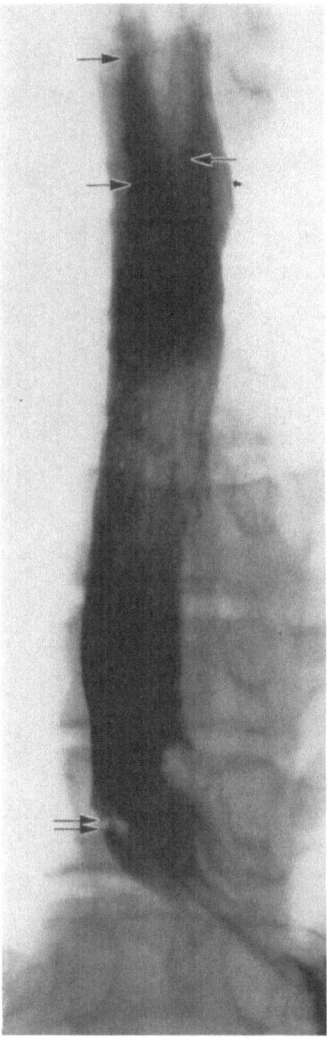

Fig. 95. Extensive esophagitis in a patient with chronic renal insufficiency. The esophagus appears atonic, the mucosal pattern is abnormal and there are penetrating ulcers (→). In the esophagogastric region, the mucosal folds of gastric aspect are hypertrophic (⇉)

epithelium (Barrett ulcer) (Fig. 98 C). A marginal ulcer is usually associated with a localized stricture and may be more or less masked by a local inflammatory reaction due to the contiguous lesions of chronic esophagitis. It may be located high in the gullet, even near the level of the aortic arch, if the esophagus is lined with columnar epithelium or if there is a brachyesophagus with intrathoracic stomach. The ulcer may be penetrating and may perforate into the mediastinum or into adjacent thoracic organs. A penetrating ulcer may be irregularly outlined and, if it is associated with an esophageal or peri-esophageal inflammatory reaction, it may mimic an ulcerating carcinoma. A benign esophageal ulcer usually occurs as a complication of gastroesophageal reflux and regresses after

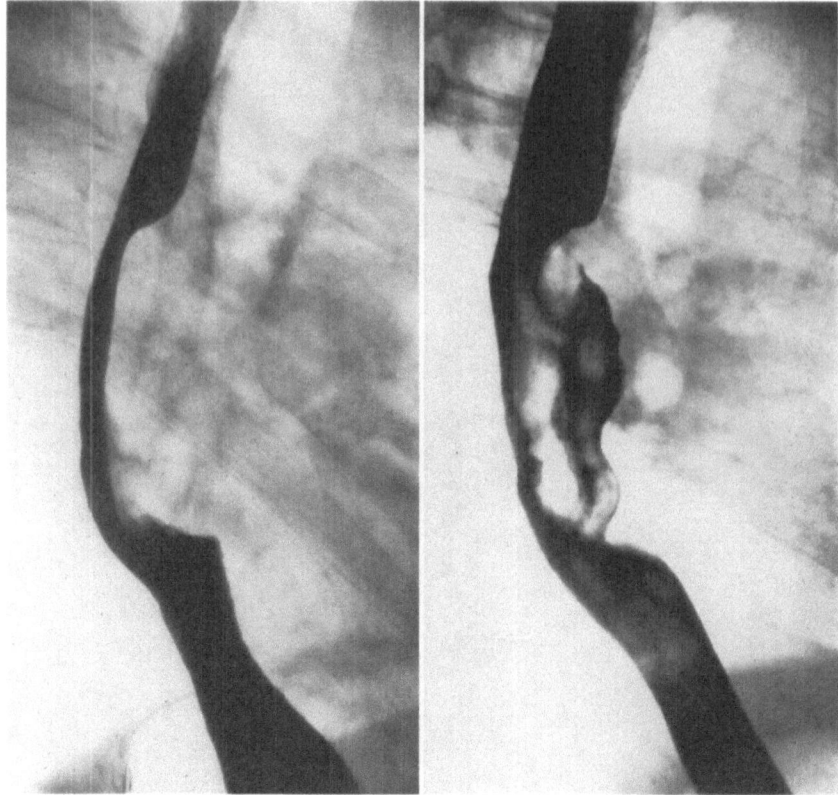

A   Fig. 96   B

Fig. 96 A and B. Metastatic bronchial carcinoma invading the middle esophagus. Initially the filling defect (A) was sharply outlined; two months later, it had changed into a typical "meniscus sign" (B)

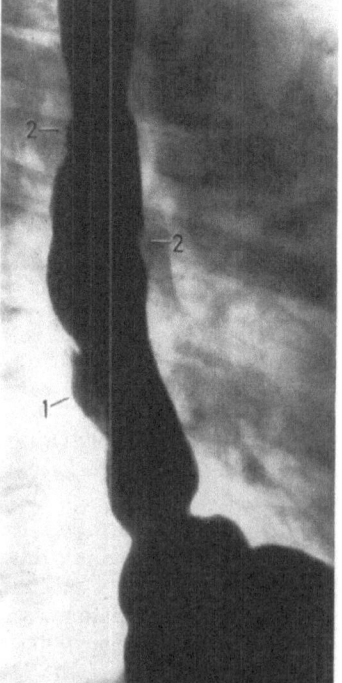

Fig. 97. Hiatus hernia and reflux esophagitis in a 57-year old patient. There is a niche with ulcer collar (1) caused by a benign ulcer and marginal irregularities (2) due to reflux esophagitis

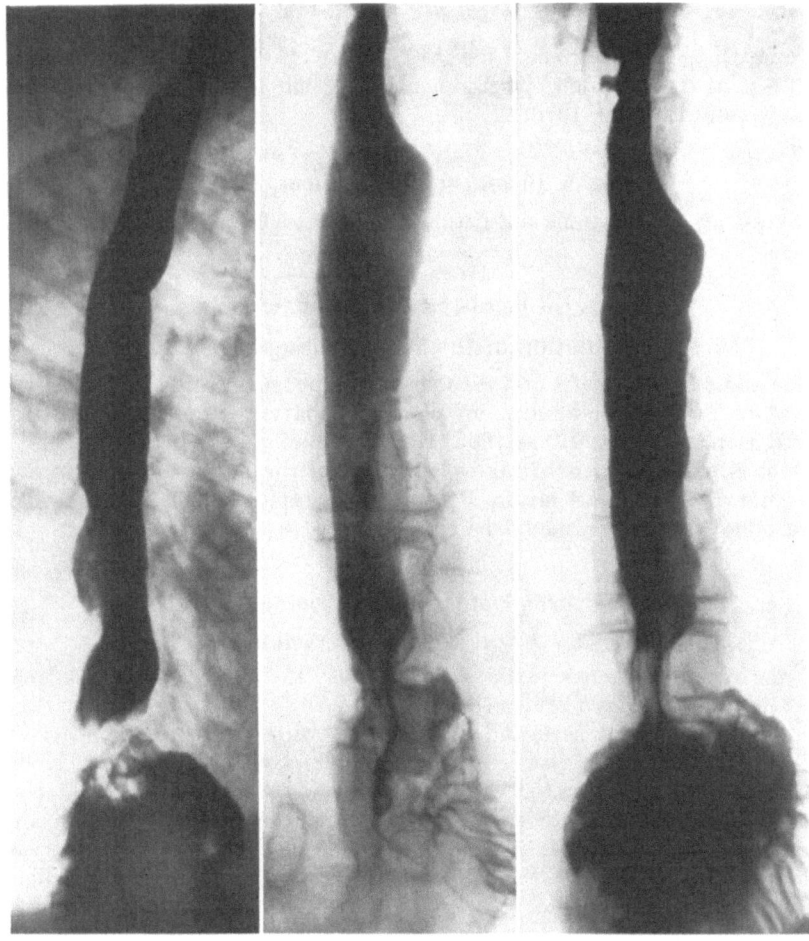

A   B   C

Fig. 98 A–C

Fig. 98 A–C. Esophagus lined with columnar epithelium up to the level of the aortic arch and associated with a hiatus hernia in a 61-year old patient. In the esophageal segment lined with columnar epithelium a 3 cm long oval ulcer can be seen in both the lateral (A) and frontal projections (B). In addition there is a marginal ulcer at the squamocolumnar mucosal junction (C)

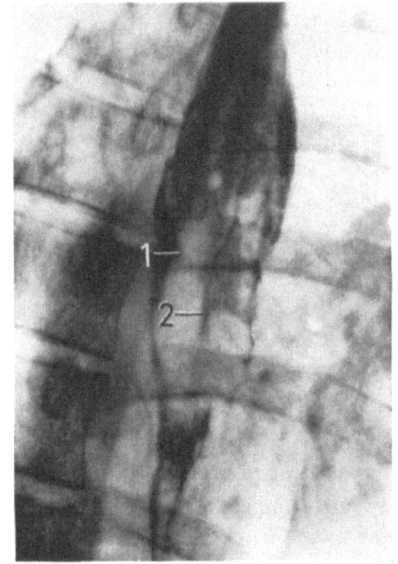

Fig. 99. Endoscopic removal of a swallowed fish bone revealed, at the site of impaction, a localized swelling of the esophageal wall surrounding a linear mucosal ulceration. These findings were confirmed by subsequent X-ray examination, which showed a poorly delineated filling defect (1) and a linear barium fleck (2)

correction of the reflux. Benign ulcerations may also be observed in other conditions, such as trauma due to foreign bodies (Fig. 99) and in patients with Crohn's disease (Kemp Harper, 1970).

3.5.2.5. Diverticula, Perforations, Fistulas

Diverticula, perforations and fistulas are discussed in the appropriate sections.

3.6. Special Procedures
3.6.1. Examination of the Pharyngoesophageal Region

The radiological study of the pharyngoesophageal region includes an anatomical and a dynamic analysis of pharynx, pharyngoesophageal junction and cervical esophagus (Bachman, 1963; Seaman, 1967a). For detail studies of this region it is recommended to take plain films of the neck before beginning the examination with contrast media. Because of the rapid changes during swallowing the standard techniques should be complimented by special procedures.

3.6.1.1. Examination without Contrast Material
3.6.1.1.1. Technique of Examination

Plain films of the neck permit to distinguish the air-filled pharynx from the surrounding soft tissues and vertebral structures. On lateral views the aryepiglottic folds can be seen and the thickness of the prevertebral space can be appreciated. To enhance the contrast on the films either the Bucky technique at high voltage is used, or a low voltage technique without grid. The first technique is widely applied because it permits to enhance the contrast between air and surrounding tissues (Fig. 54). The second technique better visualizes the osseous structures and is therefore the technique of choice to detect faint radiopaque calcifications or foreign bodies. On both the anteroposterior and lateral projections the X-ray beam is centered on the upper border of the thyroid cartilage, with the patient in the upright position. The focal distance will usually be 1 m with a 0.6 mm focus or 1.5 m with a 1 mm focus. The exposures are usually made while the patient holds his breath. On lateral views a better visualization of the air-filled hypopharynx is obtained if the patient keeps his head slightly extended or if he phonates the vowel "ee" which puts the tongue forwards (Seaman, 1969). In children care should be taken to make the exposures at the end of inspiration in order to avoid confusing enlargement of the prevertebral space. Additional pictures can be made while the patient is performing a modified Valsalva maneuver, which tests the distensibility of the pharyngeal walls and may reveal masses that are otherwise not visible (Bachman, 1963) (Fig. 100). Anteroposterior laminography beginning at 2 cm behind the thyroid cartilage and covering a distance of 4 cm is used to eliminate the obscuring shadows of the cervical spine (Bachman, 1963).

3.6.1.1.2. Abnormal Images

Enlargement of the prevertebral space can be caused by several pathological conditions (Fig. 101). Carcinoma of the pharyngoesophageal region is characterized by the irregular aspect of the displaced posterior pharyngeal wall.

A retropharyngeal abscess produces an enlarged prevertebral space with a convex anterior border and sometimes air in the soft tissue mass. Zenker's divertic-

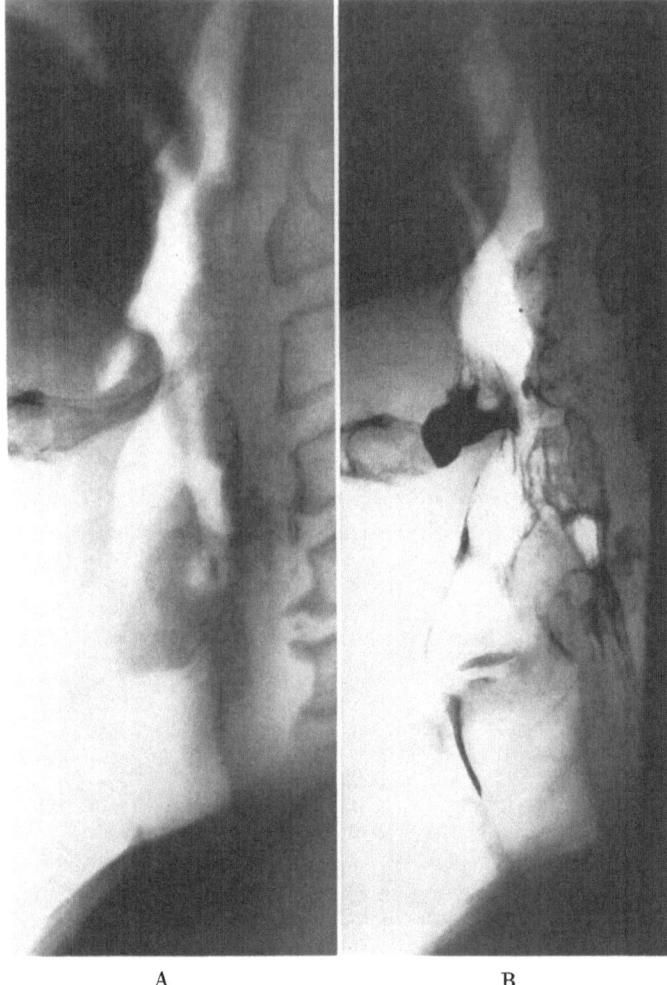

A   B

Fig. 100A and B. Fungating carcinoma of the posterior wall of the hypopharynx. The intraluminal aspect of the tumor is outlined on the plain film by a Valsalva maneuver (A) and
can also be seen after a barium swallow (B)

ulum is often associated with a fluid level in the enlarged prevertebral space.
Foreign bodies can penetrate into the retropharyngeal space and cause an abscess;
when impacted in the postcricoid area, they can cause edema of the prevertebral
space. To distinguish between air in the soft tissues around the foreign body
and air around an intraluminal foreign body, it is necessary to perform a radiological examination with contrast material. An enlarged thyroid, interposed
between the trachea and the spine, can often be recognized by the associated
calcifications. Severe cervical spondylarthrosis with osteophyte formation and
other space-occupying lesions of the cervical spine result in blurring or displacement of the radiolucent stripe of prevertebral fatty tissue (WHALEN and WOOD-
RUFF, 1970). Other causes of prevertebral space enlargement are the superior
caval vein syndrome and a parathyroid adenoma.

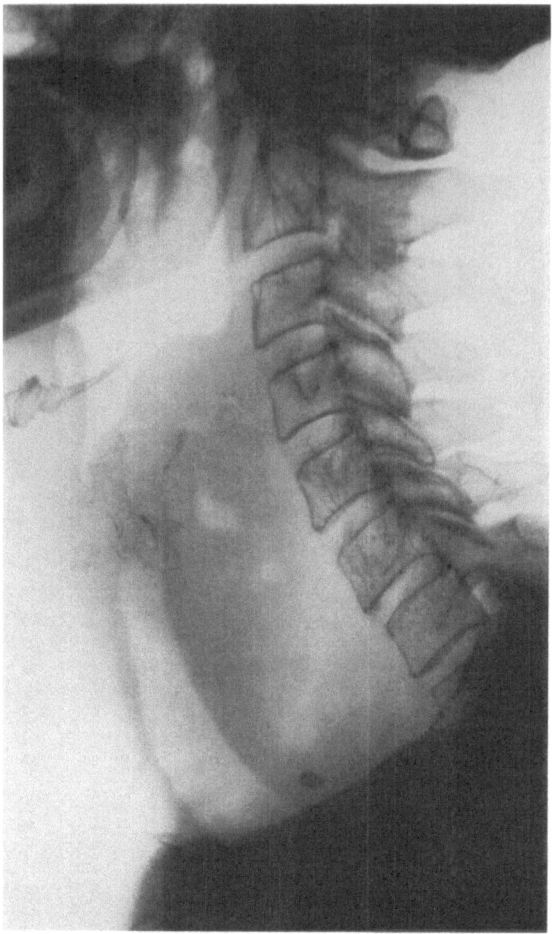

Fig. 101. Plain film of the neck showing a greatly enlarged prevertebral space with an impression on the posterior wall of the trachea and air in the soft tissue density. In this case the space-occupying lesion was a necrotizing carcinoma

3.6.1.2. Examination with Contrast Material

The conventional radiological examination of the pharyngoesophageal region consists of single pictures taken either during or after a barium swallow. The latter can be made with or without a Valsalva maneuver. In addition to antero-posterior and lateral views, pictures can be taken in the oblique position, particularly if compression of the cervical esophagus by thyroid (Kreel et al., 1965) or parathyroid tumors is suspected (Wyman and Robbins, 1954). In the lateral projection the hands are joined posteriorly and held as low as possible to avoid interference of the shoulders. In short-necked subjects an extremely oblique view yields a better visualization of pharyngoesophageal junction and cervical esophagus than the lateral position. In order to avoid tracheal aspiration in patients with swallowing difficulties the examination is best performed with small amounts of thick contrast material, with the patient lying on his back and with a horizontal X-ray beam for profile views (Ardran and Kemp, 1961).

3.6.1.2.1. Single Films of the Swallowing Act

Spot filming under fluoroscopic control is usually preferred over the Bucky technique, because it is easier to control the position of the patient and to time the exposures by means of the count-down method (Figs. 53, 57). The patient is asked to swallow a mouthful of barium at number 3 and the radiograph is taken at a previously established number. If the patient is unable to initiate swallowing at a predetermined number, the pictures should be taken during the upward movement of the thyroid. Owing to the unavoidable differences in the degree of hypopharyngeal distension from one swallow to the other, pictures should be taken of different swallows in order to obtain at least one film in maximal pharyngeal distension, which is essential for the detection of webs (WALDENSTRÖM and KJELLBERG, 1939; SCATLIFF and SCIBETTA, 1963). This technique of examination is suitable to show gross anatomic changes in the hypopharynx but is less accurate than cinefluorography to demonstrate webs and small lesions (SEAMAN, 1967b). A highly opaque liquid barium is now preferred over barium paste because it provides a large and continuous bolus of regular density (BACHMAN, 1963; SCATLIFF and SCIBETTA, 1963).

3.6.1.2.2. Single Films after Swallowing

After a single swallow of creamy barium paste the hypopharyngeal mucosa is coated with contrast material. Usually films are made in both the resting state and during a modified Valsalva maneuver to outline the contours and to test the distensibility of the hypopharynx (Figs. 60, 61). For accurate examination, contrast laryngopharyngography should be preferred.

3.6.1.2.3. Rapid Photofluorography of the Swallowing Act

Photofluorography on 70 mm films at a rate of 6 f.p.s., when started before swallowing is initiated, allows to obtain 3 to 4 successive pictures of the pharyngoesophageal region during the pharyngeal phase of swallowing (Figs. 56, 103). Three successive swallows recorded in the same projection usually yield sufficient information to evaluate the morphological appearance of hypopharynx and upper esophagus during swallowing, to demonstrate the presence of webs and small diverticula and to get an idea of the pharyngoesophageal functioning. It may also demonstrate whether laryngeal aspiration is due to weak laryngeal contraction or to overflow of pharyngeal residue. This technique should be preferred over cinefluorography for the routine recording of the swallowing act.

3.6.1.2.4. Cinefluorography of the Swallowing Act

At present cinefluorography permits the most accurate radiological evaluation of the pharyngoesophageal region during swallowing. This technique is used when simpler methods such as rapid photofluorography do not yield sufficient information, when the patient should not take a large amount of barium because of his poor general condition or the risk of aspiration and when simultaneous radiological and manometric studies are performed (SOKOL et al., 1966). Filming at a speed of 24 to 50 f.p.s. on 35 mm film with a 0.3 mm focus yields the best results.

3.6.1.2.5. Contrast Laryngopharyngography

This technique of examination requires topical anesthesia of pharynx and larynx and is designed to demonstrate the structural appearance of these organs (POWERS et al., 1957).

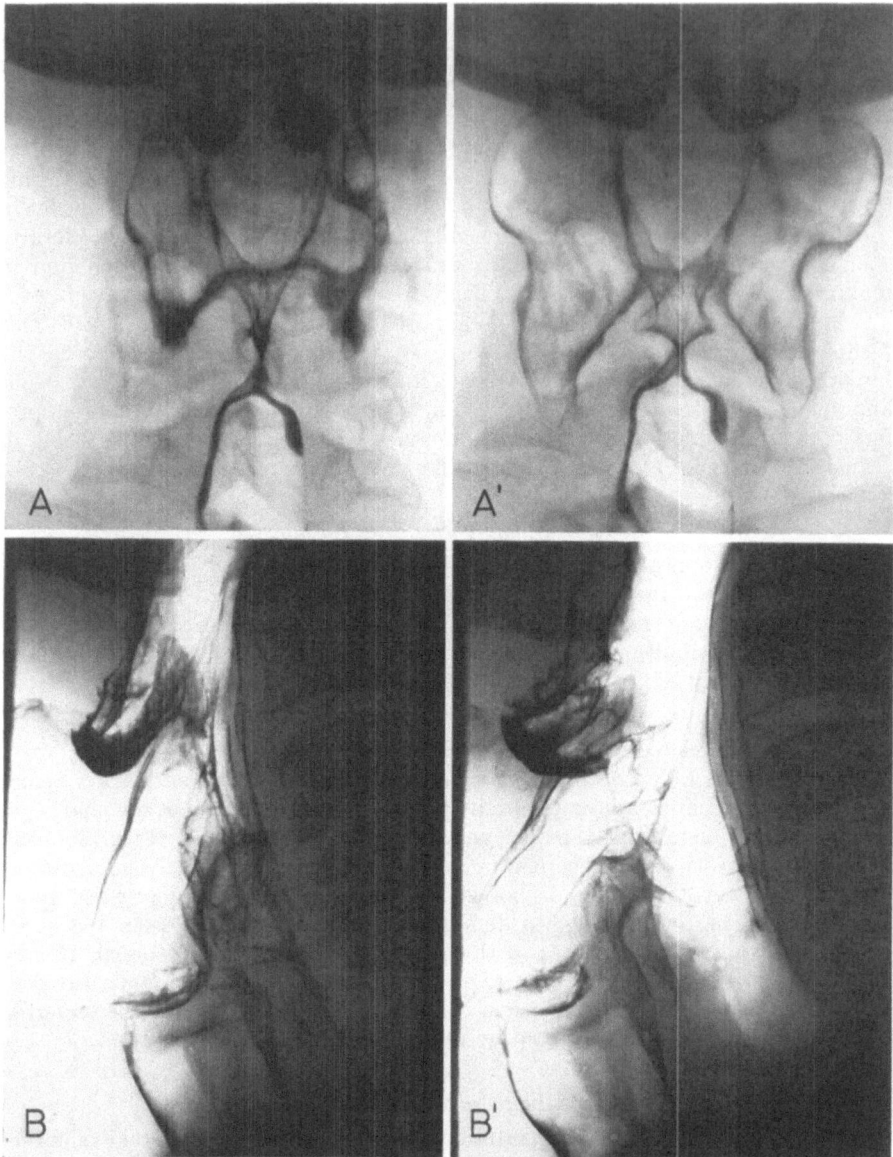

Fig. 102. Frontal (AA') and lateral views (BB') of a normal laryngopharyngogram during inspiration (A, B) and during a modified Valsalva maneuver (A'B')

A small amount of contrast material (dionosil or hytrast) is squirted on the back of the tongue and into the pharynx, fills the valleculae and the pyriform sinuses and spills into the larynx. Spot films are taken in the anteroposterior and lateral positions while the patient performs the following maneuvers: quiet inspiration through the nose, modified Valsalva maneuver, phonating the vowel "ee" and a true Valsalva maneuver. The pyriform sinuses are well visualized on the films taken during quiet inspiration and during the modified Valsalva maneuver (Fig. 102).

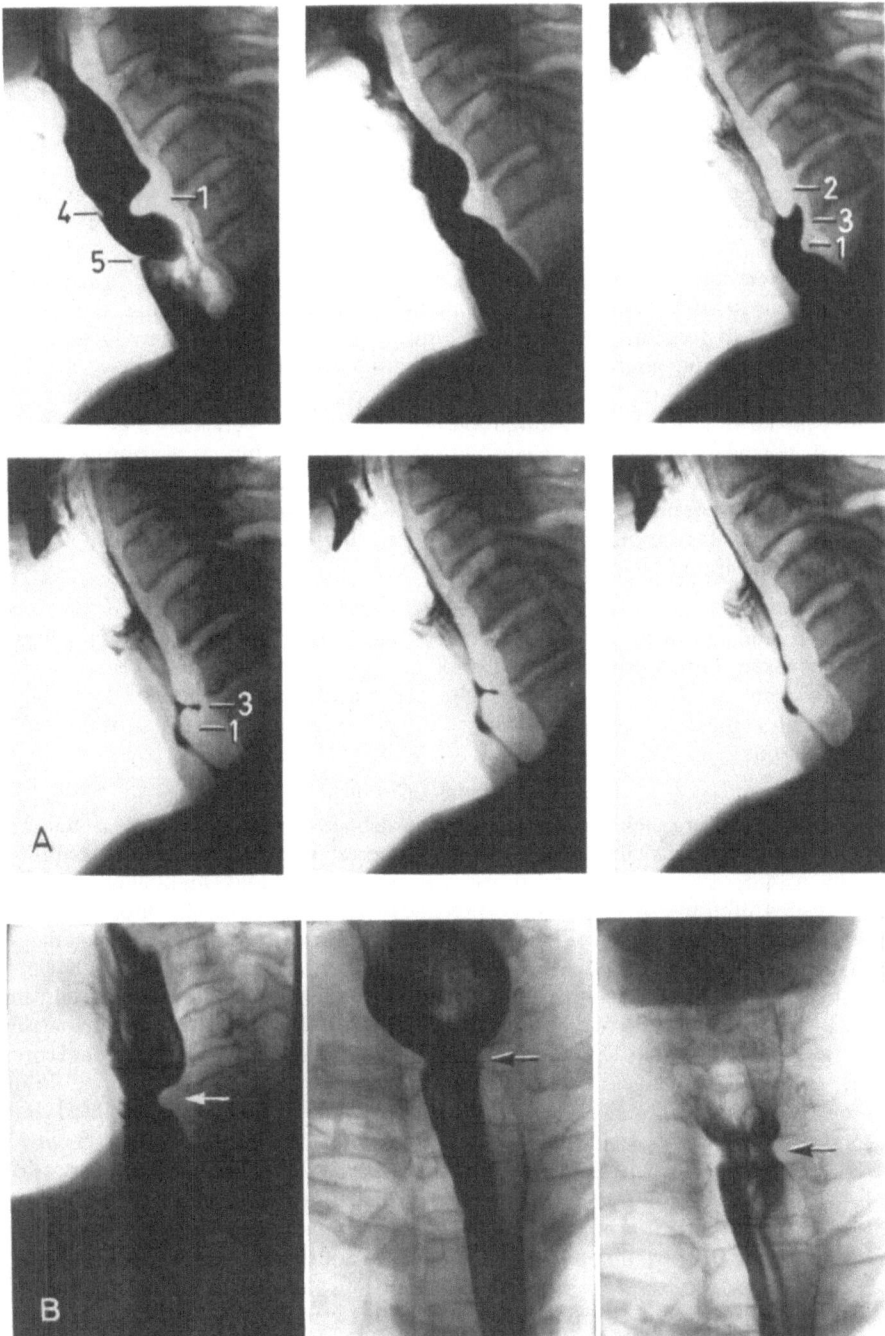

Fig. 103A and B. Photofluorographic pictures of pharynx and hypopharynx during swallow-ing. A Note a typical cricopharyngeal indentation (*1*), an indentation due to pharyngeal peristalsis (*2*), a pseudodiverticular outpouching between the two indentations (*3*), a web-like venous plexus (*4*) and an asymptomatic web (*5*). B In another patient, the cricopharyngeal indentation (←) appears on frontal views as a transversal radiolucent band

Laryngopharyngography is the method of choice to demonstrate pharyngeal carcinoma and to determine the degree of pharyngeal invasion by laryngeal carcinoma.

3.6.1.3. Abnormal Images of the Opacified Pharyngoesophageal Region
3.6.1.3.1. Cricopharyngeal Indentation

In lateral projection the cricopharyngeal indentation appears at the pharyngoesophageal junction of the posterior wall as a sharply localized, smooth indentation of hemispherical or triangular shape. In frontal view may it appear as a transversal radiolucent band. Its visualization is abnormal if it occurs before the contraction of the pharynx is complete or if it persists during the phase of pharyngeal distension. The site of the impression varies between C5 and C7, depending upon the phase of swallowing. The degree of indentation is variable and is most marked after the opaque bolus has passed. It is particularly prominent after total laryngectomy. The diagnosis is based on the persistence of a normal mucosal pattern and on the characteristic, but changing appearance of the indentation (Figs. 102, 213). Indentation of the posterior pharyngeal wall due to hyperactive peristalsis may simulate the cricopharyngeal indentation on single films. This indentation, however, is situated at a higher level and is seen to move down on serial films.

3.6.1.3.2. Filling Defects

Filling defects can be caused by various lesions including webs, benign (intramural or extramural) tumors and cysts, malignant tumors originating in the pharyngoesophageal region or larynx and intramural defects produced by foreign bodies. The typical X-ray appearance of these lesions is described in the appropriate sections.

3.6.1.3.3. Extrinsic Compression

Extrinsic compression is best seen on lateral views and appears as a smooth indentation of the barium column while mucosal pattern and wall flexibility remain intact. It can be caused by various benign and malignant lesions. Osteophytes produce indentations which move up and down the posterior wall of hypopharynx and cervical esophagus during deglutition. A retropharyngeal abscess or mass produces an impression on the posterior aspect of the barium column. Thyroid enlargement often produces a curvilinear impression on the lateral esophageal border which may predominate on either the anterior or the posterior side (Fig. 57). The impression is usually associated with a deviation of the pharyngoesophageal region except in cases of a single thyroid nodule or thyroid carcinoma. Tracheal compression or deviation is often associated but need not be pronounced. Parathyroid masses, when measuring at least 2 cm in length, may compress the lateral wall of the cervical esophagus, the trachea and, more rarely, the lower portion of the pyriform sinuses (Wyman and Robbins, 1954; Scatliff and Scibetta, 1963). Cysts or tumors of the soft tissues of the neck and metastatic adenopathies also cause impressions on hypopharynx or cervical esophagus. Rigidity and an abnormal mucosal pattern characterize the invasion of the pharyngoesophageal wall by an extrinsic malignant tumor such as a thyroid carcinoma.

3.6.1.3.4. Narrowing

An asymmetric and irregular narrowing of the hypopharynx is usually due to carcinoma. A symmetric narrowing with normal mucosal pattern may be observed after radiation therapy for laryngeal carcinoma and is related to edematous swelling of cervical soft tissues. Narrowing at the pharyngoesophageal junction is usually caused by a postcricoid carcinoma or a voluminous Zenker's diverticulum. The carcinomatous narrowing is rigid, fixed, often asymmetric and appears sinuous when the carcinoma is of the fungating type or annular and smooth when it is of the submucosal infiltrating type (TEMPLETON, 1964) (Fig. 104).

Numerous benign lesions can cause narrowing and strictures of the wall of the cervical esophagus. They are discussed in the section on benign esophageal strictures.

3.6.1.3.5. Obstruction

Obstruction in the pharyngoesophageal region results in an arrest of barium flow and in tracheal aspiration. It is usually due to a foreign body, a tumor or a Zenker's diverticulum.

3.6.1.3.6. Dilatation of the Pharynx

Dilatation of the pharynx is observed in bilateral pharyngeal palsy. The pyriform sinuses are not collapsed at rest and balloon out considerably during the modified Valsalva maneuver (ARDRAN and KEMP, 1961). After thyroidectomy the cervical esophagus enlarges and the tracheal indentation becomes more prominent (KREEL et al., 1965).

3.6.1.3.7. Diverticula and Pouches

The diverticula of the pharyngoesophageal region, including Zenker's diverticulum, and the lateral pharyngeal diverticula are discussed in the chapter on diverticula.

3.6.1.3.8. Motility Disorders of the Pharyngoesophageal Region

Pharyngoesophageal dysfunction may present as an isolated disorder or as part of a more generalized disturbance of the whole swallowing act. It results from neuromuscular disorders of peripheral or central origin, or it may be due to organic diseases of the pharyngoesophageal region itself.

The radiological signs observed in neuromuscular disorders of this region include limited ascending movement of the hyoid bone or laryngeal cartilage, failure to develop a good pharyngeal stripping wave, poorly coordinated relaxation of the cricopharyngeal muscle, spilling of barium into the airways, stasis of barium in valleculae and pyriform sinuses and absence of the primary peristaltic wave in the esophagus. The signs are aspecific and can be observed in most cases of advanced neuromuscular diseases, such as bulbar and pseudobulbar palsy poliomyelitis (Fig. 105), severe myopathies, dermatomyositis, myasthenia gravis (Fig. 202), familial dysautonomia and myotonic dystrophy. Aspiration of contrast material in the airways may be due to a defective closure of the larynx during swallowing or to stasis of barium in the pharynx when the larynx opens at the end of the swallowing act. Organic lesions of the pharyngoesophageal region such as a congenital or acquired tracheoesophageal fistula, or a pharyngeal or pharyngoesophageal obstruction may also lead to tracheal aspiration. Asymmetric swallowing, characterized by the unilateral flow of barium through the pharynx, is commonly due to carcinoma of the pyriform sinuses (Fig. 106). However, it may also be observed when the head is turned to one side, when the epiglottis descends asymmetrically, a disorder found more frequently in old people (ARDRAN and KEMP, 1961; ZAINO et al., 1970), in cases of unilateral pharyngeal

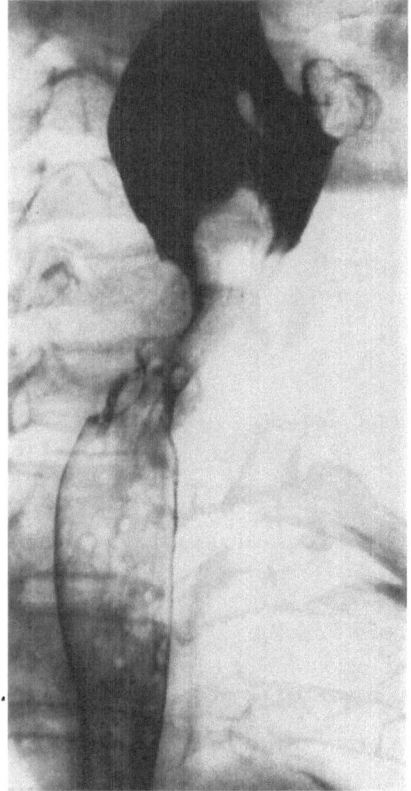
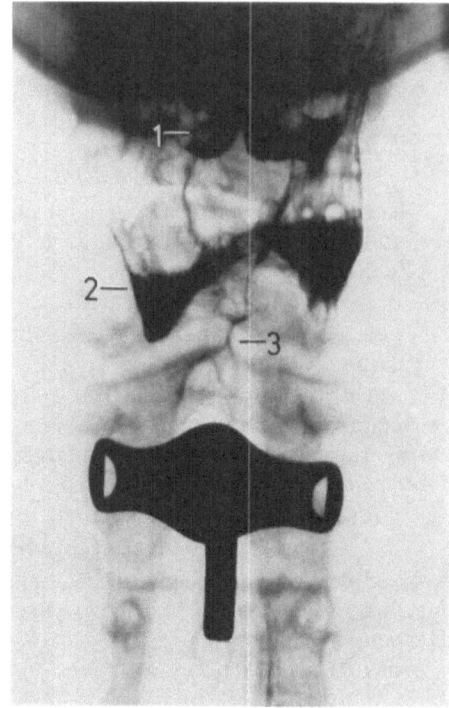

Fig. 104   Fig. 105

Fig. 104. Malignant stenosis in the pharyngoesophageal region

Fig. 105. Swallowing disorder in a case of bulbar poliomyelitis. There is stasis of contrast material in valleculae (*1*) and pyriform sinuses (*2*) and a spill-over of contrast material into the airways (*3*)

palsy (Fig. 107), and in cases of unilateral extrinsic compression by a laterally developed Zenker's diverticulum (DOHLMAN and MATTSON, 1959), or a soft tissue mass in the neck.

3.6.2. The Demonstration of Esophageal Varices

The radiological demonstration of esophageal varices by means of swallowed contrast material is a convenient method but requires special procedures if optimal results are to be obtained (NELSON, 1957; SWART, 1963; SCHATZKI, 1965). Although varices can be visualized in the upright position, they are more prominent in the recumbent position, probably as a result of the increased pressure in the superior caval vein. The technique of coating the mucosa with barium should be preferred over that which fills the esophageal lumen completely with contrast material, because the latter may empty the varices by distension of the esophageal wall and may mask them by the density of the radiopaque column (Figs. 308, 310). A satisfactory coating of the mucosa is usually achieved with

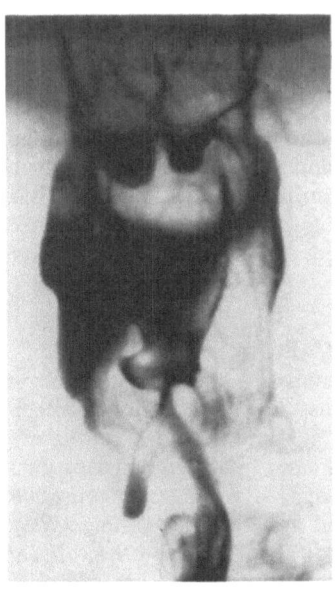

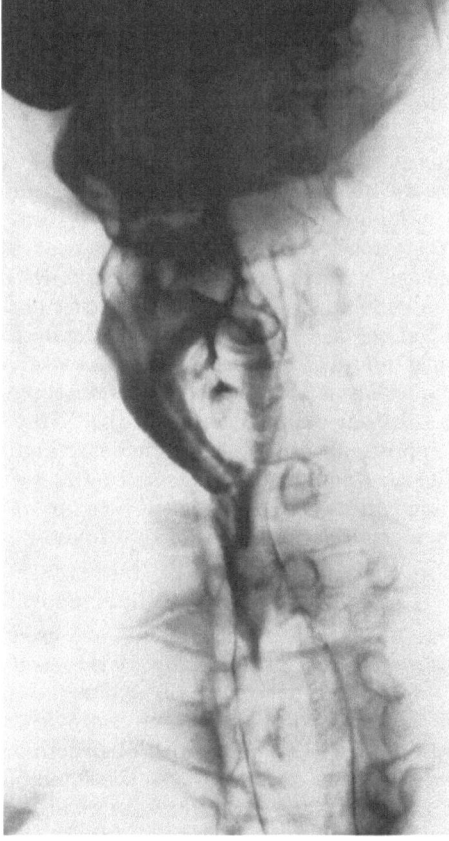

Fig. 106   Fig. 107

Fig. 106. Carcinomatous invasion of the left pyriform sinus resulting in an asymmetric flow of swallowed contrast material through the pharyngoesophageal region and a spill-over into the airways

Fig. 107. Right unilateral pharyngeal palsy due to involvement of cranial nerves (9, 11 and 12). The swallowed contrast material flows asymmetrically along the right hypotonic side of the hypopharynx

fluid concentrated barium after the simple passage of a contrast bolus. Still better results may be obtained by taking a deep breath before the bolus has reached the cardia; if the inspiration is sustained for a sufficiently long time, the ensuing retrograde flow of barium usually results in good coating of the relaxed esophagus (TEMPLETON, 1964). Creamy barium paste should be used if the liquid bolus travels through the esophagus too fast or if the mucosal coating is poor. The exposures should not be made during the contraction phase of the involved segment, because the esophageal contraction empties the varices (Fig. 309). Therefore, the patient should refrain from swallowing and the examiner should wait until the esophagus is fully relaxed and the varices are filled again; this may take as long as 20 sec after the passage of the contraction wave. To promote relaxation of the esophagus a Valsalva maneuver, repetitive swallowing and anticholinergics (DALINKA et al., 1972) may be useful. In our experience varices are also well visualized in the esophageal segment ahead of an oncoming peristaltic contraction (Fig. 306). Multiple spot films should be performed in different positions of the patient. Sometimes varices can be clearly demonstrated only if the patient is turned into the appropriate position, determined by fluoroscopy (SCHATZKI, 1965). Usually, however, varices are well demonstrated in one of the two oblique positions, most frequently in the left anterior oblique position. Cinematographic and videotape recording techniques may increase the diagnostic accuracy of the radiological examination, because they yield a higher percentage of positive results and eliminate some false positive interpretations, related to the presence of air bubbles (ADLER et al., 1964). Esophageal varices can be associated with varices in the gastric fundus or even in the duodenum, as well as with gastric and duodenal ulcer. Therefore, if esophageal varices are found, a radiological exploration of stomach and duodenum is called for. The studies of DAGRADI et al. (1971) indicate that radiological techniques are less accurate than endoscopy for the demonstration of esophageal varices. In our experience, when the X-ray technique is applied carefully there is no appreciable difference in the detecting capabilities of both methods. Indeed, small varices may be demonstrated by X-rays (Fig. 307); however, the endoscopic technique offers the advantage of being more accurate in the differential diagnosis between small varices and mucosal folds.

3.6.3. Pharmacoradiography

Several pharmacological agents are used to enhance the diagnostic accuracy of the radiological examination of the esophagus. Anticholinergics decrease the tone and the contractility of esophagus and gastroesophageal sphincter and inhibit the mucus secretion. The use of these agents has been advocated (1) to relieve "spasm" associated with obstructing esophageal lesions and consequently to obtain a better outline of both the stenosed and poststenotic segment (WRIGHT, 1965; MURRAY, 1966; GHAHREMANI et al., 1972); (2) to facilitate the differential diagnosis between achalasia and organic obstructing lesions of the cardia; (3) to evaluate more accurately non-stenosing regions of esophagitis; (4) to enhance the radiological visualization of esophageal varices (DALINKA et al., 1972); (5) to better demonstrate the presence of a lower esophageal ring (LONGIN, 1966); (6) to facilitate the radiological examination of the filled esophagus (WAHL and KEMPF, 1964) and (7) to perform double-contrast studies (SUZUKI et al., 1972; WAHL and KEMPF, 1964).

Topical anesthetic agents are sometimes used in advanced achalasia to achieve a better opacification of the narrowed segment and to help in the differential diagnosis with cancer of the cardia (NEMIR et al., 1971).

The inhalation of amyl nitrite yields inconstant results in cases of achalasia and may have undesirable side effects (TEMPLETON, 1964).

Cholinergic drugs such as Mecholyl are used in the Mecholyl test (see Pharmacological Test).

4. The Radiological Examination of the Esophagus in Children[1]

The radiological examination of children requires a special technique, mainly because they usually cannot cooperate before the age of 4. If satisfactory results are to be obtained an adequate immobilization of the child, short exposure times and an efficient way of administering the contrast material are essential.

---

[1] In cooperation with D. CLAUS.

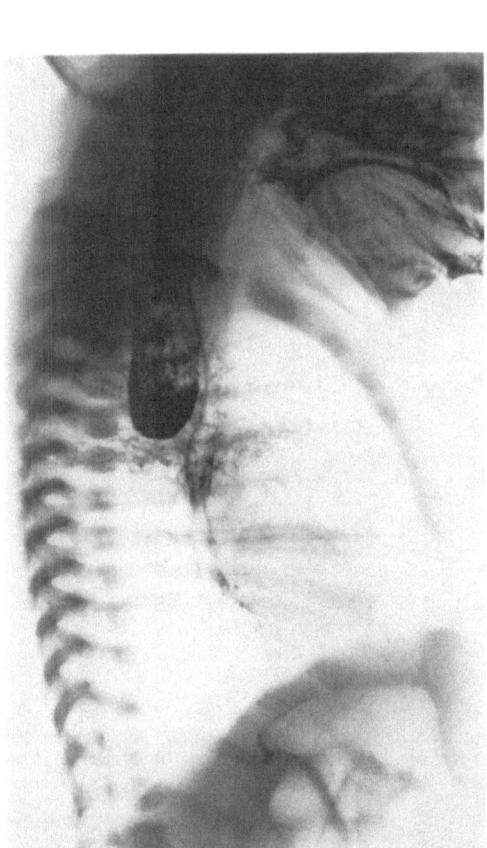
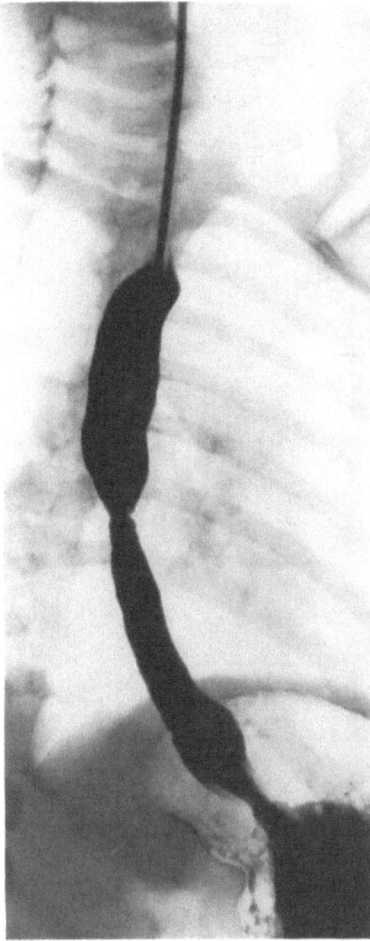

Fig. 108   Fig. 109

Fig. 108. Contrast material was administered to this newborn with esophageal atresia by means of a feeding bottle. The upper esophageal pouch is clearly outlined, but there is also aspiration of contrast material into the airways. With an adequate technique (introduction of a catheter, aspiration, injection of air or a very small amount of contrast material) this complication can be avoided

Fig. 109. A slight narrowing can be well visualized in infants if contrast material is injected through an esophageal catheter

    Various systems have been used to immobilize the child during the examination, including a compression band and sandbags, a padded board with bandages and a hanging harness.

    The apparatus developed by AIME not only secures a good immobilization but also allows the examination of the child in any position from upright to recumbent, and the rotation of the patient along the longitudinal axis. Immobilization apparatus should be constructed in such a way that the child can be watched and is easily accessible during the examination. Equipment for aspiration and reanimation

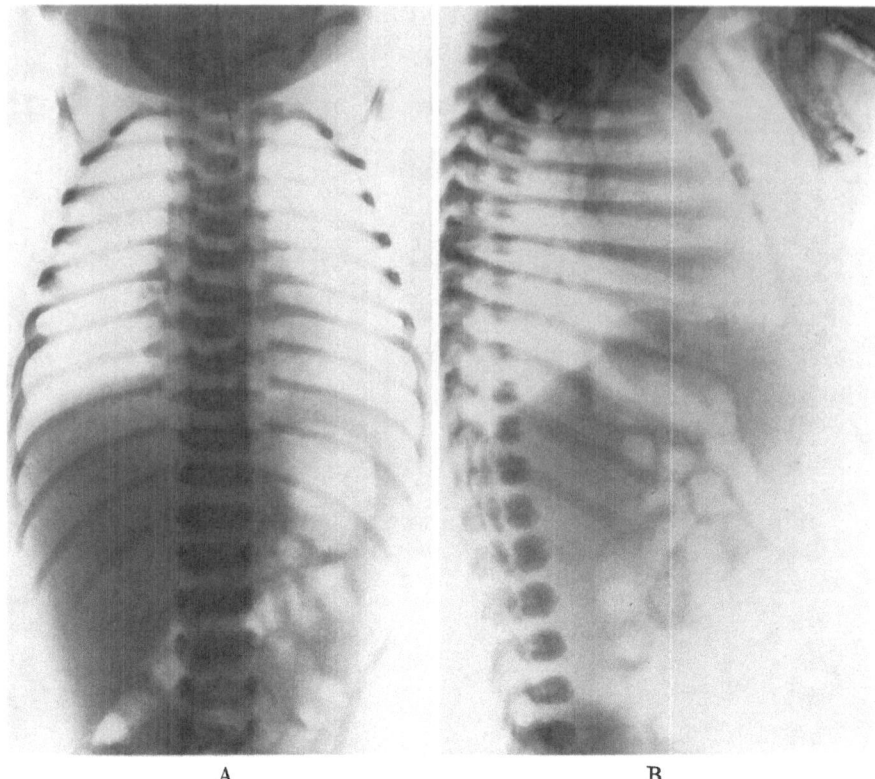

A   B

Fig. 110. Esophageal atresia with tracheoesophageal fistula. A catheter inserted in the esophagus is halted at a distance of 11 cm from the upper alveolar ridge. The diagnosis is established by the visualization of the inserted radiopaque catheter and the presence of air in stomach and bowel

must be available in case of an accident. Short exposure times, preferably not exceeding 0.01 sec, can be achieved by omitting a grid or by using a grid with a low ratio; also by means of the technique of photofluorography with the 70 mm camera.

The contrast material can be administered by means of a feeding bottle or via a radiopaque tube introduced through the nose into the esophagus. In order to avoid accidental intubation of the airways it is recommended to introduce the tube into the stomach and to withdraw it up to the desired level. The contrast material is injected by means of a syringe under fluoroscopical control. The feeding bottle cannot be used when the baby is not willing to drink and should not be used when there is risk of tracheal aspiration due to vomiting or massive regurgitation, nor in children in whom esophageal atresia is suspected (Fig. 108). Administration of the contrast material through a tube is the only technique which always permits a complete examination (Fig. 109). In aspiration-prone children, the contrast medium of choice is a difficult and controversial problem because the contrast material should not be harmful to the airways. A bronchographic contrast medium (CAFFEY, 1967; SAUVEGRAIN, 1969) or a thick suspension of barium sulfate (ARDRAN and KEMP, 1969; SAUVEGRAIN, 1969) are both

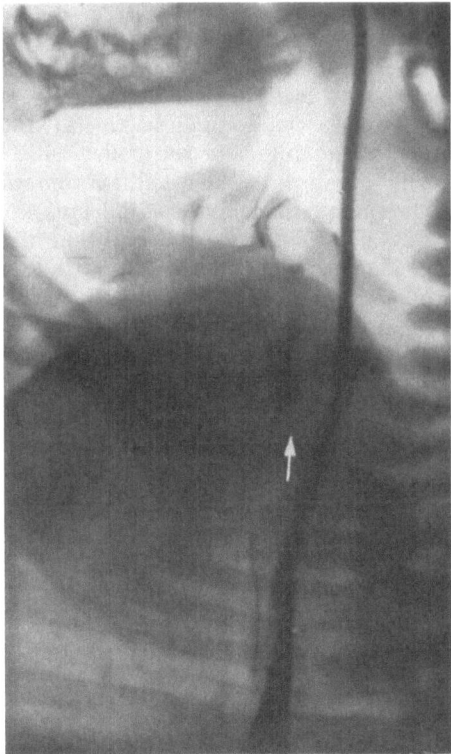

Fig. 111. This tracheoesophageal fistula (↑) was visualized by injection through a catheter of contrast material at the level of the esophageal opening of the fistula

acceptable. The latter cannot reach the small bronchi and is easily expectorated. Gastrografin must be avoided in infants, because it is dangerous if it is aspirated into the airways (REICH, 1969; FRECH et al., 1970) or if it produces a severe diarrhea in dehydrated children (HARRIS et al., 1964).

The radiological examination of the esophagus is usually performed with the child in horizontal position, rotated adequately. The supine position with horizontal beam is usually preferred to study the swallowing mechanism and to examine the cervical esophagus.

When esophageal atresia is suspected on clinical grounds, plain films of chest and abdomen may give valuable information (Figs. 286, 287 A, B, 289 A). If the upper esophagus is dilated with fluid they may show compression and forward displacement of the trachea. If there is a fistulous connection between the airways and the post-atretic gullet, they may demonstrate the presence of air in the distal esophagus or the upper gastrointestinal tract. Following these standard X-rays a radiopaque tube is gently pushed down the esophagus, and chest X-rays in the anteroposterior and lateral positions are taken (Fig. 110). This is usually sufficient to establish the diagnosis. If it is deemed necessary, 20 ml of air and/or a small amount of bronchographic contrast medium are injected into the upper pouch after aspiration of any fluid residue. The contrast material must be aspirated immediately after taking the pictures (Fig. 288 A, B). Visualization of an esophagotracheal or esophagobronchial fistula is very difficult. Usually the child is placed in the position which provides the best profile view of trachea and esophagus. Contrast material is injected through a tube at different levels of the esophagus (Fig. 111). Sometimes it may be useful to inject air at the same time (Sauvegrain, 1969) or to use the feeding bottle (Gwinn, 1969) in order to achieve a better dilatation and filling of the gullet. Most examinations of the upper digestive tract in infants are requested for abnormal regurgitation. In these circumstances the examination of the esophagus is only part of a more complete radiological investigation. After the injection of air into the stomach, gastric evacuation is evaluated; then the tube is withdrawn into the gullet to study esophageal morphology and motility; finally the pharyngoesophageal region may be studied with the use of a feeding bottle.

References

Abbott, O. A., Mansour, K. A., Logan, W. D., Symbas, P. N.: A traumatic so-called "spontaneous" rupture of the esophagus. J. thorac. cardiovasc. Surg. **59**, 67-83 (1970).

Adler, D. C., Haverback, B. J., Meyers, H. I.: Cineradiography of esophageal varices. J. Amer. med. Ass. **189**, 77-106 (1964).

Allison, P. R., Johnstone, A. S.: Oesophagus lined with gastric mucous membrane. Thorax **8**, 87-101 (1953).

Ardran, G. M.: The value of cineradiography in medicine. Brit. J. Radiol. **37**, 819-825 (1964).

Ardran, G. M., Kemp, F. N.: The radiography of the lower lateral food channels. J. Laryng. **75**, 358-370 (1961).

Ardran, G. M., Kemp, F. H.: Normal and disturbed swallowing. In: Progress in pediatric radiology, vol. 2. Basel: Karger; Chicago: Year Book 1969.

Bachman, A. L.: The radiologic study of some normal and abnormal swallowing mechanisms; aspiration phenomena and cricopharyngeus spasm. Laryngoscope (St. Louis) **69**, 947-967 (1959).

Bachman, A. L.: Methodology in the radiographic examination of the larynx and hypopharynx. N.Y. St. J. Med. **63**, 1155-1162 (1963).

Bachman, A. L., Seaman, W. B., Macken, K. L.: Lateral pharyngeal diverticula. Radiology **91**, 774-782 (1968).

Beranbaum, S. L., Lignon, A. J.: Routine gastrointestinal series with a 70-mm sequence camera. Radiology **83**, 337-341 (1964).

Berne, A. S., Gerle, R. D., Mitchell, G. E.: The mediastinum. Normal roentgen anatomy and radiologic technics. Semin. Roentgenol. **4**, 3-21 (1969).

Berridge, F. R.: The requirements in design of an X-ray table for fluoroscopic examinations. Brit. J. Radiol. **44**, 150-157 (1971).

Berridge, F. R., Friedland, G. W., Tagart, R. E. B.: Radiological landmarks at the oesophago-gastric junction. Thorax **21**, 499-510 (1966).

Berridge, F. R., McGregg, D.: The value of cinematography in the diagnosis of malignant strictures of the oesophagus. Brit. J. Radiol. **31**, 465-471 (1958).

Birken, H., Bejczy, C. I.: Eine neue Generation von Röntgenbildverstärkern. Eigenschaften und Ergebnisse. Röntgenstr. **27**, 17-25 (1972).

Bodart, P., Pringot, J.: Application of the 70 mm camera combined with a 9/5-inch image intensifier in the radiological examination of the alimentary tract. Medicamundi **13**, 69-76 (1968).

Böttger, G.: Ringförmig wachsendes Leiomyom des abdominalen Oesophagus. Chirurg **41**, 284-285 (1970).

Boijsen, E., Holm, T., Kaude, J.: Comparative angiographic studies using 70 mm intensifier fluoroscopy and serial film changer. Medicamundi **14**, 120-131 (1969).

Botden, P. J. M., Feddema, J., Vijverberg, G. P. M.: First results with experimental integrated image intensifier television system. Medicamundi **14**, 155-159 (1969).

Botha, G. S. M.: Radiological localisation of diaphragmatic hiatus. Lancet **1957 I**, 662-664.

Bouwers, A.: Improvements of radiological image quality. Radiologe **11**, 230-231 (1971).

Bouwers, A., Krebs, R.: Elektronische Methoden zur Herstellung des Röntgenbildes, Bildverstärker — Fernsehen. Handbuch der medizinischen Radiologie, Bd. I/1. Berlin-Heidelberg-New York: Springer 1968.

Bozorgi, S., Migliorelli, F. A., Cook, W. A.: Leiomyoma of the esophagus presenting as a bleeding epiphrenic diverticulum. Chest **63**, 281-284 (1973).

BRENNER, G. H.: Variations in the depth of the cervical prevertebral tissues in normal infants studied by cinefluorography. Amer. J. Roentgenol. **91**, 573–577 (1964).

BROMBART, M.: Clinical radiology of the oesophagus. Bristol: John Wright & Sons 1961.

CAFFEY, J.: Pediatric X-ray diagnosis, 5th ed. Chicago: Year Book 1967.

CALENOFF, L.: Pedunculated epidermoid carcinoma of the midesophagus. Amer. J. Roentgenol. **88**, 733–735 (1962).

CARLSSON, C., KAUDE, J.: Integral dose in 70 mm fluorography of the gastroduodenal tract. Acta radiol. (Stockh.) **7**, 84–88 (1968).

CHESNEY, D. N., CHESNEY, M. O.: Radiographic photography, 3rd ed. Oxford-Edinburgh: Blackwell Scientific Publications 1971.

CHIARI, H., WANKE, M.: Oesophagus. In: Spezielle pathologische Anatomie, Bd. 2, Teil 1. Berlin-Heidelberg-New York: Springer 1971.

CHRISTIEN, G., BOUCKE, J., COTONNEC, C.: Deux observations de compression œsophagienne par adenopathie tuberculeuse. Sem. Hôp. (Paris) **48**, 1245–1248 (1972).

CHRISTOFORIDIS, A. J., NELSON, S. W., TOMASHEFSKI, J. F.: Effects of bronchography on pulmonary function. Amer. Rev. resp. Dis. **85**, 127–129 (1962).

CIMMINO, C. V.: The esophagus. In: GOLDEN's diagnostic radiology. Baltimore: Williams & Wilkins 1969.

COLLARD, M.: Une méthode simple de laryngographie. J. belge Radiol. **47**, 31–34 (1964).

COOLEY, R. N., SCHREIBER, M. H.: Radiology of the heart and great vessels, 2nd ed. Baltimore: Williams & Wilkins 1967.

CREELY, J. J., TRAIL, M. L.: Intramural diverticulosis of the esophagus. Sth med. J. (Bgham, Ala.) **63**, 1257–1260 (1970).

CRUZE, K., BYRON, F. X., HILL, J. T.: The association of peptic ulcer and symptomatic hiatal hernia. Surgery **46**, 664–668 (1959).

DAGRADI, A. E., RODILES, D. H., COOPER, E., STEMPIEN, S. J.: Endoscopic diagnosis of esophageal varices. Amer. J. Gastroent. **56**, 371–377 (1971).

DAGRADI, A., SAUNDERS, D., STEMPIEN, S. J.: The sources of upper gastrointestinal bleeding in liver cirrhosis. Ann. intern. Med. **42**, 852–855 (1955).

DALINKA, M. K., SMITH, E. H., WOLFE, R. D., GOLDENBERG, D., LANGDON, D. E.: Pharmacologically enhanced visualization of esophageal varices by pro-banthine. Radiology **102**, 281–282 (1972).

DINSMORE, R. E., GOODMAN, D., DREYFUSS, J. R.: The air esophagogram: a sign of scleroderma involving the esophagus. Radiology 87, 348–349 (1966).

DODDS, W.J., McGLAUGHIN, P. S., GOLDBERG, H. I., DEHN, T. G.: Esophageal roentgenography using tantalum paste. Radiology **102**, 204–206 (1972).

DODGE, O. G.: The surgical pathology of gastro-oesophageal carcinoma. Brit. J. Surg. **49**, 121–125 (1961).

DOHLMAN, G., MATTSON, O.: Role of the cricopharyngeal muscle in cases of hypopharyngeal diverticula. Amer. J. Roentgenol. 81, 561–569 (1959).

DOI, H.: X-ray technique. In: Double contrast studies of the stomach. Tokyo: Bunkodo Co. 1971.

DONNER, M. W., MARGULIES, S. I.: Radiographic examination. In: Gastroesophageal reflux and hiatal hernia, p. 59-85, eds. SKINNER, D. B., BELSEY, R. H., HENDRIX, T. R., ZUIDEMA, G. D. Boston: Little, Brown & Co. 1972.

DONNER, M. W., SILBIGER, M. L., HOOKMAN, P., HENDRIX, T. R.: Acid-barium swallows in the radiographic evaluation of clinical esophagitis. Radiology 87, 220–225 (1966).

DUTREIX, J.: La fonction de transfert de modulation, espression objective de la finesse de l'image radiologique. J. Radiol. Électrol. **46**, 658–664 (1965).

EDELL, S. L.: Non-visualizing gall bladder. Brit. J. Radiol. **45**, 706 (1972).

EISEN, S., ELLIOTT, L. P.: A plain film sign of total anomalous pulmonary venous connection below the diaphragm. Amer. J. Roentgenol. **102**, 372–379 (1968).

ELMER, R. A.: 70 mm filming: Factors affecting image sharpness. Radiology 89, 420–425 (1967).

ELMER, R.A.: Practical methods for improving quality in 70 mm and 90 mm filming. Radiology **98**, 247–261 (1971).

EMBRING, G., MATTSON, O.: Barium contrast agents. Acta radiol. (Stockh.) **7**, 245–256 (1968).

ENDO, M., KOBAYASHI, S., SUZUKI, H., TAKEMOTO, T., NAKAYAMA, N.: Diagnosis of early esophageal cancer. Endoscopy **3**, 61–66 (1971).

FAGAN, C. J., PALMER, E. P.: Gastroesophageal retrograde mucosal prolapse. Amer. J. Roentgenol. **90**, 774–777 (1963).

FEDDEMA, J.: 70 mm fluorography with 9″ image intensifier mounted on a remotely controlled ring stand. Medicamundi 8, 7–13 (1962).

FEDDEMA, J., RECOURT, A., MONTE, G. L. A.: Evaluation of image quality in various methods for the recording of movement phenomena. Medicamundi **14**, 140–154 (1969).

Figley, M. M.: Mediastinal minutiae. Semin. Roentgenol. 4, 22–32 (1969).

Fisher, A. M., Kendall, B., Van Leuven, B. D.: Hodgkin's disease: a radiological survey. Clin. Radiol. 13, 115–127 (1962).

Fleischli, D. J.: Boerhaave syndrome. J. Amer. med. Ass. 198, 844–846 (1966).

Frech, R. S., Davie, J. M., Adatepe, M., Feldhaus, R., McAlister, R. T., McAlister, W. H.: Comparison of barium sulfate and oral 40% Diatrizoate injected into the trachea of dogs. Radiology 95, 299–303 (1970).

Friedland, G. W., Melcker, D. H., Berridge, F. R., Gresham, G. A.: Debatable points in the anatomy of the lower oesophagus. Thorax 21, 487–498 (1966).

Frik, W.: Ösophagus. In: Lehrbuch der Röntgendiagnostik, Bd. V. Stuttgart: Georg Thieme 1965.

Fuchs, H., Hofmann, F. W.: Ein Röntgenbildverstärker mit verbesserter Bildqualität. Ergebnisse der praktischen Erprobung mit der 70-mm-Kamera. Electromedica 39, 94–97 (1971).

Gebauer, A., Lissner, J., Schott, O.: Roentgen television. New York-London: Grune & Stratton 1967.

Ghahremani, G. G., Heck, L. L., Williams, J. R.: A pharmacologic aid in the radiography diagnosis of obstructive esophageal lesions. Radiology 103, 289–293 (1972).

Godard, J. E., McCranie, D.: Multiple leiomyomas of the esophagus. Amer. J. Roentgenol. 117, 259–262 (1973).

Goldberg, H. I., Sheft, D. J.: Esophageal and colon changes in myotonia dystrophica. Gastroenterology 63, 134–139 (1972).

Grainger, R. G., Castellino, R. A., Lewin, K., Steiner, R. N.: Hytrast: experimental bronchography comparing two different formulations. Clin. Radiol. 21, 390–395 (1970).

Gutman, E.: Posterior mediastinal calcification due to esophageal leiomyoma. Gastroenterology 63, 665–666 (1972).

Gwinn, J. L.: Tracheo-esophageal fistula with and without esophageal atresia. Special aspects. Progr. Pediat. Radiol., vol. 2. Basel: Karger; Chicago: Year Book 1969.

Harper, R. A., Tiscenco, E.: Benign tumor of esophagus and its differential diagnosis. Brit. J. Radiol. 18, 99–107 (1945).

Harris, P. D., Neuhauser, E. B. D., Gerth, R.: The osmotic effect of water-soluble contrast media on circulating plasma volume. Amer. J. Roentgenol. 91, 694–698 (1964).

Heitmann, P., Wolf, B. S., Sokol, E. M., Cohen, B. R.: Simultaneous cineradiography, manometric study of the distal esophagus, small hiatal hernias and rings. Gastroenterology 50, 737–753 (1966).

Hellekamp, J. C., Endlich, B.: First experiences with an image intensifier with electronic enlargement. Medicamundi 11, 9–14 (1965).

Hendee, W. R.: Medical radiation physics. Chicago: Year Book Medical Publishers 1970.

Hofmann, F. W.: Röntgenbildverstärker mit verbesserter Bildqualität. Röntgen-Bl. 25, 1–8 (1972).

Huddy, Ph., Griffiths, G.: Leiomyoma of the esophagus with calcification. Brit. J. Surg. 59, 239–242 (1972).

Jacobs, R. C., Gershengorn, K., Chait, A.: Dysphagia associated with a distended pulmonary vein. Brit. J. Radiol. 45, 225–228 (1972).

Jacobson, H. G., Shapiro, J. H., Popel, M. H.: Oral renografin 76%, a contrast medium for examination of the G.I. tract. Amer. J. Roentgenol. 80, 82–88 (1958).

James, A. M., Goddard, G. H.: A study of barium sulphate preparations used as x-ray opaque media. Pharm. Acta Helv. 46, 708–720 (1971).

Jansen, W.: Delcalix-S mit Isocon und Kinescopie. Odelca Mirror 8, 2–4 (1969).

Johnston, G. W., Stevenson, H. M.: Reflux esophagitis secondary to duodenal diaphragm in an adult. Thorax 21, 65–66 (1966).

Jonsson, K., Rian, R. L.: Pseudotumoral esophageal varices associated with portal hypertension. Radiology 97, 593–597 (1970).

Jorgens, J.: Cinefluorography of the gastrointestinal tract. Radiol. Clin. N. Amer. 7, 163–173 (1969).

Jutras, A., Duckett, G.: Roentgendiagnosis by remote control telefluoroscopy and cineradiography. Medicamundi 4, 77–82 (1958).

Jutras, A., Levrier, P., Longtin, M.: Étude radiologique de l'œsophage paradiaphragmatique et du cardia. J. Radiol. Électrol. 30, 373–414 (1949).

Kaude, J.: Fluorography of the gastroduodenal tract, a comparative study with 70 mm film. Acta radiol. (Stockh.) 6, 355–367 (1967).

Kaufmann, H. J.: Progress in pediatric radiology, vol. 2, Gastro-intestinal tract. Basel-New York: Karger 1969.

Kavlie, H., White, T. T.: Leiomyomas of the upper gastrointestinal tract. Surgery 71, 842–848 (1972).

KEIGHLEY, M. R. B., GIRDWOOD, R. W., IONESCU, M. I., WOOLER, G. H.: Spontaneous rupture of the esophagus. Avoidance of postoperative morbidity. Brit. J. Surg. 59, 649–652 (1972).

KELLY, J. E.: The marshmallow as an aid to radiologic examination of the esophagus. New Engl. J. Med. 265, 1306–1307 (1961).

KEMP HARPER, R. A.: New advances in radiology of the gastro-intestinal tract. In: Modern trends in diagnostic radiology, vol. 4. London: Butterworths 1970.

KENDALL, B. E., ASHCROFT, K., WHITESIDE, C. G.: A physiological variation in the barium filled gullet. Brit. J. Radiol. 35, 769–776 (1962).

KLINKHAMER, A. C.: Esophagography in anomalies of the aortic system. Baltimore, Maryland: Williams & Wilkins Cie., Amsterdam: Excerpta Medica Foundation 1969.

KRAMER, P.: Progressing gastroenterology. Esophagus. Gastroenterology 54, 1171–1191 (1968).

KREEL, L., BLOOM, R. A., PIERCY, J. E.: The barium swallow in thyroid enlargement. Brit. J. Radiol. 38, 926–933 (1965).

KÜHL, W.: X-ray image intensifiers today and tomorrow. Medicamundi 14, 132–136 (1969).

KÜHL, W., VAN OVERHAGEN, J. W. D.: A 9-inch X-ray image intensifier with variable magnification. Medicamundi 11, 1–4 (1965).

LEIGH, T. F., WEENS, H. S.: Roentgen aspects of mediastinal lesions. Semin. Roentgenol. 4, 59–73 (1969).

LESSMAN, F. P., LILIENFELD, R. M.: Gastrografin as water soluble contrast medium in roentgen examination of the G.I. tract. Acta radiol. (Stockh.) 51, 170–178 (1959).

LEVIN, A. R., FRAND, M., BALTAXE, H. A.: Left atrial enlargement. Radiology 104, 615–621 (1972).

LICHTENBERG, R., DUTREIX, J.: L'image dynamique. In: Traité de radiodiagnostic, tome 1. Paris: Masson 1969.

LONGIN, F.: Pharmakoradiographische Untersuchungen der ösophagogastrischen Übergangsregion zum Nachweis der kleinen Hiatushernie. Fortschr. Röntgenstr. 104, 389–398 (1966).

LOWMAN, R. M., GOLDMAN, R., STERN, H.: The roentgen aspects of intramural dissection of the esophagus. Radiology 93, 1329–1331 (1969).

MANDELSTAM, P., LIEBER, A.: Cineradiographic evaluation of the esophagus in normal adults. Gastroenterology 58, 32–39 (1970).

MASSHAK, R. H.: The roentgen findings of benign and malignant tumors of the esophagus. J. Mt Sinai Hosp. 23, 75–89 (1956).

MARTEL, W.: Radiologic features of esophagogastritis secondary to extremely caustic agents. Radiology 103, 31–36 (1972).

MATHESON, N. A., DUDLEY, H. A. F.: Contrast radiography, an aid to post-operative management. Lancet 1963 I, 914–917.

McCORT, J. J.: Esophageal carcinosarcoma and pseudosarcoma. Radiology 102, 519–524 (1972).

MEYERS, H. I., JACOBSON, G.: The use of water soluble contrast medium in suspected perforated peptic ulcer. Radiol. Clin. N. Amer. 2, 55–69 (1964).

MIKURIYA, S. et al.: X-ray diagnosis of the esophagus. Stomach Intest. (Tokyo) 3, 1345–1358 (1968).

MILLER, E. R.: Barium sulfate suspensions. Radiology 84, 241–251 (1965).

MONGES, H.: Considerations sur le rôle du diaphragme dans la physiologie de la continence gastro-esophagienne et sur la projection de l'hiatus œsophagien. Gastroenterologia (Basel) 82, 232–241 (1956).

MORI, P. A., BARRETT, H. A.: A sign of intestinal perforation. Radiology 79, 401–407 (1962).

MURRAY, J. P.: Buscopan in diagnostic radiology of the alimentary tract. Brit. J. Radiol. 93, 102–111 (1966).

NABEYA, K.: Early carcinoma of the esophagus. Stomach Intest. (Tokyo) 5, 1205–1213 (1970).

NADEL, J. A., DODDS, W. J., GOLDBERG, H., GRAF, P. D.: Insufflation of powdered tantalum in the esophagus, new esophagogastric technique. Invest. Radiol. 4, 57–62 (1969).

NAHUM, H., REYSSEGUIER, J. C., PRANDI, D., CONTE-MARTI, J., BENASSE, S., LORTA JACOB, J. L.: Les tumeurs benignes de l'œsophage. Ann. Radiol. 15, 581–590 (1972).

NELSON, S. W.: The roentgenologic diagnosis of esophageal varices. Amer. J. Roentgenol. 77, 599–611 (1957).

NELSON, S. W., CHRISTOFORIDIS, A. J., PRATT, P. C.: Further experience with barium sulfate as a bronchographic contrast agent. Amer. J. Roentgenol. 92, 595–614 (1964).

NELSON, S. W., CHRISTOFORIDIS, A, J., ROENIGK, W. J.: Barium suspensions versus water soluble iodine compounds in the study of obstruction of the small bowel, an experimental study of physiologic characteristics and radiographic value. Radiology 80, 252–254 (1963).

NEMIR, P., FALAHNEJAD, M., ROSE, B., JACOBOWITZ, D., FROBESE, A. S., HAWTHORNE, H. R.: A study of the causes of failure of esophagocardiomyotomy for achalasia. Amer. J. Surg. 121, 143–149 (1971).

O'Connell, N. D.: Spontaneous rupture of the esophagus. Amer. J. Roentgenol. 99, 186–203 (1967).

Ormond, R. S., Jaconette, J. R., Templeton, A. W.: The pleural esophageal reflection: an aid in the evaluation of esophageal disease. Radiology 80, 738–741 (1963).

Panaro, V. A., Leslie, E. S.: Spontaneous rupture of the esophagus. Radiology 84, 252–258 (1965).

Pitman, R. G., Fraser, G. M.: The post-cricoid impression on the esophagus. Clin. Radiol. 16, 34–39 (1965).

Pope, C. E. II: Progress in gastroenterology. The esophagus: 1967 to 1969. Gastroenterology 59, 460–476, 615–629 (1970).

Powell, K. C., Shepherd, A., Cooke, R.: Giant leiomyoma of the oesophagus. Med. J. Austr. 2, 483–484 (1971).

Powers, W. E., McGee, H. H., Jr., Seaman, W. B.: Contrast examination of the larynx and pharynx. Radiology 68, 169–178 (1957).

Prevot, R., Lassrich, M. A.: Röntgendiagnostik des Magen-Darmkanals. Stuttgart: Thieme 1959.

Rao, G. U. V.: Do high detail screens always yield better resolution than high speed screens? Amer. J. Roentgenol. 112, 812–817 (1971).

Reich, S. B.: Production of pulmonary edema by aspiration of water-soluble nonabsorbable contrast media. Radiology 92, 367–370 (1969).

Renzo, S., Di, Pereira-Duarta, R. O.: Die Bronchographie mit Barium. Fortschr. Röntgenstr. 86, 315–318 (1957).

Rogers, L. F., Puig, A. W., Dooley, B. N., Cuello, L.: Diagnostic considerations in mediastinal emphysema: a pathophysiologic-roentgenologic approach to Boerhaave's syndrome and spontaneous pneumomediastinum. Amer. J. Roentgenol. 115, 495–511 (1972).

Sakiyalak, P., Bellon, E. M., David, P., Ankeney, J. L.: Esophageal obstruction due to saccular aneurysm of the distal thoracic aorta. J. thorac. cardiovasc. Surg. 64, 959–962 (1972).

Samuel, E., Summerling, M. D.: An assessment of the use of the 70 mm camera in radiologic practice. Brit. J. Radiol. 37, 620–624 (1964).

Sandmark, S.: Influence of heavy contrast media on the demonstration of hiatus hernia and gastroesophageal reflux. Acta radiol. (Stockh.) 1, 1045–1052 (1963).

Sauvegrain, J.: The technique of upper gastro-intestinal investigation in infants and children. Progress in pediatric radiology, vol. 2, Gastrointestinal tract. Basel-New York: Karger 1969.

Scatliff, J. H., Scibetta, P.: Pharyngeal cinefluorography in clinical practice. Amer. J. Roentgenol. 90, 823–834 (1963).

Schatzki, R.: Esophagus: progress and problems. Amer. J. Roentgenol. 94, 523–540 (1965).

Schatzki, R.: Editorial: "You still have to work for it". Analysis of the impact of screen intensification. Radiology 87, 759–761 (1966).

Schatzki, R., Gary, J. E.: The lower esophageal ring. Amer. J. Roentgenol. 75, 246–261 (1956).

Schatzki, R., Harves, L. E.: The roentgenological appearance of extramucosal tumors of the esophagus. Amer. J. Roentgenol. 48, 1–15 (1942).

Seaman, W. B.: Cineroentgenographic observations of the cricopharyngeus. Amer. J. Roentgenol. 96, 922–931 (1966).

Seaman, W. B.: Examination of the pharynx. In: Alimentary tract roentgenology, vol. 1. St. Louis: Mosby 1967 a.

Seaman, W. B.: Roentgenology of pharyngeal disorders. In: Alimentary tract roentgenology, vol. 1. St. Louis: Mosby 1967 b.

Seaman, W. B.: Functional disorders of the pharyngo-esophageal junction: achalasia and chalasia. Radiol. Clin. N. Amer. 7, 113–119 (1969).

Shehadi, W. H.: Orally administered water soluble iodinated contrast media. Amer. J. Roentgenol. 83, 933–941 (1960).

Shin, C.-S., Bakst, A. A., Levowitz, B. S.: Intrathoracic goiter located in posterior mediastinum. N.Y. St. J. Med. 72, 1723–1728 (1972).

Som, M. L., Wolf, B. S., Marshak, R. H.: Narrow esophagogastric ring treated endoscopically. Gastroenterology 39, 634–638 (1960).

Sokol, E. M., Heitmann, P., Wolf, B. S., Cohen, B. R.: Simultaneous cineradiographic and manometric study of the pharynx, hypopharynx, and cervical esophagus. Gastroenterology 51, 960–974 (1966).

Staple, T. W., Margulis, A. R.: Diagnostic study of cine and conventional roentgenography in 103 patients. Radiology 82, 895–897 (1964).

Staple, T. W., Ogura, J. W.: Cine radiography of the swallowing mechanism following supraglottic subtotal laryngectomy. Radiology 87, 226–230 (1966).

STEPHAN, G.: Röntgendiagnostik des Ösophagus beim Bronchialkarzinom in Beziehung zum Tumorstadium (TNM), zur Tumorlokalisation und Histologie. Fortschr. Röntgenstr. **113**, 1–11 (1970).

STIEVE, E. F.: Zur Analyse von Bewegungsvorgängen in der Röntgendiagnostik. Odelca Mirror 8, 7–9 (1969).

STILSON, W. L.: Cinefluorography in the study of oesophagus and gastric introit. Amer. Surg. **31**, 669–678 (1965).

SUZUKI, H., KOBAYASHI, S., ENDO, M., NAKAYAMA, K.: Diagnosis of early esophageal cancer. Surgery **71**, 99–103 (1972).

SWART, B.: Die Technik der Varicendarstellung am Oesophagus. Radiologe **3**, 65–75 (1963).

SWISCHUK, L. E.: Plain film interpretation in congenital heart disease. Philadelphia: Lea & Febiger 1970.

TEMPLETON, F. E.: X-ray examination of the stomach, revised ed. Chicago-London: Chicago Univ. Press 1964.

TER-POGOSSIAN, M. M.: The physical aspects of diagnostic radiology. New York-Evanston-London: Hoeber Medical Division; Harper & Row 1967.

TOLEDO, T. M., MOORE, W. L., NASH, D. A., NORTH, R. L.: Spontaneous pneumopericardium in acute asthma: Case report and review of the literature. Chest **62**, 118–120 (1972).

TOSCH, R.: Untersuchungen über die Resorption von J 131-markiertem Gastrografin aus dem Magen-Darm-Kanal. Fortschr. Röntgenstr. **95**, 189–192 (1961).

TOWNSEND, E. J. S.: An evaluation of the 70 mm camera. Brit. J. Radiol. **42**, 950 (1969).

VANTRAPPEN, G., LIEMER, M. D., IKEYA, J., TEXTER, E. C., BARBORKA, J. C.: Simultaneous fluorocinematography and intraluminal pressure measurements in the study of esophageal motility. Gastroenterology **35**, 592–602 (1958).

VANTRAPPEN, G., TEXTER, E. C., BARBORKA, C. J., VANDENBROUCKE, J.: The closing mechanism at the gastroesophageal junction. Amer. J. Med. **28**, 564–577 (1960).

VIDNE, B., GARTI, I., ROSENBERG, V., LEVY, M. J.: Aortic arch anomalies: simplified classification. Chest **62**, 39–44 (1972).

WAHL, R., KEMPF, F.: L'isopropamide (priamide): son utilisation en tant que modificateur de comportement en gastroentérologie. J. Radiol. Électrol. **45**, 492–494 (1964).

WALDENSTRÖM, J., KJELLBERG, S. R.: The roentgenological diagnosis of sideropenic dysphagia. Acta radiol. (Stockh.) **20**, 618–638 (1939).

WEYLMAN, W. T., SIMON, H.: Mediastinal calcification. J. Amer. med. Ass. **177**, 502–503 (1961).

WHALEN, J. P., WOODRUFF, C. L.: The cervical prevertebral fat stripe. Amer. J. Roentgenol. **109**, 445–451 (1970).

WILLIAMS, J. R., BONTE, F. J.: The roentgenological aspect of nonpenetrating chest injuries. Springfield (Ill.): Charles C. Thomas 1961.

WILLSON, J. K. V., RUBIN, P. S., McGEE, T. M.: The effects of barium sulfate on the lungs, a clinical and experimental study. Amer. J. Roentgenol. **82**, 84–94 (1959).

WOLF, B. S.: Roentgenology of the esophagogastric junction. In: Alimentary tract roentgenology, vol. 1. St. Louis: C. V. Mosby Co. 1967.

WOLF, B. S.: Progress in gastroenterology. Radiology. Gastroenterology **57**, 324–338 (1969).

WOLF, B. S.: The inferior esophageal sphincter—anatomic, roentgenologic, and manometric correlation, contradictions, and terminology. Amer. J. Roentgenol. **110**, 260–277 (1970).

WOLF, B. S., KHILNANI, M. T.: Progress in gastroenterological radiology. Gastroenterology **51**, 542–559 (1966).

WOODS, R. R., CHANCE, O.: Soft tissue radiography in the diagnosis of hypopharyngeal tumors. J. Irish Med. Ass. **57**, 156–158 (1965).

WRIGHT, J. T.: Allison and Johnstone's anomaly. Amer. J. Roentgenol. **94**, 308–320 (1965).

WÜRDINGER, H.: Die Röntgendiagnostik des Magen-Darm-Kanals mit einem wasserlöslichen Kontrastmittel (Gastrografin). Med. Klin. **57**, 307–310 (1962).

WYCHULIS, A. R., FONTANA, R. S., PAYNE, W. S.: Instrumental perforations of the esophagus. Dis. Chest **55**, 184–189 (1969 a).

WYCHULIS, A. R., FONTANA, R. S., PAYNE, W. S.: Noninstrumental perforations of the esophagus. Dis. Chest **55**, 190–196 (1969 b).

WYCHULIS, A. R., WOOLAM, G. L., ANDERSEN, H. A., ELLIS, F. H.: Achalasia and carcinoma of the esophagus. J. Amer. med. Ass. **215**, 1638–1641 (1971).

WYMAN, S. M., ROBBINS, L. L.: Roentgen recognition of parathyroid adenoma. Amer. J. Roentgenol. **71**, 777–784 (1954).

ZAINO, C., JACOBSON, H. G., LEPOW, H., OZTURK, C. H.: The pharyngo-esophageal sphincter. Springfield (Ill.): Charles C. Thomas 1970.

ZBORALSKE, F. F., DODDS, W. J.: Roentgenographic diagnosis of primary disorders of esophageal motility. Radiol. Clin. N. Amer. **7**, 147–162 (1969).

Esophagoscopy

P. HOUSSET, A. SIMOENS, and CH. DEBRAY

With 16 Figures

1. Introduction

Esophagoscopy has undergone very important changes during the past 20 years. This evolution is due mainly to the development of medical esophagoscopy. When employed by gastroenterologists to an essentially diagnostic purpose, this technique differs from operative esophagoscopy, used by the oto-rhino-laryngologists for extracting foreign bodies and for some dilatation maneuvers. Likewise, the equipment has been improved. The diameter of the rigid esophagoscopes was decreased, the optical systems were perfected and cold light adapted to esophageal endoscopy. Last but not least, the finding that glass fibers transmit images and light has led to the construction of flexible esophagoscopes, or fiber esophagoscopes, which entirely transformed medical esophagoscopy. Owing to these improvements, the examination technique gradually became simpler. At present, fiber esophagoscopy is no longer the disagreeable, incomplete and even dangerous examination it used to be.

After a few recommendations valid for all endoscopic examinations we shall successively discuss the instruments and the techniques used by the gastroenterologists; the indications and the contraindications of medical esophagoscopy, and finally the accidents and incidents that may be caused by this exploration.

2. Common Recommendations for All Endoscopic Examinations

Whichever method is used, esophagoscopy necessitates the respecting of general rules, which may be summarized as follows: (1) Endoscopy demands a homogeneous team, well trained, having at its disposal a well equipped room, good endoscopic instruments and basic reanimation equipment. (2) The endoscopist must study carefully the medical and radiological documents of the patients. His action cannot be limited to a blind application of a technique. (3) The psychological preparation of the patients is as important as premedication or anesthesia. (4) The endoscopist must never overrate his skill; a failure is always to be preferred to an accident. (5) Endoscopic data are mostly subjective. Unwarranted interpretations should be avoided. (6) Every examination is subject to error. Endoscopy is no exception to this rule.

3. Equipment and Techniques

Methods vary considerably according to the type of instruments used. Rigid and flexible esophagoscopes will be discussed successively with special emphasis on the fiberscope technique, which is replacing the previous procedures.

3.1. Rigid Esophagoscopy

There are many types of rigid esophagoscopes. Only those of a small diameter used by gastroenterologists, and more particularly those with which we have gathered some experience will be discussed: the esophagoscope of S. SEGAL and DUBOIS DE MONTREYNAUD and the EDER-HUFFORD esophagoscope with flexible obturator. Similar instruments have been devised by SCHNEIDER and by KALK.

3.1.1. The Esophagoscope of Segal and Dubois de Montreynaud
(Fig. 112)

This instrument comprises a metallic tube with a diameter of 10.5 mm and a length of 45 cm. The light source is proximal, external and the cold light is transmitted to the distal extremity by means of a quartz rod. An optical system,

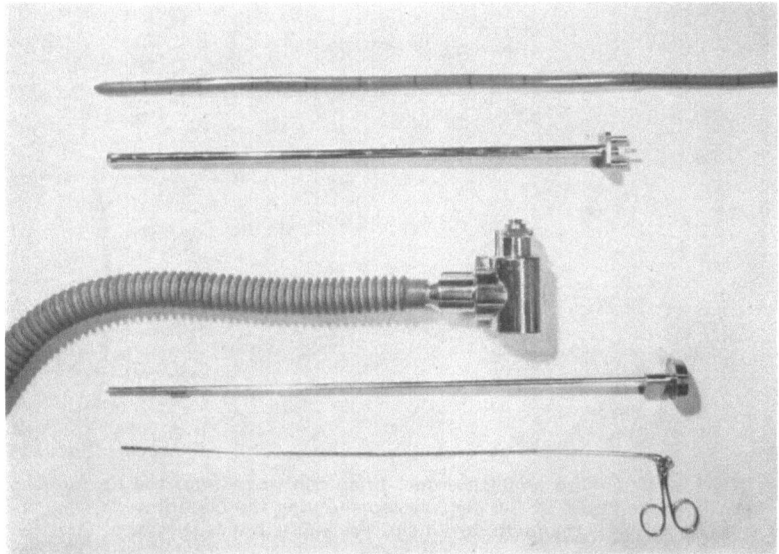

Fig. 112. Rigid esophagoscope of Segal and Dubois de Montreynaud. From top to bottom: the plastic sheath around a mercury probe, the body of the esophagoscope, the light source, the optical system inserted in the endoscopic tube and the biopsy forceps

covering a field of 60°, is inserted in the metallic tube; it is also possible to use lateral or retrograde lenses. Owing to its great optical qualities and to the intensity of its light source, this apparatus makes possible the shooting of excellent cinematographic pictures. A small tube can be inserted into this instrument for aspirating the secretions during the examination, or a biopsy forceps for taking tissue under visual control.

The technique suggested by SEGAL comprises the placement of a flexible and transparent sheath of plastic material mounted on a No. 12 mercury probe. When the probe is withdrawn the esosphagoscope can be inserted under the protection of the sheath. The patient is examined in the position adopted by the oto-rhino-laryngologists, i.e. in dorsal decubitus, the head resting on a headstall and the thorax slightly lifted with a hard cushion.

The esophagoscopy can be done under local anesthesia, but SEGAL prefers general anesthesia not only to render the exploration less painful to the patient, but also to get a better relaxation of the patient, to progress more safely and more easily and finally to study better the lower esophagus.

3.1.2. The Eder-Hufford Esophagoscope
(Fig. 113)

This endoscope is simple and of easy maintenance. It is made of a straight tube, beveled at its distal extremity, 7 or 9.5 mm in diameter and 45 or 53 cm in length, according to the model used. The endoscopic tube is fitted with two

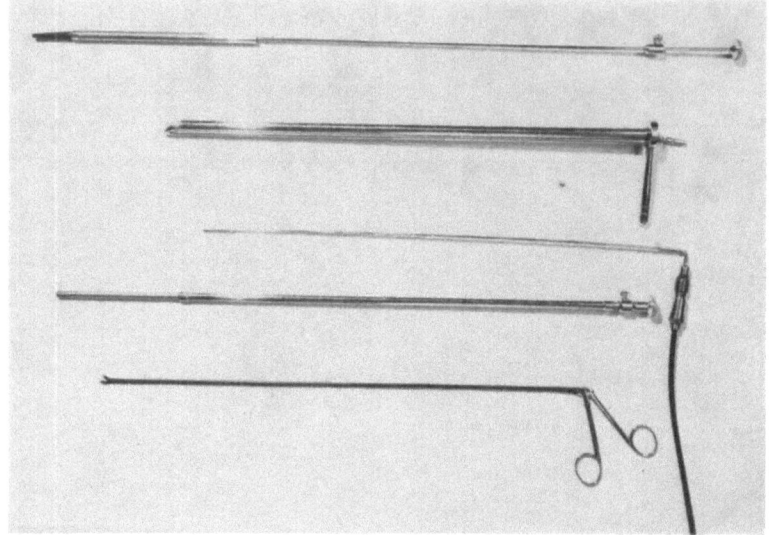

Fig. 113. Rigid Eder-Hufford esophagoscope. From top to bottom: the flexible obturator, which is placed in the lumen of the esophagoscope during the blind introduction, the endo-scopic tube, the rod with the lamp on its tip, the internal optical system, and the biopsy forceps

separate channels, one for aspiration of the secretions, the second for insertion of a lamp carrier since the instrument has distal lighting. A flexible obturator protruding several centimeter from the distal end of the esophagoscope facilitates the passage of the instrument through the upper orifice of the esophagus. The optical system comprises either a small telescope attached to the proximal extremity or a classic optical system inserted inside the esophagoscope. After premedication and local anesthesia of the tongue and the throat, the patient is placed in the position of gastroscopy, i.e. in left lateral decubitus, the head being held by an assistant.

3.1.3. Results of Rigid Esophagoscopy

The results of esophagoscopy with rigid instruments are variable and this technique involves a number of drawbacks.

First, it is a delicate technique, necessitating a well trained operator. Indeed, it requires very accurate maneuvers to get beyond the pharyngoesophageal sphincter and to straighten the curves of the gullet. These maneuvers may be dangerous when done by an inexpert person; they are liable to injure the mucosa severely and to cause bleeding which hinders vision considerably. The use of a protective sheath according to SEGAL's technique is doubtlessly a security factor; moreover the sheath is pushed a little beyond the extremity of the esophagoscope and thereby protects the object-glass from defilement. On the other hand the exploration of the lower esophagus is mostly unsatisfactory. With the Eder-Hufford apparatus, the cardia and the last few centimeters of the esophagus are usually not well visualized. Under general anesthesia with SEGAL's technique, the cardia is seen more often, but never passed beyond. Thus this technique does not allow the study of the cardia and the pericardial region of the stomach by retrograde exploration. Moreover the cardia is always seen with the mucosa pushed ahead. A final difficulty lies with the fact of accurately spotting the cardia: a slightly prolonged contraction of the lower esophagus may simulate the cardia and bring about a "false cardia" corresponding to the "false pylorus" in the stomach.

In conclusion, rigid esophagoscopy, particularly SEGAL's technique, is a "heavy" procedure, requiring hospitalization, general anesthesia and careful watching of the patient.

3.2. Flexible Esophagoscopy

3.2.1. Principle of the Fiberscopes

The fiberscopes transmit the images point by point with very tenuous and flexible glass fibers, each acting as a light conductor. Although the realization of these instruments is of recent date, their basic principle is of a long standing knowledge: that of the refracted light. If a beam of light strikes the wall of a light conductor at an angle equal or superior to the limit angle of total reflection, this beam does not get out of the conductor; striking another surface in the same conditions, the beam undergoes another reflection. Step by step this beam is transmitted on to the extremity of the light conductor. But between the discovery of these physical laws and the practical realization of the fiberscopes, many years of research elapsed.

3.2.2. Instruments

The first fiberscope was built in the U.S.A. by HIRSCHOWITZ in 1963, then modified in 1964 by Lo PRESTI. During the following years, more perfected instruments were made in Japan. Recently, the American apparatus have also been greatly improved.

We have a rather extensive experience with Lo PRESTI's initial fiberscope and we have been using for several years the fiber esophagoscope manufactured by the Japanese firm Olympus. The main features of the latter instrument (Figs. 114, 115) can be summarized as follows: Length: 660 or 850 mm, according to the model; diameter of the body: 11.9 mm; angle of forward flexion: 90°; angle of backward flexion: 90°; flexion point of instrument in relation to distal extremity: 40 mm; angle of vision: 60°; deviation of angle of vision in relation to the axis of the apparatus (fore-oblique lens): 10°; field depth (fixed focus of the apparatus: 10 to 30 mm.

The field depth is actually greater than 30 mm owing to the possibility of curving the distal end of the instrument forward or backward, and to the fact that the bending point lies 40 mm from the extremity, thus very close to it.

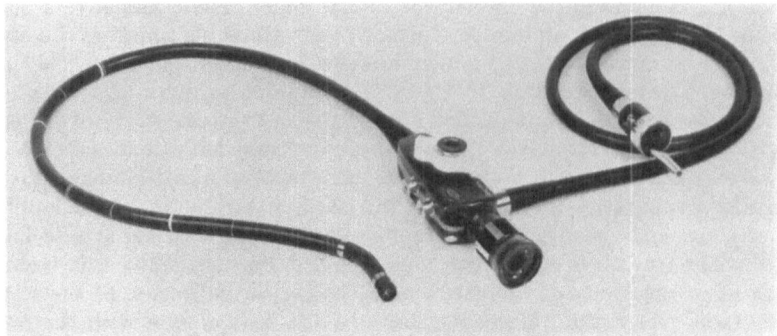

Fig. 114. Olympus fiber esophagoscope. From right to left, the cable connecting the fiber-scope with the generator, the proximal end of the apparatus with its different controls, and the flexible body of the esophagoscope which is bent slightly at its end

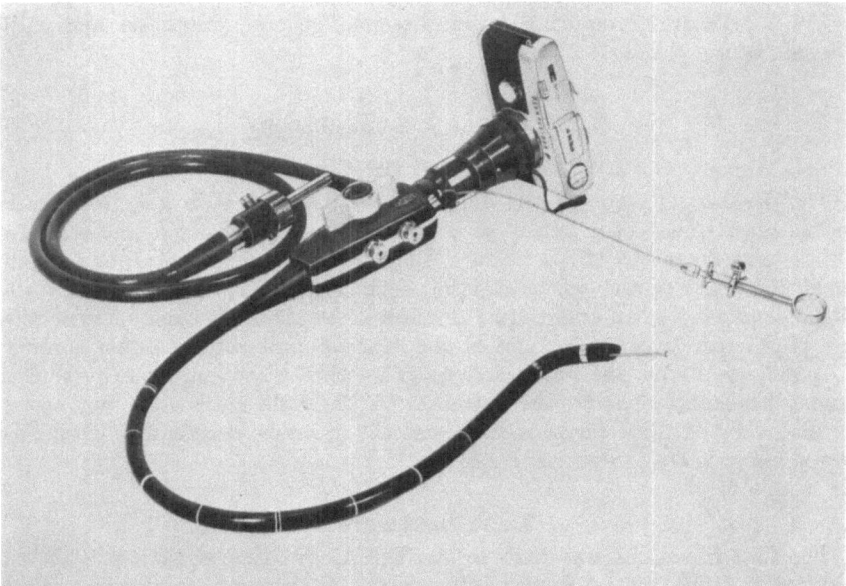

Fig. 115. Olympus fiber esophagoscope. The camera is mounted on the eye-piece. The biopsy forceps is inserted and protrudes slightly from the distal end of the apparatus

This instrument has been greatly perfected, and is equipped with devices that facilitate the examination and render some maneuvers semi-automatical.

The proximal end comprises an eye-piece for focusing on the intersection plane of the fibers on which the image forms; two push buttons (one sets off the insufflation and, if pressed to the bottom, the cleansing of the lens; the other one commands the aspiration); an operating lever for the flexion of the lower extremity with the possibility of blocking the bend in a determined position; an orifice for the introduction of the biopsy forceps.

The distal end is protected with a rubber cap. It comprises a fixed focus lens, deviating 10° in relation to the principal axis of the instrument (fore-oblique lens); an orifice for aspiration and biopsy; a channel for insufflation and cleansing, the orifice of which is directed laterally to sweep the lens; two openings in which end the two bundles of light-conducting fibers (cold light).

The body of the apparatus contains: the fiber bundles for the transmission of images; the two bundles of light-conducting fibers; the channel for aspiration and biopsy; the channel for insufflation and cleansing and the wires commanding the flection movements of the distal end.

The whole is protected by a spiraling metal sheath, covered with a second sheath of plastic material. This sheath has marks every 5 cm of its length. A permanently attached strand connects the endoscope to the light source. This strand transmits light and contains the channels for aspiration, insufflation and cleansing.

The light generator comprises a powerful lamp (an iodine lamp of 150 watts and 24 volts), a pump for insufflation and cleansing and an electronic integrator which automatically adjusts the light intensity when photographic pictures are shot. Finally, the aspiration channel can be connected to any source of vacuum. The biopsy forceps is long and flexible and has two mobile jaws.

3.2.3. Examination Technique

As every endoscopic exploration, flexible esophagoscopy is performed in 3 essential phases: preparation and positioning of the patient, insertion of the instrument, and exploration with associated maneuvers if need be.

3.2.3.1. Preparation and Positioning of the Patient

General anesthesia is seldom used except with young or fainthearted subjects, or when difficult and painful explorations have to be performed. In other cases, the patients themselves ask to be narcotized and agree to an esophagoscopy but under this condition. If narcosis is used, it is always preferable to intubate the trachea; this is no hindrance to the passing of the esophagoscope. The presence of a qualified anesthetist is obligatory. When an urgent examination has to be performed for upper gastrointestinal hemorrhage the patient must have received traditional reanimation treatment first. A gastric lavage with a rather wide tube allows the evacuation of blood clots. The injected liquid may be chilled water or physiologic serum. The lavage should be gentle and careful. It is to be continued until the liquid returns limpid or rosy. The tube is left in place, for it makes early recognition of recurrent hemorrhage possible. Customary preparation includes a thorough psychological preparation, light premedication and anesthesia of the back of the throat. Methods and products used vary considerably according to the operators. An intramuscular injection of diazepam (10 mg, Valium) and atropine (0.5 mg) is a satisfactory premedication. With careful psychological preparation of the patient a suppository composed of phenobarbital and atropine may be sufficient. Local anesthesia is obtained by rinsing the mouth and swallowing a tablespoonful of an anesthetizing jelly containing 2 g of lidocaine mixed in 100 ml of an aromatized gel (viscous xylocaine).

The patient is then placed on the examination table, in left lateral decubitus. The head is held by an assistant in slightly anterior flexion and rests on a cushion, sufficiently thick to keep the cervical spine well in the axis of the dorsal spine. During the examination the patient may put his (her) head in the position which he (she) feels to be most comfortable; hyperextension, necessary with the rigid apparatus, is no longer needed here. On the contrary, it is better to bend the head a little forward and to deflect it slightly towards the left side to allow secretions to flow out.

This is the most customary position. In fact, the fiberscope can be inserted in all positions. When an urgent examination is to be carried out at the bedside, the patient may be in sitting or half-sitting position, or in dorsal decubitus. The only important precaution is to have the patient's head slightly flexed forward at the moment of insertion. The position of the patient can be altered during the fiberscopic examination.

3.2.3.2. Insertion of the Apparatus and Exploration

The most delicate moment of the examination and the most disagreeable one for the patient is the insertion of the instrument into the throat and the passing of the pharyngoesophageal sphincter. The operator should take the distal end of the esophagoscope between the index and the middle finger of the left hand, while his right hand holds the body of the instrument between the thumb and the index; an assistant supports the proximal extremity, leaving free the lever commanding the flexion of the distal end. Indeed, the movements of this lever give precious information on the bending and then the straightening of the lower extremity of the fiberscope as it passes the pharyngoesophageal sphincter. It is sometimes required to depress the basis of the tongue with the left middle finger in order to facilitate the insertion into the throat, or to keep the distal end of the fiberscope rigid by blocking the flexion lever. All these maneuvers require some experience.

To get beyond the pharyngoesophageal sphincter the patient is asked to swallow while the instrument is inserted without forcing. Two or three swallows are sometimes needed; on swallowing the pharyngoesophageal sphincter relaxes as part of the deglutition movement.

The examination can commence as soon as the pharyngoesophageal sphincter has been passed. However, the body of the fiberscope should be protected immediately from bites, which are liable to damage it. A piece of plastic material provided to this effect is placed between the teeth of the patient (this piece must be slipped on the esophagoscope prior to insertion of the apparatus). Insufflation of air, aspiration of mucous secretions and cleansing of the lens permit to spot at once the esophageal lumen. The progression should go on slowly, smoothly, under direct vision. It is imperative to keep the esophageal lumen in the axis of progression with forward or backward bending maneuvers and with rotating movements. The exploration of the thoracic esophagus is easy. The passing of the esophagogastric junction likewise does not meet with major difficulties; it necessitates an increased backward bending movement because

Fig. 116. Normally opened cardia. Note the coarse folds of gastric mucosa reaching the esophagogastric mucosal junction

Fig. 117. Closed cardia. The esophagogastric mucosal junction is clearly visible

Fig. 118. Hiatal hernia. In the upper right, on the foreground, the cardiac border; in the background, on the left, the neck of the hernia. The gastric mucosa that covers the hernia is slightly inflamed

Fig. 119. Esophagitis above a hernia. The hiatal hernia was associated with severe esophagitis in the lower esophagus. The mucosa appeared red and showed false membranes

Fig. 120. Narrow stenosis of the lower esophagus. In this case the differential diagnosis between cancer and stenosing esophagitis is difficult. Biopsy revealed a cancer of gastric origin

Fig. 121. Typical polypoid cancer of the esophagus confirmed on biopsy

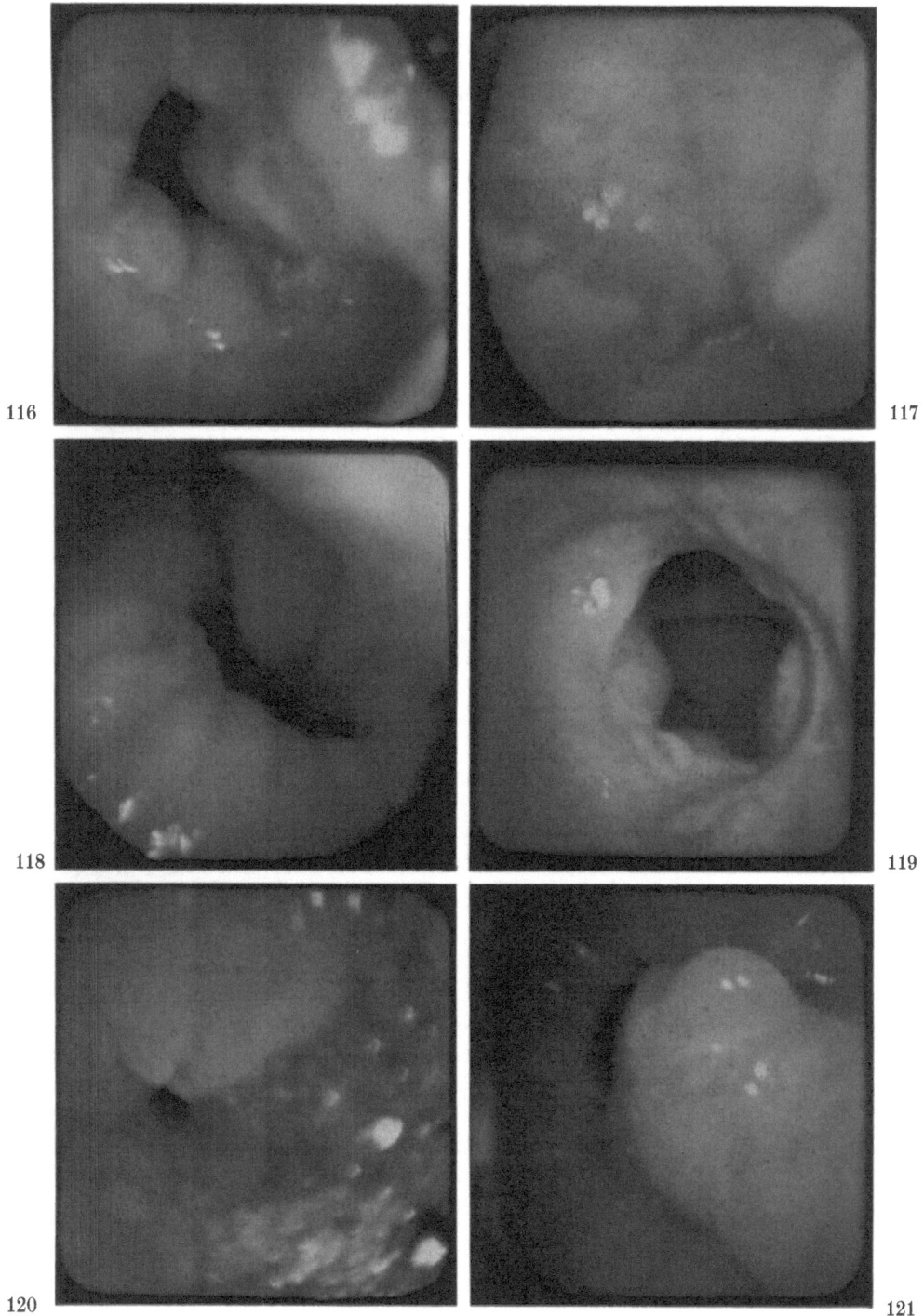

Figs. 116–121

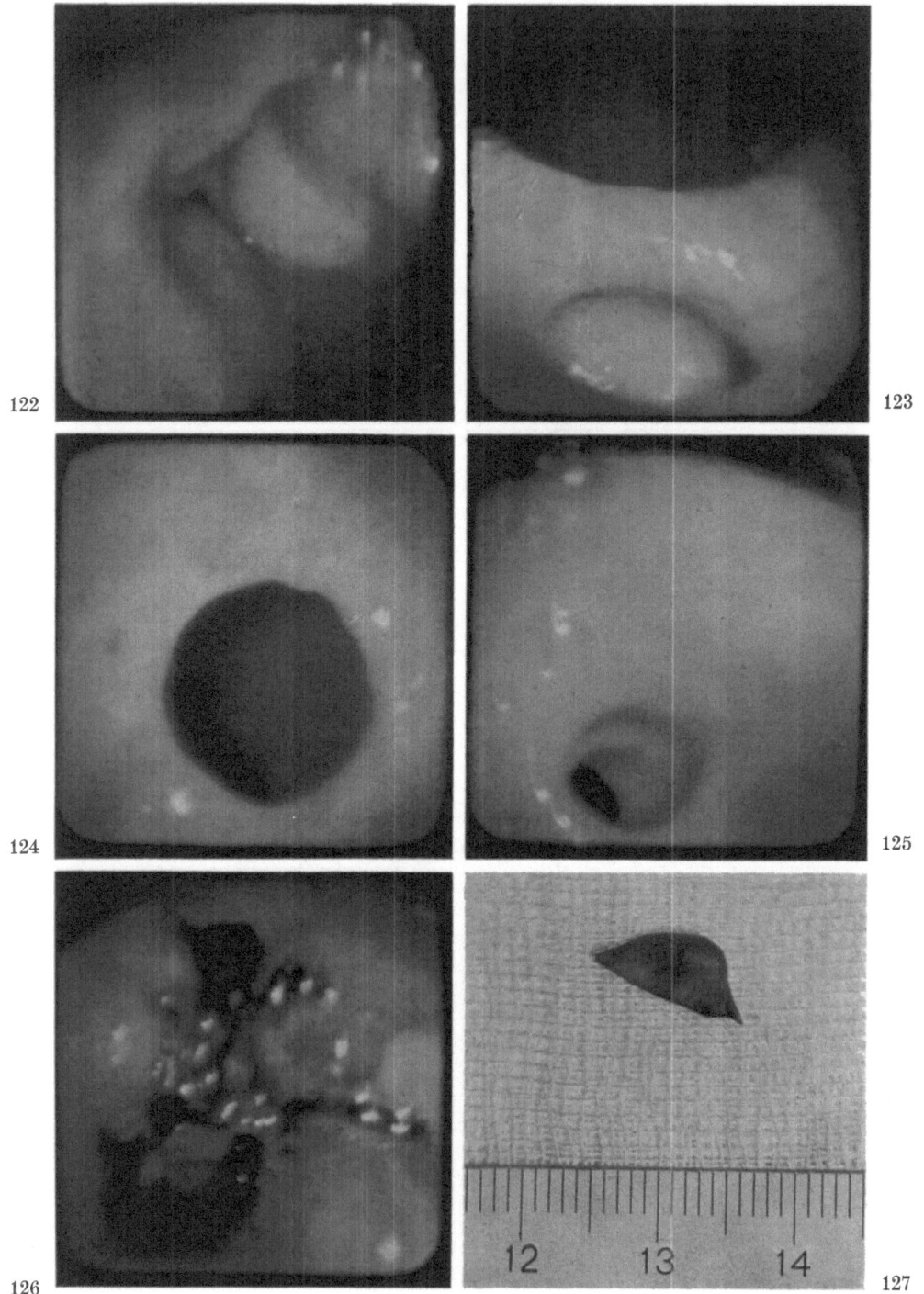

Figs. 122—127

the abdominal esophagus is directed downward and to the left. The instrument then penetrates into the gastric cavity, the exploration of which requires peculiar maneuvers which will not be described here. The exploration during the insertion of the instrument is limited to a rather swift progression under direct vision.

The safest and best exploration, which is effected during the slow withdrawal of the instrument, is the retrograde exploration. This examination permits to recognize the diaphragmatic hiatus, the esophagogastric mucosal junction, the esophagus proper and the pharyngoesophageal junction. In the normal subject, the diaphragmatic hiatus roughly coincides with the "cardia" (Figs. 116, 117). When closed, it is punctiform with converging esophageal folds. Upon relaxation it opens and forms a regular round orifice. In patients with a sliding hiatal hernia, the narrowing formed by the enlarged diaphragmatic ring looks like a round or oval orifice, permanently open; the mucosa above and below the narrowing is of the gastric type; the ring moves up and down with respiration, ruffling the mucosa as with a roller (Fig. 118). The squamocolumnar mucosal junction is easily recognizable in the normal esophagus: the gastric mucosa is thick, red-orange colored; the esophageal mucosa is thin and pale with very fine blood vessels. This junction is located at a variable distance from the incisors; it is always useful to note this distance by means of the marks to be found on any type of fiber esophagoscope. The limit between the two mucous membranes may be linear; often it looks like a geographical map with capes and gulfs. Sometimes the gastric folds reach slightly above the diaphragmatic ring and end precisely at the junction of gastric and esophageal mucosa. The esophagus proper is lined with a glossy and wan mucosa, showing sometimes small whitish elevated spots. Circular contractions slowly lift the mucosa and result in fine longitudinal folds. The pharyngoesophageal junction is mostly seen for only a short while. Indeed, the extremity of the fiberscope is very swiftly propelled upwards once the apparatus reaches the upper orifice of the esophagus.

The other possibilities of the fiber esophagoscope will not be discussed. Worth mentioning, however, is the fact that long fiber esophagoscopes (panendoscopes) allow to examine the gastric cavity, to reach the pylorus and to penetrate into the duodenal bulb. The most recent American types make it furthermore possible to explore the fundus of the stomach and the cardia by flexing the distal end over 180°.

3.2.3.3. Associate Maneuvers

During the endoscopic exploration, the operator can carry out various maneuvers, of which only still photography, cinematography and biopsy will be discussed.

With the Japanese esophagoscopes, still photography (Fig. 115) is very easy because the exposure times are automatically calculated. The photographic camera

Fig. 122. Typical esophageal varices

Fig. 123. Simple esophageal diverticulum. Normal mucosa

Fig. 124. Regular circular narrowing, located 25 cm from the incisors. Note the complete absence of inflammatory signs. Congenital malformation

Fig. 125. Non-inflammatory congenital narrowing in the lower esophagus

Fig. 126. Suture material left after upper polar gastrectomy

Fig. 127. Rabbit bone extracted via a flexible esophagoscope

is a reflex Olympus Pen special apparatus which can take 40 negatives 18 × 24 mm on a 35 mm standard film designed for 20 exposures. The film used is Ektachrome high sensitivity (125 ASA), artificial light type (Figs. 116–126). The increased light intensity required for cinematography is easily obtained with a push button on the generator. For cinematography we use a 16 mm Beaulieu camera and Ektachrome film high sensitivity (125 ASA) of the artificial light type. The camera is fitted to the eye-piece with a connecting device, especially designed for this purpose; at present a speed of 2 frames per second is used. A color television camera can be fitted onto the fiberscope, but this requires a much more powerful light generator, including a Xenon or an arc lamp.

To get good pictures, it is advisable to wash the lens and then to aspirate slightly lest the photographs and films be shot through a watery screen, which deforms the images. The application of silicone oil on the lens prior to the endoscopic examination is also a good precaution. Finally, it is wise to take many negatives to be able to select the best pictures afterwards. Biopsies can be taken easily (Fig. 115). This maneuver, which should be accurate and quick, without rudeness, requires some training. The following operations are carried out in succession: the extremity of the forceps is placed into the field of the objective, the jaws of the probe, are opened and put on the area selected for the sampling, the jaws of the forceps are closed and a tissue fragment is torn off. In some cases the esophago-fiberscope has to be straightened in order to facilitate the passage of the forceps; afterwards the end of the instrument is curbed again to enable the sampling. In this instance too, it is often required to wash, insufflate, aspirate, and, after the biopsy has been taken, to rid the objective of blood or mucus. When ulcerations are present multiple biopsies should be taken from the edge of the lesion but not from the bottom of the ulceration, lest one gets back necrotic fragments which can not be interpreted. The biopsy of tumorous folds should be as deep as possible and should be effected perpendicularly to the fold axis to get every chance of detecting a submucosal cancer. Finally, in the case of stenosing lesions the biopsy must not be taken above the stenosed area, where the lesions are aspecific; the forceps should be inserted into the stenotic segment to take a blind biopsy. In all cases the sampling must be multiple. Only a positive biopsy has a real value; if negative, it does not prove that there is no cancer.

Instead of a biopsy forceps, a catheter of plastic material may be inserted into the fiber esophagoscope. This catheter can be used to wash the esophageal wall or remove adherent mucus hindering the examination; it may help to aspirate under supervision the secretions covering a suspected lesion in view of a cytological study.

The extraction of small foreign bodies is feasible (Fig. 127) but difficult since the biopsy forceps does not allow a firm hold. The foreign body must be withdrawn into the rubber casing protecting the distal end of the fiberscope. A faint traction upon the forceps keeps the foreign body in this position while the entire apparatus is smoothly withdrawn. This maneuver is feasible only if the dimensions of the foreign body are inferior to the diameter of the fiberscope; it should be done very gently to avoid scratching of the mucosa on the way back.

3.2.3.4. Advantages and Drawbacks

The advantages of the flexible esophagoscope are manifold. Of paramount importance is the excellent tolerance by the patients, which makes possible prolonged examinations, iterative explorations for follow-up studies, and the performing of associate maneuvers, the importance of which is steadily increasing in digestive endoscopy. On the other hand the flexibility of the apparatus allows the exploration of the lower esophagus and the esophagocardial region, practically inaccessible zones to rigid esophagoscopy. Lastly, in spite of its name, the fiber esophagoscope can also be used in the examination of the stomach and the pylorobulbar region, but this will not be discussed here.

The exploration of the pharyngoesophageal sphincter remains the weak spot of esophagoscopy with flexible instruments. Indeed, the upper orifice of the esophagus is only seen at withdrawal; on the way down, the instrument is inserted blindly. Some lesions can be overlooked this way; other lesions only become manifest because of an impassible obstacle that precludes exploration and biopsy. Improvements are still to be made in this field. Other disadvantages of fiber esophagoscopy are the high cost of the instruments, their fragility, and the cost and duration of repairs.

4. Indications and Contraindications

The indications for esophagoscopy are determined by the X-ray findings. This means that one must refuse to perform any endoscopy which was not preceded by a thorough and recent X-ray examination. These indications can be summarized as follows:

If the X-rays are sufficiently typical, endoscopy is a form of complementary examination which may have the great advantage of providing a histological or biological proof of the diagnosis.

If the X-ray examination reveals suspect images, endoscopy becomes necessary. It must be carried out with the intention of first examining the suspected zones. In this way the endoscopic examination will often provide important information which, added to the clinical and radiological data, may make possible a more accurate diagnosis and indicate the most suitable treatment.

In case of negative X-ray examination and symptoms which, because of their intensity or persistence, are sufficiently alarming, an endoscopic exploration is indicated and will sometimes reveal unnoticed lesions.

Unexplained upper digestive hemorrhages are a frequent indication for endoscopic examination, which may then be urgently performed prior to any other investigation.

Finally, the extraction of small foreign bodies may also constitute an indication for medical esophagoscopy.

These are all classical indications for esophagoscopy. The difficulties inherent in rigid esophagoscopy have hampered its clinical application for quite a long time. At present, the flexible instruments allow a broader and more efficacious use of these indications. Fiber esophagoscopy has revealed the frequent incidence of peptic esophagitis (Fig. 119). It has facilitated the diagnosis of carcinoma of the lower esophagus and cardia (Figs. 120, 121). Stenosing lesions (Figs. 124, 125), diverticula (Fig. 123), and esophageal varices (Fig. 122) are easily accessible to fiberscopic examination. Lastly, the flexible esophagoscopes allow to explore surgical anastomoses after total gastrectomy, upper polar gastrectomy or partial esophagectomy (Fig. 126).

Except in cases of aortic aneurysms and severe deformities of the cervical or dorsal spine there is practically no absolute contraindication. In almost all cases an esophagoscopy may be attempted, provided that it be carried out very prudently. However, the age of the patient, his general and especially his cardiovascular condition must be taken into account in order to impose on an exhausted patient only absolutely indicated endoscopic investigations.

5. Accidents and Incidents

As any instrumental maneuver, esophagoscopy involves some risks. The rigid esophagoscopes are doubtlessly more dangerous than the flexible instruments. However, the fiberscopes can cause accidents even when handled by the best experts and several cases of perforation have been reported. The enthusiasm for this well tolerated and apparently easy technique should not be a reason to overlook the rules of prudence imperative in any esophagogastric intubation.

5.1. Accidents
5.1.1. Perforation

Perforation is the most important accident of esophagoscopy and occurs usually at the level of the cervical esophagus (see also: Iatrogenic Perforations). The clinical symptoms, appearing immediately or after a few hours' interval include continuous pain, total dysphagia and, most telling sign, emphysema at the basis of the neck. As soon as one of these symptoms becomes evident one must look for radiological signs of mediastinal emphysema. Once the diagnosis of perforation is certain, surgery is imperative to prevent suppurative mediastinitis, the evolution of which is mostly fatal. The ominous character of these esophageal perforations deserves to be stressed, but one should bear in mind that the incidence of this accident is fortunately very low and that the utilization of fiber-esophagoscopes, has diminished the odds in a remarkable fashion. In more than 4000 esophagoscopies performed up to date, we have not noted a single perforation accident, either with rigid instruments or with flexible ones. Perforation may occur during biopsy maneuvers as well; the removal of a piece of mucosa grown brittle by inflammation or tumorous invasion must always be done with much prudence.

5.1.2. Hemorrhage

Hemorrhagic accidents in esophagoscopy result from fissuring of an aortic aneurysm and laceration or biopsy of a varix. The very notion of hemostatic defects or of an anticoagulant treatment must incite to caution and forbids any biopsy maneuver. When a biopsy is followed by abnormally abundant bleeding the patient should be watched to give the appropriate treatment if necessary.

5.2. Incidents

Incidents are most likely to occur at the onset of the examination. They are rare and, as a rule, benign. Their existence, however, should not be overlooked for they may necessitate immediate maneuvers or, in certain cases, a closer postoperative watching. Failure of passing the pharyngoesophageal sphincter, respiratory spasm, abnormal pain, blood on the extremity of the esophagoscope or in the secretions expelled by the patient are the most important incidents.

5.2.1. Failure to Pass Pharyngoesophageal Sphincter

Certain maneuvers facilitate the passing of the esophageal sphincter when the deglutition movements of the patient appear insufficient. One of these maneuvers consists in the insertion of a tube prior to the introduction of the esophagoscope. This maneuver provides information concerning the permeability of the upper orifice of the esophagus and about the way of orienting the distal end of the fiberscope. Unrelenting spasm of the esophageal mouth in a nervous patient can be overcome by the intravenous injection of diazepam, in which event it is wise to watch the patient for a few hours.

5.2.2. Respiratory Spasm

Respiratory spasm is an unpredictable dramatic incident requiring the immediate withdrawal of the esophagoscope. This incident, as harmless as spectacular, mostly does not prevent the reinsertion of the esophagoscope without difficulty as soon as the subject has resumed a normal respiration rhythm.

5.2.3. Pain

Pain is a symptom of paramount importance, especially with flexible instruments. Indeed, rigid esophagoscopy is frequently painful, but fiber esophagoscopy is not or almost not. The pain must be located accurately; if it is a laterocervical pain, the orientation of the extremity of the instrument should be changed; in case of median pain, the cause lies with the passage of the pharyngoesophageal sphincter and care should be taken not to force it. When the upper orifice of the esophagus is passed, the feeling of a dorsal pain is an alarm signal indicating that the esophageal wall is being pressed by the end of the esophagoscope against the spine. This pain frequently occurs with rigid instruments and precludes the further insertion of the instrument; it is exceptional with flexible instruments and can be easily remedied by bending the distal extremity of the fiberscope. Lastly, the esophagocardial region should be passed under visual control and should not be painful. It is very important to know the duration of the pain accurately, whichever its site; if persisting, a prolonged watching of the patient is indicated. It should be pointed out that the absence of pain sensation is one of the drawbacks of endoscopy under general anesthesia.

5.2.4. Bleeding

The presence of a little blood on the distal end of the esophagoscope or in the secretions expelled by the patient is of no consequence with rigid instruments; it is exceptional with fiber esophagoscopes and should catch the attention of the operator. It might be a faint hemorrhage of dental, gingival or lingual origin but in many cases the exact origin of the bleeding is unknown. In such a case the patient must be kept under close supervision for one or two hours to trace the first symptoms of a possible, more serious complication, even if the examination was easily performed. Administration of antibiotics is justified to prevent the infection of a mucosal scratching.

In conclusion, the manufacturing of flexible esophagoscopes is the onset of a new era for esophageal endoscopy. In the past, an accessory method, far less important than radiology, esophageal endoscopy has nowadays become a primary examination method. Every gastroenterology department needs an endoscopy room, well equipped for esophagogastroscopy. The rigid esophagoscope as well as the semi-flexible gastroscope are out of date, except for special indications. At present the examinations are performed in conditions of comfort and safety beyond comparison; one should know, however, that accidents, more particularly perforations, may still occur.

References

BOCKUS, H. L.: Tests employed in the study of esophageal function and disease. In: Gastroenterology, vol. 1, p. 132, 2nd ed. Philadelphia: W. B. Saunders Co. 1963.

HIRSCHOWITZ, B. I.: A fibre optic flexible oesophagoscope. Lancet 1963 II, 388.

HOUSSET, P., PERREAU, G., DEBRAY, CH.: L'endoscopie digestive. Techniques d'exploration et de prélèvements. Rev. Prat. (Paris) 15, 459–487 (1965).

LO PRESTI, P. A., HILMI, A. M.: Clinical experience with a new foroblique fiber esophagoscope. Amer. J. dig. Dis. 9, 690–697 (1964).

Exfoliative Cytology of the Esophagus

F. VILARDELL

With 9 Figures

1. Introduction

Probably LIONEL BEALE (1867) should be credited with the first reference in the medical literature on the use of cytological methods for the diagnosis of cancer of the digestive system. In his book "The Microscope and its Application in Clinical Medicine", BEALE published several drawings of gastric and esophageal cells which he thought to be malignant. The first clinical paper in which cancer cells, obtained by a washing procedure from patients with gastric and esophageal cancer, were described according to modern criteria was published by MARINI in 1909. In spite of the importance of these observations the cytological method never became popular, perhaps because of the rapid expansion of roentgenology as a practical diagnostic procedure. The publications by PAPANICOLAOU (1942–1943) renewed the interest of several gastroenterologists for cytological methods, and in the last few years several books referring to gastrointestinal cytodiagnosis have been published (PAPANICOLAOU, 1954; BRUINSMA, 1957; SCHADE, 1960; VILARDELL, 1962; GRAHAM, 1963; NIEBURGS, 1967; GIBBS, 1968; KOSS and DURFEE, 1968; HENNING and WITTE, 1968).

In recent years, exfoliative cytology has become a valuable adjunct to endoscopy and radiology in the diagnosis of esophageal cancer, and a great variety of procedures have been recommended in order to obtain well preserved cells in sufficient numbers to provide an easy diagnosis of cancer.

2. Esophageal Cytological Techniques

The aim of all esophageal cytological techniques is to increase the number of cells which normally exfoliate from the surface of tumors, since, as COMAN (1944) already demonstrated, cancer cells lack the adhesiveness of normal epithelial cells.

2.1. Techniques Combined with Esophagoscopy

Several authors have studied cytological samples obtained at endoscopic examination. Thus ANDERSEN et al. (1949) were able to obtain diagnostic cells in cases in which biopsy had been inconclusive or negative. MESSELT (1952) achieved good results using cotton swabs over areas that looked suspicious on esophagoscopy. More recently, MILANESI and TOSI (1965) have utilized a special tube in order to wash the esophagus and aspirate its contents under direct vision. SANZ and REMENIUK (1968) reported good results by the use of cotton swabs or bougies and washing the esophagus afterwards. LANCE and GROISSIER (1965) have studied cancer cells by simply washing the esophagoscope at the end of the examination; they recovered positive samples in 68 per cent of proven cases of carcinoma.

In spite of the attractiveness of these methods, which permit the use of several diagnostic measures during one single examination (cytology, biopsy, photography, etc.) many experienced cytological laboratories still recommend cytology as an isolated procedure. They claim that with this method cells are better preserved and contamination of the smears with mucus, blood and foreign material is avoided (LANCE and GROISSIER, 1965). In our own experience, cytological material obtained through the esophagoscope is often heavily contaminated with detritus and mucus, which greatly interfere with microscopical examination. However, with the new fiber esophagoscopes we have recently obtained much better results. Cytological samples taken at fiber esophagoscopy will probably be the technique of choice in the future. In any case, cytological procedures should be performed prior to biopsy in order to avoid excessive amounts of blood and normal epidermoid cells in the smears.

2.2. Abrasive Techniques

The first instrument that has been widely employed to obtain blind cytological samples of the esophagus and stomach has been HENNING's "Zelltupfsonde" (1952). It consists of a flexible tube provided with a steel wire carrying at the distal end a foam rubber sponge. The tube is introduced into the esophagus and the sponge is pushed forward when the instrument has reached the lesion. A fine cellophane envelope, protecting the sponge from contamination with pharyngeal epithelium, is then broken, the lesion is swabbed for a few minutes and the sponge is reintroduced into the tube. Finally the sponge is rinsed with saline and the fluid centrifuged. The smears are stained with the Papanicolaou or Giemsa techniques.

AYRE and OREN (1953) introduced another type of instrument, the "gastric brush", which they utilized to obtain samples from the esophagus and stomach. It consists of a polythene tube to which a metallic capsule, about 7 cm long, is attached. Inside the capsule there is a double brush which is extruded by means of a spring mechanism. By rotating the instrument inside the esophagus or stomach, mucosal cells are abraded. The tube is then pulled out, the brush is washed with saline or Ringer's solution and the sediment obtained by centrifugation is processed according to the usual Papanicolaou technique.

NIEBURGS' brush (1956), which is mainly used for gastric cytology, can also be employed. It consists of a flexible tube containing several nylon loops which can be extruded in order to obtain mucosal material by abrasion. The loops can be reinserted into the tube after abrasion by an external mechanism.

Other abrasive instruments have been devised in recent years. DEBRAY et al. (1967) have introduced a new apparatus which they call "Cyto-rape". It consists of a Camus tube with a metallic cylinder attached to its distal extremity. This cylinder has multiple perforations. Forceful aspiration attracts small fragments of mucosa into the tube which are removed after the tube has been pulled out. HUMPHREYS et al. (1968) use for abrasion a thin aluminum foil which envelops the distal end of a gastric tube. The cellular material is recovered afterwards by washing the esophagus with saline. COHEN and FLOWERS (1969) favor the use of small brushes like the ones used for cleaning electric razors. With this simple device attached to a tube, they were able to get 32 positive results out of 34 cases of cancer of the esophagus. Several years ago, HERSHENSON (1959) obtained good results by using a cotton swab attached to a metal piano wire.

In spite of the large number of abrasive instruments available, none seems to have reached widespread popularity and in many laboratories, especially in the U.S.A., simple lavage methods are preferred.

2.3. Lavage Techniques

Washing methods are more appealing than abrasive procedures because of their simplicity and lack of risk, and because of their high percentage of accuracy (JOHNSON et al., 1955; RASKIN et al., 1959; GEPHART and GRAHAM, 1959; MacDONALD et al., 1963; PROLLA et al., 1965; BRANDBORG and WENGER, 1968).

Usually the technique consists of introducing a Levine tube into the stomach of the fasting patient. The patient drinks about 100 ml of Ringer solution which is aspirated with a 100 ml syringe. In this way a sample of the whole esophageal mucosa is obtained. Then the tube is slowly withdrawn with the patient in a recumbent position and the esophagus is washed every 5 cm. The radiologically or endoscopically suspicious areas are washed with special care. A few authors are using double lumen tubes for the simultaneous injection and aspiration of fluid (BRITSCH, 1962; GHOSSEIN and BRITSCH, 1962).

In our experience, better samples are obtained by repeatedly injecting into the esophagus small amounts of fluid (about 20 ml) rather than by using larger amounts which are often poorly tolerated by patients with obstructing lesions. Sudden distention may produce pain; one of our patients developed coronary symptoms so that the procedure had to be stopped. When there is food retention in the esophagus it is necessary to perform meticulous washings before the test.

Smears are always fixed without delay, after centrifugation of the fluid at about 1500 r.p.m. for 10 min. Angle centrifuges are particularly useful for this purpose. Membrane filtration (Millipore) has been recommended by YOUNGS and NIELSEN (1965) for esophageal cytology. At this moment they do not seem to offer real advantages over the standard procedures.

Fixation in ether-alcohol is still the routine procedure in most laboratories. To avoid shedding of the cells the fixatives may also be sprayed on the slides "spray-cyte" (NIEBURGS, 1967).

In the U.S.A. slides that are frosted on one side are often used because of their greater adhesiveness (Dakin frosted slides). The Papanicolaou stain with or without modifications is widely employed. Other strains (Giemsa, Feulgen) do not seem to have advantages for routine use.

2.4. Combined Techniques

In our department, a technique which combines abrasion with washings has been used for years (CABRE-FIOL, 1953). The instrument consists of a radiopaque, double lumen tube provided with a steel wire that ends in a rubber tip to avoid traumatic lesions. Attached to the wire is a tuft of nylon threads which are protected from contamination with mucus and pharyngeal cells by their enclosure in a small rubber cylinder. Exfoliation is done under fluoroscopy by moving the steel wire with the tuft of nylon threads several times back and forth and gently pressing its end against the esophageal walls. The esophagus is then washed with ice-cold saline or Ringer's solution through the additional tube opening (about 20 ml of fluid).

All samples, including those attached to the nylon threads and cells obtained by lavage, are centrifuged and processed according to the Papanicolaou technique.

Larger fragments may be embedded in paraffin and studied with ordinary histo-logic techniques. No accidents have been encountered with this method in more than 1 000 gastric and esophageal examinations (VILARDELL, 1968).

3. An Appraisal of Cytologic Techniques

Controversy between those who favor abrasive methods and those who prefer washing techniques is as old as digestive cytology itself. In general, washing methods have become popular because they do not require special instruments and because their results are as good or better than those of abrasive methods. Washings can be done by auxiliary personnel while abrasion requires the presence of a physician. Accidents have been reported with abrasive techniques: SASSON (1964) has described unfavorable experiences with AYRE's brush and MLECKO (1968) mentions a case of hematemesis following abrasion of the esophagus with the method of HUMPHREYS et al. (1968). Nevertheless the literature on abrasive methods continues to grow, perhaps because in some cases large amounts of cells are retrieved and rapid and impressive diagnoses of malignancy can be made. After a rather large experience with both lavage and abrasive methods it seems to us that the choice of technique is less important than the experience of the operator with his method. Meticulous care during the procedure is the most important element for success or failure. Diagnostic cells can be obtained in most cases if one succeeds in introducing a tube beyond the suspicious area. The mechanical abrasion caused by this introduction obviously plays a role also when lavage alone is utilized.

4. Normal Cytology of the Esophagus

Normal esophageal smears show almost exclusively squamous epithelial cells of the upper digestive tract: these are large, flat, sometimes wrinkled cells; their cytoplasm shows vivid colors with the Papanicolaou stain. Nuclei are small, often pycnotic. Cells of the oral cavity often contain bacteria and other inclusions in their cytoplasm which allow their differentiation from esophageal cells. When they originate in the deeper layers of the epithelium, cells are smaller. Thus parabasal cells offer the peculiar aspect of rapidly growing cells, their nuclei being larger and richer in chromatin and their cytoplasm smaller than in super-ficial squamous cells.

In a cytometric study (VILARDELL, 1962) the mean nuclear diameter of esophageal cells in 21 normal smears was 8.02μ. The chromatin of 60 per cent of the nuclei appeared homogeneous without evidence of a nucleolus. In the majority of cells, chromatin was arranged in small clumps, about 0.5μ in diameter. Nucleoli, when seen, were about 1μ in diameter. The thickness of the nuclear membrane was never greater than 0.5μ.

Besides epithelial cells of the esophagus, smears often contain ciliated cells of the bronchial epithelium as well as histiocytes from the respiratory tract.

5. Criteria for Malignancy in Esophageal Cytology

Already in the nineteenth century several authors described some charac-teristics of malignant cells. LEBERT (1851) noted the presence of large nucleoli in tumor cells and BEALE (1867) mentioned variations in size and shape of the nuclei as an important diagnostic criterion. In his paper, MARINI (1909) described gastric and esophageal tumor cells such as are seen in Fig. 128.

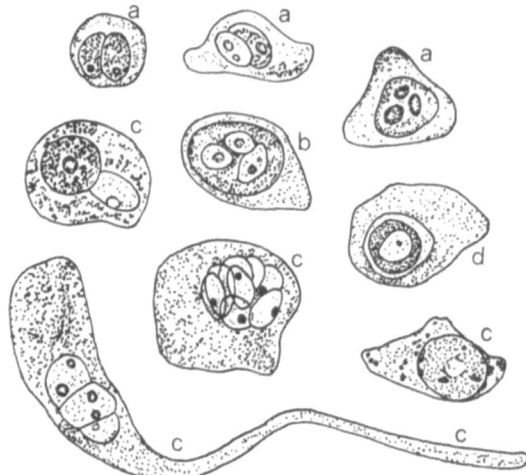

Fig. 128. Tumor cells according to Marini (1909). A multinucleated tadpole cell can be
recognized

The work of Papanicolaou (1943) established criteria for malignancy which
are universally accepted (Graham, 1963; Taylor, 1967; Nieburgs, 1967; Hughes
and Dodds, 1968; Koss, 1968). The most useful ones are listed as follows: (1) increase in the size of the nucleus; (2) nuclear/cytoplasmic ratio altered in favor
of the nucleus; (3) presence of several large nucleoli; (4) variations in size and
shape of the nuclei; (5) increase and irregular distribution of the nuclear chromatin,
which appears condensed in some areas of the nucleus and absent in others
(according to Graham, 1963, this criterion is particularly important); (6) irregular
thickening of the nuclear membrane; (7) presence of abnormal mitoses.

These criteria are applicable to all aspects of gastrointestinal cytology; however, there are some additional criteria which are useful for the diagnosis of
squamous cell carcinoma of the esophagus and which are similar to those used
in vaginal cytology. Graham (1963) described the following cell types in esophageal tumors: (1) Undifferentiated tumor cells (the cells have almost no cytoplasm). (2) "Third type" cells (Fig. 129): these are small round cells with a
dense cytoplasm and with characteristics of squamous epithelial cells. (3) "Tadpole cells" (Fig. 130): their nucleus is hyperchromatic and the cytoplasm has
an elongated shape which bears some resemblance to a tadpole. (4) Fiber cells:
these are elongated cells with a thin, very dark, fiber-like nucleus. Cells usually
appear arranged in large clusters.

These two last types of cells are characteristic of squamous cell carcinoma
but unfortunately they are rarely found in smears. According to Koss (1968)
cells with eosinophilic and keratinized cytoplasm are also diagnostic of this type
of cancer. Cells of squamous cell carcinoma are usually small (Raskin et al., 1959;
Gephart and Graham, 1959).

Although primary adenocarcinoma of the esophagus is a relatively infrequent
lesion (Turnbull and Goodner, 1968) invasion of the esophagus by cancer of
the gastric fundus is a very common finding. In these cases, tumor cells often
show in their cytoplasm mucus-secreting vacuoles which are characteristic of
glandular carcinoma. Moreover, the cells of squamous cell carcinoma can be

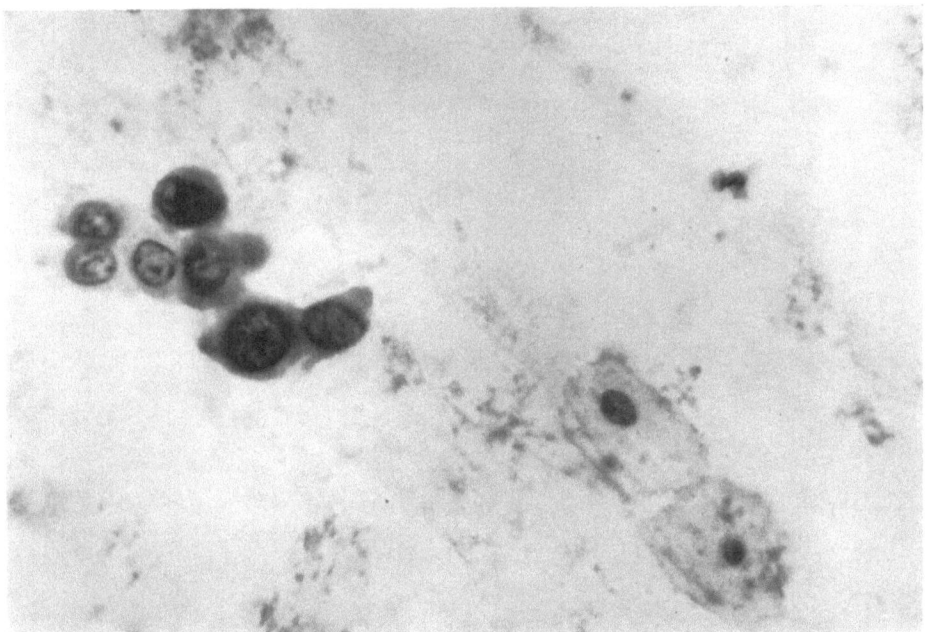

Fig. 129. Group of malignant cells of GRAHAM's "third type". On the right, two normal esophageal cells can be seen. (×150)

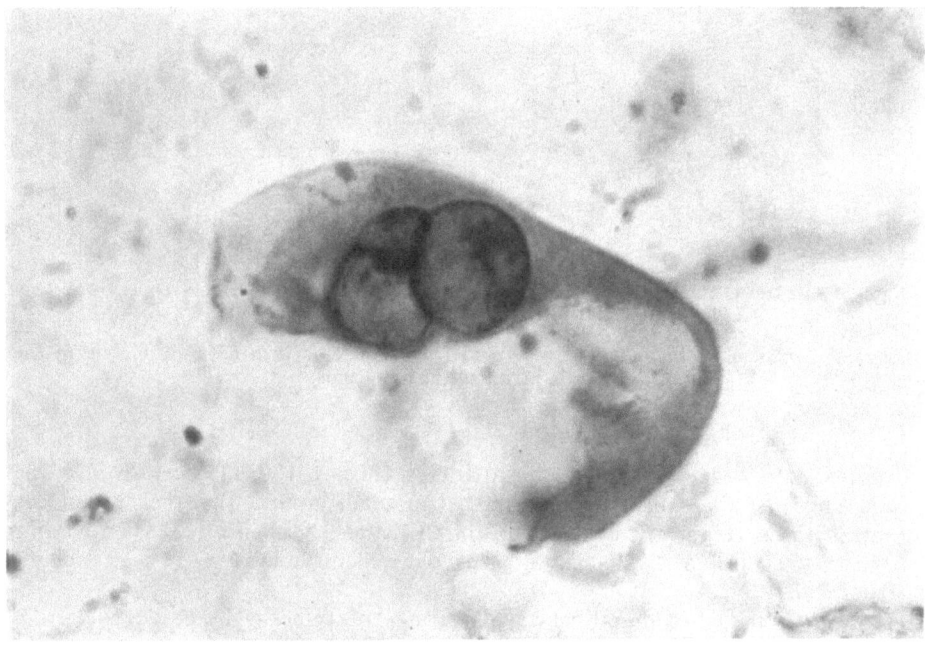

Fig. 130. Tadpole cell with several nuclei. (×850)

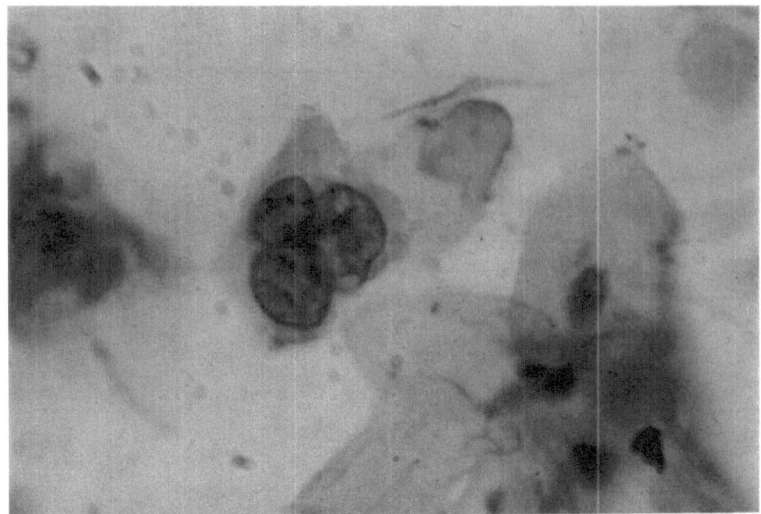

Fig. 131

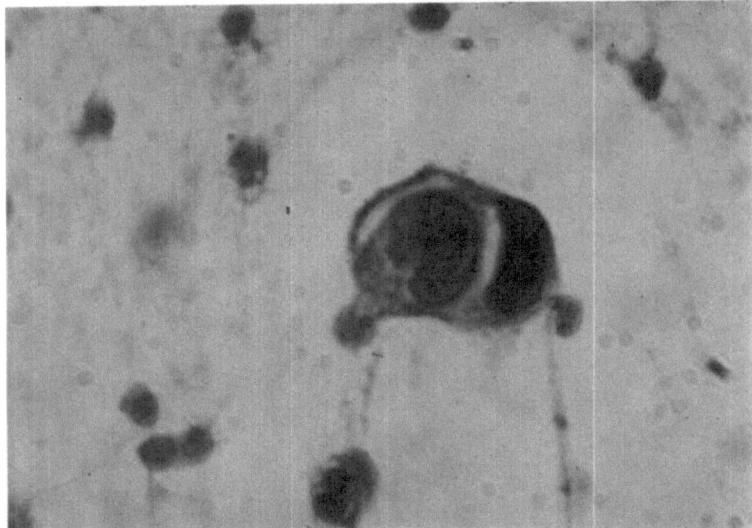

Fig. 132

Fig. 131. In the center of the picture, a group of malignant epidermoid cells are clearly recognizable; to the right, normal esophageal cells

Fig. 132. Group of malignant cells recovered from a patient with adenocarcinoma of the cardia invading the esophagus

differentiated from those of adenocarcinoma (Figs. 131, 132): they tend to be isolated rather than piled up and molded in small groups, the nucleus is more centrally located, and the cytoplasm is often sparse. Cytologically it is impossible to distinguish between primary and secondary adenocarcinoma of the esophagus (Koss, 1968).

Rubin (1961) has described some features of tumor cells exfoliating from lymphomata of esophagus and stomach. Usually these are small round cells, uniform in size, somewhat larger than lymphocytes, isolated or arranged in small groups. The cytoplasm is small, often featuring a bluish hue. One case of melanoma of the esophagus was diagnosed by Koss (1968) as an undifferentiated carcinoma since cells showed no pigmentation.

In a cytometric study of squamous cell carcinomas of the esophagus (VILARDELL, 1962) the mean nuclear diameter was 9.7 μ for tumor cells while the mean nuclear diameter of 1200 benign cells was 8.2 μ. In seven cases there were multinucleated cells and phagocytosis of tumor cells was seen in four cases. About 50 percent of tumor cells featured two or more nucleoli.

6. Cyto-Histological Correlations

There are but few data in the literature on the correlation of cellular morphology in smears and the histologic features of esophageal tumors. SCHICKENDANTZ et al. (1967) have studied 57 patients with cancer of the esophagus in whom a cytologic study had been made. They found some correlation between the degree of differentiation of exfoliated cells (fusiform cells, tadpole cells, etc.) and of neoplastic tissue. GRAHAM's third type cells were particularly frequent in tumors originating in basal layers. In 79 percent of the adenocarcinomas, pathognomonic cells were found in the smears.

In spite of these investigations, we share Koss' opinion (1968) that classifications of esophageal tumor cells are arbitrary and that they only have didactic value. Cyto-histological correlations have therefore little practical interest.

7. Indications of Esophageal Cytology

The main indication for cytologic study of the esophagus is dysphagia. Another indication is the radiological finding of stenosis in the lower third of the esophagus. Cytologic studies should be done in all patients with suspected cancer in which esophagoscopic biopsy has been negative and in cases in which esophagoscopy cannot be performed.

Cytological examinations are also very useful for the follow-up of patients with achalasia, as the incidence of carcinoma is increased in such patients. KLAYMAN (1955) has published cases of carcinoma secondary to megaesophagus which were diagnosed only by cytology. Recently, LUKASH and JOHNSON (1969) have described two cases of infiltrating carcinoma of the cardia which clinically mimicked achalasia. Both were correctly diagnosed as cancer by cytologic study.

GRAHAM (1963) stresses the importance of cytologic studies for the early diagnosis of recurrence in situ after resection of esophageal carcinoma. Cytology is also recommended in patients with the Plummer-Vinson syndrome, which may be considered as a precancerous condition (RUBIN, 1961).

8. Results of Esophageal Cytology

The results of esophageal cytology are listed in Table 4. Most studies report false negative results in less than 15 percent of their cases. Tumors of the lower third of the esophagus are often more difficult to diagnose than those of the middle third, perhaps because the latter may grow to large size without giving rise to symptoms. PROLLA et al. (1965) as well as DEBRAY et al. (1967) report that the diagnostic accuracy in cancer of the gastroesophageal junction is, in their experience, about 10 percent lower than their overall results.

Table 4. Results of cytology in the diagnosis of esophageal carcinoma

Author	Method	Number of cases with carcinoma	Positive	Results	
				dubious %	negative %
Andersen et al., 1949	Abrasion (gauze)	84	66.6	—	33.3
Johnson et al., 1955	Washings	148	69.6	12.2	18.2
Klayman et al., 1955	Washings	20	95.0	—	5.0
Raskin et al., 1959	Washings	53	94.3	—	5.7
Gephardt and Graham, 1959	Washings	64	89.0	6.0	5.0
McDonald et al., 1963	Washings	72	94.0	—	6.0
Henning et al., 1964	Abrasion	88	79.5	—	21.5
Prolla et al., 1965	Washings	64	87.5	—	11.5
Debray et al., 1967	Abrasion	98	74.0	—	26.0
Cabre-Fiol et al., 1969	Abrasion and washings	81	96.0	—	4.0

Cytology occasionally permits the diagnosis of small carcinomas at a stage when they have not yet invaded the muscularis mucosae (Imbriglia and Lopusniak, 1949). "Carcinoma in situ" of the esophagus was diagnosed by Schade (1964) in patients without clinical evidence of a tumor in whom gastric washings had been done to elucidate the etiology of a gastric ulcerative lesion. Malignant squamous epithelial cells were found and an asymptomatic carcinoma was discovered in the upper third of the esophagus, a diagnosis that was confirmed later by endoscopy and biopsy.

9. Diagnostic Errors

Besides the 10 to 20 percent of false negative results esophageal cytology may also give rise to false positive diagnoses of cancer. Fortunately these errors are not very frequent. Immature cells, resembling cancer cells, may exfoliate from the regenerating mucosa of chronic esophagitis. Dysplastic (dyskariotic) squamous cells are mostly single and characterized by a large hyperchromatic nucleus with coarse chromatin distribution, surrounded by an inconspicuous cytoplasm. Metaplastic squamous epithelial cells are smaller than cells from the intermediate or superficial squamous layers; they tend to have a rather large nucleus, surrounded by a dense, sometimes highly vacuolated peculiar cytoplasm. These cells originate in the basal layers and resemble Graham's third type tumor cells. Most of these errors are seen in peptic esophagitis but they may occur in patients with achalasia and esophagitis secondary to stasis (Gephart and Graham, 1959). These cells may disappear from the smears after intensive therapy of esophagitis (Raskin et al., 1959).

Atypical cells may also exfoliate in cases of primary ulcer of the esophagus. According to Rubin (1961), young fibroblasts originating in granulation tissue may be confused with tumor cells. Repeated cytologic studies are necessary especially if the diagnosis of cancer is based on a scarce number of cells. Antacid therapy should be administered for several days before the second examination.

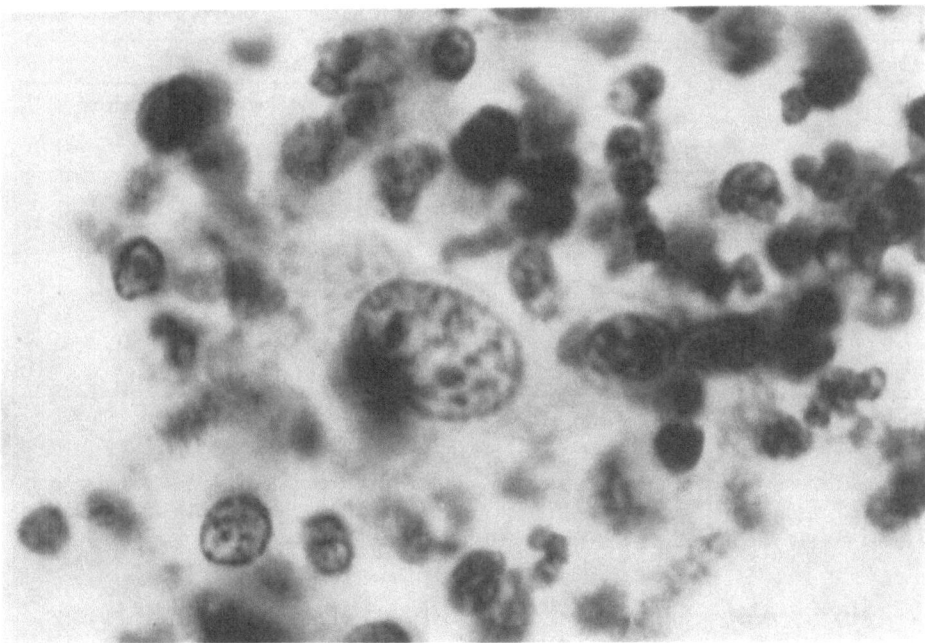

Fig. 133. Chronic esophagitis. A large nucleus showing two nucleoli. A fragmented nuclear membrane as well as an irregular distribution of the chromatin can be seen in the middle of the picture (false positive diagnosis of tumor). ($\times 950$)

In smears of inflammatory conditions of the esophagus, large numbers of polymorphonuclear leucocytes may sometimes be observed as inclusions inside epithelial cells. Their finding, however, does not preclude the presence of a tumor, since they may also be prominent in cases of malignant ulceration.

False diagnoses of cancer are likely to be made in vitamin B_{12} or folic acid deficiencies (untreated pernicious anemia, folic acid antagonist therapy, megalo-blastic anemia of pregnancy and other ill-defined nutritional deficiencies). Such cells are most readily recognized by their size, the typical folded appearance of their nuclear membrane, the small chromatin aggregates standing out on a relatively empty nuclear background (MASSEY and RUBIN, 1954) and by their normal nuclear cytoplasmic ratio.

Some degenerating benign epithelial cells may show nuclear and cytoplasmic characteristics which resemble those of tumor cells (fragmentation of the nuclear membrane, cytoplasmic vacuoles, etc.). Diagnostic errors decrease with the increasing experience of the cytologic laboratory and can be kept at an acceptable limit. In PAPANICOLAOU's laboratory, JOHNSON et al. (1955) reported false positive diagnoses of tumor in 2.2 percent of their cases. RASKIN et al. (1959) made two erroneous diagnoses among 85 patients in whom a benign lesion could be demon-strated. KIRSNER et al. (1966) reported 3 percent of errors in patients with esophagitis and BRANDBORG and WENGER (1968) made 2 false diagnoses of cancer among 63 patients with benign conditions of the esophagus. In our labora-tory, 3.8 percent of false positive results among 52 patients with achalasia, peptic esophagitis or primary ulcer of the esophagus have been reported (CABRE-FIOL et al., 1969). In one of our patients a diagnosis of carcinoma was made

Table 5. Comparision of cytology with endoscopic biopsy in the diagnosis of esophageal cancer

Author	Number of cases with carcinoma	Correct diagnosis	
		cytologic diagnosis %	positive biopsy %
JOHNSON et al., 1955	148	69.6	78.0
DEE and HANSEN, 1963	16	81.0	68.6
HENNING et al., 1964	88	79.5	83.0
PROLLA et al., 1965	64	87.5	90.9
LANCE and GROISSIER, 1965	21	68.0	80.9
COHEN and FLOWERS, 1969	34	94.0	64.7

on the basis of esophageal cytology; the esophagoscopic biopsy was also considered malignant by the pathologist; operation, however, revealed esophagitis, presumably secondary to agranulocytosis (Fig. 133).

10. Cytology Compared with Other Diagnostic Techniques

Comparative studies between cytology and other diagnostic techniques are seldom published in the literature. Several authors have reported cases in which a cytologic diagnosis of cancer was made while endoscopy had been negative or inconclusive. These observations indicate that both techniques are complementary (MESSELT, 1952; DEE and HANSSEN, 1963; HUMPHREYS et al., 1968; LUKASH and JOHNSON, 1969). Some of these observations are shown in Table 5. As a whole, cytology may add between 10 and 20 percent of positive diagnoses to those obtained by radiology and endoscopy. It is particularly useful when esophagoscopic biopsy is difficult, due to marked obstruction of the esophageal lumen or to the intramural localization of the tumor (PALMER, 1955).

11. Fluorescent Techniques in Esophageal Cytology

In an effort to obtain a rapid diagnosis of cancer without the help of highly trained personnel, several authors have tried to utilize the property of tumor cells to store fluorescent substances (Atabrine, Acridine-orange, etc.). Thus HENNING and WITTE (1968) have shown that gastric and esophageal tumor cells exhibit a marked cytoplasmic fluorescence when Atabrine is administered prior to the cytologic procedure. The cytoplasm of malignant cells shows a series of rather coarse yellowish granules under the fluorescence microscope which are

Table 6. Results of intravital fluorescence with Atabrine or Acranil in benign and malignant diseases of the esophagus (HENNING and WITTE, 1968)

Diagnosis	Number of cases	Results of fluorescence		
		positive	dubious	negative
Malignant tumors	82	56 (68%)	12	14
Benign diseases	25	2 (8%)	3	20

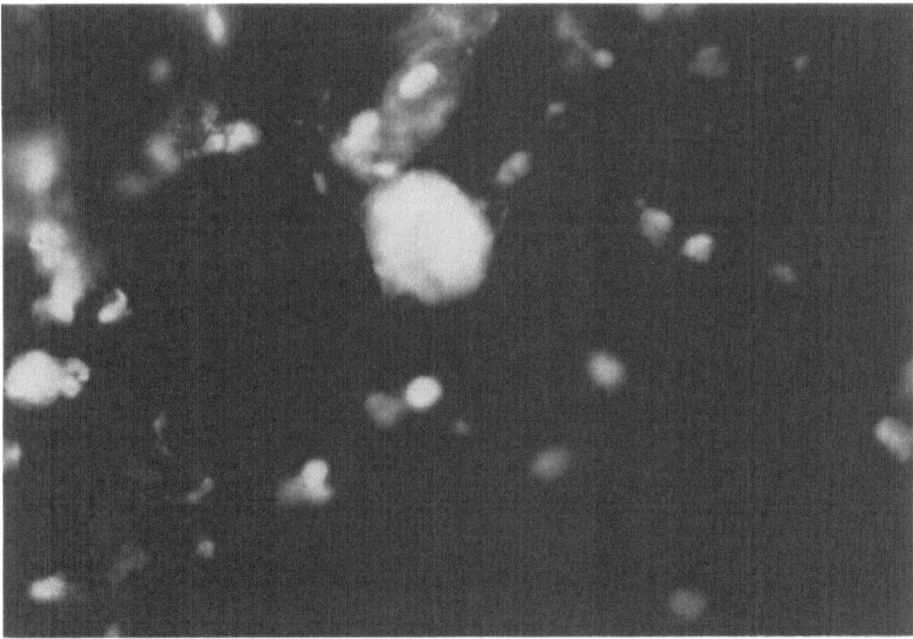

Fig. 134. Fluorescence cytology with Acridine-orange. In the middle of the picture an esoph-ageal tumor cell can be seen, showing bright fluorescence of the nucleus. Dart and Turner method. (×250)

rarely seen in benign cells (Table 6). Similar results have been reported by BASTOS and MADEIRA (1964) who have demonstrated that Atabrine forms a complex with cytoplasmic ribonucleic acid.

In a pilot study done on 30 patients (VILARDELL, 1962) using the Acridine-orange fluorescence technique of BERTALANFFY et al. (1956), a correct diagnosis of cancer was made in all five cases of esophageal tumor; the remaining 25 benign cases were correctly diagnosed with the ordinary Papanicolaou stain, while 3 false positive results were obtained with the fluorescence technique (Fig. 134). Similar experiences in gastric cytology (VILARDELL, 1964) suggest that fluores-cence methods do not have consistent advantages over the routine Papanicolaou technique, due to the considerable number of false positive results (excessive fluorescence of atypical cells) and to the necessity of reexamining with the Papa-nicolaou stain all the inconclusive cases. In spite of its potential value, more studies are needed to define clearly the real usefulness of fluorescent techniques in esophageal cytology.

12. Cytology in Benign Conditions of the Esophagus

Marked anomalies of epithelial cells of the oral cavity and the esophagus are often seen in patients with pernicious anemia. GRAHAM and RHEAULT (1954) reported an increase in the size of both the nucleus and the cytoplasm of esoph-ageal cells in 20 cases of pernicious anemia. In some instances cytoplasms measured as much as 72 μ in diameter. These observations were confirmed by MASSEY and RUBIN (1954), by MASSEY and KLAYMAN (1955), by RASKIN et al.

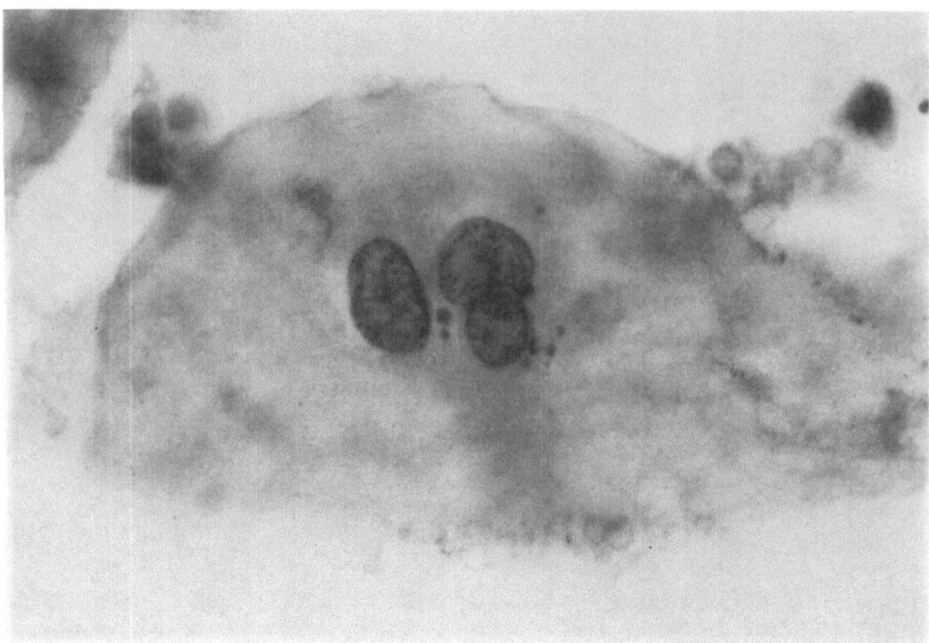

Fig. 135. Giant cells with multiple nuclei of normal characteristics. These cells are commonly observed in smears from patients with pernicious anemia and also after roentgen therapy. (× 450)

(1961) and by BRANDBORG et al. (1961). These cells appear not only in pernicious anemia but also in cases with various vitamin deficiencies (Fig. 135). They may disappear after therapy with vitamin B_{12} (RASKIN et al., 1961) or with folic acid (RUBIN, 1961). In some instances these cells may feature multiple nuclei or an increase in nuclear chromatin which may mimic malignancy. A differential trait which is of great value in our experience is the concomitant increase of the size of the cytoplasm in these atypical cells, resulting in a normal nuclear-cytoplasmic ratio (Fig. 135).

13. Effects of Roentgen Therapy on Esophageal Cells

The effects of roentgen therapy on esophageal epithelium are similar to those observed in vaginal cytology, which have been extensively investigated by GRAHAM (1963). GOLDGRABER (1956), performed serial cytologic studies in two cases of esophageal cancer treated by radiation: he observed that cells became very large, and that nuclei appeared swollen, featuring small vacuoles and scarce chromatin granules which were irregularly distributed in the nuclear background; cytoplasms were also vacuolated, exhibiting inclusions of neutrophiles, red cells or fine filaments. These cellular changes have also been described by GEPHART and GRAHAM (1959), by KOSS (1968) and by CABRE-FIOL et al. (1970) (Fig. 136). According to GOLDGRABER (1956), effects of roentgen therapy persist for 5 to 6 weeks and then disappear gradually; about 25 percent of exfoliated cells in the two cases showed some of these abnormalities after two months.

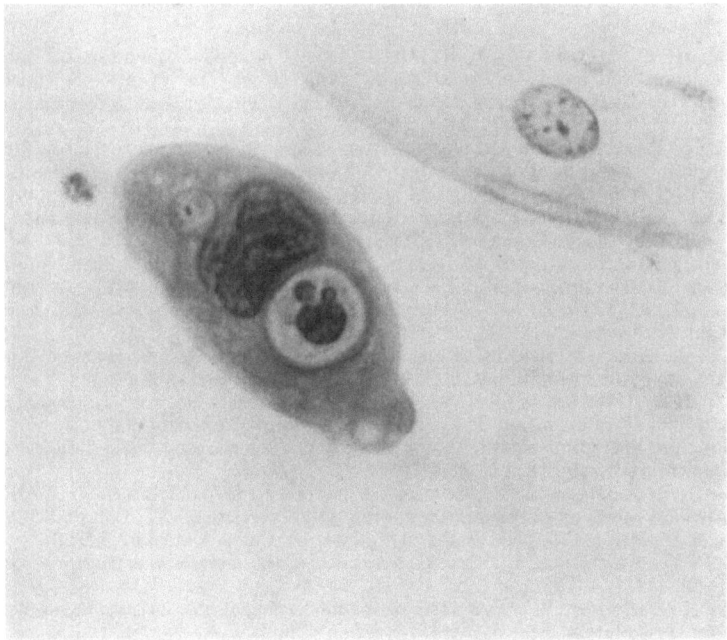

Fig. 136. Radiation therapy effect. A large cell with red cell and leukocyte inclusions. The nucleus is very large in size; it appears creased and shows little chromatin. (×950)

Attempts have been made by GRAHAM and GRAHAM (1953) to evaluate the percentage of benign cells showing radiation effects as an index of sensitivity to roentgen therapy in vaginal cytology. Similar studies by GEPHART and GRAHAM (1959) in esophageal cytology have yielded rather disappointing results. Esophageal carcinoma does not seem to be very sensitive to irradiation, and malignant cells may persist in smears in spite of clinical improvement (Koss, 1968). GRAHAM (1963) examined a group of patients submitted to roentgen therapy for esophageal cancer and found only one case with a positive sensitivity response (more than 10 percent of cells with cytoplasmic vacuoles). The number of positive responses is much greater in vaginal cytology. These cytological differences may explain in part the limited success of roentgen therapy in esophageal tumors.

14. Cytology in the Early Diagnosis of Esophageal Cancer

Unfortunately in most cases cytology only confirms the presence of a tumor which has already been diagnosed clinically or by other examinations. In spite of several papers reporting the finding of small tumors primarily diagnosed by cytology (IMBRIGLIA and LOPUSNIAK, 1949; RUBIN, 1961; SCHADE, 1964) it does not seem possible at present to establish systematic screening programs for cancer of the esophagus as they are performed in gynecologic clinics. The incidence of esophageal cancer does not justify the time and expense involved in such a program, in spite of the fact that the true aim of cytology is to discover these early tumors in the asymptomatic patient.

References

ANDERSEN, H. A., McDONALD, J. R., OLSEN, M.: Cytological diagnosis of carcinoma of the esophagus and cardia of the stomach. Proc. Mayo Clin. **24**, 245–253 (1949).

AYRE, J. E., OREN, B. G.: A new rapid method for stomach-cancer diagnosis: the gastric brush. Cancer (Philad.) **6**, 1177–1181 (1953).

BASTOS, A. L., MADEIRA, F. J.: Intravital fluorescence in oesophageal, gastric and serous-effusion exfoliated cells. Port. Acta biol. A **8**, 187–194 (1964).

BEALE, L. S.: The microscope in clinical medicine, 3rd ed. London: Churchill 1867.

BERTALANFFY, L. V., MAISIN, F., MAISIN, M.: Use of Acridine-Orange fluorescence technique in exfoliative cytology. Science **124**, 1024–1025 (1956).

BRANDBORG, L. L., TANIGUCHI, L., RUBIN, C. E.: Exfoliative cytology in nonmalignant conditions of the upper intestinal tract. Acta cytol. (Philad.) **5**, 187–190 (1961).

BRANDBORG, L. L., WENGER, J.: Cytological examination in gastrointestinal tract disease. Med. Clin. N. Amer. **52**, 1315–1328 (1968).

BRITSCH, C. J.: A new method using a double lumen tube to obtain esophageal and gastric washings for cytological studies. Acta cytol. (Philad.) **6**, 332–334 (1962).

BRUINSMA, H. A.: Over het aandeel van de cytodiagnostiek in het vroeg aantonen van carcinomen in slokdarm en maag. Thesis Utrecht. Kemink en Zoon (1957).

CABRE-FIOL, V.: Procedimiento de obtención de musetras para citología endogastrica. Rev. esp. Enferm. Apar. dig. **12**, 186–189 (1953).

CABRE-FIOL, V., OLO GARCIA, R., SUBIAS FAGES, A., PUIG-DERRAJOLS, J. M.: Efectos de la irradiación antitumoral en citología exfoliativa esofágica. XI. Congreso Nacional de Patología Digestiva. Libro de Actas y Communicaciones. Barcelona (1970).

CABRE-FIOL, V., VILARDELL, F., OLO GARCIA, R.: Citodiagnâstico esofágitico. Acta ginec. (Madr.) **20**, 111–114 (1969).

COHEN, N. N., FLOWERS, W.: Diagnosis of stenosing lesions of the esophagus using brush cytology. Gastrointest. Endoscopy **15**, 213–215 (1969).

COMAN, D. R.: Decreased mutual adhesiveness, property of cells from squamous cell carcinomas. Cancer Res. **4**, 625–629 (1944).

DEBRAY, C., HOUSSET, P., MARTIN, E., MARCHE, CL., GARAT, J.-P.: Un nouveau procédé de cyto- et d'histo-diagnostic: l'aspiration par sonde râpe ou cyto-râpe. Arch. Mal. Appar. dig. **56**, 988–989 (1967).

DEE, A. L., HANSSEN, B.: An experience in the cytopathologic diagnosis of carcinoma of the esophagus. Acta cytol. (Philad.) **7**, 236–238 (1963).

GEPHART, T., GRAHAM, R. M.: The cellular detection of carcinoma of the esophagus. Surg. Gynec. Obstet. **108**, 75–82 (1959).

GHOSSEIN, N. A., BRITSCH, C. J.: A new method with a double lumen tube as a means of obtaining esophageal and gastric washings for cytologic studies. Amer. J. clin. Path. **37**, 279–281 (1962).

GIBBS, D. D.: Exfoliative cytology of the stomach. London: Butterworths 1968.

GOLDGRABER, M. B.: The response of esophageal cancer to irradiation: a serial cytologic study of two cases. Gastroenterology **30**, 618–624 (1956).

GRAHAM, R. M.: The cytologic diagnosis of cancer. Philadelphia-New York: Saunders 1963.

GRAHAM, R. M., GRAHAM, J. B.: A cellular index of sensitivity to ionizing radiation—the sensitization response. Cancer (Philad.) **6**, 215–223 (1953).

GRAHAM, R. M., RHEAULT, M. H.: Characteristic cellular changes in epithelial cells in pernicious anemia. J. Lab. clin. Med. **43**, 235–245 (1954).

HENNING, N., WITTE, S.: Über eine neue Methode zur Zytodiagnostik der Magenkrankheiten. Dtsch. méd. Wschr. **77**, 1–4 (1952).

HENNING, N. U., WITTE, S.: Atlas der gastroenterologischen Zytodiagnostik, 2. Aufl. Stuttgart: Georg Thieme 1968.

HENNING, N., WITTE, S., BRESSEL, D.: The cytologic diagnosis of tumors of the upper gastrointestinal tract (esophagus, stomach, duodenum). Acta cytol. (Philad.) **8**, 121–128 (1964).

HERSHENSON, L. M., LERCH, V., HERSHENSON, M. A.: Esophageal cytology by a gauze-sponge smear technique. J. Amer. med. Ass. **168**, 1871–1875 (1958).

HUGHES, H. E., DODDS, T. C.: Handbook of diagnostic cytology. Edinburgh-London: E. S. Livingstone 1968.

HUMPHREYS, E. A., WOLFF, R. A., MLECKO, L. M.: "Scrape" cytology of the esophagus and stomach. Gastrointest. Endoscopy **14**, 160–161 (1968).

IMBRIGLIA, J. E., LOPUSNIAK, M.: Cytologic examination of sediment from the esophagus in a case of intra-epidermal carcinoma of the esophagus. Gastroenterology **13**, 457–463 (1949).

JOHNSON, W. D., KOSS, L. G., PAPANICOLAOU, G. N., SEYBOLT, J. F.: Cytology of esophageal washings. Evaluation of 364 cases. Cancer (Philad.) 8, 951–957 (1955).

KIRSNER, J. B., TAEBEL, D. W., COCKERHAM, L.: The present status of gastrointestinal exfoliative cytology. Proceedings 3rd World Congress of Gastroenterology 1, 528–530 Tokyo (1966).

KLAYMAN, M. I.: The diagnosis of esophageal carcinoma by exfoliative cytology, including two cases of cardiospasm associated with carcinoma of the esophagus. Ann. intern. Med. 43, 33–44 (1955).

KOSS, L. G.: Diagnostic cytology and its histopathologic bases, 2nd ed. Philadelphia: J. B. Lippincott Co. 1968.

LANCE, K. P., GROISSIER, V. W.: Utility of cells exfoliated into the esophagoscope as an aid in the diagnosis of esophageal carcinoma. Amer. J. dig. Dis. 10, 1–12 (1965).

LEBERT, H.: Traité pratique des maladies cancéreuses et des affections curables confondues avec le cancer. Paris: J. B. Baillière 1851.

LUKASH, W. M., JOHNSON, R. B.: Importance of esophageal exfoliative cytology in achalasia. Ann. intern. Med. 70, 420–421 (1969).

MACDONALD, W. C., BRANDBORG, L. L., TANIGUCHI, L., RUBIN, C. E.: Esophageal exfoliative cytology. A neglected procedure. Ann. intern. Med. 59, 332–337 (1963).

MARINI, G.: Über die Diagnose des Magenkarzinoms auf Grund der cytologischen Untersuchungen des Stuhlwassers. Arch. Verdau.-Kr. 15, 251–259 (1909).

MASSEY, B. W., KLAYMAN, M. I.: Observations on epithelial cells exfoliated from the upper gastrointestinal tract of patients with pernicious anemia, simple achlorhydria and carcinoma of the esophagus and stomach. Amer. J. med. Sci. 230, 506–514 (1955).

MASSEY, B. W., RUBIN, C. E.: The stomach in pernicious anemia: a cytologic study. Amer. J. med. Sci. 227, 481–492 (1954).

MESSELT, O. T.: Cytological diagnosis of esophagus cancer. Acta chir. scand. 103, 440–441 (1952).

MILANESI, I., TOSI, C.: La citodiagnosi nelle neoplasie maligne esofagee. Ann. Lar. Ot. Rin. Far. 44, 716–724 (1965).

MLECKO, L. M.: Hematemesis associated with "scrape" cytology. Gastrointest. Endoscopy 15, 110–111 (1968).

NIEBURGS, H. E.: Cytologic technics for office and clinic. New York: Grune & Stratton 1956.

NIEBURGS, H. E.: Diagnostic cell pathology in tissue and smears. New York-London: Grune & Stratton 1967.

PALMER, E. D.: Difficulties in diagnosis of esophageal carcinoma: failure of transesophagoscopic biopsy. Amer. J. dig. Dis. 22, 65–67 (1955).

PAPANICOLAOU, G. N.: A new procedure for staining vaginal smears. Science 95, 438–439 (1942).

PAPANICOLAOU, G. N.: Atlas of exfoliative cytology. Cambridge, Mass.: Harvard University Press 1954.

PAPANICOLAOU, G. N., TRAUT, H. G.: Diagnosis of uterine cancer by the vaginal smear. New York: The Commonwealth Fund 1943.

PROLLA, J. C., TAEBEL, D. W., KIRSNER, J. B.: Current status of exfoliative cytology in diagnosis of malignant neoplasms of esophagus. Surg. Gynec. Obstet. 121, 743–752 (1965).

RASKIN, H. F., KIRSNER, J. B., PALMER, W. L.: Role of exfoliative cytology in the diagnosis of cancer of the digestive tract. J. Amer. med. Ass. 169, 789–791 (1959).

RASKIN, H. F., PALMER, W. L., KIRSNER, J. B.: Benign and malignant exfoliated gastrointestinal mucosal cells. Arch. intern. Med. 107, 872–884 (1961).

RUBIN, C. E.: Exfoliative cytology of the esophagus. Exfoliative cytology. New York: The American Cancer Society Inc. 1961.

SANZ, C. J., REMENIUK, E.: Cytology as an aid to endocopy. Gastrointest. Endoscopy 15, 114–117 (1968).

SASSON, L.: Unfavorable experiences with the Ayre rotating stomach brush. Amer. J. dig. Dis. 9, 398–405 (1964).

SCHADE, R. O. K.: Gastric cytology. London: Edward Arnold Ltd. 1960.

SCHADE, R. O. K.: The cytologic diagnosis of tumors of the upper gastrointestinal tract (Discussion). Acta cytol. (Philad.) 8, 129–130 (1964).

SCHICKENDANTZ, G. A., COTELLA, P. J., DIAZ WALKER, N. G., CAPIZZANO, H.: Biopsia endoscópica y citologia exfoliativa en el diagnóstico de certeza del cancer del esófago. Pren. méd. argent. 51, 1575–1580 (1964).

SCHICKENDANTZ, G. A., SABAGH, R., RAMOS MEJIA, M. M., TERZANO, G.: Cytologic-histopathologic correlation in esophageal cancer. Acta cytol. (Philad.) 11, 64–67 (1967).

Taylor, R. G. W.: Practical cytology. London-New York: Academic Press 1967.

Turnbull, A. D. M., Goodner, J. T.: Primary adenocarcinoma of the esophagus. Cancer (Philad.) **22**, 915–918 (1968).

Vilardell, F.: A study of atypical cells in gastrointestinal cytology. Thesis. Philadelphia: University of Pennsylvania 1962.

Vilardell, F.: Citología por fluorescencia en el cancer digestivo. Pren. méd. argent. Suppl. 203–208 (1964).

Vilardell, F.: Re-evaluation of cytologic methods in the diagnosis of malignant lesions of the stomach. In: Progress in gastroenterology, vol. I, G. B. Jerzy Glass ed. New York-London: Grune & Stratton 1968.

Youngs, L. A., Nielsen, O. F.: Application of the membrane-filter technique to esophageal and gastric cytology. Milit. Med. **130**, 887–889 (1965).

The Manometric Examination of the Esophagus

W. Pelemans and E. C. Texter, Jr.

With 6 Figures

1. The Balloon-Kymographic Method

Hippocrates [quoted by Sanchez et al. (1953)] was probably the first to perform experimental studies of the esophagus, but it was 1747 before Fredericus Bernardus Albinus [quoted by Eykman (1903)] showed that all swallowed substances are transported into the stomach via the esophagus. The actual study of esophageal motility begins with the experiments of Arloing (1877) and especially of Kronecker and Meltzer (1883). The latter used a balloon kymographic system which was taken over, with minor modifications, by many investigators (Cannon and Washburn, 1912; Carlson, 1916; Payne and Poulton, 1927; Abbott and Pendergrass, 1936; Zeller and Burget, 1937; Ingelfinger and Abbott, 1940; Kramer and Ingelfinger, 1949; Duwez, 1950; Foulk et al., 1954).

Basically the balloon kymographic method consists of recording the volume changes that occur in a water manometer which is connected to an intraluminal balloon. This system has many inherent disadvantages (Quigley and Brody, 1950, 1952; Brody and Quigley, 1951; Code et al., 1952; Lorber and Shay, 1954; Texter et al., 1957). The balloon must be expanded if changes in its volume are to be recorded; this distension provides a local stimulus for motor activity. This method does not measure the true intraluminal pressure changes but the volume changes of a balloon, which themselves are determined by the elasticity of the balloon as well as by the different forces acting on its surface (intraluminal pressures and tension of the esophageal wall). The volume changes which occur in a balloon under the influence of increasing external pressures are not linear (Shepherd and Diamant, 1972). In addition, the range of pressures that can be measured with a balloon is limited; once the balloon has been emptied it does no longer register additional pressure. Finally a large balloon which is anchored at one site constitutes an obstruction to the swallowed liquid or bolus.

These drawbacks can be partially overcome by using miniature balloons, which can be mounted over a microtransducer or directly fixed to the distal end of an open-tipped catheter. These microballoons are used in order to allow, even in the sphincter, a sufficiently large volume displacement to activate the pressure-sensitive device (Code and Schlegel, 1958). A modification of this technique is the microballoon made of polyester, a non-distendable material, which has the advantage of preserving the original shape and diameter of the balloon (Waldeck, 1972). With this device it is possible to perform fast and reproducible pull-through measurements in the sphincter.

2. Intraluminal Pressure Measurements

The study of esophageal motility advanced considerably once devices to record intraluminal pressure changes accurately became available. Quigley and Brody and their co-workers suggested the use of open-tipped catheters instead of balloons (Quigley et al., 1950; Brody and Quigley, 1951; Quigley and Brody, 1952; Texter et al., 1957). These catheters do not obstruct the esophagus and cause but slight local stimulation. The elasticity of these catheters, made of polyethylene or polyvinyl, is minimal. They are filled with water, which serves as a pressure conductor between the esophageal cavity and the external

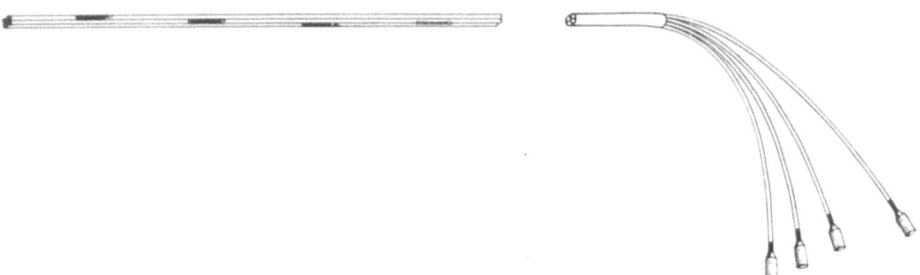

Fig. 137. 4-catheter probe, with side openings, used for esophageal motility studies. Distally from the side openings, the catheters are sealed by a metal plug. Polyethylene catheters can be held together by means of an outer silastic sheath. Polyvinyl catheters can be cemented

pressure-sensitive device. At its distal end the catheter has a terminal or lateral opening (Fig. 137); at its proximal end it is connected to an optical or electrical (strain-gauge or capacitance) manometer. Most currently used manometers are of the strain-gauge type and have a very small volume-pressure coefficient. An intraluminal change causes a slight displacement in the fluid column of the catheter, which is transduced to an electrical signal and can be registered by a recording apparatus after appropriate amplification.

The transmission of pressure via a fluid column is the weak link in this registration technique. Air bubbles in the catheter interfere with accurate measurements due to damping; inaccuracies are also caused by a catheter which is not filled to the very tip. To obviate these drawbacks the catheters are flushed intermittently or, nowadays, perfused continuously. As the detecting unit is connected to the pressure transducer via a fluid column a difference of level between the two will result in an (artificial) hydrostatic pressure. This can be greatly reduced by placing the patient in a horizontal position and the external transducer at the level of the esophagus. With the patient in a horizontal position it is also possible to use the pressure in the gastric fundus as a reference and to express changes in terms of this reference; if the hydrostatic pressure remains unchanged during the entire experiment, this way of proceeding does not influence the results. The volume of the fluid column, and the diameter, the length and the elasticity of the catheter are the main factors influencing the frequency response and the transfer characteristics of the system. Modern electromanometers have a very small volume-pressure coefficient and have reached such a degree of perfection that the frequency response of the catheter-manometer system depends almost exclusively on the characteristics of the catheter. The longer the catheter and the smaller its diameter the poorer the frequency response will be.

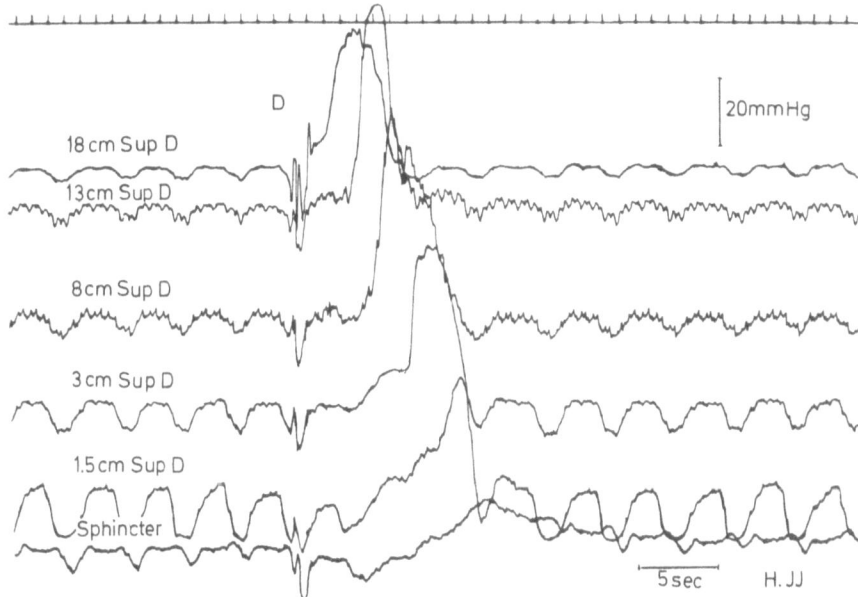

Fig. 138. Normal peristaltic wave and normal deglutition complexes. The pressures are registered simultaneously in the gastroesophageal sphincter and at 5 different levels above it. The "initial negative deflection" is visible on all the tracings. A "first positive wave" can be recognized in the upper segment (18 cm sup. D). "Second positive waves" occur in the lower esophagus (8–3 and 1.5 cm sup. D). The "terminal pressure peak" progresses in a peristaltic fashion along the esophagus. Sphincter relaxation and contraction are shown in the lower tracing. D: deglutition signal; cm sup. D: number of centimeters above P.I.P.

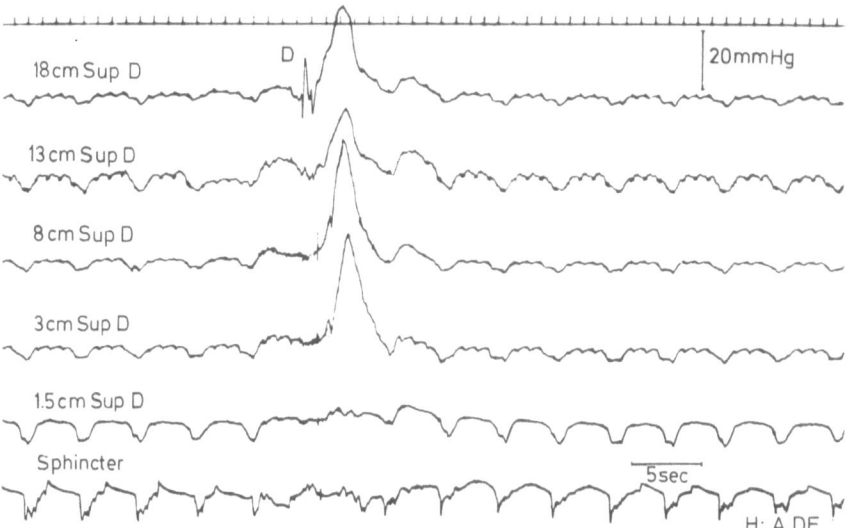

Fig. 139. Simultaneous pressure waves, appearing shortly after deglutition in a patient with achalasia. D: deglutition signal; cm sup. D: number of centimeters above P.I.P.

The small diameter of the catheters used for esophageal manometry makes it possible to combine them in a single probe and hence to measure simultaneously the pressures at different levels in the esophagus. Usually a distinction is made between the "resting pressure" and the pressure changes elicited by deglutition or occurring "spontaneously". By using a multiple catheter system the sequential, simultaneous or repetitive nature of a pressure wave can be evaluated (Figs. 138, 139). To measure the pressure profile of a sphincter the catheter can be pulled stepwise through the sphincteric segment; at each 0.5 to 1 cm interval the pressures are measured during several respiratory cycles (slow pull-through). It is also possible to withdraw the catheters rapidly and continuously through the sphincter while the respiration is held up for a moment (fast pull-through); if a perfused catheter system is used, the rate of perfusion should then be increased considerably.

3. Interpretation of Intraluminal Pressure Measurements

It soon became apparent that the different catheters of a probe pulled through the gastroesophageal sphincter often record different pressure profiles (Code and Schlegel, 1958). It was suggested that the volume of water available to activate the pressure-sensitive device might be a limiting factor when the catheter is located in a sphincter. Therefore Code and Schlegel (1958) mounted a miniature balloon over their microtransducer or on top over an open-tip catheter. The miniature balloon served to assure that an ample volume of water for displacement was present.

Most authors who performed intraluminal pressure studies with the open-tip technique used very slow perfusion (a few millimeters per hour) or intermittent flushing of the catheters in order to keep the tip of the probe open, to prevent air bubbles from developing in the catheters and to keep them completely filled to the very tip. Pert et al. (1959) realized that such a procedure may influence the measured pressure. In a closed sphincter, where the lumen is obliterated, all the gas or liquid is squeezed out, so that there is no longer a medium on which pressure can be exerted. This sustained obliteration of the lumen interferes with reliable pressure recordings. The open tip of the catheter is sealed, which means that a constant volume of water is captured and can no longer be displaced in the catheter. Such a catheter cannot function as a pressure transmitter any more, but serves rather as a long, narrow balloon (Harris and Pope, 1966). To circumvent the problem, Pert et al. (1959) perfused the catheter at the slow but continuous rate of 3 ml/hour. The pressure in the catheter mounts until the plugging of the catheter yields. At that moment the perfused fluid can escape through the distal opening and the pressure will level off. For the same reasons, and also to obviate the inconsistencies of the intermittent flushing technique, the group of Cohen also began to perfuse the catheters but the perfusion was performed under a constant hydrostatic pressure (Cohen and Wolf, 1962; Cohen et al., 1964; Cohen, 1965; Heitmann et al., 1966; Sokol et al., 1966). A similar hydrostatic system was also used by Clark and Vane (1961) in their studies on the cardia of the cat.

4. The Perfused Catheter System

The experiments of Harris, Winans and Pope (Harris and Pope, 1964; 1966; Harris et al., 1966; Winans and Harris, 1967; Pope, 1967) constituted the definite break-through of the perfusion technique.

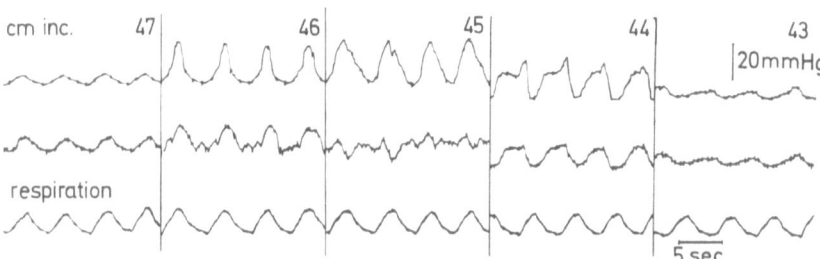

Fig. 140. Resting pressure profile through the gastroesophageal sphincter registered simultaneously with a catheter perfused at a rate of 0.6 ml/min (upper tracing) and with a non-perfused catheter (middle tracing). The recording side holes were at the same level. The recorded end-inspiratory pressure below the pressure inversion point is higher and the pressure inversion point itself is located more proximally when a perfused catheter is used

By means of pressure measurements with an open-tip catheter in the ana sphincter HARRIS and POPE (1964) were able to show that the recorded sphincter pressure is not a measurement of sphincter tone, but that it is directly related to the pressure to which the recording tip is last exposed before it enters the sphincter. Studies on an in vitro sphincter model showed that uninfused open-tip catheters underestimate sphincter force of closure whereas balloons of various size tend to overestimate the force (POPE, 1967). However, when microliter quantities of fluid were infused into an open-tip catheter via a side-arm the sphincter force of closure of this model could be measured accurately (Fig. 140). COHEN and HARRIS (1970) measured the force necessary to pull a teflon-ball with a diameter of 12 mm from the stomach into the esophagus and found a very good correlation with the yield pressure. Moreover, several studies have shown that the competence of the gastroesophageal sphincter correlates better with the yield pressure than with the resting pressure measured with uninfused catheters, although some overlapping remains (WANKLING et al., 1965; POPE, 1967; SKINNER and BOOTH, 1970; BENZ et al., 1972).

Schematically the experimental set-up can be described as follows. A number of catheters (usually three) with a lateral opening and sealed terminally, are assembled into one probe in such a way that the lateral openings are a few centimeters apart. Each catheter is connected with an electromanometer via a three-way stop-cock, to which the syringe of the infusion pump is attached via a short non-distendable catheter. The pump must be capable of delivering a constant flow in spite of considerable changes in intraluminal pressure (Fig. 141). Different authors use different perfusion rates, from 0.18 ml/min (POPE, 1967) to 1.2 ml/min (COHEN and HARRIS, 1970); some see to it that the speed of infusion does not influence the pressure in the catheter, when it is tested under atmospheric pressure.

Even with the perfusion technique there is considerable variation of results. Different groups of normal subjects yield different values; consecutive measurements on the same person, whether made over several days or during a single session may differ considerably and even different catheters of the same probe may register different results (POPE, 1967; WINANS and HARRIS, 1967; HADDAD, 1970; COHEN and HARRIS, 1970). Several explanations and hypotheses are possible. It has been established that the orientation of the lateral opening is responsible for some of the variations. According to KAYE and SHOWALTER (1971) dorsally oriented catheters register higher yield pressures than those oriented ventrally; according to WINANS (1972a) the highest pressures are registered

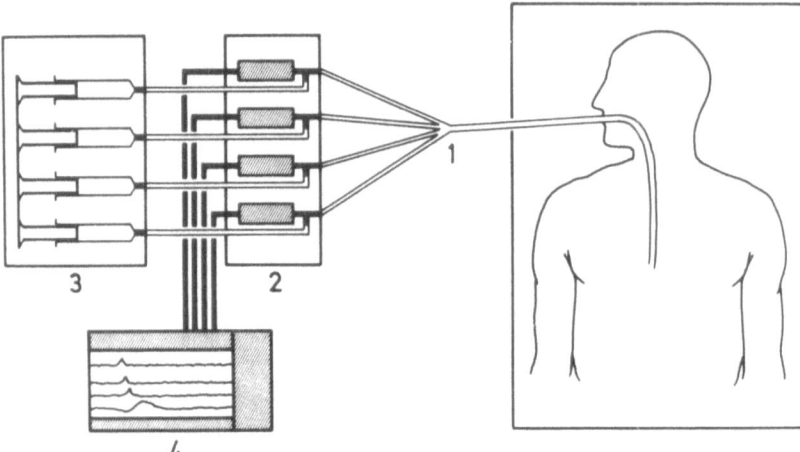

Fig. 141. Set-up for manometric measurements. *1* Probe with several catheters, to be swallowed by the subject. *2* Electro-manometers. *3* Pump for continuous perfusion. *4* Amplifiers and recording apparatus

in the left dorso-lateral zone. Furthermore, there is no uniformity in the techniques currently used (various diameters of the catheters and of the lateral openings and various perfusion rates) and in the way the results are expressed. The divergence is also partially due to differences among groups of patients studied. Finally it must be realized that the yield pressure of the gastroesophageal sphincter is influenced by hormonal and nervous factors. When a subject is studied on several occasions different sphincteric pressures may be found, but these pressures correlate fairly well with other measured parameters of sphincteric tone (pH-measurements and pull-through of a teflon ball through the sphincter) (HADDAD, 1970; COHEN and HARRIS, 1970).

The continuous perfusion technique can also be used to evaluate the force, i.e. the resistance to distension, of the upper esophageal sphincter. As this sphincter has a more or less oval shape, with its long axis oriented in a frontal plane, it was to be expected that the maximal yield pressure would be detected by the lateral opening of the catheter oriented in an anteroposterior plane (WINANS, 1972b). Inspiratory positive pressure waves are recorded in this sphincter with the perfusion technique (GOYAL et al., 1970). As electromyographic studies have shown that this is a very reactive sphincter and as the pressures registered in this sphincter by means of a continuous pull-through technique depend on the rate of infusion (RINALDO and LEVEY, 1968) the question may be raised to what extent the introduction of a perfused catheter in the sphincter elicits motor activity.

Attempts have been made to evaluate the squeeze of a contraction in the body of the esophagus by means of the perfusion technique. As the sealing of the catheter by the contraction is of short duration, the rate of perfusion must be sufficiently high to reach, in the short period of time determined by the duration of the contraction, the pressure required to break the sealing of the catheter. According to POPE (1970), a rate of 2.4 ml per minute is sufficient. However, HOLLIS and CASTELL (1972) tested ten rates of infusion, ranging from 1 to 23 ml per minute. From the hyperbolic curve, obtained by plotting the amplitude of the contraction against the infusion rate, it appears that the rate of infusion must be at least 15 ml per minute to achieve the near maximal pressure.

New techniques are being developed to improve or to compliment the current manometric methods. A force transducer has been built, which permits a better evaluation of the peristaltic force of an esophageal contraction (the "pull" of the contraction) (POPE and HORTON, 1972). Utilizing a mercury-in-Silastic strain gauge, to which a sphere has been attached, this transducer can be calibrated to measure value for force, work and power. Microtransducers of the differential transformer type (GAUER and GIENAPP, 1950) have been used for a long time in the study of esophageal motility (CODE and SCHLEGEL, 1958). More recently microtransducers of the strain-gauge type have been developed which are suitable for pressure measurements in the esophagus and allow simultaneous recording of the intraluminal pressure at different levels (Millhon-Crites, EMP-3, Motility Probe, Honeywell Model 31 esophageal probe) (Fig. 142). The experience with these new devices is still somewhat limited, but the first results seem promising and it appears likely that, because of their simplicity and accuracy, they will become the measuring device of choice (MILLHON et al., 1968; MILLHON, TEXTER, and HIGHTOWER, 1970; TEXTER et al., 1971 a, b, c; DODDS et al., 1972 a, b; HOLLIS and CASTELL, 1972). These probes eliminate the errors which can be made with external transducers, due to hydrostatic pressure. There is no fluid column and hence no damping. They also allow the separation of hydrostatic from squeeze pressure.

After a four-year experience with the motility probe (MILLHON, TEXTER, and HIGHTOWER, 1970), during which the system was compared with a conventional non-perfused system, it was concluded that the conventional system did not accurately record the amplitude of "dry swallows", an amplitude of 40 mm Hg being recorded by conventional manometry as compared with 350 mm Hg in the same subject with the probe at the same time. The probe also recorded detail not seen in the conventional tracings. No effect of damping was observed (TEXTER et al., 1971 a).

For fear that the non-perfused catheter system should be inadequate the non-perfused catheters were compared with perfused catheters and the EMP-3 probe. The internal diameter of the tubes was 0.034 inches and the perfusion rate was 40 mcl/sec as recommended by POPE (1970). These simultaneous comparative studies on more than 40 subjects and patients revealed that the probe was more accurate in assessing sphincter function. Likewise, perfusion in the body of the esophagus resulted in specious elevation of baseline pressure; perfusion at the rate recommended by POPE did not result in uniform amplitude deglutition complexes. When the tracings obtained by the EMP-3 probe were compared with tracings obtained by conventional manometry with or without perfusion, it was evident that the amplitude of the esophageal complexes was three to four times greater with the probe than those recorded with the conventional system. These differences appear to be related to the EMP-3 frequency response (over 20000 cps) and to the fact that both steady-state and squeeze pressures can be measured and differentiated simply (TEXTER et al., 1971 b, c).

Support for this view has come from the observations of HOLLIS and CASTELL (1972), who used the similarly designed Honeywell Intraesophageal Transducer Model No. 31. When comparing maximum pressure response by this probe and by a catheter system infused at a rate of 1 to 23 ml per minute, it was found that maximum amplitude was obtained with the maximum rate of infusion. They also found that the probe confirmed and recorded the same maximum amplitude as that obtained with the highest rate of infusion (i.e. 23 ml per minute)

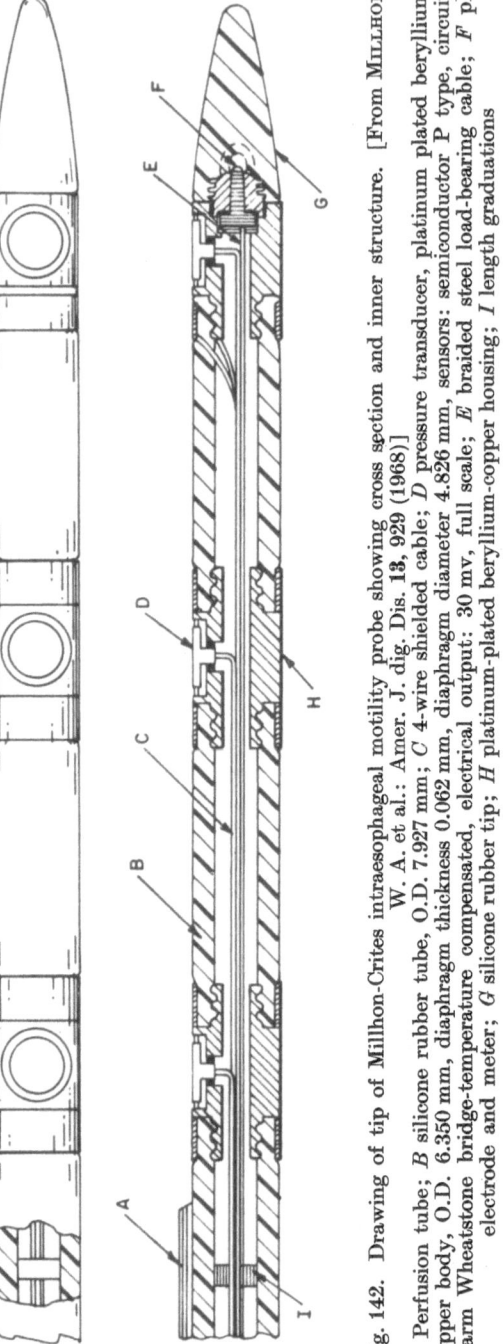

Fig. 142. Drawing of tip of Millhon-Crites intraesophageal motility probe showing cross section and inner structure. [From Millhon, W. A. et al.: Amer. J. dig. Dis. 13, 929 (1968)]

A Perfusion tube; B silicone rubber tube, O.D. 7.927 mm; C 4-wire shielded cable; D pressure transducer, platinum plated beryllium-copper body, O.D. 6.350 mm, diaphragm thickness 0.062 mm, diaphragm diameter 4.826 mm, sensors: semiconductor P type, circuit: 4-arm Wheatstone bridge-temperature compensated, electrical output: 30 mv, full scale; E braided steel load-bearing cable; F pH electrode and meter; G silicone rubber tip; H platinum-plated beryllium-copper housing; I length graduations

which is much greater than the rate used by Pope (1970). The calculated maximum response correlated very precisely with the values obtained with the direct transducer. Similar observations have been made by Dodds et al. (1972a) for pharyngeal peristalsis and esophageal peristalsis (1972b). The probe system yields information concerning the peristaltic force of esophageal contractions and also settles the controversy as to whether perfusion is necessary and what rate is the optimum one to use for various purposes.

5. The Technique of Intraluminal Pressure Measurements

In actual practice, the manometric technique to be used will depend on the purpose of the study. Therefore only those methods will be discussed which are most commonly used for diagnosis. The probe, consisting of a varying number of catheters, is introduced via the nose or the mouth into the gullet and pushed through until a number of catheter tips reach the stomach. The distance between the different recording openings and the number of catheters determines the length of the esophageal segment explored during a given swallow. The examination is performed with the patient in a supine position. The external transducers are placed at the level of the esophagus. The position of the tubes may be verified by fluoroscopy, but this is not usually necessary because the intraabdominal position can be identified by the inspiratory positive pressure swing.

Resting pressure profiles of the gastroesophageal junction are mostly obtained by withdrawing the pressure-detecting tubes by 0.5 cm increments from the stomach into the esophagus. At each interval a few breathing movements, which are representative for the resting pressure at this level, are registered. The patient is asked to breathe normally and refrain from swallowing. When the distal unit lies a few centimeters above the sphincter the pressure-detecting units are re-inserted into the stomach. The pull-through procedure is then repeated and at each recording site the patient is asked to swallow. The patient may take "dry swallows", consisting of only air and a small amount of saliva, or he may be given a few ml of water. The withdrawals are continued through the esophagus until one or more recording units have passed through the pharyngoesophageal sphincter. At each level the resting pressure is recorded, as well as the response to one or more deglutitions. The pharyngoesophageal sphincter can be explored in the same way as the gastroesophageal sphincter. A variant of this technique consists of measuring at each interval of a single pull-through both the resting pressure and the deglutitive response.

The resting pressure can be calculated and expressed in different ways. Some authors use the atmospheric pressure as a reference. The pressures in the lower sphincter and in the esophagus proper can also be expressed as pressure differences with the resting pressure in the gastric fundus. Similarly the resting pressure in the upper portion of the esophagus can be used a as reference to express the resting pressure of the pharyngoesophageal sphincter. As the resting pressure varies with respiration both the end-inspiratory and the end-expiratory pressure can be measured. The end-expiratory is the more stable value and it is therefore usually preferred. Others measure the mean pressures. The deglutitive pressure changes are measured in relation to the resting pressure in that particular segment before the swallow.

References

ABBOTT, W. O., PENDERGRASS, E. P.: Intubation studies of the human small intestine. V. The motor effects of single clinical doses of morphine sulphate in normal subjects. Amer. J. Roentgenol. **35**, 289–299 (1936).

ARLOING, F.: Application de la méthode graphique à l'étude du méchanisme de la déglutition. Thèse de Paris, 1877.

Benz, L. J., Hootkin, L. A., Margulies, S., Donner, M. W., Cauthorne, R. T., Hendricks, T. R.: A comparison of clinical measurements of gastroesophageal reflux. Gastroenterology **62**, 1–5 (1972).

Brody, D. A., Quigley, J. P.: Registration of digestive tract intralumen pressures. In: Methods in medical research, vol. 4, ed. Visscher, M. Chicago: Year Book Publishers 1951.

Cannon, W. B., Washburn, A. L.: An explanation of hunger. Amer. J. Physiol. **29**, 441 (1912).

Carlson, A. J.: The control of hunger in health and disease. Chicago: Chicago Univ. Press 1916.

Clark, C. G., Vane, J. R.: The cardiac sphincter in the cat. Gut **2**, 252–262 (1916).

Code, C. F., Hightower, N. C., Morlock, C. G.: Motility of the alimentary canal in man. Amer. J. Med. **13**, 328–351 (1952).

Code, C. F., Schlegel, J. F.: The pressure profile of the gastroesophageal sphincter in man: An improved method of detection. Proc. Mayo Clin. **33**, 406–414 (1958).

Cohen, B. R.: Cardiospasm in achalasia; demonstration of an abnormally elevated esophagogastric sphincter pressure with partial relaxation on swallowing. Gastroenterology **48**, 864 (1965).

Cohen, B. R., Lazar, H. P., Wolf, B. S., Kanowitz, H. D.: The clinical value of esophageal motility study. J. Amer. med. Ass. **187**, 819–825 (1964).

Cohen, B. R., Wolf, B. S.: Roentgen localization of the physiologically determined esophageal hiatus. Gastroenterology **43**, 43–50 (1962).

Cohen, S., Harris, L. D.: Lower esophageal sphincter pressure as an index of lower esophageal sphincter strength. Gastroenterology **58**, 157–162 (1970).

Dodds, W. J., Hogan, W. J., Reid, D. P., Stewart, E. T., Lineham, J. H., Stef, J. J., Arndorfer, R. C.: Variables affecting manometric recording of pressure amplitude during esophageal peristalsis. Gastroenterology **62**, 742 (1972b).

Dodds, W. J., Hogan, W. J., Reid, D. P., Stewart, E. T., Stef, J. J., Arndorfer, R. C.: Evaluation of pharyngeal peristalsis using a strain sensitive recording system. Gastroenterology **62**, 743 (1972a).

Duwez, Y.: La motricité de l'œsophage. Etude éxperimentale. Acta gastro-ent. belg. **13**, 961–968 (1950).

Eykman, P. H.: Der Schluckact. Pflügers Arch. ges. Physiol. **99**, 513 (1903).

Foulk, W. T., Code, C. F., Morlock, C. G., Bargen, J. A.: A study of the motility patterns and the basic rhythm in the duodenum and upper part of the jejunum of human beings. Gastroenterology **26**, 601–611 (1954).

Gauer, O. H., Gienapp, E.: A miniature pressure-recording device. Science **112**, 404–405 (1950).

Goyal, R. K., Sangree, M. H., Hersch, T., Spiro, H. M.: Pressure inversion point at the upper high pressure zone and its genesis. Gastroenterology **59**, 754–759 (1970).

Haddad, J. K.: Relation of gastroesophageal reflux to yield sphincter pressures. Gastroenterology **58**, 175–184 (1970).

Harris, L. D., Pope, C. E., II: "Squeeze" vs. resistance; an evaluation of the mechanism of sphincter competence. J. clin. Invest. **43**, 2272–2278 (1964).

Harris, L. D., Pope, C. E., II: The pressure inversion point: its genesis and reliability. Gastroenterology **51**, 641–648 (1966).

Harris, L. D., Winans, C. S., Pope, C. E., II: Determination of yield pressures: a method for measuring anal sphincter competence. Gastroenterology **50**, 754–760 (1966).

Heitmann, P., Wolf, B. S., Sokol, E. M., Cohen, B. R.: Simultaneous cineradiographic-manometric study of the distal esophagus: small hiatal hiernias and rings. Gastroenterology **50**, 737–753 (1966).

Hollis, J. B., Castell, D. O.: Amplitude of esophageal peristalsis as termined by rapid infusion. Gastroenterology **63**, 417–422 (1972).

Ingelfinger, F. J., Abbott, W. O.: Intubation studies of the human small intestine. XX. The diagnostic significance of motor disturbances. Amer. J. dig. Dis. **7**, 1–7 (1940).

Kaye, M. D., Showalter, J. P.: Manometric configuration of the lower esophageal sphincter in normal human subjects. Gastroenterology **61**, 213–223 (1971).

Kramer, P., Ingelfinger, F. J.: Motility of the human esophagus in control subjects and in patients with esophageal disorders. Amer. J. Med. **7**, 168–173 (1949).

Kronecker, H., Meltzer, S. J.: Der Schluckmechanismus, seine Erregung und seine Hemmung. Arch. Physiol. Suppl., **7**, 328–332 (1883).

Lorber, S. H., Shay, H.: Technical and physiological considerations in measuring gastrointestinal pressures in man. Gastroenterology **27**, 478–487 (1954).

Millhon, W. A., Hoffman, D. E., Jarvis, P., Cross, C. J., Millhon, J. S., Crites, N. A.: Preliminary report on Millhon-Crites intraesophageal motility probe. Amer. J. dig. Dis. **13**, 929–934 (1968).

MILLHON, W. A., TEXTER, E. C., HIGHTOWER, N. C.: Comparison of the Millhon-Crites esophageal motility probe with conventional open-tip manometry. Scientific exhibit 4th World Congress of Gastroenterology, Copenhagen, Denmark, July 12–18, 1970.

PAYNE, W. W., POULTON, E. P.: Experiments on visceral sensation. I. The relation of pain to activity in the human esophagus. J. Physiol. (Lond.) **63**, 217–241 (1927).

PERT, J. H., DAVIDSON, M., ALMY, T. T., SLEISENGER, M. H.: Esophageal catheterization studies. I. The mechanism of swallowing in normal subjects with particular reference to the vestibule (esophagogastric sphincter). J. clin. Invest. **38**, 397–406 (1950).

POPE, C. E., II: A dynamic test of sphincter strength: its application to the lower esophageal sphincter. Gastroenterology **52**, 779–786 (1967).

POPE, C. E., II: Effect of infusion on force of closure measurements in the human esophagus. Gastroenterology **58**, 616–624 (1970).

POPE, C. E., II, HORTON, P. F.: Intraluminal force transducer measurements of human esophageal peristalsis. Gut **13**, 464–470 (1972).

QUIGLEY, J. P., BRODY, D. A.: Intralumen pressures: gastrointestinal propulsion, gastric evacuation, pressure-wall-tension relationship. In: GLASER, R., Medical physics. Chicago: The Year Book Publishers 1950.

QUIGLEY, J. P., BRODY, D. A.: A physiologic and clinical consideration of the pressure developed in the digestive tract. Amer. J. Med. **13**, 73–81 (1952).

QUIGLEY, J. P., BRODY, D. A., KAY, B., LANDOLINA, W. C., McALISTER, J. H.: Accurate registration of intralumen pressures of the digestive tract by two new methods. Fed. Proc. **9**, 102 (1950).

RINALDO, J. A., LEVEY, J. F.: Correlation of several methods for recording esophageal sphincteral pressures. Amer. J. dig. Dis. **3**, 882–890 (1968).

SANCHEZ, G. C., KRAMER, P., INGELFINGER, F. J.: Motor mechanisms of the esophagus, particularly of the distal portion. Gastroenterology **25**, 321–332 (1953).

SHEPHERD, J. K., DIAMANT, N. E.: Mecholyl test: Comparison of balloon kymography and intraluminal pressure measurement. Gastroenterology **63**, 557–563 (1972).

SKINNER, D. B., BOOTH, D. J.: Assessment of distal esophageal function in patients with hiatal hernia and/or gastroesophageal reflux. Ann. Surg. **172**, 627–637 (1970).

SOKOL, E. M., HEITMANN, P., WOLF, B. S., COHEN, B. R.: Simultaneous cineradiographic and manometric study of the pharynx, hypopharynx, and cervical esophagus. Gastroenterology **51**, 960–974 (1966).

TEXTER, E. C., JR.: Motility comes of age. Amer. J. dig. Dis. **16**, 682–688 (1971 c).

TEXTER, E. C., JR., MARTIN, G. A., RAY, R. S., MILLHON, W. A.: Comparison of the EMP-3 esophageal motility probe with conventional open-tip manometry. Fed. Proc. **30**, 699 (1971 a).

TEXTER, E. C., JR., MARTIN, G. A., RAY, R. S., JR., MILLHON, W. A.: Comparison of the EMP-3 esophageal motility probe with perfused and non-perfused open-tip manometry. Rendic. R. Gastroenterol. **3**, 144 (1971 b).

TEXTER, E. C., SMITH, H. W., MOELLER, H. C., BARBORKA, C. J.: Intraluminal pressures from the upper gastrointestinal tract. I. Correlations with motor activity in normal subjects and patients with esophageal disorders. Gastroenterology **32**, 1013–1024 (1957).

WALDECK, F., JENNEWEIN, H. M., SIEWERT, R., NIEDER, B.: Manometric methods for functioned analysis of the lower esophageal sphincter (LES) and the act of swallowing. In: The function of the esophagus, ed. SØRENSEN, H. R., JEPSEN, O., PEDERSEN, S. A. Odense: Odense University Press 1973.

WANKLING, W. J., WARRIAN, W. G., LIND, J. F.: The gastroesophageal sphincter in hiatus hernia. Canad. J. Surg. 8, 61 (1965).

WINANS, C. S.: Manometric asymmetry of the lower esophageal high pressure zone. Gastroenterology **62**, 830 (1972 a).

WINANS, C. S.: The pharyngo-esophageal closure mechanism: a manometric study. Gastroenterology **63**, 768–777 (1972 b).

WINANS, C. S., HARRIS, L. D.: Quantitation of lower esophageal sphincter competence. Gastroenterology **52**, 773–778 (1967).

ZELLER, W., BURGET, G. E.: A study of the cardia. Amer. J. dig. Dis. **4**, 113–120 (1937).

pH Measurements

W. Pelemans and G. Vantrappen

With 2 Figures

1. pH Measurements in vitro

To measure the pH in vitro an indicator electrode and a reference electrode are put in the vessel containing the fluid to be examined. The glass of a glass electrode is sensitive to hydrogen ions. The potential difference between the glass and the solution is determined by the concentration of hydrogen ions in the solution when the other variables are constant. By definition the pH is equal to the negative logarithm of the concentration of the hydrogen ions; therefore the electromotive force of this electrode will depend on the pH. The reference electrode (e.g. calomel electrode) builds an electromotive force which is independent of the pH and which remains constant. Thus, the potential difference between these two electrodes is determined by the pH of the fluid. It can be measured electronically and the results can be directly read from the scale of a pH meter; if so desired they can be registered on an appropriate recording system. In order to achieve correct measurements all constituents of the solution must have the same potential. If electromechanical reasons prohibit the direct contact of the reference electrode with the solution the circuit can be closed with e.g. a salt bridge consisting of saturated KCl.

2. pH Measurements in vivo

A few changes must be made in this procedure to allow pH measurements in vivo. Small glass electrodes have been developed which can easily be introduced into the stomach and the esophagus through nose or mouth. The Beckman stomach electrode used in most studies has a diameter of 4 mm; the isolated cable connecting the electrode with the pH meter has a diameter of 2.5 mm. This electrode can be used with an ordinary pH meter. The reference electrode can be placed in different positions. HILL et al. (1961 b), HAMIT and RAYMOND (1962), OLDER et al. (1966) put the reference electrode in the mouth; BORGESKOV et al. (1966) on the back of the hand; TUTTLE et al. (1960), and KANTROWITZ et al. (1969) close the circuit by putting the patient's finger in a solution of saturated KCl containing the reference electrode. ANDERSSON and GROSSMAN (1965) connect the lumen of the esophagus with the reference electrode outside of the patient via a polyethylene catheter filled with agar and KCl. PATTRICK (1970) uses the Cambridge Instrument Company two lumen stomach electrode in which the reference electrode is placed close to the glass electrode in one unit. Theoretically it is more correct to bring the reference electrode in contact with the solution to be examined, i.e. the intraluminal content, directly or via a salt bridge. Indeed, by placing the reference electrode somewhere else a potential difference is measured which is actually the algebraic sum of the potential difference determined by the pH and the potential difference between the gut lumen and the place of the reference electrode. If the latter potential difference is constant it gives rise to a systemic error; if it is variable, such as the potential difference between gut lumen and skin, it gives rise to fluctuations in the measurements. ROVELSTAD et al. (1952) investigated how pH measurements are affected by placing the reference electrode on the skin. On the average their pH values were 0 to 0.4 pH too low in the esophagus, 0.1 to 0.5 too low in the duodenum and 0.1 to 0.6 too high in the stomach. According to their data the fluctuations of the potential difference between skin and gastrointestinal tract could give rise to a maximal error of about 1 pH unit. These relatively inaccurate measurements are not very important in the examination of the esophagus since here the mean point of interest is the occurrence or absence of reflux of gastric contents.

FEHR et al. (1966) used a pH sensitive telemetering capsule (Heidelberg capsule) in examining patients with hiatus hernia. This capsule, with a length of 20 mm and a diameter of 8 mm, contains a pH cell with an antimony electrode as indicator electrode and a silver-silver chloride electrode as reference electrode. In addition the capsule contains a transmitter whose signal varies in frequency according to the pH. This signal is received outside of the patient where it is amplified and registered on a recording system. This method offers few advantages for examination of the esophagus because it is necessary to mount the capsule on a catheter in order to locate it in the lower segment of the esophagus.

3. The Pull-through Technique

The subject is placed in dorsal decubitus and a pH electrode, sealed together with a pressure sensitive catheter, is withdrawn from the stomach into the esophagus. In normal subjects the intraesophageal pH reaches a value of 5 or more 2 cm above the pressure inversion point. This point can clearly be recognized on the pressure tracing by the sudden change in respiratory pressure swing from inspiratory positive to inspiratory negative (Fig. 143). The pH can change abruptly below or at the level of this pressure inversion point or it can mount more gradually beginning below the pressure inversion point. When the sensing device has passed the high pressure zone, a pH of more than 5 is registered throughout the esophagus (HILL et al., 1961b; MORGAN, 1962; BESANÇON et al., 1961; PICCONE et al., 1965; FEHR et al., 1966). In subjects with gastroesophageal reflux the pH profile of the esophagus is different. The change in pH does not

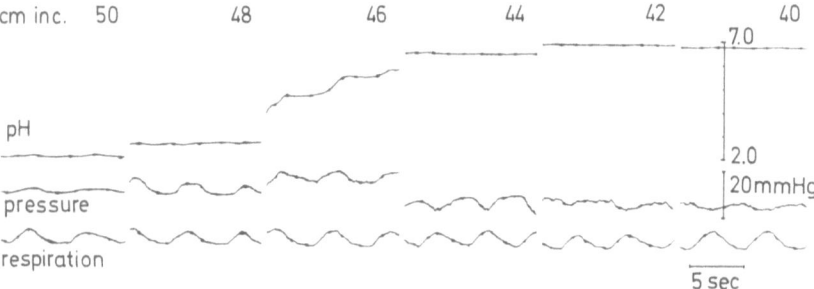

Fig. 143. Normal pH and resting pressure profile in the gastric fundus (50 cm inc.), the gastroesophageal sphincter (48–46 cm inc.) and the lower esophagus (44–42–40 cm inc.). The pH rises abruptly in the high pressure zone, and reaches a level outside the acid peptic range. (cm inc.: number of centimeters from the incisors)

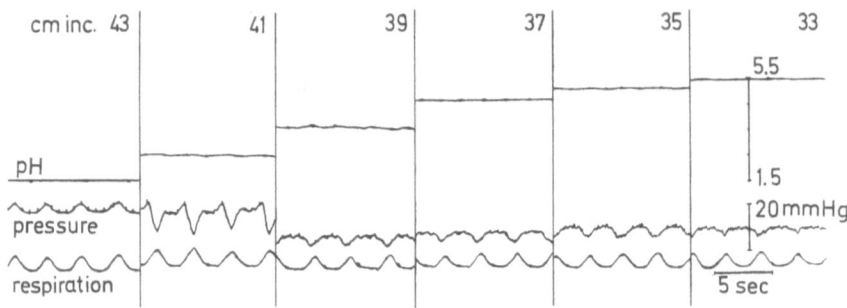

Fig. 144. pH and resting pressure profile through the gastroesophageal sphincter in a patient with severe reflux. In the lower esophagus, above the high pressure zone (39 cm inc.), pH values of 3.5 persist. More proximally there is a gradual rise of pH

take place in the high pressure zone but at varying levels in the esophagus itself (Fig. 144). Besançon et al. (1961) described two cases of reflux in which the pH of the esophagus was equal to the pH of the stomach almost as high as the pharyngoesophageal sphincter.

This pull-through technique does not appear to be sufficiently sensitive. Using this technique Besançon et al. (1961) could not find any anomaly in 12 out of 30 cases in whom reflux had been demonstrated radiologically.

Piccone et al. (1965), who had observed reflux in 50 patients, could demonstrate it by means of pH measurements in only 16 of them. The spontaneous reflux, demonstrated by the pull-through technique without any provoking maneuver except for laying down, has been considered as free reflux (Morgan, 1965). However, Piccone et al. (1965) could not find a free flow of gastric contents between stomach and esophagus in the majority of patients with such a "free reflux"; moreover all patients still had a high pressure zone, again suggesting that free acid reflux was not occurring. If during measurements using the pull-through technique the pH remains in the peptic range when the pH electrode has already passed the gastroesophageal sphincter, they use the term "long-duration reflux". According to these authors it is more likely that this reflux pattern is caused by a defective acid clearing function of the esophagus.

4. Fixed Location of pH Electrode

It is possible to demonstrate gastroesophageal reflux in a more sensitive way. The pH electrode is fixed at a constant level in the esophagus (e.g. 5 cm above the pressure inversion point) and different maneuvers are executed in order to provoke reflux. If during such maneuvers the pH drops, this demonstrates reflux at least up to the level of the electrode. In order to demonstrate reflux in this way the gastric content must be acid; if necessary the acid secretion must be stimulated in advance or HCl must be instilled in order to reach a sufficiently acid pH. Therefore, the pH of the gastric content must be tested before beginning the experiment. A whole series of maneuvers were proposed to induce reflux: the Mueller maneuver, the Valsalva maneuver, coughing, simulated singultus, inspiratory and expiratory sniffs, complete relaxation (Hill et al., 1961a, b), head-down position and abdominal compression (Fehr et al., 1966), straining at the end of both inspiration and expiration (WEBER and GREGG, 1959). According to BESANÇON et al. (1962) the procubitus position in Trendelenburg, combined with compression, yields about the same results as the decubitus dorsalis. KANTROWITZ et al. (1969) tried to provoke reflux by placing the patient in different positions (supine, left or right posterior oblique position, legs elevated). MORGAN (1962) studied the gastroesophageal pressure gradient in 10 normal persons under different circumstances. At the end of inspiration 9 out of 10 subjects had a higher pressure in stomach than in the esophagus (averaging +13.9 cm water). During deep inspiration this gradient reached an average level of 32.3 cm water. Expiratory strain against the closed glottis at full inspiration (the Valsalva maneuver) caused a higher pressure in the esophagus in two persons; the others had a positive gastroesophageal pressure gradient with a mean value of 22.2 cm water. The Mueller maneuver (inspiratory strain against the closed glottis at full expiration) caused the highest sustained gastroesophageal mean water. The maneuvers described above, therefore, provoke a variable positive gradient (49.2 cm water). A simulated singultus caused the highest gastroesophageal gradient (averaging 65.4 cm water) but this gradient was of short duration only. Voluntary coughs caused a gradient averaging 7.9 cm water, whereas inspiratory sniffs caused one of 46.3 cm and expiratory sniffs one of 17.8 cm gastroesophageal pressure gradient and are used to test the competence of the gastroesophageal junction in the prevention of reflux. It must be pointed out however, that the majority of these maneuvers cause an increase in intraabdominal pressure and not only in intragastric pressure. In normal persons i.e. in persons with an intraabdominal esophageal segment they will provoke an increase in pressure in the abdominal part of the esophagus as well as in the stomach.

Hence such maneuvers are not ideal for provoking reflux. In addition the normal closing mechanism of the gastroesophageal sphincter should not be interferred with during the experiment. If a catheter is left in place through the sphincter, e.g. to measure the gastric pressure at the same time, reflux along the catheter can occur when the gastroesophageal pressure gradient is increased (MORGAN, 1962).

5. Interpretation of Results

In normal persons this technique induces reflux only rarely. HILL et al. (1961b) found no reflux at all in normal persons. MORGAN (1962) attempted to provoke gastroesophageal reflux in 10 normal subjects but in his experiment a catheter was left in place through the gastroesophageal sphincter. Four out of 10 normal subjects had induced reflux. Of these 4 two were examined again without a catheter in the gastroesophageal sphincter and did not have reflux anymore. PICCONE et al. (1965) examined 18 asymptomatic patients. pH measurements established reflux in 3 of them; in all 3 radiological examination revealed a small sliding hernia though no radiologically demonstrable reflux.

FEHR et al. (1969) found in their 8 controls one positive test but this subject also had an abnormal pH profile in the sphincter. KANTROWITZ et al. (1969) examined 15 control patients and expressed their results semi-quantitatively. 8 subjects had no reflux, 7 had minimal reflux (i.e. one or two isolated episodes). Therefore, the occurrence of a few brief drops in pH has no clearly pathological significance.

The determination of the pH profile of the esophagus together with the ascertainment of induced reflux is a sensitive method to determine gastroesophageal reflux. Piccone et al. (1965) compared this esophageal pH test with other means of detecting gastroesophageal reflux. It appeared that the test was more sensitive than radiography, esophagoscopy and acid perfusion to obtain evidence of gastroesophageal reflux in symptomatic patients.

The method described thusfar detects acid gastroesophageal reflux and tests the competence of the gastroesophageal junction in the prevention of reflux. If reflux occurs, the duration of the pH drop is determined in part by the acid clearing function of the esophagus. The pH test gives information about the function of the gastroesophageal junction without giving information about the nature of the defect causing the reflux. Spontaneous reflux in a patient in dorsal decubitus points to a more important incompetence than induced reflux. A long-duration reflux pattern is mostly found in patients with more severe esophagitis complaints (Piccone et al., 1965). A short-duration reflux means that reflux occurs but the clearing function of the esophagus is effective. Thus the reflux pattern may yield information about the seriousness of gastroesophageal reflux. The intraluminal pH test is a very useful technique to objectively evaluate a hiatal hernia and the sphincter competence and to delineate the indications for surgical treatment more clearly; furthermore the test can also be used to evaluate the result of surgical treatment. A positive pH test proves the incompetence of the gastroesophageal junction and can be an indication of the existence of an unrecognized hiatal hernia. Whereas reflux is by no means diagnostic of esophagitis, it is an abnormal phenomenon; if there is no acid reflux with a pH within peptic range the diagnosis of peptic esophagitis is very unlikely. Finally, the demonstration of reflux may furnish helpful evidence in assigning an esophageal cause to thoracic pain. In 34 patients with thoracic pain of obscure origin tested by this method 17 were found to have reflux (Morgan and Hill, 1964).

6. The Acid Clearing Test

Gastroesophageal reflux is the most important factor in the pathogenesis of peptic esophagitis. On occasion everybody may have gastroesophageal reflux; Skinner and Camp (1967) showed that 40 percent of normal volunteers has occasional reflux; belching or singultus can provoke regurgitation even in normal persons (Morgan, 1962). The studies of Pattrick (1970) and Spencer (1968) confirm that the normal subjects also have reflux on occasion. When reflux occurs the esophagus is protected against peptic digestion by its ability to empty refluxed gastric contents. Already in 1961 Morgan found that reflux can provoke a strong esophageal contraction; he supposed that this clearing wave wipes the acid from the distal esophagus. On the other hand esophagitis may disturb the motor function of the esophagus (Besançon et al., 1962; Olsen et al., 1965; Donner et al., 1966). Booth et al. (1968) have developed a test to evaluate the acid clearing function of the distal esophagus. A pH probe and three polyvinyl tubes are introduced into the stomach. The tubes are sealed together so that their open tips are 5 cm apart and the pH probe is adjacent to the most distal opening. Under manometric control this assembly is positioned in such a way that the pH probe is situated 5 cm above the upper end of the sphincter. Via the proximal tube 15 ml of 0.1 N HCl is instilled so that the pH of the distal esophagus drops sharply. The subjects are instructed to swallow with intervals and the number of swallows required to raise the pH of the distal esophagus to pH 6.0 is observed. Once this level has been attained reflux-tests are done.

These studies indicate that in normal persons 4 to 10 swallows are needed to raise the pH of the distal esophagus to 6. The interval between two swallows did not influence the speed of the pH increase. In patients with non-specific complaints and with a hiatus hernia without reflux they obtained similar results. But the results were very different in patients with a symptomatic hiatus hernia. It took some of these 15 to 29 swallows to reach a pH of 6, others didn't even reach it after 30 swallows. This was due to different causes. In some patients the clearing effect of each swallow was minimal; in others some swallows had no clearing effect at all whereas other swallows resulted in only a small increase in pH. Two patients showed a marked increase in pH after some swallows but demonstrate reflux periodically with swallowing which lowered distal esophagus pH.

7. Protracted pH Measurements

Protracted pH measurements in humans indicate that normal persons also can have gastroesophageal reflux (SPENCER, 1968; PATTRICK, 1970). According to PATTRICK reflux is almost as common in people without symptoms of reflux as in those with symptoms during the day when the patient is standing or sitting. Sleeping on the left side does not make any clear difference. But those who suffer symptoms of reflux appear to reflux much more frequently when lying on the right side than those who do not suffer symptoms. SPENCER, however, found that during the day the period during which the esophageal pH is below 4 is longer in people with hiatus hernia. No control subjects showed any reflux at night, though this was observed in 8 of the 10 subjects with hernia.

References

ANDERSSON, S., GROSSMAN, M. I.: Profile of pH pressure and potential difference at gastro-duodenal junction in man. Gastroenterology **49**, 364–371 (1965).
BESANÇON, F., BAUJAT, J. P., DEBRAY, C.: Le reflux gastro-œsophagien: étude pH graphique et électromanographique. Sem. Hôp. Paris **38**, 1569–1576 (1962).
BOOTH, D. J., KEMMERER, W. T., SKINNER, D. B.: Acid clearing from the distal esophagus. Arch. Surg. **96**, 731–734 (1968).
BORGESKOV, S., LOCKWOOD, K., BERTELSEN, S., HASNER, E.: Simultaneous pressure and hydrogen ion measurements in the esophagus and stomach. Acta chir. scand, Suppl. **356** B, 105–112 (1966).
DONNER, M. W., SILBIGER, M. L., HOOKMAN, P., HENDRIX, T. R.: Acid barium swallows in the radiographic evaluation of clinical esophagitis. Radiology **87**, 220–225 (1966).
FEHR, H., STAVNEY, L. S., HAMILTON, T., SIRCUS, W., SMITH, A. N.: Hiatal hernia investigated by pH telemetering. Amer. J. dig. Dis. **11**, 747–752 (1966).
HAMIT, H. F., RAYMOND, B. A.: An intraluminal study of motility pressure and hydrogen ion concentration of the esophagus in various clinical conditions. Surg. Gynec. Obstet. **115**, 529–542 (1962).
HILL, L. D., CHAPMAN, K. W., MORGAN, E. H.: Objective evaluation of surgery for hiatus hernia and esophagitis. J. thorac. cardiovasc. Surg. **41**, 60–74 (1961a).
HILL, L. D., MORGAN, E. H., KELLOGG, H. B.: Experimentation as an aid in management of esophageal disorders. Amer. J. Surg. **102**, 240–253 (1961b).
KANTROWITZ, P. A., CORSON, J. G., FLEISCHLI, D. J., SKINNER, D. B.: Measurement of gastroesophageal reflux. Gastroenterology **56**, 666–674 (1969).
MORGAN, E. H.: Studies of intraluminal pressure and pH at the gastroesophageal junction. Quart. Bull. Northw. Univ. med. Sch. **36**, 258–267 (1962).
MORGAN, E. H., HILL, D.: Objective identification of chest pain of esophageal origin. J. Amer. med. Ass. **187**, 131–136 (1964).
OLDER, T. M., STABLER, V. E., AMENDOLA, F. H.: Determination of esophageal pH and intraluminal pressure. Technic and diagnostic applications. Ann. Surg. **163**, 621–628 (1966).

Olsen, A. M., Schlegel, J. F.: Motility disturbances caused by esophagitis. J. thorac. cardiovasc. Surg. 50, 607–612 (1965).

Pattrick, F. G.: Investigation of gastroesophageal reflux in various positions with a two-lumen pH electrode. Gut 11, 659–667 (1970).

Piccone, V. A., Gutelius, J. R., McCorriston, J. R.: A multiphased esophageal pH test for gastroesophageal reflux. Surgery 57, 638–646 (1965).

Rovelstad, R. A., Owen, C. A., Magath, T. B.: Factors influencing the continuous recording of in situ pH of gastric and duodenal contents. Gastroenterology 20, 609–624 (1952).

Skinner, D. B., Camp, F.: Measurement of gastroesophageal reflux in the evaluation of hiatus hernia and chest pain in fliers. Aerospace Med. 38, 846–850 (1967).

Spencer, J.: The use of prolonged pH recording in the diagnosis of gastroesophageal reflux. Brit. J. Surg. 56, 912–914 (1969).

Tuttle, S. G., Bettarello, A., Grossman, M. I.: Esophageal acid perfusion test and a gastroesophageal reflux test in patients with esophagitis. Gastroenterology 38, 861–872 (1960).

Weber, J. M., Gregg, L. A.: pH in situ of esophageal and gastric contents, with particular reference to hiatal hernia. Gastroenterology 37, 60–63 (1959).

PD Measurements

J. Janssens and G. Vantrappen

With 1 Figure

1. History

The existence of a potential difference (PD) across the wall of the gastro-intestinal tract was first described by Donne in 1834. The first PD measurements in humans were probably done by Schwyngedauw in 1928. This PD between mucosa and serosa was studied extensively in the stomach, especially in relation to acid secretion (Rehm, 1944, 1945, 1946, 1950, 1962), because it soon became apparent that the major portion of the gastric PD originates in the mucosa (Rehm, 1946). Goodman (1942) and many authors after him (Sawyer et al., 1949; Morton and Martin, 1953; Krasil'nikov and Fishzon-Ryss, 1964) have tried to use PD registrations in the human stomach as a diagnostic tool. According to their description a DC-component in the electrogastrogram seems to correspond to the PD across the gastric mucosa and seems to be disturbed in cases of ulcer or carcinoma. They also found an AC-component, which is probably the reflection of the slow-waves of the gastric muscle layer. The clinical results, however, were less convincing than at first hoped for. Spontaneous fluctuations of the tracings, even in normal subjects, and the interference of liquid junction potentials strongly reduce the diagnostic usefulness of the examination (Durbin, 1967).

Nevertheless, the interest in the PD measurements kept increasing among physiologists; Ussing et al. (1960) and Schultz and Zalusky (1964) pointed to the importance of the PD for the intestinal transport of electrolytes. Davenport et al. (1964) showed that the integrity of the gastric mucosa is essential for a normal PD and that PD measurements can be an indication of the presence of mucosal damage. The measurements were also done in the small intestine (Schultz and Zalusky, 1964) and in the colon (Soergel et al., 1966) especially in relation to the transport of electrolytes. Dennis et al. (1959) noticed that the PD values are not the same in different parts of the gastrointestinal tract. The PD changes rather abruptly at the pylorus (Rovelstad et al., 1952; Andersson and Grossman, 1965) and at the gastroesophageal junction (Greenwood et al., 1965; Helm et al., 1961, 1965); they were used by these authors to localize these structures in vivo.

2. The Origin of the Potential Difference

Across the wall of the entire gastrointestinal tract there exists a PD, the mucosal side being negative to the serosal. Table 7 gives the PD values of the gut in man (Geall et al., 1968, 1969); it shows that the PD reaches its highest value at the secreting part of the stomach. The mechanisms which are responsible for the origin and maintenance of the PD are not yet completely understood.

Table 7. Mean transmural potential differences in human G.I. tract (mucosal side)

Distal esophagus	$-11.8\,\mathrm{mV} \pm\ 2\quad\mathrm{mV}$
Stomach: corpus	$-40{,}2\,\mathrm{mV} \pm\ 2.1\,\mathrm{mV}$
antrum	$-22.8\,\mathrm{mV} \pm\ 3.1\,\mathrm{mV}$
Duodenum	$-\ 7.6\,\mathrm{mV} \pm\ 0.6\,\mathrm{mV}$
Colon: proximal	between $-16.5\,\mathrm{mV}$ and $48.5\,\mathrm{mV}$
sigmoid	$-28.1\,\mathrm{mV} \pm\ 1.6\,\mathrm{mV}$
rectum	$-16.1\,\mathrm{mV} \pm\ 1.2\,\mathrm{mV}$

After Geall et al., 1968; Geall et al., 1969.

One widely used technique to study these mechanisms measures the ion fluxes in the absence of an electrochemical gradient. Both the serosal and mucosal side of the preparation are put in an identical solution and the PD is kept at zero by an external source of current. The intensity of this short-circuit current, delivered by the outside source to keep the PD at zero, is a measure of those ion fluxes that are independent of any electrochemical gradient. Using this technique in studies on isolated frog stomach Hogben (1951, 1955) found that the short-circuit current was very nearly equal to the transport of Cl ions in excess of that secreted as HCl. He concluded that, at least in the frog stomach, the PD finds its origin in the secretion of Cl ions by the gastric mucosa. Heinz and Durbin (1957) demonstrated that metabolic inhibition or severe damage of the mucosa eliminates almost completely the difference between the experimentally determined conductance of Cl ions and the conductance calculated on the supposition that all Cl⁻ fluxes are passive. This led them to conclude that at least part of the Cl⁻ transport must be active. This active Cl⁻ transport is localized at the mucosal side of the gastric wall (Cotlove et al., 1959).

Previous data (Rehm, 1944; Rehm et al., 1955) seemed to indicate that the PD across the stomach wall in dogs was strongly influenced by stimulation of the acid secretion. Histamine stimulation lowers the PD from 65 mV to 35 mV (mucosal side negative). From the data of Rehm et al. (1955), Durbin (1967) calculated that the value of the short-circuit current before and during stimulation of the acid secretion remains virtually constant; thus it may be concluded that the secretion of acid inhibits the mechanism responsible for the origin of the PD only very slightly. A considerable portion of the PD changes after histamine stimulation are probably caused by diffusion potentials between HCl in the tubuli and in the mucosal solution. In the frog gastric mucosa also, the influence on the short-circuit current of the stimulation of the acid secretion with histamine or of inhibition of this secretion with thiocyanate appears minor (Durbin and Heinz, 1958).

Although the origin of the PD across the gastric wall of a frog can almost completely be explained by the active secretion of Cl ions, this mechanism certainly cannot explain all facts observed in the mammalian preparations. In mammals absorption of Na ions probably plays a very important role in the origin of the PD. The in vitro experiments of Wright (1962) indicate that the gastric mucosa of the rabbit fetus absorbs NaCl and produces a potential difference. This PD disappears if the mucosal solution does not contain Na ions; in the rat stomach in vitro also the PD disappears if Na⁺ is replaced by choline. The replacement of Cl⁻ in the solution by sulfate does not have the same effect (Cummins and Vaughan, 1965).

In addition, CUMMINS and VAUGHAN (1965) showed that a higher Na^+ concentration in the solution increases the PD across the stomach wall, but with an ever increasing Na^+ concentration the PD approaches a limit; this suggests a pump system saturated by an increasing Na^+ concentration. They also were able to demonstrate ATP-ase activity in the gastric mucosa of the rat, which they consider an indication for the existence of a Na^+ pump (DUNHAM and GLYNN, 1961).

Although these data stress the extreme importance of an active Na^+ absorption for the origin of the PD in mammals, in some of these animals active Cl secretion also plays a role in the mechanism of the PD. SHOEMAKER et al. (1966) showed that in the guinea-pig gastric mucosa the net active Cl^- secretion equated the short-circuit current; in this preparation there was no evidence of an active Na^+ absorption. SERNKA and HOGBEN (1969), however, could not confirm these data and found an active transport for both Na^+ and Cl^- in the guinea pig. Similarly KITAHARA (1967) showed an active transport of both Na^+ and Cl^- in the non-secreting gastric mucosa of the cat. The experiments of CODE et al. (1963) indicate how the combined operation of both mechanisms can build up the PD. They examined the influence of the intraluminal pH on the PD across the gastric wall and found that in dogs a lowering of the pH was associated with a lowering of the Na^+ absorption and an increase of the Cl^- secretion. KITAHARA et al. (1969) confirmed these observations and showed the existence in several mammals of a whole range of possibilities, from situations in which the PD across the gastric wall is almost completely caused by active Na^+ absorption (fed dogs), to situations in which the active Cl^- secretion dominates (fasted cats).

The few human stomach preparations which KITAHARA et al. (1969) could study fell between both extremes. HOGBEN (1962) had found that in the frog gastric mucosa the pH at the site of transport can be much lower than the pH of the bulk solution; they consider this a possible explanation of the difference between the PD mechanism found in frogs (almost exclusively active Cl^- secretion) and that found in mammals (in most animals predominantly active Na^+ absorption); the low pH at the site of transport in frogs is supposed to be responsible for the PD mechanism of the Cl pattern.

In mammals the Na^+ transport seems to play an important role in the origin of the PD along the total length of the gastrointestinal tract. BOSACKOVA and CRANE (1965) and FORDTRAN and DIETSCHY (1966) showed this in experiments on the small intestine of animals. The importance of active Na^+ absorption for the origin of the PD in the colon was demonstrated in rats by CURRAN and SCHWARTZ (1960), in dogs by COOPERSTEIN and BROCKMAN (1959) and in guinea pigs by USSING and ANDERSEN (1956). Finally, DEVROEDE and PHILLIPS (1969) showed that in humans also the colon mucosa absorbs Na^+ against a concentration gradient. For the esophagus no similar experiments have been performed as far. Yet the correlation between the presence of different esophageal glandular structures and the PD pattern suggests that here also the PD is determined by secretion and absorption mechanisms.

3. Techniques of PD Measurements

In PD measurements one measures the difference in potential between two places e.g. between mucosa and serosa of the stomach. Although method and apparatus used for this purpose are very similar to those used for pH measurements, a few essential differences exist between both techniques. PD measurements measure the difference between the "total" potentials of two places, while pH measurements measure the difference between the "total" potential in one place (reference electrode) and that part of the potential caused by the concentration of H⁺ in another location (exploring electrode). Therefore, two identical electrodes are used in PD measurements and both must be able to measure the "total" potential. In pH measurements, on the other hand, the detection electrode must be sensitive only to H⁺ (a glass electrode). As a consequence the potential difference can be read directly from a volt meter in PD measurements whereas in pH measurements the recorded potential difference must be converted into pH units by means of comparative measurements in buffers with known pH.

Because the potential differences registered in PD measurements are so small, the technique requires electrodes with a very low resistance and a volt meter with a very high impedance. Though metal electrodes have a low resistance, they are not commonly used in PD measurements because the metal in contact with the tissues gives rise to a junction potential with a battery effect. Therefore non-polarizable electrodes are used, mostly metal-metal salt-salt junctions, e.g. silver-silverchloride electrodes (Ag–AgCl–KCl) or calomel half-cells (Hg–HgCl–KCl). Calomel electrodes are quite stable and appropriate for PD measurements. Because these calomel half-cells are usually too large to be introduced directly into the gastrointestinal tract, they are connected with the site of detection via an ionic bridge (a catheter filled with an ionic solution). Most authors use a saturated KCl solution in agar (3%) (Andersson and Grossman, 1965; Greenwood et al., 1965; Geall et al., 1968, 1969, 1970; Grantham et al., 1970), because K⁺ and Cl⁻ have the same mobilities so that the potentials caused by the concentration gradient of K⁺ and Cl⁻ in the salt bridge cancel each other almost completely and because the agar gives the salt bridge a sufficient stability. Some authors (Meckeler and Ingelfinger, 1967) use a KCl solution without agar but apply a small sponge on top of the catheter to prevent leaking. Because a relatively high concentration of KCl causes mucosal lesions, Hernandez and Beck (1969) prefer a Ringer solution rather than KCl as a salt bridge. The values measured with this technique are on the average 28 percent lower than those obtained by KCl in agar. In addition they perfuse their catheters to assure a good contact between the salt bridge and the mucosa and to avoid air bubbles in the catheter, which interrupt the salt bridge.

The location of the reference electrode is important to interpret the obtained PD values. In earlier PD measurements in man (Helm et al., 1965) the reference electrode was applied to the skin (both the calomel reference electrode and the finger of the patient were dipped in a saturated KCl solution). If the PD between mucosa and serosa is to be measured, however, the reference electrode must be placed in the blood stream. Indeed Geall et al. (1970) showed that various parts of the peritoneum are equipotential with venous blood whereas a significant potential difference exists between venous blood and skin (about +40 mV) (Andersson and Grossman, 1965; Grantham et al., 1970). This potential difference changes with the emotional state of the patient (Edelberg, 1963), and this partially explains the fluctuations in earlier PD measurements which applied the reference electrode on the skin. Different techniques are used to avoid these interfering skin potentials: abraded skin, lancet puncture and subcutaneous needle.

Table 8 (Grantham et al., 1970) gives the different values of the PD between gastric or esophageal mucosa and various reference places. The value obtained by lancet puncture of the forearm is almost equivalent to the intravenous value.

Table 8. PD in mV (mean ± SEM)

Reference electrode	Exploring electrode	
	gastric mucosa	esophageal mucosa
Finger	+ 10,2 ± 3.1	+ 25.6 ± 2.9
Unabraded skin, volar forearm	− 6.8 ± 4.6	+ 11.9 ± 3.7
Abraded skin, volar forearm	− 21.8 ± 2.9	+ 1.6 ± 1.8
Lancet puncture, volar forearm	− 27.8 ± 2.6	− 4.3 ± 2.5
Subcutaneous	− 32.3 ± 3.6	− 9.5 ± 2.2
Intravenous	− 32.2 ± 3.4	− 9.8 ± 2.3

For routine purposes this technique has the great advantage that it simplifies the sterile conditions which are required when blood is taken as reference site (SCHLEGEL, 1971).

4. PD Measurements in the Esophagus

The potential difference across the gastric wall of humans is about 35 mV, the mucosal side being negative. In the distal esophagus the potential difference is much lower, about 10 mV; here also the mucosal side is negative. Using the earlier method, with the unabraded skin of the finger as reference point, HELM et al. (1965) noted an average PD of 7.5 mV in the stomach, lumen negative, whereas in the esophagus just above the gastroesophageal sphincter, the PD was even positive, with a mean of 15.6 mV. In view of the marked difference between the PD of stomach and esophagus HELM et al. (1965) wondered if it was not possible to use this technique to localize the gastroesophageal junction. By means of simultaneous registrations of intraluminal pressures and of the PD they showed that the PD change commences about 2 cm below the respiratory reversal point, the greatest change occurring at or just below that point. In certain cases the PD change was rather abrupt, in others it occurred over a few cm with more or less pronounced fluctuations (Fig. 145). These data were confirmed by HERNANDEZ and BECK (1969), who showed that the PD reversal started 1 cm below the beginning of the high pressure zone and reached its maximum 4 cm proximally.

In patients with hiatal hernia the PD pattern at the level of the gastro-esophageal junction is comparable with the pattern found in normal persons, both as to magnitude in change and to change in polarity. However, the localization of the PD reversal has moved upward, proximally of the pressure inversion point, whereas in normals it lays astride this point (HELM et al., 1965). GREEN-WOOD et al. (1965) obtained similar results in dogs with surgically induced hiatal hernia. BECK and HERNANDEZ (1969) confirmed the results of HELM et al. (1965) and added that in patients with hiatal hernia the PD transition zone was longer than in normal controls. All these data suggest that the PD reversal zone is linked with the transition between gastric and esophageal mucosa. Already HELM et al. (1965) and GREENWOOD et al. (1965) noticed on direct inspection of dogs during surgery that the maximal PD change was localized within 5 mm of the border between gastric and esophageal mucosa. MECKELER and INGEL-FINGER (1967) confirmed these data for humans by means of suction biopsies,

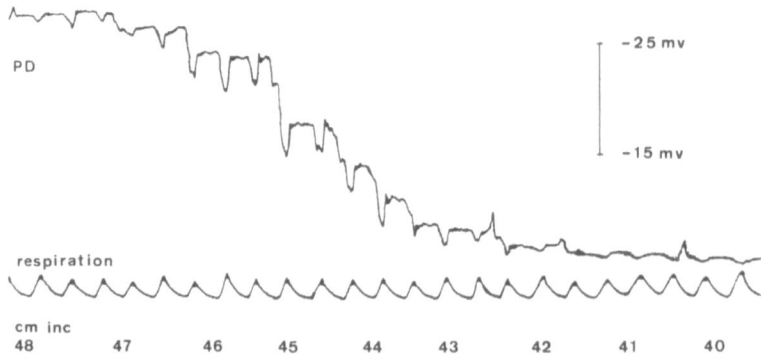

Fig. 145. PD measurement in stomach, gastroesophageal sphincter and esophagus. The reference electrode was placed in the blood stream

taken simultaneously with the PD measurements at the level of the electrode and 2.5 cm distally. In 12 out of 18 cases the PD change coincided with the transition between columnar and squamous cell epithelium. Even more remarkable was the fact that parietal cells were absent in all biopsies taken at the end point of maximal change in PD, whereas these cells were present 2.5 cm distally. Hence they concluded that the change in PD at the gastroesophageal junction coincided with the disappearance of the parietal cells at the transition of gastric and esophageal mucosa. This conclusion was also partially based on the results of VILLEGAS (1962), who had used microelectrodes in the bullfrog gastric mucosa to show that the potential difference between the outer and inner surfaces of the parietal cells was equal to the normal transmucosal PD. The finding that in some persons the PD transition at the gastroesophageal junction is more gradual than in others was ascribed by MECKELER and INGELFINGER (1967) to the existence in these persons of a more extensive zone of junctional epithelium (a simple columnar cell epithelium devoid of parietal cells [ADLER, 1963]). This hypothesis is supported by the observations of BECK et al. (1969a) and VIDINS et al. (1971), who studied the PD pattern in patients with a lower esophagus lined by columnar epithelium (Barrett's syndrome). In the most typical cases they found a first PD drop at the gastroesophageal junction. The PD in the zone with Barrett's epithelium was more negative than the PD in the normal distal esophagus. A second PD drop, after which a normal esophageal PD value was reached, was found at the transition between columnar and squamous cell epithelium. BECK and HERNANDEZ (1969) studied the PD across the esophageal wall in patients with ulcerations of the body of the esophagus and found that the transmural potential difference changed over ulcerating lesions of the esophagus. Withdrawal of the PD probe under esophagoscopic control caused a negative deflection in the region of the ulcer in all cases. In a majority of them (7 out of 10) this negative deflection could also be demonstrated when the normal technique of withdrawing the PD probe blindly centimeter by centimeter from the stomach through the esophagus was used. In the other 3 cases esophagoscopic control showed the ulcer to be so small that probably the potential difference of the normal surrounding mucosa interfered with the negative deflection. From these data BECK and HERNANDEZ (1969) inferred that the lengthening of the PD transitional zone at the gastroesophageal junction in patients with hiatal hernia may be explained by the presence of inflammatory tissue and ulceration in the lower esophagus. However, invasion of the distal part of the esophagus by gastric mucosa in patients with hiatal hernia, as described by ALLISON and JOHNSTONE (1953), may also be responsible for the lengthening of the PD reversal zone.

In patients with esophagitis BECK et al. (1969a) and VIDINS et al. (1971) found a negative deflection of the PD over the inflamed area, analogous to the findings of BECK and HERNANDEZ (1969) in patients with esophageal ulcerations. A negative deflection was also recorded in patients with esophageal carcinoma. In both instances the PD value at the level of the esophageal lesions is probably due to an abnormally functioning esophageal mucosa.

BECK et al. (1969b) studied the PD at the level of the upper esophageal sphincter in man and found a PD change (mucosal side more negative), which started just proximally of the beginning of the high pressure zone in the upper esophagus. This PD change extended over about 5 cm; in the pharynx the PD again reached values comparable with the PD in the esophageal body. Histological examinations revealed that the glandular pattern in this zone is different from the pattern in the esophageal body. In the body of the esophagus glands of the mucus type are scattered in the submucosal layer but not in the lamina propria. They can be colored by both components of the AB-PAS staining. In the upper esophagus, at the level of cricopharyngeal muscle, glands of the cardiac type are present in the lamina propria in close proximity with the overlying epithelium. They are PAS-positive and are stained only a little by the Alcian blue component of the AB-PAS staining. Perhaps the difference in depth and in secretory function between these glands and those of the esophageal body causes the drop in PD at the level of the upper esophageal sphincter.

References

ADLER, R. H.: Collective review, hiatal hernia and esophagitis. Int. Abstr. Surg. **116**, 1–15 (1963).

ALLISON, P. R., JOHNSTONE, A. S.: The oesophagus lined with gastric mucous membrane. Thorax **8**, 87–101 (1953).

ANDERSSON, S., GROSSMAN, M. I.: Profile of pH, pressure and potential difference at gastroduodenal junction in man. Gastroenterology **49**, 364–371 (1965).

BECK, I. T., HERNANDEZ, N. A.: Transmural potential difference in patients with hiatus hernia and oesophageal ulcer. Gut **10**, 469–476 (1969).

BECK, I. T., McELLIGOTT, T. F., HERNANDEZ, N. A.: Transmural potential difference at the level of the upper esophageal sphincter in man. Amer. J. dig. Dis. **14**, 456–462 (1969b).

BECK, I. T., SZIVEK, J., FOX, J. E.: Computerized analysis of motility and transmural potential difference changes at the level of the gastro-esophageal junction, body of the esophagus and upper sphincter in health and disease. Gastrointestinal motility, p. 10–25. Stuttgart: Georg Thieme; New York-London: Academic Press 1969a.

BOSACKOVA, J., CRANE, R. K.: Studies on the mechanism of intestinal absorption of sugars. IX. Intracellular sodium concentrations and active sugar transport by hamster small intestine in vitro. Biochim. biophys. Acta (Amst.) **102**, 436–441 (1965).

CODE, C. F., HIGGINS, J. A., MOSS, J. C., ORVIS, A. L., SCHOLER, J. F.: The influence of acid on the gastric absorption of water, sodium and potassium. J. Physiol. (Lond.) **166**, 110–119 (1963).

COOPERSTEIN, I. L., BROCKMAN, S. K.: The electrical potential difference generated by the large intestine: its relation to electrolyte and water transfer. J. clin. Invest. **38**, 435–442 (1959).

COTLOVE, E., GREEN, N. D., HOGBEN, C. A. M.: Localization of chloride transport in the gastric mucosa. Fed. Proc. **18**, 31 (1959).

CUMMINS, J. T., VAUGHAN, B. E.: Ionic relationships of the bioelectrogenic mechanism in isolated rat stomach. Biochim. biophys. Acta (Amst.) **94**, 280–292 (1965).

CURRAN, P. F., SCHWARTZ, G. F.: Na, Cl and water transport by rat colon. J. gen. Physiol. **43**, 555–571 (1960).

Davenport, H. W., Warner, H. A., Code, C. F.: Functional significance of gastric mucosal barrier to sodium. Gastroenterology 47, 142–152 (1964).

Dennis, W. H., Canosa, C., Rehm, W. S.: Potential difference across the pyloric antrum. Amer. J. Physiol. 197, 19–21 (1959).

Devroede, G. J., Phillips, S. F.: Conservation of sodium, chloride and water by the human colon. Gastroenterology 56, 101–109 (1969).

Donne, A.: Recherches sur quelques unes des propriétés chimiques des sécrétions, et sur les courants électriques qui existent dans les corps organisés. Ann. Chim. Phys. 57, 398–416 (1834).

Dunham, E. T., Glynn, I. M.: Adenosinetriphosphatase activity and the active movements of alkali metal ions. J. Physiol. (Lond.) 156, 274–293 (1961).

Durbin, R. P.: Electrical potential difference of the gastric mucosa. In: Handbook of physiology, ed. by C. F. Code and W. Heidel, section IV, chapter 49. American Physiological Society, Washington, D.C. 1967.

Durbin, R. P., Heinz, E.: Electromotive chloride transport and gastric acid secretion in the frog. J. gen. Physiol. 41, 1035–1047 (1958).

Edelberg, R.: Electrophysiologic characteristics and interpretation of skin potentials. In: Technical Documentary Report SAM TDR 63–95, U.S. Air Force Electron Syst. Div., Nov. 1963, p. 1–10.

Edmonds, C. J.: The gradient of electrical potential difference and of sodium and potassium of the gut contents along the caecum and colon of normal and sodium depleted rats. J. Physiol. (Lond.) 193, 571–588 (1967).

Fordtran, J. S., Dietschy, J. M.: Water and electrolyte movement in the intestine. Gastroenterology 50, 263–285 (1966).

Geall, M. G., Code, C. F., McIlrath, D. C., Summerskill, W. H. J.: Measurement of gastrointestinal transmural electric potential difference in man. Gut 11, 34–37 (1970).

Geall, M. G., McIlrath, D. C., Phillips, S. F., Code, C. F., Summerskill, W. H. J.: Measurement of the transmucosal potential difference of stomach in unanesthetized man. Gastroenterology 54, 1235 (1968).

Geall, M. G., Spencer, R. J., Phillips, S. F.: Transmural electrical potential difference of the human colon. Gut 10, 921–923 (1969).

Goodman, E. N.: Improved method of measuring the potential difference across the human gastric membranes and its clinical significance. A preliminary report. Surg. Gynec. Obstet. 75, 583–592 (1942).

Grantham, R. N., Code, C. F., Schlegel, J. F.: Reference electrode sites in determination of potential difference across the gastroesophageal junction. Proc. Mayo Clin. 45, 265–274 (1970).

Greenwood, R. K., Schlegel, J. F., Helm, W. J., Code, C. F.: Pressure and potential difference characteristics of surgically created canine hiatal hernia. Gastroenterology 48, 602–611 (1965).

Heinz, E., Durbin, R. P.: Studies of the chloride transport in the gastric mucosa of the frog. J. gen. Physiol. 41, 101–117 (1957).

Helm, W. J., Code, C. F., Summerskill, W. H. J.: Simultaneous identification of the gastroesophageal junction by pH, potential difference and pressure. Gastroenterology 40, 805 (1961).

Helm, W. J., Schlegel, J. F., Code, C. F., Summerskill, W. H. J.: Identification of the gastroesophageal mucosal junction by transmucosal potential in healthy subjects and patients with hiatal hernia. Gastroenterology 48, 25–35 (1965).

Hernandez, N. A., Beck, I. T.: Gastroesophageal transmural potential difference measured by a new constant infusion method. The effect of skin scarification on this potential difference. Amer. J. dig. Dis. 14, 206–216 (1969).

Hogben, C. A. M.: The chloride transport system of the gastric mucosa. Proc. nat. Acad. Sci. (Wash.) 37, 393–395 (1951).

Hogben, C. A. M.: Active transport of chloride by isolated frog gastric epithelium: origin of the gastric mucosal potential. Amer. J. Physiol. 180, 641–649 (1955).

Hogben, C. A. M.: Ultrastructure and transport across epithelial membranes. New York Heart Symposium. Circulat. Res. 26, 1179 (1962).

Kitahara, S.: Active transport of Na^+ and Cl^- by in vitro nonsecreting cat gastric mucosa. Amer. J. Physiol. 213, 819–823 (1967).

Kitahara, S., Fox, K. R., Hogben, A. M.: Acid secretion, Na^+ absorption and the origin of the potential difference across isolated mammalian stomachs. Amer. J. dig. Dis. 14, 221–238 (1969).

Krasil'nikov, L. G., Fishzon-Ryss, Y. I.: Interpretation of electrogastrogram and its variants in healthy persons during digestion. Fed. Proc. 23 (Suppl.), 901–904 (1964).

Meckeler, K. J. H., Ingelfinger, F. J.: Correlation of electric surface potentials, intraluminal pressures, and nature of tissue in the gastroesophageal junction of man. Gastroenterology 52, 966–971 (1967).

Morton, H. S., Martin, W. S.: The electrogastrograph. Some clinical applications. Rev. Gastroent. 20, 37–53 (1953).

Rehm, W. S.: The effect of histamine and HCl on gastric secretion and potential. Amer. J. Physiol. 141, 537–548 (1944).

Rehm, W. S.: The effect of electric current on gastric secretion and potential. Amer. J. Physiol. 144, 115–125 (1945).

Rehm, W. S.: Evidence that the major portion of the gastric potential originates between the submucosa and the mucosa. Amer. J. Physiol. 147, 69–77 (1946).

Rehm, W. S.: A theory of the formation of HCl by the stomach. Gastroenterology 14, 401–417 (1950).

Rehm, W. S.: Acid secretion, resistance, short-circuit current and voltage-clamping in frog's stomach. Amer. J. Physiol. 203, 63–72 (1962).

Rehm, W. S., Dennis, W. H., Schlesinger, H.: Electrical resistance of the mammalian stomach. Amer. J. Physiol. 181, 451–470 (1955).

Rovelstad, R. A., Owen, C. A., Jr., Magath, T. B.: Factors influencing the continuous recording of in situ pH of gastric and duodenal contents. Gastroenterology 20, 609–624 (1952).

Sawyer, P. N., Rhoads, J. E., Panzer, R.: An evaluation of electrogastrography in the diagnosis of gastric cancer. Surgery 26, 479–487 (1949).

Schlegel, J. F.: American Gastroenterological Association. Postgraduate course "The esophagus". Bal Harbour, Florida, May 1971, p. 36–37.

Schultz, S. G., Zalusky, R.: Ion transport in the isolated rabbit ileum. I. Short-circuit current and Na fluxes. J. gen. Physiol. 47, 567–584 (1964).

Schwyngedauw, J.: Sur l'existence d'une difference de potentiel variable entre la bouche et l'estomac au cours de la sécrétion gastrique. C. R. Soc. Biol. (Paris) 98, 1431–1432 (1928).

Sernka, T. J., Hogben, C. A.: Active ion transport by isolated gastric mucosae of rat and guinea pig. Amer. J. Physiol. 217, 1419–1424 (1969).

Shoemaker, R. L., Sachs, G., Hirschowitz, B. E.: Secretion by guinea pig gastric mucosa in vitro. Proc. Soc. exp. Biol. (N.Y.) 123, 824 (1966).

Soergel, K. H., Whalen, G. E., Geenen, J. E., Gustke, R. F.: Potential difference of the intact human intestine during active and passive transport (Abstr.). J. Lab. clin. Med. 68, 1018 (1966).

Ussing, H. H., Andersen, B.: In: Proceedings of the Third International Congress of Biochemistry, Brussels 1955, p. 434–440. New York: Academic Press 1956.

Ussing, H. H., Kruhøffer, P., Taysen, J. H., Thorn, N. A.: The alkali metal ions in biology. In: Handbuch der experimentellen Pharmakologie (Suppl.). Edited by A. Heffter and W. Heubner, vol. 13, p. 59. Berlin-Heidelberg-New York: Springer 1960.

Vidins, E. I., Fox, J. E., Beck, I. T.: Transmural potential difference (PD) in the body of the esophagus in patients with esophagitis, Barrett's epithelium and carcinoma of the esophagus. Amer. J. dig. Dis. 16, 991–999 (1971).

Villegas, L.: Cellular location of the electrical potential difference in frog gastric mucosa. Biochim. biophys. Acta (Amst.) 64, 359–367 (1962).

Wright, G. H.: Net transfers of water, sodium chloride and hydrogen ions across the gastric mucosa of the rabbit foetus. J. Physiol. (Lond.) 163, 281–293 (1962).

The Acid Infusion Test

W. PELEMANS and G. VANTRAPPEN

The acid perfusion test was originally designed as a test for esophagitis and a means to differentiate pain of esophageal origin from that of angina pectoris (BERNSTEIN and BAKER, 1958; BERNSTEIN et al., 1962). When perfusion of the esophagus with 0.1 N HCl elicited the patient's symptoms, the test was said to be positive and was taken as evidence for the esophageal origin of these symptoms. It was suggested that these symptoms were due to esophagitis. Later studies (SIEGEL and HENDRIX, 1963) seemed to indicate that the acid perfusion procedure correlates more closely with heartburn than with the presence of esophagitis. A negative test does not exclude and a positive test does not prove the presence of esophagitis. Recent evidence seems to indicate that the acid perfusion test permits an objectivation of heartburn and helps, in evaluating patients with atypical symptoms, to determine whether the symptoms may be of esophageal origin.

1. Procedure

The test is performed by perfusing acid and control solution through a plastic catheter placed in the esophagus or stomach. The tube is first inserted into the stomach, gastric contents are aspirated and the distal tip of the tube is then withdrawn to a position somewhere at the junction of the upper and middle third of the esophagus (approximately 27 cm from the incisors). The patient is sitting in a chair. The perfusion catheter is led over one shoulder and connected via a three-way stop-cock to the test solution behind the patient so that the solution can be changed without the patient's knowledge. Initially a 0.9 percent NaCl or a 5 percent glucose solution is perfused at a rate of 100 to 120 drops per minute for 15 min.

After the control period the perfusion is switched to 0.1 N HCl at the same rate for a period of 30 min or until the patient spontaneously complains of pain. Clinically important symptoms are persistent and usually increase in severity as long as the acid perfusion is continued. The rate of perfusion may be doubled after 15 min if the patient does not complain of any discomfort. The acid perfusion test is negative if HCl does not produce symptoms, if the pain elicited by HCl infusion is different from the patients spontaneous symptoms, or if the NaCl or glucose solution causes the patient's typical sensations. The production of atypical symptoms during the perfusion of the control solution should not necessarily be regarded as a negative test, provided that the patient's own symptoms are elicited by the acid perfusion. To be positive the patient's symptoms should be exactly duplicated during the acid perfusion and not during the perfusion of control solution. In addition it should be possible repeatedly to relieve and reproduce the typical symptoms by changing the perfusion solution.

The acid delivered into the esophagus obviously enters the stomach as well. Several criteria have been used to differentiate the gastric and esophageal origin of the symptoms.

1. Midline pain and burning extending above the level of the xiphoid is presumably of esophageal origin. If the test produces pain in the upper abdomen additional criteria can be used to determine the origin of this pain.

2. The rapid disappearance of symptoms after cessation of acid administration favors their esophageal origin. Cessation of acid delivery for a few minutes will not significantly alter the intragastric milieu but would be expected to remove the acid stimulus from the esophagus.

3. Similarly, the rapid disappearance of symptoms after administration of small doses of antacids suggests an esophageal rather than a gastric origin of the symptoms.

4. The repetitive production and relief of symptoms is a strong argument in favor of esophageal disease.

5. If there is doubt about the gastric or esophageal origin of upper abdominal symptoms, acid can be delivered directly into the stomach. If the pain is of esophageal origin the intragastric infusion of acid should not produce the patient's spontaneous symptoms, whereas the intraesophageal acid perfusion does produce this symptoms.

2. Hazards of the Test

Administration of HCl into the respiratory tract can be avoided by placing the tube first into the stomach, followed by withdrawal to the desired level in the esophagus and by the initial control delivery of NaCl or glucose.

In patients with heart disease, glucose solution is used in place of the saline control solution. If the test is used to differentiate angina pectoris from esophageal pain it should be kept in mind that the procedure may produce anginal pain. Although BERNSTEIN and BAKER (1958) reported that the acid perfusion test does not precipitate cardiac symptoms or electrocardiographic changes, BENNETT and ATKINSON (1966) noted anginal pain during the perfusion of the control solution in 2 out of 11 patients with angina pectoris.

The acid perfusion test was performed in 16 patients with a history of gross gastrointestinal hemorrhage less than 3 months before the test. Recurrence of any gross bleeding episode was not observed (BERNSTEIN and BAKER, 1958).

Esophagoscopy, done on the morning following the test, failed to reveal macroscopic lesions of the esophageal mucosa in any of the 14 patients that were examined (BERNSTEIN and BAKER, 1958). Several studies indicate that the test may be performed in normal subjects without causing any symptoms (BERNSTEIN and BAKER, 1958; BERNSTEIN et al., 1962; SIEGEL and HENDRIX, 1963). BENNETT and ATKINSON (1966), but ATKINSON and BENNETT (1968), however, reported that about 50 percent of their normal control subjects had pain during the acid infusion. It has been shown in cats that the infusion of HCl (pH 1 to 1.3) into the esophagus can produce esophagitis (GOLDBERG et al., 1969).

3. The Mechanism of Pain

The mechanism of pain induced by acid perfusion remains controversial. SIEGEL and HENDRIX (1963) studied a group of 25 patients with clinical symptoms of esophagitis and 25 controls. Acid perfusion did not produce symptoms in any of the controls. In all cases where esophageal symptoms were induced, motor abnormalities were observed in the lower esophagus, i.e. increased amplitude and duration of peristaltic contractions, spontaneous non-progressive esophageal contractions and increased esophageal tone. Only 4 of the 25 controls

Table 9. Peptic esophagitis and the acid infusion test

Diagnostic Criteria	Authors	Number of patients	Number of positive te tests
Clinical diagnosis of esophagitis	TUTTLE et al., 1960	79	64
	BERNSTEIN et al., 1962	100	58
	SIEGEL and HENDRIX, 1963	25	25
	BENNETT and ATKINSON, 1966	29	28
	AFFOLTER, 1966	34	32
	ATKINSON and BENNETT, 1968	40	39
	ISMAIL-BEIGI et al., 1970	27	27
		334	273 (81%)
Clinical diagnosis of esophagitis + positive esophagoscopy	BERNSTEIN et al., 1962	21	15
	SIEGEL and HENDRIX, 1963	20	20
	ISMAIL-BEIGI et al., 1970	14	14
		55	49 (89%)
Clinical diagnosis of esophagitis + positive esophagoscopy + positive biopsy	SIEGEL and HENDRIX, 1963	15	15
	ISMAIL-BEIGI et al., 1970	13	13
		28	28 (100%)
Clinical diagnosis of esophagitis + negative esophagoscopy	BERNSTEIN et al., 1962	25	15
	SIEGEL AND HENDRIX, 1963	5	5
	ISMAIL-BEIGI et al., 1970	6	6
		36	26 (72%)
Clinical diagnosis of esophagitis + negative esophagoscopy + negative biopsy	SIEGEL and HENDRIX, 1963	2	2
	ISMAIL-BEIGI et al., 1970	1	1

developed motor disorders, which, however, were not associated with symptoms. From these observations it was concluded that disordered motor function plays a role in the production of pain induced by acid perfusion of the esophagus. TUTTLE et al. (1961) and ATKINSON and BENNETT (1968) could not demonstrate any constant motor changes associated with pain induced by acid. It was also observed that a sodium bicarbonate infusion will relieve the pain without bringing about any striking changes in motility and, conversely, that the anticholinergic drug propantheline will abolish motility without necessarily relieving the pain. From these observations it was concluded that motor disorders do not form an integral part of the pain mechanism.

Observations pertinent to the evaluation of the esophageal acid perfusion test are summarized in Table 9. Originally the test was designed as a clinical test of esophagitis (BERNSTEIN and BAKER, 1958). There is a fairly good correlation indeed between the symptoms of esophagitis and the acid perfusion test.

The test was positive in 81 percent of 334 patients in whom a diagnosis of esophagitis was made on the basis of their clinical symptoms (TUTTLE et al., 1960; BERNSTEIN et al., 1962; SIEGEL and HENDRIX, 1963; BENNETT and ATKINSON, 1966; AFFOLTER, 1966; ATKINSON and BENNETT, 1968; ISMAIL-BEIGI et al., 1970). When the clinical diagnosis of esophagitis was confirmed by esophagoscopy, the test was positive in 89 percent of 55 patients (BERNSTEIN et al., 1962; SIEGEL and HENDRIX, 1963; ISMAIL-BEIGI et al., 1970). When the clinical diagnosis of esophagitis was confirmed by both endoscopic and microscopic examination, the test was found to be positive in all 28 cases reported (SIEGEL and HENDRIX, 1964; ISMAIL-BEIGI et al., 1970).

These observation should not be interpreted as evidence indicating that the acid perfusion test correlates perfectly with esophagitis. The patients in the above mentioned studies were all selected on the basis of fairly good clinical evidence of esophagitis.

A "false positive test" was found in 72 percent of 36 patients in whom esophagoscopy could not confirm the clinical diagnosis of esophagitis (BERNSTEIN et al., 1962; SIEGEL and HENDRIX, 1963; ISMAIL-BEIGI et al., 1970). Moreover, the test was found to be "falsely positive" in 3 patients in whom the clinical diagnosis could not be confirmed by esophagoscopy and biopsy. Similarly, false negative tests have been observed in asymptomatic patients in whom lesions of esophagitis were found to be present at both esophagoscopy and biopsy (SIEGEL and HENDRIX, 1965). The absence of symptoms in these patients has been ascribed to the effect of treatment or to destruction of sensory fibers in the mucosa.

The value of the acid perfusion test as a clinical tool would be rather negligible if it were limited to an objectivation of the symptoms of heartburn. The studies of BERNSTEIN et al. (1958), BENNETT and ATKINSON (1966) and SKINNER and BOOTH (1970), however, indicate that the acid perfusion procedure is a valuable test to determine whether aspecific thoracic and retrosternal pain or upper abdominal pain may be of esophageal origin. When a patient develops pain of the same nature as his spontaneous pain during the acid perfusion and not during the perfusion of the control solution, the esophageal origin of the pain is quite probable. It may be concluded that the acid perfusion test allows to objectivate the symptom of heartburn and that it seems a useful, reliable technique for establishing whether or not the patient's symptoms have an esophageal component.

References

AFFOLTER, H.: Die Rolle der Säureperfusion in der Diagnostik der Refluxösophagitis. Gastro-enterologia (Basel) **106**, 157–164 (1966).

ATKINSON, M., BENNETT, J. R.: Relationship between motor changes and pain during esophageal acid perfusion. Amer. J. dig. Dis. **13**, 346–350 (1968).

BENNETT, J. R., ATKINSON, M.: The differentiation between oesophageal and cardiac pain. Lancet **1966 II**, 1123–1127.

BERNSTEIN, L. M., BAKER, L. A.: A clinical test for esophagitis. Gastroenterology **34**, 760–781 (1958).

BERNSTEIN, L. M., FRUIN, R. C., PACINI, R.: Differentiation of esophageal pain from angina pectoris: role of the esophageal acid perfusion test. Medicine (Baltimore) **41**, 143–162 (1962).

BERNSTEIN, L. M., PACINI, R., FRUIN, R. C., GORVETT, E.: Esophagitis as a cause of upper abdominal pain. J. Amer. med. Ass. **168**, 27–33 (1958).

GOLDBERG, H. I., DODDS, W. J., GEE, S., MONTGOMERY, C., ZBORALSKE, F.: Role of acid and pepsin in acute experimental esophagitis. Gastroenterology **56**, 223–230 (1969).

ISMAIL-BEIGI, F., HORTON, P. F., POPE, C. E.: Histological consequences of gastroesophageal reflux in man. Gastroenterology **58**, 163–174 (1970).

SIEGEL, C. I., HENDRIX, T. R.: Esophageal abnormalities induced by acid perfusion in patients with heartburn. J. clin. Invest. **48**, 686–695 (1963).

SKINNER, D. B., BOOTH, D. J.: Assessment of distal esophageal function in patients with hiatal hernia and/or gastroesophageal reflux. Ann. Surg. **172**, 627–637 (1970).

TUTTLE, S. G., BETTARELLO, A., GROSSMAN, M. I.: Esophageal acid perfusion test and a gastro-esophageal reflux test in patients with esophagitis. Gastroenterology **38**, 861–872 (1960).

TUTTLE, S. G., RUFIN, F., BETTARELLO, A.: The physiology of heartburn. Ann. intern. Med. **55**, 292–300 (1961).

Pharmacological Tests

J. JANSSENS and J. HELLEMANS

With 2 Figures

KRAMER and INGELFINGER (1949) were the first to describe the oversensitivity of the achalatic esophagus to parasympathomimetic drugs. In their balloon-kymographic studies (a balloon of 40 cm³ was used as an oncometer to detect esophageal volume) they found in achalatic patients a lumen-obliterating esophageal contraction in response to a dose of Mecholyl (methacholine; acetyl-beta-methylcholine) which has little effect upon the normal esophagus. Other cholinergic drugs such as Urecholine (Bethanechol; carbaminoyl-β-methylcholine) (OLSEN and CREAMER, 1957) or Neostigmine (KRAMER et al., 1956) were found to have a similar effect.

These data were confirmed in manometric studies with open-tip catheters (BUTIN et al., 1953; HIGHTOWER et al., 1954): in most patients with achalasia of the cardia the resting pressure in the esophagus increases by 20 cm of water or more 1 to 2 min after a subcutaneous or intramuscular injection of 5 to 10 mg of Mecholyl. Usually these spastic contractions disappear after 5 to 10 min but sometimes they can last up to half an hour (Fig. 146). The hypersensitive reaction to Mecholyl can also be visualized radiologically (Fig. 147). Many patients experience severe substernal cramps which disappear spontaneously after a while or can be terminated by the administration of atropine. Some patients with achalasia of the cardia react positively on administration of as little as 1.5 mg of Mecholyl, but 6 mg seems to be the optimal dose (KRAMER and INGELFINGER, 1951). Practically, 2 to 3 mg of Mecholyl are administered subcutaneously or intramuscularly; if after 25 min no reaction occurs, another 2 to 3 mg is added, and this is repeated until a total dose of 6 to 10 mg is reached, unless a positive response occurs earlier (KRAMER et al., 1967 b). The reaction of the achalatic esophagus to Mecholyl has been interpreted as a manifestation of CANNON's law of denervation (1949): "When in a series of efferent neurons a unit is destroyed, an increased irritability to chemical agents develops in the isolated structure or structures, the effect being maximal in the part directly denervated". Indeed, in achalasia of the esophagus the parasympathetic innervation is interrupted by degeneration of the plexus of Auerbach. The degenerative lesions of Auerbach's plexus are more marked in the dilated portion of the esophagus than in the sphincteric region (CASSELLA et al., 1964), and there is a greater reduction in acetylcholinesterase activity in the body of the esophagus than in its distal portion (TROUNCE et al., 1957; ADAMS et al., 1960–1961).

The effect of Mecholyl on the esophagus was studied in esophageal diseases other than achalasia as well. In patients with Chagas' disease, CASTRO and GROSSI (1963) found a positive Mecholyl test in 92 percent of the cases. As the disease progresses the response to Mecholyl is reduced so that the most severely affected patients have no reaction at all.

KRAMER et al. (1963–1967 b) studied the effect of Mecholyl on the esophagus in patients with diffuse spasm. They distinguished between patients with "symp-

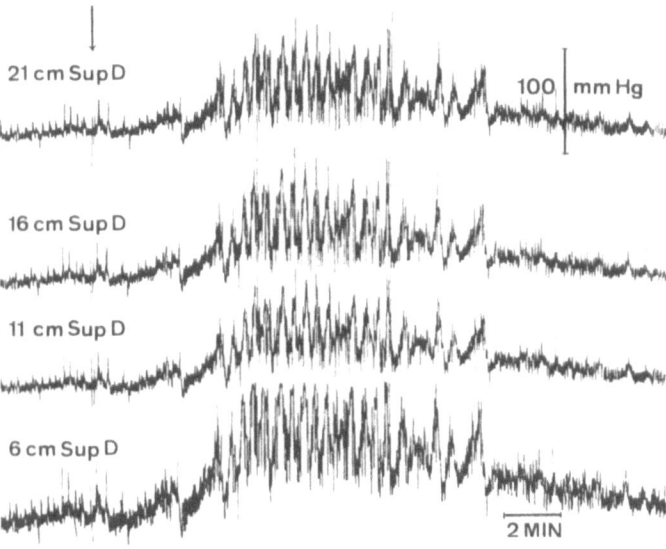

21 cm Sup D

100 mm Hg

16 cm Sup D

11 cm Sup D

6 cm Sup D

2 MIN

Fig. 146. Mecholyl test in a patient with achalasia. About 5 min after the injection of 5 mg of Mecholyl, simultaneous pressure peaks of high amplitude appear and last for about 15 min

tomatic diffuse spasm", (patients with a radiologically abnormal esophagus suggestive of diffuse spasm who also had esophageal complaints) and patients with "asymptomatic diffuse spasm", (who had similar radiological abnormalities but had no esophageal symptoms). Eleven out of fourteen patients with symptomatic diffuse spasm showed a positive Mecholyl response on balloon-kymography, though less pronounced than the response found in patients with achalasia. Of the group of patients with asymptomatic diffuse spasm none had a positive response. CREAMER et al. (1958) found that of their series of 23 patients with diffuse esophageal spasm, only three had a positive Mecholyl test and of these three two were not quite convincing. The influence of Mecholyl was also studied in patients with an obstruction at the level of the distal esophagus (KRAMER and INGELFINGER, 1951). Although a few patients had a somewhat more pronounced response than normals, a clearly positive response was never found. In cases of systemic sclerosis involving the esophagus, the Mecholyl test was negative (KRAMER and INGELFINGER, 1951). KRAMER et al. (1967) examined 10 patients with presbyesophagus and found the response to be normal. Though not all patients with achalasia of the cardia have a positive Mecholyl test (VAN-TRAPPEN, 1961; CODE and SCHLEGEL, 1969), it seems that the test is positive in the vast majority of the achalasia cases and negative in cases of other esophageal diseases. KRAMER et al. (1963–1967b) were the only ones to find a clearly positive response in most patients with "symptomatic diffuse spasm". Therefore the question must be raised whether this should not be ascribed to differences in methods of measuring esophageal motility. CODE and his co-workers used open-tip catheters in their manometric studies, while KRAMER's group used a fairly large balloon as an oncometer. Another possible explanation may be that the difference is simply a matter of semantics: perhaps KRAMER's "symptomatic diffuse spasm" and CODE's "vigorous achalasia" are terms applicable to the same group of patients. On the other hand it is quite possible that a positive

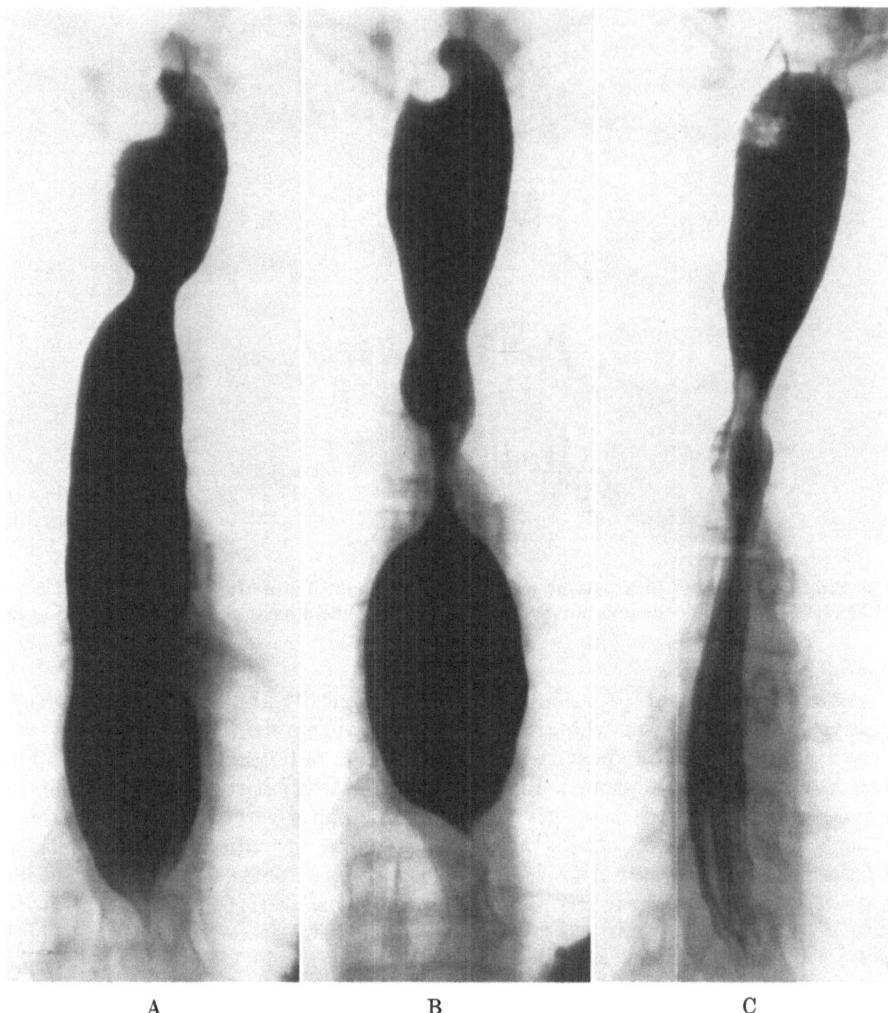

A   B   C

Fig. 147A–C. Mecholyl test in a patient with achalasia. Contractions appear 2 min after the injection of Mecholyl (A), become forceful after 3 min (B) and almost obliterate the lumen after 5 min (C)

Mecholyl response can be found in patients with "symptomatic diffuse spasm" because diffuse spasm and achalasia are not always clearly distinguishable (Hogan et al., 1969). Cases of diffuse spasm have already been described that later evolved into achalasia of the cardia (Schroder et al., 1963; Kramer et al., 1967a).

In recent years the Mecholyl test has become less popular as a diagnostic test of achalasia. Code and Schlegel (1969) described some cases with a positive Mecholyl response in which the severe substernal pain was not terminated by the administration of atropine. Intraluminal pressure measurements are less troublesome and the motor abnormalities they register in esophagus and gastro-esophageal sphincter are fairly characteristic for achalasia and form an equally reliable basis for the diagnosis of this disease.

References

ADAMS, C. W. M., BRAIN, R. H. F., ELLIS, F. G., KAUNTZE, R., TROUNCE, J. R.: Achalasia of the cardia. Guy's Hosp. Rep. 110, 191–236 (1961).

ADAMS, C. W. M., MARPLES, E. A., TROUNCE, J. R.: Achalasia of the cardia and Hirschsprung's disease. The amount and distribution of cholinesterases. Clin. Sci. 19, 473–481 (1960).

BUTIN, J. W., OLSEN, A. M., MOERSCH, H. J., CODE, C. F.: A study of esophageal pressures in normal persons and patients with cardiospasm. Gastroenterology 23, 278–293 (1953).

CANNON, W. B., ROSENBLUETH, A.: The supersensitivity of denervated structures. A law of denervation, p. 185. New York: MacMillan Co. 1949.

CASSELLA, R. R., BROWN, A. L., JR., SAYRE, G. P., ELLIS, F. H., JR.: Achalasia of the esophagus. Pathologic and etiologic considerations. Ann. Surg. 160, 474–486 (1964).

CASTRO, L. P. DE, GROSSI, C. A.: O teste do mecolil no diagnostico da aperistalsis do esofago. Rev. goiana Med. 9, 3 (1963).

CODE, C. F., SCHLEGEL, J. F.: In: Achalasia of the oesophagus, by F. H. ELLIS, JR. and A. M. OLSEN, Chapter III: Physiologic studies, p. 57–58. Philadelphia-London-Toronto: W. B. Saunders Co. 1969.

COHEN, B. R., GUELRUD, M.: Cardiospasm in achalasia: demonstration of supersensitivity of the lower esophageal sphincter (Abstract). Gastroenterology 60, 769 (1971).

CREAMER, B., DONOGHUE, F. E., CODE, C. F.: Patterns of esophageal motility in diffuse spasm. Gastroenterology 34, 782–796 (1958).

HEITMANN, P., ESPINOZA, J.: Oesophageal manometric studies in patients with chronic Chagas disease and megacolon. Gut 10, 848–851 (1969).

HEITMANN, P., ESPINOZA, J., CSENDES, A.: Physiology of the distal esophagus in achalasia. Scand. J. Gastroent. 4, 1–11 (1969).

HELLEMANS, J.: Invloed van de leeftijd op de motorische functie van de slokdarm. Tielt (Belgium): Lannoo 1970.

HIGHTOWER, N. C., JR., OLSEN, A. M., MOERSCH, H. J. A.: A comparison of the effects of acetyl-beta-methylcholine chloride (Mecholyl) on esophageal intraluminal pressure in normal persons and patients with cardiospasm. Gastroenterology 26, 592–600 (1954).

HOGAN, W. J., CAFLISCH, C. R., WINSHIP, D. H.: Unclassified oesophageal motor disorders simulating achalasia. Gut 10, 234–240 (1969).

JOHNSTONE, A. S.: Diffuse spasm and diffuse muscle hypertrophy of lower esophagus. Brit. J. Radiol. 33, 723–735 (1960).

KRAMER, P., FLESHLER, B., MCNALLY, E.: The pathophysiology of symptomatic "curling" or so-called "diffuse spasm". 2nd World Congress of Gastroenterology, Munich 1962, vol. 1, p. 57–59. Basel-New York: S. Karger 1963.

KRAMER, P., FLESHLER, B., MCNALLY, E., HARRIS, L. D.: Oesophageal sensitivity to mecholyl in symptomatic diffuse spasm. Gut 8, 120–127 (1967b).

KRAMER, P., HARRIS, L. D., DONALDSON, R. M., JR.: Transition from symptomatic diffuse spasm to cardiospasm. Gut 8, 115–119 (1967a).

KRAMER, P., INGELFINGER, F. J.: II. Cardiospasm, a generalized disorder of esophageal motility. Amer. J. Med. 7, 174–179 (1949).

KRAMER, P., INGELFINGER, F. J.: Esophageal sensitivity to Mecholyl in cardiospasm. Gastroenterology 19, 242–253 (1951).

KRAMER, P., INGELFINGER, F. J.: Esophageal sensitivity to Mecholyl in cardiospasm. Gastroenterology 54, 771–773 (1968).

KRAMER, P., INGELFINGER, F. J., ATKINSON, M.: The motility and pharmacology of the esophagus in cardiospasm. Gastroenterologia (Basel) 86, 174–178 (1956).

OLSEN, A. M., CREAMER, B.: Studies of oesophageal motility with special reference to the differential diagnosis of diffuse spasm and achalasia (cardiospasm). Thorax 12, 279–289 (1957).

PADEN, P. A.: Corkscrew esophagus. U.S. armed Forces med. J. 5, 1371–1374 (1954).

ROTH, H. P., FLESHLER, B.: Diffuse esophageal spasm. Ann. intern. Med. 61, 914–923 (1964).

SCHRODER, S., ACHORD, J. L., ROGERS, J. V., JR.: Achalasia preceded by noncardiospastic diffuse esophageal spasm: A cineriadographic study (Abstract). Gastroenterology 44, 849 (1963).

SHEINMEL, A., PRIVITERI, C. A., POPPEL, M. H.: A study of the effect of certain drugs on curling of the esophagus: a preliminary report. Amer. J. Roentgenol. 62, 807–813 (1949).

TROUNCE, J. R., DEUCHAR, D. C., KAUNTZE, R., THOMAS, G. A.: Studies in achalasia of the cardia. Quart. J. Med. 26, 433–443 (1957).

VANTRAPPEN, G.: Slokdarmmotiliteit. Brussel: Arscia Uitg. N.V. 1961.

Electromyography of the Esophagus

J. HELLEMANS, G. VANTRAPPEN, and J. JANSSENS

With 14 Figures

1. Introduction

Electromyographic examination of skeletal muscles with extracellular detection techniques has already been in clinical use for a long time. Several diseases of the muscles and their innervation cause a typical and often diagnostic electromyographic pattern. It may therefore be anticipated that the electromyographic exploration of the gastrointestinal tract also will come to clinical use. The electrical activity of stomach, small intestine and colon of animals has been studied intensively, both in vivo and in vitro, and has yielded important data on the regulation of the contraction patterns in these organs. Electromyographic examination of the esophagus, however, is of quite recent date. CHRISTENSEN and DANIEL (1966) used an in-vitro technique to study the electrical activity in strips of the longitudinal and circular muscle layer of the distal feline esophagus and found that spike potentials, which were sometimes superposed on slow waves, could be recorded upon contraction of these muscles. ROMAN (1966, 1967) studied the peristaltic mechanism of the sheep esophagus and observed that deglutition produced spike potentials which occurred immediately before the muscle contraction. These data were later confirmed by DOUGHERTY et al. (1971). INOUYE (1966) studied the electrical activity of the esophagus of dogs and cats under general anesthesia. The esophageal deglutitive activity could not be studied under these experimental conditions. In addition to spontaneous spiking activity in the cricopharyngeal muscle, this author also noticed spike potentials in the lower segment of the esophagus, coinciding with inspiration. After vagotomy he found signs of denervation (fibrillation potentials, positive sharp waves) and of regeneration (giant potentials, polyphasic potentials).

ARIMORI et al. (1965, 1966, 1970), using chronically implanted electrodes, studied the electrical pattern of the canine esophagus at rest and after deglutition, and found that upon deglutition a wave of action potentials proceeded down the esophagus, followed immediately by the contraction wave. In the gastroesophageal sphincter they found a continuous phasic activity which disappeared immediately after deglutition. They considered this disappearance to be related to the sphincteric relaxation. After deglutition they noticed in the sphincter a burst of action potentials which preceded the sphincteric contraction. Independent studies by HELLEMANS and VANTRAPPEN (1967) yielded analogous results. These authors described in detail the burst of deglutitive action potentials, which moved down the esophagus in a peristaltic way and was exactly correlated in time with the final peak of the deglutitive pressure complex (Fig. 148). In addition they described the phenomenon of the deglutitive electrical inhibition. At the level of the gastroesophageal sphincter, however, no slow waves were found at rest. HELLEMANS et al. (1968) studied the electrical activity of the esophagus of cats and monkeys. The esophagus of these animals resembles that of

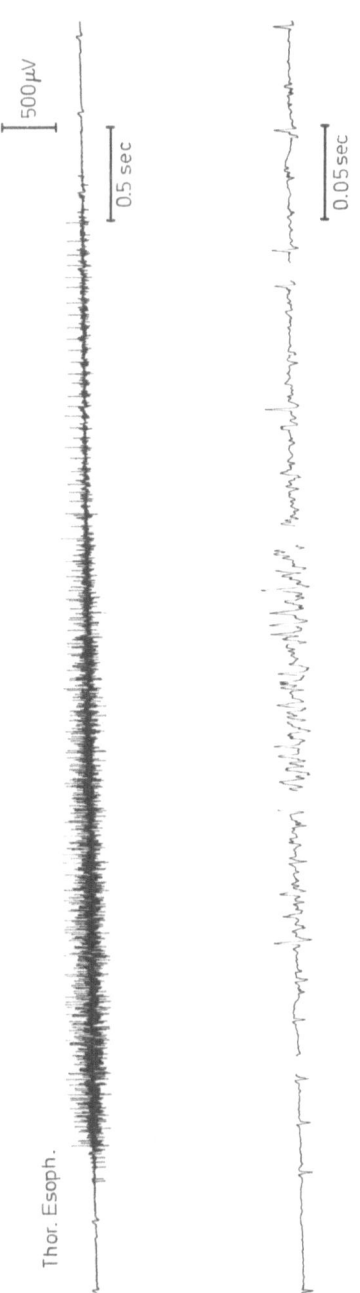

Fig. 148. E.M.G. of deglutitive contraction of the canine thoracic esophagus. The lower trace shows portions of the same spike burst, recorded at a higher speed, to illustrate the consecutive phases of the deglutitive electrical activity (single, intermediary, interferential, intermediary and second single tracing)

man, in that it consists of striated muscle in the upper segments, and of smooth muscle in the lower segments. They recorded two types of action potentials corresponding to the two types of muscles. At the transitional zone between the smooth and striated muscles the deglutitive spike burst contained both types of action potentials. ROMAN and TIEFENBACH (1971), and TIEFENBACH and ROMAN (1972) obtained comparable tracings in the smooth musculature of the cat and monkey esophagus. In cats they observed after vagotomy a certain degree of spontaneous activity which could be compared to the pendular movements of the small intestine.

In the study of the animal esophagus the electromyographic technique has already been perfected to such an extent that in certain experiments some authors (ROMAN and CAR, 1970; JEAN, 1972; JANSSENS et al., 1973) prefer it to intraluminal pressure measurements to register the esophageal activity. The electromyographic study of the human esophagus remains in a considerably less advanced stage, mainly because registration poses serious problems, as it is necessary to detect the electrical activity from the mucosal side. Already in 1964 STOICHITA and BROSTEANO published electromyographic tracings of the human esophagus, recorded by means of an intraluminal probe containing surface electrodes. GOODMAN et al. (1966) published similar tracings, obtained with a similar technique. They described a slow wave which develops almost simultaneously with the deglutition complex. Studies by CHRISTENSEN (1967) and by HELLEMANS (1970), however, demonstrated that the physiological significance of these recordings is highly doubtful.

Movement of the intraluminal probe during esophageal contractions may cause significant artifacts. To prevent such movements, MONGES et al. (1968) and HELLEMANS et al. (1970b) devised a capsule containing two or more pins which can be firmly fixed against the esophageal wall by applying a negative pressure through a hole in the capsule. With this technique valid electromyographic tracings can be recorded in the striated as well as in the smooth muscle portion of the human esophagus. It also offers the possibility of locating the zone of transition between both muscle types. TOKITA et al. (1970) obtained electromyographic tracings of the human esophagus by means of an intraluminal probe with ring electrodes, which allowed simultaneous registration at different levels. Once the probe has been swallowed, it can be curved so as to bring it in closer contact with the esophageal wall. This technique also allowed the authors to distinguish the activities of striated and smooth muscles.

2. Registration Method

The best electromyographic tracings of the human esophagus thusfar were obtained by means of an intraluminal capsule with needle electrodes which was sucked against the esophageal wall. MONGES et al. (1968) used a rubber capsule containing two silver electrodes at a distance of 4 mm; via a catheter, ending in the center of the capsule, a negative pressure can be applied, which sucks the capsule against the esophageal wall. The capsule devised by HELLEMANS et al. (1970b) (Fig. 149). consists of plexiglass and contains 4 to 8 platinum covered stainless steel needles with a length of 4 mm and a diameter of 0.1 mm at the top. Via an external switching device it is possible to choose a number of bipolar combinations; thus the distance between the recording electrodes can be 2, 4 or 6 mm and a longitudinal, circular or oblique direction of detection can be chosen. An open tip catheter, which ends in the middle of the capsule, allows the intraluminal pressure to be measured at the level of the EMG capsule. The electrical activity is recorded on a multichannel recording apparatus using a preamplifier of high-ohmic differential input (>10 MOhm). To prevent artificial base line oscillations it is mostly necessary to use a time constant, which will

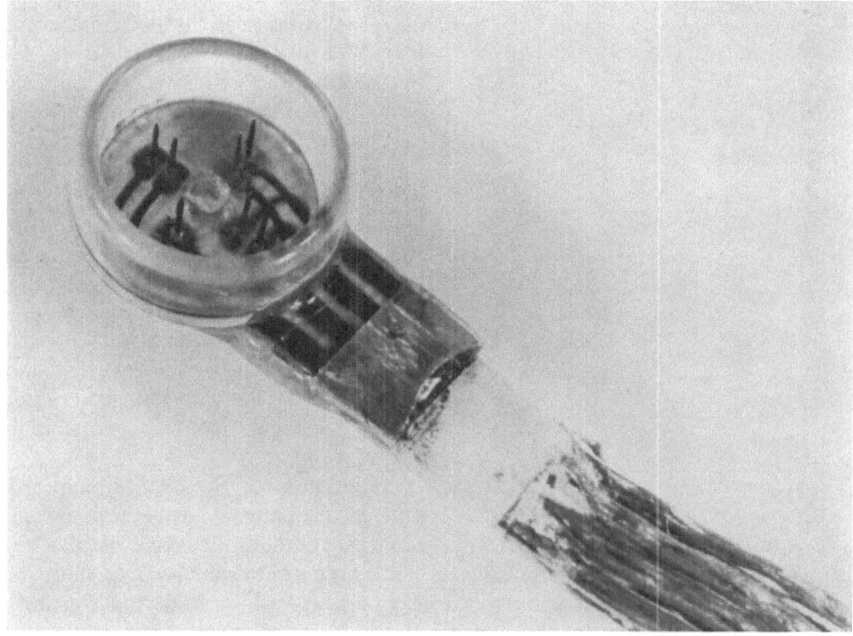

Fig. 149. Suction capsule for recording electrical activity in the human esophagus

be of the order of 0.3 to 0.015 sec if spike potentials are to be recorded. This time constant must be much greater (1 to 5 sec) if slow phenomena are to be detected.

3. The Electromyographic Tracings

In the description of the results obtained with this technique the esophagus will be arbitrarily divided into 5 segments. Furthermore, a distinction will be made between the electrical phenomena of the esophagus at rest and the deglutitive electrical activity.

3.1. The Pharyngoesophageal Sphincter

A continuous spiking activity was recorded in the pharyngoesophageal sphincter "at rest". The richness of the tracing and the number of spikes with a different configuration (i.e. the number of muscle units in action) depend on the

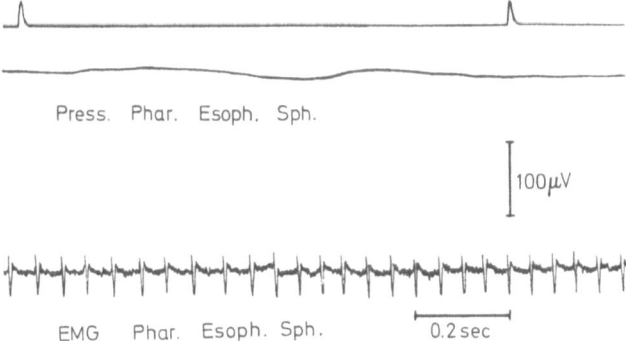

Fig. 150. E.M.G. recorded in human pharyngoesophageal sphincter with bipolar intraluminal suction electrode. Striated muscle spikes of a constant configuration are present in the resting state, the intrasphincteric pressure (Press. Phar. Esoph. Sph.) remaining constant

degree of contraction of the sphincter at a given moment. Sometimes spikes of a constant configuration follow each other at a regular interval as long as the intrasphincteric pressure remains constant (Fig. 150).

If the intraluminal pressure increases, a richer tracing appears, composed of different types of spikes. The spike potentials have the typical appearance of striated muscle spikes. The continuous spiking activity in the sphincter may be due in part to the presence of the distending capsule, which may elicit a reflex contraction of the cricopharyngeal muscle. The same phenomenon is observed in dogs and monkeys; with needle electrodes chronically implanted in the cricopharyngeal muscle, a continuous spiking activity can be recorded, the richness of the tracing depending on the degree of alertness of the animal. If it is very quiet or almost asleep, there may sometimes be a total absence of spiking activity or an absence of spiking during expiration and a very poor tracing during inspiration. Similar observations were made by LEVITT et al. (1965) who studied the influence of the degree of anesthesia on the spiking activity in the cricopharyngeal muscle of dogs. During light anesthesia some spiking activity was observed on inspiration, whereas all spiking activity in the sphincter disappeared during deep anesthesia.

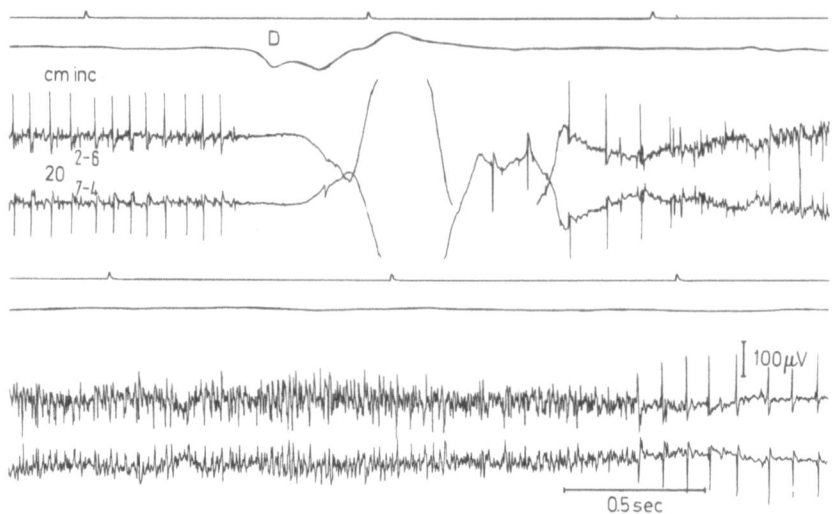

Fig. 151. Deglutitive inhibition of electrical activity in the human pharyngoesophageal sphincter recorded with bipolar intraluminal suction electrode. The continuous spiking activity, recorded in the "resting" sphincter, is inhibited by a deglutition (D) (cm inc.: number of centimeters from the incisors)

Upon deglutition the continuous spiking activity in the pharyngoesophageal sphincter is immediately and completely inhibited for 0.2 to 0.8 sec; this interruption is followed immediately by the deglutitive spike burst (Hellemans, 1970; Vantrappen and Hellemans, 1970). Sometimes a slight increase in the rhythm of the continuous spiking activity is observed just before the inhibition. The phenomenon of electrical inhibition of the pharyngoesophageal sphincter coincides with the fall of intraluminal pressure that accompanies sphincter relaxation (Fig. 151). The spike burst which accompanies the deglutitive contraction of the sphincter is qualitatively comparable to that occurring in the striated muscle of the esophagus just below the sphincter. It is discussed in Section 3.2. The increase of the intraluminal pressure in the cricopharyngeal sphincter seems to be closely correlated with the richness of the tracing. When the intraluminal pressure wave returns slowly to the base-line pressure, a burst of electrical activity of long duration is recorded, which lasts as long as the intrasphincteric pressure wave and becomes progressively poorer as the pressure slowly decreases.

3.2. The Striated Muscle Segment of the Esophagus

At rest neither spike potentials nor slow waves are observed in this segment of the esophagus. After deglutition, however, a burst of striated muscle spikes occurs (Fig. 152), which is comparable to the deglutitive spike burst in the canine esophagus (Hellemans and Vantrappen, 1967; Arimori et al., 1965, 1966, 1970), or in that segment of the monkey and cat esophagus which consists entirely of striated muscles (Hellemans et al., 1968).

The tracing begins with a series of rhythmic spikes of identical configuration. This single tracing is soon followed by an intermediary tracing, in which spikes of different configurations are interposed among these single spikes. Then there is a rapid transition from an intermediary to an interferential tracing, in which

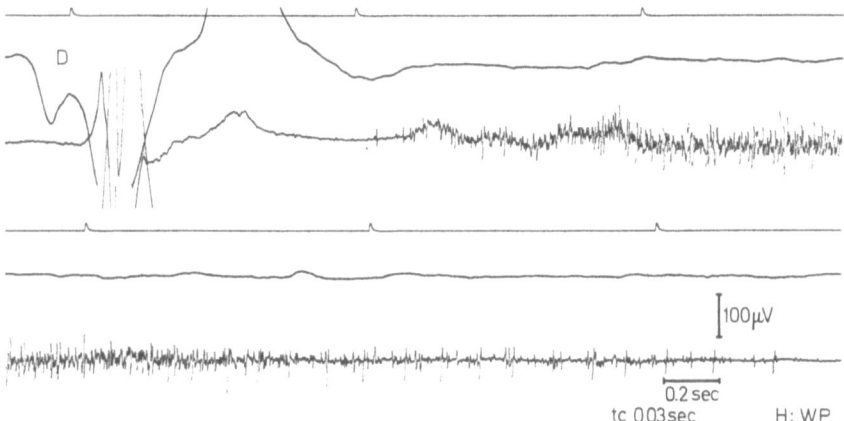

Fig. 152. E.M.G. of deglutitive contraction recorded in the striated muscle portion of the human esophagus with bipolar intraluminal suction electrode. Upper tracing: deglutition signal (D)

spikes become so numerous that, due to the confluence and summation of spikes, the base-line disappears and oscillations of markedly increased amplitude ensue. Subsequently, the number of spikes per unit of time again decreases, giving rise to a short second intermediary and a final single tracing, which usually lasts longer than the initial single tracing. The rhythm and configuration of the spikes recorded with this technique can best be analyzed on a single tracing; the action potentials show as biphasic spikes occurring rhythmically at a rate of 10 to 15 per sec with a duration of 8 to 10 msec. Recordings in the canine esophagus by means of chronically implanted bipolar needle electrodes at a distance of 2 mm show the spike rhythm of the single tracing to be much faster than in man (about 40 per sec), whereas the duration of the action potentials is shorter (about 5 msec) (HELLEMANS and VANTRAPPEN, 1967). Almost identical results are obtained in the striated muscle segment of monkeys (HELLEMANS et al., 1968) (Table 10).

At this level of the human esophagus there is a close relation between deglutitive action potentials and the mechanical response, the spike burst lasting until the final peak of the deglutitive pressure complex reaches the base-line pressure (MONGES et al., 1968; HELLEMANS, 1970).

3.3. The Transitional Zone between Striated and Smooth Muscles

At a distance of 2 to 6 cm below the pharyngoesophageal junction, the musculature of the human esophagus gradually changes from striated to smooth muscles. This corresponds to the electromyographic observations that two types of spike potentials can be recorded at a distance of 24 to 25 cm from the upper incisors (HELLEMANS et al., 1970b, 1971) (Fig. 153). In between deglutitions there is no spontaneous activity in this zone, but after deglutition a burst of action potentials occurs, often beginning and sometimes also ending with spikes of the striated muscle type. An identical electromyographic pattern is recorded in the esophagus of monkeys at a level where the longitudinal layer was found to consist mainly of striated muscles and the circular coat mainly of smooth

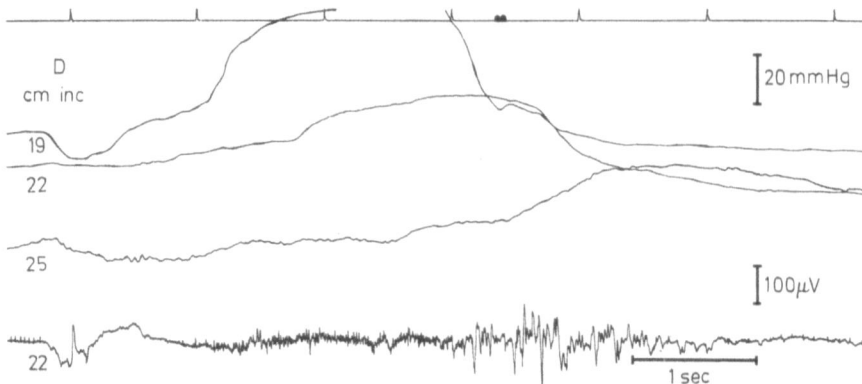

Fig. 153. E.M.G. registered in the human esophagus with bipolar intraluminal suction electrode in the transitional zone between striated and smooth muscle portions at 22 cm from
the incisors (cm inc.). Simultaneous intraluminal pressure measurements at 19, 22 and 25 cm
from the incisors. The electrical tracing shows two types of spike potentials

muscles (HELLEMANS et al., 1968). As the striated muscle fibers of the human
esophagus reach further distally in the longitudinal than in the circular layer,
this spike sequence suggests that the longitudinal layer contracts before the
circular coat.

Spikes of the smooth muscle type can easily be distinguished from those
originating in the striated muscles; their characteristics are described in Section 3.4.
How information is transmitted from the striated to the smooth muscle segment
remains unknown. Under certain circumstances both types of spikes no longer
occur in their normal sequence but appear to be disconnected. Thus HELLEMANS
et al. (1968) noticed that in monkeys secondary peristaltic contractions in this
zone consist only of smooth muscle spikes (without an associated striated muscle
component), and that anticholinergics disconnect the normal sequence (HELLE-
MANS, 1970).

3.4. The Smooth Muscle Segment of the Esophagus

At rest neither spike potentials nor slow waves are observed in the smooth
muscle portion of the human esophagus (MONGES et al., 1968; HELLEMANS et al.,
1970b). Deglutition elicits a burst of action potentials which have characteristics
entirely different from those originating in the striated esophageal muscles
(MONGES et al., 1968; HELLEMANS et al., 1970b). Smooth muscle spikes have
a greater amplitude and a markedly longer duration. Usually the tracing consists
of a mixture of spikes with different configurations. Sometimes one type returns
more or less regularly (Fig. 154). The rhythm of spiking in these tracings varies
between 3.2 and 4 per sec and the duration of the individual spikes is between
80 and 200 msec when bipolar electrodes are used with an interelectrode distance
of 6 mm. In the most distal part of the esophagus their rhythm is slower still
(2.7 sec) and their duration longer (about 200 msec) (Table 10). This type of
tracing resembles fairly well the burst of deglutitive spikes recorded in the
smooth muscle portion of the cat and monkey esophagus (HELLEMANS et al.,
1968; ROMAN and TIEFENBACH, 1971; TIEFENBACH and ROMAN, 1972), except
that the rhythm is faster and the duration considerably shorter in these animals
(HELLEMANS, 1970) (Table 10).

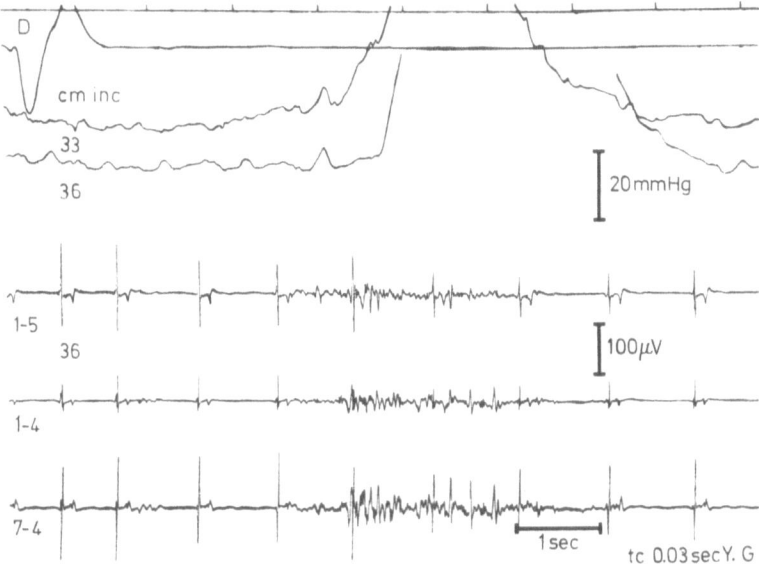

Fig. 154. E.M.G. recorded in the smooth muscle portion of the human esophagus with bipolar intraluminal suction electrode at 36 cm from the incisors (cm inc.). *1–5* E.M.G. detected in longitudinal direction; distance between needle electrodes 4 mm. *1–4* E.M.G. detected in oblique direction; distance between needle electrodes 3.75 mm. *7–4* E.M.G. detected in circular direction; distance between needle electrodes 5 mm. Simultaneous intraluminal pressure measurements at 33 and 36 cm from the incisors. Upper tracing: deglutition signal (*D*)

Table 10

	Rhythm/sec	Duration in msec
Striated muscle		
Dog	34–45	4–6
Man	10–15	8–10
Smooth muscle		
Monkey	6–9	16–40
Man	2,7–4	80–200

On electromyographic tracings recorded in the human esophagus by means of an intraluminal suction capsule, the initial spikes of the deglutitive response appear most clearly if the detection needles of the electrode are placed along the longitudinal axis of the esophagus; the final spikes are clearer if they are placed in a circular direction. It is not yet known whether this pattern corresponds to the α and β spikes described by ROMAN and TIEFENBACH (1971) and by TIEFENBACH and ROMAN (1972). According to these authors the action potentials originating in the longitudinal layer of the smooth muscle esophagus of cats and monkeys can be recognized as α spikes, those of the circular layer as β spikes. The gradual increase and the subsequent gradual decrease in amplitude and rhythm of the spikes, characteristic of the deglutitive response

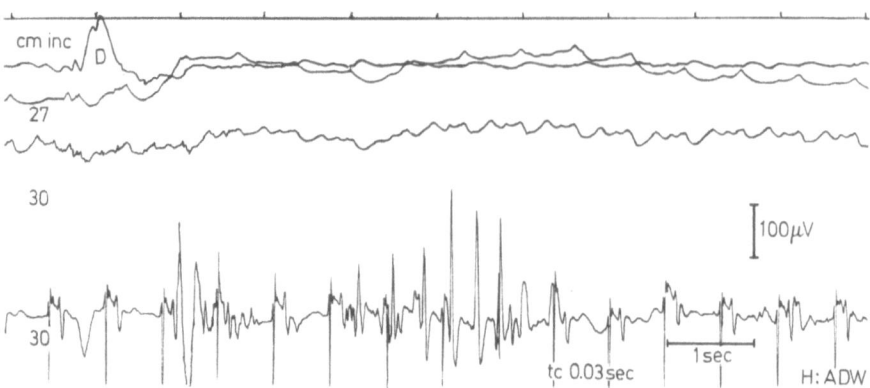

Fig. 155. E.M.G. registered in the human esophagus with bipolar intraluminal suction electrode at 30 cm from the incisors (cm inc.). Simultaneous intraluminal pressure measurements at 27 and 30 cm from the incisors. Swallowing induced a tracing of single smooth muscle spikes, which was associated by only a small increase in intraluminal pressure

of the striated muscle portion of the esophagus, are not observed in the burst of smooth muscle spikes.

Simultaneous manometric and electromyographic studies in this segment (HELLEMANS, 1970) indicate that swallowing often elicits repetitive pressure waves or pressure waves which show a second small rise of pressure, just before the descending limb of the main deglutitive pressure peak reaches the base-line pressure, and that both pressure changes are associated with action potentials. It is not impossible that these additional pressure phenomena are due to the presence of an intraluminal recording capsule, which may act as a foreign body eliciting secondary peristaltic contractions.

Rhythmic spikes of identical configuration can be observed in this segment of the esophagus, both in men and in animals. This suggests that the smooth muscles are organized in functional units just as the striated muscles. Exceptionally the burst of deglutitive electrical activity consists entirely of a series of identical spikes (Fig. 155); such a deglutitive response produces only a small increase in intraluminal pressure, probably because only one functional unit participates in the contraction.

Simultaneous recordings of intraluminal pressures and electrical activity indicate that the spike burst precedes the pressure wave by 1.33 ± 0.06 sec in young people and by 1.70 ± 0.12 sec in older subjects. In contrast with the response in the striated muscle esophagus, smooth muscle action potentials never occur after the peak pressure of the deglutitive pressure complex has been reached. This seems to indicate that during the return to the base-line pressure the smooth muscle is no longer contracting actively.

In addition to the burst of electrical activity which accompanies the main deglutitive contraction, a few spikes are often observed which occur immediately after the act of swallowing and are clearly separated from the main deglutitive spike burst; they can best be registered with the detection needles of the recording electrode located along the longitudinal axis. These spikes coincide with the first positive wave of the deglutitive pressure complex (see Physiology 3.2.2.2.).

The second positive wave is not accompanied by action potentials (HELLEMANS, 1970).

3.5. The Gastroesophageal Sphincter

The physiological characteristics of the gastroesophageal sphincter are quite different from those of the esophagus proper. At rest, in the absence of any deglutition, it is closed by a tonic contraction, which can be recorded manometrically as a high resting pressure. Deglutition causes a relaxation of this segment, followed by a contraction which is weaker and lasts longer than the contraction of the esophagus proper. It was to be expected that these differences would be reflected in the electromyographic recordings. In their experiments

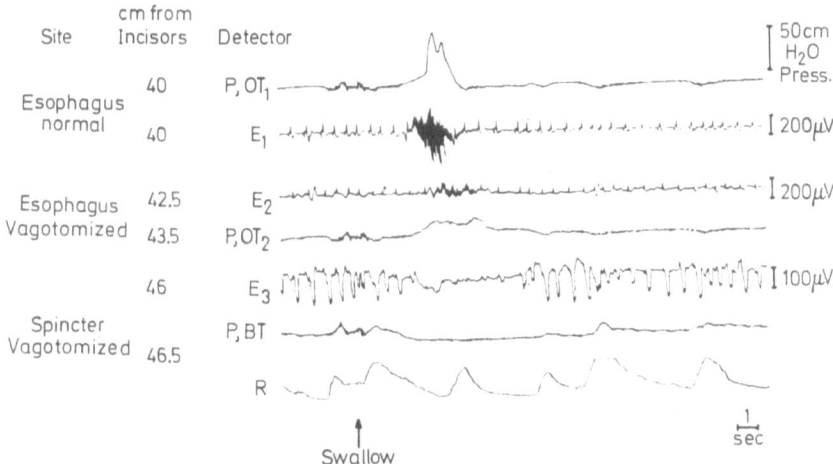

Fig. 156. Simultaneous recordings of pressure (*P*) and electrical activity in a dog with subhilar vagotomy. The slow phasic activity observed in the sphincter disappears after swallowing and returns to preswallow pattern with return of sphincteric pressure (*P, BT*).
[From ARIMORI et al., Amer. J. dig. Dis. **15**, 191 (1970)]

on dogs with chronically implanted electrodes, ARIMORI et al. (1970) described in this zone small phasic changes of electrical potential, which are independent of deglutition and occur at a rate of 1.4 to 2.1 per sec. This activity could best be recorded in the distal part of the gastroesophageal sphincter. This slow phasic electrical activity was nearly always diminished or abolished by a deglutition and this phenomenon coincided with the sphincteric relaxation (Fig. 156). Consequently the authors connected these slow electrical phenomena with the increased resting pressure in the gastroesophageal sphincter and assumed that they were generated by the circular muscle layer, which consists of smooth muscle fibers in the dog (MANN and SHORTER, 1964). Analogous slow waves were also observed by THOMAS and EARLAM (1972) in their in vitro studies on the sphincteric zone of the canine esophagogastric segment. The deglutitive spike burst in the canine gastroesophageal sphincter, as described by ARIMORI et al. (1970), consisted of action potentials which occurred at a markedly slower rhythm than in more proximal parts of the esophagus and which lasted considerably longer. These differences were interpreted by the authors as a result of the changes the striated muscle fibers of the canine esophagus undergo as they participate in the construction of the sphincter. In their experiments on dogs with chronically implanted electrodes HELLEMANS and VANTRAPPEN (1967) could not register slow phasic waves in the gastroesophageal sphincter; they were unable to demonstrate an electrical equivalent of the resting tone and of the relaxation of the sphincter. Moreover, the postdeglutitive spikes in the sphincter were not clearly different from the spikes originating more proximally in the esophagus; at most the over-all duration of the spike burst was somewhat longer in the sphincter.

Analogous results were obtained in the gastroesophageal sphincter of cats and monkeys (HELLEMANS et al., 1968). Neither spontaneous electrical activity nor any electrical equivalent of the sphincteric relaxation could be recorded from this smooth muscle sphincter. The deglutitive spike burst was entirely comparable to that occurring in the immediately proximal segment.

The electromyographic pattern of the human gastroesophageal sphincter is poorly known thusfar, mainly because of the technical problems recording poses in a high pressure zone, where it is difficult to fix a capsule. The studies of MONGES et al. (1968) do not allow a clear description of the electrical phenomena in the human gastroesophageal sphincter. HELLEMANS (1970) found neither spontaneous activity nor any electrical equivalent of the sphincteric relaxation. The deglutitive burst of action potentials in the sphincter consisted of spikes which, on the whole, were indistinguishable from those in the smooth muscle esophagus. As in cats and monkeys the duration of the deglutitive spike burst in the human gastroesophageal sphincter was not noticeably longer than in other parts of the smooth muscle esophagus, although the duration of the positive pressure wave in the sphincter clearly exceeded that in the esophagus proper. Apparently the mechanism responsible for the slow relaxation of the gastroesophageal sphincter after a contraction still escapes our current electromyographic techniques.

4. The Deglutitive Inhibition

If swallows are taken in rapid succession, no peristaltic wave appears until after the last swallow, because a new deglutition inhibits the activity of the previous swallow. This phenomenon of deglutitive inhibition has a clear electromyographic equivalent. In dogs, which have an esophagus consisting almost entirely of striated muscle, a deglutition inhibits all spiking activity in the thoracic esophagus for a period of 0.2 to 0.3 sec; after this short interruption the spiking activity continues normally (HELLEMANS and VANTRAPPEN, 1967). This inhibition occurs almost simultaneously over the whole length of the esophagus, including the gastroesophageal sphincter. In the cricopharyngeal sphincter and in the cervical esophagus of dogs, a second deglutition causes all electrical activity produced by a previous swallow to disappear entirely and definitively (Fig. 157); this is accompanied by a fall of pressure. Though the esophagus of monkeys consists of striated muscles in its proximal segment and of smooth muscles in its distal portion, the pattern of deglutitive inhibition is the same over the whole length of the gullet (HELLEMANS et al., 1968). A second deglutition causes an immediate and definitive halt of all spike activity, both in the striated and in the smooth esophageal segment, as well as in the gastroesophageal sphincter (Fig. 158). In humans, a distinction must be made between the smooth and striated muscle segments of the esophagus (HELLEMANS, 1970; VANTRAPPEN and HELLEMANS, 1970; HELLEMANS et al., 1970a; VANTRAPPEN et al., 1971). In the cricopharyngeal sphincter and in the zone where the spike burst consists entirely of striated muscle spikes, deglutition results in the immediate disappearance of all spiking activity, both spontaneous and deglutitive, and is accompanied by a decrease in intraluminal pressure. Swallowing also inhibits the spiking activity in the transitional zone where striated and smooth muscle are intermingled. In the distal segment, which consists of smooth muscles, the pattern

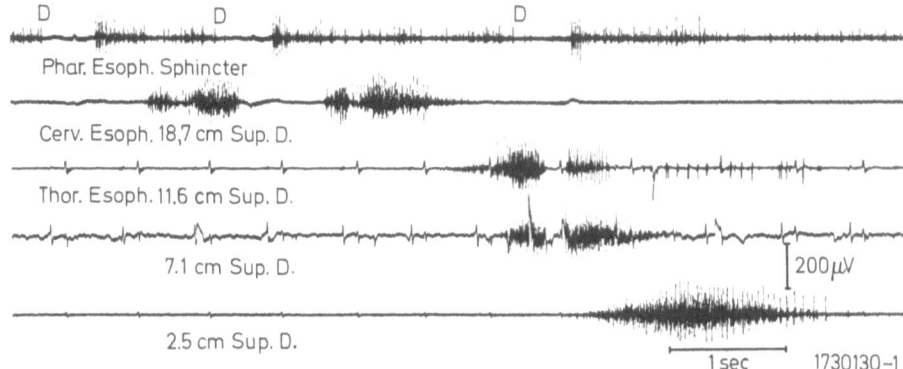

Fig. 157. Deglutitive inhibition of electrical activity in canine esophagus. The recordings were made with chronically implanted bipolar needle electrodes. Deglutition (D) results in a complete inhibition of the continuous spiking activity of the pharyngoesophageal sphincter and of the spiking activity elicited by a previous swallow in the cervical esophagus. In the thoracic esophagus, however, deglutition produces only a short interruption of the spiking activity of a previous deglutition

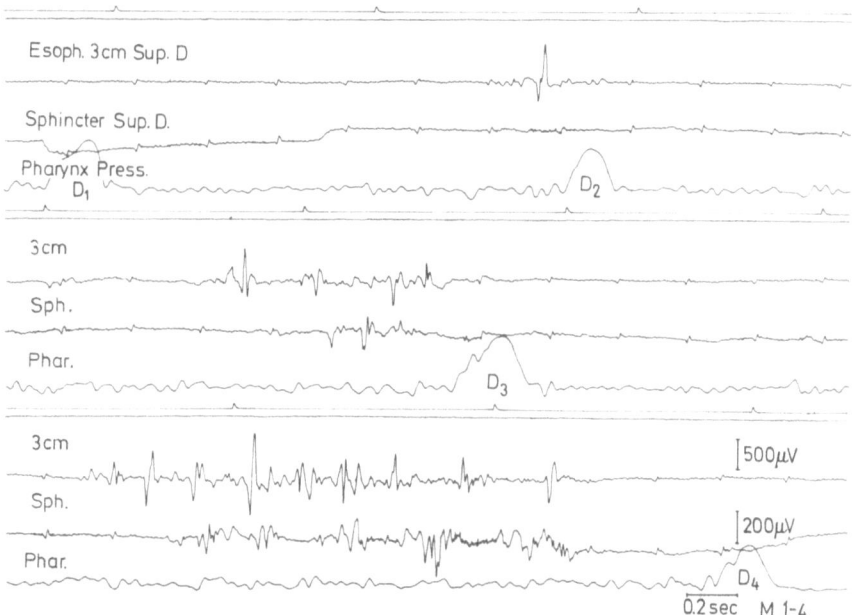

Fig. 158. E.M.G. recorded in the smooth muscle portion of the monkey esophagus with chronically implanted bipolar needle electrodes. Continuous record of successive deglutitions $(D_1–D_2–D_3–D_4)$. D_2 and D_3 occur during the burst of spike activity elicited by the preceding swallow and result in inhibition of this spike burst. Sup. D: supradiaphragmatic

is different. If the second deglutition occurs immediately before or during the initial phase of a spike burst, it does not interrupt the spiking activity in this esophageal segment; yet the distal progression of the spike burst is halted and the deglutitive pressure wave does not proceed further distally (Fig. 159).

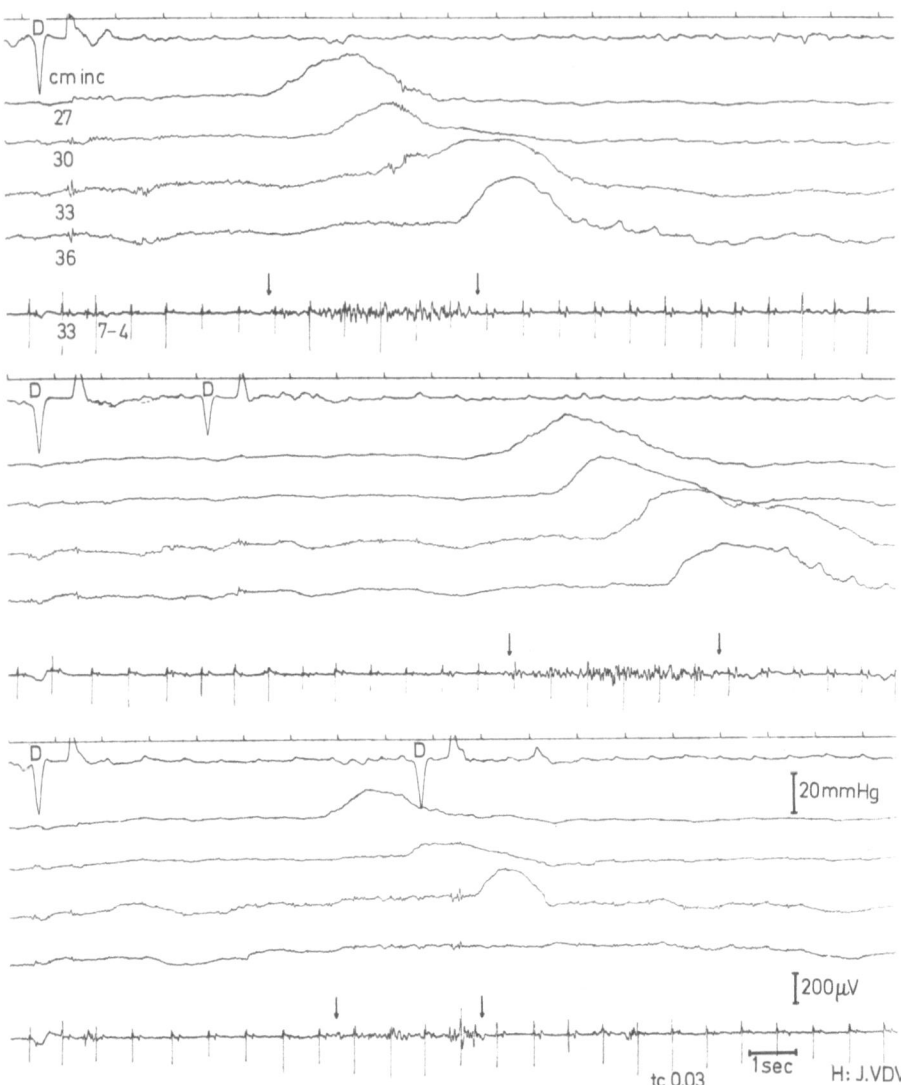

Fig. 159. Deglutitive inhibition in the human esophagus. Simultaneous intraluminal pressure measurements (at 27, 30, 33 and 36 cm from the incisors) and E.M.G. at 33 cm from the incisors. Upper part: normal deglutitive response. Middle part: a deglutition 3.5 sec after a previous swallow eliminates the deglutitive response to the first deglutition. Lower part: if the second deglutition occurs during the spike burst of a previous swallow, it does not inhibit the spiking activity in this esophageal segment but the distal progression is halted. Upper line is deglutition (D) signal

5. Electromyography in Esophageal Diseases

Electromyography of the human esophagus is still so much in its initial stage that it has not yet been applied to the study of esophageal diseases. Yet a few experiments have been carried out on animals under conditions that approach certain esophageal diseases. Inouye (1966) studied the electrical activity of the

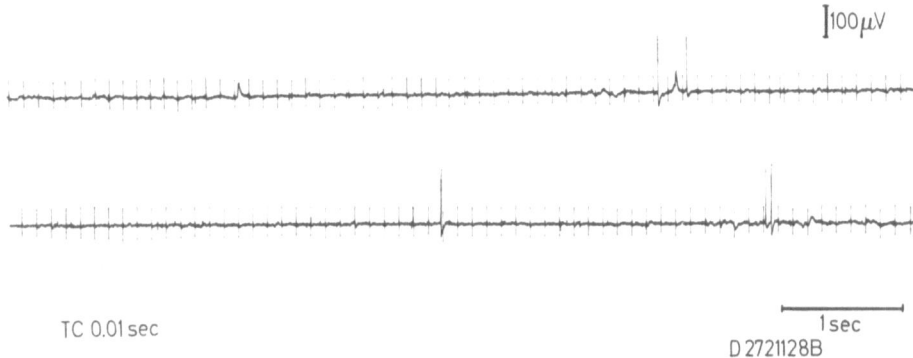

Fig. 160. Rhythmic fibrillation potentials (8.3/sec) in the canine thoracic esophagus, 30 days after unilateral cervical vagotomy

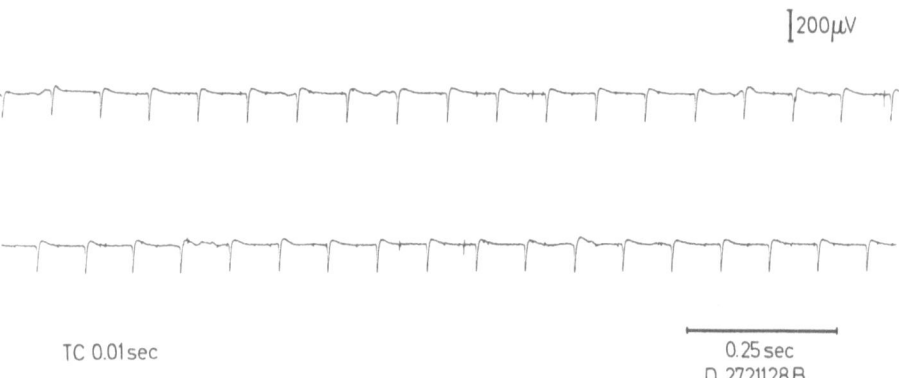

Fig. 161. Positive sharp waves in the canine esophagus after unilateral cervical vagotomy. *TC* time constant

esophagus of dogs and cats after uni- and bilateral cervical vagotomy. The tracings were registered by means of needle electrodes, inserted into the esophageal wall during general anesthesia via an esophagoscope. After an interval of 8 to 10 days in dogs and of 10 to 14 days in cats he found fibrillation potentials and positive sharp waves over a long stretch of the esophagus. Signs of reinnervation, such as giant motor unit potentials, nascent motor unit potentials and polyphasic potentials appeared after 9 weeks in dogs and after 12 weeks in cats. Analogous results were obtained by PELEMANS et al. (1973) (Figs. 160, 161). ROMAN and TIEFENBACH (1971) performed a series of acute experiments in cats to study the effect of vagotomy. An electrical activity of weak amplitude was observed, which was independent of any peristalsis and was accompanied by contractions of the longitudinal muscle layer of the esophagus. These contraction waves moved both in an oral and in an aboral direction and reminded the authors of the pendular movements of the small intestine.

HELLEMANS (1970) studied the effect of anticholinergics on human esophageal motility. The disturbances found on manometry resemble those of diffuse spasm of the esophagus or of the presbyesophagus. Moreover, he observed that the progression of the peristaltic contraction was disturbed at the zone of transition between striated and smooth musculature. Electromyographic studies in monkeys confirmed this observation. After the administration of anticholinergics the deglutitive electrical activity of striated and smooth esophageal musculature in the transitional zone appeared no longer to be coordinated; it seemed as if anticholinergics cause a functional disconnection of both types of esophageal muscles. It has not yet been established whether or not similar disturbances occur at the transitional zone of patients with diffuse spasm.

TOKITA et al. (1970) described the electromyographic pattern of a patient with "idiopathic dilatation of the esophagus". Deglutition produced a spike burst progressing in a peristaltic way. The administration of Mecholyl resulted in the appearance of "frequent sporadic spike discharges" from the mid- as well as from the lower esophagus. A fit of pain after esophagoscopy was associated with a spike salvo of low amplitude and high frequency in the abdominal esophagus of this patient. This spiking activity increased after deglutition and disappeared entirely when the pain was over. The authors correlated this abdominal spiking pattern with cardiospasm. The data of TOKITA et al. (1970) need further confirmation, as they pertain to only one case. Moreover, there are major differences between the tracings of normals given by TOKITA et al. (1970) and those given by MONGES et al. (1968) and HELLEMANS (1970). Perhaps they are due to differences in recording techniques.

References

ARIMORI, M., CODE, C. F., SCHLEGEL, J. F., STURM, R. E.: Electrical activity of the canine esophagus and gastroesophageal sphincter: its relation to intraluminal pressure and movement of material. Amer. J. dig. Dis. 15, 191–208 (1970).

ARIMORI, M., SCHLEGEL, J. F., CODE, C. F.: Action potentials of esophagus and gastroesophageal sphincter in dogs. Physiologist 8, 103 (1965).

ARIMORI, M., SCHLEGEL, J. F., CODE, C. F., STURM, R.: Relationships between electrical activity and intraluminal pressure and movement of material in the esophagus. Fed. Proc. 25, 514 (1966).

CHRISTENSEN, J.: Electrical activity of the esophagus. Gastroenterology 52, 903–904 (1967).

CHRISTENSEN, J., DANIEL, E. E.: Electric and motor effects of autonomic drugs on longitudinal esophageal smooth muscle. Amer. J. Physiol. 211, 387–394 (1966).

DOUGHERTY, R. W., HILL, K. J., COOK, H. M., RILEY, J. L.: Electromyographic and pressure studies of the esophagus of the sheep. Amer. J. vet. Res. 32, 1247–1252 (1971).

GOODMAN, E. N., FLOOD, C. A., SANDLER, B. T., SULLIVAN, M. R.: A method of studying motility in the esophagus by recording electrical potentials. Amer. J. dig. Dis. 11, 958–962 (1966).

HELLEMANS, J.: The influence of aging on the motor function of the esophagus. Thesis, Tielt (Belgium): Lannoo 1970.

HELLEMANS, J., VANTRAPPEN, G.: Electromyographic studies on canine esophageal motility. Amer. J. dig. Dis. 12, 1240–1255 (1967).

HELLEMANS, J., VANTRAPPEN, G., JANSSENS, J., PELEMANS, W.: Deglutitive inhibition of the human esophagus. 4th World Congress of Gastroenterology, Copenhagen, July 1970, Advance Abstracts p. 192 (1970a).

HELLEMANS, J., VANTRAPPEN, G., JANSSENS, J., PELEMANS, W., VALEMBOIS, P.: Electromyographic and manometric studies of the transitional zone between striated and smooth esophageal muscle. Rendic. R. Gastroenterol. 3, 138 (1971).

HELLEMANS, J., VANTRAPPEN, G., VALEMBOIS, P., JANSSENS, J., VANDENBROUCKE, J.: Electrical activity of striated and smooth muscle of the esophagus. Amer. J. dig. Dis. 13, 320–334 (1968).

HELLEMANS, J., VANTRAPPEN, G., VANDENBROUCKE, J.: The electrical activity of the human esophagus. Gastroenterology 58, 959 (1970b).

INOUYE, T.: Electromyographic investigation of the esophagus in animals. Laryngoscope (St. Louis) 76, 1502–1519 (1966).

JANSSENS, J., VALEMBOIS, P., VANTRAPPEN, G., HELLEMANS, J., PELEMANS, W.: Is the primary peristaltic contraction of the canine esophagus bolus dependent? Gastroenterology 65, 750–756 (1973).

JEAN, A.: Localisation et activité des neurones déglutiteurs bulbaires. J. Physiol. (Paris) **64**, 227–268 (1972).

LEVITT, M. N., DEDO, H. H., OGURA, J. H.: The cricopharyngeal muscle, an electromyographic study in the dog. Laryngoscope (St. Louis) **75**, 122–136 (1965).

MANN, C. V., SHORTER, R. G.: Structure of the canine esophagus and its sphincters. J. surg. Res. **4**, 160–163 (1964).

MONGES, H., SALDUCCI, J., ROMAN, C.: Etude électromyographique de la contraction œsophagienne chez l'homme normal. Arch. franç. Mal. App. dig. **57**, 545–560 (1968).

PELEMANS, W., VANTRAPPEN, G., HELLEMANS, J., VALEMBOIS, P., JANSSENS, J.: Denervation potentials in the canine esophagus. Proceedings of the 4th International Symposium on Gastrointestinal Motility. Banff, Canada, 1973 September. In press.

ROMAN, C.: Contrôle nerveux du péristaltisme œsophagien. J. Physiol. (Paris) **58**, 79–108 (1966).

ROMAN, C.: La commande de la motricité œsophagienne et sa régulation. Thèse Doct. Sci. Nat., Marseille, 1967.

ROMAN, C., CAR, A.: Déglutitions et contractions œsophagiennes réflexes obtenues par la stimulation des nerfs vague et laryngé supérieur. Exp. Brain Res. **11**, 48–74 (1970).

ROMAN, C., TIEFENBACH, L.: Motricité de l'œsophage à musculeuse lisse après bivagotomie. Etude électromyographique (E.M.G.). J. Physiol. (Paris) **68**, 733–762 (1971).

STOICHITA, S., BROSTEANO, E.: Le contrôle nerveux de la motilité œsophagienne à l'état normal et pathologique. Etude électromanométrique et radiocinématographique. Données concernant l'enrégistrement de l'activité électrique œsophagienne. Courant d'action. 7e Congrès International de Gastroenterologie, vol. II, p. 87. Bruxelles: Imprimerie des Sciences 1964.

THOMAS, P. A., EARLAM, R. J.: Electrical activity of the isolated perfused canine gastroesophageal junction. Gastroenterology **62**, 821 (1972).

TIEFENBACH, L., ROMAN, C.: Rôle de l'innervation extrinsèque vagale dans la motricité de l'œsophage a musculeuse lisse: étude électromyographique chez le chat et le babouin. J. Physiol. (Paris) **64**, 193–226 (1972).

TOKITA, T., TASHIRO, K., KATO, K.: Electromyography of the esophagus and its clinical applications. Acta oto-laryng. (Stockh.) **70**, 269–278 (1970).

VANTRAPPEN, G., HELLEMANS, J.: Espohageal motility. Rendic. R. Gastroenterol. **2**, 7–19 (1970).

VANTRAPPEN, G., HELLEMANS, J., PELEMANS, W., JANSSENS, J.: Electromyographic and manometric studies of the deglutitive inhibition in the esophagus. Rendic. R. Gastroenterol. **3**, 139 (1971).

Chapter 3

Motility Disturbances of the Esophagus

Achalasia

G. VANTRAPPEN and J. HELLEMANS

With 27 Figures

1. Definition

Esophageal achalasia can be defined as a disease of unknown etiology, characterized by absence of peristalsis in the body of the esophagus and failure of the gastroesophageal sphincter to relax in a normal way in response to swallowing (ELLIS and OLSEN, 1969).

The first description of a patient with achalasia was given by Sir THOMAS WILLIS in the earlier Latin edition of the Pharmaceutice Rationalis (1674). The patient was treated by having him push the food down into the stomach by means of a whale-bone rod with a little round button of sponge fixed to the top of it. HOFFMAN (1733) described a case of esophageal spasms provoked by cold beverage and by emotional factors such as "exuberant love and unnatural desires". The patient described by PURTON (1821) had severe dysphagia which was intermittent at the onset of the disease. Postmortem examination showed that the esophagus was largely distended and the cardiac orifice much contracted. After the publication of MAYO (1828) the disease became better known. In 1877 ZENKER and VON ZIEMSSEN were able to find 17 cases reported in the literature and added one case of their own. By 1904 VON MIKULICZ estimated that 100 cases had been reported. In 1921 THIEDING collected a total of 315 cases in the world literature.

Various names have been used to describe this disease: cardiospasm, achalasia, aperistalsis of the esophagus, megaesophagus, esophageal dystonia, idiopathic dilatation of the esophagus, "cardiospasme réactionnel", simple ectasia of the esophagus, proventriculosis, phrenospasm, hiatus esophagismus, dilatatio ingluviformis, esophagi dilatatio fusiformis, dolichoesophagus, cardiaparalysis, and dysphagia paradoxa. The most common terms are achalasia, cardiospasm, megaesophagus and aperistalsis of the esophagus. The terminological confusion is due to poor knowledge of the etiology. The term "achalasia" stresses the failure of the gastroesophageal sphincter to relax. It was first used by HURST, who at that time was still called HERTZ (HERTZ, 1914), on suggestion of Sir COOPER PERRY. The term cardiospasm was used by HUSS (1842) and later by VON MIKULICZ (1882, 1904) because the condition was thought to represent spasm at the cardia. The names "megaesophagus" and "aperistalsis" stress the disorders of the esophagus proper.

2. Incidence

2.1. Age Distribution

Achalasia can be found at any age from the neonate to the elderly. At the time of treatment of the achalasia most patients are between 40 and 60 (Plummer and Vinson, 1921; Moersch, 1929; Olsen et al., 1953; Vantrappen et al., 1971).

Achalasia in children is a very rare disorder. Only 5% of the patients with achalasia have the onset of symptoms before 14 years of age and of this group only half have the diagnosis of achalasia established by 14 years of age. Children of less than 14 to 15 years of age constituted 1.7% of the 691 patients of Moersch (1929), 2.8% of the 601 patients of Olsen et al. (1953), 4.6% of the 259 patients of Kawashima (1962) and 3.1% of the 287 patients of Tachovsky et al. (1968). Children less than 10 years of age account for approximately 1.5% of all achalasia patients (Olsen et al., 1953; Barrett, 1964; Felderhof, 1965). Achalasia can occur in the very young; cases have been described in infants 4 weeks of age (Girdany, 1963; Magilner and Isard, 1971), 6 weeks of age (Barlow, 1961), and below the age of one year (King, 1955; Barlow, 1961; Clagett, 1961; Swenson and Oeconomopoulos, 1961; Redo and Bauer, 1963; Sing et al., 1969; Dayalan et al., 1972). Even if the diagnosis is made at a later age symptoms may occasionally go back to the age of less than one (Langmead, 1920; Payne et al., 1961; Tachovsky et al., 1968; Kumar and Madan, 1969).

In adults the incidence of achalasia is distributed fairly evenly over all ages, without a gap which would suggest a congenital form affecting children and another acquired form affecting later ages, although this has been suggested (Thibert et al., 1965). Even in old people cases of achalasia with a short history can be found (Olsen et al., 1953; Vantrappen et al., 1971) suggesting that the disease can begin in old age.

2.2. Sex Distribution

Males and females tend to be equally affected by achalasia. Out of 2148 patients reported in a number of papers from North America, several European countries and Japan, 49,8% were man and 50.2% woman (Plummer and Vinson, 1921; Olsen et al., 1953; Kawashima, 1962; Kurlander et al., 1963; Zenker and Rueff, 1963; Barrett, 1964; Felderhof, 1965; Affolter and Voegeli, 1969; Akuamoa, 1971; Douvlaris, et al. 1971; Effler et al., 1971; Vantrappen et al., 1971).

2.3. Geographical Distribution and Incidence

The incidence of achalasia has been estimated to be in the range of 1 per 100000 population per year. In Rochester, Minnesota, the average incidence rate was 0.6 per 100000 population per year (Earlam et al., 1969), in Liverpool 1 per 100000 per year (Rickham and Boeckman, 1963) and in Lund 1–2 per 100000 per year (Malm, 1951), indicating that achalasia remains a rare disease.

Most cases were described in Europe and in North America, both in Blacks and in Caucasians (Kurlander et al., 1963; Schindler, 1965; Ellis and Olsen, 1969). But the disease also occurs in Japan (Kawashima, 1962; Okamoto et al., 1964), in Africa (Katz and Sender, 1959; Carayon et al., 1965; Chabal and Mensah, 1965) and in India (Ahmed, 1964). The South American Chagas' disease is a separate entity having another pathogenesis.

3. Achalasia in Animals

Congenital hereditary esophageal dilatation has been described in several breeds of dogs. German shepherd dogs seem to be affected most often (HOF-MEYR, 1966; CLIFFORD and GYORKEY, 1967; EARLAM et al., 1967a). The disease is also found in great danes (LACROIX, 1949; KIESEL, 1951), in greyhounds, (SPY, 1963), in wire fox terriers (STRATING and CLIFFORD, 1966; OSBORNE et al. 1967), in cocker spaniels (BARONTI, 1950), in dachshunds (KITCHEN et al., 1963), in Boston terriers (SCHNELLE, 1950), in dobermans (HOFMEYR, 1966) and in several other breeds and mongrel dogs (HOFMEYR, 1966; CLIFFORD and GYORKEY, 1967). Up to 1966 EARLAM et al. (1967a) found 44 cases of achalasia in dogs de-scribed in the literature; in the same year HOFMEYR (1966) published 32 cases of his own. The disease is probably transmitted as a 1-locus, 2-allele autosomal model with phenotypic dominance of the achalatic allele (OSBORNE et al., 1967). Sometimes entire litters can be affected (SPY, 1963). Congenital dilatation of the esophagus, which closely resembles achalasia, was also found in cats (CLIFFORD et al., 1971) and in mice (FERNANDES, 1968).

In a few instances the intramural ganglion cells of dogs affected by achalasia were studied. According to some (CLIFFORD and GYORKEY, 1967; CLIFFORD and PIRSCH, 1971) their number is normal; according to others (EARLAM et al., 1967a) they are absent; still others (HOFFER et al., 1967) report a decrease in the number of ganglion cells, which, as in humans, becomes more pronounced with the duration of the disease. A decreased number of cells of the nucleus ambiguus was found in canine achalasia (CLIFFORD et al., 1971). One study of a cat affected with achalasia could not establish marked lesions of the intramural plexus (CAWLEY and GENDREAU, 1969).

In most reports of animal achalasia the diagnosis is based mainly on the symptoms of regurgitation of food, on the radiological observation of a dilated esophagus filled with stagnating food, and on autopsy findings. Manometric studies were done in only a few cases (HOFFER et al., 1967; EARLAM et al., 1967a) and showed that both relaxation of the gastroesophageal sphincter and peri-staltic contraction of the esophagus were absent. More recent motility studies on young "achalatic" dogs, however, show important differences with human achalasia (DIAMANT, et al. 1972). Motor activity, usually peristaltic, was present in the lower half to one third of the esophagus and was absent in the upper part. The body of the esophagus did not show hypersensitivity to Mecholyl and the sphincter remained capable of relaxing completely. Other observations also sug-gest that this disease may not be the same as human achalasia (SOKOLOVSKY, 1972); among them the apparently congenital nature of the disorder and the reappearance of peristalsis, after some time, by feeding in a vertical position. At least some of the cases described as achalasia seem to be due to immaturity of the nervous system rather than to irreversible lesions. In some dogs conserva-tive treatment resulted in clinical improvement, but not in a return to normal peristalsis on fluoroscopy (CLIFFORD and MALEK, 1969).

4. Etiology and Pathogenesis

4.1. Genetic Factors

In animals (dogs, cats, mice) with achalasia a hereditary form seems to exist which may affect several litters from a very early age. The question may be raised, however, whether this is real achalasia (see 3. Achalasia in Animals).

In humans also rare cases of achalasia have been reported, affecting different members of the same family. However, the role of heredity in human achalasia is difficult to assess because of the small number of cases reported. In addition, some of these cases became symptomatic at a rather late age (Kilpatrick and Milles, 1972). The disease has been found in mother and daughter (Kilpatrick and Milles, 1972), in twins (Nagler et al., 1963), and in siblings (Di Bello and Zilli, 1960; Tyce and Brough, 1962; Thibert et al., 1965; Polonsky and Guth, 1970). In some families 3 (Ellis and Olsen, 1969) or even 4 children (Cloude et al., 1966) were affected. Dayalan et al. (1972) reported on one family in which at least 3 and perhaps as many as 7 out of the 8 children were affected at the age of less than one. The parents were not affected, but there was a high degree of consanguinity in the ancestors. An autosomal recessive trait was proposed as the hereditary mechanism.

The age distribution also certainly does not suggest a defect from birth. The cases in which the complaints start at a very early age are quite rare. Symptoms beginning at old age are found at least as frequently (Akuamoa, 1969; Vantrappen et al., 1971). The solution of the problem could come from manometric studies of normal subjects who later develop the clinical picture of achalasia; such studies could establish whether there were significant motility disturbances in the esophagus before the onset of symptoms. As of now there is no evidence of genetic factors in the large majority of patients; the familial occurrence of achalasia, however, cannot be denied.

4.2. Neuromuscular Abnormalities

4.2.1. Anatomical Lesions

Except for Chagas' disease, the cause of achalasia remains unknown. The discussion of its etiology is necessarily limited to a description of the lesions found at four different levels of the neuromuscular system: the nuclei of the brainstem, the vagal fibers, the intramural nervous plexus and the muscle fibers.

4.2.1.1. The Nuclei of the Brainstem

Kimura (1929) examined the brainstem of three achalasia patients and found that the nerve cells of the dorsal motor nucleus of the vagus were decreased in number or absent, and that the caudal portion of the nucleus ambiguus showed signs of degeneration. Similarly, Cassella et al. (1964), studying two achalasia patients, found that the number of cells in the dorsal motor nucleus had decreased by half, and that cytological changes had affected many of the remaining cells. Similar abnormalities have been described in Chagas' disease (Lopes et al., 1969) and in dogs with achalasia (Clifford et al., 1971).

4.2.1.2. Vagal Nerve Fibers

Cassella et al. (1965) studied the fine structure of vagal branches to the esophageal plexus in 9 patients with achalasia and found lesions resembling Wallerian degeneration. Both myelinated and non-myelinated structures were involved. The axoplasm exhibited either swelling with fragmentation and dispersion of neurofilaments or contraction with indistinct neurofilaments. Discontinuities were found in axon-Schwann membranes and mesaxons. Myelin disrupture was a common feature. Smith (1970) also found fragmentation of the vagal nerve fibers. All achalasia patients studied by Cassella et al. (1965) had some vagal lesions but the degree of involvement was variable. If vagal dysfunction plays a role in the etiology of achalasia other parameters of such a dysfunction should be present. In some patients there is impairment of reflex gastric secretion in response to insulin (IORDANSKAIA, 1962; WOOLAM et al., 1967), suggesting that some achalasia patients have vagal dysfunction of the stomach.

4.2.1.3. The Intramural Nerve Plexus

For a long time lesions of Auerbach's plexus have been held responsible for the motility disorders of achalasia (BROWN KELLY, 1912; HURST, 1924; RAKE, 1926, 1927; LENDRUM, 1937). Degeneration and diminution in number of ganglion cells have been reported by several authors (CROSS, 1952; TROUNCE et al., 1957; ADAMS et al., 1960; CASSELLA et al., 1964; OKAMOTO et al., 1964; MISIEWICZ et al., 1969).

The changes described range from infiltration of Auerbach's plexus by mononuclear cells to total replacement by scar tissue. The associated intramural nerve fibers are also involved (OKAMOTO et al., 1964). These changes are most prevalent in the body of the esophagus, ganglion cells being present in the distal esophagus, though in reduced numbers (TROUNCE et al., 1957; WANKE and KRICKE, 1962; CASSELLA ct al., 1964). It is as yet uncertain whether these degenerative changes are the primary lesions, since numerous apparently normal cells are found in some cases and since the most severe lesions seem to occur in patients with a long history or a decompensated atonic esophagus (CROSS, 1952; TROUNCE et al., 1957; CASSELLA et al., 1964). It is also uncertain whether these degenerative lesions can be secondary to vagal denervation. BINDER et al. (1968) found plexus degeneration subsequent to vagotomy in monkeys, but BURGESS et al. (1972) could not confirm this finding in cats. Transsynaptic degeneration, however, seems to occur in the colon (SMITH, 1970).

According to SMITH (1970) the ganglion cells which are left are argyrophobe, whereas the argyrophil cells disappear entirely. The latter would act as a controlling device coordinating peristalsis and stimulating the argyrophobe cells which produce acetylcholine, which in turn fires the muscle fibers. The loss of the argyrophil cells may have the same clinical effect as the disappearance of all the neurons.

4.2.1.4. Smooth Muscle

Usually the muscle of the distal narrowed esophagus is of normal thickness, whereas the dilated part has a thick wall due to hypertrophy of the circular muscle coat. Sometimes the wall of the esophageal body is thin and the circular muscle coat as well as the muscularis mucosae show extensive fibrosis (WANKE and ALNOR, 1963). On electron microscopy three types of smooth muscle cell changes are observed in the achalatic smooth muscle specimens. Most prominent is the detachment of myofilaments from the surface membranes of the cells (cellular autolysis) (CASSELLA et al., 1965). Normally the myofilaments end in specialized "grapple plaques" by which adjacent cells are firmly fixed together. These plaques are deficient in achalasia patients (HARMAN et al., 1962; CASSELLA et al., 1965). Sometimes cellular atrophy is noted, and occasionally cellular hypertrophy occurs. The changes are found mainly in the junctional zone between the dilated and the distally narrowed segment of the esophagus. They are thought to represent the picture of denervation atrophy (CASSELLA et al., 1964).

One can only speculate as to where the primary lesions are located. Involvement of the brainstem has been demonstrated, but the number of cases in which it was found is insufficient to be certain that it is always present. If the primary lesions are to be found in the brainstem or in the vagal nerve one has to accept the existence of transsynaptic degeneration, which has not been definitely proven. Moreover, this mechanism would not explain the lymphocytic infiltration in and around the ganglion.

There is no doubt that lesions of the intramural plexus are often present in achalasia, but these seem to become more severe in the course of the disease. Esophageal aganglionosis can therefore not be the primary lesion, especially not as it is also less marked in the distal segment. Smith (1970) assumes selective involvement of the argyrophil cells in the initial stage of the disease. If this is correct these lesions could play a role in the pathogenesis of achalasia.

Of course it is possible that a single cause such as a virus or an autoimmune process affects several structures. This would explain why it is so difficult to cause achalasia in animals by destroying a given structure. Neither destruction of the nuclei in the brainstem (Higgs et al., 1965), nor vagus sections in dogs or in animals with smooth esophageal muscles, such as monkeys or cats, mimic achalasia perfectly (Carveth et al., 1962; Higgs and Ellis, 1965; Binder et al., 1968; Burgess et al., 1972). Various techniques have been used to provoke an achalasia-like picture by destroying the ganglion cells in Auerbach's plexus. Carbon dioxide snow (Alnor, 1958), irradiation (Kimura, 1929) or a 5% phenol solution (Deloyers and Loygue, 1956) destroy ganglion cells, but also damage smooth muscle. Prolonged administration of DFP (di-isopropylfluorophosphate) in dogs results in esophageal aperistalsis (Harris et al., 1960), but permanent damage to the neural tissue does not usually occur and the Mecholyl test remains negative.

The effect of ischemia (Corelli et al., 1957; Culligan, 1959; Sato et al., 1963) and of a combination of ischemia and mercuric chloride (Okamoto et al., 1964, 1967) is also less selective than one might have hoped. Moreover, the initially disordered motor function improves in a later period, during which, however, the loss of ganglion cells is most severe (Earlam et al., 1967b).

The most various and ingenious techniques to mimic achalasia in experimental animals by producing anatomical lesions have not solved the problem where the primary lesions of achalasia are located. Perhaps some day the conclusion will be that in achalasia as well as in Chagas' disease a single agent affects several structures. A neurotoxic virus or an autoimmune process have been suggested as possible causes (Smith, 1970).

4.2.2. Pharmacological Defects

There is pharmacological evidence that the dilated portion of the achalatic esophagus is denervated, whereas the longitudinal muscle coat of the narrow segment has preserved some of its postganglionic innervation. This is the expected result of persistence of some ganglia in the lower segment and absence of ganglia in the upper segment (Ellis, 1962a, b).

Trounce et al. (1957) and Adams et al. (1960, 1961) found the acetylcholinesterase activity to be decreased and the response to nicotine to be normal in the lower segment of the achalatic esophagus. The response to a cholinesterase inhibitor is preserved in vitro (Misiewicz et al., 1969) as well as in vivo (Cohen et al., 1972). The achalatic sphincter is hypersensitive to the indirectly acting gastrin (Cohen et al., 1971) and moderately hypersensitive to cholinergic drugs (Cohen et al., 1972). This seems to indicate that ganglia are still present and that the postganglionic cholinergic fibers are still sufficiently intact to produce acetylcholine. The defective relaxation of the achalatic lower esophageal sphincter may be related to the absence of inhibitory β-adrenergic nervous activity, though normal β-receptors are present (MISIEWICZ et al., 1969). The denervation is more complete in the dilated portion of the gullet. That this part of the esophagus is hypersensitive to cholinergic agents, such as Mecholyl, has been known for a long time and is in accordance with Cannon's law of denervation. It is explained, at least partially, by the ganglionic deficit, which results in marked decrease of the cholinesterase activity.

5. Clinical Features

5.1. Symptoms and Signs

Dysphagia for liquids and solids is the most prominent symptom and is present in nearly all patients (Fig. 162). It is not always mentioned by the patient

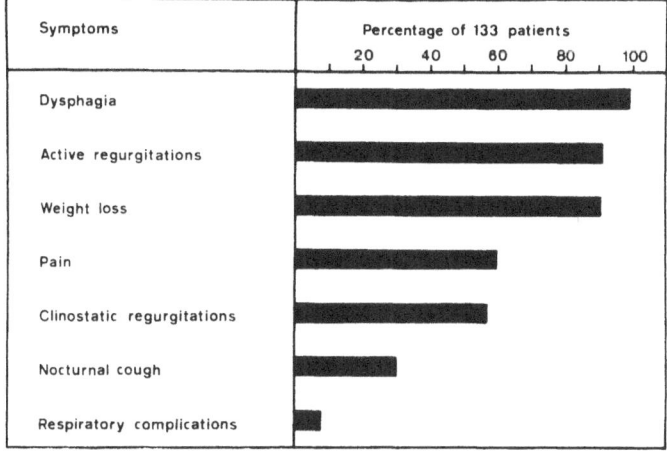

Fig. 162. Symptoms in achalasia patients. [From VANTRAPPEN et al.: Gut **12**, 268 (1971)]

(LAWRANCE and SHOESMITH, 1959), probably because some patients realize that they have had dysphagia only after treatment has improved the esophageal function. Exceptionally the patient may deny dysphagia (VANTRAPPEN et al., 1971). 69% of the patients have more trouble with solids than with fluids, 25% do not notice any difference at all and only 7% experience more trouble with liquids than with solids (VANTRAPPEN et al., 1971). Typically the patient feels that food is sticking low in the substernal or subxyphoid region, and that it passes suddenly into the stomach. Sometimes he learns to force it into the stomach by drinking or by small tricks such as a Valsalva maneuver or certain movements of the thorax.

At the time of treatment 91% of our patients had dysphagia during each meal, 7% had daily dysphagia and only 2% had dysphagia a few times a week. Others (AKUAMOA, 1969) found dysphagia in only 66% of their patients but mention additional symptoms such as retrosternal oppression, food stop and regurgitation.

The degree of the swallowing difficulties varies considerably from day to day especially in the initial stage of the disease. Many patients admit they have more trouble when they are rushed or nervous and some eat much more easily alone than in company. However, from this it should not be inferred that these patients are neurotic (Olsen et al., 1957). The type of food also is important. Apples are liable to produce symptoms; cold beverages may produce painful spasms.

Regurgitation is the second most common symptom (Sanderson et al. 1970). Active prandial or postprandial regurgitation occurs in 91% of the patients, whereas regurgitation in the recumbent position is present in only 57% of the patients (Vantrappen et al., 1971). Regurgitation may be first noted as soiling of the pillow slip (Olsen et al., 1953). It seems to be the most frequent symptom in children (Tachovsky et al., 1968). In the initial stage of the disease active prandial or postprandial regurgitation (which the patient may mistake for vomiting) may alleviate the substernal discomfort. Therefore, some patients provoke it voluntarily. Later, when the esophagus becomes more distended, considerable quantities of food and fluid may accumulate in the esophagus, which can be regurgitated at varying intervals after meals. The regurgitated food is undigested and non-acid. When the esophagus is markedly dilated stasis of even large quantities of food is tolerated fairly well and the degree of dysphagia may decrease, but such patients risk regurgitation during sleep. This results in nocturnal coughing spells in 30% of the patients and in bronchopulmonary complications (lung abscesses, bronchopneumonia or bronchiectasis from esophageal spill-over) in 5% (Sanderson et al., 1970) to 7.5% of the patients (Vantrappen et al., 1971).

Substernal pain was experienced by 60% of our patients at some time during the course of the disease. Attacks of cramp-like substernal pain not related to meals, not infrequently occurring at night, and often radiating to the neck or the back, are present in 46% of the patients. Olsen et al. (1953) give a somewhat lower figure (29%). Pain occurs especially in the initial stage of the disease and in cases of vigorous achalasia (Olsen et al., 1957; Sanderson et al., 1967). It may disappear later when the esophagus distends further.

The degree of weight loss is related to the severity of the dysphagia. In some cases extreme cachexia may be found. Exceptionally vitamine deficiencies have been described (Ellis and Olsen, 1969) and hyperbilirubinemia due to starving in patients with Dubin-Johnson syndrome can be observed (personal observations). At the time of treatment 91% of our patients had lost weight; 12% had lost over 10 kg.

Anemia also has been observed (Olsen et al., 1953). Hemorrhage is a rare symptom occurring in 2.5% of the patients (Olsen et al., 1953). Although it may be due to esophagitis it should primarily rise the suspicion of carcinomatous degeneration.

Cases of achalasia with minimal complaints have been described. Apparently some patients tolerate the disturbances so well that they wait for years to seek medical advice (Lawrance and Shoesmith, 1959). This is especially true for older patients. In these cases the main symptoms are recurring pulmonary infections combined with a poor general condition. In 2 of our older patients the diagnosis was made on a chest X-ray which revealed a widened mediastinum.

In infants and children achalasia often goes unrecognized (Moersch, 1929). The respiratory symptoms of achalasia in childhood are particularly important. Nocturnal regurgitation is extremely common and the condition may be mistaken for chronic pulmonary infection (Payne et al., 1961; Ellis and Olsen, 1969). Feeding problems and vomiting in infants may be due to numerous other conditions, more frequent than achalasia; the symptoms of achalasia in infants may therefore be ascribed to other causes if no X-ray and/or manometric examinations are performed.

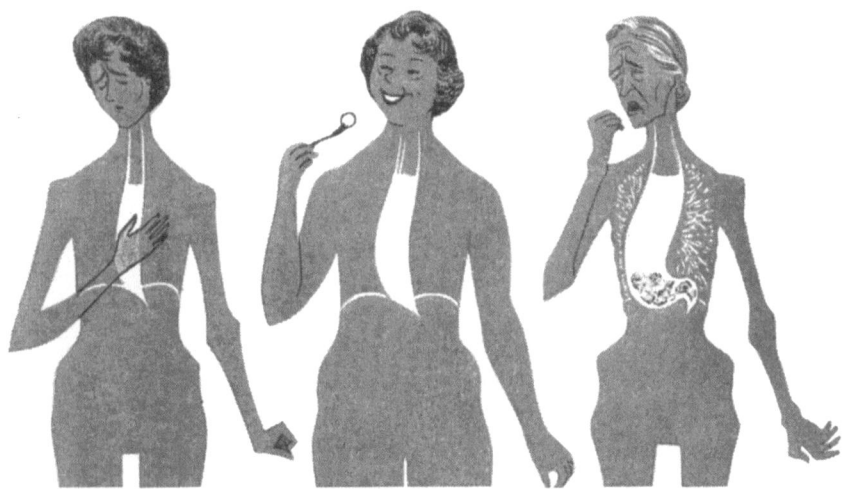

Fig. 163. Clinical evolution of achalasia patients as diagrammatically presented by ADAMS et al. [Guy's Hosp. Rep. **110,** 191 (1961)]

The symptoms of achalasia may vary in the course of the disease. Schematically the natural history has been subdivided into three stages (ADAMS et al., 1961) (Fig. 163). The initial stage is characterized by pain, dysphagia, and regurgitation. Symptoms are often connected with emotional stress situations and especially in this stage the disease may go unrecognized. The compensated stage is characterized by distension of the esophagus and improvement of the symptoms of pain and dysphagia. The motility disorders, however, do not improve. The stage of decompensation occurs after an evolution of many years. The esophagus has become enormously distended and the tricks the patients learned are no longer sufficient to push the food down into the stomach. Weight loss, cachexia, spill-over into the airways and a continuous feeling of oppression in the thorax cause by a huge esophagus characterize this stage.

There are many exceptions to this classification. Although there is a relation between the caliber of the esophagus and the mean duration of the symptoms (VANTRAPPEN et al., 1971), and although roentgenological progression of the disease does exist, the relation between the duration of the disease, the symptoms and the radiological appearance of the esophagus is rather variable (OLSEN et al., 1953). ELLIS and OLSEN (1969) use the terms compensated and decompenasted achalasia in a somewhat different meaning from ADAMS et al. (1961). In what they call a compensated phase, muscular hypertrophy may take place. Although contractions are not peristaltic, there is enough motor activity in the esophagus to force the cardia. In the period of decompensation the esophagus is virtually inactive and a progressive dilatation and subsequent elongation occur. On manometric examination deglutitive pressure waves are no longer observed. This classification is based mainly on radiological data. But the relation between clinical symptoms and degree of esophageal dilatation is also variable. A patient may die of the disease without his gullet becoming greatly enlarged and another, who has had a megaesophagus for years, may be in "reasonably good health" (BARRETT, 1964).

5.2. Vigorous Achalasia
(Fig. 164)

SANDERSON et al. (1967) selected, mainly on the basis of manometric data, a group of 72 patients with symptoms of both achalasia and diffuse spasm. As in the case of achalasia these patients complain of dysphagia, regurgitation and food stasis but the majority also had moderate to severe pain reminiscent

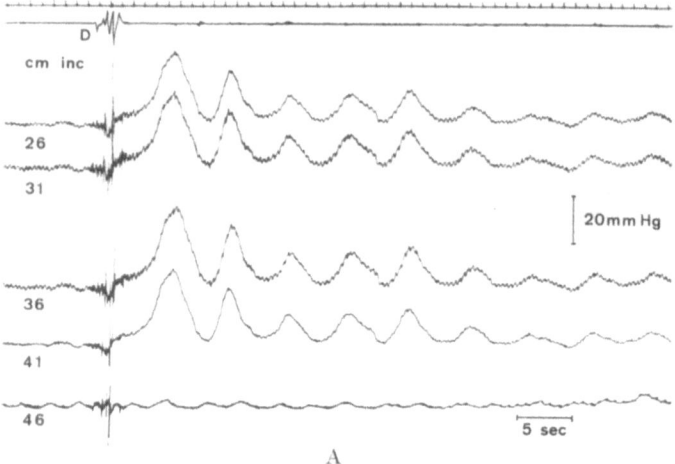

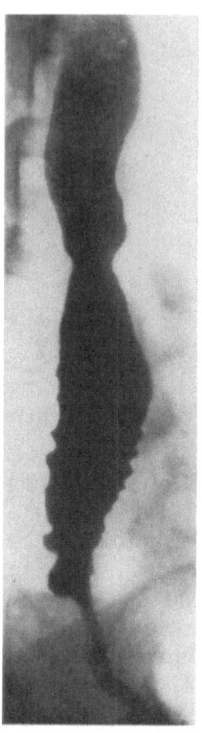

Fig. 164. A Manometric recording in a case of "vigorous achalasia". Swallowing (D) provokes simultaneous repetitive contractions (cm inc:cm from the incisors). B X-ray of the esophagus of the same patient shows tertiary contractions

of diffuse spasm. This pain is often more distressing than other symptoms and can be associated with meals or swallowing, or it can occur independently. In a few patients the esophagus is distended, a radiological picture which is not found in cases of diffuse spasm. Segmental spasm of the lower half of the esophagus is very common. In this series of 72 patients the spectrum of radiographic appearances was quite variable and the interpretation of the same case sometimes varied between diffuse spasm and achalasia. Manometrically, simultaneous und repetitive pressure waves of high amplitude occur after deglutition. No peristalsis is present, but sphincteric relaxations occur in 82% of the cases although they are weak or incomplete. This condition therefore occupies an intermediate place between achalasia and diffuse spasm. It is distinguished from typical achalasia by the segmental spasms, which can be observed both radiologically and manometrically, and which are responsible for the pain and for the absence or slight degree of esophageal dilatation.

"Vigorous achalasia" is manometrically different from diffuse spasm by the total absence of peristalsis, even in the proximal segment of the esophagus, by the absence of normal sphincteric relaxations and by the hypersensitivity to Mecholyl. In contrast with cases of diffuse spasm these patients nearly always have obstruction and frequently retention. It is unlikely that "vigorous achalasia" corresponds to the initial stage of achalasia since the symptoms and signs remain consistent over a long period of time. This condition is probably not a special entity, but rather a less common manifestation of achalasia.

ADAMS (1964) has coined the term "amyenteric achalasia of the esophagus" to describe a condition characterized by a wide esophagus and by the absence of resistance to the passage of an esophagoscope through the sphincter; whether this really constitutes a separate form of achalasia is doubtful.

6. Technical Examinations
6.1. Radiology
6.1.1. Plain Chest Film

In the initial stages of the disease the chest X-rays are normal. A dilated esophagus may show up on a postero-anterior chest X-ray as a widening of the mediastinum; the upper right mediastinal border then becomes convex and displaced to the right (Fig. 165). When the esophagus is markedly dilated the mediastinal widening may even appear to the right of the heart as an elongated convex arch (Fig. 166). On lateral chest films a markedly distended esophagus, containing a large amount of residue and air, may result in an anterior displacement of the trachea and in an air-fluid level behind the trachea (Fig. 167). The

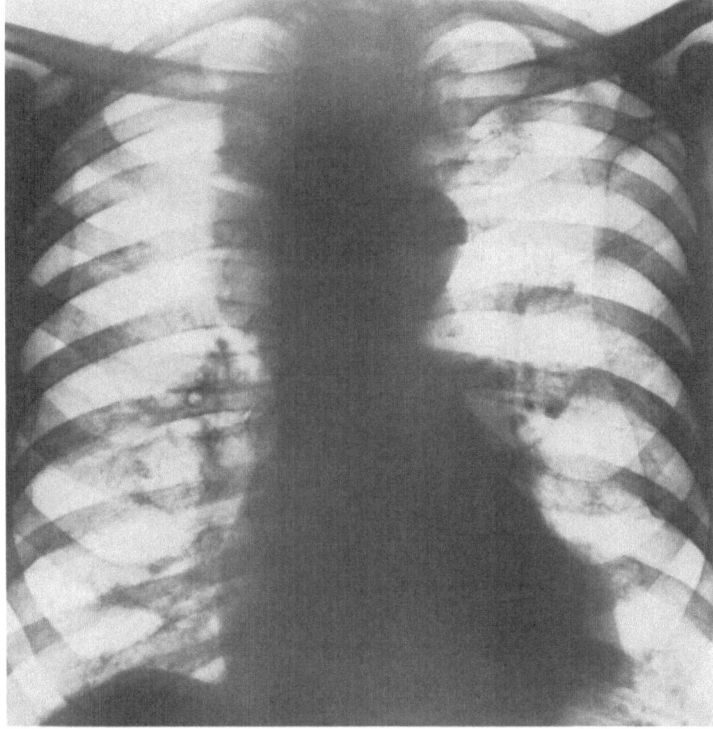

Fig. 165. Plain chest film in an achalasia patient with grossly dilated esophagus, which has widened the upper mediastinum to the right

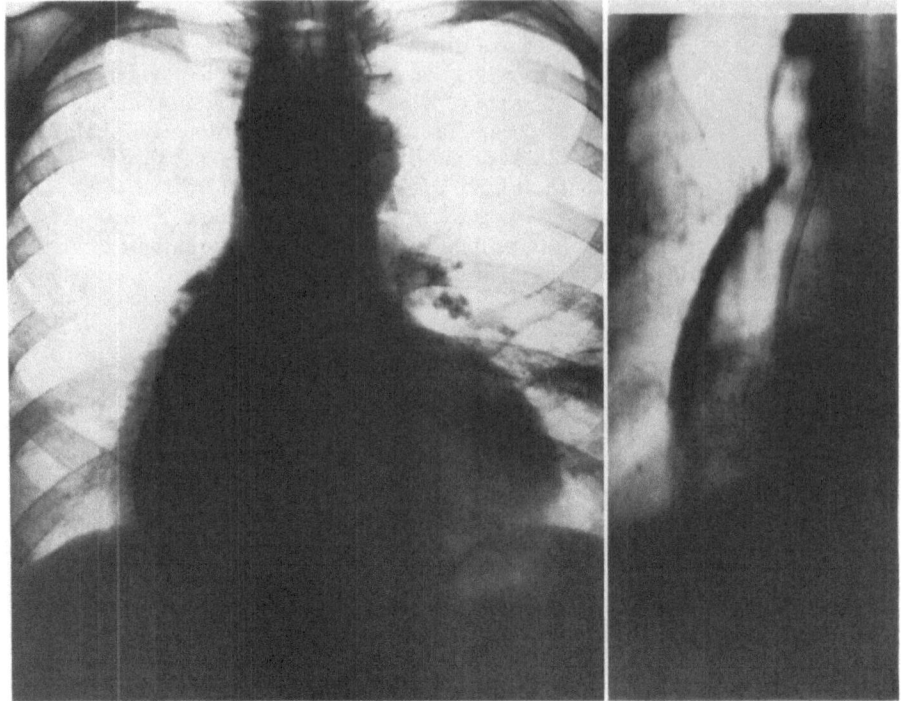

A   Fig. 166   B

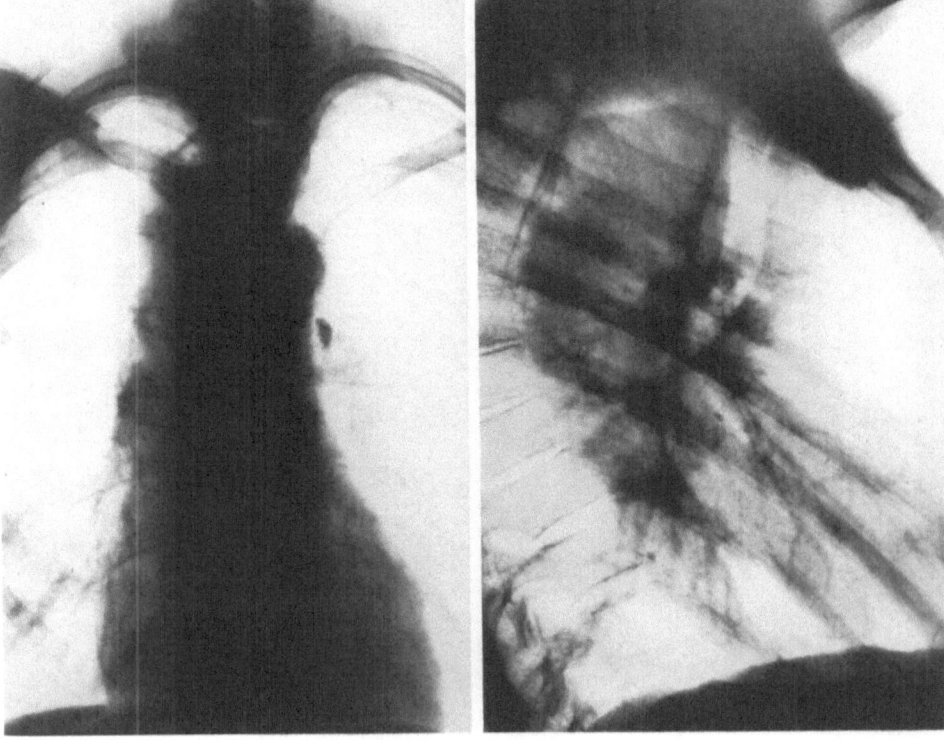

A   Fig. 167   B

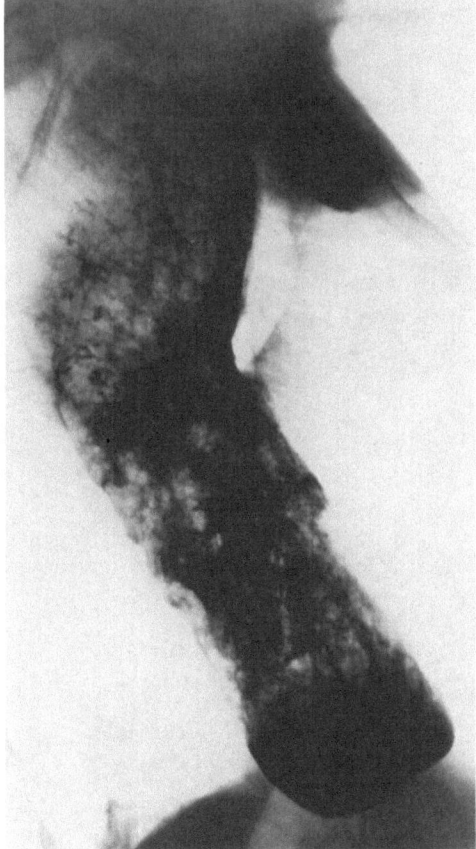

Fig. 167 C

Fig. 166 A and B. Plain chest film of an achalasia patient with grossly dilated esophagus. A Antero-posterior view, made after the esophagus has been filled with contrast medium. Marked widening of the "cardiac shadow" and slight widening of the upper mediastinum by the dilated esophagus. B Laminogram made after the dilated esophagus has been emptied and insufflated with air via a tube. The thickening of the wall, suggested by picture (A), is clearly visualized

Fig. 167. A Chest X-ray of an achalasia patient with grossly dilated esophagus. The mediastinum is widened and there is a fluid level in the upper part of the gullet. B Same patient, lateral view. Abnormal shadow in the middle mediastinum and fluid level in the upper part of the gullet. The trachea is displaced ventrally. C Same patient, the esophagus has been filled with contrast medium

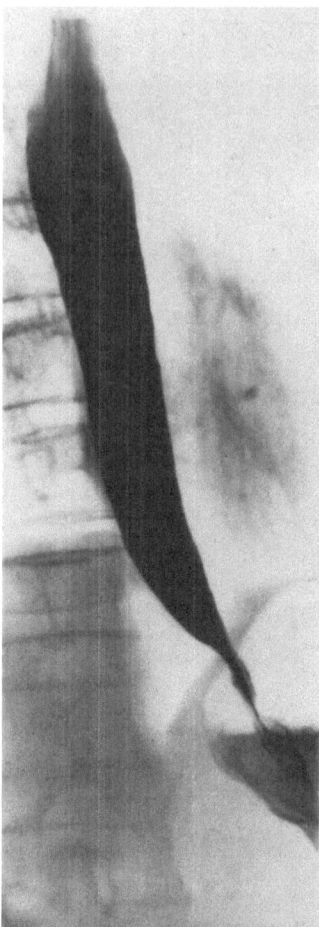

Fig. 168. Minimal dilatation in a case of beginning achalasia

gastric air bubble is usually absent because the swallowed air is held up in the
esophagus by the stagnating fluid. The chest X-ray may also show signs of
pulmonary complications due to spill-over into the airways.

6.1.2. Radiological Examination with Contrast Medium

The radiological appearance of the esophagus in achalasia is variable. The
constant symptom is loss of peristalsis. In addition the lower esophageal segment
opens insufficiently and incompletely, and the body of the esophagus undergoes
a progressive distension. Four degrees of achalasia have been distinguished mainly
on the basis of the extent of the dilatation (Olsen et al., 1953; Carlson, 1969).

6.1.2.1. Minimal Achalasia (Fig. 168)

In this stage the esophagus still has its normal caliber and there is no stasis.
The progression of the barium is hindered by vigorous disorganized contractions
in the lower third of the esophagus, whereas, according to Templeton (1944),

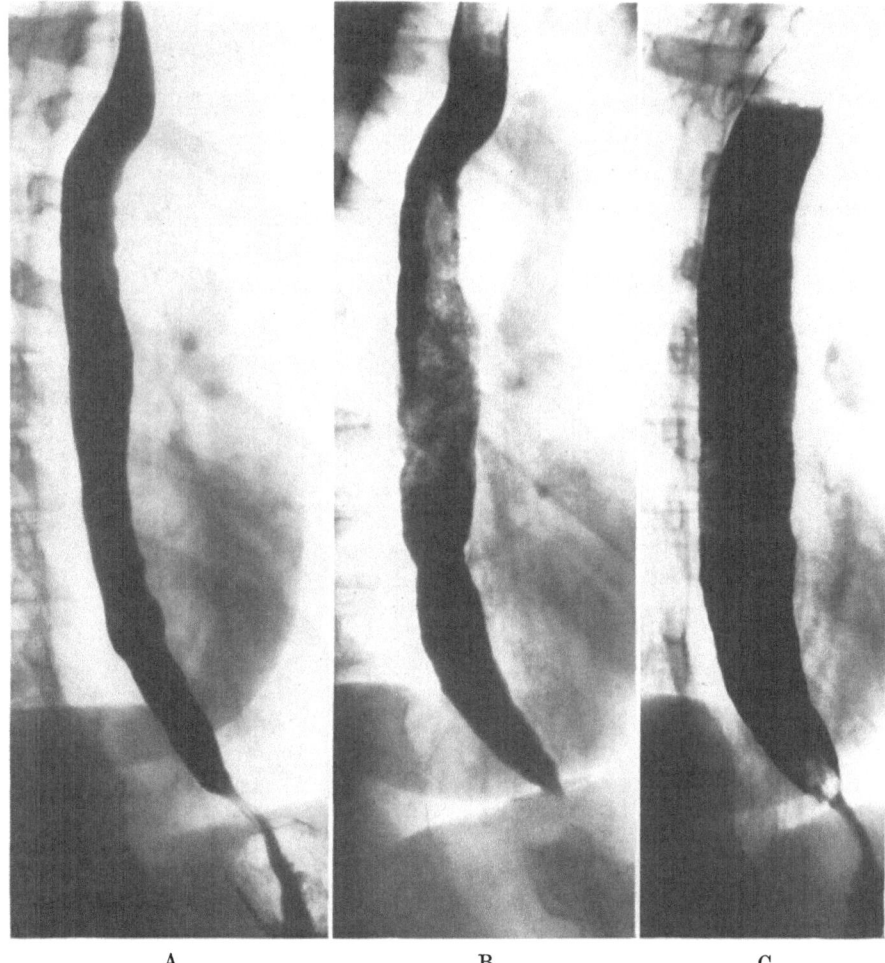

A   B   C

Fig. 169 A—C. Spontaneous evolution of achalasia. Progressive increase of the esophageal
diameter. A 30. 3. 1955. B 22. 11. 1955. C 27. 11. 1956

peristalsis is still present in the upper third of the esophagus. These disturbances
can best be demonstrated in the recumbent position which eliminates the influence of gravity. The gastroesophageal sphincteric segment opens insufficiently,
but this is not as apparent as in later stages because the body of the esophagus
is not yet dilated. In this stage the differential diagnosis with diffuse spasm is
difficult. CARLSON (1969) reported a case, thought to be diffuse spasm at the
first examination, which turned out to be a typical achalasia 7 years later.

6.1.2.2. Mild Achalasia (Fig. 169)

The retention becomes more marked and some dilatation takes place. Uncoordinated tertiary contractions are still present but peristaltic contractions
are lacking and the middle segment of the gullet becomes slightly dilatated,
giving rise to a fusiform esophagus. Often the gastric air bubble remains present.

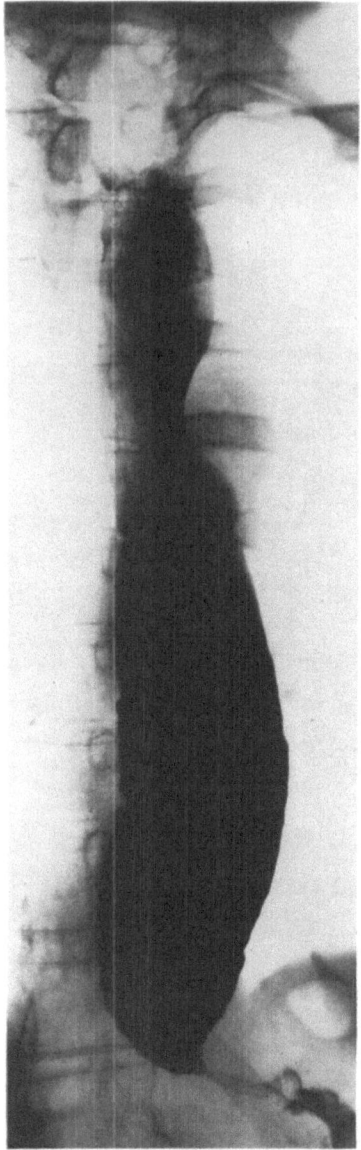

Fig. 170

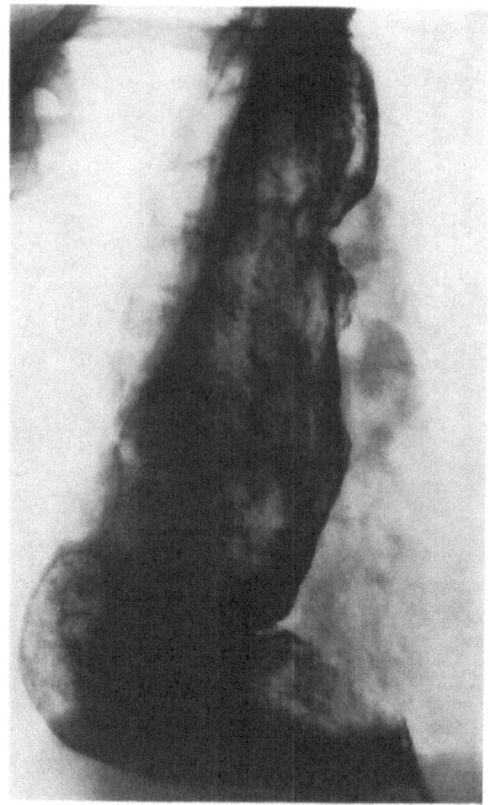

Fig. 171

Fig. 170. X-ray picture of classical achalasia

Fig. 171. Severe achalasia with markedly widened
and elongated esophagus

6.1.2.3. Moderate Achalasia (Fig. 170)

After months or years the esophagus becomes dilated over its total length,
from the pharyngoesophageal sphincter down to the gastroesophageal sphincter.
The absence of sphincteric relaxations gives rise to typical radiological appearances, which are described in the next paragraph (6.1.2.4.). There is considerable
stasis and in the upright position a barium-fluid and a fluid-air level can be seen.
When the esophagus has not been emptied before, the swallowed barium sinks
through this stagnating fluid and accumulates in the lower part of the eso-

phageal body. The disappearance of the air bubble from the stomach may give a collapsed appearance to the gastric fundus.

6.1.2.4. Severe Achalasia (Fig. 171)

The esophagus not only becomes very wide (up to 10 cm) but also elongated. This elongation results in a tortuous sigmoid shaped esophagus and/or in a kink in the upper third of the gullet. Food and stagnating fluid float on the barium and may falsely suggest a filling defect caused by a tumor.

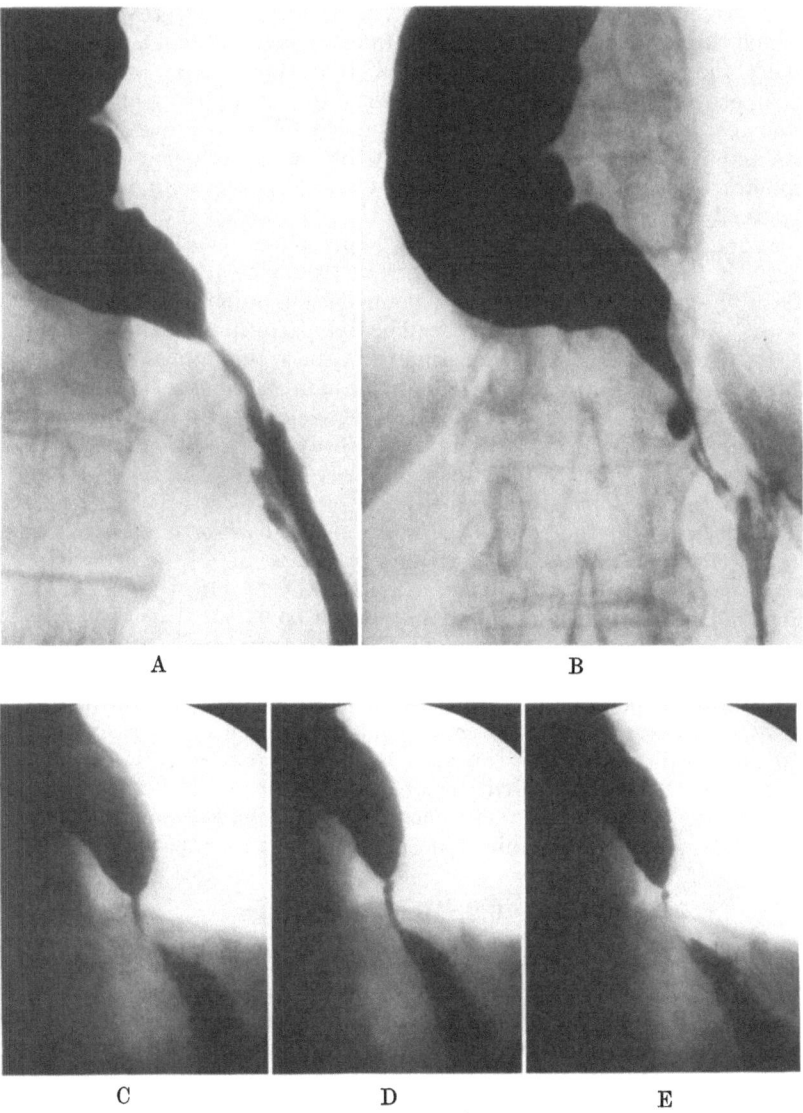

A   B

C   D   E

Fig. 172A—E. Morphological variants of the terminal esophageal segment in achalasia. A Classical picture, showing progressive tapering of the cardia. B Intermittently an asymmetrical pseudodiverticulum is seen in the narrowed segment of this patient. C, D and E A small fusiform dilatation appears intermittently in the terminal esophageal segment of this patient

The incidence of food residue, of esophageal elongation and of disappearance of the air bubble from the gastric fundus increases with an increasing esophageal diameter but they may also occur in patients with a slightly dilated esophagus. In our patients the esophageal diameter varied from 34 to 95 mm, with a mean of 55 mm. The esophagus was slightly dilated ($<$ 5 cm) in 38% of the patients, moderately dilated (5 to 8 cm) in 55% and severely dilated ($>$ 8 cm) in 7%. OLSEN et al. (1953) found minimal achalasia in 12%, mild achalasia in 44%, moderate achalasia in 28% and a markedly dilated gullet in 16% of their cases.

Contrasting with the mostly wide esophageal body the terminal segment is narrow. This segment is 1 to 3 cm, rarely 6 cm long. In severe cases no barium passes and the segment is not visualized. In other cases a small amount of barium may pass and penetrate into the stomach, the caliber of the esophagus is seen to be tapering down gradually and to terminate in a string-like passage into the stomach. The transition from the distended to the narrow segment is often smooth and even. In about 20% of the patients the lower narrow segment shows a symmetrical or asymmetrical dilatation, delineated proximally by a constriction and gradually tapering down distally (VAN GOIDSENHOVEN et al., 1963) (Fig. 172). The proximal contraction ring probably corresponds to the lower esophageal sphincter of Lerche or to the A-ring of Wolf (WOLF et al., 1958).

When the undilated portion is asymmetric, a unilateral outpouching may create an ulcer-like picture. But the mucosal pattern is unaltered and shows three fine mucosal fields. The transition from the wide esophagus to the narrow vestibule takes place in a smooth conical fashion. Although small irregularities may be caused by retention esophagitis, irregularities in the outline of this transition or an angular transition must always suggest an organic stenosis (carcinoma). As stagnating food may give rise to false images it is necessary first to remove the esophageal residue.

On fluoroscopy in the recumbent position the barium is seen to penetrate into the stomach only with great difficulty or not at all. In the upright position, the esophageal lumen fills until the weight of the barium opens the sphincter wide enough for a small amount of barium to spurt into the stomach. There is no peristalsis; simultaneous or uncoordinated contractions progressively disappear as the esophagus becomes more distended. After the administration of Mecholyl uncoordinated activity increases markedly, the caliber of the esophagus decreases due to a massive contraction and the barium is usually regurgitated.

The narrow distal segment can open not only under the influence of gravity but also under that of amyl nitrite or of an effervescent solution such as Seidlitz powder (STEIN, 1963). An organic stenosis such as a carcinoma has a more fixed diameter. To exclude an organic stenosis bougienage may be useful.

6.2. Manometry

6.2.1. Resting Pressures in the Gastroesophageal Sphincter

Manometric studies with non-perfused open-tip catheters reveal that the mean resting pressure profile of the gastroesophageal sphincter in achalasia is almost identical to that observed in normal subjects. This similarity applies to the localization and extent of the zone of elevated pressure as well as to the individual and mean pressure values (CREAMER et al., 1957; CODE et al., 1968; VANTRAPPEN et al., 1963; CREAMER, 1968; VANTRAPPEN et al., 1971). Similar results were obtained with miniature balloons (CODE et al., 1958) and with miniature electromagnetic pressure transducers (CREAMER et al., 1957). In view of this data the name "cardiospasm" was abandoned but later BESANÇON et al. (1962) reintroduced it as "cardiospasme réactionnel" by which they meant that the pressure in the achalatic sphincter increases upon filling the esophagus with fluids.

Using a perfused catheter system some found a normal end-expiratory resting pressure in patients with achalasia (HEITMANN et al., 1969: 11.5 mm Hg). COHEN's results, however (COHEN, 1965; COHEN et al., 1971, 1972), reveal a markedly increased sphincteric pressure in achalasia patients. In our experience many patients with typical achalasia have normal yield pressures in their gastro-esophageal sphincter, those with a hyperactive esophagus an elevated yield pressure. As the perfusion techniques do not measure the resting pressure but the yield pressure necessary to force the sphincter, this elevated pressure could correspond to BESANÇON's "cardiospasme réactionnel". The high pressure has been ascribed to hypersensitivity to gastrin. Serum gastrin levels are not elevated in patients with achalasia (COHEN et al., 1971) and the sphincteric pressures can be reduced to normal by acidification of the gastric antrum, which inhibits gastrin secretion (COHEN et al., 1971).

6.2.2. Resting Pressure in the Esophagus

The resting pressure in the esophagus is higher than normal. The end-expiratory resting pressure is as high as the fundic pressure; the end-inspiratory resting pressure is only 3 mm lower than the fundic pressure instead of 20 to 24 mm (CREAMER et al., 1957; EDWARDS and ROWLANDS, 1959; VANTRAPPEN et al., 1963). This high resting pressure is mostly ascribed to stasis of food, fluid and air in the esophagus. The resting pressure in the esophagus markedly decreases after effective treatment.

6.2.3. The Deglutitive Response in the Gastroesophageal Sphincter

As the term achalasia indicates, the relaxation of the gastroesophageal sphincter is deficient. Most authors find the relaxations to be rare (CODE et al., 1958;

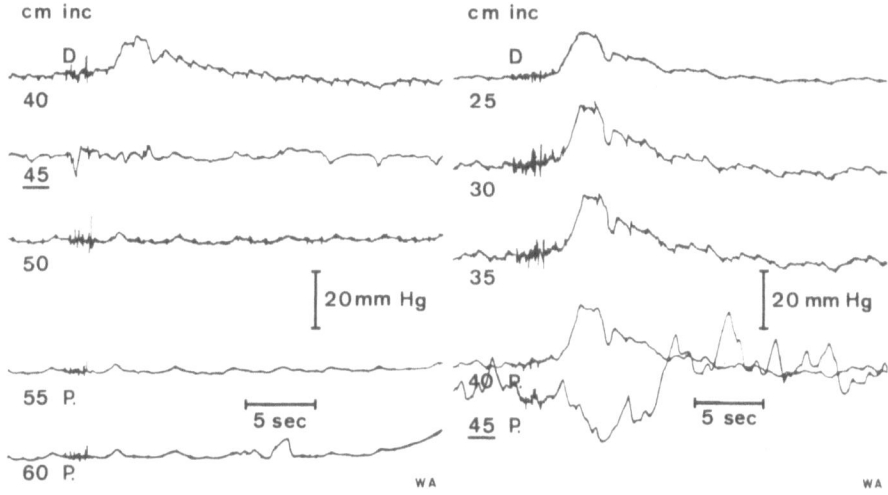

Fig. 173. Manometric recording in an achalasia patient. Left: the catheter at 45 cm from the incisors (cm inc.) is located in the high pressure zone. Non-perfused catheter and no fall in pressure following deglutition (D). Right: the catheter at 45 cm from the incisors (cm inc.) is located in the high pressure zone. The lower two catheters were perfused continuously. After deglutition there is a distinct fall in pressure at 45 cm (D). This relaxation, however, is not complete

VANTRAPPEN, 1961) and if they occur they are not infrequently abnormal, the fall in pressure being of significantly shorter duration and of lesser amplitude than it is in health (CREAMER et al., 1957; CODE et al., 1958; VANTRAPPEN et al., 1963; CODE, 1969). These rare relaxations are terminated by premature sphincter contractions. In the lower portion of the sphincter a decrease in pressure upon deglutition is more frequent but here also it is short (ELLIS and OLSEN, 1969). Relaxations are observed more frequently when constantly infused catheter systems are used but the fall in pressure is mostly short and incomplete and does not reach the level of the fundic pressure (COHEN, 1965; HEITMANN et al., 1969) (Fig. 173). The deglutitive contractions begin about 3 sec after swallowing so that the period of passage through the sphincter is shortened. The amplitude and duration of the sphincteric contractions, however, are normal (CREAMER et al., 1957; VANTRAPPEN et al., 1963).

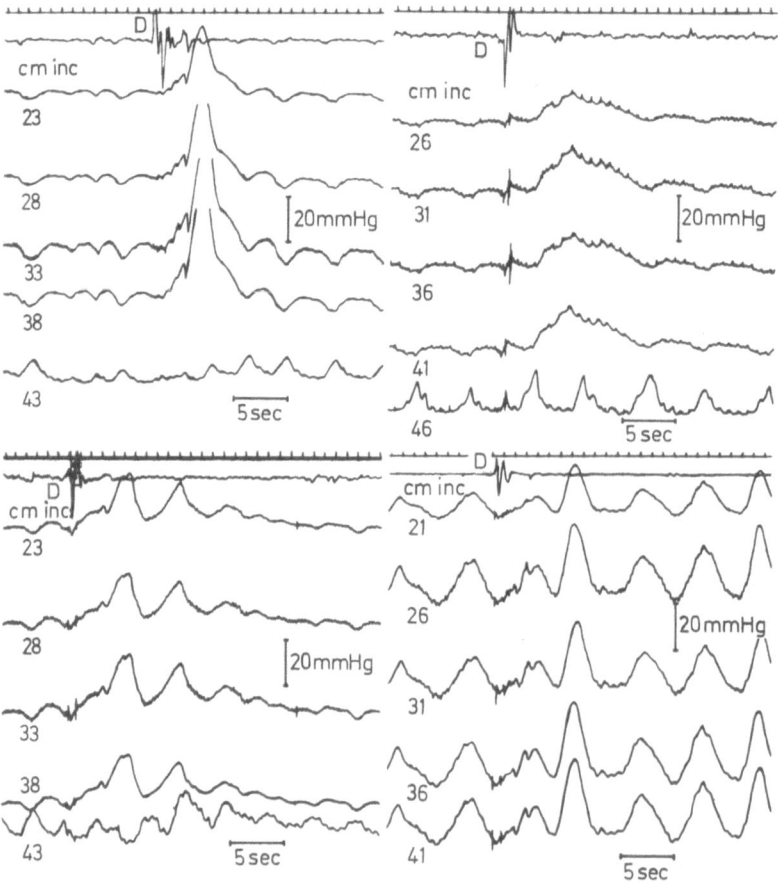

Fig. 174. Types of esophageal pressure wave in achalasia. Upper left: simultaneous contraction, beginning very soon after deglutination (D). The amplitude is still high. Upper right: low and wide simultaneous waves. Lower left: simultaneous repetitive contractions. Lower right: continuous activity (cm inc.: centimeters from the incisors)

6.2.4. Deglutitive Responses in the Esophagus

Deglutition does not cause peristaltic contractions but results in pressure waves which occur simultaneously and often repetitively over the entire length of the esophagus (Fig. 174). These pressure waves usually occur earlier than normal, shortly after deglutition. It is remarkable that the sphincter contracts a little bit later than the distal segment of the esophagus. The simultaneous character of the pressure waves registered in a widely distended esophagus does not necessarily indicate that the contraction itself occurs simultaneously over the whole length of the esophagus. In a widely distended organ any contraction that does not obliterate the lumen will be recorded as a pressure wave which occurs simultaneously over the whole common cavity. Deglutition waves in the markedly distended achalatic esophagus often have a lesser amplitude and a longer duration than normal; correspondingly they often have a different configuration from normal complexes and appear to be feeble waves with a slow rise, a gradual fall and a small amplitude (Fig. 174). In vigorous achalasia the contractions are relatively strong and almost always repetitive; their strength is nearly equal to that in health. When the esophagus is very large deglutitive pressure waves are no longer recorded (NORTON and SULTAN, 1968; SULTAN and NORTON, 1969). This is partially due to the weak contractions of the esophageal muscle in this stage of the disease and partially to the extreme dilatation of the organ, which makes adequate manometry impossible. In a few cases non-simultaneous uncoordinated pressure waves are recorded. Spontaneous activity may also be observed (Fig. 175). In some patients it is virtually continuous. After careful aspiration of the esophagus and after treatment by dilatation it decreases (BUTIN et al., 1953; HIGHTOWER et al., 1954; VANTRAPPEN et al., 1963). This suggests that spontaneous activity is related to the degree of obstruction and retained materials (HIGHTOWER, 1955). Spontaneous waves are more frequently seen in vigorous achalasia (see 5.2.).

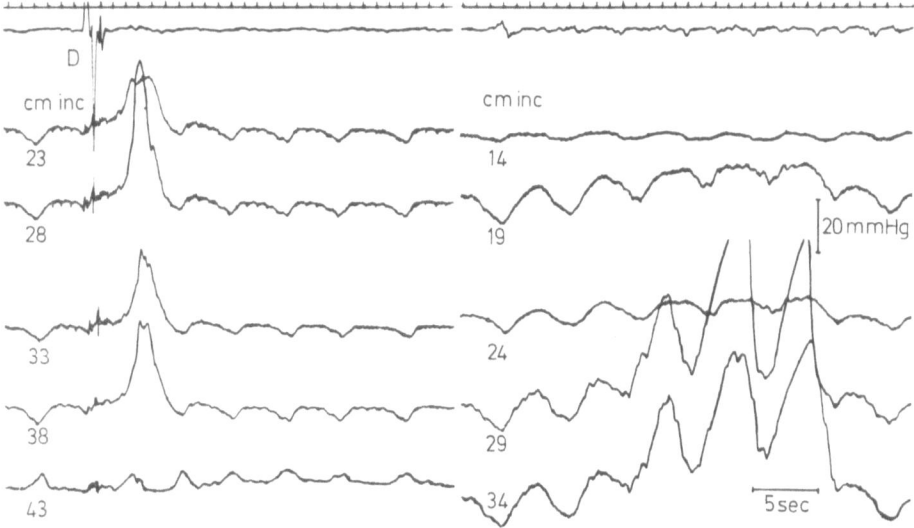

Fig. 175. Manometry in achalasia. Left: simultaneous contraction and absence of sphincteric relaxation after deglutition. Right: spontaneous activity

6.3. Mecholyl Test

The injection of acetyl-beta-methylcholine chloride (Mecholyl) in a dose of
6 to 10 mg has been shown by Kramer and Ingelfinger (1949 b, 1951) to give
a dramatic response of the achalatic esophagus. When administered to normal
subjects Mecholyl does not cause a significant response (Kramer and Ingelfinger, 1951; Kramer et al., 1956). In these subjects the resting pressure does
not increase after Mecholyl although more peristaltic activity may be recorded
because salivation and swallowing are stimulated (Creamer, 1968). In patients
with achalasia, however, Mecholyl produces a painful, tonic, lumen-obliterating
contraction of the esophagus beginning after 1 to 2 min and lasting up to 30 min.
This contraction can be recorded nicely by a balloon kymographic system. On
manometric studies the basic pressure of the esophagus is seen to increase 20 cm
of water or more (Butin et al., 1953) and simultaneous repetitive pressure waves
are superposed on it. The resting pressure in the gastroesophageal sphincter
also increases (Heitmann et al., 1969; Cohen and Guelrud, 1971) and abnormal
sphincteric relaxations are more frequent (Heitmann et al., 1969). Radiologically
the esophagus is seen to contract forcefully in a non-propulsive fashion and
barium is forced back into the upper esophagus and into the mouth. At the time
of the tonic contraction the patient frequently experiences substernal pain, which
mostly improves upon the administration of atropine. Mecholyl often causes
generalized cholinergic reactions such as hypersalivation and perspiration in
patients with achalasia. Other cholinergic drugs such as bethanechol (Olsen
and Creamer, 1957) or neostigmine (Kramer et al., 1956) have an effect similar
to that of Mecholyl. The Mecholyl test is not necessarily positive in all cases
of achalasia; cases of extreme dilatation sometimes do not react. The Mecholyl
test may be falsely positive. Gastric carcinoma involving the esophageal myenteric
plexus can produce an achalasia-like picture with a positive Mecholyl test (Ingelfinger, 1964; Kolodny et al., 1968; Herrera et al., 1970). Hypersensitivity
to Mecholyl has also been reported in a number of patients with symptomatic
diffuse esophageal spasm (Creamer et al., 1958; Kramer et al., 1967a; Kramer,
1970).

In cases of Chagas' disease with esophageal aperistalsis the Mecholyl test
is positive in 92% of the cases (Castro and Grossi, 1963). As the disease progresses the response to Mecholyl may be so reduced that the most severely
affected patients have no reaction at all (Castro and Grossi, 1963). The Mecholyl
test is positive in half of the patients with Chagas' disease without dysphagia
or without radiographic changes of the esophagus (Vieira and Godoy, 1963).

6.4. Cytological Examination

Cytological examination is especially valuable to demonstrate infiltrating
carcinomas, which can occur at any moment of the evolution, even several years
after successful treatment. Therefore, it has been proposed to repeat this examination every six months in achalasia patients above 30 (Cliffton, 1970).

6.5. Endoscopic Examination

Endoscopy does not contribute significantly to establish the diagnosis of
achalasia or to differentiate achalasia from other motor disorders. Combined
with biopsy esophagoscopy may be useful to exclude carcinomatous degeneration
(see 8.1.), to differentiate achalasia from carcinoma of the cardia (see 7.1.2.),
and to establish the degree of stasis esophagitis. Esophagoscopy may reveal

reddening and thickening of the esophageal mucosa plus varying amounts of mucus and retained secretions. Small superficial erosions appear. The epithelium regenerates in an attempt to cover the denuded areas and hyperplasia results in the formation of small nodules resembling verrucae (JUST-VIERA and HAIGHT, 1969). In extreme cases the mucosa offers a polypoid aspect and bleeds easily, so that a carcinoma must be excluded. Occasionally larger ulcerations may occur. Papillomas and leukoplakia have also been found (ELLIS and OLSEN, 1969).

7. Differential Diagnosis

7.1. Other Causes of Megaesophagus

7.1.1. Chagas' Disease

7.1.1.1. Acute Phase

Current knowledge about Chagas' disease of the gastrointestinal tract has been reviewed extensively by KÖBERLE (1968) and EARLAM (1972b). The disease is caused by a trypanosoma prevalent in South America. This trypanosoma is also found on the North American continent but there it does not usually cause Chagas' disease. The disease is not found in Europe, Asia and Africa. In some regions of Brazil, however, the complement fixation test for trypanosomiasis is found to be positive in 10 to 25% of the population. At least 7 million people are affected by the disease.

The disease may begin as an acute illness in childhood and if the patient survives, chronic Chagas' disease may manifest itself 30 to 40 years later. The trypanosomes are transmitted by a bug (triatoma) or other insects which bite and leave infected feces near the skin wound. The patient may rub this bitten area, introducing the parasites into the wound or may contaminate the conjunctivae. Other routes of infection are transfer of parasites through the placenta, or, exceptionally, by maternal milk, blood transfusions or laboratory accidents. After a week a local inflammatory reaction with acute regional lymphadenitis develops. The parasites soon reach the blood. The acute phase of the disease is characterized by general malaise, fever, muscular pains, anorexia, local signs (usually unilateral swelling of the orbit) and later on by hepatosplenomegaly and generalized edema. The intracellular development of the parasites gives rise to a leishmania pseudocyste, from which new trypanosomas are released into the circulation. The parasite develops preferentially in muscle cells and produces a neurotoxic substance which is released when the pseudocyst is broken down. It is therefore not surprising that mainly the ganglion cells in muscles are affected. Ganglion cells are lost equally throughout the bowel, except in the stomach where the loss is less pronounced. Encephalopathies and myelopathies occur and there is a reduction in the number of cells in the dorsal motor nucleus of the vagus. The destruction of ganglion cells seems to be limited to the acute phase of the disease. The greater the destruction of ganglion cells, the shorter is the life expectancy. This explains why at autopsy patients surviving to old age have more ganglion cells than patients with Chagas' disease who die earlier after the acute phase. The parasitemia disappears within 10 weeks. Already in the first few weeks antibody formation begins. The Machado-Guerreiro complement fixation test usually remains positive throughout life. Xenodiagnosis is a method of having laboratory-bred triatomid bugs feed on patients and examining the insects 40 days later for the presence of T. Cruzi in the intestinal tract. This test is positive in only about 20 per cent of chronic cases.

7.1.1.2. Chronic Chagas' Syndrome

A majority of the patients develops, after a latency period of 10 to 30 years, the symptoms of chronic Chagas' syndrome. The lesions result primarily from the destruction of ganglion cells during the acute phase of the disease. In a series of 800 autopsy cases, 746 had heart lesions, 182 megacolon, 158 megaesophagus, 40 enlarged bronchi, 13 megagaster, 20 megaduodenum, 3 megajejunum, 5 mega-gallbladder, 3 megacystis and 2 had megaureter (KÖBERLE, 1968). In 12 cases megaesophagus was the only lesion found. The seminal vesicles, the salivary glands and the pancreas may be involved as well. 87% of the deaths in Chagas' syndrome are due to cardiopathy. Sudden deaths are common in young people. In endemic areas football teams always have a few extra players on the side line "because not infrequently some players die suddenly during the match" (KÖBERLE, 1968).

7.1.1.3. Megacolon

The colon is often affected by Chagas' disease, especially the sigmoid. The rectum is often involved. Disordered motility can already be noticed before dilatation. Lengthening is usually seen before any increase in diameter although both occur in extreme cases. The outstanding symptom is chronic obstipation, bowel movements occurring at intervals of 8 days to 5 or 6 months. The capacity of the colon may be as large as 30 to 40 liters! The most common complications are fecal obstruction, perforation and volvulus of the sigmoid. Pathological examination reveals a decrease in the number of ganglion cells and degeneration

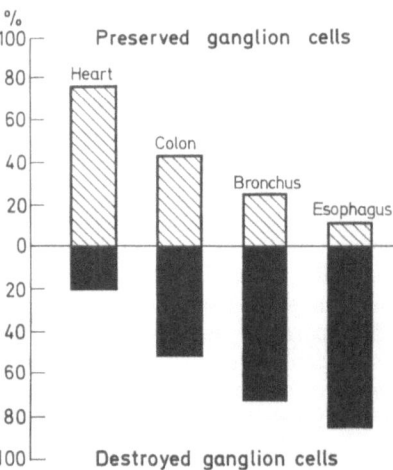

Fig. 176. Ganglion cell loss (in black) required for dilatation of heart, colon, bronchus and esophagus in Chagas' disease. [From KÖBERLE, F.: Adv. Parasitol. **6**, 63 (1968)]

of ganglion cells throughout the large intestine. The colon enlarges when the ganglion cell loss surpasses a critical limit of 55% (KÖBERLE, 1963; SMITH, 1967) (Fig. 176). The enlarged denervated colon in Chagas' disease is hypersensitive to cholinergic agents (VIEIRA et al., 1963, 1964). Muscle thickening, most marked in the circular muscle layer, is observed in the early stage of the disease (TODD et al., 1969).

7.1.1.4. Megaesophagus

Several degrees of esophageal involvement in chronic Chagas' disease have been described. The clinical, radiological and manometric picture of the symptomatic megaesophagus is similar to that of achalasia. The most common symptoms are dysphagia (99%), usually of a progressive character, pain on swallowing (52%), regurgitation in a recumbent position (57%), aspiration bronchopneumonia and coughing (26%), malnutrition (70%), eructation (41%), singultus (38%), sensation of fulness (32%), heartburn (70%) and hypertrophy of the salivary glands, particularly of the parotic glands (KÖBERLE, 1968). Esophageal ulcers, bleeding, perforations and fistulas, leukoplakia and possibly carcinomatous degeneration can be complications due to stasis of food (FERREIRA-SANTOS, 1961).

Table 11. Number of nerve cells in an esophageal ring segment 1 mm high

	Upper part	Middle part	Lower part
Normal esophagus	445	778	1003
Chagas' syndrome normal esophagus	122	261	391
Chagas' disease megaesophagus	0.1	1.5	2.7

Radiologically, four degrees of esophageal dilatation can be recognized. Group I (15.6%) is characterized by a normal esophageal diameter and a small retention of contrast material, group IV (13%) by a dolichomegaesophagus. Groups II (47%) and III (24%) are intermediate; in the latter the dimensions of the esophagus are greater but its muscular activity is smaller (DE REZENDE, 1963). Other classifications are based on the diameter of the esophagus (FERREIRA-SANTOS, 1968).

On manometric examinations peristaltic waves are absent or disordered and the sphincteric relaxations impaired (PINOTTI et al., 1968).

Up to 35% of patients with chronic Chagas' disease have an abnormal esophagus (BRASIL, 1955). In half of the cases the patient is between 20 and 39 years old at the onset of symptoms, but 17% have symptoms before the age of 14 (DE REZENDE, 1968). Disordered motor activity and dysphagia can already be observed a few months after the acute phase (DE REZENDE and ROSSI, 1958).

The number of ganglion cells in cases with megaesophagus is diminished to nearly zero (KÖBERLE, 1959) (Table 11). It has been suggested that the total number of ganglion cells must be reduced by at least 50% to produce a functional disturbance and by 90% to produce megaesophagus (KÖBERLE, 1963, 1968) (Fig. 176). As in achalasia, the denervated muscle is hypersensitive to acetylcholine-like substances. The Mecholyl test is positive, except when the esophagus is extremely dilated. As in the colon, the circular muscle is thickened much more than the longitudinal muscle. The muscularis mucosae is hypertrophic as well. The wall may be as thick as 10 mm.

The differential diagnosis with typical achalasia constitutes a problem only in regions where Chagas' disease is found and can be based on the fact that Chagas' disease usually involves other organs as well (heart, colon, parotic glands, etc.). The Machado-Guerreiro complement fixation test is positive in 90 to 95% of the patients with esophageal and/or colon involvement (FERREIRA-SANTOS, 1961; DE REZENDE, 1963). A great number of patients with chronic Chagas' disease seem to have minor esophageal involvement without complaints or without dilatation of the gullet. In patients with chronic Chagas' disease and an apparently normal esophagus KÖBERLE (1959) found the number of ganglino cells to be diminished throughout the esophagus. The administration of Mecholyl to asymptomatic patients often results in an increase of pressure in the gastro-esophageal sphincter as well as in an increased non-deglutitive activity in the esophagus (VIEIRA and DE GODOY, 1963; DE GODOY and VIEIRA, 1963; HEITMANN and ESPINOZA, 1969). In this stage esophageal peristalsis and gastroesophageal sphincteric relaxation are still normal (PINOTTI et al., 1968; HEITMANN and ESPINOZA, 1969). The disordered sphincteric motility seems to correlate better with dysphagia than with esophageal dilatation.

7.1.2. Esophageal Cancer

Malignant tumors can cause two different kinds of problems in relation to the diagnosis of achalasia. First there is the possibility of carcinomatous degenera-tion (see 8.1.). Such cancers can develop at any level of the esophagus. They cause very late symptoms when they are located in the widely dilated esophageal body and are hard to diagnose radiologically if they are located in or below the sphincteric zone. Second, carcinoma of the lower esophagus or gastric cardia extending into the esophagus can result in a stenosis of the distal esophagus, which may mimic achalasia (Fig. 177) (MARSHAK and ELLIASOPH, 1957; ROTH

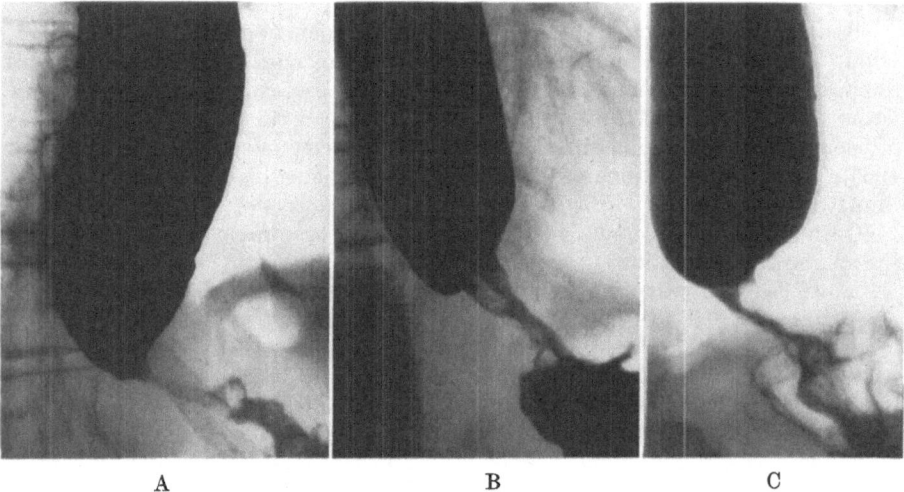

A   B   C

Fig. 177A—C. Differential diagnosis between achalasia and carcinoma. A Achalasia: pro-gressive narrowing of the cardia with smooth margins and intact mucosal folds. B Carcinoma of the cardia: irregular narrowing of the cardia; the mucosa appears nodular. C Carcinoma of the cardia. The differential diagnosis is based on the irregularity of the left antero-lateral margin

and STEIN, 1963; SEAMAN et al., 1963). In such cases the history is usually short. On radiological examination the esophagus is not very wide, an air bubble is present in the gastric fundus and the mucosal folds at the cardia are irregular or interrupted. Other signs include deviation of the barium flow in the gastric fundus by the presence of a tumorous mass and a rigid asymmetric narrowing of the cardia. Extensive tumors of the gastric fundus may become manifest by encroachment on the air-filled fundus, an increased soft tissue thickness between fundus and diaphragm or deformity of the fundal contour (SEAMAN et al., 1963). NEMIR and FROBESE (1962) and ROTH and STEIN (1963) advocate the use of an effervescent powder, which is said to cause evacuation in cases of achalasia but not in cases of cancer. However, this is not a very reliable test because rapid emptying after ingestion of Seidlitz powder can occur also in cases of carcinoma (HERRERA et al., 1970). Manometric studies can be useful. Carcinoma leaves peristalsis in the proximal part of the esophagus intact, and the Mecholyl test is mostly negative. Whenever there is any doubt, endoscopy, biopsy and cytological examination are indicated, although even these examinations can be negative in cases of infiltrating tumors (KOLODNY et al., 1968). On rare occasions neoplastic invasion of the esophageal wall can closely mimic the manometric pattern of achalasia and cause a positive Mecholyl test (ROTH and STEIN, 1963; KOLODNY, et al. 1968; HERRERA et al., 1970). This is ascribed to invasion and damage of Auerbach's plexus in the esophagus. An infiltrating carcinoma can also mimic the manometric picture of a hypertensive sphincter (DEBRAY et al., 1962). Exceptionally an organic stenosis due to stricture or to a benign tumor such as leiomyoma or fibrolipoma can give a radiological image resembling that of achalasia (MOERSCH, 1952; BERNATZ et al., 1958).

7.1.3. Rare Causes of Esophageal Dilatation

Marked dilatation of the esophagus has been observed in patients intoxicated with Yperite during World War I. Although an organic stenosis of the cardia was present in most patients, the esophageal dilatation seemed to be out of proportion with the degree and the duration of this stenosis, and the dilatation was ascribed to the neurotoxic effect of this war gass (WORMS and LEROUX-ROBERT, 1934).

A megaesophagus with a smooth distal narrowing has been found in children with familial dysautonomia (Riley-Day syndrome) but in these patients esophageal peristalsis is preserved (JOSEPH and JOB, 1963). Amyloidosis may cause a megaesophagus which closely resembles achalasia both on radiological and manometric examination (MILLER, 1969). A megaesophagus associated with megacolon has been found in morphine addicts (HILLEMAND, 1955). Moderate esophageal dilatation can also be due to an organic obstruction in the distal segment of the esophagus. Finally bulbar paralysis can cause an atonic esophagus.

7.2. Other Causes of Aperistalsis

Scleroderma has sometimes been taken for achalasia and has been treated as such (HANNA, 1972). However, in scleroderma the gastroesophageal sphincter is usually patent until reflux esophagitis and stenosis occur, and the degree of esophageal dilatation is moderate (OLSEN et al., 1953). Cutaneous manifestations or Raynaud phenomena sometimes appear years after the onset of the dysphagia (RODNAM and FENNEL, 1962). Manometry may yield important diagnostic clues. The proximal part of the esophagus, consisting of skeletal muscle, is usually not involved (CREAMER et al., 1956; CODE and SCHLEGEL, 1963; STEVENS et al., 1964). Peristaltic activity may be intact over the entire length of the gullet, but the contractions may also be weak and peristaltic, or weak and simultaneous, or absent in the distal esophageal segments. The tone of the gastroesophageal sphincter is decreased, sphincteric relaxations are present but contractions are weak. The Mecholyl test is negative (KRAMER and INGELFINGER, 1951; CODE et al., 1958).

Disorders of esophageal motility have been described in dermatomyositis (DONOGHUE et al., 1960), myotonia dystrophica (FISCHER et al., 1965; SIEGEL et al., 1966), multiple sclerosis (Daly et al., 1962; Fischer et al., 1965), hypothyroidism (Christensen, 1967), diabetes (Mandelstam and Lieber, 1967; Mandelstam et al., 1969) and alcoholic neuropathy (Winship et al., 1968). But these patterns can easily be differentiated from achalasia.

7.3. Achalasia-like Disorders

Some patients show the clinical and radiological picture of achalasia but do not fulfill the manometric criteria for the diagnosis. Vantrappen et al. (1963) found that pneumatic dilatations resulted in the appearance of rare peristatic

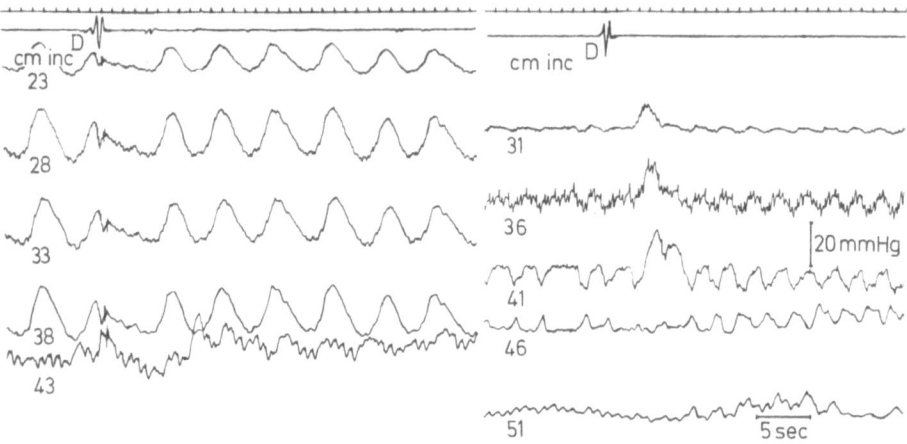

Fig. 178. Left: manometry of achalasia before dilatation. Simultaneous contractions only; spontaneous activity. Right: manometry of the same patient after dilatation. The tracing is much more quiet. Rare progressive contractions reappear in addition to the expected simultaneous contractions. The lower two catheters are perfused (1.2 ml/min)

contractions in a few patients who had only simultaneous contractions and a typical radiological picture of achalasia before treatment (Fig. 178). Hogan et al. (1969) described 4 untreated patients with a dilated esophagus which strongly suggested achalasia. At some time during the motility study they still had peristaltic contractions, mainly in the upper segment of the esophagus. Secondary peristalsis also was noted in two patients. Sanderson et al. (1967) mentioned 3 patients which they excluded from their series of vigorous achalasia because of an occasional peristaltic wave. Moersch et al. (1957) coined the term dyschalasia to describe 3 patients with an incomplete picture of achalasia. Two of these 3 patients still had peristaltic contractions in the upper segment of the esophagus and a radiological picture suggestive of achalasia. Perhaps these cases may be considered as transitions between diffuse spasm of the esophagus and achalasia. This then would be an argument for the hypothesis that both conditions actually represent only one disease. If non-perfused catheters are used to study achalasia patients, no relaxations are found in the upper part of the gastroesophageal sphincter. Using this technique Code (1959) found relaxations in the distal portion after about one third to one half of the swallows in 80% of patients with achalasia. But also in the upper part an occasional brief decline of pressure is observed (Vantrappen et al., 1963; Code and Schlegel, 1969; Hogan et al., 1969). In some patients relaxations begin abnormally late (Beck

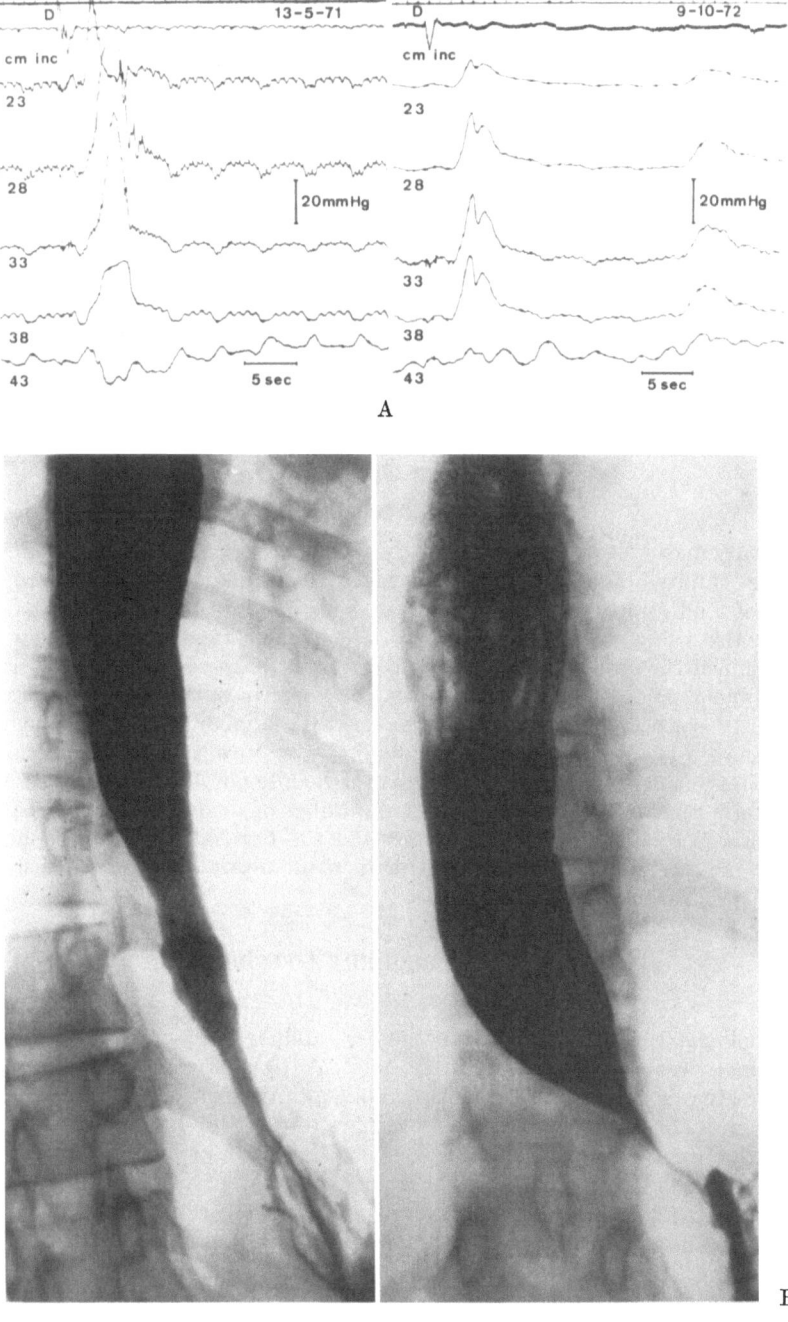

Fig. 179. A Evolution from diffuse spasm to achalasia. On 13. 5. 71 the patient was examined manometrically because of dysphagia. Some peristaltic contractions and fairly many sphincteric relaxations were still present. After a follow-up period of one year under medical therapy she had developed the typical manometric picture of achalasia. B Radiological evolution in the same patient. Left: radiological picture in 1971 showing "spastic" narrowing of the distal third of the esophagus and the persistence of an air buble in the gastric fundus. Right: radiological image in october 1972, showing a classical achalasia picture

et al., 1966; Hogan et al., 1969). This has been described as dyschalasia (Beck et al., 1966). Many of these atypical cases had a positive Mecholyl test (Moersch et al., 1957; Vantrappen et al., 1963; Beck et al., 1966; Hogan et al., 1969). Unfortunately prolonged follow-up studies are lacking. These cases raise the problem whether or not they are the initial stages of a disease which later evolves toward a complete picture of achalasia. Some observations are in favor of this hypothesis. A 56-year old patient with dysphagia was examined in May 1971. At that time she still had peristaltic contractions and some sphincteric relaxations. No treatment was instituted and the patient was reexamined in October 1972. On manometric examination only simultaneous contractions were found and the sphincteric relaxations had become quite abnormal (Fig. 179). We observed three other patients in whom the diagnosis of achalasia was considered on the first manometric examination although they had a fairly large number of apparently normal sphincteric relaxations. When they were reexamined about six months later a more typical manometric picture of achalasia was found, and they were treated successfully.

7.4. Diffuse Spasm

Symptomatic diffuse spasm is mostly characterized by substernal pain, which does not improve over the years and which is frequently not related to meals. Stasis of food and regurgitation are rare. Usually the esophagus is not dilated; instead there is a diffuse narrowing or a segmental type of contraction in the lower half of the gullet. On manometric examination peristaltic waves are found in the upper part of the esophagus. In the lower part the deglutitive response frequently consists of simultaneous waves with a high amplitude and a long duration. A variable number of swallows, however, results in contractions which maintain their peristaltic nature down to the distal end of the esophagus. Normal sphincteric relaxations are found after a number of deglutitions. The (partially) peristaltic character of the contractions and the presence of normal sphincteric relaxations after deglutition are the main manometric signs which distinguish diffuse spasm from vigorous achalasia.

7.5. Post-Vagotomy Dysphagia
(see also p. 367)

Dysphagia can occur after transthoracic and, to a lesser extent, after transabdominal vagotomy (Dagradi et al., 1962; Andersen et al., 1966; Edwards, 1970; Blackman et al., 1971). This complication is seen in one to two percent of patients who have had vagotomy (Pierandozzi and Ritter, 1966). Mostly the symptoms subside after a while, so that the surgical trauma with edema and subsequent fibrosis seem to play a role in a number of cases. However, on manometry Andersen et al. (1966) found simultaneous contractions in the lower esophagus and absence of relaxation in 5 out of 8 patients. On radiological examination also a picture not unlike achalasia has been observed (Pierandozzi and Ritter, 1966; Dahm, 1968).

7.6. Differential Diagnosis in Children

In the newborn a syndrome has been described which resembles achalasia both radiologically and clinically but differs from true achalasia in that the symptoms are not prolonged and that conservative treatment with either gastric intubation or antispasmodics has been successful. This entity has been termed spasm of the cardia, achalasia of the newborn and neuromuscular incoordination at the cardia in the newborn (BIRNBERG, 1929; SEGAR and STOEFFLER, 1930; VAN DER BOGERT, 1933; HAAS, 1941; THOMSON, 1950; REDO and BAUER, 1963).

Since a manometric examination is not so frequently performed in infants many other and more frequent causes of obstruction and vomiting must also be thought of, such as esophageal stricture, pyloric stenosis, congenital diaphragmatic hernia, other congenital malformations, foreign bodies, etc.

8. Complications and Associated Diseases

8.1. Carcinoma

8.1.1. Incidence

The association between achalasia and malignant esophageal tumors has been known for a long time and appears to have been described first by FAGGE in 1872. The literature on this subject has been summarized by DEBRAY et al. (1968), who collected 69 cases, and by JUST-VIERA and HAIGHT (1969), who collected 167 cases. The incidence of carcinoma in achalasia patients is about 4% (109 carcinomas among 2609 patients collected from the literature) (see Table 12). This is clearly higher than its incidence in the general population. The figures given vary considerably. Some authors observed very few instances of esophageal

Table 12. Esophageal carcinoma in achalasia patients

Authors	Number of cases of achalasia	Number of carcinoma	Percentage
Achalasia			
HILLEMAND and VIGUIE (1957)	700	18	2.6
LAGACHE and SOORS (1958)	45	2	4.4
MICHAUD (1958)	81	2	2.5
JOSKE and BENEDICT (1959)	180	3	1.7
SANTY et al. (1958)	180	7	3.9
LAWRANCE and SHOESMITH (1959)	118	3	2.5
ELLIS (1961)	69	7	10.1
LEROUX and WRIGHT (1961)	55	2	3.6
FELDERHOF (1965)	94	4	4.3
BOITEL (1963)	30	5	16.7
BARRETT (1964)	120	7	5.8
SILBER (1965)	35	5	14.3
BELSEY (1966)	133	9	6.8
JUST-VIERA et al. (1967)	148	5	3.4
AKUAMOA (1969)	101	3	3
DEBRAY et al., (1968)	62	4	6.5
LORTAT-JACOB (1968)	212	17	8
PIERCE et al. (1970)	110	3	2.7
GRIMES et al. (1970)	136	3	2.2
	2609	109	4.1
Chagas' disease			
CAMARA-LOPES (1961)	90	7	7.8
RESANO (1948)	400	10	2.5
FERREIRA-SANTOS (1961)	57	6	10.5
	547	23	4.2

carcinoma in their achalasia patients (PLUMMER and VINSON, 1921; OLSEN et al., 1953; VANTRAPPEN et al., 1966); others give rather high percentages (SILBER, 1965). In Chagas' disease also carcinoma is found frequently (4.2% of 547 cases collected from the literature) (see Table 12). The incidence of carcinoma in autopsy series is much higher (RAKE, 1931, 3 out of 15; LAWRANCE and SHOE-SMITH, 1959, 3 out of 12; ELLIS, 1961, 7 out of 24; FELDERHOF, 1965, 4 out of 11).

8.1.2. Age and Sex Distribution

As for esophageal carcinoma not associated with achalasia mainly men are affected. The survey of DEBRAY et al. (1968) reports 54 men and 15 women, that of JUST-VIERA and HAIGHT (1969) 78 men versus 28 women. These carcinomas occur at an early age. The averages given are 50 years (DEBRAY et al., 1968) or 48 years (JUST-VIERA and HAIGHT, 1969) as compared with 62 years for non-achalasia patients.

8.1.3. Pathology

The most common tumor found in achalasia is a squamous cell carcinoma. The literature mentions 68 squamous cell carcinomas versus 7 adenocarcinomas, one carcinosarcoma and one undifferentiated carcinoma (JUST-VIERA and HAIGHT, 1969). In the 109 patients in whom the location of the tumor was mentioned, it arose in the upper third of the esophagus in 4, in the middle third in 56 and in the lower third in 42 patients. In 7 patients the tumor involved two or more segments (JUST-VIERA and HAIGHT, 1969).

8.1.4. Pathogenesis

Cancer develops mostly in patients with a long history of achalasia, usually 17 to 20 years (WILLIAMS, 1956; DEBRAY et al., 1968; JUST-VIERA and HAIGHT, 1969). Esophagitis due to stasis is said to play a major role (RAKE, 1931). A Heller operation does not seem to prevent the evolution to carcinomatous degeneration in all cases. Even patients who underwent an early and successful myotomy may develop cancer (DEBRAY et al., 1968). DI BELLO and ZILLI (1960) found achalasia and cancer in several members of one family.

8.1.5. Signs and Symptoms

The diagnosis is very difficult and is usually made beyond the stage of curability (SELIGER et al., 1972). The tumor has to reach very large dimensions before it can obstruct a widely dilated esophagus. Moreover there is a tendency to ascribe the patient's complaints to his achalasia. The most frequent symptoms noted by JUST-VIERA and HAIGHT (1969) are weight loss, return of dysphagia and change of its character, continuous discomfort or pain, arrest of swallowed food at a specific, usually substernal site, cough, regurgitation, blood loss and anemia, and foul odor. The diagnosis must be suspected particularly when the symptoms occur after an apparently successful treatment, when the discomfort becomes continuous or when pain or bleeding develop (JUST-VIERA et al., 1967). Cytological examinations can yield positive results even if all other tests are negative (KLAYMAN, 1955).

8.1.6. Treatment

Although it has not been proven conclusively that food stasis causes cancer, most authors recommend early treatment of achalasia. Whether this will be sufficient to prevent a carcinomatous degeneration is as yet uncertain. Once a cancer has developed it must be treated in the usual way. The results, however, are very poor because of the late diagnosis and the rapid spread of these cancers.

8.2. Esophagitis

Food stasis causes esophagitis due to chemical and bacterial irritation. Exceptionally this may result in loss of blood. Hemorrhage, however, should primarily suggest cancer.

8.3. Bronchopulmonary Complications

Pulmonary symptoms occur in more than 10% of the patients (VINSON, 1924; ANDERSEN et al., 1953) and are mainly due to spill-over. They can be prominent in children (MOERSCH, 1929; PAYNE et al., 1961). Uni- or bilateral aspiration pneumonia, bronchiectasis, lungabscesses, pulmonary fibrosis and tuberculosis are the most frequent complications.

8.4. Perforation

Exceptionally spontaneous rupture (BENEDICT and GRILLO, 1962) and esophago-esophageal fistula formation (KNAUER et al., 1970) have been reported in patients with achalasia.

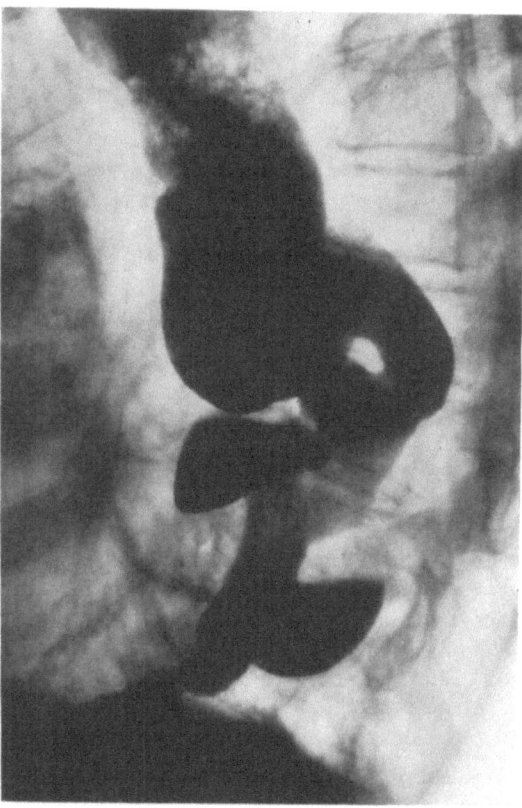

Fig. 180. Achalasia with multiple pulsion diverticula

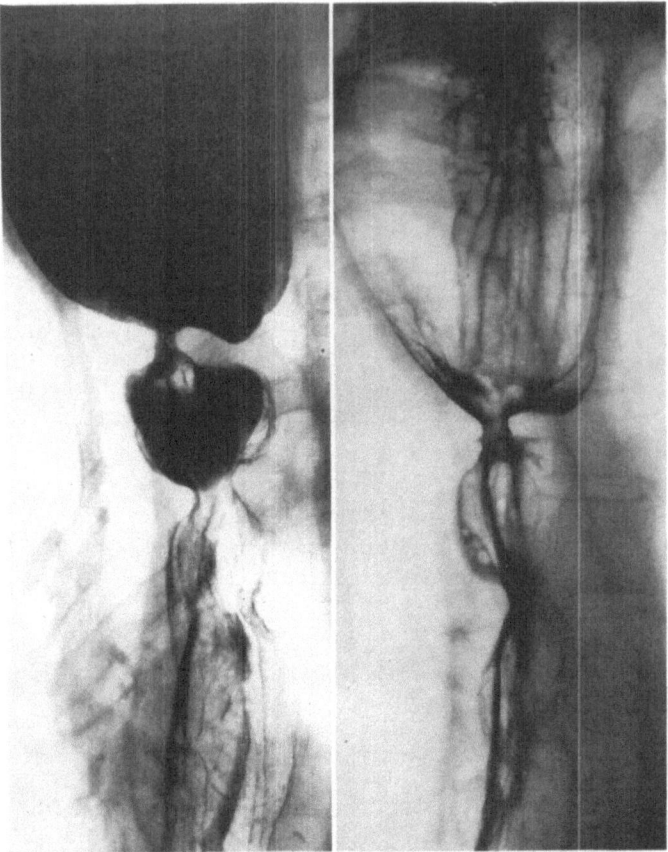

Fig. 181. Benign stenoses in the middle third of the esophagus in an achalasia patient. The strictures were found more than 4 years ago and until now no signs of carcinoma have been found on repeated esophagoscopy

8.5. Associated Conditions

Hiatal hernia is rarely combined with achalasia (Olsen et al., 1953; Binder et al., 1965). Sometimes traction diverticula of the mid-esophagus are found but pulsion diverticula in the lower third of the gullet are more common (Fig. 180) (Olsen et al., 1953). Other associated conditions have been reported in achalasia patients: an esophageal web about 5 cm above the diaphragm (Salzman, 1965), benign esophageal stenosis (Fig. 181), a thymoma (Demos et al., 1966) and arthralgias (Allison, 1950; Adams et al., 1961), In a 38-year-old patient with achalasia an atrioventricular block developed whenever the esophagus was distended by food (Rosch et al., 1969).

Pregnancy has been observed in the course of achalasia (Bloomfield, 1963; Karjalainen, 1964). If the symptoms are sufficiently severe, a pregnant woman may be treated by forceful dilatation.

9. Natural History

Although achalasia is a benign condition susceptible to treatment, it shortens life. ELLIS (1961) followed 69 patients for 10 to 25 years, during which period 28 died. Though some patients surpassed their normal life expectancy the majority did not. The onset of the disease at an early age appears to be associated with a limited survival period. Causes of death included carcinoma of the esophagus (8), cachexia (5) and causes apparently not related to the esophagus (11). One of the latter, however, died as a consequence of pneumonia, perhaps due to aspiration of esophageal contents.

10. Treatment

The current methods of treatment aim at improving the passage of food into the stomach by weakening the insufficiently relaxing sphincter. This can be achieved by stretching it forcefully (dilatation) or by dividing the circular muscle (cardiomyotomy). Theoretically it should be possible to decrease the resistance of the sphincter by medication. Whatever treatment is chosen the sphincteric function should be preserved sufficiently to prevent reflux. None of our current methods is capable of restoring the normal function of the esophagus.

10.1. Medical and Psychiatric Therapy

Current medical therapy can obtain at most temporary symptomatic relief, before more efficient treatment is instituted. Hyoscine-N-butylbromide (Buscopan) in a dose of 20 to 40 mg administrated I.V. improves the evacuation of the esophagus. Radiologically it opens the region of the cardia (WRIGHT, 1961); manometrically it decreases the sphincteric pressure (EDWARDS, 1964). But even in large doses by mouth it has no useful therapeutic effect (EDWARDS, 1964). Hexamethonium appears to be incapable of lowering the sphincter tone in cases of achalasia (SLESINGER et al., 1953; EDWARDS, 1964). Although β-adrenergic agents cause the circular muscle layer of the sphincter to relax, isopropyl noradrenaline does not affect the sphincter of the achalasia patient (EDWARDS, 1964). The in vitro studies of MISIEWICZ et al. (1968, 1969) show that the β-adrenergic inhibitory activity is lost in the muscles of the achalatic sphincter. Sympathectomy, formerly advocated by KNIGHT (1934), is also inefficient. It should be possible to reduce the lower esophageal sphincter tone in achalasia by inhibition of either gastrin release or gastrin effect (COHEN et al., 1971); whether this is clinically useful must still be demonstrated. Although it is now generally agreed that emotional instability is not a feature of the typical achalasia patient, nervous patients may derive benefit from sedatives. How hypnosis can lastingly improve achalasia (KLUMBICS, 1963) is as obscure as the therapeutic approach itself. The only medical treatment which seems valid nowadays is the administration of nitroglycerine in order to stop painful spasms.

10.2. Dilatations

Temporary relief of the dysphagia can be obtained by passing a mercury bougie, an olive dilator, or an esophagoscope through the cardia. The relief is quite temporary and incomplete, yet real. To obtain good, long term results a forceful dilatation of the sphincter is necessary. Several methods are currently used.

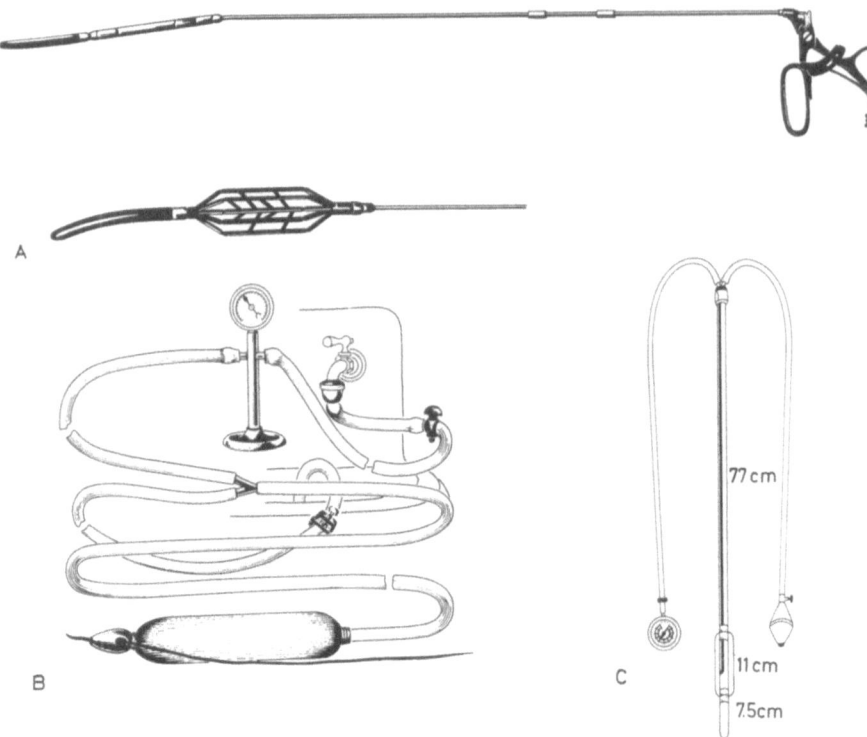

Fig. 182 A—D. Different types of dilators. A Starck dilator. B Plummer system. C Browne-
McHardy balloon. (After Ellis and Olsen: Achalasia of the esophagus, p. 125, 126 and 129.
Philadelphia: W. B. Saunders Co. 1969.) D Dilator used by the authors (Sippy system).
1 Nylon thread, to which a weighting mercury-filled latex bag is attached. 2 Metal wire, to
be passed over the nylon thread into the stomach. 3 Olive-tipped bougie. 4 Flexible wire
spiral. 5 Inner latex balloon. 6 Outer latex balloon. 7 Tube for air insufflation. 8 Nylon bag,
limiting the maximal diameter. 9 Covering latex balloon

10.2.1. Types of Dilators

10.2.1.1. Mechanical System (Fig. 182)

The Starck dilator (Fig. 182 A) is a device with expanding metal arms. The
expanding part is introduced at the level of the cardia and the sphincter is dilated
manually. The advantage of the system is that one can feel the moment the
sphincter yields. Its disadvantage is that the diameter of the dilator is not exactly
known, which makes it necessary to feel manually how far the dilator must be
expanded. The rigidity of most instruments precludes their use in the treatment
of the elongated sigmoid-shaped esophagus (Starck, 1924; Crump et al., 1952;
Schindler, 1956).

10.2.1.2. Hydrostatic System

The Negus hydrostatic dilator (Thomson, Negus et al., 1955) is introduced
through a large esophagoscope into the cardia, where the balloon is expanded.
The Plummer (1908) system (Fig. 182 B) has been used extensively by the Mayo
group. The instrument consists of a stomach tube with side openings. Three bags
are mounted over the end of the tube: an inner rubber, a middle silk and an
outer rubber bag. The silk bag limits the maximal diameter of the dilator to

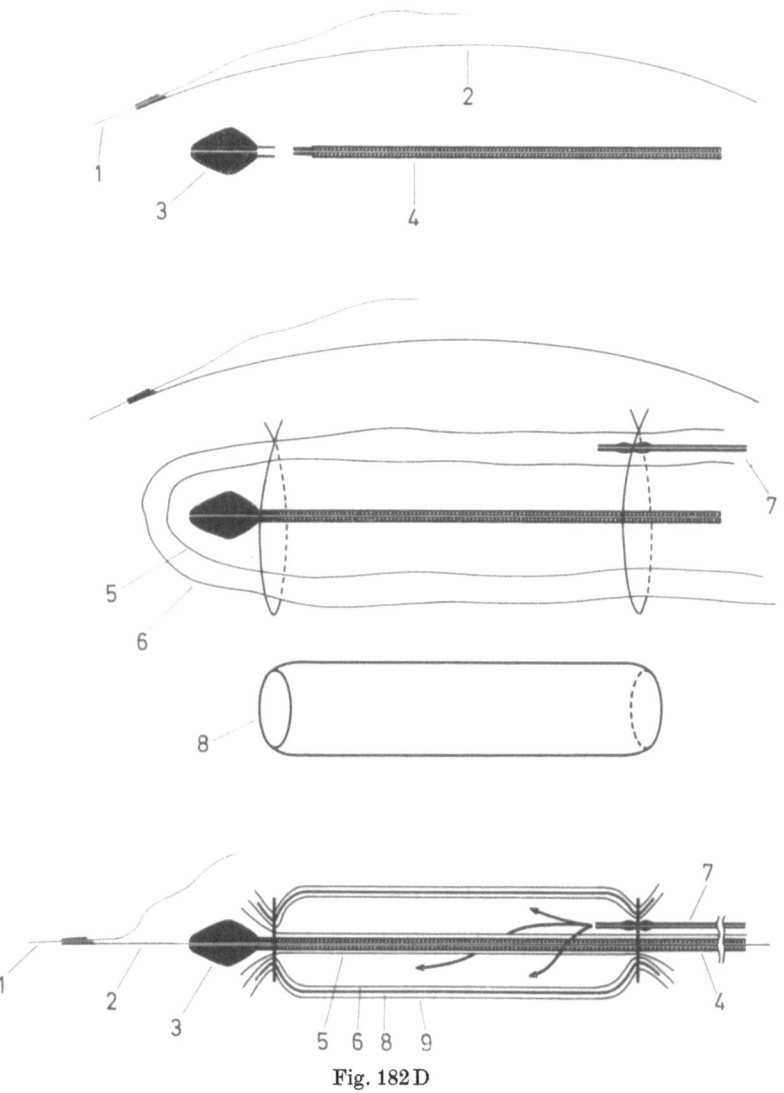

Fig. 182 D

3.6 cm. A flexible whale bone staff is passed through the rubber tube and a 41 F olive-tipped metal bougie is attached to the threaded end of the whale bone staff. The dilator is passed over a previously swallowed thread to avoid perforation. The correct position is determined in advance, not by fluoroscopy, but by measuring the distance between upper incisors and cardia by means of a 41 F olive-tipped bougie attached to a whale bone. Once positioned in the cardia, the dilator is connected to a water source and pressure gauge. The bag is slowly filled until a pressure of 18–22 feet of water is reached.

10.2.1.3. Pneumatic System

The TUCKER bag (1939) and the BROWNE-McHARDY bag (1939) (Fig. 182 C) are cylindrical balloons consisting of a silk and rubber bag coated with radiopaque material. The maximal diameter is 3 cm. The Tucker instrument is a mercury filled rubber tube on which the bag is mounted. The balloon is inflated to a fairly high pressure until the constriction at the level of the cardia disappears. The high pressure is maintained for 30–60 sec and then released. A few moments later the bag is reinflated. Disappearance of the constriction at 300 mm Hg or less is taken as evidence of successful dilatation. If necessary the procedure is repeated a second time during the same session (BENNETT and HENDRIX, 1970). The Browne-McHardy bag is almost the same instrument but it contains a mercury-filled tip. The Mosher bag (MOSHER and McGREGOR, 1928) has a maximum diameter of 3.6 cm, but as used by NANSON (1962) is inflated only to 15 psi which does not expand it fully.

It may be difficult to introduce these instruments into the cardia when the esophagus is widely dilated and sigmoid-shaped. BERGAN (1952) therefore mounted the bag around an esophagoscope.

The Sippy bag has been used by VANTRAPPEN et al. (1963, 1971) and by KURLANDER et al. (1963) (Fig. 182 D).

Typical for this method is the relatively low pressure (300 mm Hg) which is used to inflate the balloon and the fact that the procedure is spread over several sessions, using a progressively larger balloon. The technique we use can be summarized as follows (VANTRAPPEN et al., 1963, 1971). Before dilatation the patient swallows a mersilene string, weighted by a mercury-filled latex bag. Once the bag reaches the small bowel, it anchors and the string becomes a guide for the passage of the dilator. A metal wire with an eye at the end is threaded over the string into the stomach and provides a rigid guide for the safe passage of the dilator. The correct position is checked by fluoroscopy. When in place the balloon is insufflated to a pressure of 200 mm Hg for the first minute, than to 300 mm Hg for an additional minute. Initially a balloon with a diameter of 3 cm is used. A smaller balloon is used if the patient underwent a recent cardiomyotomy. At subsequent dilatations, the diameter of the balloon is increased to 3.5, 3.8, 4.2, 4.5 and rarely to 5 cm. Two to four dilatations are usually necessary. The mean number of dilatations per patient is 3.2. The criteria used to determine the number of dilatations include disappearance of dysphagia, mostly already after the first dilatation, ease in emptying the esophagus on fluoroscopy and broadening of the previously narrow lower esophageal segment. Whenever possible manometric criteria are used, i.e. complete or almost complete disappearance of the high pressure zone above the pressure inversion point. This criterium is based in the observation that a successful treatment of achalasia, either by myotomy or by dilatation, is characterized manometrically by the disappearance of the supradiaphragmatic high pressure zone (OLSEN et al., 1957; VANTRAPPEN, 1961). Manometric studies in a large group of carefully evaluated patients have demonstrated the validity of this criterium (VANTRAPPEN et al., 1971).

This method has the advantage that a flexible instrument is used, which is passed over a guiding wire. The method can be applied even when the esophagus is very tortuous; in some cases it may be desirable to omit the metal wire and simply to pass the balloon over the swallowed thread. The diameter of the balloon and hence the distending force can be adapted to each patient.

10.2.2. Preventive Measures

Before the dilatations are performed an organic obstruction at the cardia must be excluded by esophagoscopy or by mounting a 41 F olive-tipped metal bougie on top of the dilator. A fluid diet is given for a couple of days and the esophagus is evacuated in order to prevent aspiration pneumonia during the insertion of the dilator. The dilatation is performed with the patient in the upright position. If he is too weak to stand he is asked to sit down, because the sometimes abundant mucus secretions are hard to expel and can penetrate into the airways in the recumbent position. If the pain is too severe the dilatation is interrupted. If the patient is unable to cooperate sufficiently the dilatation is renounced. Mostly the pain disppaears or diminishes considerably within two minutes after the dilatation is finished. Analgetics are not given in order not to mask alarming reactions of the patient. A small amount of blood on the dilator as it is retracted is normal, and does not indicate a complication. As a rule the patients must refrain from drinking or eating for two hours after the dilatation. If the pain persists for a longer time a perforation may have occurred. In that case it is of the utmost importance that the patient does not take anything by mouth and is given antibiotics as soon as possible. If the patient's condition is good two hours after the dilatation no other measures are necessary.

10.2.3. Results

10.2.3.1. Immediate Results

The immediate results of forceful dilatations are excellent. Already after the first dilatation there is a considerable improvement of the dysphagia. From 1955 to 1968 we treated 138 patients (VANTRAPPEN et al., 1971). By the end of the treatment all stated that they were able to eat without distress. Regurgitation also had disappeared completely. The attacks of substernal pain did not always disappear immediately; in some cases it took several weeks before a relief was obtained, although the cramp-like pain was less severe than before the dilatation. Most patients gained weight rapidly.

10.2.3.2. Immediate Complications

In the 320 patients we treated until now with pneumatic dilatations the mortality rate was zero. Severe pain reactions with fever and occasionally pleural effusion were observed in 14 patients (4.4%), 7 of whom (2.2%) were found to have a perforation (Fig. 183). An empyema was drained surgically in two of them: one suffered from active Hodgkin's disease and was being treated with cytostatic drugs; in the other the perforation went unrecognized for some time and she was allowed to eat. Six of these perforations were localized in the distal segment of the esophagus. The seventh perforation occurred at the level of the hypopharynx. The seven other patients who developed pain, fever and a pleural effusion did not have a radiologically demonstrable perforation. In an other patient ECG signs of pericarditis without symptoms were observed after the dilatation. Bleeding requiring a transfusion of one pint of blood occurred in two patients. A third patient developed a small hemorrhage, for which transfusion was not deemed necessary. Aspiration pneumonia after the dilatation occurred in one patient.

OLSEN et al. (1951) mentioned 10 perforations in a series of 452 cases (2.2%). Two patients died, but this was before the advent of antibiotics. Two others underwent a thoracotomy and 6 recovered with conservative treatment. Moreover, 21 patients suffered severe epigastric or substernal pain several hours after the dilatation; some of them had fever, but there were no other sings of perforation. BENNETT and HENDRIX (1970) mentioned 3 perforations after 61

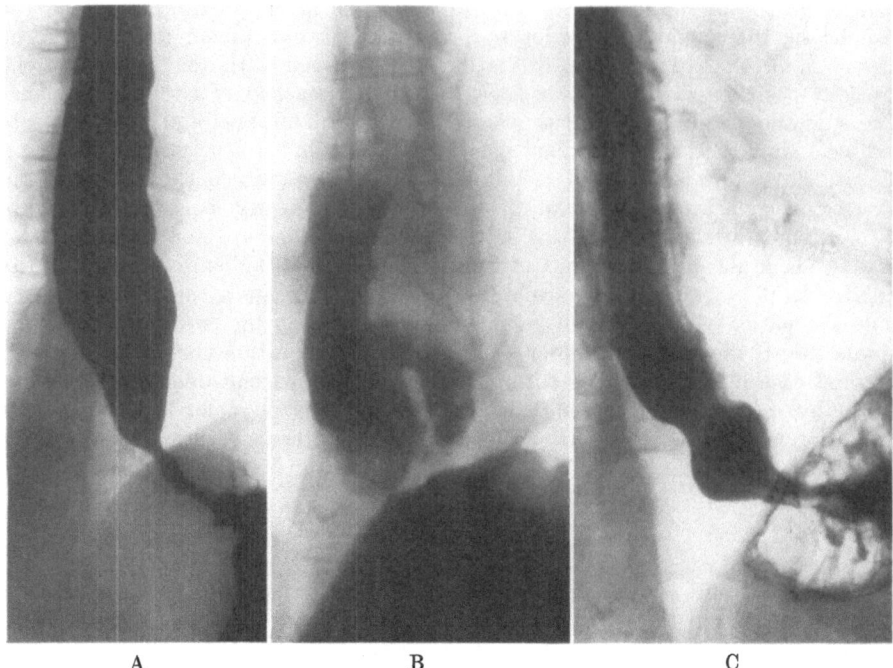

A   B   C

Fig. 183. A Achalasia before dilatation. B Perforation of the supradiaphragmatic esophageal segment after pneumatic dilatation. C Three weeks after B: the perforation has healed under conservative therapy

dilatations (4.9%) on 51 patients. Sanderson et al. (1970) reviewed the experience of the Mayo Clinic after 1950: 4.4% of the 408 patients developed major complications; 10 clearly had perforations which required surgical repair and drainage; 4 others probably had perforations: 3 had pleural effusion and one mediastinal emphysema; 4 others developed pleuritic chest pains and fever. Eight of the 90 patients treated by Kurlander et al. (1963) had prolonged chest pain and/or fever. These two symptoms were considered evidence of paraesophageal mediastinitis. All recovered uneventfully without a surgical procedure.

Schindler (1956) treated 84 patients with a Starck dilator. Three of them developed fever and two gastric lesions which required laparotomy. No fatalities occurred. Nemir et al. (1971) had 3 perforations in 40 patients; two of them died. Bennett (1968) mentioned two perforations in a series of 51 patients (3.9%). Sawyers and Foster (1967a, b) however, had 6 perforations in 64 patients (9.4%).

From these observations it appears that about 4% of the patients develop perforation or a left pleural effusion. In most of them the complication is limited to a pleural effusion with fever, which disappears rapidly after the administration of antibiotics. However, surgical repair is indicated for a few of them. Since antibiotics have become available the mortality has been almost zero in many large series (Starck, 1952; Olsen et al., 1951; Kurlander, 1963; Sanderson et al., 1970; Vantrappen et al., 1971).

A perforation must be suspected if the pain does not diminish 30 to 60 min after the dilatation or if it tends to become worse. Cramp-like pains similar to the attacks the patient experienced spontaneously before the treatment are not alarming. If the pain irradiates to the back or towards the left lower thorax, or if respiration becomes painful, a perforation must be suspected.

These patients should be watched very closely. After a few hours the breath sounds may diminish and palpation in the upper epigastrium may become painful. The radiographic picture may show a blurring of the left costophrenic sinus or a manifest pleural effusion. Hydropneumothorax occurred only once in our series and was associated with air in the mediastinum. According to ELLIS and OLSEN (1969) subcutaneous emphysema is frequently observed after perforation of the esophagus. In our series we noticed it only in the one patient who had a per-foration at the level of the hypopharynx. After a few hours the patient develops fever and leucocytosis and he looks severely ill. Whenever a patient experiences prolonged or abnormally severe pain after dilatation peroral feeding is stopped and treatment with antibiotics is started. If the pain continues onto the next day without evident signs of perforation, a radiographic examination with gastrog-rafin is performed to check whether there is a perforation. If not, peroral feeding is resumed as soon as the fever has passed. If there is a perforation, antibiotics, analgesics and parenteral feeding are continued. Pleural aspiration or continuous suction with a drain are sometimes indicated. The majority of these patients improve considerably after about three days of conservative therapy. After that, food may be administered through a gastric tube. This therapy is not started right away since it may cause vomiting in some patients. If a surgical repair of the perforation is deemed necessary it is best to perform it shortly after the accident. Residual abscesses of mediastinum or pleural cavity may require subsequent surgical drainage. Bleeding is rare and does not usually cause serious problems. It has been observed in 14 out of 1261 patients (OLSEN et al., 1951; KURLANDER et al., 1963; SANDERSON et al., 1970; VANTRAPPEN, unpublished results). Aspiration pneumonia may be caused during the insertion of the balloon. A fluid diet, correct positioning of the patient and perhaps the previous introduction of an olive-tipped metal bougie can usually prevent this complication.

10.2.3.3. Late Results

In 1970 we evaluated the late results of the 138 patients we treated with pneumatic dilatation at least three years before (VANTRAPPEN et al., 1971). The mean duration of the follow-up period was 6.6 years. The clinical evaluation of these patients was based upon the incidence and degree of dysphagia, retro-sternal pain, regurgitation and weight loss. They were subdivided into 4 groups according to the following criteria. Group I, excellent results, includes those patients who are completely free of symptoms. Group II, good results, consists of those patients who experience dysphagia or pain of short duration only oc-casionally: less than once a week there is a hesitancy of food retrosternally, lasting from a few seconds to a couple of minutes, and disappearing on drinking some fluid; there is no weight loss and no regurgitation. Group III comprises the moderate results. These patients experience dysphagia at least once a week. The sensation of food sticking in the esophagus does not last longer than a few minutes and does not prevent the patient from continuing and finishing his meal. It is not accompanied by regurgitation and weight loss. The patients are markedly improved as compared with the pre-treatment situation. Group IV, poor results. These patients have regularly dysphagia accompanied by regurgitation or daily retrosternal pain.

Table 13. Late results of pneumatic dilatations in 133 patients. Figures in parentheses give the number of patients who have had two or three series of dilatations

	Before treatment		Late after treatment	
	number of patients	%	number of patients	%
Group 1. Excellent	—	—	60 (2)	45.1
Group 2. Good	—	—	42 (5)	31.6
Group 3. Moderate	14	10.5	23 (6)	17.3
Group 4. Poor	119	89.5	8 (3)	6

Follow-up data were obtained on 133 of the 138 patients treated during that period.

Excellent or good results (Group I and II) were obtained in 76.7% of the patients. Moderate results in 17.3% and poor results in 6% (Table 13). If the same criteria are applied to the pre-treatment condition of the patients, 90% of them belong to Group IV and 10% to Group III. 94% of the patients were significantly improved by the treatment.

The radiological examinations indicate that the dilatations resulted in an immediate and sustained reduction in the diameter of the esophagus (Figs. 184 to 186). A return to normal was observed only if the esophageal diameter before treatment was not larger than 70 mm (Table 14). The mean diameter of the lower esophageal sphincter increased from 2 mm before to 9 mm late after treatment ($p < 0.005$). The elongation and tortuosity of the esophagus were hardly affected. Solid food remnants after an overnight fast were observed in 53 cases before and in 14 late after pneumatic dilatation. Before treatment the gastric air bubble was absent in 86% of the patients, late after treatment in only 8.4%. The best results were obtained in patients over the age of 45, in patients with a history of more than 5 years' duration, and in patients with a moderately dilated gullet. To obtain these results 16 patients had to undergo 2 or 3 series of dilatations. In 71.5% of the cases excellent or good results were obtained after a single series. Treatment of recurrences was successful in only 7 out of 16 cases, and thus seems to be less efficient.

Olsen et al. (1951) evaluated the results of hydrostatic dilatations in 452 cases. The follow-up period was 4 years or more. Satisfactory results were obtained in 69.2% of their cases (i.e. the patients had no dysphagia or only occasional or transient difficulty with swallowing). In their series also, patients who did

Table 14. Diameter of esophagus in 116 patients with achalasia before, immediately after and late after treatment

Diameter (mm)	Before treatment		Immediately after treatment		Late after treatment	
	number	mean	mean	range	mean	range
<40	18	35	27,6	16–38	28.1	18–42
40–49	30	44	34.3	20–48	33.6	23–60
50–59	23	53.2	35.4	26–50	33.3	19–45
60–69	20	63	45	27–71	49.3	30–78
70–79	16	72	41.7	33–60	51	32–89
80–89	3	81	53.3	43–70	67	50–80
90–99	3	91.7	76.7	70–90	66.3	62–70
≥100	3	103.3	73.7	55–90	72	41–100

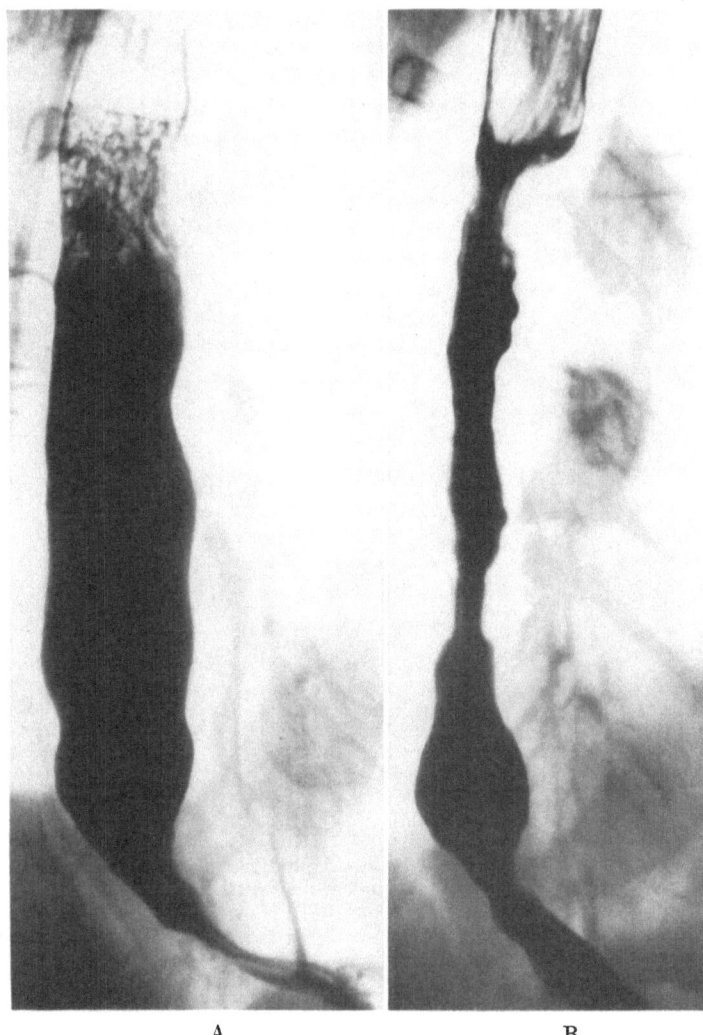

A   B

Fig. 184A and B. Achalasia with a moderately dilated esophagus before (A) and after (B) pneumatic dilatation

not respond satisfactorily to the initial course of treatment were less likely to obtain good results following a second course. A third treatment was successful in only 19.1% of the cases. The moderately dilated esophagus responded better to treatment than the slightly dilated gullet.

SANDERSON et al. (1970) obtained 65% excellent or good results in their series of 408 patients at the Mayo Clinic after 1950; 81% of the patients were improved 1 year or more after treatment. 50 patients underwent a subsequent Heller myotomy because of the persistence or recurrence of major symptoms. Patients who had dilatation therapy because of persisting symptoms after myotomy were excluded from the study. 23% of the patients treated were lost for follow-up.

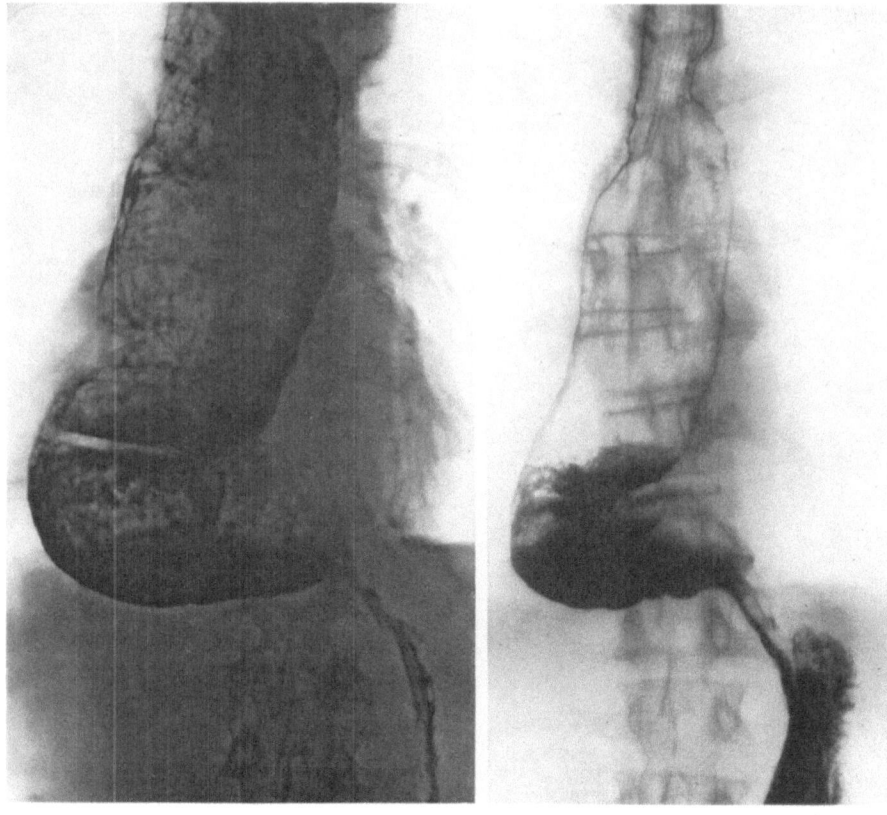

A   B

Fig. 185 A and B. Achalasia with markedly dilated and tortuous esophagus before (A) and after (B) pneumatic dilatation

The results of forceful dilatations reported in the literature vary rather widely. Much depends on the criteria used and on the duration and thoroughness of the follow-up studies. If the follow-up period is short, e.g. one year, recurrences which take place later are not taken into account. Follow-up studies based on mailed questionnaires are less valid then those based on personal interview and examination of the patients. The percentage of treated patients comprised in the follow-up studies is also important. In the policy of SANDERSON et al. (1970) and of LAWRANCE and SHOESMITH (1959) usually only one dilatation is performed and if it fails a Heller operation is done at once; under these circumstances dilatation gives good results in only 60% of the patients. After repeated dilatations good results can be expected in about 80% of the cases (OLSEN et al., 1951; NANSON, 1966; VANTRAPPEN et al., 1971; DOUVLARIS et al., 1971). KURLANDER et al. (1963) were successful after a variable number of pneumatic dilatations in 84% of the patients.

Both better and poorer results were reported (SCHINDLER, 1956; BECK et al., 1960; LAWRANCE and SHOESMITH, 1959; SAWYERS and FOSTER, 1967a). As is true for surgical therapy the most brilliant results are reported in series with a short or incomplete follow-up and in studies with vague or broad criteria.

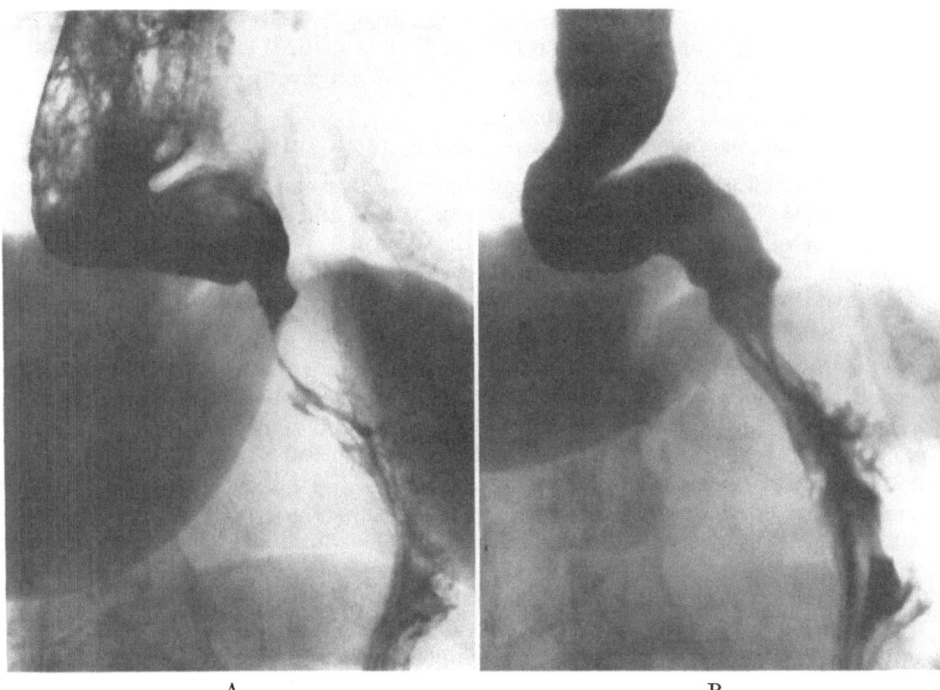

A   B

Fig. 186. A Achalasia before dilatation. B Same lower esophageal segment after pneumatic dilatation

10.3. Surgical Treatment
10.3.1. Techniques

Before cardiomyotomy became the standard procedure a whole series of operations were performed more or less successfully.

10.3.1.1. Operations Based on the Theory of "Idiopathic Dilatation"

Before the importance of the gastroesophageal sphincteric dysfunction was realized interventions were done to narrow the caliber of the dilated esophagus (REISINGER, 1907; MEYER, 1911), to shorten the gullet (TUFFIER, 1922; FREEMAN, 1923; VON HACKER, 1926; CIAGLIA and SEGAL, 1962) or to free the gullet from surrounding diaphragmatic structures which were thought to cause the obstruction at the cardia (ROEPKE, 1914; GRÉGOIRE, 1923, 1924). Still recently a longitudinal excision of the redundant sigmoid loop of a megaesophagus was performed in addition to a myotomy (NICKS, 1968).

10.3.1.2. Operations Based on the Theory of a Disturbance in Esophageal Innervation

Both vagotomy and sympathectomy have been attempted. Vagotomy was done in order to eliminate the motor innervation of the gullet and thus to abolish the alleged cardiospasm (SAUERBRUCH, 1921; PIERI, 1932). KNIGHT (1934) showed that in cats bilateral vagotomy led to an achalasia-like condition and that sympathetic denervation prevents the "cardiospasm" effect of vagotomy. Recently these observations have been partially confirmed by Burgess et al. (1972). Craig et al. (1934) and Knight (1935) and Nuboer (1939) treated a few patients with sympathectomy, but the results were moderate and of short duration.

10.3.1.3. Operations Aimed at Decreasing the Resistance at the Cardia

10.3.1.3.1. Instrumental and finger dilatation through a gastrostomy (Gottstein, 1904; Mikulicz, 1904; Schloffer, 1919) and dilatation by finger invagination of the anterior stomach wall (Wakeley, 1916) were hardly more effective than peroral bougienage and were rather dangerous. Retrograde dilatation over a thread via a gastrostomy was also attempted with little success (Martin, 1901).

10.3.1.3.2. Early surgical attempts to completely distroy or bypass the gastroesophageal sphincter were effective in relieving the stasis, but unavoidably resulted in a high incidence of reflux esophagitis and stenosis. Procedures such as the Wendel cardioplasty (1910), the extramucosal cardioplasty (Girard, 1915), or the gastroesophagostomy according to Heyrovsky (1911, 1913) or modifications designed to avoid spur formation (Lambert, 1913; Backer-Gröndahl, 1916; Keller, 1928) have been abandoned for that reason. Already in 1922 Finsterer pointed to the relation between gastroesophageal reflux and esophagitis and warned against the late consequences of such interventions. In the English literature it was mainly Maingot (1944, 1949) who stressed the advantages of esophagomyotomy and emphasized the disturbing complications following esophagogastrostomy and cardioplasty. Barrett and Franklin (1949) documented 25 personal cases, 19 of whom had undergone esophagogastrostomy and 6 a Wendel cardioplasty. Because of the high incidence of esophagitis, which was responsible for the poor late results, they preferred a Heller myotomy.

Excision of the acid secreting area of the stomach together with removal of the redundant portion of the lower esophagus (Wangensteen, 1951) has been abandoned (Wangensteen, 1957) because of bile esophagitis and pernicious anemia in some of the patients.

Recently a modified Thal procedure has been proposed for the treatment of far advanced cases of achalasia and of patients treated unsuccessfully by a Heller or Wendel procedure (Hatafuku et al., 1972). A longitudinal full-thickness incision is made on the narrow segment 5 to 6 cm above and 1 to 2 cm below the gastroesophageal junction. The esophageal defect is patched by pulling the fundus over it. By enclosing the reconstructed esophagus in a fold of the gastric fundus, a one-way valve is constructed. Hirashima and Sato (1970) described an analogous technique of "esophagocardioplasty with gastric patch".

10.3.1.3.3. The Heller myotomy and its modifications.
This procedure was already proposed by Gottstein in 1901 but was first performed by Heller in 1913 and published in 1914. Planning to perform a cardioplasty he was struck by the gross appearance of the distal esophagus and the cardia. He did not find any macroscopic lesion at the level of the cardia but a zone of narrowing, thought to be due to some type of spastic contraction. In analogy with the pyloromyotomy performed for the treatment of pylorospasm he transected the longitudinal and circular muscle layer of the lower esophagus over a distance of about 8 cm down to the esophagogastric junction. Because the result of an anterior myotomy was insufficient he added a second, posterior incision. The result was very good. The technique was not very well received in his own country. In 1921 he was aware of only 16 cases who had

been treated in this manner with this technique, either by himself or by others. After the report of PAYR in 1929 the Heller myotomy became the operation of choice in France (DELBERT, 1929), Belgium, the Netherlands (ZAAYER, 1919) and Italy (LUSENA, 1932).

Several modifications have been introduced. The most important one has been to limit the procedure to one, anterior incision (DE BRUINE GROENEVELDT, 1918; ZAAYER, 1923). To facilitate the transection of the whole muscle layer without touching the mucosa, the incision was made over the finger inserted through a gastrostomy (AMBRUMJANZ, 1930) or over an inflated Foley bag (WANGENSTEEN, 1957). Other additional interventions were proposed as well: sympathectomy, by way of a left splanchnicectomy (DUBOURG, 1949) or by way of resection of the left splanchnic and the dorsal sympathetic nerve (FONTAINE and FRANK, 1950), vagotomy (BOLOT et al., 1949; HEPP, 1949), and freeing the distal esophagus; none of these have turned out to be essential additions to the myotomy.

Additional procedures have also been proposed to prevent reflux esophagitis: vagotomy with and without pyloroplasty (MERENDINO, 1956), pylorotomy alone (HAWTHORNE et al., 1956; NEMIR and FROBESE, 1962; FROBESE et al., 1964), pyloroplasty (WANGENSTEEN, 1957; ROOT and WANGENSTEEN, 1962), gastropexy (BOEREMA, 1958), esophago-cardiofundopexy (to restore the angle of His) (RUDLER, 1950; LORTAT-JACOB et al., 1956; SANTA et al., 1956a, b), fundoplication (DOR et al., 1962; NISSEN and ROSSETTI, 1962), Belsey repair (BELSEY, 1966; CROSS, 1971) and suturing the gastric fundus over the exposed distal esophageal mucosa (JEKLER and LHOTKA, 1967).

ELLIS (ELLIS and OLSEN, 1969) limits the procedure to an ordinary myotomy down to the mucosa, from a few millimeters below the esophagogastric junction up to 6–12 cm above it. The muscle wall is dissected laterally from the mucosa, so that approximately half or more of the circumference of the esophageal mucosa is free, permitting it to protrude freely through the incision. The easiest approach is a left thoracotomy. Vagus branches as well as diaphragmatic attachments are left intact as much as possible. If necessary, the esophagogastric junction is fixed in a firm position with interrupted sutures in the phrenoesophageal membrane and subsequently by narrowing the hiatus by means of a suture approximation of the diaphragmatic crura posteriorly.

Although most authors use the thoracic approach, others prefer a laparotomy, which permits an additional drainage operation or a fundopexy (LORTAT-JACOB et al., 1956; SANTY et al., 1956a, b; STEICHEN, HELLER et al., 1960; NEMIR and FROBESE, 1962; JEKLER and LHOTKA, 1967; LAGACHE et al., 1970).

10.3.1.4. Operations to Replace Part of the Esophagus by Intestine

After resection of the distal segment of the esophagus the continuity of the intestinal tract can be restored by a Roux anastomosis of a jejunal loop with the esophagus, while the proximal end of the stomach is closed (BARRETT and FRANKLIN, 1949). AGUIRRE et al. (1963) also reported 5 such cases with good results in all. However, the procedure has many of the disadvantages of a total gastrectomy. Depending on the extent of the dilatation, surgeons have interposed jejunum (MERENDINO and DILLARD, 1955) or colon (COUTO and ALDROVANDO, 1966) to replace the resected esophagus and to restore the continuity of esophagus and stomach. This operation can be performed after failure of a Heller's operation or in patients who developed reflux esophagitis subsequent to a cardiomyotomy.

10.3.2. Results and Complications of Heller's Myotomy

10.3.2.1. Results

The Heller operation yields good results in 64 to 88% of the patients. Ellis and Olsen (1969) collected from the literature 1906 cases of different follow-up periods (Suermondt, 1953; Mattos, 1955; de Vernejoul et al., 1956; Delannoy and Soots, 1956; Santy et al., 1956a, b; Gammelgaard et al., 1956; Deloyers and Loygue, 1956; Malm, 1956; Acheson and Hadley, 1958; Tuttle et al., 1958; Cecconi, 1959; Douglas and Nicholson, 1959; Lawrance and Shoe-smith, 1959; Ferguson and Burford, 1960; Rudler, 1960; Barlow, 1961; Ellis, 1962a; Barrett, 1964; Frobese et al., 1964; Benedict, 1964; de Bella 1965; Lortat-Jacob, 1965; Belsey, 1966; Helsingen et al., 1967). Improvement was obtained in 83.6% of the patients, whereas no improvement or even deterioration occurred in 11.6%. The mortality rate was 1.4%. In more recent series the number of failures tends to be somewhat lower still (Grimes et al., 1970; Effler et al., 1971). Ellis and Olsen (1969) evaluated the results of Heller's operation in a series of 268 patients; the follow-up period varied from 1 to 17.5 years, with a mean of 5.5 years. The result was excellent in 47%, good in 36% and fair in 11% of their cases (fair, i.e. the patient continued to have some dysphagia and heartburn in excess of what might be considered normal); 6% of the patients did not improve, or developed a recurrence.

Myotomy brings immediate relief; if it does not the persistent dysphagia is mostly due to incomplete section of the circular muscle. In such cases Ellis and Olsen (1969) dilated the cardia, often successfully, with a 45 F bougie. Four of the 95 patients of Effler et al. (1971) derived no initial benefit from the esophagomyotomy, and failed to improve with subsequent bougienage. Recurrence may also take place if the continuity of the myotomized muscle is restored by scar formation; in some cases the myotomy scar is barely visible at reoperation (Lagache et al., 1970; Patrick et al., 1971). Recurrences may take place as late as 5 years after the operation (Patrick et al., 1971). Great care must therefore be taken that the mucosa can pout freely through the myotomy (Fig. 187). This can be achieved by removing a strip of muscle tissue (Lortat-Jacob, 1956; Chesterman, 1965), or by dissecting the mucosa from the esophageal wall over about half the circumference of the esophagus (Ellis and Olsen, 1969). Recurrences can be treated by a second myotomy or by pneumatic dilatations. We have been successful with the latter in 12 cases, but it requires great care in ascertaining that no organic stenosis is present at the cardia. Palmer (1972) obtained good results with a Starck dilator in 7 out of his 9 patients.

Another cause of failure is too short a myotomy. Distally the myotomy must be extended half a centimeter across the esophagogastric junction so that the gastric mucosa is exposed just barely. The incision should be carried cephalad 7 to 9 cm from the esophagogastric junction well over the dilated, thickwalled portion of the esophagus to ensure complete relief of the obstructing suprahiatal portion of the sphincter (Gammelgaard et al., 1956; Ellis and Olsen, 1969; Nemir et al., 1971). Silber (1965) however, makes his incision on the esophageal side only 2 to 2.5 cm long. Still others (Grimes et al., 1970) make an incision as long as 12 to 15 cm, beginning at the level of the inferior pulmonary vein. When the myotomy is too short it can be lengthened in either direction. A distal lengthening entails the risk of sphincter incompetence. Proximal lengthening does not always yield the desired result (Patrick et al., 1971).

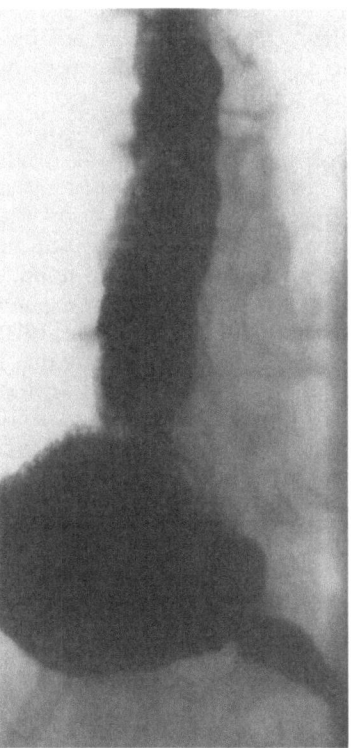

Fig. 187. Outpouching of the right contour of the lower esophagus after a myotomy for achalasia

The published results are widely divergent, which is due to a number of factors. The duration of the follow-up period plays a certain role (BARRETT, 1964; MILROY, 1969). Though it is often assumed that after 5 years a good result of a Heller operation may be considered permanent, it may take many years for a peptic stenosis to develop. One year after the operation BARKER and FRANKLIN (1971) noted 28 excellent results out of 30; but among the 14 patients who were followed up for more than 10 years, only 5 had no complaints and 5 had developed severe reflux esophagitis. In the series of PATRICK et al. (1971) 5 of the 6 patients who developed peptic stenosis after myotomy had been doing well for a period of two months to 7 years. Late complications, after 5 years or more, have been mentioned also by BARLOW (1961), BARKER and FRANKLIN (1971), WINGFIELD and KARWOWSKI (1972). Another factor which determines the quality of the result is the stage of the disease at the time of treatment: nearly all agree that the better results are obtained before the development of a large sigmoid esophagus (JEKLER et al., 1964; NEMIR et al., 1971; WINGFIELD and KARWOWSKI, 1972). The initial impression of GAMMIE et al. (1958) and TON (1961) that an early operation favors reflux has not been confirmed, so that most authors advocate treatment as soon as the diagnosis has been established. In large series such as that of ELLIS and OLSEN (1969) esophagomyotomy has had a high success rate, nearly independent of age, sex, previous treatment, duration of symptoms and stage of the disease. Undoubtedly, other factors contribute to the divergence of the reported results. The method of evaluation (by means of a mailed question-naire or a personal interview, complimented or not by objective examinations), the criteria for classifying the results and the percentage of patients lost for follow-up (dead or alive) must influence the success rate.

Most failures are due to the development of reflux esophagitis, especially when the dysphagia occurs late after treatment (JEKLER and LHOTKA, 1967; ELLIS and OLSEN, 1969). Periesophageal fibrosis has also been described as a cause of symptoms after myotomy (LAGACHE et al., 1970; EFFLER et al., 1971). If dysphagia recurs after a successful Heller operation the possibility of carcinom-atous degeneration should always be kept in mind. For even an early and successful Heller operation does not completely exclude the risk of developing a carcinoma (SAUBIER et al., 1970; REES et al., 1970; GRIMES et al., 1970). Moreover, some patients seem to be rather intractable by any method of treat-ment. If failures of forceful dilatations are dilated again, the results of the second course are clearly inferior to those of the initial course (OLSEN et al., 1953; VAN-TRAPPEN et al., 1971). If such failures are treated by myotomy the results are also less favorable than those of a Heller operation performed as a primary procedure. ELLIS and OLSEN (1969) noted that 11 of their 16 patients with poor results had undergone previous dilatations. They ascribe this to the periesoph-ageal fibrosis due to dilatation; however, patients who suffer a perforation during dilatation tend to do well once they have recovered, though they must have extensive fibrosis. If failures of a Heller procedure are treated by a second myotomy the results are inferior to those of a primary Heller operation. PATRICK et al. (1971) performed a second myotomy on 11 patients 5 months to 11 years after the first operation. One died while undergoing a concomitant pyloroplasty; the result was poor in one, fair in another. The latter two patients were precisely those in whom the primary myotomy was still quite visible. Other surgeons were also rather unsuccessful with a second Heller operation (SAWYERS and FOSTER, 1967a, b; LAGACHE et al., 1970).

10.3.2.2. Complications

In their series of 300 patients ELLIS and OLSEN (1969) reported one death and 11 significant complications. One patient developed a subphrenic abscess, another a mediastinal abscess and three an empyema, which necessitated an open drainage for two of them and a decortication for the third. In all these patients the mucosa was perforated accidentally. Another patient developed postoperative pneumonia and two a massive postoperative atelectasis which required bronchoscopic management. There were two significant wound infections.

The same authors collected from the literature 1906 cases of myotomy and found a mortality rate of 1.4%. There have also been case reports of patients who later died from malnutrition or at a second intervention (BARLOW, 1961; HELSINGEN et al., 1967; PATRICK et al., 1971). The most important early com-plication of Heller's myotomy is the inadvertent perforation of the mucosa at the time of the intervention. Such a perforation is closed with one or two sutures; some surgeons cover the sutured mucosal defect with a pedicled flap of diaphragmatic muscle (PETROVSKY, 1962; JEKLER et al., 1964), with a dia-phragmatic muscle patch (TRINCAS, 1954) or with a fundoplication (ROSSETTI, 1963). WINGFIELD and KARWOWSKI (1972) advocate air insufflation in the eso-phagus during the intervention to ensure that the mucosa is intact. If an empyema results, it must be drained as soon as possible, and peroral feeding must be stopped. Other complications include left phrenic nerve paralysis, massive hemorrhage and necrosis of stomach and esophagus due to herniation and strangulation (REES et al., 1970).

The most important late complication is reflux esophagitis (DUBOURG et al., 1962; ELLIS and COLE, 1965; PATRICK et al., 1971). According to some authors this is most likely to happen if the myotomy is lengthened too far distally. FERGUSON and BURFORD (1960) and ELLIS (PATRICK et al., 1971) insist that it must not reach further than 0.5 cm across the esophagogastric junction. Others (NEMIR and FROBESE, 1962; EFFLER et al., 1971) find it good practice to carry the myotomy below the esophagogastric junction into the anterior wall of the stomach for 1 to 2 cm. An other predisposing factor is hiatal hernia, which may have been present before the myotomy or may have developed postoperatively, due to extensive mobilization of the supporting structures of the cardia at the time of operation (RAVITCH, 1958; FROBESE et al., 1961; ELLIS and OLSEN, 1969). Therefore, any deliberate incisions in the diaphragm or the phrenoesophageal ligament should be avoided.

Stasis in the stomach is thought to favor the development of esophagitis (HERRON et al., 1957) so that it is wise to keep the vagus intact (BARLOW et al., 1961). Others perform a pyloroplasty or a pylorotomy to prevent stasis, but this requires an abdominal approach (BURFORD and LISCHER, 1956; HAWTHORNE et al., 1956; NEMIR and FROBESE, 1962). The severity of this complication has led a number of surgeons to perform an antireflux operation together with the myotomy (see 10.3.1.3.). An already existing hernia must definitely be reduced.

Fortunately, the incidence of peptic esophagitis after a Heller operation is lower than that of gastroesophageal reflux, as is indicated by Tables 15 and 16. A very high incidence was found by HAWTHORNE and NEMIR (1953). Roentgenoscopically 11 of their 21 patients (52%) were shown to have reflux. In 1956 HAWTHORNE et al. reported that 21% of their 34 patients had esophagitis associated with dysphagia, pain, or hemorrhage. In more recent publications of this group (NEMIR et al., 1971), 40% of the patients turned out to have reflux if this was especially looked for, and 13 patients (18%) had esophagitis with strictures. JEKLER et al. (1964), who treated 21 patients with myotomy, had 2 patients with reflux resulting in stenosis and one with sustained heartburn. HELSINGEN et al. (1967) also report a high incidence of reflux, 9 out of 46 patients; 2 required additional surgery, and 1 of them died of peritonitis subsequent to it. Dysphagia due to stricture may appear years after the operation (PATRICK et al., 1971).

Table 15. Incidence of gastroesophageal reflux after myotomy

Author	Number of myotomy patients	Number of patients with G.E. reflux
HAWTHORNE et al. (1956)	21	11
LORTAT-JACOB (1956)	75	10
DELOYERS and LOYGUE (1956)	146	24
SANTY et al. (1956)	168	12
BROWSE and CARTER (1961)	15	1
BARLOW (1961)	59	21
ELLIS (1962)	33	5
ELLIS and COLE (1965)	56	17
HELSINGEN et al. (1966)	56	8
HELSINGEN et al. (1967)	46	9
BENNETT and HENDRIX (1970)	54	12
MILROY (1969)	19	7
PAYNE et al. (1960)	49	2

Table 16. Incidence of reflux esophagitis after myotomy

Authors	Number of myotomy patients	Number of patients with esophagitis	Strictures (if mentioned)
Hawthorne et al. (1956)	35	7	
Dubourg et al. (1962)	48	12	3
Michaud (1952)	145	5	
Payne et al. (1960)	96	4	0
Ferguson and Burford (1960)	44	4	
Ellis and Cole (1965)	50	9	4
Barlow (1961)	59	6	6
Helsingen et al. (1967)	46	2	1
Ellis and Olsen (1969)	256	10	6
Bennett and Hendrix (1970)	51	6	
Rees et al. (1970)	59	9	1
Sawyers and Foster (1967)	22	5	1
Jekler et al. (1964)	21	3	2
Barker and Franklin (1971)	14	5	5
Nemir et al. (1971)	74	13	3
Wingfield and Karwowski (1972)	25	4	3

The treatment of severe reflux esophagitis following a Heller myotomy is difficult. Medical treatment should first be attempted; strictures can be relieved by bougienage at regular intervals. In some cases major surgery will be required. Ellis et al. (1958) suggested proximal gastric resection with antrectomy. Rapant and Doubravsky (1961) showed that Heyrowsky's esophagofundostomy in combination with either distal gastrectomy or vagotomy and pyloroplasty can yield equally good results. For patients in good condition resection of the diseased portion of the esophagus and proximal gastrectomy with interposition of either a jejunal loop (Merendino and Dillard, 1955) or a colon segment (Montenegro and Cutait, 1958; Neville and Clowes, 1963) tends to become the treatment of choice. The use of fundoplication with esophagogastrostomy after conservative resection for esophageal stricture has been advocated by Bombeck et al. (1970). An other procedure which can be performed is the modified Thal-operation (Hatafuku et al., 1972) or an esophagocardioplasty with gastric patch (Hirashima and Sato, 1970). Intraesophageal pH measurements indicate that these two procedures are capable of preventing reflux. For patients in poor condition surgery is often limited to a simple Finney pyloroplasty (Burford and Lischer, 1956).

There have been reports of herniation through a diaphragmatic counter incision (Gammie et al., 1958). Another complication was the development of a paraesophageal hiatal hernia (Hawthorne et al., 1956) which may sometimes be combined with incarceration and necrosis of the stomach (Havard, 1963).

10.4. Sphincteric Pressures after Treatment

After efficient treatment the pressure in the gastroesophageal sphincter is lowered. Forceful dilatation weakens the sphincter; in its supradiaphragmatic portion the high pressure zone is almost entirely abolished, but below the hiatus there remains a high pressure zone (Olsen et al., 1957). In patients who will turn out to be failures after dilatation, the end-expiratory resting pressure measured at the completion of the treatment remains high; if the treatment

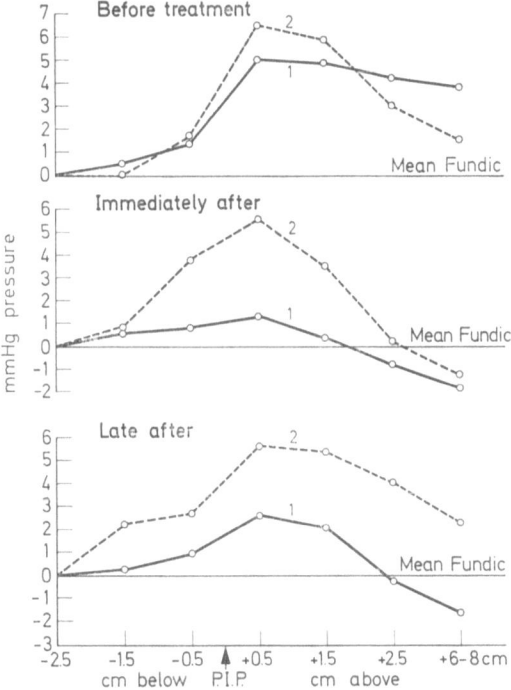

Fig. 188. Mean end-expiratory resting pressure in the lower esophageal sphincter of achalasia patients, before (upper diagram), immediately after (middle diagram), and late after treatment (lower diagram). Continuous lines indicate patients with satisfactory results; broken lines patients with unsatisfactory results or recurrences. [From VANTRAPPEN et al.: Gut **12**, 268 (1971)]

turns out to be a success, the supradiaphragmatic high pressure zone is abolished at the end of treatment and the pressure remains low during the follow-up period (VANTRAPPEN et al., 1971) (Fig. 188). COHEN and LIPSHUTZ (1971) and HEITMANN (1971), using perfused catheters, also found the sphincteric pressure of achalasia patients to be lowered to one third of its original value after pneumatic dilatation.

The sphincter pressure of normal dogs (McVEY et al., 1963; ELLIS et al., 1967) and of achalasia patients (ELLIS et al., 1967; ELLIS and OLSEN, 1969) decreases significantly after myotomy whereas the pressure in the distal part of the sphincter is partially preserved. In patients who developed reflux after cardiomyotomy the sphincter pressure is lowered more than in those without reflux (ATKINSON and SUMERLING, 1959).

10.5. Myotomy or Forceful Dilatation?

A large number of authors radically opt for myotomy. EFFLER et al. (1971) consider dilatations to be a "non-productive phase of therapy that offers little more than short-term relief". DUGAN (1970) feels that dilatation should be reversed for rural areas in which no thoracic surgeon is available. Others are less outspoken, though they also consider the Heller myotomy as the treatment of choice for achalasia; among them are NEMIR (NEMIR and FROBESE, 1962;

Nemir et al., 1971), the Mayo group (Payne et al., 1961; Clagett, 1967; Ellis et al., 1967; Ellis and Olsen, 1969; Sanderson, 1970), Lawrance and Shoe- smith (1959), Ravitch (1970), and Grimes et al., (1970). However, some of the arguments against dilatation are hardly valid. Thus it is claimed that dilatations are unsafe and dangerous (Barlow, 1961; Effler et al., 1971; Wingfield and Karwowski, 1972) with an overall mortality of 9.4% (Dugan, 1970), whereas cardiomyotomy is termed a safe, uncomplicated procedure with negligible morbidity (Effler et al., 1971). It is also claimed that to be effective dilatation requires a dilator capable of expanding to a diameter of 5 to 7 cm (Chester- man, 1965). In addition the results of dilatations are alleged to be poor as well as temporary. In the best hands, it is stated, reasonable results approach 60%, but the percentage does not represent the long term outlook; thus the majority of the patients require multiple dilatations so that the clinical picture is one of obstruction recurring between dilatations and the patient is unable to lead a normal life (Effler et al., 1971). Some authors state that the bag cannot always be engaged in the narrow segment (Barrett, 1964). This may be especially difficult if a rigid instrument such as the Starck dilator is used (Hafter, 1969). It is also said that a patient recovers more rapidly after a myotomy and Van- trappen is cited as belonging "to the increasing number of surgeons that recognize surgery as the primary treatment for achalasia" (Wingfield and Karwowski, 1972).

It is true that a Heller myotomy has become a safe procedure. Ellis and Olsen (1969) arrived at an over-all mortality figure of 1.4% in the literature, but in their own series the figure was only 0.3%. The mortality rate of forceful dilatation is also very low: in our own series of 320 cases treated with pneumatic dilatations it was zero despite the numerous poor risk cases; also in that of Sanderson et al. (1970) (408 patients, treated with hydrostatic dilatations) and in that of Starck (1952) who treated 1134 patients with this method. The two deaths in the series of 452 patients treated by Olsen et al. (1951) occurred at a time when antibiotics were not available. In expert hands, both procedures have a low mortality rate.

The results of the Heller myotomy are very good if the technique is applied correctly. Ellis and Olsen (1969) obtained 83% good results and 6% failures, after a follow-up period of 1 year, or more, but late failures do occur (Barrett, 1964; Barker and Franklin, 1971). If one is willing to treat each patient up to three times, the results of forceful dilatations are comparable to those of myotomy. Good results were obtained in 77% (Vantrappen et al., 1971), 80% (Olsen et al., 1953), 84% (Kurlander et al., 1963), 73% (Douvlaris et al., 1971), 85% (Benedict, 1964) and 94 %(Hafter, 1969) of the patients. If the patient is treated only once, good results are obtained in 60 to 75% of the cases (Olsen et al., 1951; Sanderson et al., 1970; Vantrappen et al., 1971).

A definite disadvantage of forceful dilatations is the lack of control of the sphincteric resistance during the dilatation itself, which may lead to perforation but also to insufficient dilatation, resulting in unsatisfactory improvement of the dysphagia or short-term recurrence. In our experience sphincteric pressure measurements have proven to be a useful criterium in determining to which diameter the dilatation should be carried out. An advantage of dilatation is that it rarely leads to reflux and almost never to peptic stenosis. Dilatation failures may subsequently undergo a successful myotomy, though multiple dilatations make the procedure more difficult. The poor results of the Heller myotomy are only partially due to an insufficient transection of the muscle layer; at least half of them are caused by the development of reflux esophagitis, which often necessitates a more complex operation, associated with higher morbidity and mortality. Reflux esophagitis may manifest itself years after a myotomy, so that a good result one year after the intervention definitely cannot be considered permanent.

A comparative evaluation of forceful dilatation and Heller's myotomy, based on rigorous criteria, has not yet been carried out. Failures occur with both methods but it is unclear to what extent they are inherent to the method itself, or the result of imperfect application of the method. BENNETT (1970), BENNETT and HENDRIX (1970) and ELLIS and OLSEN (1969) compared the late results of dilatation and myotomy, using the same criteria for both methods. BENNETT and HENDRIX (1970) found the results to be better for the 54 patients who had undergone dilatations than for the 48 patients treated by myotomy. However, the follow-up of the dilated group was shorter than that of the surgically treated patients. Conversely, the Mayo group obtained superior results with the modified Heller myotomy, but in this study the follow-up of the surgical group was shorter.

The diagnosis of cancer developing in an achalatic esophagus is difficult. Carcinomatous degeneration is easily discovered at thoracic surgery and lingering doubts about the benign or malignant nature of esophageal abnormalities must be solved by surgical exploration. However, these carcinomas may develop after surgery and the hope that the problem of carcinomatous degeneration in achalasia will be solved by systematic recourse to myotomy is an illusion.

There is no doubt that myotomy is the treatment of choice for some categories of patients. The inability of children to cooperate is a contraindication for dilatation; the Heller myotomy yields good results (PAYNE et al., 1961; TACHOVSKY et al., 1968) and should be preferred. It can be performed on very young children (KING, 1955; RAVEN, 1961; SWENSON and OECONOMOPOULOS, 1961; KEITA et al., 1964; BETTEX and SCHÄRLI, 1966; POLONSKY and GUTH, 1970; MAGILNER and ISARD, 1971; DAYALAN et al., 1972). For the same reason forceful dilatation is contraindicated for psychotic patients (VANTRAPPEN et al., 1971). If a carcinoma is suspected surgical therapy is certainly indicated. A myotomy may also be preferred if the achalasia is associated with a hiatal hernia or an epiphrenic diverticulum.

A thoracic intervention, however, is more dangerous for older and poor risk patients.

In the absence of these contraindications we advocate forceful dilatation as the primary treatment, because the results, including the long-term results, are comparable to those of a myotomy, the mortality rate is virtually nihil, the procedure is simple in expert hands, and the risk of severe peptic esophagitis is very small. Moreover, for old and poor risk patients dilatation is less dangerous than a Heller operation and at the present time even an expert surgeon apparently still must face the prospect of reflux esophagitis developing in some of his patients.

References

ACHESON, E. D., HADLEY, G. D.: Cardio-myotomy for achalasia of the cardia; the experience of the Middlesex and Harefield Hospitals up to 1955. Brit. med. J. 1958 I, 543–553.
ADAMS, C. W. M., BRAIN, R. H. F., ELLIS, F. G., KAUNTZE, R., TROUNCE, J. R.: Achalasia of the cardia. Guy's Hosp. Rep. 110, 191–236 (1961).
ADAMS, C. W. M., MARPLES, E. A., TROUNCE, J. R.: Achalasia of the cardia and Hirschsprung's disease: the amount and distribution of cholinesterases. Clin. Sci. 19, 473–481 (1960).
ADAMS, H. D.: Amyenteric achalasia of the esophagus. Surg. Gynec. Obstet. 119, 251–256 (1964).

AFFOLTER, H., VOEGELI, R.: Erfahrungen mit der pneumatischen Kardiadilatation bei der Achalasie. Schweiz. med. Wschr. **93**, 547–549 (1969).

AGUIRRE, C., SORIA, F., HALABI, M.: Treatment of megaesophagus by Roux-en-y esophago-jejunostomy. Surgery **54**, 856–860 (1963).

AHMED, H. U.: Carcinoma oesophagus as a complication of achalasia cardia (report of a case). Indian J. Surg. **26**, 559–562 (1964).

AKUAMOA, G.: Achalasia oesophagi and associated diseases. Acta chir. scand. **135**, 421–427 (1969).

AKUAMOA, G.: Achalasia oesophagi. Results of the Heller operation. Acta chir. scand. **137**, 782–788 (1971).

ALLISON, P. R.: Discussion on treatment of achalasia of the cardia. Proc. roy. Soc. Med. **43**, 425–429 (1950).

ALNOR, P.: On the pathogenesis of cardiospasm: an experimental study. J. thorac. cardiovasc. Surg. **36**, 141–155 (1958).

AMBRUMJANZ, G.: Über eine Modifikation der Hellerschen Operation beim Kardiospasmus (Abstr.). Zbl. ges. Chir. Grenzgeb. **50**, 747–748 (1930).

ANDERSEN, H. A., HOLMAN, C. B., OLSEN, A. M.: Pulmonary complications of cardiospasm. J. Amer. med. Ass. **151**, 608–612 (1953).

ANDERSEN, H. A., SCHLEGEL, J. F., OLSEN, A. M.: Postvagotomy dysphagia. Gastroint. Endosc. **12**, 13–18 (1966).

ATKINSON, M., SUMERLING, M. D.: The competence of the cardia after cardiomyotomy. Gastroenterologia (Basel) **92**, 123–134 (1959).

BACKER-GRÖNDAHL, N.: Cardiaplastik ved cardiospasmus. Nord. Kirurgisk Forenings **11**, 236–240 (1916).

BARKER, J. R., FRANKLIN, R. H.: Heller's operation for achalasia of the cardia. A study of the early and late results. Brit. J. Surg. **58**, 466–468 (1971).

BARLOW, D.: Problems of achalasia. Brit. J. Surg. **48**, 642–645 (1961).

BARONTI, A. C.: Congenital esophageal dilatation in a cocker puppy. N. Amer. Vet. **21**, 666–667 (1950).

BARRETT, N. R.: Achalasia of the cardia: reflections upon a clinical study of over 100 cases. Brit. med. J. **1964 I**, 1135–1140.

BARRETT, N. R., FRANKLIN, R. H.: Concerning the unfavourable late results of certain operations performed in the treatment of cardiospasm. Brit. J. Surg. **37**, 194–202 (1949).

BECK, I., BALLEM, M., BOURNE, R., McKENNA, R.: Le traitement du méga-oesophage fonctionnel (cardiospasme): lacération musculaire forcée utilisant l'instrument pneumatique de Browne et McHardy sous contrôle fluoroscopique. Un. med. Can. **89**, 1371–1382 (1960).

BECK, I. T., HERNANDEZ, N. A., SOLYMAR, J.: Dyschalasia: a variant or early phase of achalasia? A review of motor disturbances in achalasia with reference to late relaxation of the lower esophageal sphincter. Canad. med. Ass. J. **95**, 941–946 (1966).

BELLO, B. DI, ZILLI, L.: Associazione di cancro e megaesofago in due fratelli. Acta chir. ital. **16**, 267–294 (1960).

BELSEY, R. H. R.: Functional disease of the esophagus. J. thorac. cardiovasc. Surg. **52**, 164–188 (1966).

BENEDICT, E. B.: Bougienage, forceful dilatation, and surgery in treatment of achalasia. A comparison of results. J. Amer. med. Ass. **188**, 355–357 (1964).

BENEDICT, E. B., GRILLO, H. C.: Spontaneous rupture of megaesophagus in achalasia. J. thorac. cardiovasc. Surg. **44**, 272–277 (1962).

BENNETT, J. R.: Treatment of achalasia by pneumatic dilatation of the cardia (abstract). Gut **9**, 727 (1968).

BENNETT, J. R.: The treatment of achalasia. A comparison of pneumatic dilatation and cardiomyotomy. 4th World Congress of Gastroenterology Copenhagen, Denmark, 12th–18th July 1970, p. 191. The Danish Gastroenterological Association, 1970.

BENNETT, J. R., HENDRIX, T. R.: Treatment of achalasia with pneumatic dilatation. Mod. Treatm. **7**, 1217–1228 (1970).

BERGAN, F.: Discussion. Acta chir. scand. **103**, 464–466 (1952)

BERNATZ, P. E., SMITH, J. L., ELLIS, F. H., JR., ANDERSEN, H. A.: Benign, pedunculated intraluminal tumors of the esophagus. J. thorac. cardiovasc. Surg. **35**, 503–512 (1958).

BESANÇON, F., JANIN, B., DEBRAY, C.: Le méga-oesophage, cardiospasme réactionnel. Données électromanographiques et cinéradiométriques. Sem. Hôp. Paris **38**, 1555–1564 (1962).

BETTEX, M., SCHÄRLI, A.: Achalasie und Megaoesophagus im Kindesalter. Z. Kinderchir. **3** (Suppl.), 28–35 (1966).

BINDER, H. J., BLOOM, D. L., STERN, H., SOLITARE, G. B., THAYER, W. R., SPIRO, H. M., POINDEXTER, E. R.: The effect of cervical vagectomy on esophageal function in the monkey. Surgery **64**, 1075–1083 (1968).

BINDER, H. J., CLEMETT, A. R., THAYER, W. R., SPIRO, H. M.: Rarity of hiatus hernia in achalasia. New Engl. J. Med. **272**, 680–682 (1965).

BIRNBERG, T. L.: Cardiospasm in new-born infant. Amer. J. Dis. Child. **38**, 1183–1195 (1929).

BLACKMAN, A. H., RAKATANSKY, H., NASRULLA, H. M., THAYER, W. R.: Transabdominal vagectomy and lower esophageal function. Arch. Surg. **102**, 6–8 (1971).

BLOOMFIELD, R. D.: Pregnancy and achalasia. Amer. J. Obstet. Gynec. **86**, 1074–1078 (1963).

BOEREMA, I.: Gastropexia anterior geniculata for sliding hiatus hernia and for cardiospasmus. J. int. Coll. Surg. **29**, 533–547 (1958).

BOGAERT, F. VAN DER: "Cardiospasm" in new-born. Arch. Pediat. **50**, 585–588 (1933).

BOITEL, Y.: L'achalasie du cardia; aspects radiologiques et radio-cinématographiques. Thèse Lausanne. Bâle: Karger 1963.

BOLOT, CHALLIOL, NEGRE: Trois cas de cardiospasme oesophagien traités par cardiotomie extramuqueuse de Heller associée à la neurotomie sousdiaphragmatique des deux pneumogastriques. Mém. Acad. Chir. **75**, 574–578 (1949).

BOMBECK, C. T., COELHO, R. G. P., NYHUS, L. M.: Prevention of gastroesophageal reflux after resection of the lower esophagus. Surg. Gynec. Obstet. **130**, 1035–1043 (1970).

BRASIL, A.: Aperistalsis of the esophagus. Rev. Bras. Gastroenterol. **7**, 21–44 (1969).

BROWNE, D. C., McHARDY, G.: A new instrument for use in esophagospasm. J. Amer. med. Ass. **113**, 1963–1964 (1939).

BROWN KELLY, A.: Stenose at the lower end of the oesophagus, with special reference to those of spastic origin. Brit. med. J. **1912 II**, 1049–1053.

BROWSE, N. L., CARTER, S. J.: The late results of Heller's operation in the treatment of achalasia. Brit. J. Surg. **49**, 59–63 (1961).

BÜHLER-VIERA, C.: The endemic South American megaesophagus. Pharmacologic study. IInd World Congress of Gastroenterology, Munich 1962, **1**, 75–78 (1963). ed. S. Karger, Basel.

BURFORD, T. H., LISCHER, C. E.: Treatment of short esophageal hernia with esophagitis by Finney pyloroplasty. Ann. Surg. **144**, 647–652 (1956).

BURGESS, J. N., KELLY, K. A., SCHLEGEL, J. F., ELLIS, F. H., JR.: Effect of esophageal mucosal denervation on the motility of the canine esophagus. J. surg. Res. **9**, 605–610 (1969).

BURGESS, J. N., SCHLEGEL, J. F., ELLIS, F. H., JR.: The effect of denervation on feline esophageal function and morphology. J. surg. Res. **12**, 24–33 (1972).

BUTIN, J. W., OLSEN, A. M., MOERSCH, H. J., CODE, C. F.: A study of esophageal pressures in normal persons and patients with cardiospasm. Gastroenterology **23**, 278–293 (1953).

CAMARA-LOPES, L. H.: Carcinoma of the esophagus as a complication of mega-esophagus; an analysis of seven cases. Amer. J. dig. Dis. **6**, 742–756 (1961).

CARAYON, A., PERQUIS, P., COURBIL, L. J.: Résultats de six opérations d'Heller pour mégaoesophage chez l'Africain. Bull. Soc. méd. Afr. noire Langue franç. **10**, 699–701 (1965).

CARLSON, H. C.: Roentgenologic manifestations. In: Achalasia of the esophagus (ELLIS F. H., JR. and OLSEN, A. M., eds.), chapt. 5, p. 105–121. Philadelphia-London-Toronto: W. B. Saunders Co. 1969.

CARVETH, S. W., SCHLEGEL, J. F., CODE, C. F., ELLIS, F. H.: Esophageal motility after vagotomy, phrenicotomy, myotomy and myomectomy in dogs. Surg. Gynec. Obstet. **114**, 31–42 (1962).

CASSELLA, R. R., BROWN, A. L., JR., SAYRE, G. P., ELLIS, F. H., JR.: Achalasia of the esophagus: pathologic and etiologic considerations. Ann. Surg. **160**, 474–486 (1964).

CASELLA, R. R., ELLIS, F. H., JR., BROWN, A. L.: Fine-structure changes in achalasia of the esophagus. I. Vagus nerves. Amer. J. Path. **46**, 279–288 (1965).

CASTRO, L. P. DE, GROSSI, C. A.: O teste do mecolil no diagnostico da aperistalsis do esofago. Rev. goiana Med. **9**, 3–19 (1963).

CAWLEY, A. J., GENDREAU, C. L.: Esophageal achalasia in a cat. Canad. vet. J. **10**, 195–197 (1969).

CECCONI, F.: La cardiomiotomia extra-mucosa secondo Heller nel trattamento del cosidetto „megaesofago idiopatico". Arch. Ital. Chir. **85**, 135–152 (1959).

CHABAL, J., MENSAH, A.: Le traitement chirurgical du méga-oesophage idiopathique en Afrique. Bull. Soc. méd. Afr. noire Langue franç. **10**, 163–167 (1965).

CHESTERMAN, J. T.: Observations on aspects of achalasia cardiae. Brit. J. Surg. **52**, 601–604 (1965).

CHRISTENSEN, J.: Esophageal manometry in myxedema (abstract). Gastroenterology **52**, 1130 (1967).

CIAGLIA, P., SEGAL, G.: Segmental esophagectomy: Ancillary procedure for advanced megaesophagus with sigmoid elongation. J. thorac. cardiovasc. Surg. **44**, 44–52 (1962).

CLAGETT, O. T.: Achalasia: Dilatation or myotomy? J. thorac. cardiovasc. Surg. **53**, 757–758 (1967).

CLIFFORD, D. H., GYORKEY, F.: Myenteric ganglial cells in dogs with and without achalasia of the esophagus. J. Amer. vet. med. Ass. **150**, 205–211 (1967).

CLIFFORD, D. H., MALEK, R.: Diseases of the canine esophagus due to prenatal influence. Amer. J. dig. Dis. **14**, 578–602 (1969).

CLIFFORD, D. H., PIRSCH, J. G.: Myenteric ganglial cells in dogs with and without hereditary achalasia of the esophagus. Amer. J. vet. Res. **32**, 615–619 (1971).

CLIFFORD, D. H., SOIFER, F. K., WILSON, C. F., WADDELL, E. D., GUILLOUD, G. L.: Congenital achalasia of the esophagus in four cats of common ancestry. J. Amer. vet. med. Ass. **158**, 1554–1560 (1971).

CLIFFTON, E. E.: Treatment of cancer of the esophagus. Mod. Treatm. **7**, 1261–1283 (1970).

CLOUDE, D. T., JR., WHITE, R. F., LINKNER, L. M., TAYLAR, L. C.: Surgical treatment of esophageal achalasia in children. J. pediat. Surg. **1**, 137–144 (1966).

CODE, C. F.: The physiologic basis of some disorders of motor function of the esophagus. Postgrad. Med. **26**, 265–271 (1959).

CODE, C. F., CREAMER, B., SCHLEGEL, J. F., OLSEN, A. M., DONOGHUE, F. E., ANDERSEN, H. A.: An atlas of esophageal motility in health and disease. Springfield, Illinois: Charles C. Thomas, Publisher 1958.

CODE, C. F., SCHLEGEL, J. F.: The physiological basis of some motor disorders of the esophagus. In: Surgical Physiology of the Gastro-intestinal Tract (Proceedings of a symposium held in the Royal College of Surgeons of Edinburgh, 1st and 2nd June 1962), p. 1–19, SMITH, A. N. (ed.), Edinburgh: Royal College of Surgeons of Edinburgh 1963.

CODE, C. F., SCHLEGEL, J. E.: Physiologic studies. In: Achalasia of the esophagus (ELLIS, F. H., JR., and OLSEN, A. M., eds.), chapt. 3, p. 44–63. Philadelphia-London-Toronto: W. B. Saunders Co. 1969.

COHEN, B. R.: "Cardiospasm" in achalasia: Demonstration of an abnormally elevated esophagogastric sphincter pressure with partial relaxation on swallowing (abstract). Gastroenterology **48**, 864 (1965).

COHEN, B. R., GUELRUD, M.: Cardiospasm in achalasia: demonstration of supersensitivity of the lower esophageal sphincter (abstract). Gastroenterology **60**, 769 (1971).

COHEN, S.: The hormonal regulation of lower esophageal sphincter competence. Digestion **6**, 231–240 (1972).

COHEN, S., FISHER, R., TUCH, A.: The site of denervation in achalasia. Gut **13**, 556–558 (1972).

COHEN, S., LIPSHUTZ, W.: Quantitation of lower esophageal sphincter (L.E.S.) dysfunction in achalasia: an objective guide to therapy (abstract). Gastroenterology **60**, 650 (1971).

COHEN, S., LIPSHUTZ, W., HUGHES, W.: Role of gastrin supersensitivity in the pathogenesis of lower esophageal sphincter hypertension in achalasia. J. clin. Invest. **50**, 1241–1247 (1971).

CORELLI, D., CANCIULLO, D., PANEBIANCO, G.: Cardiospasmo sperimentale con alterazione dei plessi nervos iintramurali dell' esofago epicardiocardiale. Ann. ital. Chir. **34**, 144–155 (1957).

COUTO, D., JR., ALDROVANDO, J.: Tratamento cirúrgico do megaesófago pela esofagectomia parcial e interpasicao de segmento de cólon. Folha med. **53**, 913–921 (1966).

CRAIG, W. M., MOERSCH, H. J., VINSON, P. P.: Treatment of intractable cardiospasm by bilateral cervicothoracic sympathetic ganglionectomy. Report of a case. Proc. Mayo Clin. **9**, 749–753 (1934).

CREAMER, B.: Motor disturbances of the esophagus. In: Handbook of physiology, Section 6, Alimentary canal, vol. IV, Motility, chapt. 109, p. 2331–2343, by CODE, C. F. (ed.). Washington, D.C.: American Physiological Society 1968.

CREAMER, B., ANDERSEN, H. A., CODE, C. F.: Esophageal motility in patients with scleroderma and related diseases. Gastroenterologia (Basel) **86**, 763–775 (1956).

CREAMER, B., DONOGHUE, F. E., CODE, C. F.: Pattern of esophageal motility in diffuse spasm. Gastroenterology **34**, 782–796 (1958).

CREAMER, B., OLSEN, A. M., CODE, C. F.: The esophageal sphincters in achalasia of the cardia (cardiospasm). Gastroenterology **33**, 293–301 (1957).

CROSS, F. S.: Pathologic changes in megaesophagus (esophageal distonia). Surgery **31**, 647–653 (1952).

CROSS, F. S.: Discussion of Reoperation for achalasia of the esophagus. PATRICK, D. L., PAYNE, W. S., OLSEN, A. M., and ELLIS, F. H., JR.: Arch. Surg. **103**, 122–128 (1971).

CRUMP, A. C., FLOOD, C. A., HENNIG, G. C.: Results of medical treatment of idiopathic cardiospasm. Gastroenterology **20**, 30–38 (1952).

CULLIGAN, J. A.: Attempts to produce cardiospasm in the cat. Thesis, Graduate School, University of Minnesota, 1959, quoted by Earlam, R. J. (1967).

DAGRADI, A. E., STEMPIEN, S. J., SEIFER, H. W., WEINBERG, J. A.: Terminal esophageal (vestibular) spasm after vagotomy. Arch. Surg. **85**, 955–968 (1962).

DAHM, K.: Der Kardiospasmus — eine seltene Komplikation nach beidseitiger selectiver gastraler Vagotomie. Zbl. Chir. 49, 1717–1721 (1968).

DALY, D. D., CODE, C. F., ANDERSEN, H. A.: Disturbances of swallowing and esophageal motility in patients with multiple sclerosis. Neurology (Minneap.) 12, 250–256 (1962).

DAYALAN, N., CHETTUR, L., RAMAKRISHNAN, M. S.: Achalasia of the cardia in sibs. Arch. Dis. Childh. 47, 115–118 (1972).

DE BELLA, E.: Il trattamento chirurgico del cardiospasmo (osservazioni cliniche e risultati dell' intervento di Heller in 172 casi). Arch. Chir. Torace 22, 59–76 (1965).

DEBRAY, C. H., BESANÇON, F., JANIN, B.: Le diagnostic de «l'hypertonie ensentielle du cardia». Syndrôme électromanographique similaire dans 4 cas de cancer. Sem. Hôp. Paris 38, 1565–1568 (1962).

DEBRAY, CH., LEYMARIOS, J., ETIENNE, J. P., CUQ, J. P.: Les cancers développés sur méga-oesophage idiopathique. Arch. Mal. Appar. dig. 57, 5–24 (1968).

DE BRUINE GROENEVELDT, J. R.: Over cardiospasmus. Ned. T. Geneesk. 62, 1281–1282 (1918).

DELANNOY, E., SOOTS, G.: A propos des résultats éloignés de l'opération de Heller. Ass. franç. Chir. 58, 139–142 (1956).

DELBERT, P.: Mégaoesophage: opération par voie abdominale. Mém. Acad. Chir. 55, 481–482 (1929).

DELOYERS, L., LOYGUE, J.: Résultats éloignés du traitement du mégaoesophage. Ass. franç. Chir. 58, 23–132 (1956).

DEMOS, N. J., YADUSKY, R. J., TIMMES, J. J., POULOS, P. P.: Thymoma associated with megaesophagus. A case report. J. thorac. cardiovasc. Surg. 51, 708–713 (1966).

DIAMANT, N. E., SZEZEPANSKI, M. M., MUI, M. Y.: Esophageal "achalasia" in the dog: manometric characteristics of body and sphincters (abstract). Gastroenterology 62, 741 (1972).

DI BELLO, B., ZILLI, L.: Associazione di cancro e megaesofago in due fratelli. Acta chir. ital. 16, 267–294 (1960).

DONOGHUE, F., WINKELMANN, R., MOERSCH, H.: Esophageal defects in dermatomyositis. Ann. Otol. (St. Louis) 69, 1139–1145 (1960).

DOR, J., HUMBERT, P., DOR, V., FIGARELLA, J.: L'intérêt de la technique de Nissen modifiée dans la prévention du reflux après cardiomyotomie extramuqueuse de Heller. Mém. Acad. Chir. 88, 877–883 (1962).

DOUGLAS, K., NICHOLSON, F.: The late results of Heller's operation for cardiospasm. Brit. J. Surg. 47, 250–253 (1959).

DOUVLARIS, G., CHATZITHEODOROU, G., PETMEZAKIS, J.: Der Megaoesophagus und seine Therapie mit Dilatator nach Starck. H.N.O. 19, 159–160 (1971).

DUBOURG, G.: Dix-sept méga-oesophages traités par l'opération de Heller. Arch. Mal. Appar. dig. 38, 425–431 (1949).

DUBOURG, G., FONTAN, F., GOURDON, A.: Oesophagite peptique après opération de Heller. Ann. Chir. Thorac. Cardiovasc. 1, 1649–1651 (1962).

DUGAN, D. J.: Discussion of: Achalasia of the Esophagus, GRIMES, O. F., STEPHENS, H. B., and MARGULIS, A. R.: Amer. J. Surg. 120, 198–202 (1970).

EARLAM, R. J.: A vascular cause for aganglionic bowel: a new hypothesis. Amer. J. dig. Dis. 17, 255–261 (1972a).

EARLAM, R. J.: Gastrointestinal aspects of Chagas' disease. Amer. J. dig. Dis. 17, 559–572 (1972b).

EARLAM, R. J., ELLIS, F. H., JR., NOBREGA, F. T.: Achalasia of the esophagus in a small urban community. Mayo Clin. Proc. 44, 478–483 (1969).

EARLAM, R. J., SCHLEGEL, J. F., ELLIS, F. H., JR.: Effect of ischemia of lower esophagus and esophagogastric junction on canine esophageal motor function. J. thorac. cardiovasc. Surg. 54, 882–831 (1967b).

EARLAM, R. J., ZOLLMAN, P. E., ELLIS, F. H., JR.: Congenital oesophageal achalasia in the dog. Thorax 22, 466–472 (1967a).

EDWARDS, D. A. W.: The nervous control of intestinal motility and its relation to the mecha-nism of the cardiac sphincter. 7e Congrès intern. Gastro-entérologie, Vol. II, 52–72, Bruxelles 1964.

EDWARDS, D. A. W.: Postvagotomy dysphagia. Lancet 1970 II, 90–92.

EDWARDS, D. A. W., ROWLANDS, E. N.: Physiological observations in achalasia and their significance in methods of treatment. Gastroenterologia (Basel) 92, 114–123 (1959).

EFFLER, D. B., LOOP, F. D., GROVES, L. K., FAVALORO, R. G.: Primary surgical treatment for esophageal achalasia. Surg. Gynec. Obstet. 132, 1057–1063 (1971).

ELLIS, F. G.: In: Achalasia of the cardia. By ADAMS, C. W. M., BRAIN, R. H. F., ELLIS, F. G., KAUNTZE, R., TROUNCE, J. R. Guy's Hosp. Rep. 110, 191–236 (1961).

ELLIS, F. G.: The aetiology and treatment of achalasia of the cardia. Ann. roy. Coll. Surg. Engl. **30**, 155–182 (1962a).

ELLIS, F. G.: Autonomic response in the esophagus. In: Surgical physiology of the gastro-intestinal tract. Proceedings of a symposium held in the Royal College of Edinburgh, 1st and 2nd June 1962b, p. 28–35, by SMITH, A. N., (ed.). Edinburgh: Royal College of Surgeons of Edinburgh 1963.

ELLIS, F. G., COLE, F. L.: Reflux after cardiomyotomy. Gut **6**, 80–84 (1965).

ELLIS, F. H., JR., ANDERSON, H. A., CLAGETT, O. T.: Treatment of short esophagus with stricture by esophagogastrectomy and antral excision. Ann. Surg. **148**, 526–536 (1958).

ELLIS, F. H., JR., KISER, J. C., SCHLEGEL, J. F., EARLAM, R. J., McVEY, J. L., OLSEN, A. M.: Esophagomyotomy for esophageal achalasia: experimental, clinical and manometric aspects. Ann. Surg. **166**, 640–655 (1967).

ELLIS, F. H., JR., OLSEN, A. M.: Achalasia of the esophagus. In: Major problems in clinical surgery, vol. IX. Philadelphia-London-Toronto: W. B. Saunders Co. 1969.

FAGGE, C. H.: A case of simple stenosis of the oesophagus, followed by epithelioma. Guy's Hosp. Rep. **17**, 413f. (1872).

FELDERHOF, J.: Achalasia van de cardia. Proefschrift. Utrecht: Schotanus en Jens, Utrecht N.V. 1965.

FERGUSON, T. B., BURFORD, T. H.: An evaluation of the modified Heller operation in the treatment of achalasia of the esophagus. Ann. Surg. **152**, 1–9 (1960).

FERNANDES, G.: Description of an inbred mouse colony and its management in India. 19th Ann. Meet., Am. A. Lab. Anim. Sci., Las Vegas, Nev., Oct. 22, 1968; cited by CLIFFORD, D. H., and MALEK, R.: Diseases of the canine esophagus due to prenatal influence. Amer. J. dig. Dis. **14**, 578–602 (1969).

FERREIRA-SANTOS, R.: Aperistalsis of the esophagus and the colon (mega-esophagus and mega-colon) etiologically related to Chagas' disease. Amer. J. dig. Dis. **6**, 700–726 (1961).

FERREIRA-SANTOS, R.: In: Doenca de Chagas. Brazil: J. R. Cancado 1968.

FINSTERER, H.: Zur Therapie des Kardiospasmus und der Kardiastenose (Oesophago-Gastro-anastomose). Wien. klin. Wschr. **35**, 471f. (1922).

FISCHER, R. A., ELLISON, G. W., THAYER, W. R., SPIRO, H. M., GLASER, G. H.: Esophageal motility in neuromuscular disorders. Ann. intern. Med. **63**, 229–248 (1965).

FONTAINE, R., FRANK, P.: La cardio-oesophagotomie extra-muqueuse élargie par voie intra-thoracique et associée à la résection des splanchnique et sympathique dorsaux gauches dans le traitement du méga-oesophage: A propos de 6 cas personnels. Mém. Acad. Chir. **76**, 216–223 (1950).

FREEMAN, L.: An operation for the relief of cardiospasm associated with dilatation and tortuosity of the oesophagus. Ann. Surg. **78**, 173–175 (1923).

FROBESE, A. S., HAWTHORNE, H. R., NEMIR, P., JR.: Reflections on the surgical management of achalasia of the esophagus. Amer. J. Surg. **107**, 249–252 (1964).

FROBESE, A. S., STEIN, G. N., HAWTHORNE, H. R.: Hiatal hernia as a complication of the Heller operation. Surgery **49**, 599–605 (1961).

GAMMELGAARD, A., IVERSEN, J., THOMSEN, G.: Cardiospasm, results of Heller's operation. Acta chir. scand. **111**, 98–107 (1956).

GAMMIE, W. F. P., JENNINGS, D., RICHARDSON, J. E.: Cardiomyotomie (Heller's operation) for oesophageal achalasia. Lancet **1958 II**, 917–920.

GIRARD, M.: Discussion. Rev. méd. Suisse rom. **35**, 280–281 (1915).

GIRDANY, B. R.: Esophagus in infancy: congenital and acquired disease. Radiol. Clin. N. Amer. **1**, 557–569 (1963).

GODOY, R. A. DE, VIEIRA, C. B.: Diagnostico da esophagopatia chagásia chrônica assinto-matica nao ectasia. Rev. goiana Med. **9**, 117–124 (1963).

GOIDSENHOVEN, G. E. VAN, VANTRAPPEN, G., VERBEKE, S., VANDENBROUCKE, J.: Treatment of achalasia of the cardia with pneumatic dilatations. Gastroenterology **45**, 326–334 (1963).

GOTTSTEIN, G.: Technik und Klinik der Oesophagoskopie. Mitt. Grenzgeb. Med. Chir. **8**, 57–152 (1901).

GOTTSTEIN, G.: Die operative Behandlung des Cardiospasmus. Zbl. Chir. **31**, 1362–1363 (1904).

GRÉGOIRE, R.: Résultat au bout d'un an d'une intervention pour dilatation idiopathique de l'oesophage. Section du diaphragme par voie thoraco-abdominale extra-séreuse. Oesophago-gastroplastie. Mém. Acad. Chir. **49**, 1322–1323 (1923).

GRÉGOIRE, R.: Pathogénie et traitement de la dilatation idiopathique de l'oesophage. Arch. Mal. Appar. dig. **14**, 455–469 (1924).

GRIMES, O. F., STEPHENS, H. B., MARGULIS, A. R.: Achalasia of the Esophagus. Amer. J. Surg. **120**, 198–202 (1970).

HAAS, S. V.: Relief of cardiospasm in the newborn by administration of atropine sulfate. Amer. J. Dis. Child. **62**, 1118–1123 (1941).

HACKER, V. VON: Cited by VON HACKER, V., and LOTHEISSEN, G.: Chirurgie der Speiseröhre. In: VON BRUNS, P., Neue Deutsche Chirurgie, Bd. 34, S. 292. Stuttgart, Germany: Ferdinand Enke 1926.

HAFTER, E.: Le traitement de l'achalasie du cardia par la dilatation forcée. Act. Hepatogastroenterol. 5, A 193–A 196 (1969).

HANNA, S. M.: A case of scleroderma presenting as cardiospasm (achalasia of the oesophagus). Postgrad. med. J. 48, 236–238 (1972).

HARMAN, J. W., O'HEGARTY, M. T., BYRNES, C. K.: The ultrastructure of human smooth muscle. I. Studies of cell surface and connections in normal and achalasia esophageal smooth muscle. Exp. molec. Path. 1, 204–228 (1962).

HARRIS, L. D., ASHWORTH, W. D., INGELFINGER, F. J.: Esophageal aperistalsis and achalasia produced in dogs by prolonged cholinesterase inhibition. J. clin. Invest. 39, 1744–1751 (1960).

HATAFUKU, T., MAKI, T., THAL, A. P.: Fundic part operation in the treatment of advanced achalasia of the esophagus. Surg. Gynec. Obstet. 134, 617–624 (1972).

HAVARD, C.: Para-esophageal hernia of the stomach complicating Heller's operation. Thorax 18, 139–143 (1963).

HAWTHORNE, H. R., FROBESE, A. S., NEMIR, P., JR.: The surgical management of achalasia of the esophagus. Ann. Surg. 144, 653–666 (1956).

HAWTHORNE, H. R., NEMIR, P., JR.: The surgical management of achalasia of the esophagus. Gastroenterology 25, 349–358 (1953).

HEITMANN, P.: The immediate effect of pneumatic dilatation on intraluminal yield pressures in achalasia of the oesophagus. Rendiconti Rom. Gastro-enterol. 3, 141–142 (1971).

HEITMANN, P., ESPINOZA, J.: Oesophageal manometric studies in patients with chronic Chagas disease and megacolon. Gut 10, 848–851 (1969).

HEITMANN, P., ESPINOZA, J., CSENDES, A.: Physiology of the distal esophagus in achalasia. Scand. J. Gastroent. 4, 1–11 (1969).

HELLER, E.: Extramuköse Kardioplastik beim chronischen Kardiospasmus mit Dilatation des Oesophagus. Mitt. Grenzgeb. Med. Chir. 27, 141 (1914).

HELLER, E.: Discussion. Verh. dtsch. Ges. Chir. 45, 144–146 (1921).

HELSINGEN, N., JR.: Gastroesophageal reflux as a complication of the Heller operation. Acta chir. scand., Suppl. 356 B, 96–98 (1966).

HELSINGEN, N., JR., LINAKER, O., KRISTIANSEN, O.: Achalasia cardiae: results of Heller's operation. Acta chir. scand. 133, 35–39 (1967).

HEPP, J.: A propos de vingt cas de mégaoesophage. Mém. Acad. Chir. 75, 508–511 (1949).

HERRERA, A. F., COLON, J., VALDES-DAPENA, A., ROTH, J. L. A.: Achalasia or carcinoma ? The significance of the Mecholyl test. Amer. J. dig. Dis. 15, 1073–1081 (1970).

HERRON, P. W., THOMAS, G. L., MERENDINO, A.: Experimental approach to cardiospasm: appraisal of Finney pyloroplasty in prevention of esophagitis, following Heller myotomy. J. thorac. Surg. 34, 609–614 (1957).

HERTZ, A. F.: Achalasia of the cardia. Quart. J. Med. 8, 300–308 (1914).

HEYROVSKY, H.: Discussion. Verh. dtsch. Ges. Chir. 40, 286–287 (1911).

HEYROVSKY, H.: Casuistik und Therapie der idiopathischen Dilatation der Speiseröhre: Oesophagogastroanastomose. Langenbecks Arch. klin. Chir. 100, 703–715 (1913).

HIGGS, B., ELLIS, F. H., JR.: The effect of bilateral supranodosal vagotomy on canine esophageal function. Surgery 58, 828–834 (1965).

HIGGS, B., KERR, F. W. L., ELLIS, F. H., JR.: The experimental production of esophageal achalasia by electrolytic lesions in the medulla. J. thorac. cardiovasc. Surg. 50, 613–625 (1965).

HIGHTOWER, N. C., JR.: Esophageal motility in health and disease. Dis. Chest 28, 150–169 (1955).

HIGHTOWER, N. C., JR., OLSEN, A. M., MOERSCH, H. J., SCHLEGEL, J. F.: A comparison of the effect of acetyl-beta-methylcholine chloride (mecholyl) on esophageal intraluminal pressure in normal persons and patients with cardiospasm. Gastroenterology 26, 592–600 (1954).

HILLEMAND, P.: Manifestations digestives au cours des atteintes du système nerveux central. Thèse Paris: Ed. Foulon 1955.

HILLEMAND, P., VIGUIE, R.: A propos du méga-oesophage et de son étiopathogénie. Actual. hépato-gastr.-entérol., Hôtel Dieu, Paris: Masson 1957.

HIRASHIMA, T., SATO, H.: Evaluation of a method for reconstruction of the esophagogastric junction, and the application to achalasia. Ann. Surg. 172, 897–901 (1970).

HOFFER, R. E., VALDES-DAPENA, A., BAUE, A. E.: A comparative study of naturally occurring canine achalasia. Arch. Surg. 95, 83–88 (1967).

HOFFMAN, F.: Dissertatio inauguralis medica de spasmis gulae inferioris et de nausea. Halle 1733.

Hofmeyr, C. F. B.: An evaluation of cardioplasty for achalasia of the oesophagus in the dog. J. small Anim. Prac. 7, 281–301 (1966).

Hogan, W. J., Caflisch, C. R., Winship, D. H.: Unclassified oesophageal motor disorders simulating achalasia. Gut 10, 234–240 (1969).

Hurst, A. F.: Essays and addresses on digestive and nervous diseases and on Addison's anaemia and asthma. New York: Paul B. Hoeber, Inc. 1924.

Huss, M.: Dilatatio oesophagi in gluve formis. Hygea 4, 296 (1842).

Ingelfinger, F. J.: Mecholyl test in achalasia of esophagus. In: Yearbook of Medicine 1964–1965, p. 506. Chicago, Ill.: Yearbook Medical Publishers 1964.

Iordanskaia, N. I.: Functional disorders of the vagus nerves in cardiospasm. Vestn. Klin. Grekov. 88, 24–28 (1962).

Jekler, J., Lhotka, J.: Modified Heller procedure to prevent postoperative reflux esophagitis in patients with achalasia. Amer. J. Surg. 113, 251–254 (1967).

Jekler, J., Lhotka, J., Borek, Z.: Surgery for achalasia of the esophagus. Ann. Surg. 160, 793–800 (1964).

Joseph, R., Job, J.-C.: Dysautonomie familiale et mégaoesophage. Arch. franç. Pédiat. 20, 25–33 (1963).

Joske, R. A., Benedict, E. B.: The role of benign esophageal obstruction in the development of carcinoma of the esophagus. Gastroenterology 36, 749–755 (1959).

Just-Viera, J. O., Haight, C.: Achalasia and carcinoma of the esophagus. Surg. Gynec. Obstet. 128, 1081–1095 (1969).

Just-Viera, J. O., Morris, J. D., Haight, C.: Achalasia and esophageal carcinoma. Ann. thorac. Surg. 3, 526–538 (1967).

Karjalainen, A. O.: Achalasia of the oesophagus in association with pregnancy. Acta obstet. gynec. scand. 43, 19–27 (1964).

Katz, J., Sender, A.: Cardiospasm in an African: A case report. S. Afr. med. J. 33, 1079–1080 (1959).

Kawashima, S.: In: Panel-Discussion: Achalasia of Esophagus. Proc. 2nd World Congress of Gastroenterology, Munich 1962. 1, 3–45 (1963).

Keita, A., Nguyen Buu Trieu, Kroumova, N.: A propos d'un cas de cardiospasme chez un nourrisson de huit mois traité avec succès par l'opération de Heller. Bull. Soc. méd. Afr. noire Langue franç. 9, 354–358 (1964).

Keller, W. L.: Operative relief of cardiospasm where dilatation has failed. Ann. Surg. 88, 58–64 (1928).

Kiesel, G. K.: Congenital esophageal dilatation in a Great Dane puppy. Cornell Vet. 41, 36–37 (1951).

Kilpatrick, Z. M., Miller, S. S.: Achalasia in mother and daughter. Gastroenterology 62, 1042–1046 (1972).

Kimura, K.: The nature of idiopathic esophagus dilatation. Jap. J. Gastroent. 1, 199–207 (1929).

King, R.: Achalasia of Esophagus. Amer. Surg. 21, 39–44 (1955).

Kitchen, R. A., Kehler, W. H., Henthorne, J. C.: Megaesophagus in a dog. J. Amer. vet. med. Ass. 143, 1106–1107 (1963).

Klayman, M. I.: The diagnosis of esophageal carcinoma by exfoliative cytology, including two cases of cardiospasm associated with carcinoma of the esophagus. Ann. intern. Med. 43, 33–44 (1955).

Klumbies, G.: Psychotherapeutische Behandlungsergebnisse bei Oesophagus-Achalasie. Proc. 2nd World Congress of Gastroenterology, Munich 1962. 1, 106–108 (1963).

Knauer, C. M., McLaughlin, W. T., Mark, J. B. D.: Esophago-esophageal fistula in a patient with achalasia. Gastroenterology 58, 223–228 (1970).

Knight, G. C.: The relation of the extrinsic nerves to the functional activity of the oesophagus. Brit. J. Surg. 22, 155–168 (1934).

Knight, G. C., Adamson, W. A. D.: Achalasia of the cardia. Proc. roy. Soc. Med. 28, 891–897 (1935).

Köberle, F.: Die Chagaskrankheit — ihre Pathogenese und ihre Bedeutung als Volksseuche. Z. Tropenmed. Parasit. 10, 236–268 (1959).

Köberle, F.: Enteromegaly and cardiomegaly in Chagas' disease. Gut 4, 399–405 (1963).

Köberle, F.: Chagas' disease and Chagas' syndrome: the pathology of American trypanosomiasis. Advanc. Parasitol. 6, 63–116 (1968).

Kolodny, M., Schrader, Z. R., Rubin, W., Hochman, R., Sleisenger, M. H.: Esophageal achalasia probably due to gastric carcinoma. Ann. intern. Med. 69, 569–573 (1968).

Kramer, P.: Diffuse esophageal spasm. Mod. Treatm. 7, 1151–1162 (1970).

Kramer, P., Fleshler, B., McNally, E., Harris, L. D.: Oesophageal sensitivity to Mecholyl in symptomatic diffuse spasm. Gut 8, 120–127 (1967a).

KRAMER, P., HARRIS, L. D., DONALDSON, R. M., JR.: Transition from symptomatic diffuse spasm to cardiospasm. Gut 8, 115–119 (1967 b).

KRAMER, P., INGELFINGER, F. J.: I. Motility of the human esophagus in control subjects and in patients with esophageal disorders. Amer. J. Med. 7, 168–173 (1949 a).

KRAMER, P., INGELFINGER, F. J.: II. Cardiospasm, a generalized disorder of esophageal motility. Amer. J. Med. 7, 174–179 (1949 b).

KRAMER, P., INGELFINGER, F. J.: Esophageal sensitivity to Mecholyl in cardiospasm. Gastroenterology 19, 242–253 (1951).

KRAMER, P., INGELFINGER, F. J., ATKINSON, M.: The motility and pharmacology of the esophagus in cardiospasm. Gastroenterologia (Basel) 86, 174–178 (1956).

KUMAR, R., MADAN, M. S.: Cardiac achalasia. Report of a case in a 4-year old child. Indian J. Pediat. 36, 399–401 (1969).

KURLANDER, D. J., RASKIN, H. F., KIRSNER, J. B., PALMER, W. L.: Therapeutic value of the pneumatic dilator in achalasia of the esophagus: long-term results in sixty-two living patients. Gastroenterology 45, 604–613 (1963).

LACROIX, L. J.: Congenital dilatation of the esophagus. N. Amer. Vet. 30, 29–30 (1949).

LAGACHE, G., SOORS, G.: Cancer sur méga-oesophage: à propos de deux observations. Ann. Chir. 12, 739–742 (1958).

LAGACHE, G., COMBEMALE, B., EL HASSAR, S.: Une statistique de 53 opérations de Heller pour mégaoesophage idiopathique. Lille méd. 15, 647–651 (1970).

LAMBERT, A. V. S.: Oesophago-gastrostomy for cardiospasm. Ann. Surg. 58, 415–418 (1913).

LANGMEAD, F.: Notes of a case of oesophagectasis in an infant, with radiograms. Proc. roy. Soc. Med., Study Dis. Child. section 13, 43–46 (1920).

LAWRANCE, K., SHOESMITH, J. H.: A review of the treatment of cardiospasm. Thorax 14, 211–215 (1959).

LENDRUM, F. C.: Anatomic features of the cardiac orifice of the stomach with special reference to cardiospasm. Arch. intern. Med. 59, 474–511 (1937).

LERCHE, W.: The esophagus and pharynx in action. Springfield: C. C. Thomas 1950.

LEROUX, B. T., WRIGHT, J. T.: Cardiospasm. Brit. J. Surg. 48, 619–633 (1961).

LOPES, E. R., TAFURI, W. L., CHAPADEIRO, E.: Estudo morfologico e quantitativo dos núcleos dorsal do vago e hipoglosso em Chagásicos crônicos com e sem megaesôfago. Rev. Inst. Med. trop. S. Paulo 11, 123–129 (1969).

LORTAT-JACOB, J. L.: El Cardiospasmo. Cirurg. Ginec. Urol. 19, 453–461 (1965).

LORTAT-JACOB, J. L.: Discussion in: Les cancers développés sur méga-œsophage idiopathique. Par DEBRAY, CH., LEYMARIOS, J., ETIENNE, J.-P., et CUQ, J.-P. Arch. franç. Mal. Appar. dig. 1, 5–24 (1968).

LORTAT-JACOB, J.-L., BINET, J.-P., MAILLARD, J.-N.: La prévention des hémorragies digestives après opération de Heller. Ass. franç. Chir. 58, 162–164 (1956).

LUSENA, G.: La chirurgia dell' esofago. IX Congr. Soc. Int. Chir. 1, 641–700 (1932).

MAGILNER, A. D., ISARD, H. J.: Achalasia of the esophagus in infancy. Radiology 98, 81–82 (1971).

MAINGOT, R.: Extramucous oesophagocardiotomy in cardiospasm. Postgrad. med. J. 20, 278–282 (1944).

MAINGOT, R.: The surgery of cardiospasm. Postgrad. med. J. 25, 197–202 (1949).

MALM, A.: Cardioplasty in the surgical treatment of achalasia of the esophagus. A critical review founded on experimental studies. Scand. J. clin. Lab. Invest., Suppl. 1, 1–89 (1951).

MALM, A.: A 10-year report of operated achalasia of the esophagus. Gastroenterologia (Basel) 86, 208–210 (1956).

MANDELSTAM, P., LIEBER, A.: Esophageal dysfunction in diabetic neuropathy-gastroenteropathy. J. Amer. med. Ass. 201, 582–586 (1967).

MANDELSTAM, P., SIEGEL, C. I., LIEBER, A., SIEGEL, M.: The swallowing disorder in patients with diabetic neuropathy-gastroenteropathy. Gastroenterology 56, 1–12 (1969).

MARSHAK, R. H., ELIASOPH, J.: Cardiospasm or carcinoma? The roentgen findings. Amer. J. dig. Dis. 2, 11–25 (1957).

MARTIN, E.: Zur chirurgischen Behandlung des Cardiospasmus und der spindelförmigen Speiseröhrenerweiterung. Mitt. Grenzgeb. Med. Chir. 8, 226–246 (1901).

MATTOS, J. O.: Tratamento cirúrgico do megaesôfago por "esfincterectomia esofagocardia". Ass. Paul. Med. Cir. 70, 351–360 (1955).

MAYO, H.: Dilated oesophagus. London Med. Gaz. 3, 121 (1828).

McVEY, J. L., SCHLEGEL, J. F., ELLIS, F. H., JR.: Gastroesophageal sphincteric function after the Heller myotomy and its modifications. An experimental study. Bull. Soc. Int. Chir. 5–6, 419–423 (1963).

MERENDINO, K. A.: Important side-issues in the treatment of cardiospasm. Arch. Surg. 73, 1047–1049 (1956).

Merendino, K. A., Dillard, D. H.: The concept of sphincter substitution by an interposed jejunal segment for anatomic and physiologic abnormalities at the esophagogastric junction with special reference to reflux esophagitis, cardiospasm and esophageal varices. Ann. Surg. 142, 486–506 (1955).

Meyer,W.: Impermeable cardiospasm successfully treated by thoracotomy and esophagoplication. J. Amer. med. Ass. 56, 1437–1438 (1911).

Michaud, P.: L'oesophage. Actualités hépato-gastro-entérologiques de l'Hôtel-Dieu. Paris: Masson 1958.

Mikulicz, J. von: Ueber Gastroskopie und Oesophagoskopie (Abstr.). Mitt. Vereins Aerzte Nied. Oest. Wien 8, 23–28 (1882).

Mikulicz, J. von: Zur Pathologie und Therapie des Cardiospasmus. Dtsch. med. Wschr. 30, 17–19, 50–54 (1904).

Miller, R. H.: Amyloid disease—an unusual cause of megalo-oesophagus. S. Afr. med. J. 43, 1202–1203 (1969).

Milroy, E.: Achalasia of the cardia. The long term results of Heller's operation. W. Indian med. J. 18, 65–81 (1969).

Misiewicz, J. J., Waller, S. L., Anthony, P. P., Gummer, J. W. P.: Pharmacology and histopathology of the cardiac sphincter in achalasia. Gut 9, 726–727 (1968).

Misiewicz, J. J., Waller, S. L., Anthony, P. P., Gummer, J. W. P.: Achalasia of the cardia: pharmacology and histopathology of isolated cardiac sphincteric muscle from patients with and without achalasia. Quart. J. Med. 38, 17–30 (1969).

Moersch, H. J.: Cardiospasm in infancy and in childhood. Amer. J. Dis. Child. 38, 294–298 (1929).

Moersch, H. J.: Problems in differential diagnosis of lesions of the lower portion of the esophagus and the cardia. Ann. Otol. 61, 976–986 (1952).

Moersch, H. J., Code, C. F., Olsen, A. M.: Dyschalasia of the esophagus. Coll. Papers Mayo Clin. 49, 19–27 (1957).

Montenegro, E. B., Cutait, D. E.: Construction of a new esophagus by means of transverse colon and its application for caustic atresia, carcinoma, and varices of the esophagus. Surgery 44, 785–794 (1958).

Mosher, H. P., McGregor, G. W.: A study of the lower end of the esophagus. Ann. Otol. 37, 12–70 (1928).

Nagler, R. W., Schwartz, R. D., Stahl, W. M., Jr., Spiro, H. M.: Achalasia in fraternal twins. Ann. intern. Med. 59, 906–910 (1963).

Nanson, E. M.: Treatment of cardiospasm by the expanding bag technique. Canad. Med. Ass. J. 86, 1107–1111 (1962).

Nanson, E. M.: Treatment of achalasia of the cardia. Gastroenterology 51, 236–241 (1966).

Nemir, P., Jr., Fallahnejad, M., Bose, B., Jacobowitz, D., Frobese, A. S., Hawthorne H. R.: A study of the causes of failure of esophagocardiomyotomy for achalasia. Amer. J. Surg. 121, 143–149 (1971).

Nemir, P., Jr., Frobese, A. S.: The modified Heller operation for achalasia of the esophagus. Surg. Chir. N. Amer. 42, 1407–1418 (1962).

Neville, W. E., Clowes, G. H., Jr.: Surgical treatment of the complications resulting from cardioesophageal incompetence. Dis. Chest 43, 572–581 (1963).

Nicks, R.: Surgical treatment for mega-oesophagus. Brit. J. Surg. 55, 525–530 (1968).

Nissen, R., Rossetti, M.: La fundoplication et la gastropexie dans le traitement chirurgical de l'insuffisance du cardia et de la hernie hiatale: indications, technique et résultats. Ann. Chir. 16, 825–836 (1962).

Norton, R.-A., Sultan, M.: Esophageal contractility and diameter in achalasia. Lahey Clin. Found. Bull. 17, 117–119 (1968).

Nuboer, J. F.: Sympathectomie bij cardiospasmus (achalasie). Demonstr. van 3 patiënten. Ned. T. Geneesk. 83, 592 (1939).

Okamoto, E., Iwasaki, T., Kakutani, T., Ueda, T.: Selective destruction of the myenteric plexus: its relation to Hirschsprung's disease, achalasia of the esophagus and hypertrophic pyloric stenosis. J. Pediat. Surg. 2, 444–454 (1967).

Okamoto, E., Iwasaki, T., Ueda, T., Takeda, Y.: Pathogenesis of cardiospasm: clinical and experimental studies. Med. J. Osaka Univ. 14, 245–274 (1964).

Olsen, A. M., Creamer, B.: Studies of oesophageal motility, with special reference to the differential diagnosis of diffuse spasm and achalasia (cardiospasm). Thorax 12, 279–289 (1957).

Olsen, A. M., Ellis, F. H., Jr., Creamer, B.: Cardiospasm (achalasia of the cardia). Amer. J. Surg. 93, 299–307 (1957).

Olsen, A. M., Harrington, S. W., Moersch, H. J., Andersen, H. A.: The treatment of cardiospasm: analysis of a twelve-year experience. J. thorac. cardiovasc. Surg. 22, 164–187 (1951).

OLSEN, A. M., HOLMAN, C. B., ANDERSEN, H. A.: The diagnosis of cardiospasm. Dis. Chest **23**, 477–498 (1953).

OSBORNE, C. A., CLIFFORD, D. H., JESSEN, C.: Hereditary esophageal achalasia in dogs. J. Amer. vet. med. Ass. **151**, 572–581 (1967).

PALMER, E. D.: Treatment of achalasia when the Heller operation has failed. Amer. J. Gastroent. **57**, 255–260 (1972).

PATRICK, D. L., PAYNE, W. S., OLSEN, A. M., ELLIS, F. H., JR.: Reoperation for achalasia of the esophagus. Arch. Surg. **103**, 122–128 (1971).

PAYNE, W. S., ELLIS, F. H., JR., OLSEN, A. M.: Achalasia of the esophagus. Arch. Surg. **81**, 411–418 (1960).

PAYNE, W. S., ELLIS, F. H., JR., OLSEN, A. M.: Treatment of cardiospasm (achalasia of the esophagus) in children. Surgery **50**, 731–735 (1961).

PAYR, E.: In: Discussion on surgical treatment of cardiospasm. Zbl. Chir. **56**, 1303 (1929).

PETROVSKY, B. V.: Cardiospasm and its surgical correction. Ann. Surg. **155**, 60–71 (1962).

PIERANDOZZI, J. S., RITTER, J. H.: Transient achalasia. A complication of vagotomy. Amer. J. Surg. **111**, 356–358 (1966).

PIERCE, W. S., MacVAUGH, H., JOHNSON, J.: Carcinoma of the esophagus arising in patients with achalasia of the cardia. J. thorac. cardiovasc. Surg. **59**, 335–339 (1970).

PIERI, G.: Sulla cura del cardiospasmo. IX. Congr. Soc. Int. Chir. **1**, 778–779 (1932).

PINOTTI, H. W., RAIA, A., NETTO, A. C., BETTARELLO, A.: The sphincter of the lower esophagus in various stages of mega-esophagus provoked by Chagas' disease. Arg. Gastroent. **5**, 51–58 (1968).

PLUMMER, H. S.: Cardiospasm: with a report of forty cases. J. Amer. med. Ass. **51**, 549–554 (1908).

PLUMMER, H. S., VINSON, P. P.: Cardiospasm: a report of 301 cases. Med. Clin. N. Amer. **5**, 355–369 (1921).

POLONSKY, L., GUTH, P. H.: Familial achalasia. Amer. J. dig. Dis. **15**, 291–295 (1970).

PURTON, T.: An extraordinary case of distension of the oesophagus, forming a sac, extending from two inches below the pharynx to the cardia orifice of the stomach. London Med. Phys. J. **46**, 540–542 (1921).

RAKE, G. W.: A case of annular muscular hypertrophy of the oesophagus (achalasia of the cardia without oesophageal dilatation). Guy's Hosp. Rep. **76**, 145–152 (1926).

RAKE, G. W.: On the pathology of achalasia of the cardia. Guy's Hosp. Rep. **77**, 141–150 (1927).

RAKE, G. W.: Epithelioma of the esophagus in association with achalasia of the cardia. Lancet **1931 II**, 682.

RAPANT, V., DOUBRAVSKY, J.: Ellisova Operace y Chirurgii Pokrocilé Achalasie Jienu. Rozhl. Chir. **40**, 613–617 (1961).

RAVEN, R. W.: Achalasia of the oesophagus in children. Brit. med. J. **1961 II**, 1614–1615.

RAVITCH, M. M.: In: Achalasia of esophagus (TUTTLE, W. M., R. T. CROWLEY, and R. J. BARRETT). J. thorac. Surg. **36**, 453–462 (1958).

RAVITCH, M. M.: Why the Heller operation is preferred to dilatation in achalasia of the esophagus. Med. Tms (N.Y.) **98**, 149–151 (1970).

REDO, S. F., BAUER, C. H.: Management of achalasia in infancy and childhood. Surgery **53**, 263–269 (1963).

REES, J. R., THORBJARNARSON, B., BARNES, W. H.: Achalasia: results of operation in 84 patients. Ann. Surg. **171**, 195–201 (1970).

REISINGER, M.: Ueber die operative Behandlung der Erweiterung des Oesophagus. Verh. dtsch. Ges. Chir. **36**, 86–88 (1907).

RESANO, J. H.: Commentaires sur les œsophagopathies de diagnostic difficile. Ann. Oto-laryng. (Paris) **65**, 1 (1948).

REZENDE, J. M. DE: The endemic South American mega-esophagus. Clinical aspects of endemic megaesophagus. Proc. 2nd World Congr. of Gastroenterology, Munich 1962, 1, 69–74 (1963).

REZENDE, J. M. DE: In: Doenca de Chagas. Brazil: R. J. Cancado 1968.

REZENDE, J. M. DE, ROSSI, A.: Comprometimento do esôfago no moléstia de Chagas. Rev. goiana Med. **4**, 9 (1958).

RICKHAM, P. P., BOECKMAN, C. R.: Achalasia of the esophagus in young children. Clin. Pediat. (Philad.) **2**, 676–681 (1963).

RODNAN, G. P., FENNELL, R. H., JR.: Progressive systemic sclerosis sine scleroderma. J. Amer. med. Ass. **180**, 665–670 (1962).

RÖPKE: Zur Operation des Oesophagospasmus. Verh. dtsch. Ges. Chir. **43**, 121–122 (1914).

RÖSCH, W., BACHMANN, K., OTTENJAN, R.: Asystolischer Herzstillstand bei Achalasie. Dtsch. med. Wschr. **94**, 2191–2194 (1969).

Root, H. D., Wangensteen, O. H.: Cardiospasm and its treatment. Arch. Surg. **85**, 594–599 (1962).

Rossetti, M.: Ösophagocardiomyotomie und Fundoplicatio: Eine physiologische Operation bei Cardiospasmus und Megaoesophagus. Schweiz. med. Wschr. **93**, 925–931 (1963).

Roth, J. L. A., Stein, G. N.: Achalasia (Cardiospasm). In: Gastroenterology, Bockus, H. L. (ed.), vol. I, chap. 10. Philadelphia-London: W. B. Saunders Company 1963.

Rudler, J. C.: In discussion «Inconvénients de l'oesophagogastrostomie dans les échecs de l'opération de Heller», of Lortat-Jacob, J. L. Arch. Mal. Appar. dig. **39**, 524–527 (1950).

Rudler, J. C.: Pour l'opération de Heller (oesophago-cardiomyotomie extra-muqueuse), Helv. chir. Acta **27**, 411–420 (1960).

Salzman, A. J.: Lower esophageal web associated with achalasia of the esophagus. N.Y. J. Med. **65**, 1922–1925 (1965).

Sanderson, D. R., Ellis, F. H., Jr., Olsen, A. M.: Achalasia of the esophagus: results of therapy by dilation, 1950–1967. Chest **58**, 116–121 (1970).

Sanderson, D. R., Ellis, F. H., Jr., Schlegel, J. F., Olsen, A. M.: Syndrome of vigorous achalasia: Clinical and physiologic observations. Dis. Chest **52**, 508–517 (1967).

Santy, P., Michaud, P., Latreille, R.: Le traitement du mégaoesophage par l'opération de Heller; résultats de 168 interventions. Lyon Chir. **51**, 513–522 (1956a).

Santy, P., Michaud, P., Latreille, R.: Le traitement du mégaoesophage par l'opération de Heller; résultats de 179 interventions. Ass. franç. Chir. **58**, 133–139 (1956b).

Santy, P., Michaud, P., Viard, H.: Cancer sur méga-oesophage. Lyon chir. **54**, 354–367 (1958).

Sato, H., Akihama, M., Tanaka, T., Igararshi, M., Yamagata, S., Huruhashi, M., Hasegawa, K., Hunabashi, W., Hoshino, M., Yoshida, K.: Studies on idiopathic esophagus dilatation with special reference to the compression interruption method with a glass plate and the carbolic acid-injecting method used as intermuscular nervous plexus destroying methods. (Abstr.) Jap. J. Gastroent. **1**, 71–72 (1963).

Saubier, E., Chalencon, J.-F., Beaulieux, J.: Réinterventions chirurgicales après opération de Heller pour mégaoesophage essentiel (à propos de cinq observations). Lyon méd. **223**, 883–891 (1970).

Sauerbruch, F.: Discussion. Verh. dtsch. Ges. Chir. **45**, 149 (1921).

Sawyers, J. L., Foster, J. H.: Surgical considerations in the management of achalasia of the esophagus. Ann. Surg. **165**, 780–785 (1967a).

Sawyers, J. L., Foster, J. H.: Surgical treatment of achalasia. Dis. Chest **52**, 310–314 (1967b).

Schindler, R.: Observations on cardiospasm and its treatment by brusque dilatation. Ann. intern. Med. **45**, 207–215 (1956).

Schindler, R.: Two unusual cases of achalasia. Gastroint. Endosc. **12**, 10–11 (1965).

Schlesinger, M. H., Steinberg, H., Almy, T. P.: The disturbance of esophageal motility in cardiospasm: studies of autonomic stimulation and autonomic blockade of the human esophagus, including the cardia. Gastroenterology **25**, 333–348 (1953).

Schloffer: Cited by Pamperl, R., Zur operativen Behandlung des Kardiospasmus. Dtsch. Z. Chir. **148**, 206–227 (1919).

Schnelle, G. B.: Radiology in small animal practice. 2nd ed. Evanston, Ill.: North Am. Vet. 1950.

Seaman, W. B., Wells, J., Flood, C. A.: Diagnostic problems of esophageal cancer: relationship to achalasia and hiatus hernia. Amer. J. Roentgenol. **90**, 778–791 (1963).

Segar, L. H., Stoeffler, W.: Cardiospasm in new-born infant. Amer. J. Dis. Child. **39**, 354 (1930).

Seliger, G., Lee, T., Schwartz, S.: Carcinoma of the proximal esophagus. A complication of long-standing achalasia. Amer. J. Gastroent. **57**, 20–25 (1972).

Siegel, C.-I., Hendrix, T. R., Harvey, J. C.: The swallowing disorder in myotonia dystrophica. Gastroenterology **50**, 541–550 (1966).

Silber, W.: Achalasia. Lancet **1965 II**, 1287–1289.

Singh, H., Gupta, H. L., Sethi, R. S., Khetarpal, S. K.: Cardiac achalasia in childhood. Postgrad. med. J. **45**, 327–335 (1969).

Smith, B.: The myenteric plexus in Chagas' disease. J. Path. **94**, 462–463 (1967).

Smith, B.: The neurological lesion in achalasia of the cardia. Gut **11**, 388–391 (1970).

Sokolovsky, V.: Achalasia and paralysis of the canine esophagus. J. Amer. vet. med. Ass. **160**, 943–955 (1972).

Sorsdahl, O. A., Gay, B. B., Jr.: Achalasia of the esophagus in childhood. Amer. J. Dis. Child. **109**, 141–146 (1965).

Spy, G. M.: Megaloesophagus in a litter of greyhounds. Vet. Rec. **75**, 853–855 (1963).

Starck, H.: Die Behandlung der spasmogenen Speiseröhrenerweiterung. Münch. med. Wschr. **71**, 334–336 (1924).

STARCK, H.: Die Krankheiten der Speiseröhre. Darmstadt: Dr. W. Steinkopff 1952.

STEICHEN, F. M., HELLER, E., RAVITCH, M. M.: Achalasia of the esophagus. Rec. Adv. Surg. 17, 846–876 (1960).

STEIN, G. N.: Roentgenologic diagnosis. In: Gastroenterology, BOCKUS, H. L. (ed.), vol. I, p. 158–164. Philadelphia and London: W. B. Saunders Company 1963.

STEVENS, M. B., HOOKMAN, P., SIEGEL, C. I., ESTERLY, J. R., SHULMAN, L. E., HENDRIX, T. R.: Aperistalsis of the esophagus in patients with connective tissue disorders and Raynaud's phenomenon. New Engl. J. Med. 270, 1218–1222 (1964).

STRATING, A., CLIFFORD, D. H.: Canine achalasia with special reference to heredity. Southwest Vet. 19, 135–136 (1966).

SUERMONDT, W. F.: Achalasia of the cardia. Arch. chir. neerl. 5, 59–63 (1953).

SULTAN, M., NORTON, R.: Esophageal diameter and the treatment of achalasia. Amer. J. dig. Dis. 14, 611–618 (1969).

SWENSON, O., OECONOMOPOULOS, C. T.: Achalasia of the oesophagus in children. J. thorac. cardiovasc. Surg. 41, 49–59 (1960).

TACHOVSKY, T. J., LYNN, H. B., ELLIS, F. H., JR.: The surgical approach to esophageal achalasia in children. J. pediat. Surg. 3, 226–231 (1968).

TEMPLETON, F. E.: X-ray examination of the stomach. Chicago: Chicago Univ. Press 1944,

THIBERT, F., CHICOINE, R., CHARTIER-RATELLE, G., THIBODEAU, L.-P., COLLIN, P.-P., COLLU. R.: Forme familiale de l'achalasie de l'oesophage chez l'enfant. Un. méd. Can. 94, 1293–1300 (1965).

THIEDING, F.: Ueber Cardiospasmus. Atonie und „idiopathische" Dilatation der Speiseröhre. Bruns' Beitr. klin. Chir. 121, 237–300 (1921).

THOMSON, J.: Neuro-muscular incoordination at the cardia in the newborn. Arch. Dis. Child. 25, 52–60 (1950).

THOMSON, S., NEGUS, V. E., BATEMAN, G. H.: Disease of the nose and throat. In: A Textbbok for Students and Practitioners. Ed. 6, p. 776. London: Cassel and Company Ltd. 1955.

TODD, I., PORTER, N. H., MORSON, B. C., SMITH, B., FRIEDMAN, C. A., NEAL, R. A.: Chagas' disease of the colon and rectum. Gut 10, 1009–1014 (1969).

TON, J. G.: Selective surgery for achalasia. Arch. chir. neerl. 13, 27–40 (1961).

TRINCAS, M.: Una variante alla esofagomiotomia (operazione di Heller). Minerva chir. 9, 1089–1901 (1954).

TROUNCE, J. R., DEUCHAR, D. C., KAUNTZE, R., THOMAS, G. A.: Studies in achalasia of the cardia. Quart. J. Med., N.S. 26, 433–443 (1957).

TUCKER, G.: Cardiospasm: A pneumatic-mercury dilator. Ann. Otol. 48, 808–816 (1939).

TUFFIER, M.: Dilatation de l'oesophage. Méga-oesophage. Opération: Résultat fonctionnel suivi sur radiographie, huit mois après. Bull. Mém. Acad. Chir. (Paris) 48, 446–450 (1922).

TUTTLE, W. M., CROWLEY, R. T., BARRETT, R. J.: Achalasia of the esophagus: further thoughts on surgical management. J. thorac. cardiovasc. Surg. 36, 453–459 (1958).

TYCE, F. A., BROUGH, W.: The appearance of an undescribed syndrome and the inheritance of a family. Psychiat. Res. Rep. Amer. psychiat. Ass. 15, 73–79 (1962).

VANTRAPPEN, G.: Slokdarmmotiliteit. Brussel: Arscia uitg. N.V. 1961.

VANTRAPPEN, G., HELLEMANS, J., DELOOF, W., VALEMBOIS, P., VANDENBROUCKE, J.: Treatment of achalasia with pneumatic dilatations. Gut 12, 268–275 (1971).

VANTRAPPEN, G., HELLEMANS, J., VALEMBOIS, P., VANDENBROUCKE, J.: De behandeling van achalasia. Acta chir. belg. 65, Suppl. II, 25–40 (1966).

VANTRAPPEN, G., GOIDSENHOVEN, G. E. VAN, VERBEKE, S., BERGHE, G. VAN DEN, VANDENBROUCKE, J.: Manometric studies in achalasia of the cardia, before and after pneumatic dilations. Gastroenterology 45, 317–325 (1963).

VERNEJOUL, R. DE, DOR, J., GRISOLI, J., HENRY, E., FLEURY, R., EYMERY, J.: La place de l'opération de Heller dans le méga-œsophage, ses modalités techniques, ses résultats éloignés. Ass. franç. Chir. 58, 151–155 (1956).

VIEIRA, C. B., GODOY, R. A. DE: Resposta motora do esôfago nao ectásico a agentes colinergicos na moléstia de Chagas. Rev. goianna Med. 9, 21–28 (1963).

VIEIRA, C. B., GODOY, R. A. DE, CARRIL, C. F.: Hypersensitivity of the large intestine to cholinergic agents in patients with Chagas' disease and megacolon. Rev. bras. Gastroent. 16, 41–48 (1964).

VINSON, P. P.: The diagnosis and treatment of cardiospasm. J. Amer. med. Ass. 82, 859–861 (1924).

WAKELEY, C. P. G.: A case of hiatal oesophagismus in a man aged thirty-six years. Brit. med. J. 1916I, 589–590.

WANGENSTEEN, O. H.: A physiologic operation for mega-esophagus: (dystonia, cardiospasm, achalasia). Ann. Surg. 134, 301–315 (1951).

WANGENSTEEN, O. H.: Technique of achieving an adequate extramucosal myotomy in megaoesophagus (achalasia, cardiospasm, dystonia). Surg. Gynec. Obstet. 105, 339–347 (1957).

Wanke, R., Alnor, P. C.: Die morphologischen Grundlagen der Achalasia Oesophagei. Studies in Surgery Malmö, 135–144 (1963).

Wanke, R., Kricke, E.: Operative Behandlung der Achalasia (Sclerosis) Cardiae, zugleich ein Beitrag zur Morphologie. Dtsch. med. Wschr. 87, 1036–1040 (1962).

Wendel, W.: Zur Chirurgie des Oesophagus. Langenbecks Arch. klin. Chir. 93, 311–329 (1910).

Williams, J. L.: Carcinoma of the oesophagus as a complication of achalasia of the cardia. Thorax 11, 268–274 (1956).

Willis, T.: Pharmaceutice rationalis sive diatriba de medicamentorum operationibus in humano corpore. London-Hagae Comitis: 1674.

Wingfield, H. V., Karwowski, A.: The treatment of achalasia by cardiomyotomy. Brit. J. Surg. 59, 281–284 (1972).

Winship, D. H., Caflisch, C. R., Zboralske, F. F., Hogan, W. J.: Deterioration of esophageal peristalsis in patients with alcoholic neuropathy. Gastroenterology 55, 173–178 (1968).

Wolf, B. S., Marshak, R. H., Som, M. L., Brahms, S. A., Greenberg, E. I.: The gastroesophageal vestibule on roentgen examination; differentiation from the phrenic ampulla and minimal hiatal herniation. J. Mt Sinai Hosp. 25, 167–200 (1958).

Woolam, G., L. Maher, F. T., Ellis, F. H., Jr.: Vagal nerve function in achalasia of the esophagus. Surg. Forum 18, 362–365 (1967).

Worms, G., Leorux-Robert, J.: Les séquelles oesophagiennes des intoxications par les gaz de combat: contribution à l'étude pathogénique des grandes dilatations de l'oesophage. Presse méd. 1, 646–649 (1934).

Wright, J. T.: Buscopan and oesophageal achalasia. Brit. J. Radiol. 34, 113–119 (1961).

Zaayer, J. H.: Cardiospasme en andere slokdarmaandoeningen. Zbl. Chir. 46, 57–60 (1919).

Zaayer, J. H.: Cardiospasm in the aged. Ann. Surg. 77, 615–617 (1923).

Zenker, F. A., Ziemssen, H. von: Krankheiten des Oesophagus. Ziemssen's Handbuch der speziellen Pathologie und Therapie, Bd. 7, 17 (1877).

Zenker, R., Rueff, F. L.: Ergebnisse der Behandlung des Kardiospasmus. Münch. med. Wschr. 105, 1437–1442 (1963).

Diffuse Esophageal Spasm

G. Vantrappen and J. Hellemans

With 3 Figures

1. Definition

The first clinical description of esophageal spasm was given by Osgood in 1889, but the term diffuse spasm of the lower part of the esophagus was used for the first time by Moersch and Camp in 1934. Diffuse spasm is a neuromuscular motor disorder of the esophagus characterized by substernal distress or dysphagia or both, by the roentgenographic appearance of localized non-progressive contractions and by an increased incidence of non-peristaltic and often huge pressure waves on manometric recordings (Fleshler, 1967; Kramer, 1970). To denote these radiological and manometric abnormalities in an asymptomatic patient the term asymptomatic diffuse spasm has been proposed (Kramer, 1970). The disorder is less diffuse than its name might suggest. Generally the distal segment of the esophagus is affected over a variable extent, whereas the proximal segment remains normal.

The disease has been described under various names, such as localized esophageal spasm, ladder spasm, segmental spasm, rosary bead esophagus, spastic pseudoverticulosis, corkscrew esophagus, hysterical spasm and muscular hypertrophy of the esophagus. Most cases of hypertensive gastroesophageal sphincter (Code et al., 1960; Vantrappen et al., 1960; Vantrappen, 1961) or of the hypercontracting sphincter (Garrett and Godwin, 1969) belong to this entity.

Most authors consider diffuse spasm as a separate entity (Fleshler, 1967; Kramer, 1970). According to others it is no more than a clinical syndrome with multiple causes and non-specific reactions of the esophageal musculature (Bennett and Hendrix, 1970; Bennett et al., 1970). According to Edwards (1971) the separation of achalasia and diffuse spasm is "a man-made distinction of a God-given disease".

2. Incidence

Although diffuse spasm can occur at any adult age, commonly individuals over 50 are affected (Creamer et al., 1958; Fleshler, 1967; Kramer, 1970). No sexual predisposition can be defined (Fleshler, 1967; Rider et al., 1969; Kramer, 1970). The typical patient is a very nervous person and his complaints are clearly related to emotional stress (Moersch and Camp, 1934; Ellis and Olsen, 1969). The disease is 5 times less frequent than achalasia (Craddock et al., 1966), though precise data are not available. In our department where the diagnosis of diffuse spasm is made according to fairly strict criteria, the ratio diffuse spasm-achalasia is even lower.

3. Pathology

Hypertrophy of the longitudinal and especially of the circular esophageal muscle coat and of the muscularis mucosae has been observed (Sloper, 1954; Johnstone, 1960; Ellis et al., 1964; Cassella, 1965; Nicks et al., 1968; Ferguson et al., 1969). There may be degenerative changes of the myofilaments in the smooth muscle cells (Cassella et al., 1965). The muscular layer may become as thick as 2 cm (Gillies et al., 1967) but muscular thickening is not observed in all patients (Paden, 1954) and may occur without symptoms (Bennett and Hendrix, 1970). The spasm of the longitudinal muscles may draw up the cardia through the hiatus (Nicks et al., 1968). Auerbach's plexus is preserved (Roth and Fleshler, 1964; Craddock et al., 1966) but focal infiltration of chronic inflammatory cells in and sometimes around the plexus has been found (Nicks et al., 1968). Hence the reason why the Mecholyl test is positive in some cases of symptomatic diffuse spasm remains unknown (Creamer et al., 1958; Kramer et al., 1962, 1967a) (see achalasia 6.3.). In one case sparsity of Meissner's plexus has been described (Paden, 1954). Electron microscopic examination of 4 severe cases of diffuse spasm has shown degeneration in the esophageal branches of the vagus nerves and generalized degenerative changes of the wallerian type in many axons (Cassella et al., 1965). The generalized character of these vagal changes contrasts with the focal involvement in cases of achalasia.

4. Symptoms

The clinical picture is quite variable from one patient to the other. Symptoms may even by absent. If they are present, dysphagia and pain are most prominent. Of the 46 patients with severe symptoms reported by Ellis et al. (1964), 15 had pain only, 24 pain and dysphagia and 7 dysphagia only. The degree of dysphagia varies considerably; some patients experience rare discomfort whereas others suffer from severe dysphagia at each meal. The dysphagia is frequently provoked by cold or carbonated beverages or by sticky boluses (such as meat) and is clearly influenced by psychological factors. A bolus may become impacted and this may block further attempts to swallow for minutes to hours (Creamer, 1968). An impaction, however, suggests the presence of an organic stenosis; whenever impaction occurs, such a lesion must be looked for carefully. Generally the bolus is arrested only for a short time and the fasting esophagus does not contain any residue. In contrast with achalasia, diffuse spasm does not usually lead to regurgitation in the recumbent position, to vomiting or to weight loss. Some patients, however, experience such pain that they fear to eat and therefore lose weight (Gillies et al., 1967).

The substernal distress is often intense. It may be a substernal cramp or it may radiate to neck and arms like cardiac pain (Moersch and Camp, 1934; Vantrappen et al., 1959, 1960; Schmidt et al., 1962; Garrett and Godwin, 1969). The pain may appear during meals, but is usually not related to the intake of food and may even appear at night, awakening the patient. Exceptionally a vagovagal syncope occurs during eating. A patient has been described in whom drinking ginger ale could elicit a nodal cardiac rhythm (Kopald et al., 1964). The evolution of the disease may span years without deterioration.

5. Technical Examinations

The diagnosis is made by means of radiological and manometric examination. Other techniques (endoscopy, intraluminal pH measurements, etc.) are used to detect other conditions such as organic obstruction or reflux.

5.1. Radiology

Not infrequently routine X-rays of the esophagus are interpreted as normal though radiological abnormalities are noticed on reviewing the pictures or on repeating the examination (ROTH and FLESHLER, 1964). ELLIS et al. (1964) reported on 46 patients who experienced such severe discomfort that they were treated surgically; yet esophageal roentgenography yielded negative results in 24 patients and in 6 others a small diaphragmatic hernia was the only abnormality. Cases in whom no radiological abnormalities were found are also mentioned by CREAMER et al. (1958), JOHNSTONE (1960) and GILLIES et al. (1967). There is little relation between the severity of the symptoms and the radiological deformity (JOHNSTONE, 1960). With an appropriate technique, aimed at discovering motility disorders (examination of the patient in a recumbent position using a sufficient amount of contrast material, and cinematographic or video recording of several swallows), abnormalities will usually be found in patients with diffuse spasm. In some patients an otherwise normal examination may yield markedly abnormal results if it is carried out during an attack of pain (JOHNSTONE, 1960). The most common disorder to escape attention is a diffuse narrowing of a long esophageal segment. Most abnormalities are found in the lower half of the gullet. The abnormal contractions result in a variety of radiological images which can all be called "curling" and which are all manifestations of the same disorder (MOERSCH and CAMP, 1934).

In some cases they cause a fine rippling of the contour of the lower esophagus; in others there is a marked segmental symmetrical indentation with longitudinal shortening, which has been called segmental spasm. In extreme cases, the picture shows a corkscrew esophagus with deep asymmetrical contractions, separated by functional outpouchings, which may mimic diverticula (KRAMER, 1967a) (Fig. 189). Real diverticula may also occur and it is not unlikely that the motor disorders favor their development. Sometimes there is a diffuse narrowing of the lower half or third of the esophagus, which then empties in a systolic rather than in a peristaltic fashion (ROTH and FLESHLER, 1964). The frequent association between diffuse spasm and hiatus hernia is ascribed to esophageal shortening by the massive contractions (ELLIS et al., 1964; CREAMER, 1968).

The transport of the contrast material through the esophagus depends on several factors, one of which is the moment the simultaneous contractions appear. Sometimes the peristaltic contraction runs its normal course down to the cardia but is followed in the distal segment by the simultaneous appearance of a series of contraction rings. This disorder does not usually affect the propulsion of the bolus. Mostly, however, the primary peristaltic wave reaches only the level of the arch of the aorta when the lower half of the esophagus suddenly becomes distorted by simultaneous segmental contractions which capture the bolus or push it into different directions (MOERSCH and CAMP, 1934; CREAMER et al., 1958; McNALLA and KATZ, 1967). In contrast with achalasia the esophagus does not dilate or widens only slightly, regardless of the duration of the symptoms, and there is no food residue in the fasting gullet. As in achalasia the thickening of the esophageal wall may be visible on X-rays (JOHNSTONE, 1960).

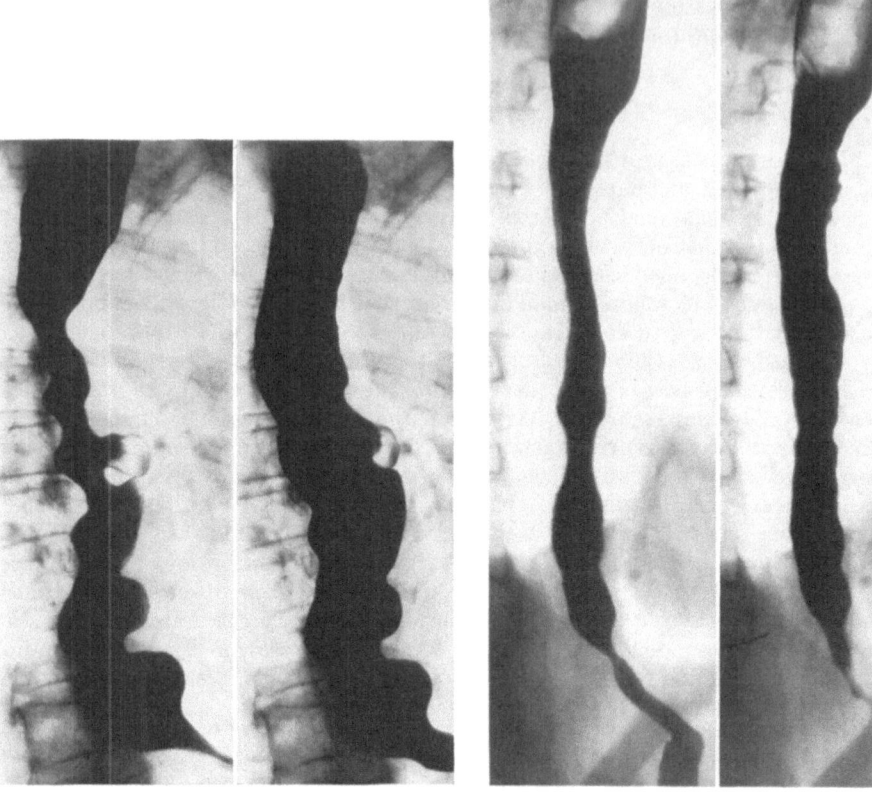

A   B

Fig. 189 A–C. Different and changing radiological patterns seen in patients with diffuse spasm of the esophagus. In addition to the tertiary contractions, there is a pulsion diverticulum in A, and a small hiatal hernia in C. Note the diffuse narrowing of the lower two thirds of the esophagus in B, a patient with severe symptoms

5.2. Manometric Examinations

In a few patients the abnormal segment is limited to the gastroesophageal sphincter. Generally, however, the motor disorder affects the distal third or two thirds of the esophagus. The proximal segment is often normal (Creamer et al., 1958) though it may be involved as well, albeit to a lesser degree (Gillies et al., 1967).

A characteristic motility pattern has been described by Creamer et al. (1958). The deglutitive response in the distal segments of the esophagus is characterized by the occurrence of simultaneous (non-sequential) pressure peaks, of repetitive and biphasic waves (i.e. several pressure peaks in response to a single deglutition) and of giant waves (with an abnormally high amplitude and long duration) (Fig. 190). These contractions are not necessarily painful; very abnormal tracings can be recorded at a moment when a patient is asymptomatic. Spontaneous activity can also be present.

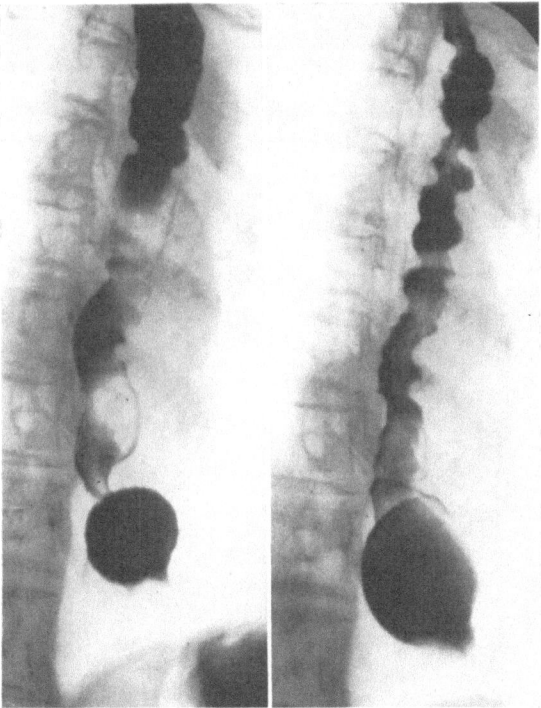

Fig. 189 C

In some patients swallowing a water bolus will provoke the typical motility disorders more readily than dry swallows (CREAMER et al., 1958).

Usually the esophagus retains its capability of producing peristaltic contractions. The primary peristaltic contraction may progress down to the cardia in a normal way, to be followed in the lower segments by simultaneous and even repetitive contraction waves. In other cases the primary peristaltic wave dies out in the middle esophagus, to be replaced in the lower segments by simultaneous, repetitive and/or giant pressure peaks (FLESHLER, 1967; CREAMER, 1968; KRAMER, 1970). In a few cases of so-called symptomatic diffuse spasm, the Mecholyl test is positive; in cases of asymptomatic diffuse spasm it is always negative (see Achalasia 6.3.) (KRAMER et al., 1967a).

The pressure in the gastroesophageal sphincter, measured with the perfusion technique, has been found by some to be increased (KRAMER, 1970; BOMBECK et al., 1972); by others to be normal (HEITMANN, 1971). The same controversy already existed before the introduction of the perfusion technique. CREAMER et al. (1958) found increased pressures and a wider band of high pressure especially if a hiatal hernia was associated (OLSEN and CREAMER, 1957); others found normal resting pressures (GILLIES et al., 1967). HEITMANN (1971) pointed out that the gastroesophageal sphincteric pressure is often increased in hernia patients and therefore excluded these cases from his series, whereas 14 out of the 16 patients of CREAMER et al. (1958) and 18 out of the 28 patients of BOMBECK et al. (1972) had a hernia. The incidence of deglutitive relaxations is decreased and the relaxations are often incomplete. In contrast with achalasia, however, some

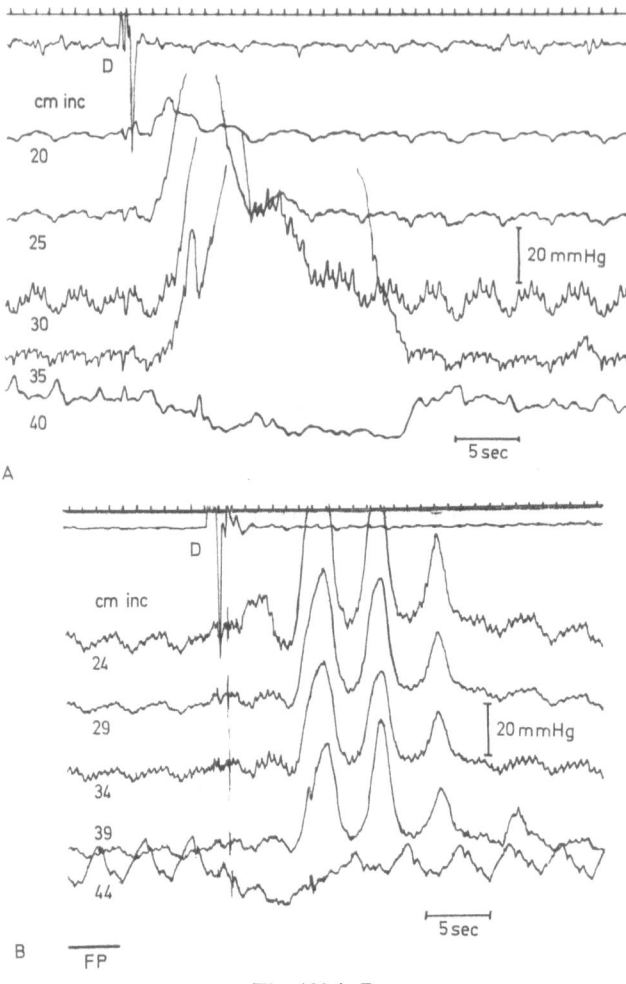

Fig. 190 A–B

Fig. 190. Different manometric patterns observed in diffuse spasm of the esophagus. In C
and D there is "spontaneous" activity

normal relaxations can still be observed (Kramer, 1970). The sphincter contractions are mostly normal (Heitmann, 1971) though sometimes premature
(Olsen and Creamer, 1957). Diffuse spasm of the esophagus usually affects
larger portions of the gullet, including the gastroesophageal sphincter, though
in some cases it is limited to the sphincter; this problem is discussed in 6.2.

The basis for symptom production has been studied by combined cineroentgenography and manometry (Roth and Fleshler, 1964). Esophageal emptying
was adequate in the presence of large waves if the peaks of pressure were distally
sequential. These waves did not cause any symptoms. Emptying was inefficient,
even in the presence of small waves, when the pressure peaks occurred irregularly.
A prolonged but moderate elevation of pressure was noted in the one patient
who had an episode of pain during the study (Roth and Fleshler, 1964).
Creamer et al. (1958) have also had the occasion to measure the intraluminal

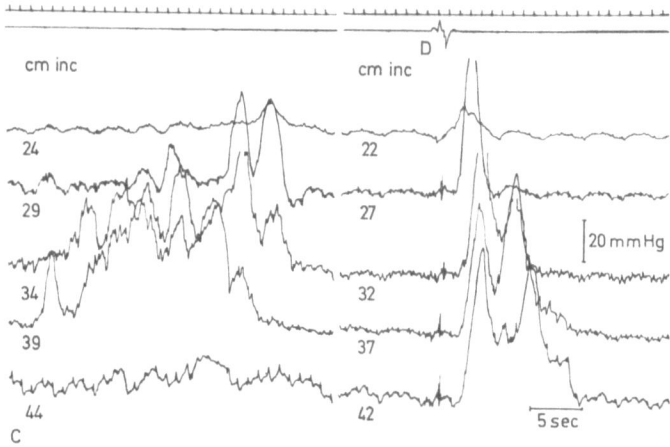

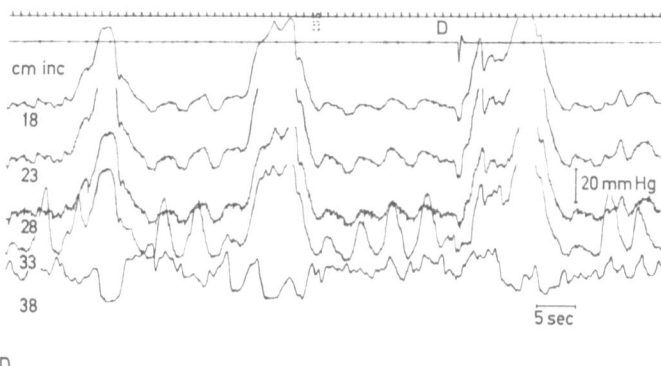

Fig. 190 C–D

pressures during an attack of pain. In their patient the pain was associated with a prolonged and marked increase in pressure. Neither the X-ray pictures nor the pressure tracings allow to distinguish between symptomatic and asymptomatic diffuse spasm (ROTH and FLESHLER, 1964). Abnormal sphincter responses may also produce symptoms, as is seen in symptomatic cases of hypertensive sphincter (VANTRAPPEN, 1961; CODE et al., 1960).

6. Related Conditions

6.1. Idiopathic Muscular Hypertrophy of the Lower Esophagus

In rare instances the musculature of the lower half of the esophagus is greatly and diffusely thickened while the lumen is of a normal diameter. SLOPER (1954) collected 25 cases and added 7 of his own; the study of GUICHARD et al. (1963) deals with 65 cases. The majority are men in their sixth and seventh decade, but the significance of this observation is diminished by the fact that in 30 of the 32 cases of SLOPER (1954) the presence of an esophageal lesion was unsuspected until revealed at necropsy. Muscular hypertrophy of the esophagus has also been described in children, sometimes associated with hypertrophy of the heart. Some 12 cases have been described of both hypertrophy of the esophagus and of the pylorus (SLOPER, 1954; GUICHARD et al., 1963). The histological finding consists of simple hypertrophy of all muscular coats, particularly of the inner muscle layer. The intramural plexus is normal or exhibits slight degenerative changes (PEISON, 1971).

It is reasonable to accept that this syndrome is identical with or closely related to diffuse spasm. It is difficult, however, to prove this because in many cases the hypertrophy is an autopsy finding, and in most instances data about the motility of the esophagus before death are lacking. There have been but a few cases in which pathological as well as clinical and radiological observations are available (SLOPER, 1954; JOHNSTONE, 1960; BOQUIEN et al., 1963).

6.2. The Hypertensive Sphincter

Diffuse spasm of the esophagus can be associated with a hypertensive or hyperactive gastroesophageal sphincter but this sphincteric disorder can also occur as an isolated condition (VANTRAPPEN et al., 1960; CODE et al., 1960; ELLIS et al., 1964). Hiatal hernia is thought to be a predisposing factor (GARRETT and GODWIN, 1969; HEITMANN, 1970). According to CODE et al. (1960) the manometric criteria of hypertonicity are pressures exceeding 140 cm of water when measured with a 5 mm balloon-covered pressure transducer, or pressures in excess of 40 cm of water when measured with an uninfused open tip catheter (CODE et al., 1960). Theoretically it might be possible to distinguish between hypertensive sphincters (high resting pressure), hyperreacting sphincters (deglutitive contractions of high amplitude) and hypercontracting sphincters (deglutitive contractions of long duration). However, there is too much overlap between these parameters to consider them as separate entities.

The isolated sphincteric disorder can produce clinical symptoms, particularly substernal or high epigastric pain and sometimes dysphagia (VANTRAPPEN et al., 1959; ELLIS et al., 1964; GARRETT and GODWIN, 1969). VANTRAPPEN (1961) described 7 patients with attacks of substernal or high epigastric pain, unrelated to meals or physical exertion and not associated with heartburn or dysphagia. Both the end-expiratory and the end-inspiratory pressures were significantly higher than in cases of diffuse spasm; the sphincter relaxations were normal; but the contractions were stronger and of a considerably longer duration as compared with diffuse spasm. The peristalsis was only slightly disturbed, significantly less than in the usual case of diffuse spasm.

High resting pressures and prolonged sphincteric contractions can also be observed in organic diseases, such as carcinoma of the cardia (VANTRAPPEN, 1961; DEBRAY et al., 1962; SEREBRO et al., 1970).

7. Diagnosis

Numerous other conditions can produce motor disorders of the esophagus resembling diffuse spasm, so that the problem has been raised whether diffuse spasm exists as an identity (BENNETT and HENDRIX, 1970). An organic obstruction at the cardia (stricture, neoplasm, lower esophageal ring etc.) may result

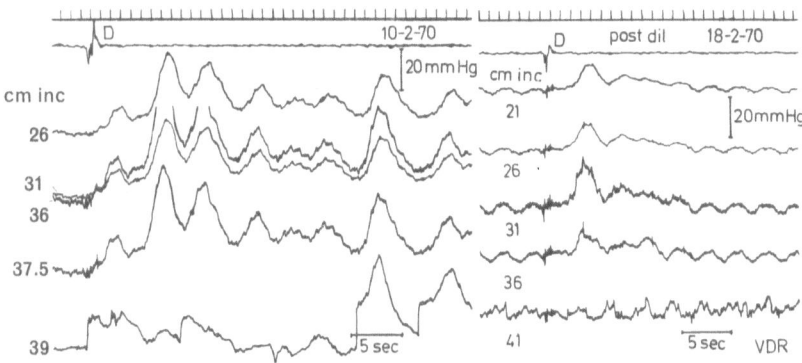

Fig. 191. Diffuse spasm before and after pneumatic dilatation

in a disordered motility pattern simulating that of idiopathic diffuse spasm (SCHATZKI, 1965). Before the diagnosis of diffuse spasm can be made, obstruction at the cardia must therefore be excluded. The motility disorder usually disappears when the obstruction is eliminated (KELLEY, 1968). It should be noted, however, that in cases of diffuse spasm also, the motility tracing may look significantly less disordered after pneumatic dilatation of the cardia (Fig. 191).

Neural damage by carcinomatous infiltration cannot only mimic achalasia (see achalasia 7.1.2.) but also diffuse spasm without causing an obstruction (SEREBRO et al., 1970). Esophagitis induced by reflux or by ingestion of corrosive agents can provoke localized non-progressive and repetitive contractions (CREAMER, 1955; BESANÇON et al., 1962; SIEGEL and HENDRIX, 1963; ATKINSON and BENNETT, 1968). Motility disturbances are also observed in patients with asymptomatic hiatal hernia (KELLEY, 1965). Diffuse spasm and reflux esophagitis cannot always be distinguished on the basis of the subjective complaints, although BOMBECK et al. (1972) have emphasized some differences between the symptoms of spasm, esophagitis and the combination of both. Manometry, however, may permit the distinction, the sphincter pressure being decreased in cases of reflux. The acid infusion test may be a valuable aid for the diagnosis of gastroesophageal reflux esophagitis (see acid infusion test 3).

The differential diagnosis of diffuse spasm and atypical or vigorous achalasia presents more difficulties (see achalasia 5.2.). The difference between the conditions described as symptomatic diffuse spasm, vigorous achalasia, dyschalasia and achalasia is not always very clear and may be somewhat artificial. Cases have been reported evolving from diffuse spasm to achalasia (SCHRODER et al., 1963; KRAMER et al., 1967b). We have observed several cases in whom the few peristaltic contractions still left at a first examination later disappeared, and who eventually came to present the typical manometric and radiological picture of achalasia (Fig. 179). Presbyesophagus, diabetic and alcoholic neuropathy, scleroderma, amyotrophic lateral sclerosis and neurological diseases also can disturb the normal motility pattern and provoke simultaneous and repetitive contractions (such disorders are not infrequently found even in normal subjects particularly under abnormal experimental conditions, e.g. prolonged manometry). But in all these diseases the giant pressure waves of high amplitude and long duration are lacking and the repetitive contractions appear as 2, sometimes 3, rarely 4 or more pressure waves. In cases of diffuse spasm, 5 or more pressure peaks are commonly observed, as well as a higher degree of spontaneous activity. If the presence of a few simultaneous repetitive waves is considered sufficient to make a diagnosis of diffuse spasm, it is hard to delineate this condition, but if it is limited to cases characterized by giant pressure waves, strongly repetitive contractions, "spontaneous" activity and/or clear sphincteric disorders, diffuse spasm is markedly different from the motility disorders mentioned above.

Manometrically established motor disturbances may be visible on routine X-rays but can better be visualized on dynamic studies using cinematography or videorecording (McNally and Katz, 1967).

As long as angina pectoris has not been excluded as carefully as possible, the diagnosis of diffuse spasm should be made with caution.

8. Treatment

8.1. Medical Treatment

Medical treatment is superfluous in asymptomatic cases and disappointing, both for the patient and the physician, in symptomatic ones. It is important to inform the patient about the nature of his disease and to assure him of its benign character. He should be advised to avoid food and drink that provoke the symptoms and to eat slowly, but he is likely to answer that he is been doing this for months. Medical treatment consists of sedative and "spasmolytic" drugs. Diazepam (Valium) combines both these effects. Anticholinergics are not indicated because they worsen the disturbance of the peristaltic contractions and favor reflux, which can trigger motor disturbances. Spasmolytic drugs, acting directly on the muscle cell, should be preferred. Nitroglycerine and nitrites do stop an attack of pain, but the tolerated dose is low because of the headache they produce.

8.2. Dilatation

If patients with severe symptoms respond poorly to medical therapy, we resort to pneumatic dilatations, using the same technique as for achalasia patients. In our limited experience the results are clearly less favorable than in achalasia though occasionally excellent clinical results are obtained, associated, on manometry, with a markedly less disordered motility pattern. Nine patients were treated sucussfully by Rider et al. (1969) but several dilatations were required. One patient became symptomless and gradually developed normal esophageal contractions after pneumatic dilatations (Bennett et al., 1970). Craddock et al. (1966) observed a temporary improvement after a dilatation, which sometimes consisted only of simply passing a Negus esophagoscope.

8.3. Surgical Treatment

Patients with severe complaints, in whom other methods of treatment failed, can benefit from a long esophagomyotomy (Craddock et al., 1966; Gillies et al., 1967). The incision must be extended to just above the level of involvement, which can be determined by manometry (Ellis, 1969; Brindley, 1972). This operation can be completed by a procedure aimed at reconstructing a competent sphincter (Brindley, 1972). Ellis et al. (1964) mentioned 67% good or excellent results in 40 patients, but the follow-up was only one year. On radiological examination, the myotomy produces a widening of the esophageal lumen. On manometry the sphincteric pressure decreases and weak simultaneous pressure waves are seen instead of giant contractions (Ellis et al., 1964). The repetitive and spontaneous activity also diminishes. It thus seems that not only pneumatic dilatation but also long esophageal myotomy is less successful in the treatment of diffuse spasm than in that of achalasia. The limited number of reports in recent literature seems to indicate that the procedure is not widely accepted.

References

ATKINSON, M., BENNETT, J. R.: Relationship between motor changes and pain during esophageal acid perfusion. Amer. J. dig. Dis. 13, 346–350 (1968).

BENNETT, J. R., DONNER, M. W., HENDRIX, T. R.: Diffuse esophageal spasm: return to normality. J. Hopk. med. J. 126, 217–224 (1970).

BENNETT, J. R., HENDRIX, T. R.: Diffuse esophageal spasm: a disorder with more than one cause. Gastroenterology 59, 273–279 (1970).

BESANÇON, F., BAUJAT, J. P., DEBRAY, C.: Le reflux gastroesophagien: étude pH-graphique et électromanographique. Sem. Hôp. Paris 38, 1569–1576 (1962).

BOMBECK, C. T., BATTLE, W. S., NYHUSS, L. M.: Spasm in the differential diagnosis of gastroesophageal reflux. Arch. Surg. 104, 477–483 (1972).

BOQUIEN, Y., DUPON, H., GORDEEFF, A., HARDY, M., CORNET, E.: Myomatoses diffuses de l'oesophage. Etude anatomo-clinique de cinq cas traités chirurgicalement. Ann. Chir. Thor. Car. 2, C 1351–1365, CT 383–397 (1963).

BRINDLEY, G. V.: Discussion on: C. T. BOMBECK et al., Spasm in the differential diagnosis of gastroesophageal reflux. Arch. Surg. 104, 477–483 (1972).

CASSELLA, R. R., ELLIS, F. H., JR., BROWN, A. L.: Diffuse spasm of the lower part of the esophagus. Fine structure of esophageal smooth muscle and nerve. J. Amer. med. Ass. 191, 379–382 (1965).

CODE, C. F., SCHLEGEL, J. F., KELLEY, M. L., JR., OLSEN, A. M., ELLIS, F. H., JR.: Hypertensive gastroesophageal sphincter. Proc. St. Meet. Mayo Clin. 35, 391–399 (1960).

CRADDOCK, D. R., LOGAN, A., WALBAUM, P. R.: Diffuse oesophageal spasm. Thorax 21, 511–517 (1966).

CREAMER, B.: Oesophageal reflux. Lancet 1955 I, 279–281.

CREAMER, B.: Motor disturbances of the esophagus. In: Handbook of physiology, sect. 6, Alimentary canal, vol. IV, Motility, ed. C. F. CODE, p. 2331–2343. Washington, D.C.: Amer. Physiol. Soc. 1968.

CREAMER, B., DONOGHUE, F. E., CODE, C. F.: Pattern of esophageal motility in diffuse spasm. Gastroenterology 34, 782–796 (1958).

DEBRAY, C. H., BESANÇON, F., JANIN, B.: Le diagnostic de «l'hypertonie essentielle du cardia». Syndrôme électromanographique similaire dans 4 cas de cancer. Sem. Hôp. Paris 38, 1565–1568 (1962).

EDWARDS, D. A. W.: Personal communication 1971.

ELLIS, F. H., JR.: Discussion on: T. B. FERGUSON et al., Giant muscular hypertrophy of the esophagus. Ann. thorac. Surg. 8, 209–219 (1969).

ELLIS, F. H., JR., OLSEN, A. M.: Achalasia of the esophagus. In: Major problems in clinical surgery, vol. IX. Philadelphia: W. B. Saunders Co. 1969.

ELLIS, F. H., JR., OLSEN, A. M., SCHLEGEL, J. F., CODE, C. F.: Surgical treatment of esophageal hypermotility disturbances. J. Amer. med. Ass. 188, 862–866 (1964).

FERGUSON, T. B., WOODBURY, J. D., ROPER, C. L., BURFORD, T. H.: Giant muscular hypertrophy of the esophagus. Ann. thorac. Surg. 8, 209–218 (1969).

FLESHLER, B.: Diffuse esophageal spasm. Gastroenterology 52, 559–564 (1967).

GARRETT, J. M., GODWIN, D. H.: Gastroesophageal hypercontracting sphincter. J. Amer. med. Ass. 208, 992–998 (1969).

GILLIES, M., NICKS, R., SKYRING, A.: Clinical, manometric, and pathological studies in diffuse oesophageal spasm. Brit. med. J. 1967 II, 527–530.

GUICHARD, A., TOMMASI, M., ROCHET, M.: A propos d'un nouveau cas de pachyœsophage. (Myomatose diffuse de l'œsophage.) Arch. Anat. Path. 11, 180–185 (1963).

HEITMANN, P.: Die Hiatusgleithernien mit einem hypertonischen gastro-ösophagealen Verschlußmechanismus. Dtsch. med. Wschr. 95, 824–829 (1970).

HEITMANN, P.: Der idiopathische diffuse Ösophagusspasmus. Dtsch. med. Wschr. 96, 1668–1675 (1971).

JOHNSTONE, A. S.: Diffuse spasm and diffuse muscle hypertrophy of lower esophagus. Brit. J. Radiol. 33, 723–735 (1960).

KELLEY, M. L.: Deglutitive pressure responses in the gastroesophageal sphincters of symptomatic hiatal hernia patients. Amer. J. dig. Dis. 10, 582–595 (1965).

KELLEY, M. L.: Intraluminal manometry in the evaluation of malignant disease of the esophagus. Cancer (Philad.) 21, 1011–1018 (1968).

KOPALD, H. H., ROTH, H. P., FLESHLER, B., PRITCHARD, W. H.: Vagovagal syncope; report of a case associated with diffuse spasm. New Engl. J. Med. 271, 1238–1241 (1964).

KRAMER, P.: Diffuse esophageal spasm. In: Modern Treatment. Management of esophageal disease, ed. BAYLESS, T. M., p. 1151–1162. New York: Harper & Row 1970.

KRAMER, P., FLESHLER, B., McNALLY, E.: The pathophysiology of symptomatic "curling" or so-called "diffuse spasm". In: Proc. 2nd World Congr. of Gastroenterology, Munich 1962, 1, 57–59. Basel and New York: Karger 1963.

KRAMER, P., FLESHLER, B., McNALLY, E., HARRIS, L. D.: Oesophageal sensitivity to Mecholyl in symptomatic diffuse spasm. Gut 8, 120–127 (1967a).

KRAMER, P., HARRIS, L. D., DONALDSON, R. M., JR.: Transition from symptomatic diffuse spasm to cardiospasm. Gut 8, 115–119 (1967b).

McNALLY, E. F., KATZ, I.: The roentgen diagnosis of diffuse esophageal spasm. Amer. J. Roentgenol. 99, 218–222 (1967).

MOERSCH, H. J., CAMP, J. D.: Diffuse spasm of the lower part of the esophagus. Ann. Oto-Rhinol. 43, 1165–1173 (1934).

NICKS, R., GILLIES, M., SKYRING, A.: Diffuse muscular spasm. (Diffuse muscular hypertrophy of the oesophagus.) Bull. Soc. int. Chir. 6, 637–648 (1968).

OLSEN, A. M., CREAMER, B.: Studies of oesophageal motility, with special reference to the differential diagnosis of diffuse spasm and achalasia (cardiospasm). Thorax 12, 279–289 (1957).

OSGOOD, H.: A peculiar form of esophagism. Boston med. Surg. J. 120, 401–405 (1889).

PADEN, P. A.: Corkscrew esophagus. U. S. A. F. Med. J. 5, 1371–1374 (1954).

PEISON, B.: Idiopathic muscular hypertrophy of the lower esophagus and pylorus in an adult. Chest 59, 682–687 (1971).

RIDER, J. A., MOELLER, H. C., PULETTI, E. J., DESAI, D. C.: Diagnosis and treatment of diffuse esophageal spasm. Arch. Surg. 99, 435–440 (1969).

ROTH, H. P., FLESHLER, B.: Diffuse esophageal spasm. Clinical, radiological and manometric observations. Ann. intern. Med. 61, 914–923 (1964).

SCHATZKI, R.: Esophagus: progress and problems. The Caldwell lecture 1964. Amer. J. Roentgenol. 94, 523–540 (1965).

SCHMIDT, C. D., JONES, H. D., HUNT, J. C., CODE, C. F., ANDERSON, M. W., ANDERSON, H. A.: The value of the esophageal motility test in the evaluation of thoracic pain problems. Dis. Chest 41, 303–314 (1962).

SCHRODER, S., ACHORD, J. L., ROGERS, J. V.: "Achalasia" preceded by non-cardiospastic diffuse esophageal spasm. A cineradiographic study (Abstract). Gastroenterology 44, 849 (1963).

SEREBRO, H. A., VENKATACHALAM, B., PRENTICE, R. S. A., NEUMAN, H. W., BECK, I. T.: Possible pathogenesis of motility changes in diffuse esophageal spasm associated with gastric carcinoma. Canad. med. Ass. J. 102, 1257–1259 (1970).

SIEGEL, C. I., HENDRIX, T. R.: Esophageal motor abnormalities induced by acid perfusion in patients with heartburn. J. clin. Invest. 42, 686–695 (1963).

SLOPER, J. C.: Idiopathic diffuse muscular hypertrophy of the lower esophagus. Thorax 9, 136–146 (1954).

VANTRAPPEN, G.: Slokdarmmotiliteit. Thesis. Brussel: Arscia Uitg. 1961.

VANTRAPPEN, G., DERSTAPPEN, G. VAN, VANDENBROUCKE, J.: The syndrome of the hypertonic gastroesophageal sphincter. Proceedings of the Internat. Congr. of Gastroenterology, Leiden 1960, 377–384. Amsterdam: Excerpta med. 1960.

VANTRAPPEN, G., GOIDSENHOVEN, G. VAN, DERSTAPPEN, G. VAN, VANDENBROUCKE, J.: L'importance des études électromanométriques pour le diagnostic et le traitement de l'achalasie et de l'hypertonie du cardia. Acta chir. belg. 58 (Suppl. 2), 54–63 (1959).

Post-Vagotomy Dysphagia

D. A. W. Edwards

With 1 Figure

1. Definition

Post-vagotomy dysphagia can be defined as a partial or complete obstruction to the passage of solid food and sometimes of liquid from esophagus to stomach, developing after the vagus nerve has been sectioned in the region of the esophagogastric junction.

2. Incidence

Mild symptoms lasting a few days or weeks may occur in 33% of a surgeon's patients (BANK et al., 1966) but 10 to 15% is a common incidence (BRUCE and SMALL, 1959; WILLIAMS and COX, 1969). Severe prolonged dysphagia is uncommon; the incidence varies from one surgeon to another, some do not observe it, others appear to recognize it as often as 1% (DAGRADI et al., 1962). It may occur after transabdominal, transthoracic, selective or truncal vagotomy.

3. Symptoms

A curious and characteristic feature of the natural history is that dysphagia usually develops between the 7th and 14th post-operative day; sometimes the onset is as early as the 3rd day, sometimes as late as 3 weeks. The first unusual sensation is of food moving slowly past an obstruction. Within a few meals most solids impact within a few seconds of swallowing, often with pain which persists until the food moves on or is regurgitated. Pain is less evident if the esophagus is dilated. Liquids pass easily at this time, indicating that the channel is still open; but within a few more days, drinking may also become difficult and only saliva and sips of water may be retained. There is no pain at other times. Hot drinks or alcohol do not sting, suggesting there is no esophagitis, although the retention of hot fluid in the esophagus may feel uncomfortably warm. Regurgitation, often called vomiting, may follow all attempts to eat or even drink, until the esophagus dilates or the channel opens again.

In most instances, the dysphagia spontaneously disappears in days or weeks, occasionally worsening to and remaining a severe dysphagia for solids and sometimes, in addition, a dysphagia for liquids.

4. Etiology and Pathogenesis

The syndrome is clearly the result of the operation *for* vagal section. Whether it is the result *of* vagal section has been disputed. Some reports in the literature (HARRIS and MILLER, 1960; DAGRADI et al., 1962; PIERANDOZZI and RITTER, 1966; GUILLORY and CLAGETT, 1967) describe the condition as esophageal "spasm" or achalasia, or "cardiospasm", implying that the muscle is in an abnormal state of contraction or stating that its nerve supply has been damaged so that there is no reflex relaxation of the lower esophageal sphincter with swallowing, the so-called "neurogenic" dysphagia. Others believe that esophagitis is a possible cause because esophagoscopy and biopsy have sometimes shown inflammation of the mucosa, although this might have been the result of stagnation of esophageal contents (BRUCE and SMALL, 1959; GUILLORY and CLAGETT, 1967). SILBER (1969) emphasizes that pre-operative abnormality, for example stricture or esophageal "spasm" with or without hiatus hernia, may result in post-operative dysphagia, but this is a comment on the doctor's pre-operative acumen rather than of the cause of post-vagotomy dysphagia. The other suggested etiology is periesophageal edema, hemorrhage or fibrosis (BRUCE and SMALL, 1959; GUILLORY and CLAGETT, 1967; SILBER, 1969; EDWARDS, 1970).

Dysphagia for liquids means total closure of the lumen, either by a rigid process, or one which can be forced open by an appropriate intraesophageal pressure. Dysphagia for solids but not liquids means a narrowed but still open tube. The dysphagia is unlikely to be a direct consequence of nerve section, because it does not occur immediately after the operation. The suggestion that the late onset is because the esophagus is not sufficiently challenged by food and drink until a week or two after operation cannot be the whole explanation because many patients are known to have eaten and drunk without difficulty for some days before the onset of the dysphagia, which, after its onset, worsens for days or weeks before stabilizing or improving.

In the patients examined by manometry by EDWARDS (1970), a normal relaxation of the sphincter segment was observed after a swallow; the subsequent after-swallow contraction was also found to be normal. Immediately above the sphincter, the wall was capable of contracting sequentially to produce a normal peristaltic response. The innervation mediating both relaxation and contraction was therefore intact and the muscle responded normally to its neural stimuli. ANDERSON et al. (1966), by contrast, found two types of response: (1) a lack of relaxation of the cardiac sphincter in response to a swallow together with atonicity of part of the esophagus, and which they attributed to damage to the nerve supply; and (2) a normal relaxation of the sphincter together with a normal or increased esophageal muscle tone. In the second type they attributed the dysphagia to either esophagitis starting from the mucosal surface, or periesophageal edema or fibrosis. It is difficult to explain the recorded lack of relaxation except by artifact, or by infiltration or damage to the circular muscle layer, or by damage to the nerve supply to the cardiac sphincter. Section of the vagal fibers seems the least likely explanation because (1) the nerve supply to the muscle layers seems to be from the vagal plexus and the knife cuts distal and superficial to these intramural fibers, otherwise the condition would be much more frequent. (2) GUILLORY and CLAGETT (1967) claim that dysphagia due to denervation resolves spontaneously but do not suggest how renervation occurs so quickly and successfully. (3) Dysphagia should be maximal immediately after the operation instead of developing and worsening some time later.

"Spasm" has been postulated as the cause of the narrowing but this is a description of the state of contraction of the muscle rather than of the cause of the contraction. If the muscle is in spasm, its state of contraction can still be modified by neural stimuli in those which show relaxation on swallowing.

Esophagitis, as a lesion which starts as inflammation or destruction of the mucosal surface and extends outwards to develop thickening or fibrosis

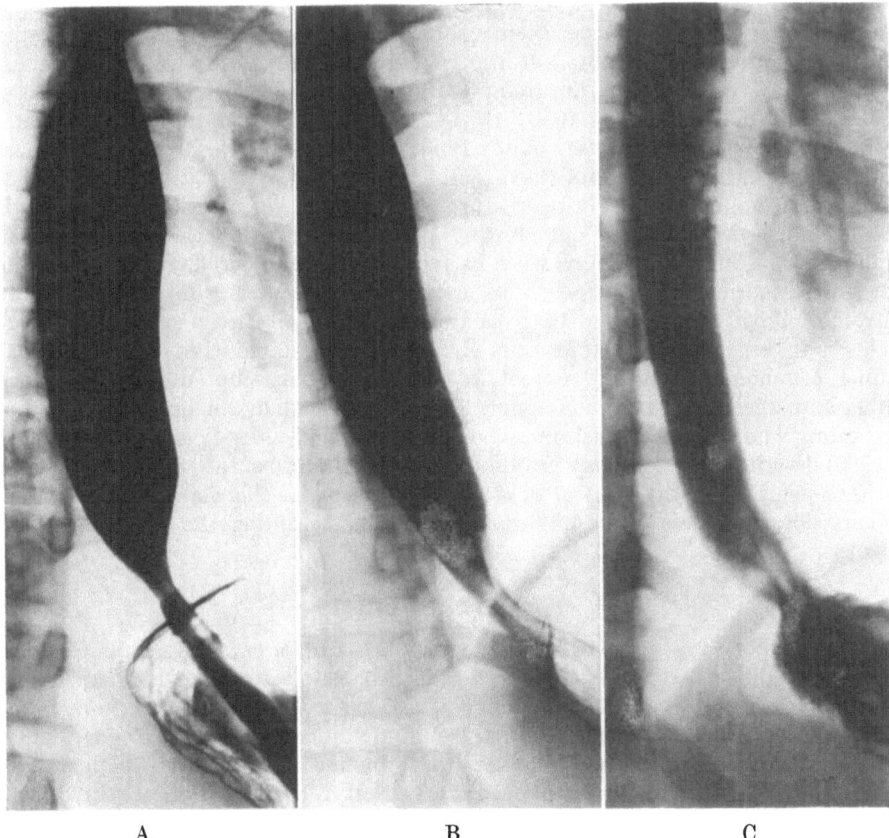

A   B   C

Fig. 192 A–C. Esophagograms of a patient with post-vagotomy dysphagia. A Picture taken 10 days after abdominal vagotomy. The esophagus has an "achalasia-like" appearance. B One month later, the patient was almost asymptomatic but the esophagogram was still abnormal. C On a control examination two years later the patient remained asymptomatic and the esophagus was normal

of the wall, seems an unlikely cause. The vagotomy itself should not involve the mucosa and there is no good evidence that reflux is precipitated by the vagotomy itself. Esophagoscopy almost always fails to reveal any lesion of the mucosa although the lumen may be firmly closed. Patients do not complain of hyperesthesia to hot drinks or alcohol in contrast to subjects with esophagitis. The presence of a nasogastric tube post-operatively is not the explanation because some patients have not been intubated and post-intubation dysphagia of this type is much less common than post-vagotomy dysphagia. These processes could hardly be attributed specifically to the operation of vagotomy.

Radiology can demonstrate a normal peristaltic wave in the esophagus and this wave can be seen to flow into and through the narrowed segment, demonstrating the capacity of the wall to contract. A variable length of the lower end of the esophagus, not always coincident with the extent of the lower esophageal sphincter, is seen to fail to open fully when the subject swallows barium (Fig. 192). The restriction of bore may be slight, or complete, and the appearance is of some restricting cylinder or cone with a variable resistance to stretch.

The resemblance to achalasia on still films is due to (1) retention of barium after a swallow in those who have dysphagia with liquids, and (2) the smooth taper from open to closed lumen; but the dynamic appearance is clearly different.

There are reports of a fibrotic or granulomatous sheath being found around the wall (Bruce and Small, 1959; Guillory and Clagett, 1967; Rabiah and Elliott, 1968; Postlethwait et al., 1969; Williams and Cox, 1969). The most likely explanation which fits the natural history and reported findings is that tissue damage, sustained during the process of sectioning the vagus nerve, leads to edema or a hematoma outside and perhaps infiltrating the outer layer of muscle. This hematoma may suck in more serum and swell, or may become organized, shrink and produce a periesophageal cuff with a high resistance to stretch, or be reabsorbed so that elasticity is regained after a period of weeks. This is in accord with Dagradi et al. (1962) who found that dysphagia was much commoner among the patients of surgeons who attempted to section every fiber and were likely to produce much local trauma, than among the patients of surgeons who caused the minimum of local damage. Guiney and McDermott (1960) describe a foreign body granulomatous reaction to suture material together with a neuroma of the cut end of the vagus causing a constriction of the lumen. There does not seem to be any good reason for accepting the other suggested causes.

5. Treatment

The milder forms recover spontaneously. If, after a few days, liquid can be drunk steadily at a reasonable speed, the tube is elastic enough to open and serious persistent dysphagia is unlikely, although solid food may impact for several days or weeks. A semi-solid or liquid diet should be taken. Reports quote the use of so-called anti-spasmodic drugs, lignocain in methyl cellulose gel, glyceryl trinitrite and intravenous hyoscine butyl bromide but no convincing evidence of their efficiency is given; nor is it likely, from what knowledge of the etiology that we have, that any "anti-spasmodic" or other drugs supposedly acting in a clinically significant way on smooth muscle or on the autonomic nervous system will be of any benefit.

When dysphagia for liquids is present, esophagoscopy and repeated dilatation by bougie or pneumatic or hydrostatic bag is usually helpful, allowing liquid food to be retained until recover occurs (Harris and Miller, 1960; Dagradi et al., 1962). Rarely a thoracotomy for removal of the fibrous sheath or a modified cardiomyotomy or a Thal procedure is necessary (Bruce and Small, 1959; Thal et al., 1965; Guillory and Clagett, 1967). It seems likely that most examples will spontaneously recover, but if hydration and nutrition become inadequate, dilatation should be tried as the first step.

References

Adloff, M., Kohler, J. J., Weiss, A. G.: Dysphagie après vagotomie sous-diaphragmatique. Acta gastro-ent. belg. **31**, 873–882 (1968).

Anderson, H. A., Schlegel, J. F., Olsen, A. M.: Postvagotomy dysphagia. Gastroint. Endosc. **12**, 13–18 (1966).

Bank, S., Marks, N., Louw, J. H.: Gastric secretory patterns after vagotomy. Lancet **1966 II**, 548.

Bruce, J., Small, W. P.: Dysphagia following vagotomy. J. roy. Coll. Surg. Edinb **4**, 170–178 (1959).

Dagradi, A. E., Stempien, S. J., Seifer, H. W., Weinberg, J. A.: Terminal esophageal vestibular spasm after vagotomy. Arch. Surg. **85**, 955–968 (1962).

DAHM, K.: Le cardiospasme: une complication rare après vagotomie sélective. Acta gastroent. belg. **31**, 883–888 (1968).

EDWARDS, D. A. W.: Post vagotomy dysphagia. Lancet **1970 II**, 90–92.

GUILLORY, J. R., CLAGETT, O. T.: Post vagotomy dysphagia. Surg. Clin. N. Amer. **47**, 833–839 (1967).

GUINEY, E. J., MACDERMOTT, E. N.: Benign stricture of the esophagus following gastroenterostomy and vagotomy. J. int. Coll. Surg. **33**, 297–299 (1960).

HARRIS, J., MILLER, C. M.: Cardiospasm following vagotomy. Surgery **47**, 568–570 (1960).

PIERANDOZZI, J. S., RITTER, J. H.: Transient achalasia. A complication of vagotomy. Amer. J. Surg. **111**, 356–358 (1966).

POSTLETHWAIT, R. W., KIM, S. K., DILLON, M. L.: Esophageal complications of vagotomy. Surg. Gynec. Obstet. **128**, 481–488 (1969).

RABIAH, F. A., ELLIOTT, H. B.: Intramural hematoma of the esophagus. An unusual complication of vagotomy. Amer. J. dig. Dis. **13**, 925–928 (1968).

SILBER, W.: Post vagotomy dysphagia. S. Afr. med. J. **43**, 803–805 (1969).

THAL, A. P., HATAFUKU, T., KURTZMAN, R.: New operation for distal esophageal stricture. Arch. Surg. **90**, 464–472 (1965).

WILLIAMS, J. A., COX, A. G.: After vagotomy. London: Butterworths 1969.

Presbyesophagus

J. HELLEMANS and G. VANTRAPPEN

With 5 Figures

The motility disturbances associated with old age are called presbyesophagus (SOERGEL et al., 1964; ZBORALSKE et al., 1964). Although swallowing difficulties of various origin are not infrequently found in old people, presbyesophagus is rarely symptomatic.

1. Pharynx

The pharyngeal lumen of elderly subjects often appears dilated and thin-walled, both when filled with air in the resting stage and with barium while swallowing. On anteroposterior views there is apt' to be asymmetry of filling and the lateral walls of the pahrynx bulge prominently (RAMSEY et al., 1955).

2. Esophagus

It has been known for a long time, both from radiological and manometric studies, that the incidence of non-peristaltic contractions increases in old age (TEMPLETON, 1944; INGELFINGER, 1958; PIAGET and FOUILLET, 1959; HELLE-MANS et al., 1963). ZBORALSKE et al. (1964) examined cineradiographically 41 nonagenarians. Approximately 90% of the subjects revealed radiographic evidence of impaired peristaltic activity; in one third of them no peristalsis was observed. However, this does not prove that the esophagus was unable to respond in a peristaltic way, because the incidence of primary peristalsis is underestimated on cineradiography (SOERGEL et al., 1964). About 60% of the nonagenarians exhibited delayed esophageal emptying when examined in the supine position. In these patients the esophagus was often moderately dilated (ZBORALSKE et al., 1964 (Fig. 193). Similar observations were made by MANDELSTAM and LIEBER (1970), who found that the primary peristaltic wave was impaired in 50% of their octagenarians and in 80% of their nonagenarians. The primary wave was classified impaired when it was absent or markedly reduced in amplitude, when it did not result in effective esophageal emptying, or when it traversed only a short segment of the esophagus. Before the age of 70, impairment of esophageal function was observed only rarely.

Manometric studies by means of a set of 3 open-tipped non-perfused catheters were performed by SOERGEL et al. (1964), who studied the motility of the distal half of the esophagus in 15 nonagenarians. Spontaneous activity occurred in almost half the of subjects although it was rarely an outstanding phenomenon. Only 51% of the swallows resulted in peristaltic contractions of the lower half of the esophagus. This reduced incidence of peristalsis was accompanied by an increase in non-progressive contractions occurring in 45% of the deglutitions. 12% of all deglutitions were followed by repetitive non-progressive contractions.

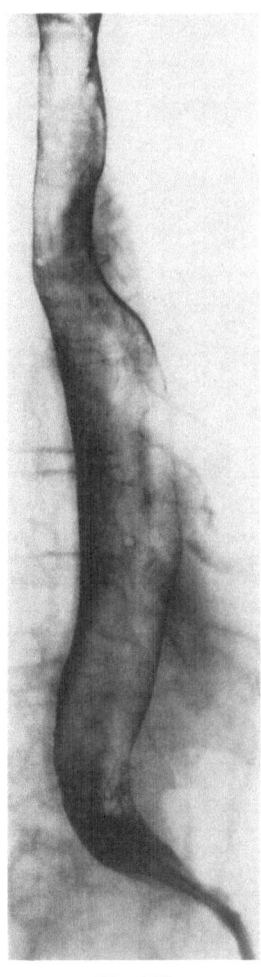

Fig. 193

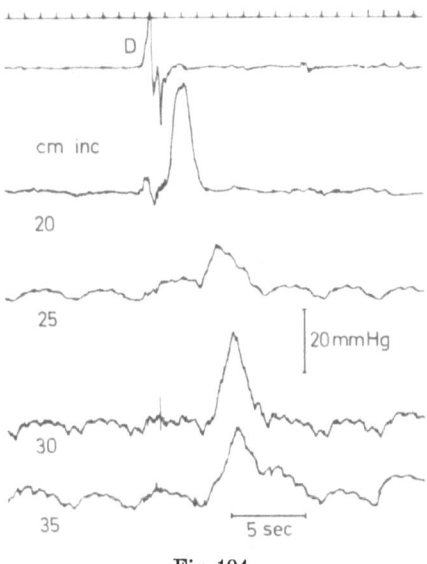

Fig. 194

Fig. 193. X-ray of a "presbyesophagus" showing a slightly dilated gullet, and an abnormally persistent double contrast

Fig. 194. Peristaltic contraction in the upper part of the esophagus (20–25 and 30 cm from the incisors) changing into a simultaneous "tertiary" contraction (30, 35 cm inc.)

The lower esophageal sphincter relaxed after only 44% of the swallows. Another abnormality was the entirely intrathoracic position of the lower esophageal high-pressure zone, noted in 7 of the 15 subjects. This is probably related to the high incidence of hiatal hernia in the elderly.

HELLEMANS (1970) performed extensive manometric studies on the influence of age on esophageal motility. The disturbances found in the presbyesophagus are most marked in the lower third and less obvious in the middle third, whereas in the upper third of the esophagus the peristaltic contraction is normal (Fig. 194). These motor disorders are found from the age of 50 onwards. In the lower third of the esophagus the incidence of non-peristaltic simultaneous waves increases from about 12% of the swallows in the younger age group (20–34 years), to about 42% in the older age group (65 or more) (Table 17). The incidence of repetitive waves progressively increases with increasing age from 2 to 14% of the swallows. There is an increased incidence of both the first negative deflection and the second positive wave of the deglutition complex; the former is probably

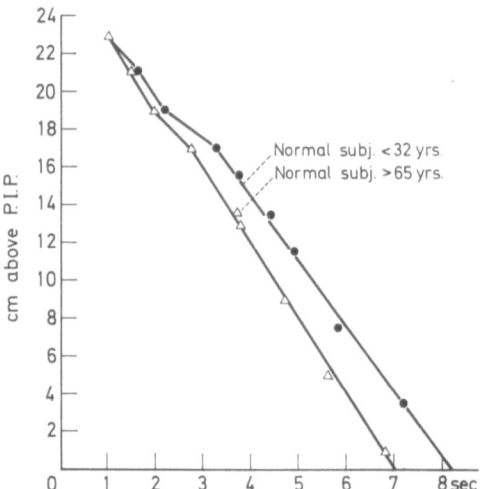

Fig. 195. Scheme indicating the progression of the peristaltic contractions along the esophagus. Distance is given in cm above the pressure inversion point (P.I.P.) in the lower esophageal sphincter. The proximal sphincter can be located at 23 cm above the P.I.P. Time is given in seconds after the deglutition signal, activated by laryngeal movements. The progression of the peristaltic contraction is slowed down in the zone of transition from striated to smooth muscle; this effect is less marked in old than in young subjects

Table 17

Age groups	Incidence of (in percentage of deglutition complexes analysed)				
	Peristaltic waves	Simult. waves	Repetitive	Negat. defl.	Sec. pos. waves
20–34 years (23 subj.; 418 deglut.)	88	12	2	13	20
35–49 years (21 subj.; 365 deglut.)	85	15	5	18	13
50–64 years (21 subj.; 477 deglut.)	64	36	10	42	24
65 or more (24 subj.; 504 deglut.)	58	42	14	43	37

due to changes in the mechanical characteristics of the thorax, the latter to less efficient sphincter relaxations (VANTRAPPEN and HELLEMANS, 1967).

Similar abnormalities are found in the middle third of the esophagus, albeit to a lesser degree.

The mean progression velocity of the primary peristaltic contraction in old people is similar to that in younger subjects, except for a short segment located 4 to 6 cm below the pharyngoesophageal sphincter (Fig. 195). In younger subjects the mean progression velocity is 3.44 ± 0.45 cm/sec in the upper esophagus and 3.53 ± 0.44 cm/sec in the lower portion. In the vestibulum, the progression velocity decreases again. In the elderly, these velocities are somewhat higher

Terminal peak pressures at different levels of the esophagus in young and old subjects

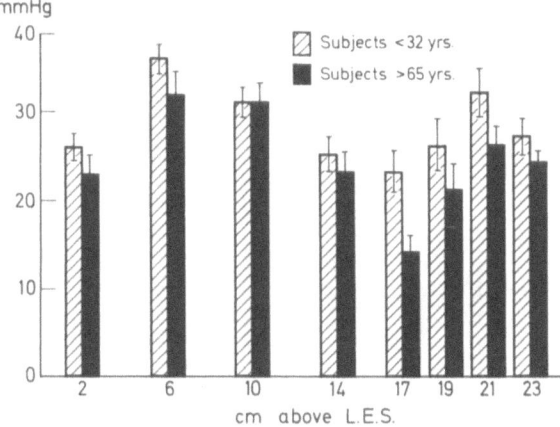

Fig. 196. Diagram indicating that the amplitude of the deglutitive peristaltic pressure waves in old subjects is similar to that in young persons, except for a short segment, which probably corresponds to the zone of transition from striated to smooth musculature

(4.25 ± 0.75 cm/sec and 4.00 ± 0.79 cm/sec; $p > 0.05$). In the segment located between 4 and 6 cm below the pharyngoesophageal sphincter the progression velocity in younger subjects is significantly lower than in the adjacent segments (1.87 ± 0.15 cm/sec; $p < 0.001$). The zone in which the progression velocity of the primary peristaltic wave is slowed down corresponds to the segment where, on electromyography, both smooth and striated muscle cell spikes can be detected. The slow-down effect of this segment is less marked in older subjects, in whom the peristaltic wave traverses this zone at a speed of 2.56 ± 0.29 cm/sec, which is significantly higher than in younger subjects ($p < 0.05$). Immediately beyond this segment 13% of the contractions become simultaneous in old subjects (HELLEMANS, 1970).

A second age-induced change in this transitional zone is the localized weakening of the peristaltic contraction. The pressure of the terminal peak of the deglutition complex in this zone, extending from 17 to 21 cm above the gastroesophageal sphincter, is significantly lower in old subjects as compared to young persons (Fig. 196).

Another characteristic of the presbyesophagus is the fact that the alterations produced by a swallow last longer in the presbyesophagus than in the esophagus of young subjects. If two swallows are taken at an interval of 10 sec, the deglutition complex following the second swallow is often impaired, both in young and in old subjects. Its amplitude is on the average only 70% of the wave produced by the first swallow and the percentage of non-peristaltic contractions is increased. However, at an interval of 12 to 14 sec, the second deglutition complex is much less impaired in young than in old subjects (Fig. 197).

3. Gastroesophageal Sphincter

The main abnormality of the gastroesophageal sphincter in older people is a decreased incidence of relaxation after swallowing, whereas the sphincter

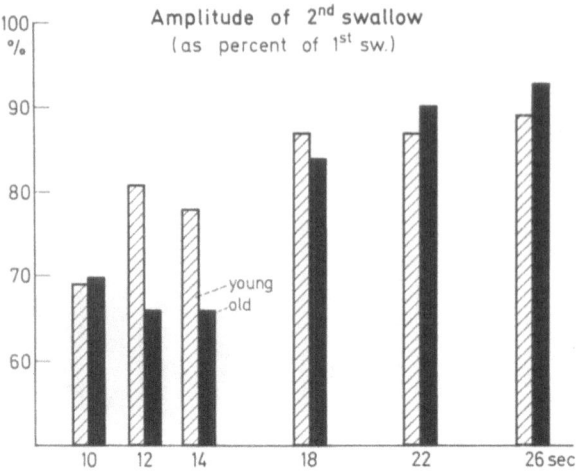

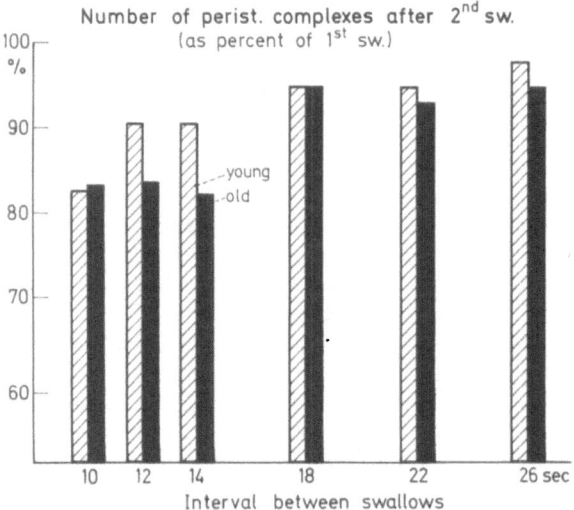

Fig. 197. When 2 swallows are taken in succession, the response to the second swallow is impaired in relation to that of the first deglutition: the amplitude of the pressure peaks is lower (upper part) and the incidence of peristaltic contractions is decreased (lower part). This effect lasts longer in old than in young subjects

contractions are normal. Soergel et al. (1964) found that the lower esophageal high pressure zone is displaced into the thorax; however, if old patients known to have hiatal hernia are excluded from the study, the only abnormality found is that the high pressure zone is slightly lengthened (Hellemans, 1970). Although reflux esophagitis occurs more frequently in the aged, the intrasphincteric resting pressure of the presbyesophagus is not decreased (Soergel et al., 1964; Hellemans, 1970).

4. Nature of the Lesions

The localization of the lesions causing the motility disturbances of the presby-esophagus is as yet uncertain. Lesions of the brainstem mainly cause disturbances of pharynx and striated muscles, and only occasionally of the distal segment of the esophagus. The disorders associated with diabetes and alcoholism, which are generally ascribed to peripheral neuropathy, are quite similar to those of the presbyesophagus and also affect the proximal part of the esophagus to a lesser degree. Peripherally acting anticholinergics can provoke in young adults many of these disturbances, such as non-peristaltic repetitive contractions and disordered sphincter relaxations. However, the increased progression velocity in the transitional zone between striated and smooth muscles cannot be reproduced by anticholinergics, which have the opposite effect of slowing down the progression at that level (HELLEMANS et al., 1969).

There are no pharmacological signs of denervation, the Mecholyl test being negative (ZBORALSKE, 1965). According to some authors the number of ganglion cells is normal (ELLIS and OLSEN, 1969); however, the careful counts by KÖBERLE (1968) show that the number of ganglion cells decreases with increasing age and that in nonagenarians the number is halved (Table 18). The numerical diminution of nerve cells occurs uniformly over the entire length. The functional implications of these findings are still uncertain.

Table 18. Number of ganglion cells in a 1 mm ring of the distal esophagus (mean of 10 subjects)

15–30 years	1 200
30–45 years	1 050
45–60 years	900
60–75 years	750
75–90 years	620
90 or more	550

It is also unknown whether the esophageal muscle itself undergoes important changes in old age. The techniques of electromyography which are currently available do not show any changes in spiking activity in old subjects as compared to young people.

References

ELLIS, F. H., JR., OLSEN, A. M.: Achalasia of the esophagus. In: Major problems in clinical surgery, vol. IX. Philadelphia-London-Toronto: W. B. Saunders Co. 1969.

HELLEMANS, J.: Invloed van de leeftijd op de motorische funktie van de slokdarm. Thesis, Tielt (Belgium): Lannoo 1970.

HELLEMANS, J., VANTRAPPEN, G., VANDENBROUCKE, J.: L'influence de l'âge sur la motilité gastro-intestinale. 6th Intern. Congr. Geriatrics, Copenhagen (1963).

HELLEMANS, J., VANTRAPPEN, G., VANDENBROUCKE, J.: The effect of anticholinergics on the activity of the smooth and striated esophageal muscle. Rendic. R. Gastroenterol. 1, 130 (1969).

INGELFINGER, F. J.: Esophageal motility. Physiol. Rev. 38, 533–584 (1958).

KÖBERLE, T.: Chagas' disease and Chagas' syndrome: the pathology of American trypano-somiasis. Advanc. Parasitol. 6, 63–116 (1968).

MANDELSTAM, P., LIEBER, A.: Cineradiographic evaluation of the esophagus in normal adults. A study of 146 subjects ranging in age from 21 to 90 years. Gastroenterology 58, 32–39 (1970).

Piaget, F., Fouillet, J.: Le pharynx et l'œsophage sénile. J. Méd. Lyon **955**, 951–967 (1959).

Ramsey, G. H., Watson, J. S., Gramiak, R., Weinberg, S. A.: Cinefluorographic analysis of the mechanism of swallowing. Radiology **64**, 498–518 (1955).

Soergel, K. H., Zboralske, F. F., Amberg, J. R.: Presbyesophagus: esophageal motility in nonagenarians. J. clin. Invest. **43**, 1472–1479 (1964).

Templeton, F. E.: X-ray examinations of the stomach. Chicago: Chicago Univ. Press 1944.

Vantrappen, G., Hellemans, J.: Studies on the normal deglutition complex. Amer. J. dig. Dis. **12**, 255–266 (1967).

Zboralske, F. F.: The esophagus in the geriatric patient. Radiol. Clin. N. Amer. **3**, 321–330 (1965).

Zboraslke, F. F., Amberg, J. R., Soergel, K. H.: Presbyesophagus: Cineradiographic manifestations. Radiology **82**, 463–467 (1964).

Esophageal Motility in Neonatal Infants

J. De Schryver and J. Hellemans

1. Introduction

A neonate is able to perform a coordinated swallowing act (Crump et al., 1958). Swallowing occurs already in 12 week old fetuses (Hooker, 1952, 1954) and from the 23rd week on the fetus drinks amniotic fluid (Pritchard, 1965). The innervation of the esophagus starts early. According to Smith and Taylor (1972) neuroblasts reach the embryological esophagus before the 10 mm stage. Jit (1955) has shown that Auerbach's plexus appears at the 13 to 14 mm stage and Meissner's plexus at 21 mm.

Infants perform the swallowing act in a manner which differs from that of adults (see Physiology 3.1.3.3.).

2. Normal Motility

2.1. Mouth and Pharynx

Sucking in infants produces negative pressures in the mouth. In premature infants with a birth weight of 2000 to 2400 g and in full-term infants these negative pressures reach −5 to −15 mm Hg between 1 to 12 hours after birth. At three days these negative pressures are stronger still (Gryboski, 1965) and infants of 5 weeks to 7 months may build negative pressures of −44 to −184 mm Hg (Colley and Creamer, 1958). In between his sucking movements, the neonate builds positive pressures of 5 to 20 mm Hg (Gryboski, 1965). In older infants the pressure returns to its basic level or a negative plateau of −15 to −44 mm Hg perists (Colley and Creamer, 1958).

The deglutitive pressure waves in the pharynx of premature and full-term infants reach 15 to 30 mm Hg 12 hours after birth (Gryboski, 1965); in infants between the age of 5 weeks and 7 months these waves have an amplitude of 22 to 73 mm Hg (Colley and Creamer, 1958).

2.2. Esophagus

2.2.1. The Esophagus at Rest

2.2.1.1. Pharyngoesophageal Sphincter

The pharyngoesophageal sphincter is located 7 to 9 cm from the lips of the neonate (Gryboski, 1965). Under the age of 1, its length is only 0.5 to 1 cm; it gradually increases to a length of about 3 cm in older children (Colley and Creamer, 1958; Gryboski et al., 1963; Gryboski, 1965). The mean resting pressure, measured with or without continuous perfusion, reaches 22 to 29 mm Hg above the pressure in the esophagus (COLLEY and CREAMER, 1958; LIND et al., 1966). According to GRYBOSKI et al. (1963) the resting pressure during the first 5 days of life is significantly lower than in older children.

2.2.1.2. Esophageal Body

In premature and full-term infants the esophageal resting pressure is 0 to 6 mm Hg lower than the fundic pressure (GRYBOSKI, 1965). This pressure gradient progressively increases with age (STRAWCZYNSKI et al., 1964). KEHRER and OESCH (1971) found a gradient of 5 to 11 mm Hg in children between 1 and 20 months old.

On radiological examination the esophagus of neonates appears wide and atonic (LASSRICH, 1959).

2.2.1.3. Gastroesophageal Sphincter

In full-term infants the sphincter is located at 12 to 17.5 cm from the lips (GRYBOSKI, 1965). Several authors found it to be located at or above the level of the pressure inversion point in 70 to 90% of all infants (GRYBOSKI et al., 1963; STRAWCZYNSKI et al., 1964; GRYBOSKI, 1965). This percentage decreases with age. These data are in accordance with the radiological observations of WILLICH (1971) and with the post-mortem findings of BOTHA (1958) which showed that neonates generally have no intraabdominal esophagus. The sphincter has a length of 0.5 to 1 cm until the age of 1, and later increases progressively (GRYBOSKI et al., 1963; STRAWCZYNSKI et al., 1964; GRYBOSKI, 1965; KEHRER and OESCH 1971).

There is general agreement that the resting pressure of the sphincter increases with age but the exact time at which this occurs is controversial. According to GRYBOSKI et al. (1963) an important pressure increase occurs after 6 days; according to STRAWCZYNSKI et al. (1964) between 2 weeks and 1 month and according to WILLICH (1971) only after the second month. Using a continuous perfusion technique, ESPINOZA and HEITMANN (1971) found a mean gastro-esophageal yield pressure of 21.5 mm Hg (range 5 to 50 mm of Hg) in 65 out of 70 children; in the 5 others, all under 6 months, there was no high pressure zone. Neonates commonly regurgitate small quantities of food, which does not lead to weight loss or malnutrition. During the first 5 days it occurred in 38% of the 1100 children studied by KEITEL and ZIEGRA (1961). Apart from the absence of an intraabdominal esophagus there are no peculiar anatomical findings in most cases. Regurgitation usually disappears during the first year of life, with or without conservative therapy. In a small number of patients it persists and surgical intervention is necessary to prevent complications (FERGUSON, 1971; VOS and BOEREMA, 1971). The resting pressure in the lower esophageal sphincter of these regurgitating children is below normal (GRYBOSKI et al., 1963; WILLICH, 1971).

Radiological studies have demonstrated that some infants have a patulent and incompetent sphincter (NEUHAUSER and BERENBERG, 1947). This condition has sometimes been called chalasia. These functional abnormalities may be attributed to a delay in the development of adequate sphincter tone (GRYBOSKI et al., 1963; STRAWCZYNSKI et al., 1964), as suggested by the observation that the neural differentiation of the cardia lags behind that of the pylorus and the ileocecal sphincter (LORENZ, 1962).

2.2.2. Deglutition

2.2.2.1. Pharyngoesophageal Sphincter

In full-term infants deglutition results in a relaxation of the pharyngo-esophageal sphincter beginning 0.1 sec after the onset of the positive pressure wave in the pharynx. The pressure fall of 3 to 10 mm Hg is followed by a positive pressure wave of 5 to 20 mm Hg (GRYBOSKI, 1965).

2.2.2.2. Esophageal Body

According to COLLEY and CREAMER (1958), the peristaltic pressure waves in infants between 1 and 7 months old have an amplitude of 15 to 29 mm Hg, a duration of 2 to 4 sec and a progression velocity of 0.7 to 4 cm/sec. The esophageal response to deglutition is uncoordinated in premature and full-term neonates, as is demonstrated by the frequent occurrence of simultaneous contractions and biphasic waves. It can be shown, both radiologically and mano-metrically, that the peristaltic performance improves with age (LASSRICH, 1959; GRYBOSKI et al., 1963; GRYBOSKI, 1965). In children of less than 2 years, esophageal peristaltic pressure waves progress into the stomach over a distance of a few cm (GRYBOSKI et al., 1963).

2.2.2.3. Gastroesophageal Sphincter

The relaxation of the gastroesophageal sphincter in neonates results in a fall of pressure of 3 to 20 mm Hg and lasts for 0.5 to 1 sec. It is followed by an in-crease in pressure of 5 to 15 mm Hg, continuing for 0.5 to 1.5 sec. After a few days the relaxation is shortened (GRYBOSKI, 1965). As in adults, the duration of the relaxation is increased when measured with a perfused catheter system (ESPINOZA and HEITMANN, 1971).

References

BOTHA, G. S. M.: The gastroesophageal region of infants. Arch. Dis. Childh. **33**, 78–94 (1958).

COLLEY, J. R. T., CREAMER, B.: Sucking and swallowing in infants. Brit. med. J. **1958 II**, 422–423.

CRUMP, E. P., GORE, P. M., HORTON, C.: The sucking behaviour in premature infants. Hum. Biol. **30**, 128–132 (1958).

ESPINOZA, J., HEITMANN, P.: The gastroesophageal sphincter in the first year of life (abstract). Gastroenterology **60**, 773 (1971).

FERGUSON, C. F.: Esophageal dysfunction and other swallowing difficulties in early life. Ann. Otol. (St. Louis) **80**, 541–548 (1971).

GRYBOSKI, J. D.: The swallowing mechanism of the neonate. I. Esophageal and gastric motility. Pediatrics **35**, 445–452 (1965).

GRYBOSKI, J. D., THAYER, W. R., SPIRO, H. W.: Esophageal motility in infants and children. Pediatrics **31**, 382–395 (1963).

HOOKER, D.: The prenatal origin of behavior (Porter Lectures, Ser. 18). 143 pp. Lawrence, Kan.: Univ. of Kansas Press 1952.

HOOKER, D.: Early human fetal behavior, with a preliminary note on double simultaneous fetal stimulation. Ass. Res. nerv. Dis. **33**, 98–113 (1954).

JIT, I.: The development of the nerve supply of the human oesophagus and stomach. J. Anat. Soc. India **4**, 55–68 (1955); in: Excerpta med. (Amst.), Sect. I, 1522 (1958).

KEHRER, B., OESCH, A.: Motility studies of the terminal esophagus in hiatus hernia in childhood. Z. Kinderchir. **10**, 345–358 (1971).

KEITEL, H. G., ZIEGRA, S. R.: Regurgitation in the full-term infant: a controlled clinical study. Amer. J. Dis. Child. **102**, 749–750 (1961).

LASSRICH, M. A.: Zur Entwicklung der motorischen Funktionen des oberen Verdauungs-traktes. In: LINNEWEH, F., Die physiologische Entwicklung des Kindes. Berlin-Göttingen-Heidelberg: Springer 1959.

LIND, J. F., BLANCHARD, R. J., GUYDA, H.: Esophageal motility in tracheoesophageal fistula and esophageal atresia. Surg. Gynec. Obstet. **123**, 557–564 (1966).

LORENZ, J.: Observations comparatives sur l'innervation intramurale du cardia, du pylore et de la valvule iléo-coecale chez l'homme normal au cours de l'âge. Z. mikr.-anat. Forsch. **68**, 540–563 (1962).

NEUHAUSER, E. B. D., BERENBERG, W.: Cardio-esophageal relaxation as a cause of vomiting in infants. Radiology **48**, 480–483 (1947).

PRITCHARD, J. A.: Deglutition by normal and anencephalic fetuses. Obstet. and Gynec. **25**, 289–297 (1965).

SMITH, R. B., TAYLOR, I. M.: Observation on the intrinsic innervation of the human foetal oesophagus between the 10-mm and 140-mm crown-rump length stages. Acta anat. (Basel) **81**, 127–138 (1972).

STRAWCZYNSKI, H., BECK, I. T., MCKENNA, R. D., NICKERSON, G. H.: The behavior of the lower esophageal sphincter in infants and its relationship to gastroesophageal regurgita-tion. J. Pediat. **64**, 17–23 (1964).

VOS, A., BOEREMA, I.: Surgical treatment of gastroesophageal reflux in infants and children. J. Pediat. Surg. **6**, 101–111 (1971).

W ILLICH, E.: The function of the cardia in childhood. Progr. Pediat. Surg. **3**, 141–167 (1971)

Motor Disorders Due to Collagen Diseases

J. Hellemans and G. Vantrappen

With 2 Figures

1. Progressive Systemic Sclerosis

1.1. Definition and General Data

Progressive systemic sclerosis is a generalized disease of unknown origin, involving many organs (Goetz, 1945; Tuffanelli and Winkelmann, 1961). It produces hardness of the skin, fibrosis, loss of smooth muscle of internal organs and progressive loss of visceral and cutaneous functions (Winkelmann, 1971). Muscles, bones, heart, lungs, mucous membranes and the gastrointestinal tract may be involved. Several types of systemic sclerosis have been described: (1) Acrosclerosis is the more common form of systemic scleroderma (95%). It is characterized by Raynaud's phenomenon, which is often the initial symptom. The disease usually begins on the hands and later spreads to other structures. The incidence in women is 2.6 to 2.9 times that in men (Leinwand et al., 1954; Tuffanelli and Winkelmann, 1961; D'Angelo et al., 1969; Poirier and Rankin, 1972). (2) Acute diffuse scleroderma, or malignant scleroderma, is a rare condition (5% of the patients with systemic sclerosis), characterized by generalized cutaneous sclerosis and usually beginning centrally. It has a rapid onset and course, and a poor prognosis. Raynaud's phenomenon is absent. Malignant scleroderma affects as many men as women.

About 75% of the cases of systemic sclerosis are diagnosed between the ages of 30 and 60 (Poirier and Rankin, 1972). The average annual age-specific mortality has been estimated at about 1 per million for males, 2.2 per million for white females and 6.6 per million for negro females (Masi and D'Angelo, 1967). The characteristic pathological lesions include proliferation of collagen and vascular changes (Leinwand et al., 1954). In contrast with lupus erythematosus or dermatomyositis there is no or only minimal inflammatory cell infiltration and no evidence of proliferation of fibroblasts (Winkelmann, 1971). No abnormalities of collagen structure or metabolism have been found (Fisher and Rodnan, 1960; Rasmussen et al., 1964; Winkelmann, 1971). The collagen in scleroderma contains more hexosamine than normal and the levels of hexosamine in blood and urine are elevated as well. This may account for the increased water binding and edema (Fleischmajer and Krol, 1967; Winkelmann, 1971). The blood vessels of the affected organs show concentric intimal proliferation, hyperplasia of the media with reduplication of the elastic fibers and adventitial sclerosis (Bianchi et al., 1966). A characteristic feature is the widespread microangiopathy resulting in a disappearance of many capillaries. The remaining capillaries frequently show thickening and reduplication of the basement membrane, and thickening and degeneration of the endothelium (Norton and Nardo, 1970).

Usually the symptoms begin insidiously. The cutaneous lesions generally precede the visceral symptoms and begin at the hands with subsequent involvement of face, neck and chest. After an initial period of edema a widespread symmetrical leathery induration develops which binds the skin tightly to the subcutaneous tissues. These lesions are followed by atrophy, pigmentation and ulcerations, especially of the hands and fingers; soft tissue calcification in the fingers and absorption of the terminal phalanges, shortening the fingers, also occur (Kemp Harper and Jackson, 1965; Bianchi et al., 1966). Furthermore, calcium may be deposited in pressure areas such as elbows, knees and buttocks. The periodontal membrane is widened in 10 to 36% of the cases (Farmer et al., 1960; Kemp Harper and Jackson, 1965). Patchy reticulated pigmentation and teleangiectasia of the skin are frequently observed, particularly on the face and upper trunk (Cullinan, 1953). Arthralgias occur in the majority of cases at some time in the course of the disease (Orabona and Albano, 1958). Systemic sclerosis involves mainly the small joints and may suggest rheumatoid arthritis, but there is no pannus formation in the synovial membrane (Rodnan, 1962) and the articular bone destruction typical of arthritis is lacking.

The esophagus is affected in 50 to 80% of the cases. Whereas gastric lesions are rare, radiological abnormalities of the small intestine, particularly the duodenum, are found in 42% of the patients (Bluestone et al., 1969; Poirier and Rankin, 1972). A decreased motility, thickening of the mucosal folds with "wire spring" appearances when the loops are not distended with barium, dilatation, segmentation and dilution or flocculation of barium are the most typical radiological images (Kemp Harper and Jackson, 1965; Peachey et al., 1968). Between 20 and 57% of the patients have symptoms referable to the small intestine (Reinhardt and Barry, 1962; Heinz et al., 1963; Bluestone et al., 1969). Steatorrhea, if present, is usually moderate and caused by bacterial overgrowth (Greenberger et al., 1967; Bluestone et al., 1969). The reported incidence of colon involvement varies from 10 to 50%, although most patients have no complaints related to the colon (Hale and Schatzki, 1944; Kemp Harper, 1953; Gondos, 1960; Kaufmann et al., 1968). Large mouth square neck diverticula on the antimesenteric border give the colon a typical asymmetrical aspect (Hale and Schatzki, 1944; Kemp Harper and Jackson, 1965). These diverticula are interspersed with areas of rigidity. Later the entire colon wall becomes involved and atonic and the diverticula disappear.

Respiratory symptoms are due to alveolocapillary block and pulmonary fibrosis, especially in the lower half of the lungs (Bianchi et al., 1966; D'Angelo et al., 1969). Repeated infections, respiratory insufficiency, hypoxemia without CO_2-retention and pneumothorax can complicate the condition.

Heart failure is rarely due exclusively to replacement of myocardium with fibrous tissue. Pulmonary hypertension contributes to the right-sided, and systemic hypertension to the left-sided heart failure. Pericardial effusion is occasionally present.

Involvement of the kidneys is frequent and may lead to renal lesions which are indistinguishable from those of malignant hypertension. Malignant hypertension may complicate the course of the disease and rapidly progressing renal insufficiency is a cause of death in between 5 and 20% of the patients. Mixed collagenoses occur in 4% of the patients (Poirier and Rankin, 1972). Rare instances of combined scleroderma and systemic lupus erythematosus with a positive LE cell phenomenon have been described (Tuffanelli and Winkelmann, 1962; Bianchi et al., 1966; Clark et al., 1971 b; Winkelmann, 1971).

The disease can also be associated with dermatomyositis, rheumatoid arthritis, Sjögren's syndrome and Hashimoto's thyroiditis.

The sedimentation rate is increased in two thirds of the patients and mild microcytic anemia may be found. Mild hypergammaglobulinemia is present in about half of the patients (BIANCHI et al., 1966). Immunoglobulin studies have failed to demonstrate changes specific for scleroderma. The rheumatoid factor is present in one third of the cases. LE cells are rarely found (CLARK et al., 1971b). Antinuclear factors have been found in 55 to 78% of the patients (BECK et al., 1963; POIRIER and RANKIN, 1972). Urinary creatine and hydroxyproline excretion is increased due to destruction of muscle tissue and increased collagen turnover.

The prognosis of the disease is rather poor, with 30% of the patients dying within 5 years and 40% within 10 years (TUFFANELLI and WINKELMANN, 1961). No specific treatment is available and the evolution of the internal lesions is hard to influence. Vasodilating drugs such as α-adrenergic blocking agents, α-methyldopa, ganglion blocking agents, nicotinic acid and intravenous procaine are administered to combat vasospasms and Raynaud's phenomenon. Intra-arterial reserpine improves Raynaud's phenomenon and has been reported to normalize esophageal motility (ABBOUD et al., 1967; WILLERSON et al., 1970). Griseofulvine also seems to influence favorably Raynaud's phenomenon (WINSHIP, 1970). The results of adrenal corticosteroids and A.C.T.H. are not convincing, but when the systemic sclerosis is rapidly progressive, or when it is associated with sclerodermatomyositis or lupus erythematosus, some improvement may be expected from this therapy (WINSHIP, 1970; WINKELMANN, 1971; WINKELMANN et al., 1971). Apparently, renal failure rapidly leading to death may be precipitated by the administration of steroids (RODNAN et al., 1957; WINKELMANN et al., 1971). Salicylates and potassium p-aminobenzoate have been tried to reduce sclerosis and inflammation (ZARAFONETIS, 1961; WINKELMANN et al., 1971). Patients with scleroderma and lupus may derive some benefit from antimalarial drugs as such as 4-aminoquinidine. Alkylating agents have also been tried. The limited experience of recent years seems to indicate that Leukeran can arrest the general evolution of the disease as well as the deterioration of esophageal function (MACKENZIE, 1970; BRINDLEY and TEXTER, 1972). Melphalan is indicated for patients with scleromyxedema when abnormal proteins or polysaccharides are present (WINKELMANN et al., 1971). Antimetabolites such as thioguanine seem to have little effect (DEMIS et al., 1964). Azathioprine improved 8 of the 21 patients of JANSEN et al. (1968) but had no effect on esophageal function. Edema-reducing agents such as potassium p-aminobenzoate (ZARAFONETIS, 1959), disodium E.D.T.A. (KLEIN and HARRIS, 1955; NELDNER et al., 1962), and ε-aminocaproic acid (WINKELMANN et al., 1971) resulted in cutaneous improvement in individual patients. As a result of its lathyrogenic action, penicillamine softens the skin (WINKELMANN et al., 1971). Hormonal therapy with sodium dextrothyroxin (MILLER et al., 1959), progesterone (HOLZMANN and KORTING, 1968), estrogen and relaxin (CASTEN and BOUCEK, 1958) has also be attempted.

1.2. Esophageal Involvement in Progressive Systemic Sclerosis

1.2.1. Incidence

The esophagus has been reported abnormal in 50 to 80% of patients with scleroderma examined by radiology and/or by manometry (MAHRER et al., 1954; FARMER et al., 1960; TUFFANELLI and WINKELMANN, 1961; RODNAN, 1963; TREACY et al., 1963; KEMP HARPER and JACKSON, 1965; ATKINSON and SUMMER-

Ling, 1966; Siegel et al., 1966; Saladin et al., 1966; Clark and Fountain, 1967; D'Angelo et al., 1969; Garrett et al., 1971). Exceptionally the esophagus may be involved in the absence of any skin lesions (Lindsay et al., 1943; Olsen et al., 1945; Rodnan and Fennell, 1962; Hanna, 1972).

The severity of the esophageal involvement does not correlate with the degree of other visceral or skin lesions and the involvement of the esophagus has no prognostic significance. Some patients dying from scleroderma have mild esophageal changes whereas in others the skin lesions improved while the esophageal disorders deteriorated (Farmer et al., 1960; Garrett et al., 1971).

1.2.2. Pathology

It has not yet been established whether the disordered esophageal motility is due to muscular atrophy and sclerosis or to a defect of the intramural innervation. Raynaud's phenomenon correlates fairly well with the presence or absence of esophageal motility disturbances in patients with collagen diseases (Olsen et al., 1945; Bourne, 1949; Stevens et al., 1964; Willerson et al., 1970), although the importance of the arteriolar and capillary changes has been stressed (Norton, 1970). However, in large series of patients with progressive systemic sclerosis the presence or absence of Raynaud's phenomenon does not seem to influence the development of motor disorders of the esophagus (Garrett et al., 1971; Poirier and Rankin, 1972). About 50 to 60% of the patients with scleroderma and abnormal esophageal motility have dysphagia (Tuffanelli and Winkelmann, 1961; Saladin et al., 1966; Tatelman and Keech, 1966; Winship, 1970; Garrett et al., 1971). Esophageal symptoms may be absent despite radiologic or manometric evidence of a disordered motility (Leinwand et al., 1954; Kemp Harper and Jackson, 1965; Saladin et al., 1966). In contrast with the skin lesions the disordered esophageal motility rarely improves (Garrett et al., 1971) and 2 to 3% of the patients develop esophageal stricture due to reflux esophagitis (Kemp Harper and Jackson, 1965; Poirier and Rankin, 1972). The low pressure in the sphincter and the decreased clearing activity of the esophagus which are frequently associated with scleroderma (36 to 50%) favor the development of reflux esophagitis (Olsen et al., 1945; Atkinson and Summerling, 1966; Garrett et al., 1971).

Histologic studies of the esophagus have shown that the smooth muscle coats are atrophied with minimal fibrous replacement (Dornhorst et al., 1954; Treacy et al., 1963; Atkinson and Summerling, 1966; D'Angelo et al., 1969). The submucosal space may be thickened by sclerodermatous infiltration and inflammatory infiltrate (Leinwand et al., 1954; Goldgraber and Kirsner, 1957; Bianchi et al., 1966; Atkinson and Summerling, 1966). In most cases collagen deposition is not very abundant and is not considered the cause of the muscle atrophy (D'Angelo et al., 1969). The small blood vessels of the esophagus are involved by lesions similar to those found elsewhere. Chronic inflammation of the mucosa of the lower esophagus results in thickening, leukoplakia, ulceration and eventually fibrous replacement with stenosis (Leinwand et al., 1954; Atkinson and Summerling, 1966; Brindley and Texter, 1972). These changes are ascribed in part to the scleroderma itself, and in part to the accompanying reflux esophagitis. The striated muscle fibers are remarkably well preserved and atrophic smooth muscle cells have been found intermingled with unaffected striated muscle fibers. The atrophy of the smooth muscle itself is not uniform throughout the esophagus (Treacy et al., 1963). It is unlikely that muscle atrophy is responsible for the motor disturbances which are seen in the early stages of the disease.

The sphincteric smooth muscle contracts normally on direct stimulation (COHEN et al., 1972). Motor disturbances can occur in the absence of visible histologic changes. In other collagenous diseases similar motor disorders have been observed without any accompanying atrophy of the musculature (SALADIN et al., 1966). Although in most cases the intramural ganglion cells appear normal (BEVANS, 1945; TREACY et al., 1963; ATKINSON and SUMMERLING, 1966; D'ANGELO et al., 1969), the loss of peristaltic progression, the occurrence of motor disorders without muscle atrophy and pharmacological observations suggest that neural dysfunction plays a role (TREACA et al., 1963; COHEN et al., 1972). Obviously, atrophy is important for the aperistalsis in later stages of the disease.

1.2.3. Radiological Examination

In advanced cases the involved esophagus appears somewhat dilated and may contain air (Fig. 69), recognizable on plain chest films (DINSMORE et al., 1966). The air esophagogram is most frequently seen in the distal esophagus and is best shown on a lateral view. Deglutition results in a normal peristaltic wave in the cervical esophagus but further distally peristalsis weakens or dies out altogether. Occasionally deglutition is followed by tertiary contractions. Esophageal emptying in the recumbent position is greatly delayed, which constitutes an early sign of sclerodermic involvement (LINDSAY et al., 1943; DORN-HORST et al., 1954; KEMP HARPER and JACKSON, 1965). Cineradiography may show disorders which go unrecognized on routine barium esophagograms (POIRIER and RANKIN, 1972). Shortening of the esophagus may result in a hiatus hernia of moderate size (NESCHIS et al., 1970). The gastroesophageal sphincter is frequently seen to be patulous (WINSHIP, 1970), and gastroesophageal reflux is common in scleroderma (Fig. 198); it may even lead to esophagitis, ulceration or stricture formation. A curious cobblestone appearance, resulting from leukoplakia, has also been described (KEMP HARPER, 1953).

1.2.4. Manometric Examination

Intraluminal pressure measurements reveal the motor disturbances of systemic sclerosis more readily than radiology (BOYD et al., 1954; NESCHIS et al., 1970). On manometry, 80% of the patients are found to be abnormal (GARRETT et al., 1971). As scleroderma affects primarily smooth muscle and leaves striated muscle intact, peristalsis usually remains normal in the upper, striated muscle portion of the esophagus. In 103 patients, all of whom were examined on two different occasions, GARRETT et al. (1971) found no manometric evidence of involvement of this upper segment. In the smooth muscle portion, however, the pressure peaks become weak, often simultaneous, and eventually disappear (Fig. 199) (DORNHORST et al., 1954; CODE et al., 1958; TREACY et al., 1963; ATKINSON and SUMMERLING, 1966; KAUFMANN et al., 1968; GARRETT et al., 1971). The Mecholyl test is negative (KRAMER and INGELFINGER, 1951; HIGHTOWER et al., 1954). The resting pressure in the gastroesophageal sphincter is often below normal (CREAMER et al., 1956; ATKINSON and SUMMERLING, 1966; SALADIN et al., 1966; HEITMANN and ESPINOZA, 1968; KAUFMANN et al., 1968; COHEN et al., 1972). If the high pressure zone in the distal esophagus is lacking an increase in intragastric pressure, produced by abdominal compression, will be transmitted into the esophagus (HEITMANN and ESPINOZA, 1968). The sphincter may fail to contract after deglutition (CREAMER et al., 1956). In moderately advanced cases the sphincter contracts reasonably well in response to direct stimuli such as Mecholyl but insufficiently to indirect stimulation by gastrin (COHEN et al., 1972).

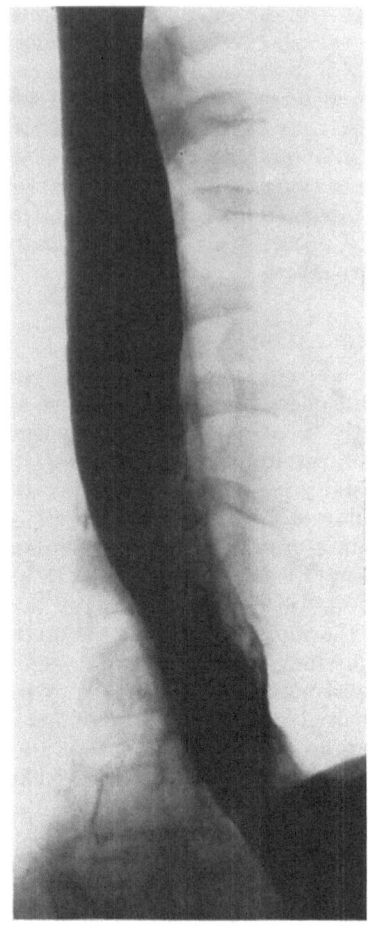

Fig. 198

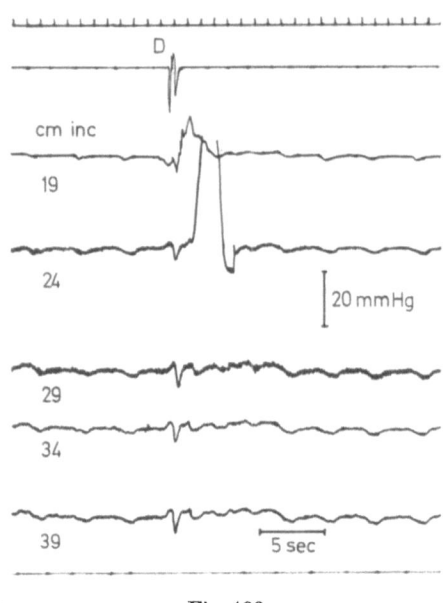

Fig. 199

Fig. 198. Esophageal scleroderma. Massive gastro-esophageal reflux of barium through a patulous sphincter into a dilated and aperistaltic esophagus

Fig. 199. Scleroderma involving the esophagus. Normal peristaltic contraction in the upper part, absence of deglutitive response in the lower part

In far advanced cases the smooth muscle is markedly atrophied (Treacy et al., 1963; D'Angelo et al., 1969) and the lower esophageal sphincter no longer contracts on direct stimulation (Cohen et al., 1972). In the course of the disease the motility disorders either remain unchanged or deteriorate (Garrett et al., 1971).

1.2.5. Differential Diagnosis

The motility disorders observed on radiology or manometry are not pathognomonic by themselves but must be interpreted within their clinical context. Yet tracings characterized by low amplitude pressure waves and loss of peristaltic progression in the distal segments of the esophagus, by low pressures in the gastroesophageal sphincter and by normal peristaltic waves in the proximal segments suggest the diagnosis (Creamer et al., 1956). When the esophagus is dilated and atonic the differential diagnosis with achalasia must be made (Winship, 1970). The persistence of normal peristaltic waves in the upper esophagus, the low resting pressure in the gastroesophageal sphincter, the negative Mecholyl test, and signs of systemic sclerosis in other locations generally permit the differential diagnosis. In some cases it may be difficult to distinguish the tracings from those found in diffuse spasm, in presbyesophagus or in diabetic neuropathy. The differentiation from lupus erythematosus and other collagenous diseases is based on clinical, histological and biochemical data. Dermatomyositis, progressive muscular dystrophy, oculopharyngeal muscular atrophy and myasthenia gravis involve the striated musculature and may be diagnosed by their typical clinical symptoms, pharmacological tests (e.g. Tensilon test in the case of myasthenia) and histological lesions.

1.2.6. Treatment

The treatment of the sclerodermatous involvement of the esophagus constitutes only part of the therapy of systemic sclerosis (see 1.1.). Intraarterial reserpine restored normal motility in 2 of the 5 patients with Raynaud's phenomenon treated by WILLERSON et al. (1970). One of these had Raynaud's disease, the other systemic lupus erythematosus and Raynaud's phenomenon but neither had scleroderma. TAUBENHAUS and LEV (1951) reported the reappearance of peristaltic waves in one patient after 3.5 months of cortisone therapy, but such an effect could not be confirmed by others (ZION et al., 1955). Urecholine is said to improve esophageal propulsion, but more detailed studies are required (ZARAFONETIS, 1959; LORBER and ZARAFONETIS, 1963). Preliminary studies suggest that chlorambucil (Leukeran) may prevent the progressive deterioration of esophageal dysfunction and may even restore esophageal peristalsis (MACKENZIE, 1970; BRINDLEY and TEXTER, 1972).

Dysphagia due to reflux esophagitis should be treated by antacids (WINSHIP, 1970). If the dysphagia is due to stricture formation, relief may be obtained by mechanical dilatation.

In a few patients with scleroderma of the esophagus corrective surgery may become necessary to control reflux or to treat a narrow stricture. The stenosed segment of the esophagus should be managed either by a modified Thal procedure with fundoplication, or by resection of the stricture and interposition of an achlorhydric gastric tube, jejunum or colon graft (BRINDLEY and TEXTER, 1972).

2. Systemic Lupus Erythematosus

In contrast with systemic sclerosis only 10 to 25% of the patients with systemic lupus erythematosus have an impaired esophageal motility. The disturbances are similar to those observed in systemic sclerosis, although generally less pronounced (STEVENS et al., 1964; TATELMAN and KEECH, 1966). About 6% of the patients have dysphagia (HARVEY et al., 1954). Radiological examination may reveal slight dilatation, atony and impaired peristalsis with slow evacuation (GOULD and DAVES, 1958; KEATS, 1961). TATELMAN and KEECH (1966) examined radiologically 28 cases of systemic lupus erythematosus and found 1 case of aperistalsis, and 4 with slight to moderate decrease in peristalsis, accompanied by some esophageal dilatation. On manometric examination similar motility disturbances were found in about one fourth of the patients (STEVENS et al., 1964; SALADIN et al., 1966; WILLERSON et al., 1970).

3. Polymyositis — Dermatomyositis

Polymyositis encompasses a group of disorders in which muscular weakness is the principal clinical feature. On pathological examination inflammatory and degenerative changes are found in the muscles. About one-half of the cases are linked either with one of the collagen diseases or with a malignant tumor.

The remainder develop as isolated primary myopathies or occur in conjunction with skin manifestations (dermatomyositis) (Pearson, 1969). Females are affected about twice as commonly as males.

More than 60% of dermatomyositis and polymyositis patients complain of high dysphagia (Christianson et al., 1956; Donoghue et al., 1960; Pearson, 1969). The degree of dysphagia parallels the course and severity of the muscle involvement. Both may improve with steroids. As the pharyngeal muscles are deficient, tracheal aspiration and nasal reflux frequently occur. Dysphagia referable to the lower esophagus is rare. Radiological examination often reveals pooling of barium in the valleculae and pyriform sinuses and sometimes nasal reflux or aspiration of barium. The cricopharyngeal muscle is atonic, a feature which may help to differentiate this condition from involvement by cerebrovascular accidents or poliomyelitis (Seaman, 1969). Air may be seen in the upper flaccid segment of the gullet. In the distal esophagus peristalsis is often weak or absent (Donoghue et al., 1960; O'Hara et al., 1967). Hernia, reflux esophagitis, erosions and ulcerations occur but are less frequent than in scleroderma.

On manometric studies the contractions in the pharynx and in the upper sphincter are weak (Creamer et al., 1956; Stevens et al., 1964). Peristalsis in the lower segment is disturbed and weak; often simultaneous pressure waves occur after deglutition (Creamer et al., 1956; Donoghue et al., 1960; Saladin et al., 1966). The lower esophageal sphincter pressure is decreased (Creamer et al., 1956). Initially the motility disturbances are most prominent in the proximal segment, while the distal segment can still be normal. The patient described by O'Hara et al. (1967) at first had difficulties of swallowing with tracheal aspiration and pharyngeal reflux; only after two years had a generalized loss of esophageal motility developed. Similarly, a severely disturbed motility in the proximal esophagus with a normal motility in the distal gullet was observed by Grünebaum and Salinger (1971) on radiological examination and by Stevens et al. (1964) on manometric study.

4. Related Syndromes

Sjögren's syndrome may produce dysphagia, mucosal atrophy and strictures of the esophagus (Hradsky et al., 1967). Dryness of the esophagus is the most important cause of this dysphagia but the semilunar strictures of the anterior wall in the postcricoid area may also produce swallowing difficulties. The mucosa of the upper third to upper half of the esophagus is pale and friable.

Patients with Raynaud's phenomenon apparently free of other symptoms of collagen disease frequently have aperistalsis of the esophagus (Creamer et al., 1956; Stevens et al., 1964; Saladin et al., 1966; Willerson et al., 1970), a decreased lower esophageal sphincter pressure (Creamer et al., 1956; Cohen et al., 1972) and poor sphincteric contractions (Creamer et al., 1956). The response of the sphincter to gastrin stimulation is less than normal (Cohen et al., 1972). The upper sphincter, however, is normal. Clark and Fountain (1967) found that motility disturbances in patients with Raynaud's phenomenon are usually a sign of associated systemic sclerosis or another connective tissue disorder. None of their 13 patients with Raynaud's disease had aperistalsis.

References

Abboud, F. M., Eckstein, J. W., Lawrence, M. S., et al.: Cited by Willerson, J. T., R. H. Thompson, P. Hookman, J. Herdt, and Decker, J. L.: Reserpine in Raynaud's disease and phenomenon: short-term response to intra-arterial injection. Ann. intern. Med. 72, 17–27 (1970).

ATKINSON, M., SUMMERLING, M. D.: Oesophageal changes in systemic sclerosis. Gut **7**, 402–408 (1966).

BECK, J. S., ANDERSON, J. R., GRAY, K. G., ROWELL, N. R.: Antinuclear factor and precipitating autoantibodies in progressive systemic sclerosis. Lancet **1963 II**, 1188–1190.

BEVANS, M.: Pathology of scleroderma, with special reference to the changes in the gastrointestinal tract. Amer. J. Path. **21**, 25–51 (1945).

BIANCHI, F. A., BISTUE, A. R., WENDT, V. E., PURO, H. E., KEECH, M. K.: Analysis of twenty-seven cases of progressive systemic scleroderma (including two with combined systemic lupus erythematosus) and a review of the literature. J. chron. Dis. **19**, 953–977 (1966).

BLUESTONE, R., MacMAHON, M., DAWSON, J. M.: Systemic sclerosis and small bowel involvement. Gut **10**, 185–193 (1969).

BOURNE, W. A.: Oesophageal lesions in sclerodactyly. Lancet **1949 I**, 392–394.

BOYD, J. A., PATRICK, S. I., REEVES, R. J.: Roentgen changes observed in generalized scleroderma. Report of sixty-three cases. Arch. intern. Med. **94**, 248–258 (1954).

BRINDLEY, G. V., TEXTER, E. C., JR.: Scleroderma of the esophagus. Texas Med. **68**, 74–80 (1972).

CALNE, D. B., SHAW, D. G., SPIERS, A. S. D., STERN, G. M.: Swallowing in parkinsonism. Brit. J. Radiol. **43**, 456–457 (1970).

CASTEN, G. G., BOUCEK, R. J.: Use of relaxin in the treatment of scleroderma. J. Amer. med. Ass. **166**, 319–324 (1958).

CHRISTIANSON, H. B., BRUNSTING, L. A., PERRY, H. L.: Dermatomyositis: unusual features, complications, and treatment. Arch. Derm. Syph. (Chic.) **74**, 581–589 (1956).

CLARK, J. A., WINKELMANN, R. K., McDUFFIE, F. C., WARD, L. E.: Synovial tissue changes and rheumatoid factor in scleroderma. Mayo Clin. Proc. **46**, 97–103 (1971 a).

CLARK, J. A., WINKELMANN, R. K., WARD, L. E.: Serologic alterations in scleroderma and sclerodermatomyositis. Mayo Clin. Proc. **46**, 104–107 (1971 b).

CLARK, M., FOUNTAIN, R. B.: Oesophageal motility in connective tissue disease. Brit. J. Derm. **79**, 449–452 (1967).

CODE, C. F., CREAMER, B., SCHLEGEL, J. F., OLSEN, A. M., DONOGHUE, F. E., ANDERSEN, H. A.: An atlas of esophageal motility in health and disease. Springfield, Ill.: Ch. C. Thomas Publ. 1958.

COHEN, S., FISHER, R., LIPSHUTZ, W., TURNER, R., MYERS, A., SCHUMACHER, R.: The pathogenesis of esophageal dysfunction in scleroderma and Raynaud's disease. J. clin. Invest. **51**, 2663–2668 (1972).

CREAMER, B., ANDERSEN, H. A., CODE, C. F.: Esophageal motility in patients with scleroderma and related diseases. Gastroenterologia (Basel) **86**, 763–775 (1956).

CULLINAN, E. R.: Scleroderma (Diffuse systemic sclerosis). Proc. roy. Soc. Med. **46**, 507–511 (1953).

D'ANGELO, W. A., FRIES, J. F., MASI, A. T., SHULMAN, L. E.: Pathologic observations in systemic sclerosis (scleroderma). Amer. J. Med. **46**, 428–440 (1969).

DEMIS, D. J., BROWN, C. S., CROSBY, W. H.: Thioguanine in the treatment of certain autoimmune, immunologic and related diseases. Amer. J. Med. **37**, 195–205 (1964).

DINSMORE, R. E., GOODMAN, D., DREYFUSS, J. R.: The air esophagogram: a sign of scleroderma involving the esophagus. Radiology **87**, 348–349 (1966).

DONOGHUE, F., WINKELMANN, R., MOERSCH, H.: Esophageal defects in dermatomyositis. Ann. Otol. **69**, 1139–1145 (1960).

DORNHORST, A. C., PIERCE, J. W., WHIMSTER, I. W.: The esophageal lesion in scleroderma. Lancet **1954 I**, 698–699.

FARMER, R. G., GIFFORD, R. W., HINES, E. A., JR.: Prognostic significance of Raynaud's phenomenon and other clinical characteristics of systemic scleroderma: a study of 271 cases. Circulation **21**, 1088–1095 (1960).

FISHER, E. R., RODNAN, G. P.: Pathologic observations concerning the cutaneous lesion of progressive systemic sclerosis: an electron microscopic, histochemical and immunohistochemical study. Arthr. and Rheum. **3**, 536–545 (1960).

FLEISCHMAJER, R., KROL, S.: Chemical synthesis of the dermis in scleroderma. Proc. Soc. exp. Biol. (N.Y.) **126**, 252–256 (1967).

GARRETT, J. M., WINKELMANN, R. K., SCHLEGEL, J. F., CODE, C. F.: Esophageal deterioration in scleroderma. Mayo Clin. Proc. **46**, 92–96 (1971).

GOETZ, R. H.: The pathology of progressive systemic sclerosis (generalized scleroderma) with special reference to changes in viscera. Clin. Proc. **4**, 337–392 (1945).

GOLDGRABER, M. B., KIRSNER, J. B.: Scleroderma of the gastrointestinal tract—a review. Arch. Path. **64**, 255–265 (1957).

GONDOS, B.: Roentgen manifestations observed in progressive systemic sclerosis (Diffuse scleroderma). Amer. J. Roentgenol. **84**, 235–247 (1960).

GOULD, D. M., DAVES, M. L.: A review of roentgen findings in systemic lupus erythematosus (S.L.E.). Amer. J. med. Sci. 235, 596–610 (1958).

GREENBERGER, N. J., RUPPERT, R. D., TZOGOURNIS, M.: Use of medium chain triglycerides in malabsorption. Ann. intern. Med. 66, 727–734 (1967).

GRÜNEBAUM, M., SALINGER, H.: Radiologic findings in polymyositis-dermatomyositis involving the pharynx and upper oesophagus. Clin. Radiol. 22, 97–100 (1971).

HALE, C. H., SCHATZKI, R.: The roentgenological appearance of the gastrointestinal tract in scleroderma. Amer. J. Roentgenol. 51, 407–420 (1944).

HANNA, S. M.: A case of scleroderma presenting as cardiospasm (achalasia of the oesophagus). Postgrad. med. J. 48, 236–238 (1972).

HARVEY, A. M., SHULMAN, L. E., TUMULTY, P. A., CONLEY, C. L., SCHOENRICH, E. H.: Systemic lupus erythematosus: review of the literature and clinical analysis of 138 cases. Medicine (Baltimore) 33, 291–437 (1954).

HEINZ, E. R., STEINBERG, A. J., SACKNER, M. A.: Roentgenographic and pathologic aspects of intestinal scleroderma. Ann. intern. Med. 59, 822–826 (1963).

HIGHTOWER, N. C., OLSEN, A. M., MOERSCH, H. J.: Comparison of effects of acetyl-beta-methylcholine chloride (Mecholyl) on esophageal intraluminal pressure in normal persons and patients with cardiospasm. Gastroenterology 26, 592–600 (1954).

HOLZMANN, H., KORTING, G. W.: Die Behandlung der Sklerodermie. Dtsch. med. Wschr. 93, 1721–1722 (1968).

HRADSKÝ, M., HYBÁŠEK, I., ČERNOCH, V., SAZMOVÁ, V., JURAN, J.: Oesophageal abnormalities in Sjögren's syndrome. Scand. J. Gastroent. 2, 200–203 (1967).

JANSEN, G. T., BARRAZA, D. F., BALLARD, J. L., HONEYCUTT, W. M., DILLAHA, C. J.: Generalized scleroderma. Treatment with an immunosuppressive agent. Arch. Derm. (Chic.) 97, 690–698 (1968).

KAUFMANN, H. J., BRAVERMAN, I. M., SPIRO, H. M.: Esophageal manometry in scleroderma. Scand. J. Gastroent. 3, 246–254 (1968).

KEATS, T. E.: The collagen diseases: a demonstration of the non-specificity of their extra-pulmonary manifestations. Amer. J. Roentgenol. 86, 938–943 (1961).

KEMP HARPER, R. A.: The radiological manifestations of diffuse systemic sclerosis (scleroderma). Proc. roy. Soc. Med. 46, 512–521 (1953).

KEMP HARPER, R. A., JACKSON, D. C.: Progressive systemic sclerosis. Brit. J. Radiol. 38, 825–834 (1965).

KLEIN, R., HARRIS, S. B.: Treatment of scleroderma, sclerodactylia and calcinosis by chelation (E.D.T.A.). Amer. J. Med. 19, 798–807 (1955).

KRAMER, P., INGELFINGER, F. J.: Esophageal sensitivity to Mecholyl in cardiospasm. Gastroenterology 19, 242–253 (1951).

LEINWAND, I., DURYEE, A. W., RICHTER, M. N.: Scleroderma (based on a study of over 150 cases). Ann. intern. Med. 41, 1003–1041 (1954).

LINDSAY, J. R., TEMPLETON, F. E., ROTHMAN, S.: Lesions of the esophagus in generalized progressive scleroderma. J. Amer. med. Ass. 123, 745–750 (1943).

LORBER, S. H., ZARAFONETIS, C. J. D.: Esophageal transport studies in scleroderma. Amer. J. med. Sci. 245, 654–667 (1963).

MACKENZIE, A. H.: Prolonged alkylating drug therapy is beneficial in systemic scleroderma. Amer. Rheumatism Assoc. Detroit, June (1970).

MAHRER, P. R., EVANS, J. A., STEINBERG, I.: Scleroderma: relation of pulmonary changes to esophageal changes. Ann. intern. Med. 40, 92–110 (1954).

MASI, A. T., D'ANGELO, W. A.: Epidemiology of fatal systemic sclerosis (diffuse scleroderma): a 15-year survey in Baltimore. Ann. intern. Med. 66, 870–883 (1967).

MILLER, R. D., KEATING, F. R., JR., WINKELMANN, R. K.: Progressive systemic sclerosis: acrosclerosis with extensive visceral involvement; report of a case. Proc. Mayo Clin. 34, 58–65 (1959).

NELDNER, K. H., WINKELMANN, R. K., PERRY, H. O.: Scleroderma: an evaluation of treatment with disodium edetate. Arch. Derm. Syph. (Chic.) 86, 305–309 (1962).

NESCHIS, M., SIEGELMAN, S. S., ROTSTEIN, J., PARKER, J. G.: The esophagus in progressive systemic sclerosis. A manometric and radiographic correlation. Amer. J. dig. Dis. 15, 443–447 (1970).

NICE, C. M., MENON, A. N. K., RIGLER, L. G.: Pulmonary manifestations in collagen diseases. Amer. J. Roentgenol. 81, 264–279 (1959).

NORTON, W. L.: Comparison of the microangiopathy of systemic lupus erythematosus, dermatomyositis, scleroderma, and diabetes mellitus. Lab. Invest. 22, 301–308 (1970).

NORTON, W. L., NARDO, J. M.: Vascular disease in progressive systemic sclerosis (Scleroderma). Ann. intern. Med. 73, 317–324 (1970).

O'HARA, J. M., SZEMES, G., LOWMAN, R. M.: The esophageal lesions in dermatomyositis. Radiology 89, 27–31 (1967).

OLSEN, A. M., O'LEARY, P. A., KIRKLIN, B. R.: Esophageal lesions associated with acro-sclerosis and scleroderma. Arch. intern. Med. **76**, 189–200 (1945).

ORABONA, M. L., ALBANO, O.: Progressive systemic sclerosis (or visceral scleroderma): review of the literature and report of cases. Acta med. scand. **160** (Suppl. 333), 1–170 (1958).

PEACHEY, R. D. G., CREAMER, B., PIERCE, J. W.: Sclerodermatous involvement of the stomach and the small and large bowel. Gut **10**, 285–292 (1968).

PEARSON, C. M.: Polymyositis and related disorders. In: Disorders of voluntary muscle, ed. J. N. WALTON, 2nd ed., p. 501–539. London: J. & A. Churchill Ltd. 1969.

POIRIER, T. J., RANKIN, G. B.: Gastrointestinal manifestations of progressive systemic scleroderma based on a review of 364 cases. Amer. J. Gastroent. **58**, 30–44 (1972).

RASMUSSEN, D. M., WAKIM, K. G., WINKELMANN, R. K.: Isotonic and isometric thermal contraction of human dermis. III. Scleroderma and cicatrizing lesions. J. invest. Derm. **43**, 349–355 (1964).

REINHARDT, J. F., BARRY, W. F.: Scleroderma of the small bowel. Amer. J. Roentgenol. **88**, 687–692 (1962).

RODNAN, G. P.: The nature of joint involvement in progressive systemic sclerosis (diffuse scleroderma): clinical study and pathologic examination of synovium in twenty-nine patients. Ann. intern. Med. **56**, 422–439 (1962).

RODNAN, G. P.: Natural history of progressive systemic sclerosis (diffuse scleroderma). Bull. rheum. Dis. **13**, 301–304 (1963).

RODNAN, G. P., FENNELL, R. H., JR.: Progressive systemic sclerosis sine scleroderma. J. Amer. med. Ass. **180**, 665–670 (1962).

RODNAN, G. P., SCHREINER, G. E., BLACK, R. L.: Renal involvement in progressive systemic sclerosis (generalized scleroderma). Amer. J. Med. **23**, 445–450 (1957).

SALADIN, T. A., FRENCH, A. B., ZARAFONETIS, C. J. D., POLLARD, H. M.: Esophageal motor abnormalities in scleroderma and related diseases. Amer. J. dig. Dis. **11**, 522–535 (1966).

SEAMAN, W. B.: Functional disorders of the pharyngo-esophageal junction; achalasia and chalasia. Radiol. Clin. N. Amer. **7**, 113–119 (1969).

SIEGEL, C. I., HENDRIX, T. R., HARVEY, J. C.: The swallowing disorder in myotonia dys-trophica. Gastroenterology **50**, 541–550 (1966).

STEVENS, M. B., HOOKMAN, P., SIEGEL, C. I., ESTERLEY, J. R., SHULMAN, L. E., HENDRIX, T. R.: Aperistalsis of the esophagus in patients with connective-tissue disorders and Raynaud's phenomenon. New Engl. J. Med. **270**, 1218–1222 (1964).

TATELMAN, M., KEECH, M. K.: Esophageal motility in systemic lupus erythematosus, rheuma-toid arthritis and scleroderma. Radiology **86**, 1041–1046 (1966).

TAUBENHAUS, M., LEV, M.: Clinical and histological observations on a case of scleroderma treated with cortisone. Arch. intern. Med. **87**, 583–593 (1951).

TREACY, W. L., BAGGENSTOSS, A. H., SLOCUMB, C. H., CODE, C. F.: Scleroderma of the esophagus. A correlation of histologic and physiologic findings. Ann. intern. Med. **59**, 351–356 (1963).

TUFFANELLI, D. L., WINKELMANN, R. K.: Systemic scleroderma: clinical study of 727 cases. Arch. Derm. Syph. (Chic.) **84**, 359–371 (1961).

TUFFANELLI, D. L., WINKELMANN, R. K.: Scleroderma and its relationship to the "colla-genoses": dermatomyositis, lupus erythematosus, rheumatoid arthritis and Sjögren's syndrome. Amer. J. med. Sci. **243**, 133–146 (1962).

WILLERSON, J. T., THOMPSON, R. H., HOOKMAN, P., HERDT, J., DECKER, J. L.: Reserpine in Raynaud's disease and phenomenon: short-term response to intra-arterial injection. Ann. intern. Med. **72**, 17–27 (1970).

WINKELMANN, R. K.: Classification and pathogenesis of scleroderma. Proc. Mayo Clin. **46**, 83–91 (1971).

WINKELMANN, R. K., KIERLAND, R. R., PERRY, H. O., MULLER, S. A., SAMS, W. M.: Manage-ment of scleroderma. Proc. Mayo Clin. **46**, 128–134 (1971).

WINSHIP, D. H.: Management of esophageal problems in patients with collagen vascular disease. Modern Treatment **7**, 1241–1249 (1970).

ZARAFONETIS, C. J. D.: Treatment of scleroderma. Ann. intern. Med. **50**, 343–365 (1959).

ZARAFONETIS, C. J. D.: The treatment of scleroderma: results of potassium para-amino-benzoate therapy in 104 cases. Inflammation and diseases of connective tissue: A Hahne-mann symposium, ed. by L. C. MILLS, J. H. MOYER, p. 688–696. Philadelphia: W. B. Saunders Company 1961.

ZION, M. M., GOLDBERG, B., SUZMAN, M. M.: Corticotropin and cortisone in the treatment of scleroderma. Quart. J. Med. **24**, 215–228 (1955).

Motor Disorders Due to Muscle Disorders

G. VANTRAPPEN and J. HELLEMANS

With 3 Figures

1. Myotonic Dystrophy (Steinert's Disease)

1.1. Definition and General Data

Myotonia dystrophica is a familial disease, transmitted by an autosomal dominant gene with incomplete penetrance and variable expression. It is found most frequently in young adults of both sexes (THOMASEN, 1948; WELSH et al., 1964), but can begin from childhood (DODGE et al., 1965). The main symptoms are myotonia, i.e. the continued active contraction of a muscle persisting after the cessation of voluntary effort or stimulation, and weakness and wasting of voluntary muscles. The disease affects mainly the muscles of hands and feet, as well as the facial, ocular and oropharyngeal muscles. The most telling symptom of myotonia is a slowness of relaxation after a forceful contraction such as a handshake. The electromyographic pattern of the involved muscles is characterized by bursts of fibrillation-like potentials, elicited by insertion of the recording needle, by a slight voluntary effort or by muscle percussion (Fig. 200A). Their frequency is high at the beginning and then decreases, giving the characteristic dive-bomber sound in the loudspeaker. The dystrophic process is manifested by the short duration and the weak amplitude of the action potentials, and by the increased number of polyphasic spikes (DUMOULIN and AUCREMANNE, 1959). Smooth muscles and cardiac muscle are also frequently involved. The esophagus is the most frequently affected gastrointestinal organ; stomach, small intestine, colon and gallbladder are less often abnormal. The muscles of the uterus and of the urinary bladder can also be weakened (WELSH et al., 1964; SCHUMAN et al., 1965; HARVEY et al., 1965; GOLDBERG and SHEFT, 1972). Involvement of the internal anal sphincter is characterized by myotonic contraction instead of relaxation after rectal distension (SCHUSTER et al., 1965). On histological examination, lesions of the smooth muscle cells are found whereas the intramural nerve plexuses seem to be intact (GOLDBERG and SHEFT, 1972).

Other symptoms of myotonic dystrophy are frontal baldness, testicular atrophy, cataract, extrathyroidal hypometabolism, internal frontal hyperostosis, mental retardation, Raynaud's phenomenon and perhaps diabetes mellitus (WELSH et al., 1964). Myotonia can be treated with procainamide (4 to 6 g/day) diphenylhydantoin (0.3 to 0.6 g/day) or quinidine (0.3 to 1.5 g/day). The dysphagia can be improved with procainamide 3×500 mg/day (CASEY and AMINOFF, 1971), but the weakness of the muscles is not improved by medication.

1.2. Esophageal Involvement

In virtually all cases examined, lesions of the striated muscles of pharynx and esophagus have been found (PIERCE et al., 1965; HARVEY et al., 1965; HUGHES et al., 1965; SIEGEL et al., 1966). The histological lesions and the electro-

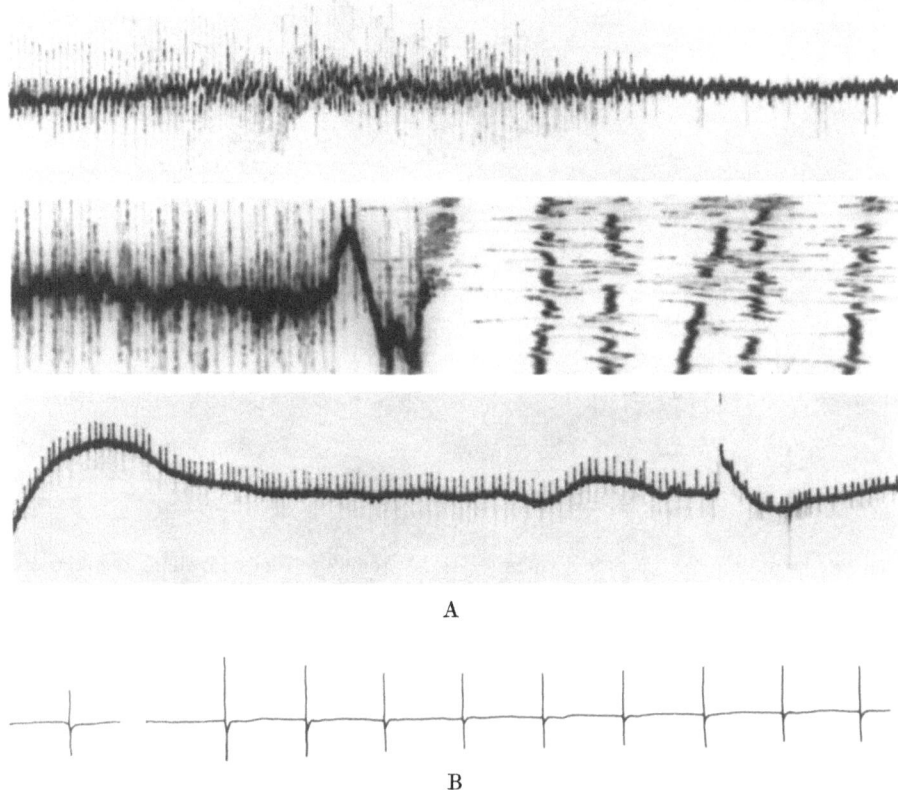

A

B

Fig. 200A and B. EMG in skeletal muscles. A Patient with myotonic dystrophy. Upper
tracing: myotonic discharge with high frequency (140 c/sec) and decreasing amplitude.
Middle tracing: "myogenic" record showing low amplitude potentials (< 500 μV) (left part);
at higher speed (right part) the potentials are very much frayed out and look like a stroke of
a brush («potentiels déchiquetés — potentials finement dentellés»). Lower tracing: rest
activity: "myogenic fibrillations" at a frequency of 110 c/sec. Amplitude: 10 μV/cm. Paper
speed: 200 msec/cm. B Patient with myasthenia gravis: the record was made in the right
M. orbicularis oculi on supramaximal stimulation at 3 c/sec. The amplitude of the 5th potential reaches 75% of the original value. (Courtesy of N. ROSSELLE, Laboratory of Electromyography, Dept. of Physical Med. and Electromyography, Akademisch Ziekenhuis St.-Rafaël
Leuven)

myographic disorders are similar to those of the myotonic skeletal muscles
(BLACK and RAVIN, 1947; CASEY and AMINOFF, 1971). Dysfunction of the smooth
esophageal musculature is found in at least half of the patients (SIEGEL et al.,
1966; HARVEY et al., 1965) and can cause dysphagia. Patients with myotonic
dystrophy may have swallowing difficulties without mentioning them (KELLEY,
1964). Hence the incidence of dysphagia is hard to estimate, but values between
30 and 50% have been reported (CHIU and ENGLERT, 1962; WELSH et al., 1964;
SCHUMAN et al., 1965).

In the striated muscle portion of the esophagus abnormalities are found
both on cineradiography (BOSMA and BRODIE, 1969; SEAMAN, 1969) and on
manometry (KRAMER et al., 1957). In early cases the radiocinematographic
pictures are often characteristic. The patient exhibits myotonia in the muscles

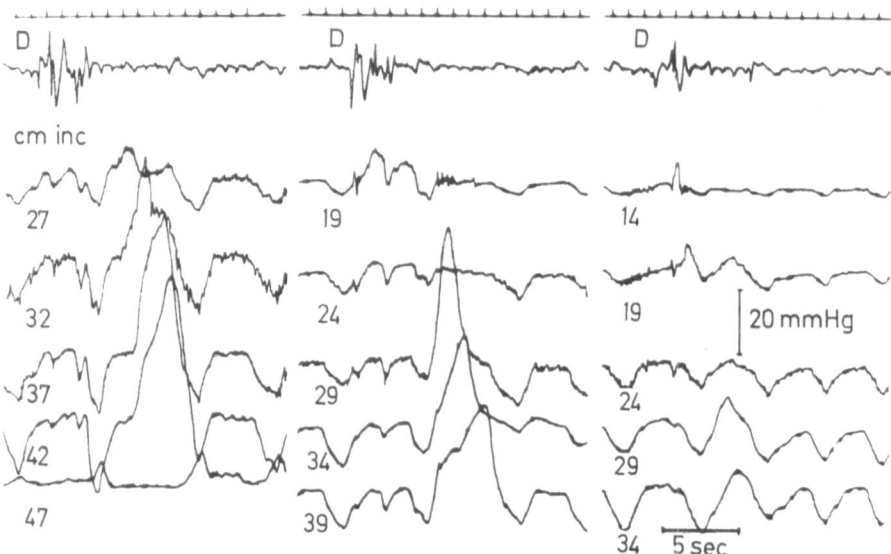

Fig. 201. Deglutitive pressures in a patient with myotonic dystrophy involving the pharynx,
the pharyngoesophageal sphincter and the upper part of the esophagus

suspending the hyoid, with sustained upward and forward displacement of the
hyoid during swallowing. The myotonic contraction of the m. tensor veli palatini
causes a sustained downward displacement of the soft palate during swallow
or speech. The myotonic distortion of the hyoid suspensory muscles occasions
compensatory displacement of the pharyngeal constrictor. The dorsal wall of
the mesopharynx protrudes abnormally (Bosma and Brodie, 1969). In more
advanced cases the lower esophagus is often, the upper esophagus rarely dilated
(Hughes et al., 1965).

There is pooling of barium in the pharynx and the pyriform sinuses (Kramer
et al., 1957), which may last for minutes (Pruzanski and Profis, 1966). Pyriform
sinuses and valleculae are frequently deformed and ballooned. In the recumbent
position, regurgitation of esophageal contents into the pharynx and nose frequently occurs (Hughes et al., 1965; Seaman, 1969). There may also be tracheal
aspiration, which may lead to severe bronchopulmonary complications (Harvey
et al., 1965; Pierce et al., 1965). The swallowing disorders are due mainly to
muscular dysfunction rather than to lack of coordination of the swallowing
mechanism itself, which may be preserved for a long time. In the lower esophagus
peristalsis is weakened to a varying extent and degree (Schuman et al., 1965).
Sometimes swallowing results in simultaneous contractions or in no contractions
at all (Pierce et al., 1965). Esophageal evacuation may be delayed for an unduly
long time; Pruzanski and Profis (1966) observed stasis of barium during
5 to 30 min in 4 out of their 21 patients.

On manometric examination, marked abnormalities were found in the pharynx
and in the esophagus, both in the striated and smooth muscles. The resting
pressure in the pharyngoesophageal sphincter is decreased, or the high pressure
zone has disappeared altogether (Pierce et al., 1965). Deglutition results in a
normally timed relaxation but the contraction waves recorded in the pharynx
and pharyngoesophageal sphincter are weaker than normal (Pierce et al., 1965;
Siegel et al., 1966) (Fig. 201). The relaxation of the muscles may require an

abnormally long time, which results in pressure waves of long duration and has been interpreted as a consequence of myotonia (SIEGEL et al., 1966). In most cases, the amplitude of the peristaltic contractions is reduced throughout the esophagus. Some patients fail to show any esophageal peristalsis in response to swallowing, and in a majority the incidence of peristaltic contractions upon deglutition is below normal (PIERCE et al., 1965; HARVEY et al., 1965; SCHUMAN et al., 1965; SIEGEL et al., 1966; GARRETT et al., 1969).

The gastroesophageal sphincter has a normal resting pressure (SIEGEL et al., 1966; GARRETT et al., 1969), a normal relaxation and a normal or prolonged contraction (GARRETT et al., 1969). As is to be expected in the case of a muscular disease, the manometric coordination remains intact for a long time (GARRETT et al., 1969) and the Mecholyl test remains negative (GOLDBERG and SHEFT, 1972). The intramural plexuses are intact on histological examination (GOLDBERG and SHEFT, 1972). The muscle atrophy affects the smooth muscle as well as the striated muscle (PRUZANSKI and HUVOS, 1967).

2. Ocular Myopathy and Oculopharyngeal Myopathy

2.1. Definition and General Data

Ocular myopathy usually begins with ptosis and progresses to complete bilateral ophthalmoplegia (WALTON and GARDNER-MEDWIN, 1969). In many cases there is progressive involvement of other muscles as well, particularly the upper facial muscles and of the muscles of neck, trunk and limbs. Ocular myopathy may be seen in patients suffering from diseases of the hereditary ataxia group, but usually it is a muscular dystrophy and the primary site of involvement is the muscle itself. The disease may involve single individuals, but it may also be familial with evidence of dominant inheritance. From this group a number of patients was separated, characterized by the late onset, the association with pharyngeal involvement and a higher incidence of affected members in their families. This variant was called oculopharyngeal myopathy (VICTOR et al., 1962; BRAY et al., 1965). Many of these were of French Canadian stock (BRAY et al., 1965; BARBEAU, 1966; MURPHY and DRACHMAN, 1968).

In these patients there is myopathy without myotonia and electromyography reveals polyphasic potentials and spikes of small amplitude and short duration (MURPHY and DRACHMAN, 1968). Unlike in myasthenia gravis the symptoms are not improved by neostigmine.

2.2. Pharyngoesophageal Involvement

About half of the patients with ocular dystrophy have swallowing difficulties which usually develop a few years after the ptosis (WALTON, 1964; ROBERTS and BAMFORTH, 1968). In patients with oculopharyngeal dystrophy the swallowing difficulties are more prominent and may precede as well as follow the ptosis (BRAY et al., 1965; LEWIS, 1966; MURPHY and DRACHMAN, 1968). Other types of progressive muscular dystrophy may also produce swallowing difficulties. On radiological examination the usual signs of pharyngeal dystrophy appear: delay in pharyngeal emptying, nasopharyngeal reflux and tracheal aspiration. The distal esophagus may be involved as well, showing uncoordinated contractions or no contractions at all (ROBERTS and BAMFORTH, 1968). On manometric examination the resting pressure in the pharyngoesophageal sphincter is normal or decreased. The deglutitive response in the body of the esophagus is often abnormal;

simultaneous contractions, weak peristalsis in the upper 7 cm and normal peristalsis in the rest of the esophagus or weak peristalsis throughout the gullet have all been described. The lower esophageal sphincter seems to function normally.

3. Myasthenia Gravis

3.1. Definition and General Data

Myasthenia gravis is a syndrome characterized by an increased muscle weakness upon repetitive contraction of involved muscles and by partial return of function when anticholinesterases are administered or when the muscle is allowed to rest (Osserman and Genkins, 1971). The neuromuscular transmission is disturbed, which can be shown electromyographically by the decline of the evoked potential in affected muscles upon nerve stimulation (Fig. 200B). But myasthenia gravis cannot be considered in terms of defective neuromuscular transmission only (Simpson, 1969). Degenerative changes of the skeletal muscle fibers and of the motor endplates have been observed (Russell, 1953; Woolf, 1966). They seem to bear no direct relationship to the severity of the loss of function (Simpson, 1969). Cardiac and smooth muscles may be affected as well. Huvos and Pruzanski (1967) described six cases of myasthenia gravis with edema, myofiber degeneration and fatty infiltration of the esophageal smooth muscle. The intramural plexuses were prominent with some concomitant abnormalities of their ganglion cells.

The disease affects 1.5 times as many women as men. The age of onset is usually between 10 and 30 years in women and between 40 and 60 in men. The most common symptoms are diplopia (73%), ptosis (84%), dysarthria (61%), dysphagia (63%) and chewing weakness (52%). Other muscles are also frequently affected (Osserman and Genkins, 1971).

3.2. Pharyngoesophageal Involvement

Swallowing dysfunction is a very frequent finding. On fluoroscopy the deterioration of pharyngoesophageal function on repeated swallowing is easily observed. There is pooling of barium in the pharyngeal sinuses associated with loss of tone and ballooning of the pharyngeal cavity (Silbiger et al., 1967; Kusin et al., 1971) (Fig. 202). The cricopharyngeal sphincter does not appear to be spastic (Donner and Siegel, 1965). Administration of prostigmine clearly improves the swallowing function (Schwab and Viets, 1941; Kramer et al., 1957; Donner and Siegel, 1965). Kusin et al. (1971) observed delayed esophageal evacuation in 8 of their 24 patients, which suggests dysfunction of the smooth musculature. On manometric examination the resting pressure in the pharyngoesophageal sphincter is decreased or the high pressure zone is entirely absent. The contraction waves of pharynx, sphincter and upper esophagus are weak (Kramer et al., 1957; Fisher et al., 1965; Moldow and Cohen, 1971). The amplitude of the contractions rapidly decreases upon repeated deglutitions (Kusin et al., 1971). This dysfunction can be partially corrected by the administration of 2 to 8 mg of edrophonium (Tensilon), a drug with anticholinesterase activity (Moldow and Cohen, 1971). Thymectomy also results in improvement of the pharyngoesophageal motility disorders. In the more distal esophagus the deglutitive response may be absent or weak; in one third of the cases simultaneous contractions have been observed (Fisher et al., 1965; Moldow and Cohen, 1971; Kusin et al., 1971). The smooth muscle dysfunction, however, is not improved by edrophonium (Moldow and Cohen, 1971).

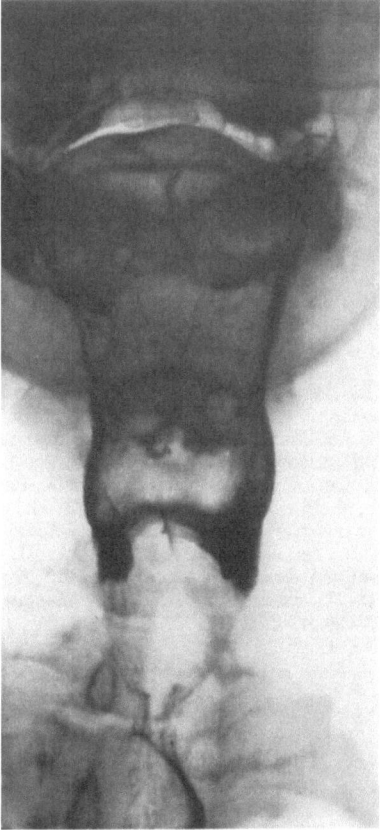

Fig. 202. Myasthenia gravis. Pharyngeal dysfunction with pooling of barium in the pyriform
sinuses after repeated swallowing

4. Endocrine Disorders of Muscle

In 90% of unselected cases of hyperthyroidism electromyographic abnormalities are found in skeletal muscle (RAMSAY, 1966). Thyrotoxicosis is frequently
accompanied by muscle weakness or wasting. Adequate treatment of the thyrotoxicosis results in full recovery. In rare cases swallowing complaints may be
prominent (LEACH, 1962). In a patient with apathic hyperthyroidism, dysphagia
and wasting of hand muscle, FISHER et al. (1965) observed "esophageal spasm",
elevated pressure and many spontaneous waves on manometry.

CHRISTENSEN (1967) performed manometric studies in 5 cases of myxedema
and observed that in the distal three quarters of the esophagus the pressure wave
was reduced, the peristaltic wave duration prolonged and the propagation velocity
decreased. Simultaneous contractions were more frequent than normal. The upper
quarter of the esophagus was unaffected. Radiologically a delayed esophageal
transit time was observed.

As in alcoholic and diabetic disorders it is uncertain whether the malfunction
is of myogenic or neurogenic origin.

References

BARBEAU, A.: The syndrome of hereditary late onset ptosis and dysphagia in French-Canada. In: Symposium über progressive Muskeldystrophie, ed. E. KUHN, p. 102–109. Berlin-Heidelberg-New York: Springer 1966.

BLACK, W. C., RAVIN, A.: Studies in myotonia dystrophica. VII. Autopsy observations in five cases. Arch. Path. **44**, 176–191 (1947).

BOSMA, J. F., BRODIE, D. R.: Cineradiographic demonstration of pharyngeal area myotonia in myotonic dystrophy patients. Radiology **92**, 104–109 (1969).

BRAY, G. M., KAARSOO, M., ROSS, R. T.: Ocular myopathy with dysphagia. Neurology (Minneap.) **15**, 678–684 (1965).

CASEY, E. B., AMINOFF, M. J.: Dystrophia myotonica presenting with dysphagia. Brit. med. J. **1971 II**, 443–444.

CHIU, V. S. W., ENGLERT, E., JR.: Gastrointestinal disturbances in myotonia dystrophica. Gastroenterology **42**, 745–746 (1962).

CHRISTENSEN, J.: Esophageal manometry in myxoedema (abstract). Gastroenterology **52**, 1130 (1967).

DODGE, P. R., GAMSTORP, I., BYERS, R. K., RUSSELL, P.: Myotonic dystrophy in infancy and childhood. Pediatrics **35**, 3–19 (1965).

DONNER, M. W., SIEGEL, C. I.: The evaluation of pharyngeal neuromuscular disorders by cinefluorography. Amer. J. Roentgenol. **94**, 299–307 (1965).

DUMOULIN, J., AUCREMANNE, CH.: Précis d'électromyographie. Paris: Librairie Maloine 1959.

FISCHER, R. A., ELLISON, G. W., THAYER, W. R., SPIRO, H. M., GLASER, G. H.: Esophageal motility in neuromuscular disorders. Ann. intern. Med. **63**, 229–248 (1965).

GARRETT, J. M., DuBOSE, T. D., JR., JACKSON, J. E., NORMAN, J. R.: Esophageal and pulmonary disturbances in myotonia dystrophica. Arch. intern. Med. **123**, 26–32 (1969).

GOLDBERG, H. I., SHEFT, D. J.: Esophageal and colon changes in myotonia dystrophica. Gastroenterology **63**, 134–139 (1972).

HARVEY, J. C., SHERBOURNE, D. H., SIEGEL, C. I.: Smooth muscle involvement in myotonic dystrophy. Amer. J. Med. **39**, 81–90 (1965).

HUGHES, D. T. D., SWANN, J. C., GLEESON, J. A., LEE, F. I.: Abnormalities in swallowing associated with dystrophia myotonica. Brain **88**, 1037–1042 (1965).

HUVOS, A. G., PRUZANSKI, W.: Smooth muscle involvement in primary muscle diseases. III. Myasthenia gravis. Arch. Path. **84**, 280–285 (1967).

KELLEY, M. L., JR.: Dysphagia and motor failure of the esophagus in myotonia dystrophica. Neurology (Minneap.) **14**, 955–960 (1964).

KRAMER, P., ATKINSON, M., WYMAN, S. M., INGELFINGER, F. J.: The dynamics of swallowing. II. Neuromuscular dysphagia of pharynx. J. clin. Invest. **36**, 589–595 (1957).

KUSIN, M. I., SMAKOW, G. M., GREBENEW, A. L., STEPENKO, A. S.: Dysphagische Störungen bei den Mystheniekranken und ihre Dynamik unter dem Einfluß der chirurgischen Behandlung (Thymektomie). Z. ges. Neurol. Psychiat. **200**, 279–290 (1971).

LEACH, W.: Generalized muscular diseases presenting as pharyngeal dysphagia. J. Laryng. **76**, 237–240 (1962).

LEWIS, I.: Late-onset muscle dystrophy: oculopharyngoesophageal variety. Canad. med. Ass. J. **95**, 146–150 (1966).

MOLDOW, R. E., COHEN, B. R.: A disorder of esophageal smooth muscle in myasthenia gravis (abstract). Gastroenterology **60**, 787 (1971).

MURPHY, S. F., DRACHMAN, D. B.: The oculopharyngeal syndrome. J. Amer. med. Ass. **203**, 1003–1008 (1968).

OSSERMAN, K. E., GENKINS, G.: Studies in myasthenia gravis: review of a twenty-year experience in over 1200 patients. Mt Sinai J. Med. **38**, 497–537 (1971).

PIERCE, J. W., CREAMER, B., MacDERMOT, V.: Pharynx and oesophagus in dystrophia myotonica. Gut **6**, 392–395 (1965).

PRUZANSKI, W., HUVOS, A. G.: Smooth muscle involvement in primary muscle disease. I. Myotonic dystrophy. Arch. Path. **83**, 229–233 (1967).

PRUZANSKI, W., PROFIS, A.: Dysfunction of the alimentary tract in myotonic dystrophy. Israel J. med. Sci. **2**, 59–64 (1966).

RAMSEY, I. D.: Muscle dysfunction in hyperthyroidism. Lancet **1966 II**, 931–935.

ROBERTS, A. H., BAMFORTH, J.: The pharynx and esophagus in ocular muscular dystrophy. Neurology (Minneap.) **18**, 645–652 (1968).

RUSSELL, D. S.: Histological changes in the striped muscles in myasthenia gravis. J. Path. Bact. **65**, 279–289 (1953).

SCHUMAN, B. M., RINALDO, J. A., JR., DARNLEY, J. D.: Visceral changes in myotonic dystrophy. Ann. intern. Med. **63**, 793–799 (1965).

SCHUSTER, M. M., Tow, D. E., SHERBOURNE, D. H.: Anal sphincter abnormalities, characteristic of myotonic dystrophy. Gastroenterology 49, 641–648 (1965).

SCHWAB, R. S., VIETS, H. R.: Roentgenoscopy of the pharynx in myasthenia gravis before and after prostigmine injection. Amer. J. Roentgenol. 45, 357–359 (1941)

SEAMAN, W. B.: Functional disorders of the pharyngo-esophageal junction; achalasia and chalasia. Radiol. Clin. N. Amer. 7, 113–119 (1969).

SIEGEL, C. I., HENDRIX, T. R., HARVEY, J. C.: The swallowing disorder in myotonia dystrophica. Gastroenterology 50, 541–550 (1966).

SILBIGER, M. L., PIKIELNEY, R., DONNER, M. W.: Neuromuscular disorders affecting the pharynx. Cineradiographic analysis. Invest. Radiol. 2, 442–448 (1967).

SIMPSON, J. A.: Myasthenia gravis and myasthenic syndromes. In: Disorders of voluntary muscle, ed. J. N. WALTON, 2nd ed., p. 541–578. London: J. & A. Churchill, Ltd. 1969.

THOMASEN, E.: Myotonia: Thomsen's disease (myotonia congenita), paramyotonia, and dystrophia myotonica: a clinical and heredobiologic investigation. 251 pp. Aarhus, Denmark: Universitets Forlaget i Aarhus 1948.

VICTOR, M., HAYES, R., ADAMS, R. D.: Oculopharyngeal muscular dystrophy. A familial disease of late life characterized by dysphagia and progressive ptosis of the eyelids. New Engl. J. Med. 267, 1267–1272 (1962).

WALTON, J. N.: Muscular dystrophy: some recent advances in knowledge. Brit. med. J. 1964 I, 1271–1274.

WALTON, J. N., GARDNER-MEDWIN, D.: Progressive muscular dystrophy and the myotonic disorders. In: Disorders of voluntary muscle, ed. J. N. WALTON, 2nd ed., p. 455–604. London: J. & A. Churchill, Ltd. 1969.

WELSH, J. D., HAASE, G. R., BYNUM, T. E.: Myotonic muscular dystrophy: systemic manifestations. Arch. intern. Med. 114, 669–679 (1964).

WOOLF, A. L.: Morphology of the myasthenic neuromuscular junction. Ann. N.Y. Acad. Sci. 135, 35–59 (1966).

Motor Disorders Due to Lesions of the Central Nervous System

J. Hellemans and G. Vantrappen

Lesions of the vagal nuclei of the brainstem may be caused by various diseases. Although disturbance of the swallowing act is one of the most prominent symptoms these lesions usually cause other neurological disorders also.

1. Brainstem Lesions

Swallowing difficulties may complicate cerebrovascular accidents affecting the brainstem. The "Wallenberg's syndrome" is characterized by contralateral paresis of arm and leg, and ipsilateral paralysis of tongue, palate and pharynx, resulting in swallowing disturbances. The occlusion may be located in the posterior inferior cerebellar artery or in the vertebral artery itself. Radiological examination of the pharyngoesophageal region reveals asymmetric swallowing with barium descending along the paralysed half of the pharynx, pharyngeal stasis, nasal regurgitation and, in some cases, poor relaxation of the pharyngoesophageal sphincter (Donner and Siegel, 1965; Lund, 1965; Silbiger et al., 1967). On manometric examination the major defect is the pharyngoesophageal sphincter where the usual decrease in pressure after deglutition is absent (Creamer, 1968). Most patients with pharyngeal palsy due to brainstem lesions recover rather quickly.

Pseudobulbar palsy may cause, in addition to swallowing difficulties, disorders of esophageal motility such as forceful simultaneous contractions, weak peristaltic waves and an atonic gastroesophageal sphincter (Fischer et al., 1965). Brainstem tumors, degenerative diseases, such as hereditary spastic ataxia, traumatic lesions and tabes may also cause swallowing difficulties (Daly et al., 1962; Silbiger et al., 1967; Walker et al., 1969). Multiple sclerosis may cause difficulties in the earliest phases of swallowing as well as sticking of food in the esophagus. The swallowing difficulties may be due to an ataxia-like disorder hampering the initiation of deglutition or to disorders of the first phases of swallowing (Daly et al., 1962). On radiocinematographic examination abnormal pharyngeal contractions were seen in 5 out of 6 patients. The manometric abnormalities were aspecific and did not correlate well with the patient's symptoms. Uncoordinated and repetitive contractions, feeble resting pressure and poor relaxation of the gastroesophageal sphincter were the most frequent disorders. The pharyngoesophageal sphincter seemed to be involved only rarely (Daly et al., 1962).

2. Poliomyelitis

Bulbar poliomyelitis is frequently accompanied by difficulty in swallowing. Among the patients having residual disability of the lower pharynx following poliomyelitis, a variety of particular impairments are found. These include laxity of the walls of the hypopharynx, persistent closure of the hypopharyngeal sphincter and abnormalities in the elevation of the larynx upon swallowing, due to weakness of the suspensory musculature or to contractions of the intrinsic or of the supporting musculature. Facilitative maneuvers of head and neck can compensate for the defective elevator mechanism upon swallowing (BOSMA, 1957 a, b). The head is characteristically tilted in the direction opposite to the side of weaker constrictor and elevator muscles, thus facilitating the elevation of the larynx on the weaker side (BOSMA, 1953). Exceptionally occlusion of the pharynx by apposition of its anterior and posterior walls between the lordotic cervical spine and the retro-displaced skeleton of the face results in total disability of speech and swallow (MERRITT et al., 1957).

Weakness of the pharyngeal constrictor muscles results in nasal reflux, pooling of secretions or swallowed boluses, and spill-over in the pharynx. In contrast with polymyositis the pharyngoesophageal sphincter remains closed in the resting state and relaxes normally.

Persistent closure of the pharyngoesophageal sphincter occurs in certain subjects having evidence of marked weakness of the constrictor and levator musculature of the pharynx. In these subjects an attempt at swallowing results in regurgitation of the bolus from the hypopharynx. Recovery from this disorder is possible.

Manometric studies in poliomyelitic patients with dysphagia indicate that the resting pressure and the relaxations of the upper esophageal sphincter are normal. The contractions of pharynx and cervical esophagus, however, are frequently deficient or absent (KRAMER et al., 1957).

3. Motor Neuron Disease

The motor neuron diseases are a group of diseases of the motor system of unknown origin, whose principal pathology is a degeneration of lower motor neurons in the spinal cord and the brainstem. Clinically several distinctive syndromes can be recognized. The most frequent form, in which muscular atrophy and hyperreflexia are combined, is called "amyotrophic lateral sclerosis". In the less frequent cases of "progressive muscular atrophy", weakness and atrophy alone exist without clinical evidence of corticospinal tract dysfunction. When the disorder affects predominantly the musculature innervated by the cranial nerves, the syndrome is called "progressive bulbar palsy". Very rarely the picture is dominated by spasticity and hyperreflexia without obvious muscular wasting; such cases are classified as "primary lateral sclerosis".

Impairment of visceral musculature and dilatation of esophagus and stomach have been reported in amyotrophic lateral sclerosis (OPPENHEIM, 1911; BOUDIN et al., 1954). The motility disorders are not limited to pharynx and tongue (BOSMA and BRODIE, 1969); the esophagus may be affected as well.

Esophageal motility was studied in 19 patients with amyotrophic lateral sclerosis who, at the time of examination, had symptoms of bulbar or pseudo-bulbar involvement. Abnormalities were found mainly in the middle and lower third of the esophagus. The amplitude of the peristaltic waves was decreased or the esophagus completely failed to respond to swallowing. In still other patients simultaneous and/or repetitive waves could be observed and in some, the resting sphincteric pressure was lowered (SMITH et al., 1957).

4. Extrapyramidal Disturbances

Parkinsonian patients often experience dysphagia (Eadie and Tyrer, 1965 a, b) which may be alleviated by L-dopa (Calne et al., 1970; Cotzias et al., 1969). Tongue tremor and hesitancy in initiating swallowing cause difficulties in bolus formation but misdirected swallowing and dysfunction of the upper esophageal sphincter also contribute to the dysphagia (Donner and Silbiger, 1966; Silbiger et al., 1967). On manometric studies various motility disturbances have been observed, such as absence of peristaltic waves, spontaneous activity and a pattern resembling diffuse esophageal spasm. In other cases no abnormalities are found (Fisher et al., 1965). Chorea may also cause pharyngeal dysfunction (Silbiger et al., 1967).

5. Stiff-man Syndrome

The stiff-man syndrome was described by Moersch and Woltman (1956) and critically reviewed by Gordon et al. (1967). This syndrome consists of symmetrical progressive stiffness and painful spasm of axial musculature, particularly of the muscles of trunk and neck, and tends to affect males in middle life. Electromyographic findings are those of continuous muscle activity at rest, the action potentials being of normal configuration. The syndrome is thought to be caused by impairment of the inhibitory control of the anterior horn cells, which is normally effected by specific interneurons of the inhibitory pathway of Renshaw (Howard, 1963; Olafson et al., 1964). Diazepam results in a dramatic symptomatic improvement (Howard, 1963; Sulway et al., 1970). Dysphagia, sometimes very severe, was observed in a few cases (Sulway et al., 1970). On radiological examination the motility disorders seemed to be located in the upper esophageal sphincter, which did not relax, and in the cervical esophagus, whereas the motility of the distal esophagus was normal (Sulway et al., 1970).

6. Dysautonomia

Familial dysautonomia (Riley-Day syndrome) is a congenital condition, frequently seen in siblings and occurring mostly in children of Jewish extraction. It is manifested by specific disturbances of the central nervous system. The most striking manifestations are disorders of autonomic functions, such as a diminished lacrimation, hyperhidrosis, transient skin blotching, abnormal swallowing reflexes, lability of blood pressure and instability of temperature control. Other features include poor motor coordination, dysarthria, relative insensivity to pain, hypoactive deep tendon reflexes and emotional instability (Riley, 1957). Sucking and swallowing difficulties are usually present from birth. Exceptionally dysphagia develops in later life (Margulies et al., 1968). These children are subject to recurrent pneumonia, presumably related to aspiration. The swallowing difficulties apparently are not caused by pharyngeal muscle weakness, but rather by delayed opening of the cricopharyngeal sphincter (Margulies et al., 1968). Linde and Westover (1962) noted that the esophagus had an atonic aspect and that esophageal emptying was delayed in the supine position, while emptying occurred promptly in the upright position. In other patients esophageal emptying is delayed even in the upright position and the radiological picture mimics that of achalasia. In two such patients a cardiomyotomy was performed and the intramural plexuses were found to be normal (Linde and Westover, 1962; Joseph and Job, 1963). Metacholine and prostigmine (Smith et al., 1965; Margulies et al., 1968) may improve some of these disorders.

Varying degrees of pylorospasm (KIRKPATRICK and RILEY, 1957; JOSEPH and JOB, 1963), small bowel distension (THIEFFRY et al., 1961) and megacolon (GROSSMAN et al., 1956) may also be present.

Dysautonomic syndromes in adults rarely cause dysphagia (SPARBERG et al., 1968). But even in patients with dysphagia the Mecholyl test is normal, suggesting that the myenteric plexus is unaffected.

References

BOSMA, J. F.: Studies of disability of the pharynx resultant from poliomyelitis. Ann. Otol. (St. Louis) **62**, 529–547 (1953).

BOSMA, J. F.: Studies of the pharynx. II. Poliomyelitic disabilities of the lower pharynx. Pediatrics **19**, 1053–1079 (1957a).

BOSMA, J. F.: Residual disability of pharyngeal area resulting from poliomyelitis. J. Amer. med. Ass. **165**, 216–221 (1957b).

BOSMA, J. F., BRODIE, D. R.: Disabilities of the pharynx in amyotrophic lateral sclerosis as demonstrated by cineradiography. Radiology **92**, 97–103 (1969).

BOUDIN, G., BARBIZET, J., HILLEMAND, B., LOTE, J.: Atonie et dilatation gastro-œsophagienne au cours de la sclérose latérale amyotrophique. Bull. Soc. méd. Hôp. Paris **2**, 641–648 (1954).

CALNE, D. B., SHAW, D. G., SPIERS, A. S. D., STERN, G. M.: Swallowing in parkinsonism. Brit. J. Radiol. **43**, 456–457 (1970).

COTZIAS, G. C., PAPAVASILIOU, P. S., GELLENE, R.: Modification of parkinsonism. Chronic treatment with L-dopa. New Engl. J. Med. **280**, 337–345 (1969).

CREAMER, B.: Motor disturbances of the esophagus. In: Handbook of physiology, sect. 6, Alimentary canal, vol. IV, Motility, ed. C. F. CODE, p. 2331–2343. Washington, D.C.: Amer. Physiol. Soc. 1968.

DALY, D. D., CODE, C. F., ANDERSEN, H. A.: Disturbances of swallowing and esophageal motility in patients with multiple sclerosis. Neurology (Minneap.) **12**, 250–256 (1962).

DONNER, M. W., SIEGEL, C. I.: The evaluation of pharyngeal neuromuscular disorders by cinefluorography. Amer. J. Roentgenol. **94**, 299–307 (1965).

DONNER, M. W., SILBIGER, M. L.: Cinefluorographic analysis of pharyngeal swallowing in neuromuscular disorders. Amer. J. med. Sci. **251**, 600–616 (1966).

EADIE, M. J., TYRER, J. H.: Alimentary disorder in parkinsonism. Aust. Ann. Med. **14**, 13–22 (1965a).

EADIE, M. J., TYRER, J. H.: Radiological abnormalities of the upper part of the alimentary tract in parkinsonism. Aust. Ann. Med. **14**, 23–27 (1965b).

FISCHER, R. A., ELLISON, G. W., THAYER, W. R., SPIRO, H. M., GLASER, G. H.: Esophageal motility in neuromuscular disorders. Ann. intern. Med. **63**, 229–248 (1965).

GORDON, E. E., JANUSZKO, D. M., KAUFMAN, L.: A critical survey of stiff-man syndrome. Amer. J. Med. **42**, 582–599 (1967).

GROSSMAN, H. J., LIMOSANI, M. A., SHORE, M.: Megacolon as a manifestation of familial autonomic dysfunction. J. Pediat. **49**, 289–296 (1956).

HOWARD, F. M., JR.: A new and effective drug in the treatment of stiff-man syndrome. Proc. Mayo Clin. **38**, 203–212 (1963).

JOSEPH, R., JOB, J.-C.: Dysautonomie familiale et mégaœsophage. Arch. franç. Pédiat. **20**, 25–33 (1963).

KIRKPATRICK, R. H., RILEY, C. M.: Roentgenographic findings in familial dysautonomia. Radiology 68, 654–660 (1957).

KRAMER, P., ATKINSON, M., WYMAN, S. M., INGELFINGER, F. J.: The dynamics of swallowing. II. Neuromuscular dysphagia of pharynx. J. clin. Inevst. **36**, 589–595 (1957).

LINDE, L. M., WESTOVER, J. L.: Esophageal and gastric abnormalities in dysautonomia. Pediatrics **29**, 303–306 (1962).

LUND, W. S.: A study of the cricopharyngeal sphincter in man and in the dog. Ann. roy. Coll. Surg. Engl. **37**, 225–246 (1965).

MARGULIES, S. I., BRUNT, P. W., DONNER, M. W., SILBIGER, M. L.: Familial dysautonomia. A cineradiographic study of the swallowing mechanism. Radiology 90, 107–112 (1968).

MERRITT, W. H., NIELSEN, M., BOSMA, J. F., GOATES, W. A., HASKINS, R., RAMSELL, C., LAMB, R. H.: Studies of the pharynx. III. Occlusion of the mesopharynx resulting from bulbar and cervical spinal poliomyelitis. Pediatrics **19**, 1080–1087 (1957).

MOERSCH, F. P., WOLTMAN, H. W.: Progressive fluctuating muscular rigidity and spasm (stiff-man syndrome). Proc. Mayo Clin. **31**, 421–427 (1956).

Olafson, R. A., Mulder, D. W., Howard, F. M.: Stiff-man syndrome: a review of the literature, report of three additional cases and discussion of pathophysiology and therapy. Proc. Mayo Clin. **39**, 131–144 (1964).

Oppenheim, H.: Text-book of nervous diseases for physicians and students, 5th ed., vol. 1, p. 220. London: T. N. Foulis 1911.

Riley, C. M.: Familial dysautonomia. Advanc. Pediat. **5**, 157–190 (1957).

Silbiger, M. L., Pikielney, R., Donner, M. W.: Neuromuscular disorders affecting the pharynx. Cineradiographic analysis. Invest. Radiol. **2**, 442–448 (1967).

Smith, A. A., Hirsch, J. I., Dancis, J.: Responses to infused methacholine in familial dysautonomia. Pediatrics **36**, 225–230 (1965).

Smith, A. W. M., Mulder, D. W., Code, C. F.: Esophageal motility in amyotrophic lateral sclerosis. Proc. Mayo Clin. **52**, 438–441 (1957).

Sparberg, M., Knudsen, K. B., Frank, S. T.: Dysautonomia and dysphagia. Neurology (Minneap.) **18**, 504–506 (1968).

Sulway, M. J., Baume, P. E., Davis, E.: Stiff-man syndrome presenting with complete esophageal obstruction. Amer. J. dig. Dis. **15**, 79–84 (1970).

Thieffry, S., Joseph, R., Martin, C., Job, J. C., Lortholary, P.: La dysautonomie familiale (syndrome de Riley-Day): symptômes habituels et manifestations atypiques. Arch. franç. Pédiat. **18**, 194–212 (1961).

Walker, J., Singer, K., Baker, P.: Disorders of esophageal motility in a family with hereditary spastic ataxia. Neurology (Minneap.) **19**, 1212–1216 (1969).

Motor Disorders Due to Peripheral Nerve Lesions

J. Hellemans and G. Vantrappen

1. Motor Disorders Associated with Diabetes

Mandelstam and Lieber (1967) found cineradiographic evidence of esophageal motor dysfunction in 12 out of 14 patients with diabetic neuropathy-gastroenteropathy. The primary peristaltic wave was found to be absent or markedly weakened, esophageal emptying was delayed when the patient was recumbent and tertiary contractions were observed. 11 of these patients had gastric motor dysfunction. On manometric examination the amplitude of the pharyngeal and esophageal pressure waves was decreased, primary peristaltic contractions were present in only 45% of the swallows, which were often followed by tertiary contractions, and the resting pressure in the gastroesophageal sphincter was lowered. Bailey et al. (1969) examined 15 diabetic patients and found similar disorders, correlating with the existence of peripheral neuropathies.

In non-selected diabetic patients some authors also found motility disorders, while others did not. Vela and Balart (1970) observed in diabetic patients without visceral neuropathy marked incoordination in the mid-esophagus together with a marked reduction of pressure in the lower esophageal sphincter. The results of studies on the lower esophageal sphincter function in diabetics are still controversial (Vela and Balart, 1970; Horgan and Doyle, 1969, 1971). Further studies using yield pressure measurements and adequate normal controls are necessary to resolve the apparent contradictions.

On cineradiographic studies, Vix (1969) found normal peristaltic contractions to be absent in one third of his diabetic patients. In patients who had had diabetes for four years or more, the incidence of this disorder was 50%. Neuropathy occurred with the same frequency in patients with normal or abnormal motility. Thusfar no consensus has been reached as to whether there is any connection between esophageal motility disorders and the presence of peripheral or even local esophageal neuropathy.

Post-mortem examination of a severely dysphagic diabetic revealed no abnormality and the esophageal myenteric plexus appeared normal (Mandelstam and Lieber, 1967). Rundles (1945), however, did find degenerative changes in the nerve trunks of the esophageal plexus in two patients with gastrointestinal symptoms, but these observations were not confirmed later (Hensley and Soergel, 1968).

There is no doubt that some diabetics have a markedly disordered motility, both of the esophagus (Mandelstam et al., 1969) and of other parts of the gastrointestinal tract. The diabetics described by Mandelstam et al. (1969), however, were pre-selected on the basis of symptoms of neuropathy-gastroenteropathy; yet only a few of these patients had esophageal symptoms. Therefore, dysphagia in the diabetic should not be ascribed to neuropathy, unless the other well-known causes have been excluded first (Goyal and Spiro, 1970).

2. Motor Disturbances Associated with Alcoholic Neuropathy

In patients with peripheral neuropathy secondary to chronic alcoholism, the peristaltic mechanism of the esophagus markedly deteriorates. Simultaneous contractions are frequent especially in the distal esophagus. The lower esophageal sphincter seems to function normally (Winship et al., 1968). Besides neuropathies, alcoholism also seems to cause myopathies (Perkoff et al., 1967) so that it may be difficult to determine whether nervous or muscular lesions are responsible for the motility disorders of the esophagus.

When performing manometric studies it is better to perfuse the catheters with water rather than with bourbon whiskey, as the latter is liable to influence the results. Peroral administration of 300 ml of 86 proof bourbon whiskey over a period of one hour (which equals the administration of 103.5 g ethanol) results in a disturbed peristaltic progression, particularly in the lower third of the esophagus. The yield pressures of upper and lower sphincters are increased. In addition, technical difficulties due to persistent singultus of the subject can be expected (Viegas de Andrade et al., 1969; Hogan et al., 1972). Fortunately motility returns to normal after about 8 hours.

References

Bailey, R., Langille, D., Sidorov, J. J.: Esophageal dysfunction in diabetes mellitus (abstract). Gastroenterology 56, 1136 (1969).

Goyal, R. K., Spiro, H. M.: Esophageal function in diabetes mellitus. Ann. intern. Med. 72, 281–282 (1970).

Hensley, G. T., Soergel, K. H.: Neuropathologic findings in diabetic diarrhoea. Arch. Path. 85, 587–597 (1968).

Hogan, W. J., Viegas de Andrade, S. R., Winship, D. H.: Ethanol-induced acute esophageal motor dysfunction. J. appl. Physiol. 32, 755–760 (1972).

Horgan, J., Doyle, J. S.: Manometric oesophageal motility studies in diabetics without neuropathy. Irish J. med. Sci. 62, 475–480 (1969).

Horgan, J. H., Doyle, J. S.: A comparative study of esophageal motility in diabetics with neuropathy. Dis. Chest 60, 170–174 (1971).

Mandelstam, P., Lieber, A.: Esophageal dysfunction in diabetic neuropathy-gastroenteropathy. Clinical and roentgenological manifestations. J. Amer. med. Ass. 201, 582–586 (1967).

Mandelstam, P., Siegel, C. I., Lieber, A., Siegel, M.: The swallowing disorder in patients with diabetic neuropathy-gastroenteropathy. Gastroenterology 56, 1–12 (1969).

Perkoff, G. T., Dioso, M. M., Bleisch, V., Klinkerfuss, G.: A spectrum of myopathy associated with alcoholism. I. Clinical and laboratory features. Ann. intern. Med. 67, 481–492 (1967).

Rundles, R. W.: Diabetic neuropathy (general review with report of 125 cases). Medicine (Baltimore) 24, 111–160 (1945).

Vela, A. R., Balart, L. A.: Esophageal motor manifestations in diabetes mellitus. Amer. J. Surg. 119, 21–26 (1970).

Viegas de Andrade, S. R., Hogan, W. J., Winship, D. H.: Esophageal motor dysfunction in man following acute alcohol ingestion (abstract). Gastroenterology 56, 1204 (1969).

Vix, V. A.: Esophageal motility in diabetes mellitus. Radiology 92, 363–364 (1969).

Winship, D. H., Caflisch, C. R., Zboralske, F. F., Hogan, W. J.: Deterioration of esophageal peristalsis in patients with alcoholic neuropathy. Gastroenterology 55, 173–178 (1968).

Emotional Disorders of the Esophagus

H. Monges and A. Hancy

With 6 Figures

1. Globus Hystericus

1.1. Definition and Generalities

Certain subjects, in general with a psychopathological background, complain about a permanent "lump" or "foreign body" in their throat. This sensation is called globus hystericus when, as is usually the case, no local lesion or motor disorder of the pharyngoesophageal region can be detected. The name indicates that the symptom is considered as a manifestation of a neurotic trouble. It has been known for a long time and was already mentioned in the Hippocratic treatises.

1.2. Clinical Findings

The symptom is found in adolescents and adults of all ages, but occurs mostly in subjects in their fifties, especially in menopausal women. The subjects always have emotional disorders (such as fear of cancer, domestical problems, etc.) and are sometimes real psychopaths. The globus sensation is described by the patient in a stereotype way and with a lot of details: his throat feels tight; in it a lump moves up and down, which may get blocked, and sometimes may give a chocking impression. The patients always localize their sensations at the same level: deep in the throat at the lower part of the neck, behind the upper portion of the sternum. The sensation is generally more a discomfort than a real pain. Subjects say they experience it either intermittently, especially during periods of nervous tension, or almost permanently. A constant factor, of considerable diagnostic value, is that the sensation disappears upon swallowing either solid food or liquids. In general patients are not aware of this fact, and are surprised to discover it. These patients often end up concentrating their attention on their "symptom" with such an intensity that it becomes a real obsession. They analyse it continuously to find the most bizarre interpretations, and keep on performing buccopharyngeal movements only to make things worse and worse.

1.3. Diagnosis

The way a subject describes his symptom may often be so typical as to suggest the diagnosis of globus hystericus. Endoscopic, radiologic and manometric examinations of the oropharynx are necessary to rule out the presence of organic lesions and motor disturbances, particularly in the pharynx and pharyngoesophageal sphincter.

Lesions that may cause sensations similar to those of a globus hystericus include chronic pharyngitis secondary to smoking, a small Zenker's diverticulum, cervical arthrosis and motor disturbances of the pharyngoesophageal region secondary to neurologic lesions or myopathies.

1.4. Interpretation

Usually globus hystericus is considered a neurotic disorder of a purely psychogenic nature. According to MALCOMSON (1966), the rich innervation of the oropharynx could explain why in anxious or moderately psychopathic persons any sensation at this level gives rise to the feeling of a lump. JONES (1938), quoted by MALCOMSON (1966), showed that the inflation of a small balloon at the level of the oropharynx always results in the sensation of a lump. SCHATZKI (1964), on the other hand, believes that a physiological mechanism rather than a psychological one is responsible for the symptom, and therefore proposes to drop the name "globus hystericus", replacing it by "globus sensation".

Repeated swallowing of saliva and, when no more saliva is available, repeated dry swallows would result in a globus sensation. However, the neurotic personality seems to be the primary cause, as anxiety or emotion creates in these objects a compelling need to swallow. Whatever the interpretation, globus hystericus always appears to be connected with a neurotic personality.

1.5. Treatment

Psychotherapeutic treatment should try to convince the subject that there is no organic lesion whatsoever. Tranquilizers and neuroleptics will be used to treat the neurotic part of the disorder. Seldom, however, will one be able to relieve the patient completely of his symptom.

2. Esophageal Belching

2.1. Definition

The noisy aspiration of air into the esophagus and its subsequent noisy rejection is called esophageal eructation. Thus the etymological sense of this term, which only implies a rejection of air, has been widened. In esophageal eructation or esophageal belching the air does not penetrate beyond the cardia and is aspirated voluntarily, although almost subconsciously, once this maneuver has become a habit. Both events often occur in series. Belching, on the other hand, consists of the rejection of swallowed air from the stomach.

2.2. Etiology

Esophageal eructation is usually observed in emotionally unstable and anxious subjects, who induce it to get relief from a sensation of epigastric fullness. The disorder is accentuated during periods of nervous tension. Hysterical persons use this phenomenon to catch the attention of their surroundings. Adolescents, particularly students living in community, may perform it as a play to amuse their friends.

2.3. Clinical Findings

Patients are usually convinced that their eructations are an involuntary phenomenon caused by some underlying disease. The voluntary nature of the disorder appears from the fact that it can be induced and stopped on command.

Often esophageal eructations become a habit and a patient may provoke them almost unconsciously. Persuaded that eructations bring some relief, some patients will repeat them again and again, thus perpetuating their problem and provoking others such as tearing, tachycardia, fainting, abdominal pain resulting from contractions of abdominal and diaphragmatic muscles, a sensation of esophageal and gastric distension, and hypersalivation. The disorder is particularly intense when on each aspiration a certain amount of air penetrates beyond the cardia, is not expelled during the next rejection, and accumulates in the stomach, causing gastric distension and finally belching. Aspiration and rejection are accompanied by sounds of a different tonality. The first is in general shorter and less sonorous, although in some cases the opposite is true. Patients usually attribute both sounds to air being expelled from their stomach.

2.4. Pathophysiology

Clinical observations indicate that esophageal eructation comprises the following maneuvers: To aspirate air the mouth is opened, the chin is slightly lowered and the neck is extended to straighten the esophagus and to facilitate the opening of the pharyngoesophageal sphincter. The subject then suddenly inhales while

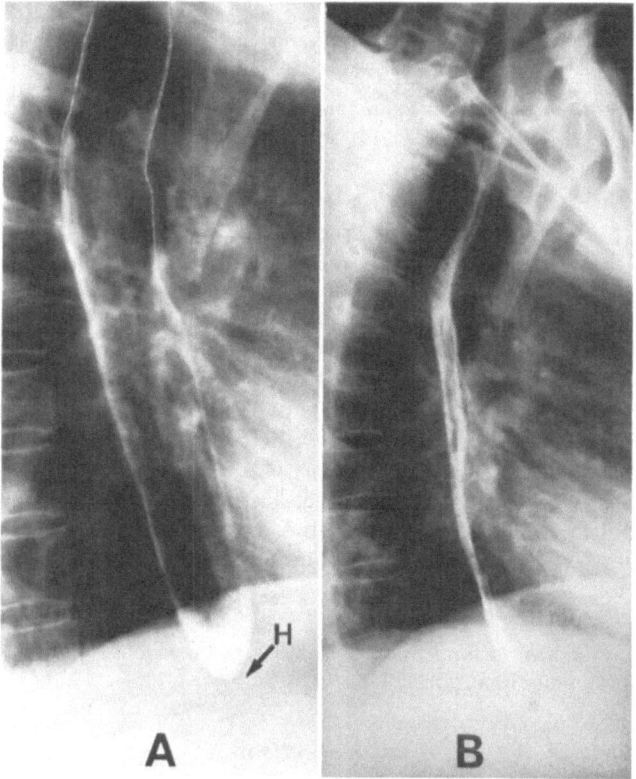

Fig. 203A and B. Esophageal belching. A Aspiration of air. The entire thoracic esophagus is distended by the aspirated air; the contraction of the hiatal ring (H) caused by inspiration against a closed glottis prevents the air from penetrating into the stomach. B Expulsion of air. During expiration, the entire gullet suddenly collapses, expelling the air through the upper esophageal sphincter

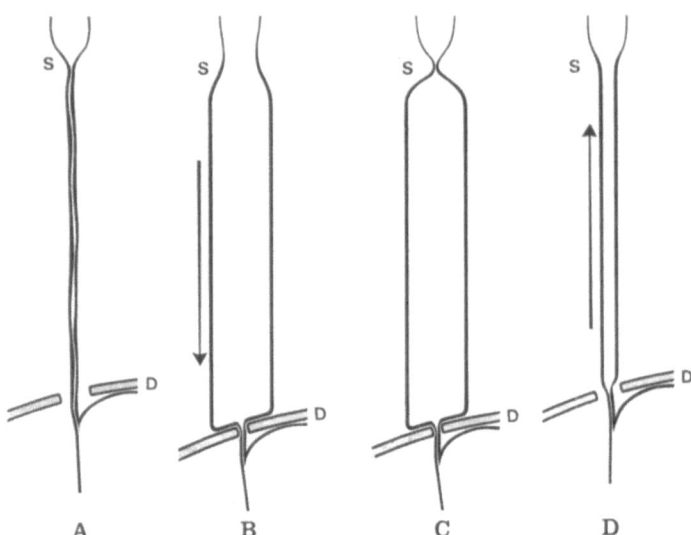

Fig. 204 A–D. Scheme showing the different phases of esophageal belching (S upper esophageal sphincter; D diaphragm). A The esophagus before the maneuver. B and C Inspiration against a closed glottis decreases the intrathoracic pressure and sucks air through the
open upper esophageal sphincter into the distended gullet. The diaphragmatic pinchcock
action prevents the air from penetrating into the stomach. C When the distended thoracic
esophagus is filled, the upper esophageal sphincter closes. D On expiration air is expelled
through the upper esophageal sphincter

the glottis is closed. This manifests itself by a lowering of the thyroid cartilage,
a depression of the fossae supraclaviculares and suprasternalis, a tightening of
the sternomastoid muscles and a projection of the thorax. The intrathoracic
vacuum thus created causes air to penetrate suddenly into the esophagus. This
aspiration is accompanied by a noise of variable intensity, resulting from the
vibration of air passing the pharyngoesophageal sphincter.

After the aspiration the subject expels the air through mouth and nose,
producing again a sound which will last for some time, depending upon the
rate of air expulsion.

Some subjects swallow after having elevated their chin and extended their
neck. The deglutition permits the opening of the upper esophageal sphincter,
and is manifested by an elevation of the thyroid cartilage. This elevation is
immediately followed by a lowering of the thyroid cartilage due to the aspiration
against a closed glottis.

Radioscopic examination, and especially radiocinematography reveal the
following phenomena (Figs. 203, 204).

a) Aspiration

Deep inspiration against a closed glottis lowers the diaphragm and abruptly
distends the thoracic esophagus over its total length, which is then "illuminated"
by the entering air. The diaphragmatic contraction caused by aspiration with
closed glottis squeezes the esophagus at the level of the hiatus, so that the air
column is generally unable to enter the stomach. The upper esophageal sphincter,

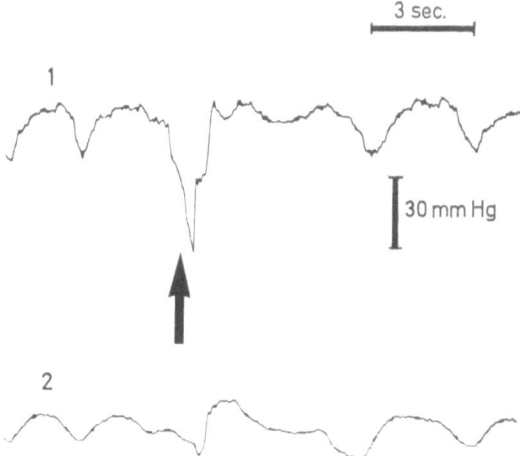

Fig. 205. Manometric registration of esophageal belching. Trace 1: Intraluminal pressure recorded in the middle third of the esophagus by means of an open-tip catheter. Trace 2: Pneumogram. The aspiration of air is accompanied by a sudden fall of intraluminal pressure in the thoracic esophagus, followed by a return to the basal pressure during the expulsion of air

which was open during aspiration, closes and because the inspiration is maintained the thoracic esophagus remains distended and filled with air.

b) Eructation

During expiration the esophagus collapses suddenly and simultaneously over its total length, while air escapes through the upper esophageal sphincter. Usually air does not enter the stomach. In some cases, however, a small amount of air gets trapped into the stomach on every aspiration; the gastric air bubble will gradually increase until the elevated pressure in the stomach causes gastric eructation.

Intraluminal pressure measurements in the middle third of the esophagus indicate that the pressure falls abruptly during aspiration, to increase again and stay at a plateau of elevated pressure during eructation (Fig. 205).

These observations indicate that in esophageal eructation the air first penetrates into the esophagus by aspiration, after an intraesophageal vacuum has been created by inspiration against a closed glottis. When the inspiratory effort is stopped, the forces that produced the distension of the esophagus are no longer active and expiration results in a collapse of the esophagus. This is associated with a noisy expulsion of air through the mouth.

2.5. Treatment

One will explain to the subject that his symptoms are not related to or caused by a serious pathological condition, but are provoked voluntarily by himself, and that he himself creates or maintains the symptoms he thinks to relieve. One will show him that he is indeed able to control the phenomenon. The symptomatic treatment will be directed against the digestive complaints which led the patient to start his bad habit. Sedatives and tranquilizers are indicated but in general, treatment fails.

3. Eructation or Belching

3.1. Definition

Eructation consists of the noisy rejection through the mouth of air from the stomach.

Deglutition of solids, liquids or saliva is always accompanied by a variable amount of air penetrating into the stomach. Rejection of part of this air is a physiological phenomenon, occurring from time to time in normal subjects, particularly in children during the postprandial period. In some subjects belching is so frequent as to become very uncomfortable. These frequent eructations may be due to an incompetent gastroesophageal sphincter mechanism, particularly in patients with a sliding hernia. Mostly, however, the disorder is related to the presence of an excessive amount of air in the stomach. Such a situation may arise in aerophagia (i.e. the excessive swallowing of air in emotionally unstable and anxious persons who are eating too rapidly or swallowing saliva excessively) or in some cases of esophageal eructation. In aerophagia as well as in esophageal belching, the gastric distension is provoked to get the relief afforded by belching. Because of the sensation of well-being associated with eructation, some patients will try to repeat it again and again.

It should be noted that the amount of air tolerated in the gastric fundus is quite variable. Some patients eructate even when the gastric air bubble is small, whereas others tolerate a large amount of air without discomfort.

3.2. Mechanism of Eructation

The mechanism of eructation has not yet been elucidated. It is difficult to study spontaneous belching by radiocinematography, because of its short duration and its infrequent occurrence. Eructations induced by insufflation of air into the stomach or by ingestion of gas-producing beverages may be different from spontaneous belching, because the degree of gastric distension required to induce these eructations is considerably greater than that of spontaneous belching. When the subject feels the desire to eructate he slowly takes in a deep breath and at the end stretches the thorax and closes the glottis (BOTHA, 1962). Then, while the glottis remains closed, gas is felt to leave the stomach, the glottis opens, expiration starts and gas escapes through mouth and nose, producing the characteristic noise and relieving the pre-existing discomfort.

The mechanism which opens the cardia during belching remains unclear. The esophagogastric pressure gradient may play a role: the inspiration followed by closure of the glottis increases the intragastric pressure and lowers the intraesophageal pressure. The increase of intragastric and intracolonic pressure during eructation indicates a contraction of the somatic muscles (McNALLY et al., 1954). BOTHA (1962) believes that the lowering of the diaphragm during inspiration will stretch the thorax, open the angle of His and move the cardia up into the hiatus. This upward movement of the cardia has been clearly demonstrated by JOHNSON (1966). According to BOTHA (1962) relaxation of the lower esophageal sphincter, mediated by extrinsic nerves, plays a very important role in the mechanism that allows air to escape from the stomach to the esophagus.

Radiological examination indicates (Fig. 206) that eructation is associated with a regression of the air bubble, a widening of the lower esophagus which now freely communicates with the stomach and a complete abolition of the angle of His.

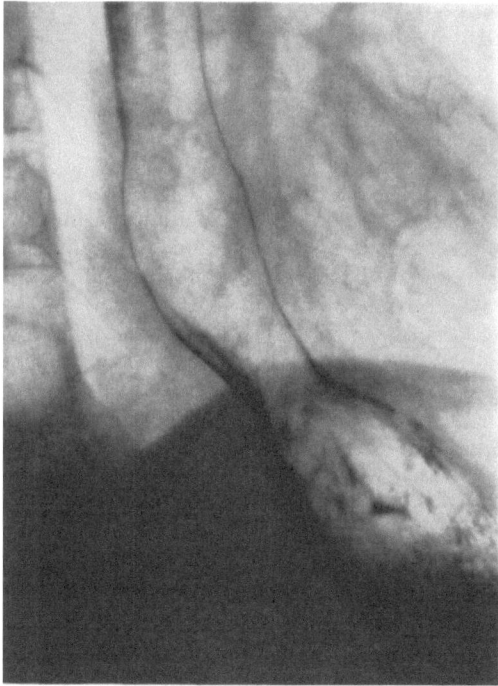

Fig. 206. Belching. The cardia is wide open, the angle of His is obtuse and the esophagus is distended by air coming from the stonach

3.3. Treatment

One should explain to the patient the nature of his disorder and reassure him that there is no serious underlying disease. Mild sedatives and tranquilizers may be helpful.

4. Merycism or Rumination

The term merycism is used to describe the voluntary act of regurgitation of gastric contents back into the mouth without nausea or vomiting. The regurgitated food is chewed and swallowed again. Thus the different stages of rumination in herbivores are accomplished. Although merycism may become a habit, the voluntary character of the phenomenon, which distinguishes it from spontaneous regurgitation and vomiting, should be stressed. Subjects who chew food after involuntary regurgitation should not be considered as merycists. Merycism was already described by ARISTOTLE and GALEN. During the last two decades its physiopathological mechanism (NEMOURS-AUGUSTE, 1953; BERNARD, 1956; MONGES et al., 1959, 1960; GEFFEN, 1966; BROWN, 1968) and the psychosomatic problems related to merycism in infancy (RICHMOND et al., 1958; FULLERTON, 1963; AUBRY et al., 1964; KREISLER, 1966) have been studied.

4.1. Merycism in Infants

Infants often regurgitate food, chew and swallow it again. Usually the phenomenon is without any clinical significance and need not be considered a serious problem. It may be hard to tell, however, whether one is dealing with a case of merycism or with spontaneous involuntary regurgitations. True merycism in infancy is a voluntary rumination which occurs regularly after feeding. It is a rare disorder of behavior but has serious consequences if not treated in the appropriate way.

4.1.1. Clinical Data

Merycism occurs usually in male, predominantly bottle-fed babies at the age of 6–8 months. In general no constitutional disorder is present. It is performed after feedings when the baby is alone or thinks he is, and is stopped as soon as he knows he is being observed.

The regurgitation is accomplished by a series of complex movements involving the pharynx as well as the thoracic and abdominal musculature. These movements are difficult to analyse, but are identical with those performed by adult merycists. After prolonged mastication, part of the food is swallowed, while part of it freely runs out of the mouth or is expectorated. Close observation indicates that regurgitation is obtained voluntarily because of the pleasure and the sensation of well-being it offers to the infant. Indeed, expression and attitude during rumination are very particular. At first tension and dissatisfaction is shown on his face, while he attempts to regurgitate. This changes to an expression of beatitude during the chewing of the regurgitated food. The infant is completely absorbed in his activities, immobilized and insensitive to the external world. Due to the continuous loss of food, rumination will quickly lead to a general malaise with serious consequences, including hypotrophism, dehydration and disorders of the electrolyte and protein balance. If not corrected by appropriate treatment, no spontaneous regression will occur and the state of denutrition will finally lead to death.

Merycism may pass unrecognized for a long time, which explains its gravity. Rumination is often mistaken for vomiting, gastroesophageal reflux or food intolerance. The diagnosis is only possible by close clinical observation which will reveal the voluntary nature of the regurgitations, starting when the child thinks to be alone, and stopping as soon one pays attention to him.

4.1.2. Interpretation

The mechanism of regurgitation in infant merycists is identical to that of adult merycists. The most interesting problem, however, is why infants start to ruminate and why they like to do it.

Neuropsychiatric studies indicate that merycism in infancy is due to disturbances in the mother-child relationship. (RICHMOND et al., 1958; FULLERTON, 1963; AUBRY et al., 1964; KREISLER, 1966). Lack of affection of the mother for her child will cause the infant to turn into himself, excluding the external world and having no object of interest and occupation other than his own body. Rumination starts as a deviated oral autoerotic instinct and becomes permanent due to the satisfaction it provides. To some extent merycism should therefore be related to other autoerotic manifestations such as thumb-sucking, continuous balancing of the head, or repeated drumming with the fingers. The somatic orientation of the symptom may result from previous libidinal experiences such as vomiting.

Arguments in favor of this interpretation are derived from observations and psychological studies of the infants' mothers. Occurring in general in babies who were breast-fed only for a very short time or not at all, merycism starts around 6–8 months, the age at which differentiated relations with its surroundings are established. At this age infants recognize their mother visually, and strongly need contact and affection. Mothers incapable of providing warm, comfortable and intimate physical care or mothers who simply dislike their babies will deprive the infant of the stimulating relationships it needs and predispose it to the disorder. The personality of the mother is almost always abnormal and/or immature (RICHMOND et al., 1958). They are psychotically regressed and have often remained in the Oedipus-stage in their relationships with their fathers (AUBRY et al., 1964). Such an interpretation is confirmed therapeutically, as the only efficacious treatment consists in the establishment of affective relationships. Playing with the child, distracting and comforting it, will free it from its autistic retreat, and restore normal psychic and social behavior.

4.1.3. Treatment

All symptomatic treatments, re-animation or dietetics are completely inefficient. The same holds for intimidation. Only after re-establishment of normal mother-infant relationships does the disorder disappear. If the child is hospitalized and merycism diagnosed, a nurse should be assigned to it to provide the special attention it needs. The nature of the disorder should be explained to the mother before returning the child to her. Sometimes the mother may need psychotherapy.

The symptom disappears always within a few days. Although other auto-erotic activities such as thumb-sucking may survive, rumination will stop completely and definitely.

4.2. Merycism in Adults

Only a few individuals are capable to regurgitate voluntarily and without effort. Often the name merycist is given to people who chew and swallow regurgitated food after meals, but who are incapable of reproducing these regurgitations on command, though they claim they are able to do so. It is difficult to be sure whether one has to do with real merycism or with regurgitation in such cases. Real merycism is extremely rare.

4.2.1. Clinical Data

Some patients practice it during the postprandial period because of the pleasure they derive from chewing and tasting their food again. Generally the patient brings up a small amount of food, part of which is immediately swallowed again; he keeps in his mouth but a few pieces which he chews again and swallows afterwards. This rumination is done sometimes after each meal and lasts for some time; it is stopped when the regurgitated material turns acid. Certain subjects who ruminate are embarrassed for social reasons, but most of them are not and derive great satisfaction from ruminating. Some say they were quite upset during the period they lost their peculiar ability. It is difficult for them to determine for how long they have been ruminating; generally they claim they have always done it. Quite often they are surprised on learning that theirs is an odd ability, for they think that everybody can regurgitate food after meals. Several cases in the same family have been reported, sometimes affecting more than one generation. One report on merycism in twins has been published (MONGES et al., 1960).

Merycism entails no clinical consequences. The individuals do not even complain about spontaneous regurgitations or heartburn. Merycism is usually considered a characteristic of markedly neurotic or psychopathic subjects; others think it is a sign of mental degeneration. In reality it is found in psychologically normal subjects, who may even be very intelligent.

Other merycists exercise their talents in public performances. Such individuals would never use their talent to regurgitate food; instead they present atonishing performances. For instance they fill their stomach with great quantities of water which they regurgitate in numerous spurts or one single stream; they swallow frogs, goldfish and other objects which they store in their stomach and bring up on request.

4.2.2. Mechanism

Merycists have no morphological anomaly of the esophagus or stomach. On radiological examination the gastric function is found to be normal and there is no gastroesophageal reflux. The merycist is incapable of analyzing or describing the movements he makes to provoke regurgitation, although he knows that certain movements will do so. When requested to ruminate the subject will immobilize himself and his expression shows he is concentrating. Suddenly he takes a deep inspiration against a closed glottis; almost at the same time his abdominal muscles contract. These movements are often accompanied by others, difficult to analyze and varying from one subject to another, though always the same in one given subject (pivoting of the thorax, shrugging of one shoulder). All these movements last for only a short moment and are followed immediately by the arrival of gastric contents in the mouth.

Few satisfactory radiological studies of merycism are available. Merycists capable to provoke regurgitation when their stomach is filled with barium are hard to find. We have been able to perform radiological and radiocinematographic studies of 4 merycists (2 cases published: Monges et al., 1959, 1960), who could regurgitate at will whether their gastric content consisted of food or barium. The same phenomena were observed in each case (Figs. 207, 208). The movements performed to provoke regurgitation (inspiration against a closed glottis and abdominal contraction) entailed a brusk thrust of the cardia into the thorax followed instantaneously by reflux of barium, which entered the esophagus and part of which reached the mouth. While it was filled with barium the esophagus was considerably distended, but no antiperistaltic contraction took place. As soon as the subject stopped the inspiration against a closed glottis and the abdominal contraction, the small temporary hiatal hernia disappeared and the barium which had not reached the mouth fell back into the stomach. Apart from the small temporary hiatal hernia during the ruminating movement the esophagogastric junctional zone was completely normal. In particular there was no hiatal hernia and no gastroesophageal reflux.

Two factors contribute to bringing the food into the mouth: the negative intrathoracic pressure produced by inspiration against a closed glottis aspirates the food into the thorax; the positive intragastric pressure caused by the contraction of diaphragmatic and abdominal muscles pushes the food upwards. Another factor is needed to provoke or facilitate the opening of the cardia, which is necessary to allow regurgitation. Without it everybody could become a merycist with a little exercise. The small temporary hiatal hernia, described above, favors the opening of the cardia (Monges et al., 1959, 1960). However, an insufficient number of radiological observations is available to state that this temporary hiatal hernia is a constant phenomenon in merycists. Maybe certain subjects manage to control the tonus of the lower esophageal sphincter and to open the

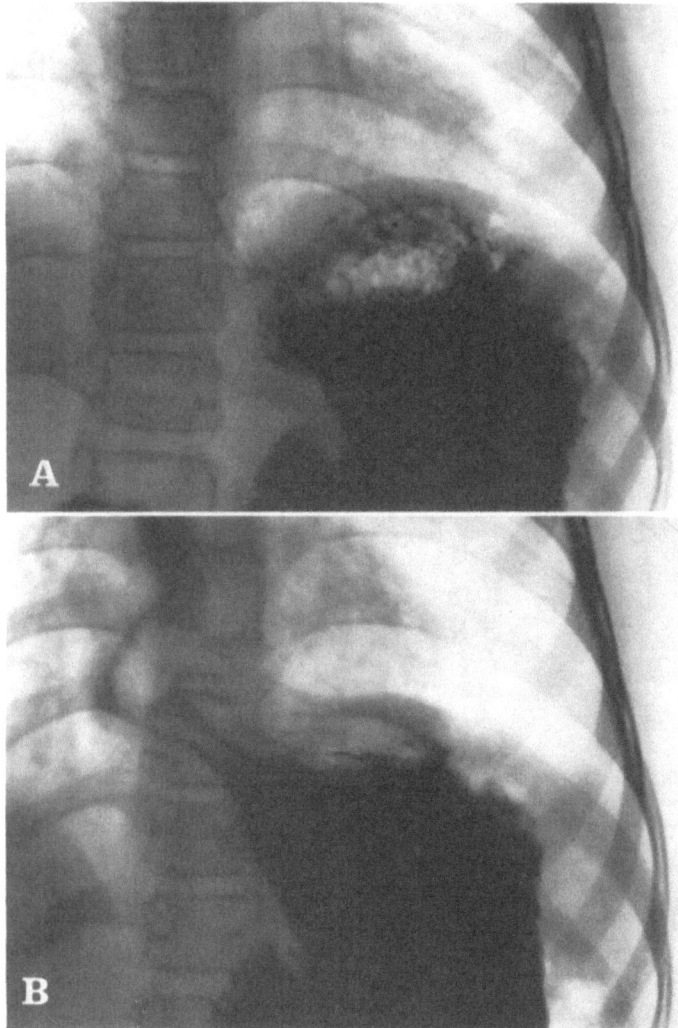

Fig. 207 A and B. Merycism. The subject is in the upright position. A Before the regurgitation the stomach has a normal radiological appearance. B During the regurgitation a small hiatal hernia is formed, the lower esophagus is twisted and displaced to the right by the cardia lodging in the hiatus, and barium flows back into the esophagus

cardia when they want to ruminate. Numerous studies on the relation between the cerebrospinal and the autonomic nervous system as well as psychosomatic studies have shown indeed that some individuals under certain circumstances are able to control this autonomic nervous system (some subjects can influence their skin temperature, their pulse, etc.).

4.2.3. Treatment

Some patients, embarrassed by their habit, ask for treatment. They should be told that they provoke their regurgitations voluntarily, though they believe

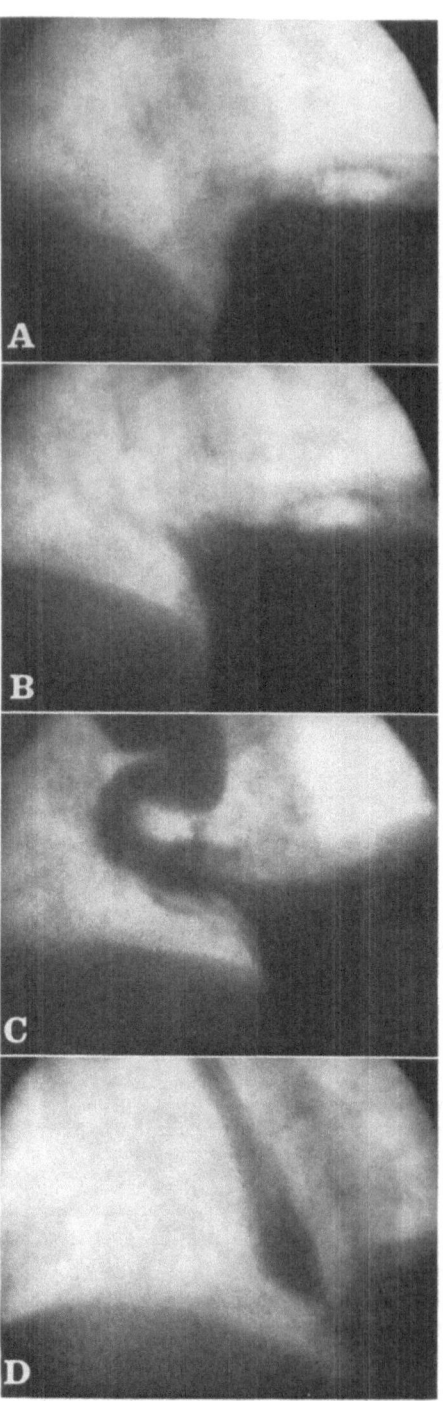

Fig. 208A–D. Radiocinematographic pictures of rumination in the same subject as in Fig. 207. The subject is in the upright left anterior oblique position. A and B Onset. The inspiration against a closed glottis and the contraction of the abdominal musculature flatten the gastric fundus and push part of the barium towards the cardia. C The cardia is propelled into the hiatus and barium flows into the esophagus. Note the torsion of the esophagus and its displacement to the right. D After the regurgitation, lower esophagus and cardia have returned to their normal position. The barium that has not been expelled through the mouth re-enters the stomach

the opposite. They must be convinced that they can refrain from performing them. Mostly, however, the merycist derives satisfaction from his condition and does not ask to be treated.

References

AUBRY, J., DALLOZ, J. C., LAJEUNESSE, B. S., DE BEAUREPAIRE, E.: Le mérycisme. Arch franç. Pédiat. **21**, 1097–1104 (1964).

BERNARD, A.: Sur le mécanisme de la rumination; rôle de l'aspiration thoracique. Arch. franç. Mal. Appar. dig. **44**, 780–785 (1955).

BERNARD, A.: Identité du mécanisme pathogénique de l'aérophagie, du mérycisme, des vomissements et de la toux émétisante. Rôle essentiel de l'aspiration thoracique. Sem. Hôp. Paris **32**, 1006–1015 (1956).

BOTHA, G. S. M.: The gastroesophageal junction. London: J. & A.Churchill, Ltd. 1962.

BROWN, W. R.: Rumination in the adult; a study of two cases. Gastroenterology **54**, 933–939 (1968).

FULLERTON, D. T.: Infantile rumination. A case report. Arch. gen. Psychiat. **9**, 595–600 (1963).

GEFFEN, N.: Rumination in man. Report of a case. Amer. J. dig. Dis. **11**, 963–972 (1966).

GUTMANN, R. A.: Les syndromes douloureux de la région épigastrique, tome II. Paris: Doin 1952.

JOHNSON, H. D., LAWS, J. W.: The cardia in swallowing, eructation, and vomiting. Lancet **1966 II**, 1268–1273.

JONES, C. M.: Digestive tract pain. New York: McMillan 1938.

KREISLER, L.: Le mérycisme. Psychiat. infantile **9**, 157–178 (1966).

MALCOMSON, K. G.: Radiological findings in globus hystericus. Brit. J. Radiol. **39**, 583–586 (1966).

McNALLY, E. F., KELLY, J. E., JR., INGELFINGER, F. J.: Mechanism of belching: Effects of gastric distension with air. Gastroenterology **46**, 254–259 (1954).

MONGES, H., LEGRE, M., VIGNOLI, R.: Aérophagie. Encyclopédie Médico-Chirurgicale, vol. Estomac-Intestin. Paris: Editions Techniques 1965.

MONGES, H., MONGES, A., COIGNET, J.: Etude d'un cas de mérycisme (avec présentation d'un film radiocinématographique). Arch. franç. Mal. Appar. dig. **48**, 364–371 (1959).

MONGES, H., MONGES, A., LEGRE, M.: Etude radiocinématographique d'un nouveau cas de mérycisme. Arch. franç. Mal. Appar. dig. **49**, 961–968 (1960).

NEMOURS-AUGUSTE, A.: Remarques cliniques et radiologiques sur 9 cas de mérycisme. Arch. franç. Mal. Appar. dig. **42**. 833–836 (1953).

RICHMOND, J. B., EDDY, E., GREEN, M.: Rumination: A psychosomatic syndrome of infancy. Pediatrics **22**, 49–55 (1958).

RIGBY, R. G.: The present status of globus hystericus. Laryngoscope (St. Louis) **62**, 401–405 (1952).

ROTH, J. L. A., BOCKUS, H. L.: Aerophagia: its etiology and syndromes and management. Med. Clin. N. Amer. **41**, 1673–1696 (1957).

SCHATZKI, R.: Globus hystericus (globus sensation). New Engl. J. Med. **270**, 676 (1964).

The Pathophysiological Basis of Gastroesophageal and Intestinoesophageal Reflux

P. Heitmann

1. The Gastroesophageal Closing Mechanism

Gastric contents are not normally present in the distal esophagus. Gastroesophageal and intestinoesophageal reflux occur when normal mechanisms fail to prevent the retrograde flow of gastric contents into the esophagus during the intervals between swallows, especially in the recumbent position. This may occur transiently under normal physiological conditions. However, the prolonged contact of gastric or intestinal secretions with the esophageal mucosa is pathological and leads to severe complications. These are due either to the chemical action of the refluxed material on the esophageal wall or to aspiration of esophageal contents into the airways.

Three main mechanisms contribute to the normal competence of the gastroesophageal junctional zone and to the avoidance of prolonged reflux: an intrinsic sphincter located in the lowermost esophagus, the relation of this structure to the hiatus, and the ability of the esophagus to clear itself rapidly from any refluxed material. The relative importance of each factor is still controversial.

The site of the barrier to reflux is normally located in the distalmost segment of the esophagus. The existence of an anatomical lower esophageal sphincter in man is not universally accepted, although special oblique or circular muscle bundle arrangements have been described (VANTRAPPEN et al., 1960; LEPOW, 1962; FRIEDLAND et al., 1966; STELZNER and LIERSE, 1968). Intraluminal pressure measurements with water-filled non-perfused catheters have shown the presence of a zone of increased resting pressure in the lower 2 to 4 cm of the esophagus. This zone was defined as the physiologic gastroesophageal sphincter (FYKE et al., 1956). This type of measurements has resulted in qualitative descriptions of gastroesophageal sphincteric behavior in normal and pathologic conditions, which were summarized by CODE and SCHLEGEL (1968) and by CREAMER (1968). However, a quantitative correlation of resting sphincteric pressure and gastroesophageal competence was not uniformly found (ATKINSON et al., 1957; CODE et al., 1962; MacLAURIN, 1963; AFFOLTER, 1964). Intraluminal pressure measurements with constantly infused catheters, which quantitate yield pressures or resistance of sphincteric zones to distension (HARRIS et al., 1966; HEITMANN et al., 1966; WINANS and HARRIS, 1967; POPE, 1967) give more reproducible information on sphincter strength. Model experiments (POPE, 1967) and experiments on the force required to pull a ball through the sphincter from the stomach into the esophagus (COHEN and HARRIS, 1970) have demonstrated the accuracy of these measurements. They have been a major contribution to a better understanding of the role of the gastroesophageal sphincter in the pathogenesis of reflux in the last few years.

Attempts to define the nature of the intrinsic gastroesophageal sphincter mechanism have stimulated investigators to study its pharmacological and electrical properties. There is evidence that alpha-adrenergic receptors mediate contraction and beta-adrenergic receptors command relaxation of this sphincter (ELLIS et al., 1960; BAILEY, 1965; CHRISTENSEN, 1968). However, the excitatory response to stimulation of alpha-adrenergic receptors is not limited to the lower esophageal sphincter (CHRISTENSEN and DANIEL, 1968), but differences in sensitivity to adrenergic agents and to gastrin account for the different behavior of the lower esophageal sphincter and the esophagus proper (CHRISTENSEN, 1970; LIPSHUTZ and COHEN, 1971). Electromyographic studies in dogs, cats, monkeys and men indicate that the resting tone of the gastroesophageal sphincter is not associated with a continuous spiking activity (HELLEMANS and VANTRAPPEN, 1967; HELLEMANS et al., 1968; VANTRAPPEN and HELLEMANS, 1970). Resistance to mechanical stretching in addition to contraction seems to define the resting activity of the human gastroesophageal sphincter (HARRIS and POPE, 1964). Sphincteric force of closure can be increased by gastrin (GILES et al., 1969; CASTELL and HARRIS, 1970), by cholinergic agents (HOOKMAN and FLEISCHER, 1969) and by metoclopramide (HEITMANN and MÖLLER, 1970); it can be decreased by atropine (LIND et al., 1968a), by carminatives (SIGMUND and McNALLY, 1969) by gastrin suppression (CASTELL and HARRIS, 1970), by secretin (COHEN and LIPSHUTZ, 1971), by cholecystokinin (COHEN and HARRIS, 1972; RESIN et al., 1972), by glucagon (JENNEWEIN et al., 1972), by prostaglandins E_1 and E_2 (GOYAL et al., 1973) and by smoking (DENNISH and CASTELL, 1971).

An increase of sphincteric force of closure occurs immediately when fundic pressure rises. A stronger barrier to reflux is created under these critical conditions (LIND et al., 1966a; HEITMANN and MÖLLER, 1970a; COHEN and HARRIS, 1971). There is strong evidence that this is a vagally mediated reflex.

Sliding hiatal hernias are a useful model for the study of intrinsic sphincteric mechanisms, as in this condition all extrinsic accessory help is excluded. In 1957, ATKINSON et al. were able to show the presence "of a sphincteric mechanism comparable in any respect to that found in the normal subject at the esophagogastric junction, although this was situated several centimeters from the diaphragmatic hiatus". This has been confirmed by manometric (WANKLING et al., 1965; HEITMANN, 1969; COHEN and HARRIS, 1970) as well as by simultaneous manometric and cineradiographic studies (VANTRAPPEN et al., 1958; HEITMANN et al., 1966). The intrathoracic sphincter may even become hypertensive and may cause dysphagia (HEITMANN, 1970). The competent intrathoracic sphincter may be a part of, and not the entire, normal gastroesophageal sphincter (WOLF et al., 1968; WOLF, 1970), but it retains its normal behavior during swallowing and its adequate response to increased fundic pressure (HEITMANN, 1969; COHEN and HARRIS, 1971). Experimental work has shown that intrathoracic displacement of the gastroesophageal junction does not induce reflux unless the lower esophageal sphincter is destroyed (MEISS et al., 1958; LIPPA and THAL, 1966; ANDERSON et al., 1967). These observations stress the importance of intrinsic mechanisms in the prevention of gastroesophageal reflux.

The intraabdominal portion of the sphincteric zone has been considered to constitute an additional anti-reflux mechanism (WOLF, 1960a; VANTRAPPEN et al., 1960; EDWARDS, 1961).

The increased average incidence of symptomatic reflux in patients with hiatal hernias and the frequency of asymptomatic short-term reflux episodes in this condition (PICCONE et al., 1965) may be due to the absence of this intraabdominal portion. The lessening of gastroesophageal reflux after location of an incompetent

junction into the abdomen (Hill, 1967; Hill et al., 1970; Csendes and Larrain, 1972) or after some type of fundoplication (Lippa and Thal, 1966; Skinner
and Belsey, 1967; Urschel and Paulson, 1967; Harrison and Norton, 1969)
shows that positive pressure surrounding the gastroesophageal sphincter may
help to restore its efficiency when it is intrinsically hypotonic and incompetent.
However, gross or absolute failure of intrinsic sphincteric activity as seen in
scleroderma cannot be replaced by extrinsic mechanisms for the prevention of
reflux. As already mentioned, sphincteric activity can be depressed pharmacologically or by gastrin suppression in normal subjects and reflux ensues in spite
of preservation of all supposedly present extrinsic factors.

Transient retrograde flow of acid material occurs normally or in the presence
of asymptomatic hiatal hernias (Kantrowitz et al., 1969; Pattrick, 1970).
The normal esophagus is protected by its ability to clear this material rapidly
with primary or secondary peristaltic contractions (Booth et al., 1968). Removal
of refluxed acid is impaired in patients with esophagitis due to poor motor
function of the distal esophagus (Affolter, 1966; Woodward, 1970). It is not
known if this motility defect is the cause or the consequence of esophagitis.

2. Conditions Associated with Gastroesophageal
or Intestinoesophageal Reflux

2.1. Sliding Hiatal Hernia

The incidence of hiatal hernia in radiological examinations depends on the
method of examination and the criteria used for diagnosis. It varies from 33 to
50% of the population (Hafter, 1957; Wolf et al., 1959; Stein and Finkelstein,
1960; Dyer and Pridie, 1968). Only 5% or less of these subjects have clinically
important gastroesophageal reflux (Kramer, 1969). Measurements of yield pressures in the displaced sphincter of hiatal hernia patients have shown that those
with a normotensive sphincteric zone are asymptomatic and have no objective
evidence of reflux. When the intrathoracic sphincter has a low yield pressure,
symptoms and signs of reflux are likely to appear (Wankling et al., 1965;
Heitmann et al., 1966; Heitmann, 1969; Cohen and Harris, 1970; Haddad,
1970).

Separation of both groups is not always neat (Bennett, 1973) and patients
with hiatal hernias whose sphincteric yield pressures are at the lower limits of
normality may have reflux esophagitis. In such cases, the loss of the abdominal
esophagus and of normal sphinctero-hiatal relations seems to be critical. The
sphincter of hiatal hernia patients maintains its ability to increase its resting
yield pressure in proportion to the increase in abdominal pressure as in normal
controls (Lind et al., 1966; Heitmann, 1969; Cohen and Harris, 1970, 1971).
When the resting sphincter pressure is low the response of the sphincter to an
increase in abdominal pressure is feeble (Cohen and Harris, 1971) and may
allow transmission of increased fundic pressure into the distal esophagus, an
obvious manometric sign of gastroesophageal reflux (Wankling et al., 1965;
Heitmann, 1969; Butterfield et al., 1972). Mechanical plugging at the level
of the hiatus may temporarily help keeping gastric contents below the diaphragm
(Edwards, 1961; Wolf, 1970) but adequate objectivation of this factor is
difficult.

In summary, a small number of people with a sliding hiatal hernia have
clinically significant gastroesophageal reflux. The functional integrity of the
displaced sphincteric area is probably the most important single factor for the

prevention of reflux in this condition. Recently, the importance of the intra-abdominal re-location of the sphincteric area for gastroesophageal competence has again been emphasized (CSENDES and LARRAIN, 1972). The reason, however, remains unclear (INGELFINGER, 1971).

2.2. Gastroesophageal Incompetence in the Absence of Demonstrable Hiatal Hernia

The exact incidence of this condition is difficult to assess, since criteria for the diagnosis of small hiatal hernias (WOLF, 1956, 1960) are not uniformly applied. Although as many as 54.5% of patients with reflux esophagitis have been reported as having this disease (PALMER, 1968), we feel that "primary incompetence of the gastric cardia" (HIEBERT and BELSEY, 1961; FIELD and STALKER, 1968; HIEBERT, 1970) is rare. Yield pressures in the gastroesophageal junctional zone are low in this condition and their relation to reflux is similar to that found in hiatal hernias (POPE, 1967; WINANS and HARRIS, 1967; HADDAD, 1970; COHEN and HARRIS, 1971). The difference between gastroesophageal reflux with and without hiatal hernia has not lost its importance, since even when reflux is determined mainly by intrinsic sphincteric mechanisms rather than by the mere presence of a hiatal hernia, surgical treatment of hiatal hernia offers a good chance for the control of reflux and its consequences (HILL et al., 1970; CSENDES and LARRAIN, 1972).

Failure to develop a normal gastroesophageal sphincteric zone in the first months of life may lead to severe reflux esophagitis in children (GRYBOSKI et al., 1963; STRAWCZYNSKI et al., 1964; GRYBOSKI, 1965). Other complications of reflux in children, such as intractable vomiting, aspiration into the airways and failure to grow, indicate the serious prognosis of this condition.

2.3. Scleroderma with Esophageal Involvement and Related Conditions

Esophageal abnormalities are present in 80 to 90% of patients with scleroderma (CREAMER et al., 1956; ATKINSON and SUMMERLING, 1966; SALADIN et al., 1966; HEITMANN and ESPINOZA, 1968). In addition to marked or complete sphincteric hypotonicity there is a loss of peristalsis and of esophageal clearing ability. Consequently severe peptic esophagitis frequently complicates this disease.

2.4. Following Myotomy for Achalasia of the Esophagus

In spite of optimistic reports on Heller's myotomy (ELLIS et al., 1967) gastroesophageal reflux complicates the course of some patients after this procedure (ELLIS and COLE, 1965; HELSINGEN, 1966; REES et al., 1970). This does not seem to happen after pneumatic dilatation of the cardia (VAN GOIDSENHOVEN et al., 1963; VANTRAPPEN et al., 1971). Some surgeons add a fundoplication to Heller's myotomy in the belief that this may prevent reflux (HILL et al., 1961; JEKLER and LHOTKA, 1967).

2.5. Vagotomy

Cervical vagotomy in monkeys induces severe motility disturbances (BINDER et al., 1968). Both subhilar and transabdominal vagotomy decrease the resting pressure of the gastroesophageal sphincter of dogs (GREENWOOD et al., 1962; ELEBUTE et al., 1966) and abolish the increase in sphincteric pressure elicited by abdominal compression (LIND et al., 1969). In man gastroesophageal reflux appears with increased frequency after vagotomy (CLARKE et al., 1965; KANTRO-WITZ et al., 1969). Although conventional pressure measurements showed no change in resting sphincteric pressure (MANN and HARDCASTLE, 1968), yield pressures indicate a significantly diminished resistance to distension and an inability of the human gastroesophageal sphincter to withstand reflux after vagotomy (HADDAD, 1970). Sphincter response to abdominal compression was significantly reduced (CRISPIN et al., 1967). Similar effects can be induced by atropine (LIND et al., 1968).

2.6. Pregnancy

Heartburn during pregnancy is probably due to acid reflux into the esophagus and associated disturbances of esophageal motor activity (NAGLER and SPIRO, 1961). LIND et al. (1968a) demonstrated that pregnant women with heartburn had a significantly lower maximal sphincteric pressure than controls or pregnant women without heartburn. This seems to be the cause of reflux and of secondary motility changes. Sphincter pressure returns to normal after delivery. The etiology is obscured by the fact that only some pregnant women show this abnormality. A similar situation has been described in the presence of increased intraabdominal pressure due to tense ascites (SIMPSON and CONN, 1968).

2.7. Gastric Operations

Resection of the esophagogastric junction with anastomosis is followed by free reflux and severe esophagitis (BOMBECK et al., 1970). Partial gastrectomy without surgical manipulation of the gastroesophageal junction may be followed by reflux with severe complications (WINDSOR, 1964; LOWE and PALMER, 1967). Removal of the main gastrin-producing area of the stomach could be pathogenetically important. Although reflux of duodenal contents into the stomach may occur normally (BENEVENTANO and SCHEIN, 1970) and could be etiologically important for the development of complications of reflux (GILLISON et al., 1969), partial gastrectomy markedly favors reflux of biliary and pancreatic secretions into the gastric remnant (LAWSON, 1964; VAN HEERDEN et al., 1969; PAYNE, 1970). In the presence of an incompetent sphincter these secretions reflux into the lower esophagus, where they are able to induce severe esophagitis (LAMBERT, 1962; MOFFAT and BERKAS, 1965).

2.8. Prolonged Gastric Intubation

Nasogastric tubes induce gastroesophageal reflux, especially in the recumbent position (NAGLER and SPIRO, 1963; VINNIK and KERN, 1964). The exact mechanism is unknown, but impairment of mechanical closure of the sphincteric area is a reasonable explanation. Severe peptic esophagitis may ensue (WALDMAN and BERLIN, 1965).

In spite of the impressive amount of clinical and experimental studies already performed, those mechanisms responsible for the pathogenesis of gastroesophageal reflux, and those capable to prevent it, will continue to stimulate research that will answer many open questions in this interesting field.

References

AFFOLTER, H.: Beitrag zur Pathophysiologie des gastro-ösophagealen Verschlusses bei Hiatusgleithernien. Gastroenterologia (Basel) **102**, 211–218 (1964).

AFFOLTER, H.: Pressure characteristics of reflux esophagitis. Helv. med. Acta **33**, 395–402 (1966).

ANDERSON, H. N., MAY, K. J., STEINMETZ, G. P., OFSTUN, M., HARRISON, H. G., LEYSE, R. M., DILLARD, D. H.: The lower esophageal intrinsic sphincter and the mechanism of reflux: experimental observations supporting a new concept. Ann. Surg. **166**, 102–108 (1967).

ATKINSON, M., EDWARDS, D. A. W., HONOUR, A. J., ROWLANDS, E. N.: The esophagogastric sphincter in hiatus hernia. Lancet **1957 II**, 1138–1142.

ATKINSON, M., SUMMERLING, M. D.: Oesophageal changes in systemic sclerosis. Gut **7**, 402–408 (1966).

BAILEY, D. M.: The action of sympathomimetic amines on circular and longitudinal smooth muscle from the isolated oesophagus of the guinea pig. J. Pharm. Pharmacol. **17**, 782–787 (1965).

BENEVENTANO, T. C., SCHEIN, C. J.: Pyloric sphincter incompetence in man. Gastroenterology **59**, 518–521 (1970).

BENNETT, J. R.: Section 5 of: Symposium on gastroesophageal reflux and its complications. Gut **14**, 246–249 (1970).

BINDER, H. J., BLOOM, D. L., STERN, H., SOLITARE, G. B., THAYER, W. R., SPIRO, H. M.: The effect of cervical vagectomy on esophageal function in the monkey. Surgery **64**, 1075–1083 (1968).

BOMBECK, C. T., COELHO, R. G. P., NYHUS, L. M.: Prevention of gastroesophageal reflux after resection of the lower esophagus. Surg. Gynec. Obstet. **130**, 1035–1043 (1970).

BOOTH, D. J., KEMMERER, W. T., SKINNER, D. B.: Acid clearing from the distal esophagus. Arch. Surg. **96**, 731–734 (1968).

BUTTERFIELD, D. G., STRUTHERS, J. E., SHOWALTER, J. P.: A test of gastroesophageal sphincter competence: the common cavity test. Amer. J. dig. Dis. **17**, 415–421 (1972).

CASTELL, D. O., HARRIS, L. D.: Hormonal control of gastroesophageal sphincter strength. New Engl. J. Med. **282**, 886–889 (1970).

CHRISTENSEN, J.: Pharmacology of the esophagus. In: Handbook of physiology, Section 6, Alimentary canal, vol. IV, Motility, chapt. 108, 2325–2330, by CODE, C. F. (ed.). Washington, D.C.: American Physiological Society 1968.

CHRISTENSEN, J.: Pharmacologic identification of the lower esophageal sphincter. J. clin. Invest. **49**, 681–691 (1970).

CHRISTENSEN, J., DANIEL, E. E.: Effects of some autonomic drugs on circular esophageal smooth muscle. J. Pharm. exp. Ther. **159**, 243–249 (1968).

CLARKE, S. D., PENRY, J. B., WARD, P.: Oesophageal reflux after abdominal vagotomy. Lancet **1965 II**, 824–826.

CODE, C. F., KELLEY, M. L., SCHLEGEL, J. F., OLSEN, A. M.: Detection of hiatal hernia during esophageal motility tests. Gastroenterology **43**, 521–531 (1962).

CODE, C. F., SCHLEGEL, J. F.: Motor action of the esophagus and its sphincters. In: Handbook of physiology, sect. 6, vol. IV, p. 1821–1839 by CODE, C. F. (ed.). Washington, D.C.: American Physiological Society 1968.

COHEN, S., HARRIS, L. D.: Lower esophageal sphincter pressure as an index of lower esophageal sphincter strength. Gastroenterology **58**, 157–162 (1970).

COHEN, S., HARRIS, L. D.: The lower esophageal sphincter. Gastroenterology **63**, 1066–1073 (1972).

COHEN, S., LIPSHUTZ, W.: Hormonal regulation of human lower esophageal sphincter competence: interaction of gastrin and secretin. J. clin. Invest. **50**, 449–454 (1971).

CREAMER, B.: Motor disturbances of the esophagus. In: Handbook of physiology, sect. 6, vol. IV, p. 2331–2343, by CODE, C. F. (ed.). Washington, D.C.: American Physiological Society 1968.

CREAMER, B., ANDERSEN, H. A., CODE, C. F.: Esophageal motility in patients with scleroderma and related diseases. Gastroenterologia (Basel) **86**, 763–775 (1956).

CRISPIN, J. S., McIVER, D. K., LIND, J. F.: Manometric study of the effect of vagotomy on the gastroesophageal sphincter. Canad. J. Surg. **10**, 299–303 (1967).

CSENDES, A., LARRAIN, A.: Effect of posterior gastropexy on gastroesophageal sphincter pressure and symptomatic reflux in patients with hiatal hernia. Gastroenterology **63**, 19–24 (1972).

DENNISH, J. W., CASTELL, D. O.: Inhibitory effect of smoking on the lower esophageal sphincter. New Engl. J. Med. **284**, 1136–1137 (1971).

Dyer, N. H., Pridie, R. B.: Incidence of hiatus hernia in asymptomatic subjects. Gut 9, 696–699 (1968).

Edwards, D. A. W.: The mechanism at the cardia. II. The antireflux mechanism: manometric and radiological studies. Brit. J. Radiol. 34, 474–487 (1961).

Ellebute, E., Kelley, M. L., Schwartz, S. I.: Pressure effects of transabdominal supradiaphragmatic vagotomy on the inferior esophageal sphincter of dogs. Surg. Gynec. Obstet. 123, 326–332 (1966).

Ellis, F., Cole, F. L.: Reflux after cardiomyotomy. Gut 6, 80–84 (1965).

Ellis, F. G., Kauntze, R., Trounce, J. R.: The innervation of the cardia and the lower esophagus in man. Brit. J. Surg. 47, 466–472 (1960).

Ellis, F. H., Jr., Kiser, J. C., Schlegel, J. F., Earlam, R. J., McVey, J. L., Olsen, A. M.: Esophagomyotomy for esophageal achalasia: experimental, clinical and manometric aspects. Ann. Surg. 166, 640–656 (1967).

Field, P., Stalker, M. J. B.: Incompetence of the cardiac sphincter without radiologic demonstration of hiatus hernia. Canad. J. Surg. 11, 412–419 (1968).

Friedland, G. W., Melcher, D. H., Berridge, F. R., Gresham, G. A.: Debatable points in the anatomy of the lower oesophagus. Thorax 21, 487–498 (1966).

Fyke, F. E., Code, C. F., Schlegel, J. F.: The gastroesophageal sphincter in healthy human beings. Gastroenterologia (Basel) 86, 135–150 (1956).

Giles, G. R., Mason, M. C., Humphries, C., Clark, C. G.: Action of gastrin on the lower esophageal sphincter in man. Gut 10, 730–734 (1969).

Gillison, E. W., Capper, W. M., Airth, G. R., Gibson, M. J., Bradford, I.: Hiatus hernia and heartburn. Gut 10, 609–613 (1969).

Goidsenhoven, G. E., Van, Vantrappen, G., Verbeke, S., Vandenbroucke, J.: Treatment of achalasia of the cardia with pneumatic dilations. Gastroenterology 45, 326–334 (1963).

Goyal, R. K., Rattan, S., Hersh, T.: Comparison of the effects of prostaglandins E_1, E_2, and A_2, and of hypovolumic hypotension on the lower esophageal sphincter. Gastroenterology 65, 608–612 (1973).

Greenwood, R. K., Schlegel, J. F., Code, C. F., Ellis, F. H., Jr.: The effect of sympathectomy, vagotomy, and oesophageal interruption on the canine gastro-oesophageal sphincter. Thorax 17, 310–319 (1962).

Gryboski, J. D.: The swallowing mechanism of the neonate. 1. Esophageal and gastric motility. Pediatrics 35, 445–452 (1965).

Gryboski, J. D., Thayer, W. R., Spiro, H. M.: Esophageal motility in infants and children. Pediatrics 31, 382–395 (1963).

Haddad, J. K.: Relation of gastroesophageal reflux to yield sphincter pressures. Gastroenterology 58, 175–184 (1970).

Hafter, E.: Die Hiatushernie, ihre Häufigkeit und klinische Bedeutung. Dtsch. med. Wschr. 82, 1709–1712 (1957).

Harris, L. D., Pope, C. E., II: "Squeeze" vs. resistance: an evaluation of the mechanism of sphincter competence. J. clin. Invest. 43, 2272–2278 (1964).

Harris, L. D., Winans, C. S., Pope, C. E., II: Determination of yield pressures: a method for measuring anal sphincter competence. Gastroenterology 50, 754–760 (1966).

Harrison, G. K., Norton, R.: Prevention of reflux from the stomach into the oesophagus. Thorax 24, 595–598 (1969).

Heerden, J. A., Van, Priestley, J. T., Farrow, G. M., Phillips, S. F.: Postoperative alkaline reflux gastritis. Amer. J. Surg. 118, 427–433 (1969).

Heitmann, P.: Der gastrooesophageale Verschlußmechanismus bei Hiatusgleithernien. Internist (Berl.) 10, 249–258 (1969).

Heitmann, P.: Die Hiatusgleithernien mit einem hypertonischen gastro-ösophagealen Verschlußmechanismus. Dtsch. med. Wschr. 95, 824–829 (1970).

Heitmann, P., Espinoza, J.: Funktionelle Störungen des Ösophagus bei Patienten mit Sklerodermie. Dtsch. med. Wschr. 93, 1960–1966 (1968).

Heitmann, P., Möller, N.: The effect of metoclopramide on the gastroesophageal junctional zone and the distal esophagus in man. Scand. J. Gastroent. 5, 621–625 (1970).

Heitmann, P., Möller, N.: Intraluminale Druckmessungen an der gastro-ösophagealen Übergangzone und am distalen Ösophagus bei gesunden Erwachsenen. Dtsch. med. Wschr. 95, 1963–1969 (1970a).

Heitmann, P., Wolf, B. S., Sokol, E. M., Cohen, B. R.: Simultaneous cineradiographic-manometric study of the distal esophagus: small hiatal hernias and rings. Gastroenterology 50, 737–753 (1966).

Hellemans, J., Vantrappen, G.: Electromyographic studies on canine esophageal motility. Amer. J. dig. Dis. 12, 1240–1255 (1967).

HELLEMANS, J., VANTRAPPEN, G., VALEMBOIS, P., JANSSENS, J., VANDENBROUCKE, J.: Electrical activity of striated and smooth muscle of the esophagus. Amer. J. dig. Dis. **13**, 320–334 (1968).

HELSINGEN, N.: Gastroesophageal reflux as a complication of the Heller operation. Acta chir. scand., Suppl. **356**, 96–98 (1966).

HIEBERT, C. A.: Primary incompetence of the gastric cardia. Amer. J. Surg. **119**, 365–371 (1970).

HIEBERT, C. A., BELSEY, R.: Incompetency of the gastric cardia without radiologic evidence of hiatal hernia. J. thorac. cardiovasc. Surg. **42**, 352–362 (1961).

HILL, L. D.: An effective operation for hiatal hernia: an eight year appraisal. Ann. Surg. **166**, 681–690 (1967).

HILL, L. D., GELFAND, M., BAUERMEISTER, D.: Simplified management of reflux esophagitis with stricture. Ann. Surg. **172**, 638–646 (1970).

HILL, L. D., MORGAN, E. H., KELLOGG, H. B.: Experimentation as an aid in management of esophageal disorders. Amer. J. Surg. **102**, 240–252 (1961).

HOOKMAN, P., FLEISCHER, J.: Cholinergic alteration of lower esophageal sphincter pressure. Gastroenterology **56**, 1169 (1969).

INGELFINGER, F. J.: The sphincter that is a sphinx. (Editorial.) New Engl. J. Med. **284**, 1095–1096 (1971).

JEKLER, J., LHOTKA, J.: Modified Heller procedure to prevent postoperative reflux esophagitis in patients with achalasia. Amer. J. Surg. **113**, 251–254 (1967).

JENNEWEIN, H. M., WALDECK, F., PRAHL, K.: Zur Beeinflussung des unteren Ösophagussphinkters durch gastrointestinale Hormone beim Hund. Leber-Magen-Darm **2**, 17–19 (1972).

KANTROWITZ, P. A., CORSON, J. G., FLEISCHLI, D. J., SKINNER, D. B.: Measurement of gastroesophageal reflux. Gastroenterology **56**, 666–674 (1969).

KRAMER, P.: Does a sliding hiatus hernia constitute a distinct clinical entity? Gastroenterology **57**, 442–448 (1969).

LAMBERT, R.: Relative importance of biliary and pancreatic secretions in the genesis of esophagitis in rats. Amer. J. dig. Dis. **7**, 1026–1033 (1962).

LAWSON, H. H.: Effect of duodenal contents on the gastric mucosa under experimental conditions. Lancet **1964 I**, 468–472.

LEPOW, H.: The anatomy of the lower esophageal vestibular complex. Jewish Mem. Hosp. Bull. **7**, 55–62 (1962).

LIND, J. F., COTTON, D. C., BLANCHARD, R., CRISPIN, J. S., DIMOPOLOS, G. E.: Effect of thoracic displacement and vagotomy on the canine gastroesophageal junctional zone. Gastroenterology **56**, 1078–1085 (1969).

LIND, J. F., CRISPIN, J. S., MCIVER, D. K.: The effect of atropine on the gastroesophageal sphincter. Canad. J. Physiol. Pharmacol. **46**, 233–238 (1968).

LIND, J. F., SMITH, A. M., MCIVER, D. K., COOPLAND, A. T., CRISPIN, J. S.: Heartburn in pregnancy — a manometric study. Canad. med. Ass. J. **98**, 571–574 (1968a).

LIND, J. F., WARRIAN, W. G., WANKLING, W. J.: Responses of the gastroesophageal junctional zone to increases in abdominal pressure. Canad. J. Surg. **9**, 32–38 (1966).

LIPPA, F. H., THAL, A. P.: Experimental reflux esophagitis. Arch. Surg. **93**, 148–152 (1966).

LIPSHUTZ, W., COHEN, S.: Physiological determinants of lower esophageal sphincter function. Gastroenterology **61**, 16–24 (1971).

LOWE, W. C., PALMER, E. D.: Esophageal stricture as a complication of gastric surgery. Amer. J. med. Sci. **254**, 342–346 (1967).

MACLAURIN, C.: The intrinsic sphincter in the prevention of gastro-esophageal reflux. Lancet **1963 II**, 801–805.

MANN, C. V., HARDCASTLE, J. D.: The effect of vagotomy on the human gastrooesophageal sphincter. Gut **9**, 688–695 (1968).

MEISS, J. H., GRINDLAY, J. H., ELLIS, F. H., JR.: The gastroesophageal sphincter mechanism. II. Further experimental studies in the dog. J. thorac. Surg. **36**, 156–165 (1958).

MOFFAT, R. C., BERGAS, E. M.: Bile esophagitis. Arch. Surg. **91**, 963–966 (1965).

NAGLER, R., SPIRO, H. M.: Heartburn in late pregnancy: manometric studies of esophageal motor function. J. clin. Invest. **40**, 954–970 (1961).

NAGLER, R., SPIRO, H. M.: Persistent gastroesophageal reflux induced during prolonged gastric intubation. New Engl. J. Med. **269**, 495–500 (1963).

PALMER, E. D.: The hiatus hernia-esophagitis-esophageal stricture complex. Twenty year prospective study. Amer. J. Med. **44**, 566–579 (1968).

PATTRICK, F. G.: Investigation of gastroesophageal reflux in various positions with a two-lumen pH electrode. Gut **11**, 659–667 (1970).

PAYNE, W. S.: Surgical treatment of reflux esophagitis and stricture associated with permanent incompetence of the cardia. Mayo Clin. Proc. **45**, 553–562 (1970).

PICCONE, V. A., GUTELIUS, J. R., McCORRISTON, J. R.: A multiphased esophageal pH test for gastroesophageal reflux. Surgery 57, 638–646 (1965).

POPE, C. E., II: A dynamic test of sphincter strength: its application to the lower esophageal sphincter. Gastroenterology 52, 779–786 (1967).

REES, J. R., THORBJARNARSON, B., BARNES, W. H.: Achalasia: results of operation in 84 patients. Ann. Surg. 171, 195–201 (1970).

RESIN, H., STERN, D. H., STURDEVANT, R. A., ISENBERG, J. I.: Effect of octapeptide of cholecystokinin on lower esophageal sphincter pressure in man. Gastroenterology 62, 797 (1972).

SALADIN, T. A., FRENCH, A. B., ZARAFONETIS, C. J. D., POLLARD, H. M.: Esophageal motor abnormalities in scleroderma and related diseases. Amer. J. dig. Dis. 11, 522–535 (1966).

SIGMUND, C. J., McNALLY, E. F.: The action of a carminative on the lower esophageal sphincter. Gastroenterology 56, 13–18 (1969).

SIMPSON, J. A., CONN, H. O.: Role of ascites in gastroesophageal reflux with comments on the pathogenesis of bleeding esophageal varices. Gastroenterology 55, 17–24 (1968).

SKINNER, D. B., BELSEY, R. H. R.: Surgical management of esophageal reflux and hiatal hernia. J. thorac. cardiovasc. Surg. 53, 33–54 (1967).

STEIN, G. N., FINKESLTEIN, A.: Hiatal hernia: roentgen incidence and diagnosis. Amer. J. dig. Dis. 5, 77–87 (1960).

STELZNER, F., LIERSE, W.: Der angiomuskuläre Dehnverschluß der terminalen Speiseröhre. Langenbecks Arch. klin. Chir. 321, 35–64 (1968).

STRAWCZYNSKI, H., BECK, I. T., McKENNA, R. D., NICKERSON, G. H.: The behavior of the lower esophageal sphincter in infants and its relationship to gastro-esophageal regurgitation. J. Pediat. 64, 17–23 (1964).

URSCHEL, H. C., PAULSON, D. L.: Gastroesophageal reflux and hiatal hernia. J. thorac. cardiovasc. Surg. 53, 21–32 (1967).

VANTRAPPEN, G., LIEMER, M. B., IKEYA, J., TEXTER, E. C., JR., BARBORKA, C. J.: Simultaneous fluorocinematography and intraluminal pressure measurements in the study of esophageal motility. Gastroenterology 35, 592–602 (1958).

VANTRAPPEN, G., TEXTER, E. C., JR., BARBORKA, C. J., VANDENBROUCKE, J.: The closing mechanism at the gastroesophageal junction. Amer. J. Med. 28, 564–577 (1960).

VANTRAPPEN, G., HELLEMANS, J.: Esophageal motility. Rendic. R. Gastroenterol. 2, 7–19 (1970).

VANTRAPPEN, G., HELLEMANS, J., DELOOF, W., VALEMBOIS, P., VANDENBROUCKE, J.: Treatment of achalasia with pneumatic dilatations. Gut 12, 268–275 (1971).

VINNIK, I. E., KERN, F.: The effect of gastric intubation on esophageal pH. Gastroenterology 47, 388–394 (1964).

WALDMAN, I., BERLIN, L.: Stricture of the esophagus due to nasogastric intubation. Amer. J. Roentgenol. 94, 321–324 (1965).

WANKLING, W. J., WARRIAN, W. G., LIND, J. F.: The gastroesophageal sphincter in hiatus hernia. Canad. J. Surg. 8, 61–67 (1965).

WINANS, C. S., HARRIS, L. D.: Quantitation of lower esophageal sphincter competence. Gastroenterology 52, 773–778 (1967).

WINDSOR, C. W. O.: Gastro-esophageal reflux after partial gastrectomy. Brit. med. Ass. J. 2, 1233–1234 (1964).

WOLF, B. S.: The roentgen diagnosis of minimal hiatal herniation. J. Mt Sinai Hosp. 23, 90–109 (1956).

WOLF, B. S.: Roentgen features of the normal and herniated esophagogastric region. Amer. J. dig. Dis. 5, 751–769 (1960).

WOLF, B. S.: The esophagogastric closing mechanism. J. Mt Sinai Hosp. 27, 404–416 (1960a).

WOLF, B. S.: The inferior esophageal sphincter — anatomic, roentgenologic and manometric correlation, contradictions, and terminology. Amer. J. Roentgenol. 110, 260–277 (1970).

WOLF, B. S., BRAHMS, S. A., KHILNANI, M. T.: The incidence of hiatus hernia in routine barium meal examinations. J. Mt Sinai Hosp. 26, 598–600 (1959).

WOODWARD, D. A. K.: Response of the gullet to gastric reflux in patients with hiatus hernia and oesophagitis. Thorax 25, 459–464 (1970).

Chapter 4

Tumors of the Esophagus

Benign Tumors and Cysts of the Esophagus

G. Vantrappen and J. Pringot

With 6 Figures

Benign tumors and cysts of the esophagus are relatively uncommon as compared with malignant conditions. Leiomyomas are the most common benign esophageal tumors; at least 562 reports of this condition have appeared in the literature.

1. Classification

From both the clinical and the pathologic standpoint, benign tumors may be divided into two large groups, the intramural and the intraluminal tumors (Totten et al., 1953).

The intramural growths are either solid tumors or cysts. The vast majority of the intramural tumors are considered as leiomyomas and are made up of varying proportions of smooth muscle and fibrous tissue. Closely related to leiomyomas are fibromas, myomas, fibromyomas and lipomyomas. Other histological types of solid intramural tumors have been described, such as lipomas, neurofibromas, hemangiomas, osteochondromas, granular cell myoblastomas and glomus tumors.

The cysts may be congenital or acquired. Congenital cysts are lined wholly or partly by columnar ciliated epithelium of the respiratory type, by glandular epithelium of the gastric type, by squamous or transitional epithelium, or epithelial lining cells may be absent. The controversial concepts on the embryologic origin of the congenital cysts has led to a variety of names, such as bronchogenic, enterogenous, esophagenic and mediastinal cysts. The acquired retention cysts probably result from obstruction of the excretory ducts of the esophageal glands.

The intraluminal polypoid or pedunculated growths usually originate in the submucosa, develop mainly in the lumen of the gullet and are covered with a normal stratified squamous epithelium. The majority of these tumors are composed of fibrous tissue of varying degrees of compactness with a rich vascular supply. Some are quite loose and myxoid (myxoma, myxofibroma), others more collagenous (fibroma) and some contain adipose tissue (fibrolipoma). These different types of tumors are frequently designated as fibrovascular polyps or simply as polyps.

The intraluminal sessile tumors originate in the mucosa and can be divided into papillomas and adenomas.

Plachta (1962) collected 333 cases of benign esophageal tumors from the literature and added 99 cases of his own. Table 19 from Plachta is presented

Table 19. Classified cases of benign tumors of the esophagus. [From Plachta, A.: American Journal of Gastroenterology 38, 639 (1962)]

	Patterson 1712 to 1932	Rose 1797 to 1932	Adams and Hoover 1933 to 1943	Moersch and Harrington 1933 to 1944	Isolated reports 1944 to 1948	Harrington 1949	Totten et al. 1953	Body and Hill 1954	Plachta 1960	Total	Incidence
Aberrant thyroid	1	0	0	0	0	0	0	0	0	1	0.2
Adenoma	2	0	1	0	0	0	0	0	1	4	0.9
Benign giant-cell tumor	0	0	1	0	0	0	0	0	0	1	0.2
Cyst	4	0	2	2	1	3	17	2	3	34	7.9
Fibroma	2	0	5	0	2	0	0	2	2	13	3.0
Fibrolipoma	0	0	0	0	1	0	0	0	0	1	0.2
Hemiangioma	1	0	0	3	1	0	0	1	3	9	2.1
Lipoma	2	0	3	0	1	0	0	0	1	7	1.6
Fibromyoma	0	0	0	0	1	0	0	0	2	3	0.7
Leiomyoma	6	0	0	32	6	6	46	9	51	156	36.0
Lipomyoma	1	0	0	0	0	0	0	0	1	2	0.4
Myoma	8	49	2	0	0	2	0	0	4	65	15.0
Myocele	0	0	0	1	0	0	0	0	0	1	0.2
Myxofibroma	1	0	0	0	1	0	0	0	0	2	0.4
Neurofibroma	0	0	1	1	1	0	0	0	1	4	0.9
Osteochondroma	0	0	1	0	0	0	0	0	0	1	0.2
Papilloma	8	0	1	3	0	0	0	0	2	14	3.2
Polyps	26	0	9	2	2	0	40	1	28	108	25.0
Unclassified	0	0	3	0	3	0	0	0	0	6	1.4
Total	62	49	29	44	20	11	103	15	99	432	

to illustrate the relative frequency of the various types of benign tumors reported up to 1962.

2. Incidence

Harrington and Moersch (1944) reviewed 7459 post-mortem examinations at the Mayo Clinic and found only 44 cases of benign esophageal tumor, as compared to 876 cases of esophageal carcinoma observed in this institution over the same period. Daniel and Williams (1950) found none in 4000 necropsies, Sweet et al. (1954) observed 4 cases in 13000 necropsies and Postlethwait and Sealy (1961) found 10 cases in 7000 autopsies. The highest autopsy incidence (0.25%) was reported by Plachta (1962) who found 49 cases in 19982 post-mortem examinations. Barrett (1964) suggested that many benign tumors are overlooked because the entire esophagus is not thoroughly examined at autopsy. Moersch and Harrington (1944) reported 15 benign esophageal tumors

among 11000 patients who had dysphagia. SCHMIDT et al. (1961) of the Mayo
Clinic found over a 15 year period 90 cases of benign esophageal tumors or cysts;
in 49 cases the lesions were removed by surgical means, and in the other 41 cases
the lesions were found at post-mortem examination. BOGEDAIN et al. (1963)
observed, during the period 1950 to 1962, 50 carcinomas and 6 leiomyomas in
a series of 3000 chest referals. The relative incidence of benign tumors and
carcinomas of the esophagus has been variably reported from 1 to 15 (JOHNSTON
et al., 1953), to 1 to 150 (WATSON et al., 1967).

3. Intramural Tumors and Cysts

3.1. Leiomyoma

Leiomyomas together with other types of myoma constitute more than 50%
of the benign esophageal tumors and cysts and can be considered as the prototype
of the benign intramural tumor of the esophagus. Therefore, leiomyomas will
be described in some detail and this clinical description may be applied to other
varieties of benign intramural tumors.

3.1.1. Age and Sex Incidence

STOREY and ADAMS (1956) analysed 85 cases of leiomyoma reported in the
literature and found that almost 90% of the surgical patients were over twenty
and under sixty years of age, the average age being 38.6 years. This is in sharp
contrast to the age incidence of esophageal carcinoma, in which the average age
of the patient at the time of diagnosis is more than 20 years higher. Leiomyoma
of the esophagus occurs in both sexes, but it is generally accepted that there
is a male preponderance of the order of 2 to 1.

3.1.2. Pathology

Some 90% of the leiomyomas are located in the lower two thirds of the esophagus. This is probably due to the fact that most leiomyomas originate in the
musculosa, which in the upper third of the esophagus is largely composed of
striated muscle (JOHNSTON et al., 1953; LEWIS and MAXFIELD, 1954; STOREY
and ADAMS, 1956; GRAY et al., 1961).

The lesions are mostly solitary, but multiple tumors have been found on
several occasions (CALMENSON and CLAGETT, 1946; BRADFORD et al., 1947; HIGGIN-
SON, 1954; SWEET et al., 1954; SCHMIDT, 1961; BARRETT, 1964; TOUMIEUX
et al., 1971) (Fig. 209). In their review of 88 cases of intramural esophageal
tumors TOTTEN et al. (1953) found eleven instances of multiple tumors; in 3 of
the autopsy cases these were leiomyomas of both esophagus and stomach.
The number of esophageal leiomyomas found in one patient varies from 2 to as
many as 14. In some rare cases the esophagus is wholly or partly studded with
tumors, a condition which has been called diffuse leiomyomatosis (LINDER and
VOGT-MOYKOPF, 1970). The cases of leiomyomatosis reported by LORTAT-JACOB
(1950) probably do not represent true esophageal neoplasms, but correspond to
muscular hypertrophy associated with motility disturbances.

Leiomyomas of the esophagus vary greatly in size and shape. Some of the
tumors removed surgically measured only 1 cm in diameter, but 4 cases have
been reported of surgically removed tumors which weighed more than 1000 g,
the largest one weighing 5000 g (KENNEY, 1953; FRANK et al., 1956; SCHMIDT
et al., 1961; TSUZUKI et al., 1971).

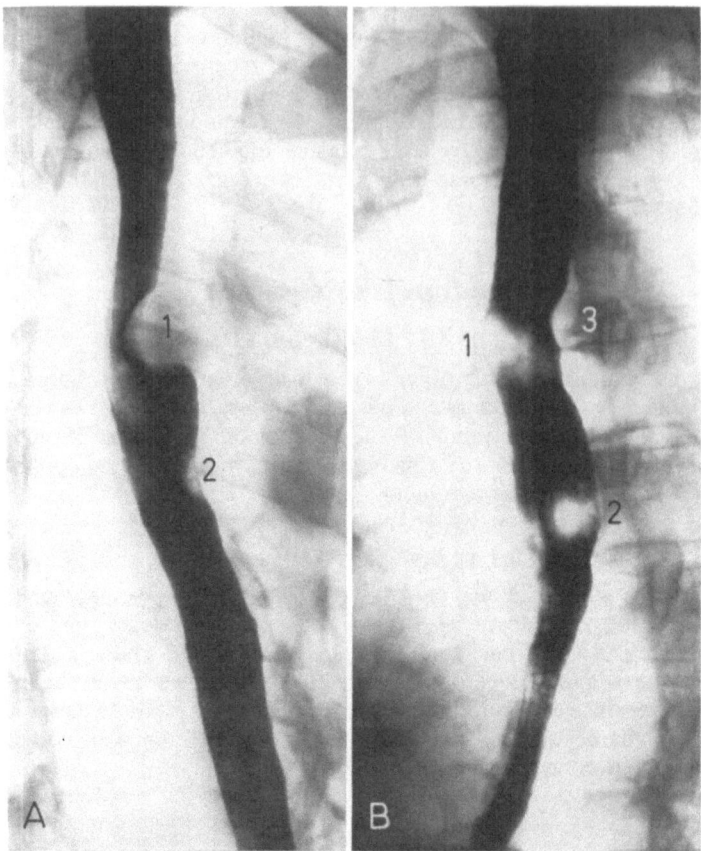

Fig. 209 A and B. Multiple leiomyomas of the middle third of the esophagus. A Two tumors are visible in the right oblique anterior view (*1*, *2*). B The third one (*3*) is demonstrated in the left oblique anterior view

Most of the tumors are spherical or ovoid, although one quarter of the cases analyzed by TOTTEN et al. (1953) were crescentic or even annular in shape. The average tumor is roughly oval in shape and measures about 6 to 8 cm in the long and 4 to 6 cm in the transverse axis. The surface of the tumor may be regular and smooth or it may be a multilobular lesion resembling uterine fibro- myomas. Most growths seem to arise in the circular or longitudinal muscle coats, but occasionally small tumors are found in the muscularis mucosae or the sub- mucosa. Most leiomyomas do not grow into the esophageal lumen; they remain intramural, with the greater mass of the tumor protruding toward the outer wall of the gullet. The tumors are sharply demarcated from the surrounding tissues and may be surrounded by a fibrous capsule. The overlying mucosa is freely movable and normal; umbilicate ulcerations, which are so typical of the mesenchymal tumors of the stomach, are not observed in esophageal leiomyomas. Histologically, the tumor shows interlacing bundles of spindle-shaped cells, con- taining intracellular myofibrils and nuclei which are narrow, long and rounded at the ends (BOGEDAIN et al., 1963). These tumors frequently contain variable amounts of fibrous tissue and may show areas of edema, hemorrhage, degenera- tion and calcification (HUDDY and GRIFFITHS, 1972) (Fig. 210).

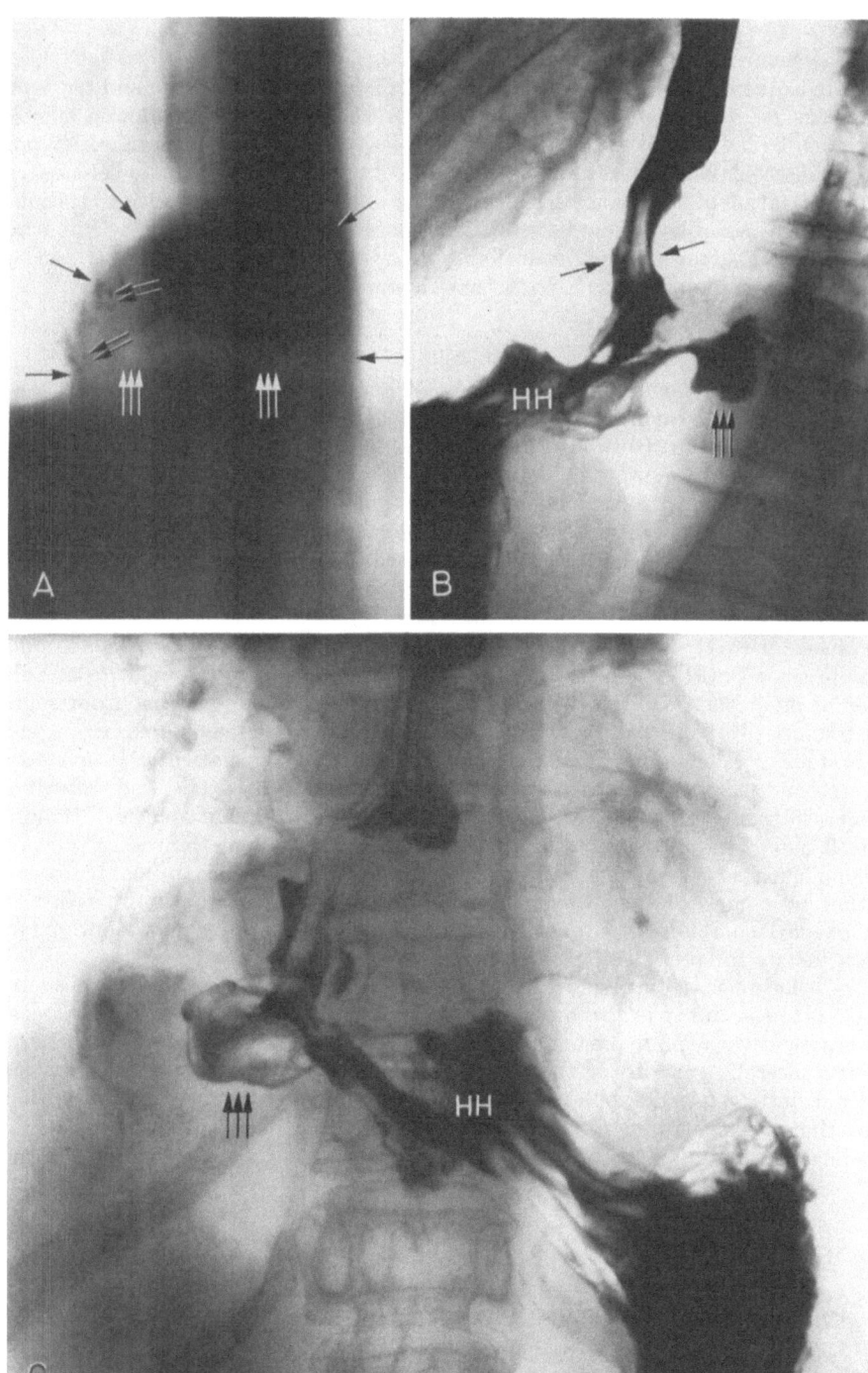

Fig. 210 A–C. Calcified leiomyoma at the esophagogastric junction and associated hiatus hernia. Laminography (A) shows the contour of the tumor (single arrow), intramural calcifications (double arrows) and an air contrast image (triple arrow). A barium meal (B, C) shows extramucosal narrowing of the lower esophagus (between single arrows), diverticular outpouching in the tumor (triple arrow) and hiatus hernia (*HH*)

The coexistence of benign tumors with other conditions has repeatedly been reported. According to Gray et al. (1961) 4.8% of the leiomyomas and leiomyo-sarcomas are associated with a hiatal hernia. Of the 88 solid intramural tumors reviewed by Totten et al. (1953) "several" cases showed an intimate association with diverticula and in 2 cases a diverticulum of the esophagus occurred elsewhere. The association of leiomyoma with carcinoma of the esophagus has led to specula-tions on a causal relationship between both conditions (Callanan, 1954; Puestow et al., 1955). According to Storey and Adams (1956) this association occurred in at least 8 of the 326 case reports they reviewed.

3.1.3. Symptoms

Patients with leiomyomas of the esophagus may be asymptomatic or may have only atypical complaints, but this appears to occur less frequently than is generally believed. Only 11 of the 82 patients reviewed by Storey and Adams (1956) were free of symptoms definitely attributable to their lesion. Neither size nor location of the tumor correlate with the degree of the symptoms.

Dysphagia and pain are the most common complaints and these two symp-toms occur more frequently together than separately. Dysphagia occurs in about 50% of the patients and is usually slowly progressive but intermittent, with long intervals of freedom of symptoms. The dysphagia is far more often caused by solids than by liquids. The degree of swallowing difficulty is usually mild, but in some patients it is so severe that it causes significant weight loss. Sub-sternal or epigastric distress during the ingestion of food, varying from slight discomfort to severe pain radiating to the back or to the shoulders, is another symptom of leiomyoma, occurring in about 51% of the patients. Respiratory symptoms such as cough, dyspnea, wheezing, choking spells and recurrent respiratory infections also occur in patients with benign esophageal tumors. In 10 out of the 82 patients of Storey and Adams (1956) they were the pre-dominant if not exclusive complaints. These symptoms are probably caused either by compression of the trachea or main stem bronchus or by reflux of esophageal contents into the airways. Choking or gagging on swallowing are occasionally the presenting complaints.

As the mucosa overlying the leiomyoma ulcerates rarely, bleeding directly related to the tumor is also observed rarely. When hematemesis or melena occur in a patient with leiomyoma one should look for another cause of the hemorrhage unless ulcerative lesions of the tumor or erosions of the overlying mucosa can be demonstrated endoscopically. Vague digestive complaints, nausea, vomiting, heartburn, bloating and flatulence are often mentioned but their relation to the esophageal tumor is uncertain.

3.1.4. Radiographic Signs

Benign tumors of the esophagus, like mediastinal space-occupying lesions, may be demonstrated on chest radiographs in anteroposterior and lateral posi-tions. Large tumors can produce a widening of the mediastinum or can be seen on routine posteroanterior chest films as a smooth and rounded or lobulated mass of increased density, bulging from one side or the other of the mediastinal shadow. This image is different from the elongated fusiform soft tissue density ensheathing a stenosing carcinomatous filling defect. Smaller benign tumors are less readily demonstrated on chest radiographs but can best be visualized on lateral views as a mass situated in the posterior mediastinum. Other signs which can be seen on plain chest radiographs are tracheal shift (Lewis and Maxfield,

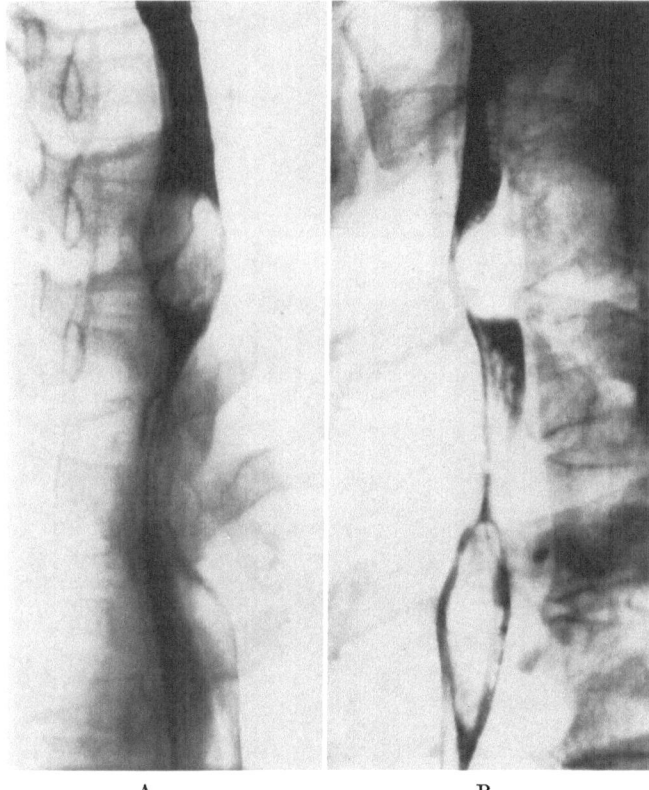

A   B

Fig. 211 A and B. Leiomyoma in the middle third of the esophagus. The sharp and smooth
contour of the filling defect and the effacement of the mucosal pattern (smear effect) are
well demonstrated on the anteroposterior view (A). Note also the abrupt onset of the smooth
filling defect, which appears to emerge from the wall at a definite angle (step effect) in the
lateral view (B)

1954) and calcification (SWEET et al., 1954; STOREY and ADAMS, 1956). Pneumomediastinum may also be used to delineate a leiomyoma of the thoracic esophagus
(PERASALO and LAUSTELA, 1955; OLBERT, 1970) but in most instances this would
seem to be a rather complicated way of diagnosing this condition.

Barium swallow examination is the most useful method to demonstrate a
leiomyoma of the esophagus. In profile the tumor appears as a smooth, semilunar or crescent-shaped filling defect which moves with swallowing, is sharply
demarcated and is covered and surrounded by normal mucosa (Figs. 211 B, 212).
The movement of the tumor with deglutition and esophageal contraction indicates
that the mass does not adhere to or does not infiltrate into the adjacent structures. The sharp angle at the proximal and distal margins, where the tumor
meets the normal esophageal wall, and the absence of ulceration, roughening
or irregularity of the mucosa are also quite characteristic. The transition from
normal mucosa to lesion is so abrupt that it has been compared to a "step effect"
(SCHATZKI and HAWES, 1942; HARPER and TISCENCO, 1945) (Fig. 211 B). A "ring
sign" has been described by HARPER and TISCENCO at the lower pole of the tumor,
at the level where the esophagus is apparently kinked against the lower border
of the growth.

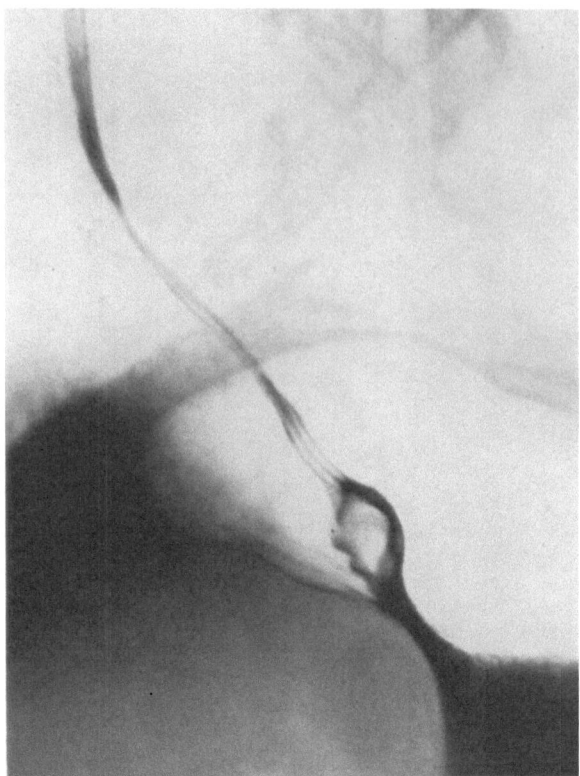

Fig. 212. Small leiomyoma at the esophagogastric junction, appearing as a smooth oval filling defect

When seen in frontal projection the submucosal tumor with its stretched mucosa protruding into the lumen of the gullet can be observed as a foldless area while the opposite wall shows normal mucosal folds (Fig. 211 A). This appearance has been described by Schatzki and Hawes (1942) as the "smear effect" and by Harper and Tiscenco (1945) as the "mold effect". During the passage of barium a smoothly outlined fork-like splitting of the barium can be observed at the level where the tumor protrudes into the esophageal lumen. The esophagus may be narrowed in one plane but stretched and widened in the opposite diameter. Dilatation of the gullet above the tumor is rare and not marked when present. An esophageal hiatus hernia or epiphrenic diverticulum may mask a leiomyoma in the distal esophagus.

3.1.5. Esophagoscopy

In any patient who has presumptive radiological characteristics of a benign esophageal tumor esophagoscopy must be performed in view of the possible coexistence of a carcinoma and as the finding of mucosal involvement will suggest malignancy of the tumor. The findings on esophagoscopic examination are quite characteristic, namely a freely movable mass which bulges into or narrows the lumen and is covered by an intact mucosa of normal appearance. As the tumor is not infiltrating the esophagoscope can usually be passed beyond the lesion without difficulty, unless the growth is completely or almost completely annular. A specimen should not be removed from the mucosa for biopsy, because this would probably increase the chance of mucosal perforation at the time of surgical enucleation, due to fibrotic fixation of the tumor to the mucosa after healing of the mucosal defect. Biopsy is justified only if roughening, irregularity or ulceration of the mucosa overlying the tumor suggest malignancy. The firm and hard mass, as often felt with the rigid esophagoscope, contrasts sharply with the soft compressible quality exhibited by cysts of esophageal or extra-esophageal origin. An intramural esophageal leiomyoma may be completely missed at esophagoscopy, due to the mobility of the tumor, which may be displaced easily by the esophagoscope so that it no longer protrudes into the lumen. Exceptionally a leiomyoma is a pedunculated lesion which cannot be distinguished from other benign pedunculated growths.

It may be wise to undertake a bronchoscopy at the same time as the esophagoscopy, in an attempt to exclude a bronchial carcinoma, because that tumor itself or metastases may produce extrinsic esophageal compression, which may mimic an intramural esophageal tumor.

3.1.6. Diagnosis

Symptomatology may be suggestive of esophageal disease. X-ray studies offer supportive evidence for a benign extramucosal or extraesophageal lesion. The radiological differential diagnosis between an intrinsic extramucosal lesion and an attached extrinsic process may be very difficult if not impossible. In both instances there may be an apparent filling defect, corresponding to a deviated esophageal segment with a slit-like lumen bulging away from a soft tissue mass; in both instances the outline of this apparent filling defect is perfectly smooth and covered by flattened mucosal folds which are intact unless the mucosa is invaded. Radiological signs which militate against a malignant or any actually attached extrinsic condition are the mobility of the mass, which moves together with the esophagus on respiration or coughing, the variation in shape and size of the distorted area and the visualization of a soft tissue mass fitting into the marginal "filling defect" on the barium-filled esophagus. The differentiation between an intrinsic extramucosal tumor and a benign sessile polypoid lesion of mucosal origin depends on the presence of a soft tissue mass with much of its outline projecting outside the outlined mucosa.

Contraction of the cricopharyngeal muscle may mimic the X-ray picture of a benign tumor. The diagnosis can easily be made when on serial X-rays the sphincter is seen to relax (Fig. 213). Elongated sausage-shaped, slightly lobulated filling defects suggest a pedunculated polyp of submucosal origin rather than a pedunculated mucosal growth, because the latter is an extremely rare esophageal lesion. It must be emphasized, however, that pedunculated mucosal growths may be malignant (BOCKUS, 1963).

Various signs can help to differentiate a benign extramucosal tumor from a carcinomatous deformity. A carcinomatous filling defect has a more irregular outline, is more or less stenosing with an elongated fusiform tissue density ensheathing the defect, has undermined margins, is covered with an erosive or ulcerated mucosa and is surrounded by thickened and abnormal mucosal folds. A benign lesion, on the other hand, is characterized by a smooth outline, the presence of a soft tissue mass bulging outside the esophageal outline, the absence of marked stenosis, the presence of a smear or mold effect and of a ring sign, and the presence of a normal mucosa overlying and surrounding the lesion.

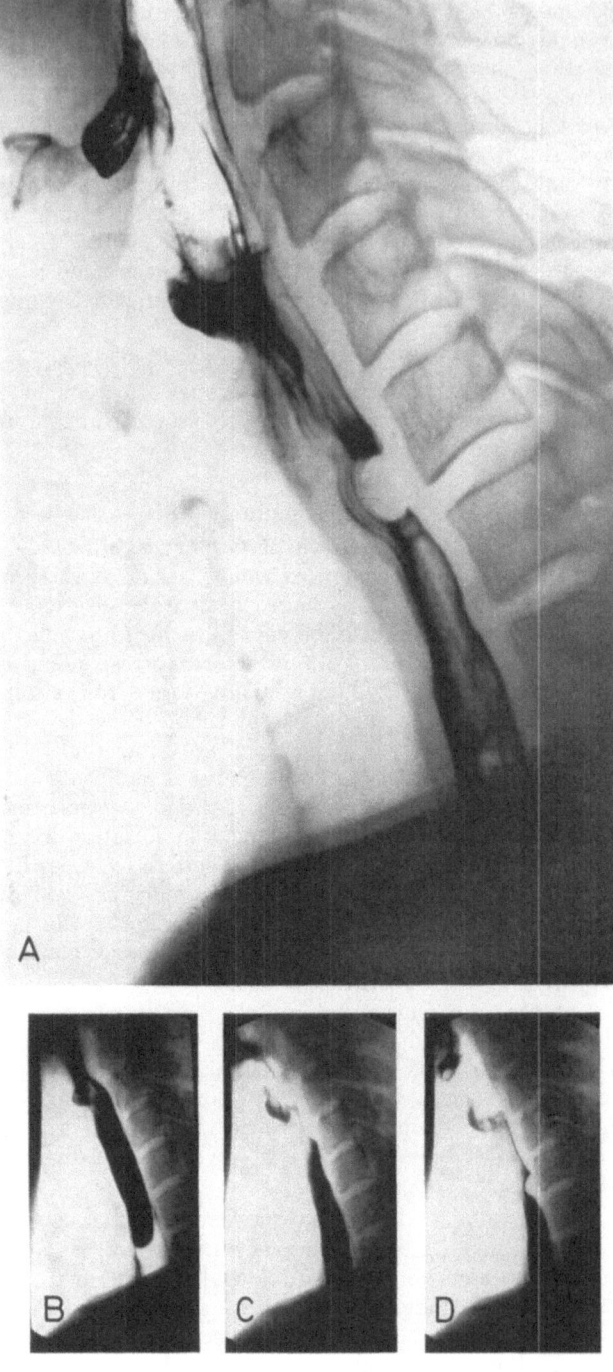

Fig. 213. A Indentation in the posterior wall of the pharyngoesophageal junction mimicking a submucosal tumor but caused by contraction of the cricopharyngeus. The 70 mm photofluorographic pictures (B, C, D) show that the indentation disappears during deglutition

The most reliable radiological signs which favor the diagnosis of primary esophageal carcinoma, even if they are discrete, are rigidity of the wall and retention of barium above the lesion due to some degree of obstruction. Esophagoscopy should be performed whenever there is doubt about the malignant or benign nature of the lesion, but biopsy is contraindicated if the overlying mucosa looks normal. A malignant tumor invading the esophagus from the outside (e.g. a bronchial carcinoma) may raise very difficult diagnostic problems. Bronchoscopy may help to rule out the possibility that a marginal filling defect is due to invasion of the mucosal wall by a bronchial carcinoma or its metastases. One should keep in mind that leiomyoma and other diseases including malignancy, diverticulum and hiatal hernia may coexist and that the recognition of this coexistence demands a thorough examination of the esophagus.

3.1.7. Complications

Intramural leiomyomas give rise to complications only rarely. Because of their extramucosal location and of the absence of the typical umbilicate ulceration so frequently seen with leiomyomas of other gastrointestinal organs, and because erosive lesions of the overlying mucosa are rare, significant hemorrhage is an exceptional complication. A case of malignant degeneration of leiomyoma to leiomyosarcoma has been reported by BIASINI (1949). In this instance a typical fibroleiomyoma of 6×4.5 cm contained a small area of leiomyosarcoma. JOHNSTON et al. (1953) and OVENS and RUSSELL (1951) also described cases in which sarcomatous change was present. Bronchopulmonary infectious complications, due to aspiration of esophageal contents into the airways, are also very uncommon.

3.1.8. Treatment

In spite of its slow growth and limited potential of malignant degeneration the tumor should be removed surgically unless there are specific contraindications. The majority of these tumors can be removed by simple enucleation. If during this procedure the mucous membrane has been opened accidentally or as a result of adhesions between the tumor and mucosa, the defect should be repaired primarily. Following removal of the lesion the outer esophageal wall can be reconstructed by closure of the attenuated muscle layer. Large defects in the esophageal wall can be supported by an omental or lung graft (NISSEN, 1949) or by a diaphragmatic pedicle or Ivalon graft (PETROVSKY and VANTSIAN, 1967). Tumors which firmly adhere to the overlying mucosa usually require local excision. Larger lesions or tumors involving the gastroesophageal region may require partial esophageal resection. Complete esophageal resection with colon interposition is indicated in cases of leiomyomas involving the entire esophagus (NAHMAD and CLATWORTHY, 1973). The location of the lesion and the extent of surgery that is anticipated will dictate the approach. Lesions of the proximal esophagus require a cervical approach or a right thoracotomy. Those in the middle are best removed from the right side, whereas the distal esophageal lesions necessitate a left thoracotomy or a thoracoabdominal approach (DILLOW et al., 1970). The mortality of enucleation is less than 2% (KAY, 1947; STOREY and ADAMS) 1956). Resection is associated with a mortality of 4.8% (GRAY et al., 1961, or more (KIRILUK, 1967).

3.2. Cysts

Enterogenous and bronchogenic cysts arise as a result of a developmental abnormality during the formation and differentiation of the lower respiratory

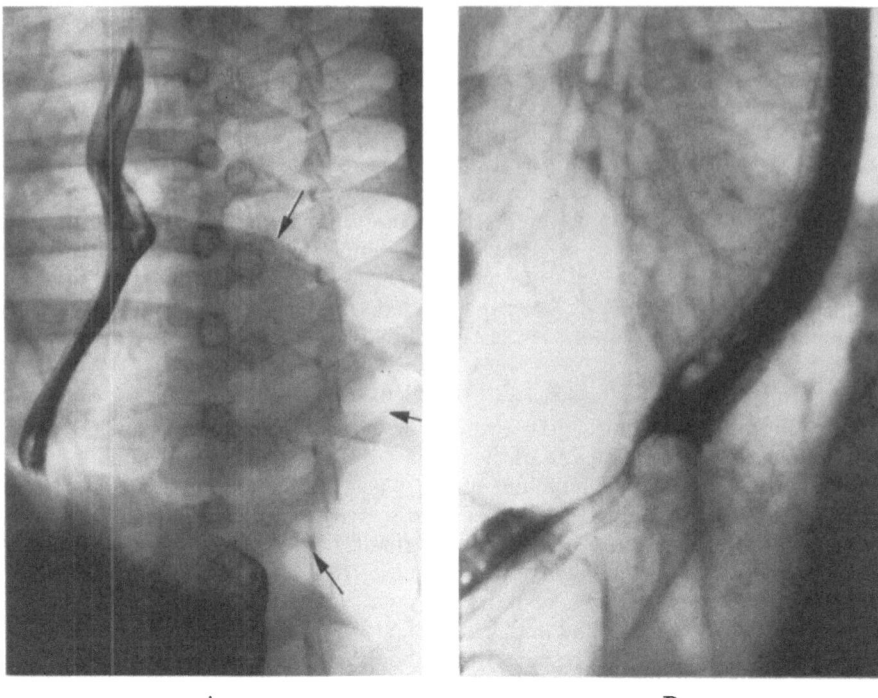

A   B

Fig. 214. A Duplication of the esophagus appearing as a cystic mass in the posterior mediastinum and producing a large indentation in the esophagus. B Small cyst in the lower esophagus appearing as a smooth filling defect with a sharp contour

tract, esophagus and stomach from the foregut (LATIMER, 1967). The complex nomenclature associated with these cysts attests to the difficulty of determining their origin. Several defects have been held responsible for their development. At the end of the second month of the embryonic life small diverticula of the foregut are found almost invariably. Instead of undergoing regression, these may persist and become pinched off to form cysts (LEWIS and THYNG, 1907, 1908). Another hypothesis holds that the nidus of a later cyst is formed by the sequestration of embryonic multipotential entodermal cells from the foregut. Failure of coalescence of the vacuoles which are formed in the solid foregut by the secretory activity of the epithelial cells is another hypothetical mechanism of cyst formation or of duplication of the esophagus (BREMER, 1944).

During its embryological development the esophagus is lined successively with simple columnar, pseudostratified, ciliated columnar and finally stratified squamous epithelium. This sequence of events probably accounts for the fact that the lining epithelium may be squamous, columnar or pseudostratified columnar, which is commonly ciliated. It should be emphasized that the presence of cilia does not necessarily indicate a respiratory origin (BOYD and HILL, 1957). Bronchogenic cysts are said to be characterized by the presence of cartilage in their wall (MYERS and BRADSHAW, 1951) whereas cysts surrounded by smooth muscle fibers have been considered as esophagenic (LATIMER, 1967). These characteristic findings are observed in a minority of instances so that differentiation of these two variaties is frequently very difficult if not impossible.

Cysts vary in size from small to very large. They are usually located intramurally in the middle or lower third of the esophagus and the majority contain mucoid material, although in some, particularly in those lined by gastric secretory epithelium, the content may be hemorrhagic (DESFORGES, 1967). The symptoms and signs of the cysts are similar to those of benign esophageal tumors (Fig. 214 A). Symptoms may be elicited by inflammation or infection of the cyst. The diagnosis depends on radiologic and endoscopic findings. Bronchographic examination is indicated whenever there are signs of bronchopulmonary infection.

Surgical excision is the treatment of choice. Most cysts can be enucleated without damage to the mucosa. The surgeon should look for fistulous tracts connecting the cyst with the airways (LACQUET et al., 1965). Segmental pulmonary resection may be indicated in these cases.

Two cases of acquired retention cysts have been reported (NESE, 1958; McCULLOUGH et al., 1970). Both occurred in the distal esophagus and were rather small (2 to 5 cm) (Fig. 214 B). One was a pedunculated lesion.

4. Intraluminal Tumors
4.1. Fibrovascular Polyp

The fibrovascular polyp is an intraluminal polypoid or pedunculated lesion, composed of varying amounts of fibrous, vascular and even adipose tissue covered by normal mucosa (STOUT, 1953). The heterogenous microscopic appearance of this growth is apparent from the varied nomenclature employed in the literature. When the fibrous elements are loose and myxoid the tumor is called myxoma or myxofibroma; when the growth contains a dense network of collagenous fibers it is called fibroma; the amount of adipose tissue may be so striking that the lesion is designated as fibrolipoma or pedunculated lipoma. Others call this lesion simply polyp (STOUT, 1953). FULLER (1963) suggests that these growths, with the exception of lipomas, should be classified as hamartomas, i.e. tumor-like but primarily non-neoplastic malformations with inborn errors of tissue development, characterized by abnormal mixtures of tissues indigenous to the part of the body where the lesion arises; frequently one or more of these tissue elements predominate over the others (WILLIS, 1958).

The fibrovascular polyps may be small lesions of about 1 cm in diameter; they may be pedunculated with a ribbon-like stalk of variable length or they may be bulky growths completely filling the esophageal lumen. Occasionally lesions of this histological type are located intramurally. Of the 40 intraluminal polyps discussed by TOTTEN et al. (1953) 29 were males and all were adults; 34 of the tumors were located in the upper third of the esophagus, and 25 of these were attached in the region of the cricoid cartilage. According to JANG et al. (1969) 56 cases have been reported in the literature.

The most common clinical features of the intraluminal polyp is dysphagia, regurgitation and weight loss. As the tumor grows very slowly these are usually late symptoms. The tumor can become so large that it compresses the trachea and causes respiratory difficulties. Epigastric and retrosternal pain of varying intensity also occur. The most dramatic manifestation of the pedunculated tumor is the regurgitation of the growth into the mouth (MINSKI, 1895). The regurgitated tumor may even cause asphyxia if it is aspirated and causes laryngeal impaction (ALLEN and TALBOT, 1957). Radiological examination shows the intraluminal tumors as oval-shaped or elongated sausage-like masses, with a smooth or lobulated surface. The area of attachment of the stalk may be identified by an indentation of the esophageal wall above the pedicle shadow. Esophagoscopy may be useful to identify the origin and size of the pedicle. When mucosal ulceration suggests malignancy a biopsy should be performed.

Pedunculated intraluminal tumors should be removed. If they are not, the ultimate outcome in many patients is poor, while only one instance of recurrence has been reported after resection of the tumor (WATSON et al., 1967).

If the lesion is not too voluminous endoscopic resection with a snare is feasible. A careful technique is required to avoid hemorrhage from blood vessels in the pedicle. Large tumors should be removed surgically through either a transcervical or a transthoracic approach.

4.2. Papillomas

Esophageal papilloma is a benign, sessile, lobulated or branching tumor consisting of central cords of fibrous tissue covered by stratified squamous mucosa (STOUT and LATTES, 1957; ADLER et al., 1959; DUBARRY et al., 1967).

In 1957, STOUT and LATTES believed that lesions called esophageal papilloma in man are the result of inflammatory processes in which the esophageal lining has been thrown into papillary folds. Since that time at least two documented cases of papilloma have been reported (ADLER et al., 1959; WEITZNER and HENTEL, 1968).

Not all wart-like protuberances or small polypoid lesions are papillomas. Localized areas of epithelial hyperplasia, granulomatous proliferation, hyperkeratosis, acanthosis and leukoplakia should not be confused with a true papilloma. Moreover, papilloma-like lesions have been observed proximal to malignancy (ADLER et al., 1959), indicating that the patient in whom the biopsy diagnosis of papilloma has been made should be carefully examined. The diagnosis of benign squamous papilloma should be made only after careful gross and histologic examination of the completely removed tumor. Although these tumors are small and asymptomatic they should be removed, because they may be precancerous lesions.

4.3. Adenomas

True adenomas of the esophageal glands are uncommon and rarely if ever produce clinical symptoms. They may resemble "pyloric glands" or they may be similar to the adenomatous polyps seen in the colon (TOTTEN et al., 1953).

5. Hemangiomas

Well-documented case reports of hemangioma of the esophagus are distinctly rare. TOTTEN et al. (1953) reviewed the literature and found no such cases. In their comprehensive review of vascular lesions of the gastrointestinal tract, GENTRY et al. (1949) found 16 benign vascular tumors of the esophagus, of which 12 were found at autopsy. Other cases have been reported by VINSON et al. (1926), by PLACHTA (1962), by RIEMENSCHNEIDER and KLASSEN (1968), by WEICHSELBAUMER (1968) and by others. From these reports it appears that X-ray therapy is inadequate to control the lesion and that observation is hazardous because of the possibility of bleeding and malignancy. Localized lesions have been resected succesfully and this would seem to be the treatment of choice if the lesion is not too extensive.

References

ADLER, R. H., CARBERRY, D. M., ROSS, C. A.: Papilloma of the esophagus. Association with hiatal hernia. J. thorac. Surg. **37**, 625–635 (1959).

ALLEN, M. S., JR., TALBOT, W. H.: Sudden death due to regurgitation of a pedunculated esophageal lipoma. J. thorac. cardiovasc. Surg. **54**, 756–758 (1957).

BARRETT, N. R.: Benign smooth muscle tumours of the oesophagus. Thorax **19**, 185–194 (1964).

BIASINI, A.: Su di un caso di fibroleiomioma dell'esofago ipobronchiale in transformazione maligna; asportazione per via transpleuro-diaframmatica ed esofago-gastrostomia guarigione. Pathologica **41**, 260–267 (1949).

BOCKUS, H. L.: Gastroenterology, vol. I. Philadelphia: W. B. Saunders Co. 1963.

BOGEDAIN, W., CARPATHIOS, J., NAJIB, A.: Leiomyoma of the esophagus. Dis. Chest **44**, 391–399 (1963).

BOYD, D. P., HILL, L. D.: Benign tumors and cysts of the esophagus. Amer. J. Surg. **93**, 252–258 (1957).

BRADFORD, M. L., MAHON, H. W., GROW, J. B.: Mediastinal cysts and tumors. Surg. Gynec. Obstet. **85**, 467–491 (1947).

BREMER, J. L.: Diverticula and duplications of the intestinal tract. Arch. Path. **38**, 132–140 (1944).

CALLANAN, J. G.: Simultaneous occurrence of simple and malignant tumors of the esophagus. J. thorac. Surg. **28**, 4–10 (1954).

CALMENSON, M., CLAGETT, O. T.: Surgical removal of leiomyomas of the esophagus. Amer. J. Surg. **72**, 745–747 (1946).

DANIEL, R. A., JR., WILLIAMS, R. B., JR.: Leiomyoma of the esophagus. J. thorac. Surg. 800–805 (1950).

DESFORGES, G.: Primitive foregut cysts. Ann. thorac. Surg. **4**, 547–577 (1967).

DILLOW, B. M., NEIS, D. D., SELLERS, R. D.: Leiomyoma of the esophagus. Amer. J. Surg. **120**, 615–619 (1970).

DUBARRY, J.-J., RICHIR, C., BERNARD, J.-P., LACOSTE, G., FAIVRE, J., BRETELLE, J.: La papillomatose de l'œsophage. Arch. franç. Mal. Appar. dig. **56**, 713–720 (1967).

FRANK, H., REINER, L., FLEISCHNER, F.: Co-occurrence of large leiomyoma of the esophagus and squamous-cell carcinoma of the thymus. New Engl. J. Med. **255**, 159–164 (1956).

FULLER, A. P.: Pedunculated hamartoma of the oesophagus. J. Laryng. **77**, 706–713 (1963).

GENTRY, R. W., DOCKERTY, M. B., CLAGETT, O. T.: Collective review; vascular malformations and vascular tumors of the gastrointestinal tract. Int. Abstr. Surg. **88**, 281–323 (1949).

GRAY, S. W., SKANDALAKIS, J. E., SHEPARD, D.: Smooth muscle tumors of the esophagus. Int. Abstr. Surg. **113**, 205–220 (1961).

HARPER, R. A. K., TISCENCO, E.: Benign tumour of the oesophagus and its differential diagnosis. Brit. J. Radiol. **18**, 99–107 (1945).

HARRINGTON, S. W., MOERSCH, H. J.: Surgical treatment and clinical manifestations of benign tumors of the esophagus with report of seven cases. J. thorac. Surg. **13**, 394–414 (1944).

HIGGINSON, J. F.: Discussion of SWEET, R. H., L. SOUTTER, and C. T. VALENZUELA: Muscle wall tumors of the esophagus. J. thorac. Surg. **27**, 13–35 (1954).

HUDDY, P., GRIFFITHS, G.: Leiomyoma of the oesophagus with calcification. Brit. J. Surg. **59**, 239–240 (1972).

JANG, G. C., CLOUSE, M. E., FLEISCHNER, F. G.: Fibrovascular polyp. A benign intraluminal tumor of the esophagus. Radiology **92**, 1196–1200 (1969).

JOHNSTON, J. B., CLAGETT, O. T., McDONALD, J. R.: Smooth muscle tumours of the oesophagus. Thorax 8, 251–265 (1953).

KAY, E. B.: Surgical lesions of the esophagus seen in an army thoracic surgery center. J. thorac. Surg. **16**, 207–214 (1947).

KENNEY, L. J.: Giant intramural leiomyoma of esophagus; case report. J. thorac. Surg. **26**, 93–100 (1953).

KIRILUK, L. B.: Leiomyoma of the esophagus. Northw. Med. (Seattle) **66**, 551–555 (1967).

LACQUET, A. M., GRUWEZ, J., STUYCK, R.: Benign lesions of the esophagus. Acta chir. belg., Suppl. **2**, 5–24 (1965).

LATIMER, R. D.: Enterogenous cysts of the oesophagus. Brit. J. Dis. Chest **61**, 136–137 (1967).

LEWIS, B., MAXFIELD, R. G.: Leiomyoma of the esophagus. Case report and review of the literature. Int. Abstr. Surg. **99**, 105–128 (1954).

LEWIS, F. T., THYNG, F. W.: Regular occurrence of intestinal diverticula in embryos of pig, rabbit, and man. Amer. J. Anat. **7**, 505–519 (1907–1908).

Linder, F., Vogt-Moykopf, I.: Diffuse Leiomyomatose des Oesophagus. Langenbecks Arch. Chir. **328**, 42–49 (1970).

Lortat-Jacob, J. L.: Myomatoses localisées et myomatoses diffuses de l'œsophage. Arch. franç. Mal. Appar. dig. **39**, 519–524 (1950).

McCullough, F. S., Klassen, K. P., Beman, F. M.: Esophageal retention cyst: an unusual entity. Ohio med. J. **66**, 576–578 (1970).

Minski, P. R.: Zur Entwicklungsgeschichte und Klinik der Polypen und polypenähnlichen Gewächse des Rachens und der Speiseröhre. Dtsch. Z. Chir. **11**, 513–585 (1895).

Moersch, H. J., Harrington, S. W.: Benign tumor of the esophagus. Ann. Otol. (St. Louis) **53**, 800–817 (1944).

Myers, R. T., Bradshaw, H. H.: Benign intramural tumors and cysts of the esophagus. J. thorac. cardiovasc. Surg. **21**, 470–482 (1951).

Nahmad, M., Clatworthy, H. W.: Leiomyoma of the entire esophagus. J. Pediat. Surg. **8**, 829–830 (1973).

Nese, G.: Benign tumors and cysts of the esophagus. Acta chir. scand. **114**, 165–171 (1958).

Nissen, R.: Bridging of esophageal defect by pedicled flap of lung tissue. Ann. Surg. **129**, 142–147 (1949).

Olbert, F.: Das Leiomyom des Ösophagus. Fortschr. Röntgenstr. **113**, 11–15 (1970).

Ovens, J. M., Russell, W. O.: Concurrent leiomyosarcoma and squamous carcinoma of esophagus. Arch. Path. (Chic.) **51**, 560–564 (1951).

Perasalo, O., Laustela, E.: Benign muscle wall tumours of the oesophagus: report of two cases. Ann. Chir. Gynaec. Fenn. **44**, 145–156 (1955).

Petrovsky, B. V., Vantsian, E. N.: Our experience in the surgical treatment of malignant and benign esophageal tumors. Surgery **62**, 833–838 (1967).

Plachta, A.: Benign tumors of the esophagus. Review of literature and report of 99 cases. Amer. J. Gastroent. **38**, 639–652 (1962).

Postlethwait, R. W., Sealy, W. C.: Benign tumors of the esophagus. Chapt. XI: Surgery of the esophagus. Springfield (Ill.): Charles C. Thomas, Publisher 1961.

Puestow, C. B., Gillesby, W. J., Powers, J. A.: Benign tumors of the esophagus. Amer. Surg. **21**, 425–433 (1955).

Riemenschneider, H. W., Klassen, K. P.: Cavernous esophageal hemangioma. Ann. thorac. Surg. **6**, 552–556 (1968).

Schatzki, R., Hawes, L. E.: The roentgenological appearance of extramucosal tumors of the esophagus: analysis of intramural extramucosal lesions of gastrointestinal tract in general. Amer. J. Roentgenol. **48**, 1–15 (1942).

Schmidt, A., Lockwood, K.: Benign neoplasms of the esophagus. Acta chir. scand. **133**, 640–644 (1967).

Schmidt, H. W., Clagett, O. T., Harrison, E. G., Jr.: Benign tumors and cysts of the esophagus. J. thorac. cardiovasc. Surg. **41**, 717–732 (1961).

Storey, C. F., Adams, W. C.: Leiomyoma of the esophagus. A report of four cases and review of the surgical literature. Amer. J. Surg. **91**, 3–23 (1956).

Stout, A. P.: Tumors of the soft tissues, sect. II, fasc. 5. Washington, D.C.: A.F.I.P. 1953.

Stout, A. P., Lattes, R.: Tumors of the esophagus, sect. V, fasc. 20. Washington, D.C.: A.F.I.P., Atlas tumor path. Fasc. 1957.

Sweet, R. H., Soutter, L., Valenzuela, C. T.: Muscle wall tumors of the esophagus. J. thorac. Surg. **27**, 13–35 (1954).

Totten, R. S., Stout, A. P., Humphreys, G. H., Moore, R. L.: Benign tumors and cysts of the esophagus. J. thorac. Surg. **25**, 606–622 (1953).

Toumieux, B., Levasseur, P., Rojas-Miranda, A., Merlier, M., Le Brigand, H.: La chirurgie des léiomyomes de l'œsophage: à propos de 12 interventions. Chirurgie **97**, 553–561 (1971).

Tsuzuki, T., Kakegawa, T., Arimori, M., Ueda, M., Watanabe, H., Okamoto, T., Akakura, I.: Giant leiomyoma of the esophagus and cardia weighing more than 1,000 grams. Dis. Chest **60**, 396–399 (1971).

Vinson, P. P., Moore, A. B., Bowing, H. H.: Hemangioma of the esophagus. Amer. J. Sci. **172**, 416–418 (1926).

Watson, R. R.: O'Connor, T. M., Weisel, W.: Solid benign tumors of the esophagus. Ann. thorac. Surg. **4**, 80–91 (1967).

Weichselbaumer, W.: Haemangioma cavernosum im Ösophagus. Mschr. Ohrenheilk. **102**, 333–340 (1968).

Weitzner, S., Hentel, W.: Squamous papilloma of esophagus. Case report and review of the literature. Amer. J. Gastroent. **50**, 391–396 (1968).

Willis, R. A.: The borderland of embryology and pathology, chapt. 9. London: Butterworths 1958.

Malignant Tumors of the Esophagus

J. G. Pearson and B. T. Le Roux

With 20 Figures

1. Esophageal Carcinoma

Nearly all primary carcinomas of the esophagus arise from its lining of stratified squamous epithelium, forming squamous cell (epidermoid) carcinoma. Rarely primary adenocarcinoma develops in the esophagus, either from ectopic gastric mucosa or from esophageal glands. (Commonly, adenocarcinoma of the stomach extends up into the esophagus.)

1.1. Incidence and Etiology

In common with most cancers, the incidence of esophageal cancer increases with age, the rate of increase being greater in older age groups (Case, 1961). There are very large geographical variations, which occur unevenly in the two sexes, the incidence usually being greater in men; and in those areas of Northern Europe where the incidence is relatively high in women this is particularly in the upper portion of the esophagus. Many factors have been found to be associated with an increased incidence of esophageal cancer but the associations are not consistently present for all groups of patients developing the disease and many of the factors are interdependent. No single factor has been identified as the main cause of the disease.

No other common human cancer shows such striking geographical variation in incidence. In men, in the Ghurjev region of Kazakhstan on the north coast of the Caspian, esophageal cancer is 200 times as common as in Nigeria, Holland, Alberta or Manitoba, and more than three times as common as lung cancer in England (Doll, 1967, 1969). The incidence of esophageal cancer is also very high, and it is the commonest cancer in men among Africans in the Transkei region of Cape Province (Burrell, 1969), in Bulawayo (Skinner, 1967), in Durban (Bradshaw and Schonland, 1969) and in the central Nyanza district of west Kenya around Kisumu (Ahmed and Cook, 1969). Within 150 miles to the west and to the east of the central Nyanza district the incidence probably falls by a factor of more than ten. Similar wide variations in incidence over a few hundred miles have been observed in Zambia (McGlashan, 1969). The disease is now common amongst Africans in all the large cities of South Africa, Southern Rhodesia, Kenya and Nyasaland but not in those in Mozambique, Northern Rhodesia, Tanganyika, Uganda or West Africa (Oettlé, 1964). Esophageal cancer is also the commonest cancer in men in the north of the Honan province in China (Li et al., 1962), in Curaçao (Hartz, 1958), and in Brazil (Pan American Health Organization, 1963). The high incidence has been observed to develop, as an epidemic, since about 1945 in parts of the Transkei (Burrell, 1969) and in Durban (Bradshaw and Schonland, 1969) and these authors and McGlashan (1969) have searched for associated environmental factors characteristic of that period. From a small series of nine esophageal cancers in Alaskan Eskimos, Hurst (1964) suspects a very high incidence in Alaskan Eskimo women, possibly associated with the prolonged chewing of wood ash-smeared seal skin used to make mukluks.

A decreasing incidence, since about 1945, of upper esophageal carcinoma associated with the Paterson-Kelly (Plummer-Vinson) syndrome in under-nourished, iron-deficient women in parts of Britain and Scandinavia has been observed in association with improved nutrition (Jacobson, 1961). In England and Wales, a marked secular decrease in mortality from cancer of the esophagus, more pronounced for males than females, has occurred over an interval of 30 years, as shown by cohort analysis. For example, at the age of 50–54, the death rate for males born around 1901 is only 27 per cent of the rate for males of the same age group born around 1871 (Case, 1961).

Of the numerous factors that have been incriminated as causes of esophageal cancer, there are rare, but occasionally strongly associated and likely predisposing factors such as lye strictures (Bigger and Vinson, 1950; Kiviranta, 1952), ionizing radiation (Goolden, 1957; Pearson, 1966), Paterson-Kelly (Plummer-Vinson) syndrome (Ahlbom, 1936, 1937), malabsorption syndrome (Wright and Richardson, 1967), previous gastric surgery (Shearman et al., 1970), and tylosis (Clarke et al., 1957; Shine and Allison, 1966); and there are, in various communities, commonly occurring and often cross-related associated factors of less easily determined etiological significance, such as malnutrition, heavy use of alcohol and tobacco (Wander and Bross, 1961), the drinking of spirits (Tuyns, 1970), betel chewing (Stephen and Uragoda, 1970), contamination by petroleum or its products of the air (Hartz, 1958) or drinking water (Morton, 1968), and the contamination of home-distilled spirits by zinc, possibly facilitating the formation of nitrosamine (McGlashan, 1969). Smithers (1961) and Ellis (1960) discuss fully the increased incidence of squamous carcinoma in the long damaged mucosa of the esophagus in patients with achalasia. Pierce et al. (1970) have reported three more such patients. Steiner (1956) found polyps of the large intestine in 17 out of 116 cases of esophageal cancer, a significantly increaesd incidence. He also confirmed numerous earlier observations of an increased incidence of second independent primary malignant tumors in the upper alimentary tract, suggesting the possibility of a common ingested carcinogen, or an increased susceptibility of the alimentary tract.

The causes of esophageal carcinoma are likely to be numerous and complex (Oettlé, 1967). Only about five per cent of the tumors arise in association with a pre-existing organic lesion (Steiner, 1956). For many of the remaining cases, in some areas malnutrition, and in others something carcinogenic, some-times consumed in alcohol, and sometimes arising from tobacco, appear likely to be important factors (Lancet Annotation, 1969).

Steiner (1956) has studied nine small symptomless esophageal cancers in cadavers and he concludes that these tumors usually arose from epithelium that tended to be atrophic and to be based on a fibrotic lamina propria. He also notes the rarity of clinically silent esophageal cancer as an incidental necropsy finding in contrast with prostatic cancer, and concludes that a prolonged in situ stage is not the rule in esophageal cancer.

1.2. Pathology

Two histological varieties of esophageal carcinoma are encountered—squamous carcinoma (Figs. 215, 216) and adenocarcinoma. The esophageal mucosa is normally lined by stratified squamous epithelium and the common carcinoma is a squamous carcinoma. SMITHERS (1956, 1961) considered that eight per cent of 314 patients with esophageal cancer had true primary adenocarcinomas of the esophagus. However, adenocarcinoma of the stomach frequently spreads up into the esophagus (Fig. 222) and he found over 70 per cent of tumors which involve the extreme lower limit of the esophagus to be adenocarcinomas.

LE ROUX (1961a) found that of 680 patients investigated for dysphagia and found to have carcinoma of the esophagus or stomach, 40 per cent had adeno-carcinoma in the proximal stomach, cardia, or lower esophagus and 60 per cent had squamous or undifferentiated carcinoma of the esophagus. Usually, adeno-carcinoma in the esophagus is in continuity with a gastric tumor. A submucous extension of a distal adenocarcinoma may ulcerate through the mucosa of the proximal esophagus.

1.2.1. Squamous Cell Carcinoma
1.2.1.1. Site

Squamous carcinoma of the esophagus is common at all levels in the organ but there is variation in site incidence with geographical area, with sex and in successive cohorts. The male-female ratio varies from 1:1 in Finland and Scotland to 10:1 in France. There is a higher incidence of the disease in the upper esoph-agus in women in Northern Europe. In most geographical areas where the incidence of the disease is very high, it is more common in men than women, but in the Transkei (BURRELL, 1969) and in Curaçao (HARTZ, 1958) the incidence in men and women is almost equal. In these latter areas the tumors showed no tendency, in either sex, to occur more frequently towards the upper end of the organ.

1.2.1.2. Size

It is unusual for the diagnosis to be made until the tumor is more than 4 cm long, not infrequently it is more than 10 cm long and occasionally it may invade the whole esophagus. It is unusual for an unulcerated tumor to cause dysphagia until more than half the circumference of the organ has been rendered inelastic by invasion of the muscle wall. Severe dysphagia does not usually occur until the whole or nearly the whole circumference has been invaded. In a series of 280 patients reported by PEARSON (1966), treated by operation or radical X-ray therapy and therefore excluding the most advanced cases with demonstrable distant spread of the disease, the mean length of the gross measurable tumor was 6.4 cm. In autopsy series, more extensive tumors may be found.

1.2.1.3. Macroscopic Appearance

The early stages of the disease are symptomless and, therefore, are rarely seen in life. By the time symptoms lead to investigation by radiography and endoscopy, the tumor presents as an ulcerating mass, an ulcer with everted margins, an excavating ulcer, an ulcerated stricture or a proliferative, partially pedunculated mass. Not uncommonly it presents as a stenosing lesion with apparently intact mucosa which is only moderately irregular, infiltration of the esophageal wall having provoked a fibrous reaction which may be the main cause of the stenosis.

1.2.1.4. Microscopic Appearance

In the esophagus squamous carcinoma is more frequently undifferentiated (Fig. 215) than it is in the oral cavity, usually Broder's Grade 3 and 4 (BURGESS

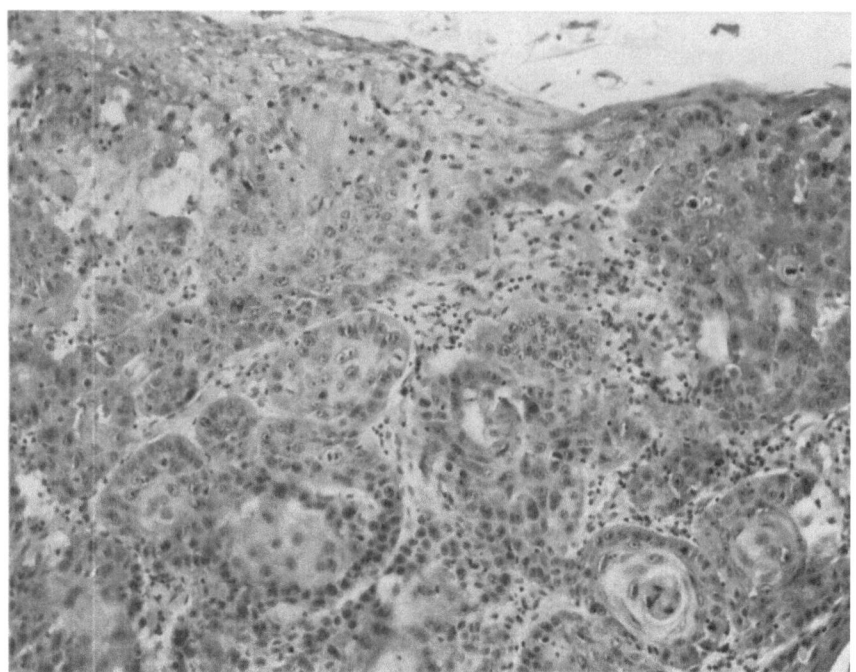

Fig. 215. Photomicrograph of a moderately undifferentiated squamous-cell carcinoma of the esophagus showing infiltrating tongues of tumor tissue in continuity with overlying squamous epithelium. In the right lower field there is a well formed "epithelial pearl". Several mitotic figures are visible (×125)

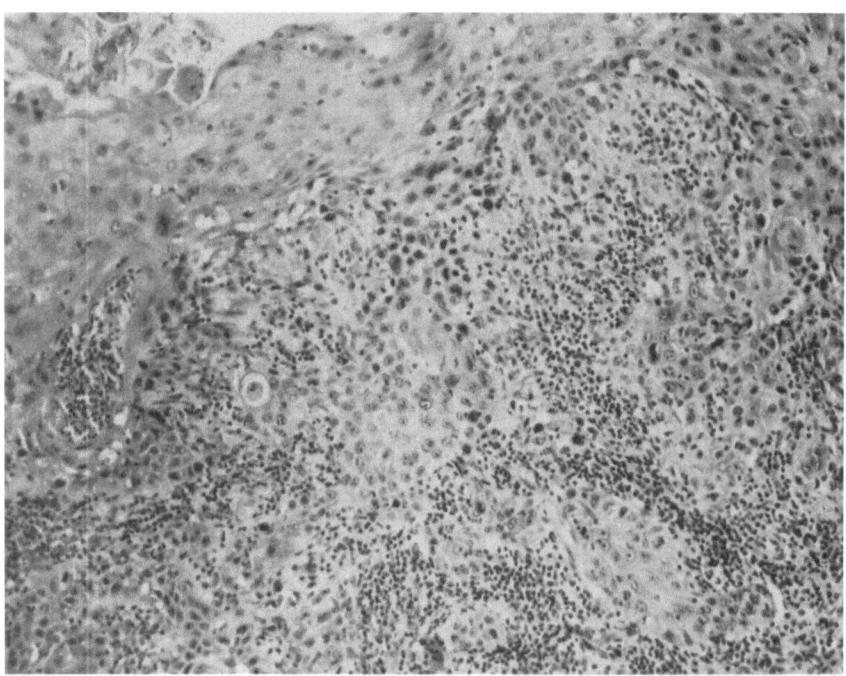

Fig. 216. Photomicrograph of squamous-cell carcinoma of the esophagus, slightly less differentiated than in Fig. 215. There is wide infiltration by inflammatory cells (×125)

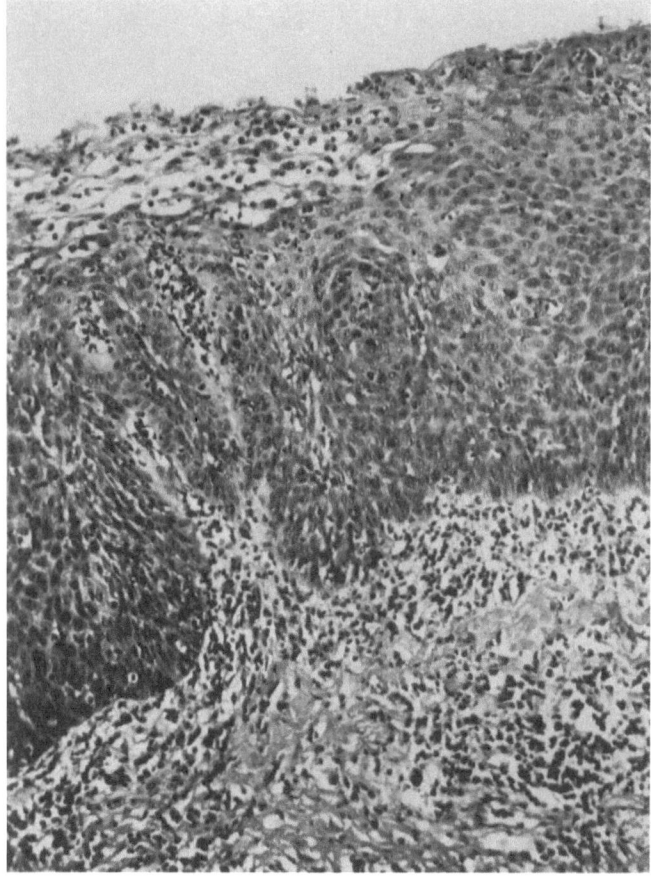

Fig. 217. Photomicrograph of thickened esophageal epithelium showing intra-epithelial carcinoma. This lay adjacent to the highly malignant squamous carcinoma shown in Fig. 218
(×125)

et al., 1951). Not infrequently only microscopy reveals the extent of submucosal
infiltration. GOWING (1961) describes and illustrates a range of appearances from
the best differentiated patterns, featuring prickle cell formation and keratinization
and sometimes showing the changes of carcinoma-in-situ for some distance along
the adjacent mucosa (Fig. 217), to poorly differentiated tumors (Fig. 218) sometimes resembling "oat-cell carcinoma" of lung and occasionally showing features
reminiscent of "basal-cell carcinoma". The amount of connective tissue ranges
from very little in relation to continuous masses of epithelial cells, to narrow
columns of tumor cells separated by abundant stroma. Frequently, marked
inflammatory cell infiltration occurs (Fig. 216).

1.2.1.5. Direct Spread

The greatest direct spread occurs in the submucosa. Preferential spread in
this layer tends to be more extensive proximally than distally (BERGMAN, 1959)

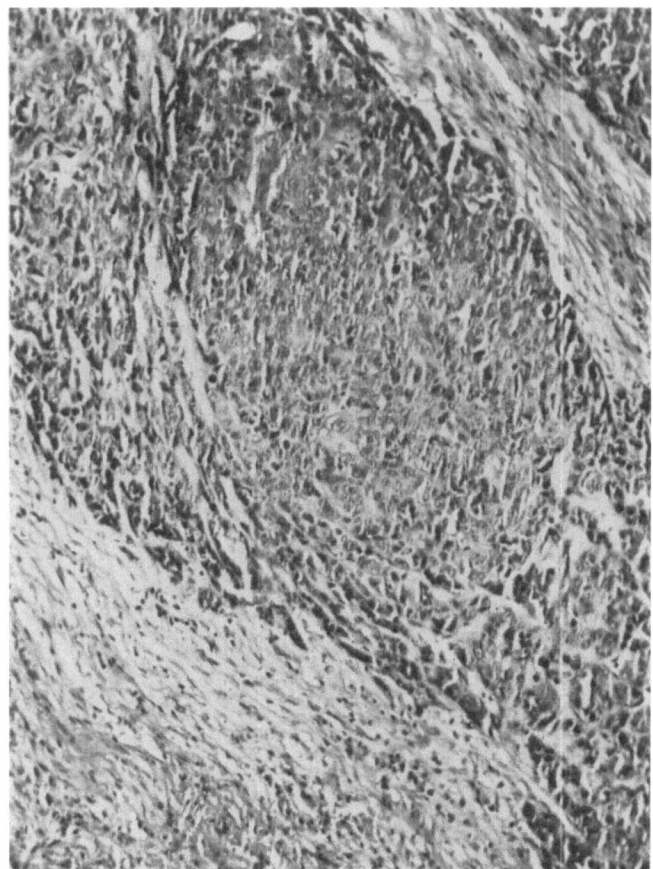

Fig. 218. Photomicrograph of a highly undifferentiated squamous-cell carcinoma of the esophagus which developed adjacent to the epithelium shown in Fig. 217 (×125)

and commonly extends more than one cm and not infrequently more than five cm beyond the naked eye margin of the tumor. The submucosal spread may be massive, or pallor of the overlying mucosa may be the only visible sign. Satellite nodules may be present. Frequently this spread may cause no visible or palpable change and be detectable only on microscopy. Local cure is infrequent unless the radiotherapist irradiates or the surgeon resects a five centimeter margin of normal seeming esophagus beyond the detectable margins of the tumor. Miller (1962) analyzed surgical experience of persistent or recurrent carcinoma at the proximal line of section of the esophagus and he concluded that a margin of twelve centimeters proximal to the detectable margin of the growth is necessary to reduce anastomotic recurrence to a really low level. It should also be noted that the submucosal layer extends proximally into the pharynx and distally into the stomach and so may the esophageal cancer, perhaps a little less distally than proximally.

By the time of diagnosis, both the circumferential and longitudinal muscle layers have usually been infiltrated and penetrated (Fig. 219) although the muscle

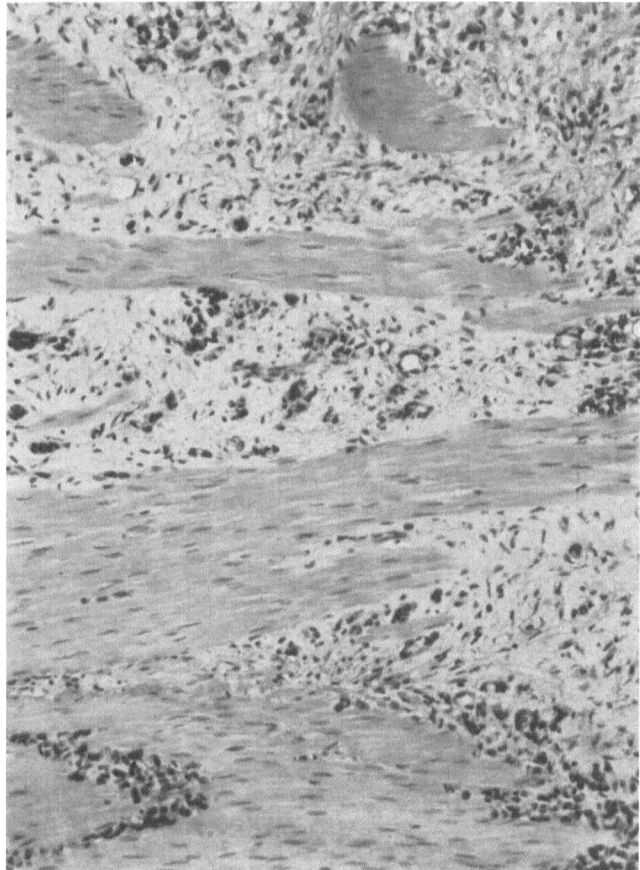

Fig. 219. Photomicrograph showing infiltration and separation of muscle fibers of the esophageal wall by a rather poorly differentiated adenocarcinoma (×125)

is less readily invaded than the submucosa. Initially the muscle layers are invaded along the pathways taken by the blood and lymphatic vessels.

The esophagus has no serosa. Once through the muscularis (Fig. 220), tumor spreads through the loose peri-esophageal adventitia to surrounding organs. Most commonly invaded are the trachea and bronchi, the lung, especially the lower lobe of either lung through the pulmonary ligament, the aortic adventitia, and also the pleura, pericardium, large veins, thyroid, recurrent laryngeal nerves, diaphragm, and left lobe of the liver, depending upon the level of the tumor. The elastic media of the aorta and the aponeuroses overlying the vertebral bodies offer, for a time, more effective barriers. The commonest mode of death of the untreated patient is a combination of starvation due to esophageal obstruction and a lung abscess or bronchopneumonia due to aspiration of liquid from the obstructed esophagus into the larynx, or through a fistulous connection between the esophagus and air passages developing through necrotic tumor. (These complications are also common following the local failure of either irradiation or surgery.)

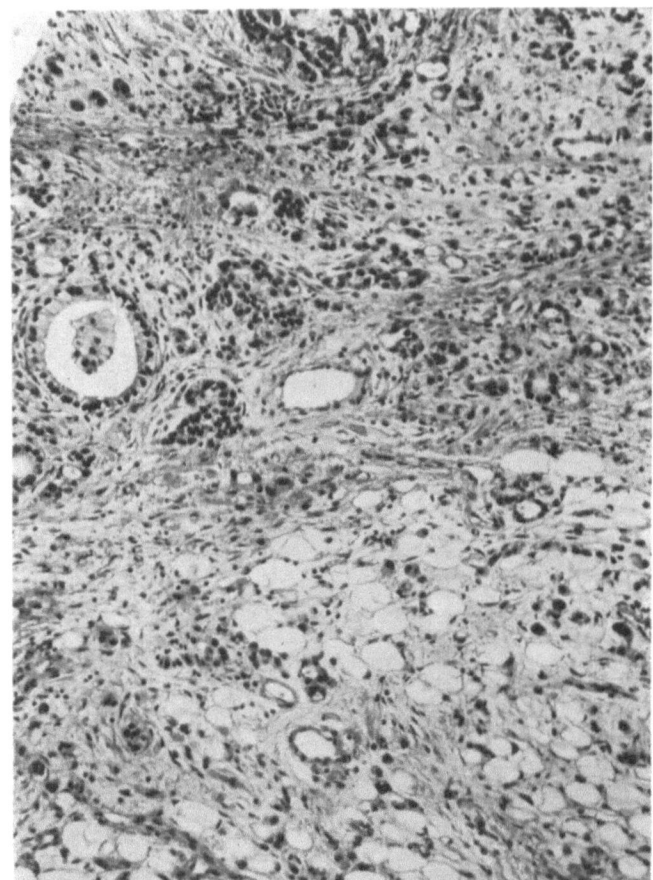

Fig. 220. Photomicrograph showing adenocarcinoma where it has invaded through the muscularis of the esophageal wall into periesophageal connective tissue (×125)

1.2.1.6. Lymphatic Metastases

Lymphatic spread occurs early in these frequently undifferentiated tumors, first into the submucosal lymphatics, then through the muscularis to the para-esophageal lymph nodes at the level of the tumor (Fig. 221), thereafter to more distant lymph nodes, although "skipping" may occur. From the upper third of the esophagus, paraesophageal, retropharyngeal, lower deep cervical, and supraclavicular nodes may be invaded. From the middle third, after invasion of local paraesophageal nodes, there is frequently invasion of quite remote nodes in the neck above, or far below the tumor around the lower esophagus. Sub-diaphragmatic nodes around the cardia and along the left gastric artery and tracheobronchial nodes extending into the hili of the lungs may also be invaded. From the lower third, beyond the local nodes, spread is commonly to below the diaphragm to the paracardial, left gastric, and celiac axis nodes. Less frequently lower third growths spread to nodes along the upper border of the pancreas and towards the hilum of the spleen, and upwards to the middle third drainage area.

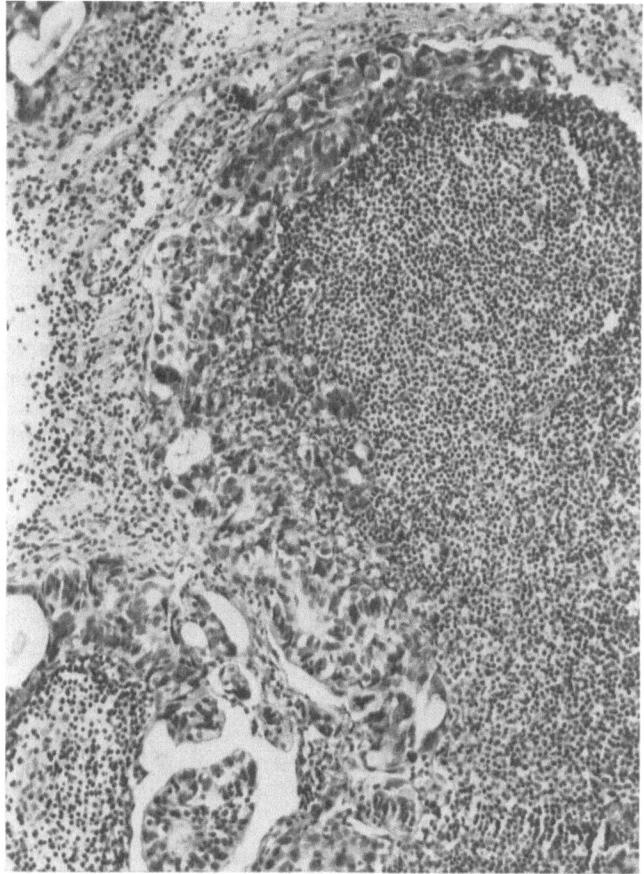

Fig. 221. Photomicrograph showing adenocarcinoma invading the peripheral sinus of a small paraesophageal lymph node (125)

LE ROUX (1961a) found histologically proved cervical glandular metastases to be the contraindication to operative treatment in 26 out of 102 patients with inoperable squamous esophageal cancer. Histological confirmation of lymph node metastases in the mediastinum or abdomen was obtained from 145 (61 per cent) of 236 patients submitted to resection for squamous carcinoma. Forty-nine of the 145 patients with proved lymph node metastases had other evidence of spread beyond the esophagus but only four patients had other spread without histologically positive lymph nodes.

1.2.1.7. Blood-Borne Metastases

The plexus of thin-walled veins in the esophageal submucosa, the periesophageal venous plexus, and the large veins situated near to the esophagus in the mediastinum direct attention to the likelihood of tumor emboli escaping into the blood-stream. However, one-third of the patients die from the local complications of the tumor without readily detectable blood-borne metastases at autopsy. Clearly, the recorded incidence of metastases is highly dependent on accessibility; whether the assessment is clinical, radiographic, at operation, or post-mortem; whether the tissue is examined with the naked eye or by microscopy. The commonest clinical evidence of blood-borne metastases is gross nodular hepatomegaly. Occasionally skin metastases are found at the time of first diagnosis. The commonest radiographically detected metastases are in the lung. Of 280 patients subjected to thoracolaparotomy for squamous esophageal cancer, Le Roux (1961a) found that 15 had liver metastases and one had a renal metastasis revealed only at operation. Of 208 patients treated by radical irradiation for squamous esophageal cancer, a number died during the following six years; Pearson (1969) attributed one quarter of the deaths to blood-borne metastases, found to occur most frequently in the liver and lungs. Amongst 1909 patients with esophageal cancer (mostly squamous carcinoma) Goodner and Turnbull (1971) reported the detection of bone metastases in the terminal three months of life in 100 patients (five per cent). In a series of 824 post-mortem examinations of patients with esophageal cancer reported from 39 institutes by Dormanns (1939), metastases were detected in the liver in 32 per cent of cases; lungs and pleura accounted for 21 per cent, bone for eight per cent, kidneys for seven percent and adrenals for three per cent.

1.2.2. Adenocarcinoma

Gowing (1961) and McPeak and Warren (1948) refer to the difficulty of determining the exact origin (whether from esophagus or stomach) of adenocarcinomas presenting in the lower end of the esophagus. Most are gastric carcinomas which have spread up (Figs. 222, 223). Estimates of the incidence of true primary adenocarcinoma of the esophagus range from a very low figure up to ten per cent (Raphael et al., 1966; Lortat-Jacob et al., 1968; Turnbull and Goodner, 1970). Smithers (1956, 1961) estimates eight per cent.

An adenocarcinoma may arise in the esophagus from the mucin-secreting tubulo-alveolar glands scattered along the whole length of the submucosa, or from the esophageal "cardiac" glands, similar in structure to the cardiac glands of the stomach and found at both the upper and lower ends of the esophagus. This type of carcinoma may also arise in one of the heterotopic patches of columnar epithelium which may be found even in the upper third, or in the lower part of the esophagus when it is lined by columnar epithelium, a condition which is arguably acquired or congenital (Allison and Johnstone, 1953; Barrett, 1958). To be distinguished from the above is a gastric adenocarcinoma lying in the thorax because it has arisen in the cardia or fundus of the stomach in association with an hiatus hernia. Azzopardi and Menzies (1962) describe four adenoid cystic tumors (cylindromas) which they argue must certainly be primary esophageal adenocarcinomas from esophageal mucus glands.

Much that has been said about squamous carcinoma is applicable to adenocarcinoma. As the latter occurs much more frequently towards the lower end of the esophagus, invasion of the trachea or bronchi is correspondingly less frequent. There are also some differences in the pattern of local growth and distant spread. Adenocarcinoma which lies astride the gastroesophageal junction usually presents as a fungating or ulcerating, fleshy tumor in the stomach and as an annular infiltrating or constrictive mass in the lower esophagus. When squamous carcinoma involves the gastroesophageal junction little spread occurs into the stomach and most are of the annular constricting variety. The abrupt, rounded distal edge of these tumors suggests that there is a barrier to further

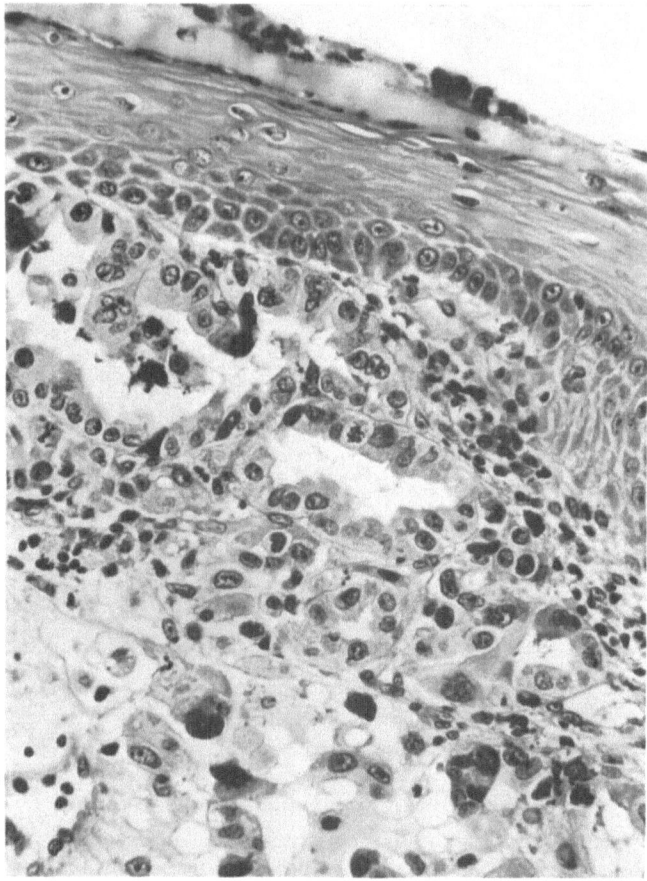

Fig. 222. Photomicrograph showing gastric adenocarcinoma which has spread up under intact squamous-cell esophageal epithelium (×312)

extension of esophageal squamous carcinoma into the stomach (DODGE, 1961). The relative resistance of the stomach to invasion by carcinoma of the adjacent esophagus is similar to the resistance of the duodenum to invasion by carcinoma of the stomach. In neither instance is resistance absolute; microscopic examination may reveal invasion beyond the apparent tumor margin. The comparative freedom with which recurrent tumor will infiltrate an artificial gastroesophageal junction, following esophagogastrectomy, suggests that the natural barrier may have been removed when the original junction was excised.

Adenocarcinoma, more frequently than squamous carcinoma, forms a bulky mass of tumor before severe narrowing of the esophageal lumen has occurred. The common mode of death from adenocarcinoma is a gradual decline from diffuse metastases, with the patient yet able to swallow, or hemorrhage from the tumor. Clinically obvious metastases are usually in the liver or cervical lymph nodes. Diffuse peritoneal metastases associated with ascites and pelvic metastases are also found, and diffuse pulmonary metastases may be recognized radiographically.

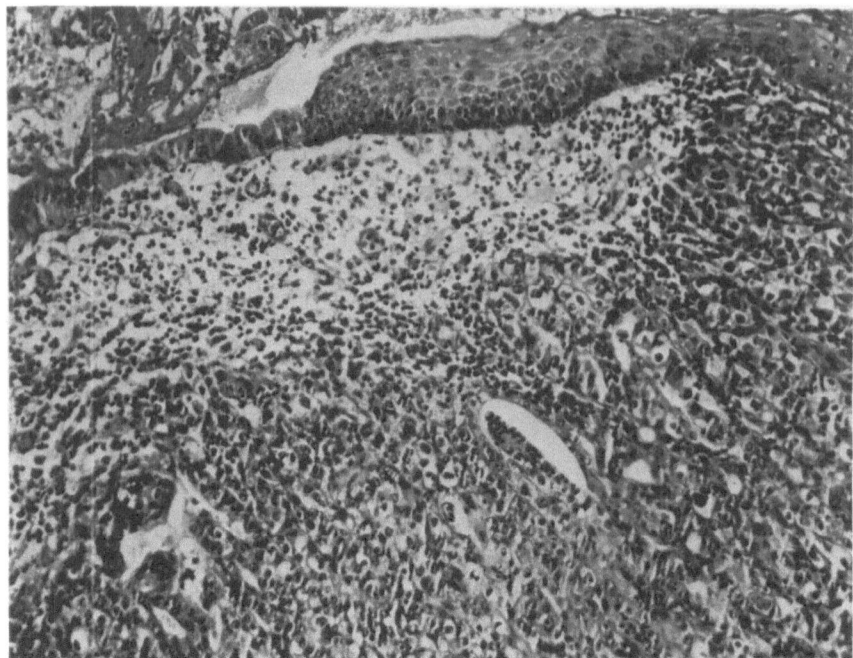

Fig. 223. Photomicrograph showing adenocarcinoma underlying the junction between gastric columnar and esophageal stratified squamous epithelium (×125)

1.2.3. Mixed Squamous and Adenocarcinoma

Mixed squamous and glandular carcinomas occur especially at the cardia. Successive biopsies may reveal adenocarcinoma and squamous carcinoma. The histogenesis of such mixed carcinomas developing across the junction of squamous and glandular epithelium points to field carcinogenesis rather than a unicellular concept of origin of the cancer. The mixed histological pattern of these tumors may be compared with that of tumors arising at other inter-epithelial junctions such as the cervix uteri and the anorectal junction. Dodge (1961) describes seven mixed tumors occurring at the esophagogastric junction and he states that they are not uncommon at this site. Two of the seven he considered to be adenocarcinomas with areas of squamous metaplasia [the only type to which Kay (1968) would apply the term adenoacanthoma], two to be muco epidermoid carcinomas, two to be examples of double histogenesis from both esophageal and gastric epithelium, and the seventh case a "collision carcinoma" caused by the growing together of initially separate gastric adenocarcinoma and esophageal anaplastic carcinoma.

1.3. Clinical Features

Natural History, Symptoms and Signs

Dysphagia, first for solids, later also for liquids, is the first symptom noticed by patients with squamous carcinoma of the esophagus in 90 per cent of the cases.

The inaccessibility of the esophagus to clinical examination and surgical management daunted surgeons for many years and, since a successful non-surgical method of treatment of this disease was not available, its natural history, untreated, is well recorded. Except in unusual circumstances—for example, when esophageal carcinoma complicates cardiospasm—dysphagia is a symptom the onset of which is likely to be remembered clearly; so it is well established that in untreated patients with esophageal carcinoma average survival from the onset of dysphagia is about eight months. Dysphagia is probably not recognized by the patient until about $2/_3$ of the circumference are infiltrated; therefore, duration of dysphagia is not synonymous with duration of the disease. Early disease is silent. Once dysphagia begins it is rapidly progressive within a period of weeks or a few months. At first solids will get stuck, not infrequently a piece of apple or meat. Once bolus obstruction has occurred it is likely to recur with increasing ease. The patient soon becomes careful to cut up his food, to restrict his diet to soft food and later to take only liquids. Then within a few weeks liquids pass more slowly and finally the patient can hardly drink at all. When obstruction of the lower esophagus is due to invasion of the esophagogastric junction by a fundal carcinoma the dysphagia tends to progress more slowly. So poorly is the public educated that patients will tolerate dysphagia for an average of four months before they seek medical advice. In Southern Africa delay is nearer eight months, dysphagia usually total, and survival after presentation measured in days or weeks, rather than months. The level at which dysphagia is appreciated need have little bearing on the site of an esophageal tumor. Obstruction is appreciated at one of three levels—in the suprasternal notch, at midsternal level or in the epigastrium. Obstruction is usually appreciated at a level proximal to the tumor and only very occasionally at a level distal to the tumor.

In addition to dysphagia, esophageal carcinoma may be the cause of pain, experienced in the epigastrium, along the costal margin anteriorly, in the suprasternal notch, the angles of the jaw, at midsternal level or between the scapulae. The pain or discomfort associated with esophageal carcinoma is usually caused by the narrowing of the lumen: it occurs within 10 sec of swallowing solids, is associated with a sensation that food is not moving on, and continues until the sense of obstruction is relieved. More rarely the patient with an ulcerated esophageal carcinoma complains of a continuous pain, which is worsened by swallowing solids or irritating liquids. Hiccup may be an obtrusive symptom. As obstruction increases, hunger and weight loss, and later thirst and dehydration develop. Regurgitation occurs, with aspiration into the air passages, coughing and choking, and not infrequently a lung abscess, causing fever, loss of weight, chest pain and cough. An esophagotracheal fistula even more rapidly produces gross lung infection. Overt bleeding, such as massive hemorrhage from erosion of aorta or pulmonary vessels is uncommon, but occult blood is present in the stools. Hoarseness may result from invasion of either recurrent laryngeal nerve. Occasionally the patient suffers foul-smelling eructation. Very occasionally, dysphagia may be preceded by stridor due to tracheal invasion, or symptoms such as jaundice due to liver metastases, or bone pain due to skeletal deposits.

On examination, there may be no abnormality; usually there is evidence of weight loss; and occasionally, even a patient with disease that is still localized and curable may be markedly emaciated, and even dehydrated. The commonest evidence of spread beyond the esophagus is enlarged, hard, lower deep cervical lymph nodes, or an enlarged, hard, nodular liver.

In patients with adenocarcinoma dysphagia is less commonly the first symptom than in patients with squamous tumor. Adenocarcinoma, especially when tumor is also present in the stomach, may cause anorexia, loss of weight, vague abdominal discomfort and even hematemesis, preceding the onset of dysphagia by three to six months.

Hiatus hernia is an accompaniment of esophageal carcinoma in approximately ten per cent of patients, and symptoms of hiatus hernia of the "sliding type" may precede those of carcinoma by many years. Distinction between peptic stricture of the esophagus and carcinoma in these patients is particularly important.

In a patient with achalasia, lye stricture, or Paterson-Kelly syndrome, a change in the nature of the dysphagia is for long not recognized. In achalasia, the esophageal lumen is wide and the tumor, which usually grows in relation to the aortic arch, can assume a large size before it noticeably obstructs the passage of food. For these reasons a carcinoma which complicates cardiospasm is rarely either operable or curable by radiation therapy.

1.4. Investigations

1.4.1. Radiology

In the investigation of dysphagia there are two essentials—the esophagus must be completely outlined with barium and must be examined with the esophagoscope. A normal esophagogram is not a reason for not undertaking esophagoscopy in a patient with dysphagia. Small tumors are sometimes not easily demonstrable radiographically and are yet a cause of symptoms. However, by the time the patient seeks aid, the tumor is usually large, impassable by the esophagoscope, and its lower limit and whole intraluminal extent better demonstrated by radiography than esophagoscopy. In addition, radiography provides a permanent visual record.

At an early stage, a carcinoma produces a persistently irregular and rigid plaque—seen best with maximal esophageal dilatation. Sometimes it is associated with feeble simultaneous contractions adjacent to the lesion, simulating a corkscrew esophagus (Cummack, 1969). Tangential viewing of the whole circumference is necessary if a small irregularity is not to be missed.

Later a marginal filling defect can be visualized if the patient is turned into the correct position. Malignant lesions tend to cause irregular but sharply demarcated filling defects which join the esophageal border at more or less sharp angles. A central ulceration in such a relatively small tumor may produce a typical meniscus sign. This image is not frequently observed because fractionated compression of the esophagus is not possible and the tumor is frequently ulcerated in several areas at the time of the radiological examination. At these later stages the tumor tends to encircle the esophagus and to cause large circumferential filling defects with one or more irregular ulcerations. A carcinoma developing mainly in the submucosa may cause a smooth annular stenosis with minor or moderate irregularity of the mucosal pattern. It may be difficult to distinguish this image from a benign fibrotic stenosis.

In the cervical esophagus, the soft tissue mass of the tumor usually displaces the trachea forwards. In the thoracic esophagus, only larger tumors give rise to a detectable soft tissue mass and tracheal displacement and narrowing. Examination in the horizontal and Trendelenburg positions is helpful in defining the lower limit of a tumor. A carcinoma at the lower end can occasionally mimic the appearances of achalasia but the main problem is to distinguish carcinoma from a peptic ulcer of the lower end of the esophagus with stricture. With carcinoma, distortion is generally more persistent, but the two lesions may be indistinguishable and, indeed, they may coexist.

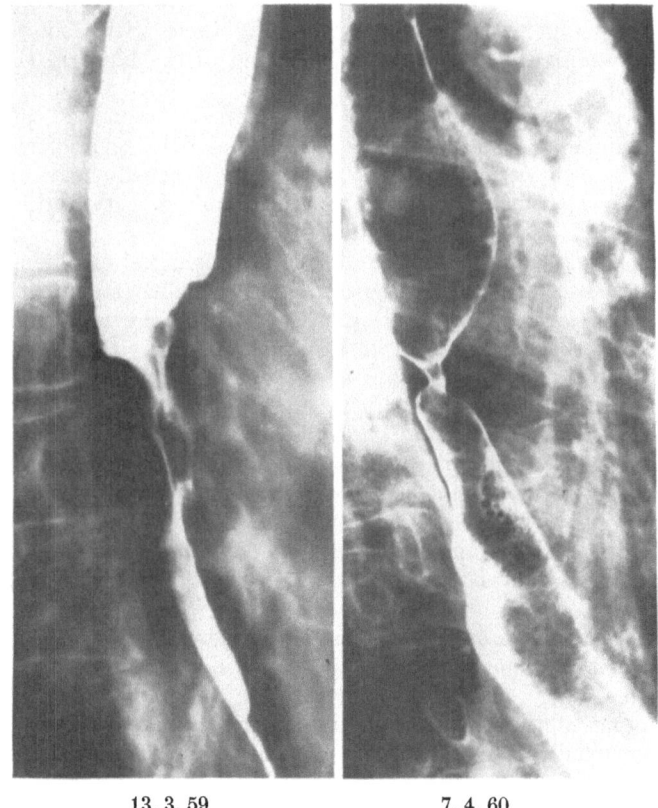

13. 3. 59   7. 4. 60

Fig. 224. A squamous esophageal carcinoma treated by megavoltage irradiation in March, 1959 leaving a short stricture, shown above in the air contrast barium film of April 1960. The patient was treated by the passage of bougies until March, 1961, and thereafter maintained weight on a semi-liquid diet. (Reproduced by courtesy of the Editor of the American Journal of Roentgenology, 1969, Vol. 105, p. 508)

Sometimes a useful double contrast can be obtained when the patient swallows air after barium (Fig. 224). If a fistula to the trachea, bronchi, mediastinum, or pleura is suspected one of the contrastmedia used for bronchography should be given rather than barium. The examination is not complete until the stomach (from which a lower esophageal carcinoma may have arisen) has also been examined, and the well distended esophageal wall remote from the tumor has also been studied for indentations due to enlarged lymph nodes.

Plain chest radiography does not usually reveal the esophageal tumor but is a necessary step in the search for metastases prior to management either by an operation or by radiotherapy. In some communities, especially in Southern Africa (LEVY, 1966), a plain chest radiograph may be the first radiographic investigation requested because symptoms may be only vaguely indicative of intrathoracic pathology without necessarily being suggestive of esophageal disease. In some patients the clinical picture is predominantly that of advancing pulmonary disease. The radiographic features on plain films which suggest esophageal carcinoma include mediastinal mass, enlargement of the esophagus, air in the esophagus, and a fluid level in the esophagus. In one series of African patients the plain chest film was abnormal in half; in those with abnormal films the abnormality was of the esophagus in half, and of the lungs in the other half.

There may be no more than an increase in the density with slight widening of the superior mediastinal shadow. An advanced lesion will, on plain films, produce a nodular or lobular bulge of the outline of the superior mediastinum—superior because in African patients the tumor is usually high in the thorax. A low esophageal tumor may be seen as a double density within the cardiac shadow.

Carcinoma does not produce the degree of esophageal enlargement observed in the late stages of achalasia of the cardia; yet a tightly stenosing tumor in the esophagus may cause considerable dilatation above the lesion which may be seen either in the posteroanterior or lateral chest films.

The normal esophagus at rest is a soft flexible tube, the walls of which are in apposition and are forced apart by the passage of food, after which they immediately fall together. When the walls are indurated by tumor they cannot come together and a stiff tube results, which, if food or liquid are not present, contains air. Air in the esophagus may indicate the presence of a foreign body; air in the cervical esophagus is seen in the lateral view of the neck with corrosive strictures and achalasia and below a hypopharyngeal carcinoma; air in the thoracic esophagus may be seen in the plain chest films in cases of esophageal carcinoma.

A fluid level, visible on a film exposed in the erect position, indicates total obstruction of the esophagus, and may be the initial radiographic presentation of a carcinoma.

Radiographs of the cervical and dorsal spine taken to reveal any anterior osteophytosis, and as an adjunct to clinical observation of lack of mobility of the spine, are a wise preliminary to rigid esophagoscopy. Radiographs of the proximal skeleton may be taken in a search for bone metastases (GOODNER and TURNBULL, 1971).

1.4.2. Endoscopy

Esophagoscopy is an essential part of the diagnostic work-up of a patient with esophageal carcinoma. Even when rigid instruments had to be used, esophagoscopy was contraindicated only if it was excessively dangerous due to causes such as rigidity of the spine, the presence of large anterior spinal osteophytes—which make perforation of the posterior wall of the cervical esophagus a grave risk—or a large aortic aneurysm (SMITH and TANNER, 1956). Since flexible fiberscopes have become available esophagoscopy is performed in almost all patients in whom an esophageal carcinoma is present or suspected, unless the procedure has become unneccessary because disease advanced beyond useful treatment has already been demonstrated by simpler means. However, fixity of the tumor is more readily appreciated using the old-fashioned, rigid esophagoscope. In addition, bronchoscopy is necessary for those patients with potentially curable carcinoma at all levels in the esophagus within reach of the trachea or bronchi to detect distortion, mucosal fixation or ulceration, or subcarinal widening due to lymph node enlargement—all additional items of information about the extent of the tumor.

The technique of esophagoscopy is described in Chapter 2 of this volume. The aim of the examination, when tumor is suspected, is to visualize the tumor; to record the level of its proximal limit and, if possible, its distal limit, as measured in centimeters from the upper alveolus; to judge its fixity by gently pressing the beak of the instrument to one side; to take washings and brushings for cytological examination (TANNER, 1961; COHEN and FLOWERS, 1969); and to take biopsies for histological examination. The vocal cords should be examined for paralysis which may be caused by tumor interrupting one or other recurrent laryngeal nerve. Isolated tumor nodules may be detected above or below the main tumor mass, due to submucosal lymphatic spread. Sometimes submucosal spread may produce a funnel-like narrowing impeding advance of the esophago-scope so that no tumor is visualized and biopsy through the normal mucosa fails to reach tumor. The more distal narrowed lumen may then be gently explored with a bougie, followed by an angled biopsy forceps with which it may be possible to feel a nodule or ulcer from which a specimen may be taken. Simple ulcers and fibrous tissue are difficult to grasp, normal mucosa tends to tear, and tumor is much easier to bite and larger fragments may be obtained. To take too deep a bite from normal esophagus or from the depths of an ulcer crater risks perforation. Progressive dilatation of the narrowed segment with bougies over a period of several days may result in a sufficient widening of the lumen to permit visualization and biopsy of the tumor. Energetic dilatation as a method of treatment of carcinoma is pointless because any benefit is transitory and the likelihood of perforation is such that the procedure is more risky than esoph-agectomy (TANNER, 1961).

TANNER (1961) states "It is a stimulus to the endoscopist in his search, to remember that when a patient first begins to complain of dysphagia over the age of 40, there is over a 90 per cent chance that the cause is a malignant lesion affecting the oesophagus". Therefore, if no abnormality is found, but the symptoms persist, repeat the examination.

1.4.3. Esophageal Cytology

The problem of exfoliative cytology in the diagnosis of esophageal malignant disease has been discussed in a previous chapter. It may suffice to re-emphasize that, in expert hands, cytology is one of the most highly productive methods of diagnosis, giving correct answers in 94 to 98 per cent of patients examined.

1.4.4. Cervical Lymph Node Biopsy

In a patient with esophageal cancer without other certain evidence of in-curability, a lymph node palpable in the neck should, in most instances, be excised for histological examination. LE ROUX (1961a) found that, of 76 patients with squamous esophageal cancer not offered operative treatment because of evidence of tumor spread remote from the primary tumor, 26 had histologically proved cervical lymph node metastases. In the absence of a palpable lymph node, it is not usual practice to perform a blind scalene node biopsy because the yield of positive findings from this procedure is so small.

1.4.5. Mediastinoscopy, Pneumomediastinography and Laparotomy

AKOVBIANTZ et al. (1965) performed mediastinoscopy on 12 patients with middle third esophageal cancer and retrieved histologically positive lymph nodes in six of the patients, and from one out of four patients with lower third tumors positive mediastinal lymph nodes were obtained in this way. Clearly some profit-less thoracolaparotomies might be prevented by prior mediastinoscopy. The mortality of the procedures is less than 0.1 per cent (ASHBAUGH, 1970) and the morbidity is low. Another technique, pneumomediastinography, has been proposed as a means of staging esophageal cancers (Holub and Simecek, 1968). A pneumomediastinum is induced through a bronchoscope and tomograms are taken soon thereafter in order to determine the extent of carcinomatous involvement of the esophageal wall and surrounding tissues. It is assumed that in this way the thickness of the lesion can be identified. Adhesions caused by previous inflammatory processes in the mediastinum may, however, mimic extensive carcinomatous involvement.

As a preliminary to an attempt at curative irradiation either mediastinoscopy or laparotomy (or diagnostic thoracotomy) will rarely be indicated because the fully irradiated volume of tissue will in any event include nearby lymph nodes, and will probably not be enlargeable to include more remote lymph nodes without the need to lower the radiation dose to an ineffective level. And should undetected remote lymphatic or indeed blood-borne spread actually be present, the irradiation given with the intent to cure will result in valuable palliation with minimal treatment morbidity, provided the dose is not excessive.

1.4.6. Other Investigations

Intraluminal manometry has been used to evaluate malignant disease of the esophagus (Kelley, 1968). Although malignancy was not associated with any characteristic findings, manometry may occasionally be useful for the differential diagnosis of achalasia and carcinoma of the esophagogastric junction, mimicking achalasia. A miniature Geiger counter, inserted through an esophagoscope may be used to measure the increased uptake of radioactive phosphorus by esophageal cancer (Belson and Lanza, 1969). The test seemed to be useful when the esophageal cancer did not have gross mucosal involvement. As false positive results may be obtained in patients with esophagitis, the diagnostic value of the test seems to be limited. Liver scan, liver function tests (BSP excretion, alkaline phosphatase and 5-nucleotidase), laparoscopy and arteriography may provide evidence that liver metastases are present.

Clearly any lesion suspicious of metastasis, in a patient being considered for potentially curative radiotherapy or surgery, will be biopsied if this can be done without unwarrantable upset to the patient.

Any necessary investigation will be carried out to determine how fit a patient is to withstand proposed major therapeutic procedures.

1.5. Prognosis

1.5.1. Factors Influencing Prognosis

The factors determining prognosis are interrelated, but there is some justification for ranking them in order of importance: (1) The balance between the aggressiveness of the tumor and the resistance of the patient. (2) Treatment. (3) Sex. (4) Site. (5) Histology. (6) Condition of the patient. (7) The community in which the patient lives.

1.5.1.1. The Balance between the Aggressiveness of the Tumor and the Resistance of the Patient

In practice, the balance between the aggressiveness of the tumor and the resistance of the patient is judged by the length of history, the extent of the primary tumor and any lymphatic or blood-borne metastases, and, where possible, the observed rate of growth. If the patient is apparently free from metastases, the smaller the tumor, in relation to the length of history, the better the prognosis.

A patient with a very small tumor and no evident metastases has a good prognosis whatever the length of history. Very occasionally, a patient with a tumor visibly ten or more centimeters in extent may be still free from lymphatic or blood-borne metastases and curable by elimination of the primary tumor, but generally the larger the primary tumor and the more rapid its rate of growth, the more extensively will it have invaded neighboring organs and metastasized via the lymphatics and blood stream. Exceptionally, long survival may follow resection even when tumor is observed in the lines of section (MACPHERSON, 1966; YOUNG-HUSBAND and ALUWIHARE, 1970). The occurrence of widespread lymphatic or blood-borne metastases from a small esophageal cancer is probably less frequent than from a small cancer of the lung or breast; however, it is unusual for an esophageal cancer to be diagnosed before it is more than four or five centimeters in visible extent. Lymph node invasion usually indicates incurable disease but occasionally long survival may occur in such cases following either resection or irradiation. In one of our patients, a squamous carcinoma of the esophagus untreated by surgery, radiation, or chemotherapy, regressed for four years following irradiation of squamous carcinoma elsewhere in the body—an excessively rare event, but a reminder of the possibility that, perhaps sometimes minute, undetectable tumor deposits, residual after surgery or radiotherapy, may be controlled or eliminated by immune mechanisms. YOUNGHUSBAND and ALUWIHARE (1970) discuss this possibility, and in their series of 77 patients treated by esophagectomy they find that histological evidence of an immunological reaction in the tumor or lymph nodes is associated with a reduced incidence of lymph node invasion and tumor extension outside the esophagus, and with longer survival.

1.5.1.2. Treatment

With rare exceptions, esophageal cancer untreated by radiation or surgery kills the patient within a year of onset of symptoms (the mean survival is eight months). The life of a frail old patient or one with extensive disease may very readily be shortened by a major surgical procedure or radiation therapy to too high a dose or too great a volume. The only hope of restoring a normal life expectancy to a patient with adenocarcinoma is by complete surgical ablation of all tumor; for a patient with squamous carcinoma, appropriate radical megavoltage radiotherapy usually gives the best chance, and should irradiation fail locally, subsequent resection may still occasionally succeed. Various other procedures may lengthen or unintentionally shorten a patient's life by a month or two but in general they should be applied only when there is a real prospect of the remaining life being enjoyable.

1.5.1.3. Sex

Independent of the other factors listed here, female patients have a better prognosis than males; in some series they are reported to have twice as good a chance of long survival as males (MUSTARD and IBBERSON, 1956; STOREY, 1962; MILLER, 1962; LEBORGNE et al., 1963; VOUTILAINEN and KOULUMIES, 1965; PEARSON, 1966; YOUNGHUSBAND and ALUWIHARE, 1970).

1.5.1.4. Site

In centers where both good surgery and good radiotherapy are available, and where collaboration between the disciplines is close, prognosis does not vary greatly with the site of the tumor in the esophagus, but tumors in the upper half of the thorax have a worse outlook because of earlier invasion of trachea, bronchi and aorta, and tumors at the upper end have a better prognosis because of the higher proportion of females. If only surgical treatment is available, prognosis is much worse in the case of upper thoracic tumors, because of the lower proportion found to be resectable at thoracolaparotomy, and the higher operation mortality. If only radiation treatment is available, the outlook is poorer for patients with lower esophageal tumors because a proportion have adenocarcinomas which respond less well to irradiation and because normal tissue tolerance limits effective irradiation below the diaphragm.

1.5.1.5. Histology

Patients with well differentiated squamous carcinoma have the best prognosis. Those with adenocarcinoma and undifferentiated carcinoma do less well because of the higher incidence of spread beyond what can be eradicated by local measures (Cox, 1957; Ellis et al., 1959; Miller, 1962).

1.5.1.6. Condition of the Patient

General frailty, especially when associated with cardiorespiratory disease, and often due to advanced age, smoking or alcoholism, or prolonged starvation, severely reduce the chance of successful major surgery, and to a lesser extent reduce the chance of curative radiation therapy. However, it must not be overlooked that a patient, even an aged patient, may be in very poor condition solely due to starvation caused by a relatively small, metastasis-free, curable esophageal carcinoma.

1.5.1.7. The Community in which the Patient Lives

Even in communities with a high standard of education and modern medical facilities patients with esophageal cancer usually present with late disease and most are in a high age group so that, with present methods of treatment, no more than one in ten is expected to be alive five years later.

In some less educated communities—even in the communities in Southern Africa in which the disease is epidemic and the esophagus is the commonest site of cancer—late presentation, too late for it to be possible to modify the course of the disease, is so general that long survival is unknown.

1.6. Treatment

Speaking to the Boston Surgical Society Turner (1931) described the attitude of most doctors to esophageal carcinoma at that time as one of studied neglect or benevolent despair. Esophagectomy was an operation introduced only to be abandoned, with an unacceptable operation mortality and life unlikely to be prolonged in those who recovered. Since that time, the results of management, either by surgery or by radiotherapy, have improved. Following sporadic success using radium bougies (Guisez and Barcat, 1909; Guisez, 1925) at the beginning of the century, there were more successes with cervical esophageal tumors following treatment with kilovoltage X-rays. In the thorax, the great advances in anesthesia and chest surgery in the 1930's made possible an effective transthoracic approach. The first successful resections with primary esophagogastric anastomosis were by Seo (1933) and Ohsawa (1933) in Japan; Adams and Phemister (1938), Garlock (1938), and Churchill and Sweet (1942) in the U.S.A.; and thereafter more widely throughout the world (Tanner and Smithers, 1961).

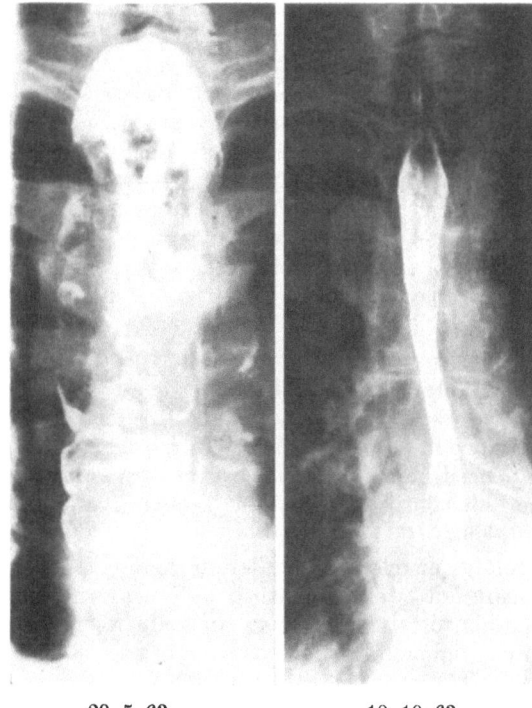

29. 5. 63   10. 10. 63

Fig. 225. A huge undifferentiated carcinoma invading nearly the whole esophagus, restored to normal function by palliative irradiation in June 1963 until death three years later from abdominal metastases

In thoracic esophageal tumors, long term survival occasionally resulted from the use of kilovoltage irradiation (NIELSEN, 1945; WATSON and BROWN, 1951; SMITHERS, 1961) but a more rewarding development in radiotherapy has been the introduction of megavoltage irradiation (BUSCHKE and CANTRIL, 1944; PIERQUIN et al., 1966; PEARSON, 1966) and telecobalt machines (MUSTARD, 1957; LOTT and SMITH, 1958; WATSON, 1963; MARCIAL et al., 1966; RIDER and MENDOZA, 1969). To this date it seems probable that the review of published work on survival of esophageal cancer carried out by TANNER and SMITHERS in 1961 is still applicable in that most successful treatment of tumors at the upper end of the esophagus has been by radiation therapy, and at the lower end by surgical resection. For manifestly incurable disease, useful palliation can not infrequently be achieved by irradiation (Fig. 225).

1.6.1. Comparison of Surgery and Radiotherapy

Comparison of the results of a method of treatment in one center with the results in other centers, and with the results of alternative methods of treatment, is fraught with difficulty. False deductions are easily made because similarly treated patients in different series are selected in different ways. Moreover, in most centers, malignant tumors in the proximal alimentary tract are treated by resection unless they are considered unsuitable for extirpation, so that alternative forms of treatment have rarely been tried in a manner fairly competitive with resection. From a scrutiny of surgical results it is clear that the elderly die as the consequence of an operation more commonly than do those who are younger; and that the operative mortality for high tumors is higher than for low tumors. It may seem an obvious deduction from these facts that the elderly must be more carefully assessed before they are submitted to an operation, and that alternative forms of management or safer operations should be found for the elderly and those with high tumors. However, in making counsels of perfection of this nature it is very easy to lose sight of the fact that the surgeon is presented with a patient unable to swallow, and, for the patient, the measure of successful treatment is the rapid relief of a symptom more distressing than most. The elderly are not less anxious to be relieved of dysphagia than are younger patients.

Deliberately palliative procedures, while they may slightly reduce initial mortality, must inevitably be followed by more frequent deaths from metastases and by a higher rate of recurrence of dysphagia. Intubation is at best an unsatisfactory maneuver, since in many instances it permits swallowing only of liquids, and even in experienced hands it carries a considerable incidence of accidental perforation of the esophagus, the inevitable sequel of which is death unless an operation is undertaken.

Modern megavoltage or telecobalt radiation therapy is an attractively benign form of management now well established as an alternative and believed by many to be preferable to resection for squamous carcinoma in the elderly and in those with high tumors. Adenocarcinoma is less suitable for irradiation. The explanation for this may be that this type of tumor is usually of gastric origin and when it produces dysphagia it is commonly extensive because it has grown from the stomach. Moreover, gastric adenocarcinoma is less sensitive to irradiation than esophageal squamous carcinoma, and there are greater technical difficulties in irradiating the larger volumes at risk below the diaphragm where also there is the problem of lower normal tissue radiation tolerance than occurs in the mediastinum. There are problems in the management of malignant dysphagia by irradiation, not the least of which are the maintenance of nutrition in the patient with severe dysphagia during irradiation, local failure of the treatment in a proportion of cases, and stricture due to the fibrous tissue which repairs the defect remaining after eradication of the tumor (Figs. 224, 226). When such a stricture occurs, it is usually amenable to management by dilatation. Provided the dose or treated volume are not excessive, radical irradiation is not a severe trial for the patient, leaves him with a normal stomach, cardia, and larynx, has been shown to be followed by survival for five or more years in some 20 per cent of those treated, and provides useful palliation for most of the others (Pearson, 1969).

The successful management of the individual case of squamous carcinoma of the esophagus by irradiation or resection depends on close cooperation between surgeon and radiotherapist. Results of treatment are most satisfactory when the element of competition for patients and results is eradicated and when the type of treatment of the individual is decided in consultation with the radiotherapist and surgeon. The management of hydration during irradiation, should this be the method of treatment selected, is also most successful when surgeon and radiotherapist collaborate.

For radiotherapy to be given a fair trial as an alternative form of management to resection, the type of patient for radiotherapy would have to be one also suitable for resection.

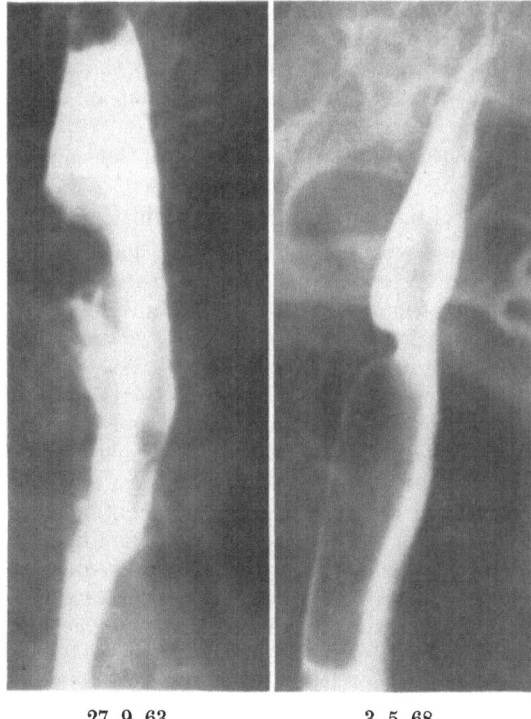

27. 9. 63   3. 5. 68

Fig. 226. A seven centimeter squamous carcinoma at the level of the suprasternal notch, presenting mainly on the posterolateral wall of the esophagus, treated by radical megavoltage irradiation in October, 1963, leaving a kink in the esophageal wall where the large malignant ulcer has been replaced by a fibrous scar. In 1968 swallowing was normal for all food except large pieces of meat

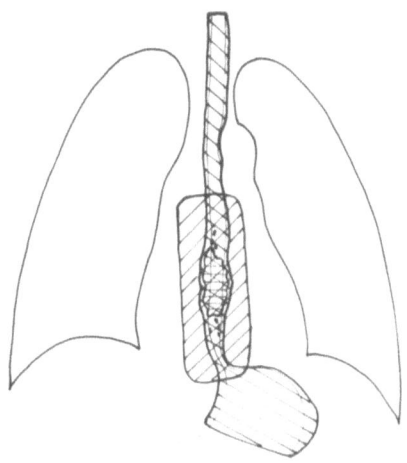

Fig. 227. Comparison of the shorter, wider volume of tissue which may be radically irradiated around an esophageal cancer with the longer but over-narrow volume removed by surgery. (Reproduced by the courtesy of the Editor of Gann, Monograph No. 9, 1970)

Radiotherapy is unlikely to control the disease over an area very much larger than that which can be resected (Fig. 227) and occasionally a resectable tumor may fail to be eradicated by irradiation. so that a considerable number of patients irradiated will be left with primary tumor or metastases, and a great alteration in long survival cannot be expected (SMITHERS and PAYNE, 1961; WATSON, 1963; LEBORGNE et al., 1963; PIERQUIN et al., 1966).

1.6.2. Anatomical Classification

For a patient fully investigated because he has an apparently localized, potentially curable, esophageal cancer, the pretreatment assessment leads to a precise anatomical description of the site, extent, and relationships of the primary tumor and its proved or suspected extensions. The traditional apportioning of a tumor to one or other third of the esophagus is too vague and not sufficiently pertinent to the main problems in management. In the course of esophagoscopy, the distance at which the various features of the tumor lie from the upper alveolus should be measured. In the average adult, the cricoid lies at 16 cm, the cardia at 40 cm, with 24 cm of esophagus between, and the lower border of the aortic arch lies at 30 cm. One of the most critical judgments is to decide whether the proximal limit of the tumor lies wholly distal to the lower border of the aortic arch, that is at more than 30 cm from the upper alveolus. Such "low" tumors have less frequently invaded irresectable structures, are more frequently operable, and the operative mortality is lower, than is the case for "high" tumors. To the surgeon, the division into "high", and "low", tumors is more useful than apportioning by thirds (SWEET, 1954; ADAMS, 1955; SMITHERS, 1957; LE ROUX, 1961a, 1962). The radiotherapist, rather than to classify by thirds, wishes to determine whether he is dealing with a small tumor at the upper end of the esophagus, which can be treated by two laterally opposed fields in the neck, or a tumor encroaching on the junctional region between neck and thorax— requiring a more sophisticated technique—or a tumor wholly confined within the thorax, which he may encompass within a suitably positioned cylindrical volume, or a tumor which extends below the diaphragm, which will probably be better excised. Other anatomical classifications may be useful to study various different problems. Division into thirds remains useful for comparisons with earlier work. Even such comparisons are bedevilled by the wide use of "thirds" which are unequal, or not clearly defined by anatomical landmarks, or are ambiguous as to whether they are thirds of the whole esophagus or of only the thoracic esophagus.

1.6.3. Radiation Therapy
1.6.3.1. Squamous Carcinoma

If cure is to be attempted, the demonstrable limits of the tumor are precisely defined (see section on Investigations, p. 460). The evidence provided by clinical, radiographic, and endoscopic examinations and by the histological examination of biopsy material falls very far short of the complete picture it would be desirable to have of the distribution of all viable malignant cells in the body. In the Edinburgh study of squamous esophageal cancer 35 per cent of the patients had demonstrable tumor of such an extent as to make any attempt at cure unwise. Of the patients subjected to thoracolaparotomy 69 per cent had evidence of tumor spread beyond the esophagus (see section on Pathology, p. 448). During the period from 1966 to the present, when curative treatment has been almost exclusively by radiotherapy, the extra information about tumor extent obtained at thoracolaparotomy was not available. In the absence of certain knowledge of remote spread, cure was attempted.

The assessment of the probable extent of spread beyond the demonstrable limits of the tumor must be based on an intimate acquaintance with the natural history of the disease and detailed knowledge of the incidence of marginal recurrence, remote lymphatic spread, and distant metastases following the use of various margins beyond the demonstrable tumor in attempts to effect local eradication (FLEMING, 1943, 1947; ALLISON and BORRIE, 1949; McCORT, 1952; BUSCHKE, 1954; SCANLON et al., 1955; WATSON et al., 1956; PIERQUIN et al., 1958, 1966; DUNLOP, 1960; MORSON, 1961; MILLER, 1962; AKOVBIANTZ et al., 1965).

Armed with this knowledge, the radiotherapist may assess the probability of any one patient's tumor being fully included within a particular target volume; and he may balance that probability against the probabilities of any one radiation dose given to that volume achieving local control of the cancer or doing intolerable damage to the patient. In practice, the need to keep the irradiated volume small enough to tolerate an adequate dose must take precedence over the need to achieve a particularly high level of probability of including all tumor. The margin treated around large tumors is less than that which can be allowed around small tumors. In the Edinburgh study (PEARSON, 1969), the most frequently used combination has been a cylindrical treated volume measuring 14×7 cm at the 80 percent isodose shell, to which has been given a mid point dose of 5100 rads in 20 equal fractions in an overall time of 28 days using a four million volt linear accelerator. Where the beam traverses lung it is essential to allow for increased transmission of radiation through this less dense tissue (LOTT and SMITH, 1958). The shape, size and positioning of the treated volume is highly individualized best to fit the volume of tissue at risk of tumor invasion, and to ensure that the spinal cord receives substantially less than 4000 rads—usually less than 3000 rads. Up until the end of 1969, 373 patients were treated in this way. Only one suffered spinal cord damage (a patient who developed a partial cord lesion, with complete symptomatic recovery after five months). Lung fibrosis was very minor in degree and rarely gave rise to symptoms. Of the 169 patients treated more than five years ago, 32 (19 per cent) survived five or more years after treatment. Six patients developed partial collapse of one or more vertebral bodies, due to radiation osteitis (Fig. 228), a complication also described by LEBORGNE et al. (1963), but in no case has this complication required any special treatment, or interfered seriously with the patient's way of life.

The examples of treatment given for this disease in Edinburgh which are referred to in this chapter have, since 1956, made use of the photon beam from a four million volt linear accelerator. An orthovoltage (less than one million volt) beam is inadequate except in the neck. Any photon beam which is sufficiently penetrating, uniform in intensity throughout its cross section, sharply defined at its margins, and of sufficiently high intensity for the daily treatment of each field to last less than one minute is suitable. These qualities must be present in sufficient degree for the irradiation to be absorbed uniformly throughout the target volume, with a sharp cut-off in radiation dose at the margin of the target volume, and the dose to all the surrounding normal tissues to be very much less. Such requirements will generally be met by a well designed four to eight million volt (or higher energy) linear accelerator, a 22 million volt (or higher energy) betatron, or a source of not less than 5000 curies of radioactive cobalt, not more than two cm in diameter, used at a source-axis distance of

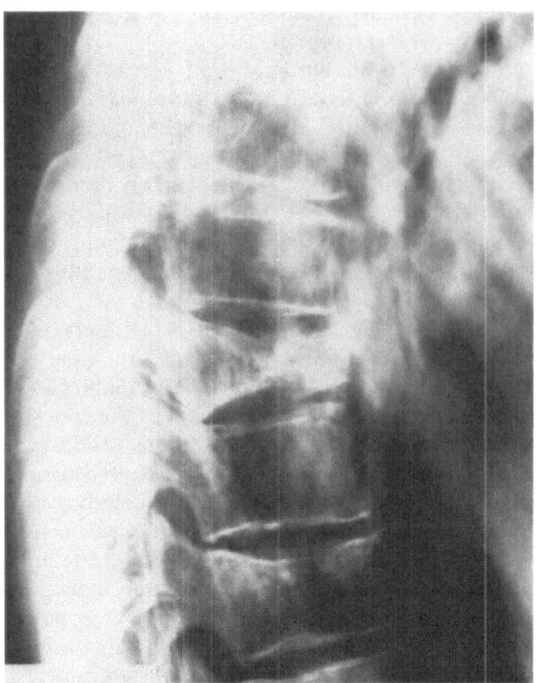

Fig. 228. Same patient as in Fig. 224—X-ray appearances of spine in October, 1962—showing irradiation osteitis of the ninth dorsal vertebra and lesser changes in the eleventh dorsal vertebra

not less than 80 cm, preferably with a beam trimmer. Whatever the source of the radiation beam, it is a great advantage to have the source and the treatment couch mounted according to the "isocentric" principle, and with great mechanical precision.

Rotation therapy is not preferable to precise fixed field techniques. A high energy electron beam has dosimetric problems in relation to lung and trachea which lead most radiotherapists to prefer a photon beam. Future techniques using neutron, pi meson, or other high energy particle beams may prove to have further advantages. For the esophagus the radium bougie or implantation techniques are outmoded because of non-uniform radiation dosage.

The great attraction of this form of radiation treatment is its wide applicability (Buschke, 1954; Pierquin et al., 1958, 1966; Smithers, 1961; Watson, 1963, 1967; Marcial et al., 1966). For the disease as it occurs in Edinburgh, 60 per cent of all patients presenting with squamous esophageal cancer can be

Fig. 229. a A squamous carcinoma irradiated in December, 1962. b At the end of the course of irradiation, showing smoothing off of the "shoulders" of the tumor. c Two months after irradiation; in February, 1963, there was still a small ulcer on the posterior aspect of the short, residual stricture. Thereafter, one gentle dilatation was carried out. d In December, 1964, the only residual abnormality was slight loss of elasticity of the esophageal wall at the original tumor site. Patient well in 1971. (Reproduced by courtesy of the Editor of American Journal of Roentgenology, 1969, Vol. 105, p. 509)

473

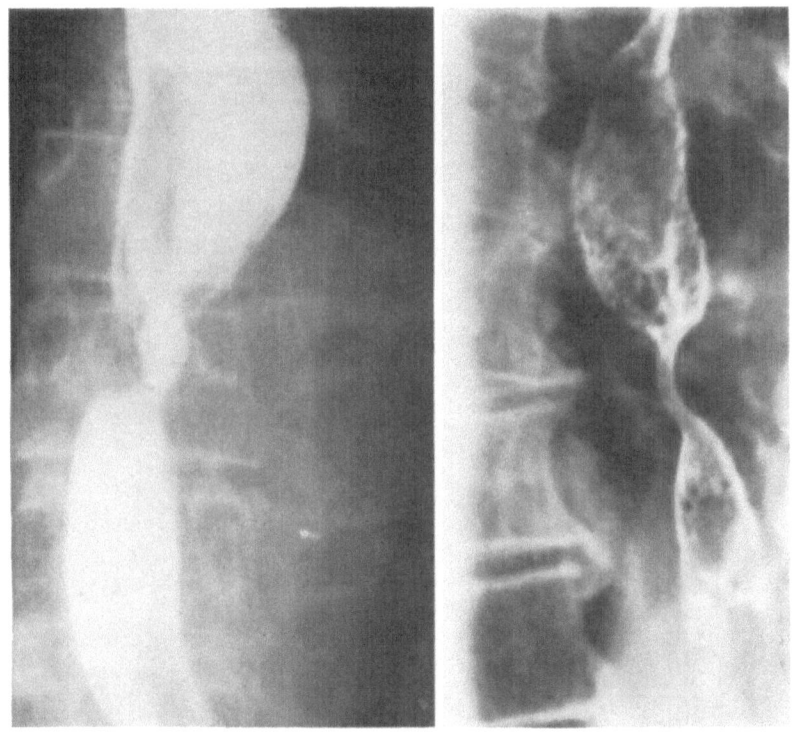

a   b

13. 11. 62   28. 12. 62

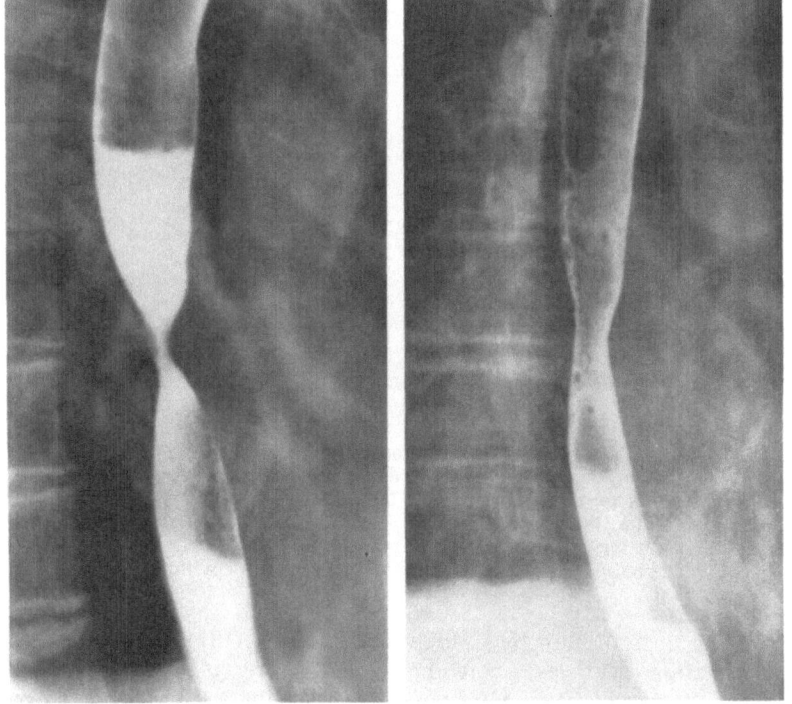

c   d

Fig. 229   21. 2. 63   3. 12. 64

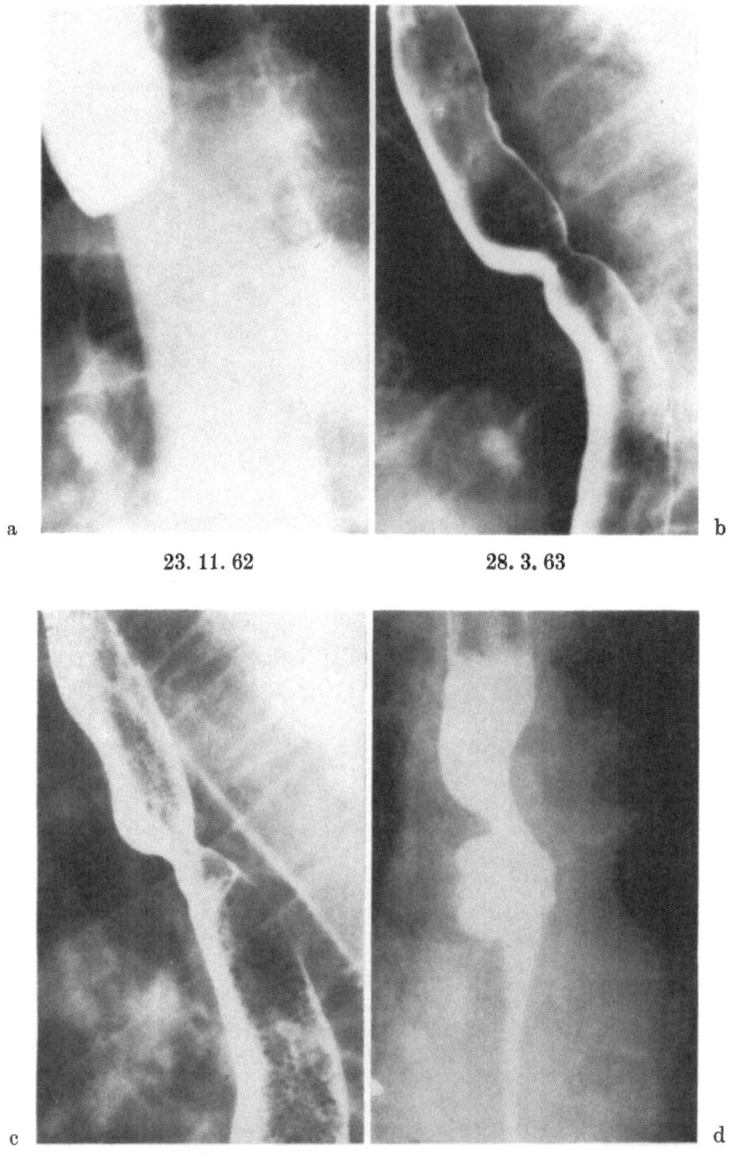

a   23. 11. 62   b   28. 3. 63

c   12. 12. 63   d   7. 7. 65

Fig. 230. a Squamous carcinoma of the mid-thoracic esophagus in an 82 year old man irradiated in December, 1962. b In March, 1963, he was gaining weight and could swallow anything except large pieces of meat. c In December, 1963, he was "almost euphagic" and leading a normal life. d In June, 1965, two and a half years after irradiation, dysphagia recurred. The appearance of locally recurrent tumor is shown in the above radiograph of the 7th July, 1965. The patient died from the local recurrence in September, 1965

offered some hope of cure by irradiation (Pearson, 1971) but in spite of such wide application, death as a consequence of the treatment is almost unknown and treatment morbidity is low. Long term survival is not good (20 per cent at five years) but better than following surgery. Even those patients who go

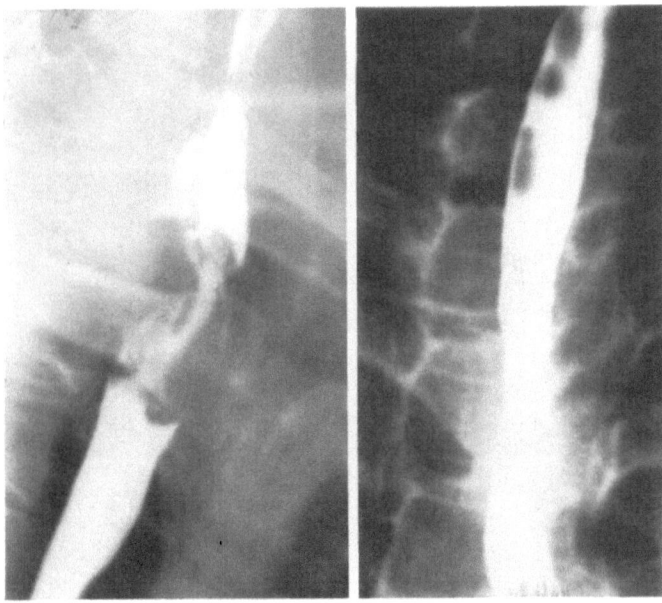

26. 8. 63   22. 12. 64

Fig. 231. Squamous carcinoma at the level of the suprasternal notch, irradiated in August, 1963, radiographically normal in December, 1964. Patient euphagic and leading a normal working life in 1971

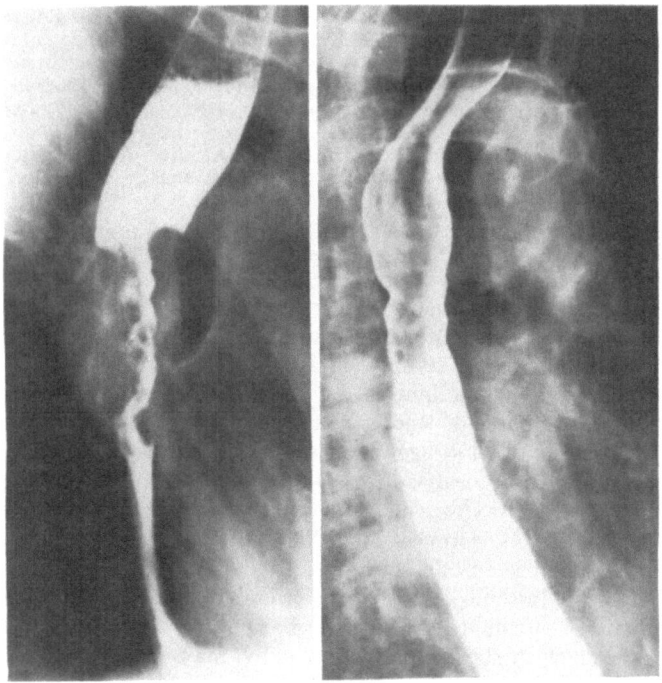

5. 10. 60   19. 10. 65

Fig. 232. Squamous carcinoma at the level of the left main bronchus in an 80 year old woman, irradiated in October, 1960 and restored to clinical normality. Re-X-rayed on the 19th of October, 1965 when treated for a new cancer, of the breast. In 1970 the patient, now aged 90, was well and apparently cured of both malignancies

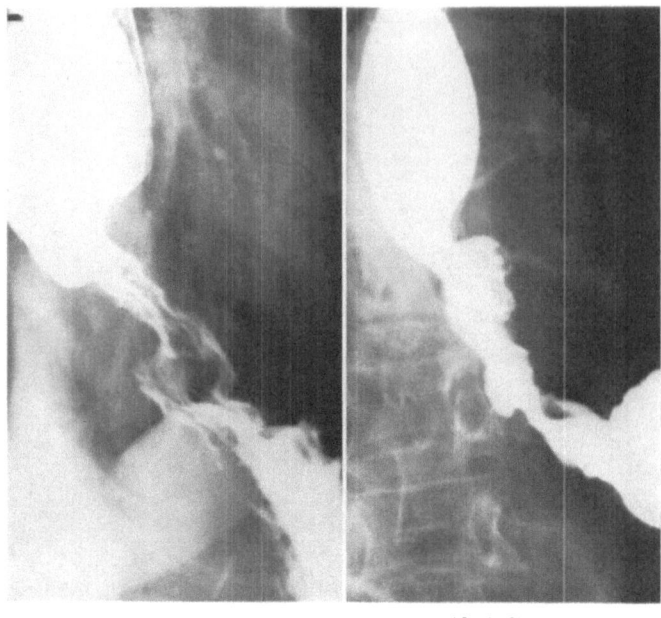

24. 8. 66   19. 4. 67

Fig. 233. An exuberant, well differentiated squamous carcinoma at the lower end of the esophagus irradiated in September, 1966, but still presenting gross residual distorsion of the esophageal lumen in April, 1967. The patient was clinically well and had regained weight. Repeated biopsies were negative but the X-ray appearance so strongly suggested the presence of recurrent cancer that an esophagogastrectomy was performed in May, 1967. In the resected specimen a 6 cm length at the lower end of the esophagus presented polypoid excrescences and ulceration within a rigid tube, but histological examination showed radiation changes with sclerosis and ulceration with no evidence of tumor (patient alive in 1970). (Reproduced by courtesy of the Editor of the American Journal of Roentgenology, 1969, Vol. 105, p. 507)

on to die from the disease have, in many cases, experienced a useful period of palliation. This type of treatment has also a number of unattractive features. It is two or three weeks after starting irradiation before useful tumor shrinkage is to be expected. Thereafter it may be another one to three months or more before the full benefit is experienced (Fig. 229). Local recurrence of the tumor (Fig. 230) occurs in about half the patients, with or without distant metastases (occasionally, a patient with a local recurrence can still be salvaged by surgery). About half of those who do not suffer a local recurrence develop distant metastases; and amongst those who develop no further sign of tumor, although a half require no further interference (Figs. 226, 231, 232), a quarter require dilatation of a fibrous stricture on one occasion (Fig. 229) and another quarter require repeated bougienage, in some cases for more than a year (Fig. 224). The diagnosis of a local recurrence of tumor following irradiation can be difficult. Occasionally, the esophagus heals with marked distortion which may simulate the radiographic appearances of persistent or recurrent tumor (Fig. 233). Occasionally, after elimination of a large tumor, simple ulceration persists (Buschke, 1954; Pearson, 1969). This is a formidable list of unattractive features distinguished only by being less disastrous than the disadvantages of primary surgical treatment (Pearson, 1969, 1971).

1.6.3.2. The Level of the Esophageal Cancer

Patients with squamous carcinoma in the upper thoracic and cervical esophagus do rather better with megavoltage irradiation than patients with low tumors (at more than 30 cm from the upper alveolus), whereas the reverse is true for surgery. Irradiation can certainly eliminate lower esophageal squamous carcinomas, but probably no more consistently so than surgical treatment

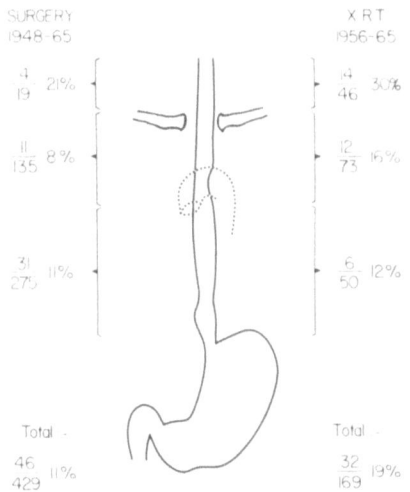

Fig. 234. The five year survival fractions and percentages of 429 patients subjected to operation from 1948–1965 and 169 patients radically irradiated from 1956–1965 are shown according to three levels: cervical esophagus, upper half thoracic esophagus, lower half thoracic esophagus (SCOTLAND)

(Fig. 234). Therefore, for a patient with a low esophageal squamous carcinoma who is an excellent operation risk, surgical treatment is probably to be preferred. If there is any doubt about the patient surviving the procedure, irradiation is certainly preferable. For high tumors, irradiation is to be preferred, with surgery held in reserve for patients known to have a local recurrence following irradiation and still without evidence of distant tumor spread.

1.6.3.3. Adenocarcinoma

Long term control by irradiation of adenocarcinoma presenting in the esophagus appears to be very rare, and even good palliation rather uncommon. Therefore, if at all possible, adenocarcinoma should be resected.

1.6.4. Surgical Treatment

In view of the frequent lack of success with any method of treatment of carcinoma of the esophagus, the most important objective must be to restore the patient's ability to swallow during his last months of life (BELSEY, 1965). The surgical technique which will be used to achieve this objective depends upon the resectability of the lesion as well as on the general condition of the patient. If both are favorable and if there are no distant metastases, a curative resection will be performed. Numerous operative techniques have been described, which can be classified as follows:

1. Resectable and good general condition:
   a) one-stage procedures:
      — excision with end-to-end anastomosis (Parker, 1949).
      — — replacement, by
      — — stomach or gastric tube (Beck, 1905)
      — — colon (Kelling, 1911)
      — — skin tube (in cases of carcinoma of the cervical esophagus) (Wookey, 1942).

The organ used to restore the continuity of the digestive tract may be brought subcutaneously, or in the retrosternal region, or it may be placed in its usual intrathoracic position, with cervical or intrathoracic anastomosis.

   b) staged interventions (these procedures are performed when the general condition of the patient is not extremely poor or when surgery is combined with radiotherapy.
      — 1. bypass; 2. resection (Luna, 1963).
      — 1. resection and gastrostomy; 2. bypass (Mahoney, 1965).
      — 1. gastrostomy; 2. resection; 3. bypass (Nakayama, 1967).

2. Irresectable or poor general condition:
      — bypass with stomach or colon, without resection.
      — intubation
      — — endoscopic (Souttar, 1924; Celestin, 1959).
      — — operative: (Mousseau, 1956).
      — bougienage.
      — gastrostomy or jejunostomy.

Some have adopted an aggressive operative approach to carcinoma of the esophagus. In their opinion metastatic involvement does not contraindicate palliative resection (Nakayama, 1967; Plested, 1968; Lortat-Jacob, 1970) because resection of the primary lesion is believed to result in improvement of the patient's general condition. Others have completely abandoned reconstructive surgery for upper esophageal carcinoma, and use bougienage to reduce dysphagia (Menguy, 1964).

High esophageal carcinomata are usually approached through a right thoracotomy, should it be decided that the treatment of choice in the individual patient is by resection. The approach for lower lesions is through a left thoracotomy. The right-sided approach is often preferred for high tumors because of the facility with which the azygos vein can be divided, without measurable detrimental effect to the patient, as opposed to the difficulty of mobilization and the indivisibility of the aortic arch on the left, medial to which high tumors usually lie. However, bleeding points around the aortic arch are difficult to reach from the right-sided approach.

The most lucid description of a technique of mobilization of the esophagus from the mediastinum, and one that satisfies the theoretical requirements which avoid dissection in the immediate extraesophageal plane is that by Logan (1962, 1963). Proximity of trachea and left recurrent laryngeal nerve preclude a satisfactory block dissection higher than the lower border of the aortic arch; below this level a block dissection, which amounts to the removal of a cylinder of tissue which encloses the tumor together with related lymph nodes and a length of normal viscus above and below the tumor, without exposure of the esophagus save at the site chosen for reconstruction, is a logical procedure.

The best functional results are obtained with the colon as an esophageal substitute, even if it is used as an antiperistaltic segment. Esophagitis is less common and the risk of leakage of the anastomosis is smaller than with the stomach. Most surgeons prefer to use the stomach as an esophageal substitute after resection of an esophageal carcinoma. The operative procedure is easier, there is no need to use intraabdominal anastomosis, and post-operative complications are few in experienced hands (PLESTED, 1968). However, in approximately 27 per cent of the patients who survive more than 6 months, reflux esophagitis will develop, and dysphagia may occur. Both the stomach and the colon are suitable to restore the continuity of the digestive tract in defects that reach as high as the cervical region. In order to avoid gastric stasis after surgery a pyloromyotomy or a pyloroplasty should be performed, as the esophageal resection is necessarily associated with a vagotomy.

1.6.4.1. Complications of Esophagogastrectomy

1.6.4.1.1. Disruption or Leakage at the Site of the Anastomosis is the commonest complication to follow esophagogastrectomy (LE ROUX and KNOTHE, 1962). Avascular necrosis of the organ used for restoration of the alimentary continuity is likely to result in death during the first four or five post-operative days. A more common sequence of events is an uneventful first post-operative week, or one complicated by intermittent low fever, followed, on the seventh to tenth post-operative day, by an increase in fever and perhaps the development of atrial fibrillation. Thereafter, there may occur a dramatic incident of sudden, severe pain in the chest or abdomen with prolonged shock, and clinical and radiographic evidence of hydropneumothorax. Intercostal drainage of the pleura, suspension of oral feeding and resuscitation generally fail to prevent death. Less dramatic evidence of leakage from the anastomosis is less usual and less often lethal. Pleural effusion or hydropneumothorax develop insidiously in the second post-operative week; thoracocentesis demonstrates that the pleural liquid is contaminated with alimentary contents; pleural drainage, with the maintenance of adequate hydration intravenously, provides the opportunity for elective definitive management. An attempt at reconstruction of the anastomosis at this juncture usually fails, and the form of management most likely to be successful is exteriorisation of the esophagus in the neck and of the stomach below the costal margin, as a gastrostomy, with restoration of alimentary continuity at leisure when all evidence of pleural infection has subsided.

The incidence of leakage from the anastomosis is greatly reduced if an esophagogastrostomy is fashioned far from the site of gastric division and closure, and if antibiotics are administered in liquid form by mouth for some days after the anastomosis has been fashioned, while other oral feeding is withheld. It is probably technically impossible to fashion an esophagogastrostomy which is watertight, and all probably seep rather than leak; if seepage is rendered innocuous and a mediastinal abscess does not form, the anastomosis is unlikely to disrupt unless the blood supply of the organ used for replacement has been jeopardized at operation.

1.6.4.1.2. Hemorrhage from Aortic Erosion may be the consequence of seepage or leakage from an esophageal anastomosis which results in the development of a mediastinal abscess without obvious disruption of the anastomosis (LE ROUX, 1961 b); fever and the development of atrial fibrillation during the second post-operative week are often the only evidence of such an event—the chest radiograph remaining normal. There is commonly a warning hemorrhage six to twenty-four hours before the patient dies from terminal hemorrhage. At post-mortem in these patients there is found a mediastinal abscess in relation to the anastomosis, in the wall of which there is the aorta or one of its intercostal branches which has been eroded by infection and which communicates directly with the alimentary tract.

1.6.4.1.3. Death from Pulmonary Infection after esophagogastrectomy is not uncommon. Aspiration pneumonia is a frequent complication of dysphagia, especially where dysphagia is nearly total. Some deaths in the post-operative period from pulmonary infection may be averted if operation is delayed whilst respiratory infection is cleared with physiotherapy and chemotherapy. This simple approach is complicated by the fact that many of these patients have total dysphagia, and, in them, aspiration may have played a significant part in the pulmonary infection. Aspiration of saliva and ingested liquids in any patient with dysphagia often passes unnoticed, the respiratory tract quickly becoming tolerant of foreign materials. In most patients who die from respiratory infection after esophagogastrectomy the pre-operative respiratory state has an important bearing on the development of the post-operative complication. Earlier recourse to tracheostomy helps to diminish mortality in relation to post-operative pulmonary infection.

In the circumstances of esophagogastrectomy for carcinoma, the distal esophageal sphincter is inevitably removed with the operative specimen. It is unsafe to rely upon the competence of the proximal esophageal sphincter, which is usually unable to retain the contents of the intrathoracic stomach if stomach has been used to restore continuity after esophagogastrectomy. For this reason, it is unsafe to lay flat, for the purpose of physiotherapy for example, a patient submitted to esophagogastrectomy because of the high probability of massive aspiration pneumonia. Even many years after esophagogastrectomy patients find it more comfortable to sleep with several pillows, and should they slip from these pillows during sleep they may wake up with a sense of suffocation, the consequence of regurgitation and aspiration into the trachea of gastric contents.

1.6.4.1.4. Pulmonary Embolism and Myocardial Infarction are causes of death in convalescence from esophagogastrectomy probably not more commonly than after any other major thoracic surgical procedure in the elderly. *Atrial fibrillation* is a common complication of thoracotomy in the aged and after esophagogastrectomy, and while it is sometimes evidence of mediastinal infection, leakage from the anastomosis, or impending hemorrhage from the aorta, it is not inevitable evidence that these catastrophes are imminent.

1.6.4.1.5. The Pleural Complications of thoracotomy are pneumothorax, hemothorax, pyothorax and chylothorax. Block dissection of the esophagus in the mediastinum exposes the thoracic duct to the risk of injury, with leakage of chyle; since both pleural spaces are commonly opened during esophagectomy, chylothorax may be right- or left-sided or bilateral. Management is by closed intercostal drainage, with supplementary feeding. This conservative regime is usually successful. Chylous liquid is recognized by its appearance—a cloudy white liquid resembling milk—and it is recognized to be different from pus by the fact that the liquid, because of its high content of fat, becomes clear when ether is added.

1.6.5. Preoperative and Postoperative Irradiation

Any local treatment, such as irradiation or surgery, will fail for those numerous patients, 80 per cent or more of all those presenting with the disease, who already have disseminated disease. But even some patients without disseminated disease are not cured, due to death as a consequence of resection, recurrence of tumor within the irradiated area, or recurrence at the margins of either the irradiated or the resected tissues. Many different combinations of irradiation and surgery have been tried in attempts to reduce these hazards. AKAKURA et al. (1970) found that during a period when surgical technique altered little, the introduction of full pre-operative irradiation to a dose of 5000 to 6000 rads in four to six weeks, followed two to four weeks later by resection, was associated with a striking improvement in resectability, reduction in the incidence of tumor at the margins of resection, and improvement in five year survival rate. NAKA-YAMA et al. (1967) report that the introduction of pre-operative irradiation giving four or five fractions of 500 rads daily, followed several days later by esophagectomy, has improved the long term survival rate of their patients. They believe that such pre-operative irradiation increases the number of patients suitable for resection, that it shrinks tumor, and facilitates resection.

On the other hand WATSON (1963, 1967), and PEARSON (1969, 1971) argue that having carried out irradiation or surgery either of which, by itself, might have cured the patient, no further assault should be made on the (usually frail and old) patient unless it is established that the initial treatment has failed.

Post-operative irradiation is probably inferior to pre-operative irradiation because after surgery the blood supply and oxygenation of residual tumor, and therefore its radiosensitivity, are believed to be less.

1.6.6. Intubation

Sir SYMONDS (1885) developed what was probably the first successful tube for endoscopic intubation of malignant esophageal strictures. His earlier tubes, of boxwood, ivory and silver, gave way to a more successful tube made of gum-elastic. Sir SOUTTAR (1924) revived SYMONDS' method using a coiled metallic tube. These tubes and those subsequently developed depended upon thrusting the tube distally through the tumor. MOUSSEAU et al. (1956) pioneered the alternative method of pulling a tube through the stricture through a high gastrotomy. All tubes which carry a circular funnel have the disadvantage that an edematous ring may form above the funnel and lead to obstruction or ulceration. CELESTIN (1959) designed an oval tube with a short, barrel-shaped funnel, which he claimed offers advantages over the V-shaped funnel of other tubes. Larger and longer tubes are said to become less easily obstructed provided that patients masticate food thoroughly. Tablets and capsules should be avoided. Sips of water taken during a meal assist the passage of solids. Before and after meals the tube is cleaned by drinking soda water or any similar effervescent drink. Intubation carries a high risk of perforation of the esophagus, even in expert hands. Intubation as an adjunct to irradiation, if dysphagia is also for liquids and the patient cannot swallow saliva, is a more rational use of the technique, but if curative irradiation appears possible, the tube should be removed as the tumor commences to shrink to avoid exacerbation of scarring and stricture due to the combination of radiation esophagitis and mechanical pressure from the tube. For those unsuitable for even palliative irradiation, skillful sedation with morphia is a more benign form of management and is no more likely to hasten death than intubation complicated by esophageal perforation.

1.6.7. Cancer Chemotherapy

Chemotherapy benefits only a small minority of patients with esophageal carcinoma and is curative in none. Therefore it is reserved for the tumor beyond further help by radiation therapy or surgery (CLINE, 1971). For squamous carcinoma of the esophagus, its use is severely limited by the absence of any sufficiently effective drug the toxicity of which does not outweigh its usefulness. Although not yet adequately investigated in the treatment of esophageal squamous carcinoma *methotrexate* has been used to treat advanced squamous carcinoma of the head and neck with useful tumor shrinkage in about 10 percent of cases, and some of these patients did not suffer unacceptable toxicity. It is possible that similar results may follow the use of methotrexate for esophageal squamous carcinoma. It is clear that any benefit to be anticipated from the use of this drug does not justify a dose which results in more than very mild toxicity. Radiation therapy and methotrexate in combination have been tried for head and neck squamous carcinoma. These experiments have not yet established whether the effect of combining the two agents is merely additive or something more than additive. Failure to respond to methotrexate, or remission after response to methotrexate (in squamous carcinoma in the head and neck) may very occasionally be followed by a useful response to an alkylating agent.

Bleomycin, discovered by Dr. H. Umezawa and his associates in 1962 in Japan, is an interesting drug which concentrates in the skin and is sometimes effective against squamous carcinoma but has various toxicity problems which have prevented its wide use. One is pneumonitis proceeding to fibrosis, which may be fatal. The effect has not proved to be sufficiently dose-related to be safely controllable. There have been a number of reports from Japan of some regression of esophageal carcinoma with bleomycin (Wada et al., 1969; Ichikawa, 1969) but considerable toxicity occurred.

For adenocarcinoma presenting in the esophagus guidance for chemotherapeutic management may be taken from experience with gastric carcinoma. For about 20 per cent of patients beyond further help by surgery or radiation therapy *5-fluorouracil* may be of benefit. Improvement may occur without toxicity occasionally for six months or longer, and only mild toxicity should be risked. A reasonable dose is 12.5 mg per kg body weight once weekly until toxicity develops or until no longer effective. If 5-fluorouracil is ineffective; or if relapse occurs, occasionally an alkylating agent may produce some response but only very mild toxicity is justifiable. For example, chlorambacil 0.1 mg per kg body weight per day is a suitable dose. Thereafter methotrexate may be tried at a dose of 0.2 mg per kg body weight daily for four days and then 0.1 mg per kg every other day until mild toxicity develops.

1.6.8. Treatment of Esophagotracheal Fistula

A patient with a fistula through tumor between the esophagus and trachea or bronchus is incurable (Martini et al., 1970; Ong and Kwong, 1970). Without treatment, most such patients die within a month. Martini reports one such fistula which healed following irradiation, the patient dying six months later without recurrence of the fistula, and Akakura et al. (1970) refer to "a few cases" in which they have observed healing of such a fistula following irradiation. Martini et al. report 40 per cent of their patients dead within one month, 87 per cent dead within six months and all dead within two years. Ong and Kwong describe the use of major surgical procedures for malignant esophagotracheal fistula in 17 patients with complete relief of symptoms for eight patients. Nine of the patients died within one month, 14 were dead within six months, and all were dead within a year.

The present authors believe that most workers in this field will choose to occlude the fistula by intubation of the esophagus, thus enabling the patient to ingest liquid and creamy soft food without aspiration into the bronchial tree for a few months before death supervenes from advance of the cancer.

1.6.9. Results of Treatment

Factors influencing prognosis have already been discussed. Treatment is one such factor. The results of treatment of esophageal cancer in a community depend on the stage of advancement of the disease when the patient seeks help more than on any other factor. The proportion suitable for an attempt at curative treatment depends on the nature of such treatment, the age and robustness of the patients and the stage of the disease, and varies from as high as 65 per cent to as low as five per cent. Perusal of the literature leads one to the somber conclusion that in no sizable population from which the whole experience of esophageal cancer is reported is the overall five year survival more than ten per cent, and in some communities it is nil. Even the overall one year survival does not exceed 33 per cent. Even a few of those who survive five years later die of recurrent cancer.

The results will be better the larger the proportion of females in the series.

1.6.9.1. Results of Surgical Management

In a center where surgery is normally the definitive treatment of esophageal cancer, and radiotherapy is either not available or is used merely as a surgical adjuvant, much depends on the experience and consequent skill gained by the individual surgeon. COLLIS (1957), who has recently reported excellent surgical results (COLLIS, 1971), has discussed the need for a team to gain experience and become proficient in this difficult field before satisfactory results can be expected. MILLER (1962) holds a similar view and writes: "in the surgery of oesophageal carcinoma, the occasional operator is likely to be at a considerable disadvantage".

Esophagogastrectomy, whether for squamous or adenocarcinoma, carries an operative mortality often as high as 30 per cent. Taking squamous and adeno-carcinoma together it is possible to reduce available figures to a percentage in the following way. Of every 100 patients with dysphagia caused by a primary tumor in the proximal part of the alimentary tract, at least 40, and in some series nearly all, will not be submitted to an operation—most of these because of metastases—, or will prove to be unsuitable for resection at thoracolaparotomy. At best, 50 or 60 patients may undergo resection, and of these some 20 may die as a consequence of the operation. Of those who survive, at least 15 will die from metastases during the first year after operation, some 20 will die subsequently from metastases and, at the most, five will survive operation for five years or longer.

Dysphagia from tumor recurrence returns before death in about a third of patients—more commonly in those in whom the original tumor was high. Those who die within the first year after resection from metastases, especially those who die with recurrence of dysphagia, derive little palliative benefit from resection, although restoration of swallowing for a limited period is probably regarded by these patients as valuable. In approximately 60 per cent of patients in whom resection is undertaken for squamous carcinoma the natural history of the disease is either shortened (in those who die from an operation), or little altered. In all others, significant palliative benefit—that is, increase in survival time from the onset of dysphagia—can be claimed (LE ROUX, 1962).

From a comparison of five large series—those of SWEET (1954), NAKAYAMA (1959), ELLIS (1960), LOGAN (1963), and LORTAT-JACOB et al. (1970)—the five year survival rate ranged from ten per cent to 15 per cent. Where distinction is made between tumors that are low and high, the five year survival rate amongst those with low tumors is nearer 20 per cent. Large series reported from Southern Africa—for example Proctor (1968)—do not include any five year survivors because, in underdeveloped countries, presentation is invariably late.

Of all patients with adenocarcinoma in the proximal part of the alimentary tract, causing dysphagia, and submitted to resection, only eight per cent are alive after five years.

1.6.9.2. Results of Management of Squamous Esophageal Cancer by Irradiation

In a center where radiotherapy is normally the definitive treatment of squamous esophageal cancer and modern megavoltage facilities are available, and where surgery is reserved for establishing the diagnosis and the management of recurrence should irradiation fail, satisfactory results are obtainable by an experienced team—again, this is a field in which the occasional practitioner is less likely to succeed. Of every 100 patients presenting with squamous esophageal cancer 35 will have cancer so extensive, or other disease so advanced, that curative treatment is not attempted; five will be treated by resection either for a lower esophageal tumor without pre-operative histological proof but believed to be an adenocarcinoma, or resected as an emergency procedure following perforation during investigation; 60 will be treated by radical megavoltage irradiation; 30 will be alive one year later and ten will live five or more years. One of the ten five year survivors will had have the esophagus resected, either initially, or following failure of irradiation.

1.6.9.3. Results of Management of Squamous Esophageal Cancer by Irradiation and Surgery

In a center where both megavoltage irradiation is available and radiotherapists and thoracic surgeons with wide experience of esophageal cancer consult fully, of every 100 patients presenting, 35 will not receive any form of curative treatment. Of the remaining 65 patients, 50, that is all who are in poor condition, or over the age of 60 years, or have tumors suspected of reaching to within 30 cm or less of the upper alveolus, will be treated by radical megavoltage irradiation; and the remaining 15 patients who are relatively young, in very good condition, and have tumors low in the esophagus will be treated by partial esophagogastrectomy. Ten patients will be alive five years later, three mainly as a consequence of surgical treatment and seven mainly as a consequence of irradiation.

If there are many more males than females presenting with the disease, the yield of long survivors will be even lower than quoted above.

In conclusion, a review of carcinoma of the esophagus, as of malignant disease in many other sites, leads one clearly to recognize that whilst highly skilled treatment can be of some avail, determination of the cause and prevention would be much more rewarding, and, failing prevention, earlier diagnosis and treatment is likely to be the most rewarding development.

2. Sarcoma

Sarcomata constitute less than one per cent of malignant tumors of the esophagus. The least uncommon is leiomyosarcoma. Rhabdomyosarcoma, fibrosarcoma, and malignant lymphoma have also been described. Stout and Lattes (1957) caution against acceptance of many of the esophageal fibrosarcomata reported in the literature.

No one team has had experience of more than a few cases of leiomyosarcoma (JACKSON, 1935; JOHNSTON et al., 1953; CAMISHION et al., 1961; GOODNER et al., 1963) and therefore observations about the nature of the disease must be somewhat tentative. It seems very probable that, compared with carcinoma, most cases of leiomyosarcoma grow less rapidly; more frequently form large polypoid or even pedunculated masses; metastasize later, more frequently by the blood stream than the lymphatics; and are rather more amenable to eradication by resection, whilst cure following irradiation is also possible. The age incidence is not clearly different from that of carcinoma and there is no obvious predilection for either sex or any particular level in the esophagus. Females have a better chance of long survival than males.

Malignant lymphomata—Hodgkin's disease, lymphosarcoma, and reticulum cell sarcoma—may occasionally involve the esophagus, very occasionally as the presenting symptom (ENNUYER et al., 1950). In such cases treatment is by irradiation if the disease is apparently localized or confined to one region, and chemotherapy or a combination of chemotherapy and irradiation if the disease is already widely disseminated. There is a possibility that reticulum cell sarcoma may present in this site, as it may do elsewhere in the body, as a truly localized malignancy curable by irradiation.

3. Pseudosarcoma and Carcinosarcoma

Both pseudosarcoma and carcinosarcoma are very rare, usually polypoid, tend to grow more slowly than carcinoma and usually pursue a less malignant course.

Pseudosarcoma presents as a polypoid mass of sarcoma-like tissue, often associated with a small area of intramucosal or invasive squamous carcinoma, which is usually confined to the base of the pedicle. STOUT and LATTES (1957) believe that such lesions behave benignly. LANE (1957) has described such tumors in the oropharynx. Tumors fitting this description do not always behave benignly, and whilst it is usually the carcinomatous element which may metastasize (DE MARCO et al., 1965), HUGHES and CRUICKSHANK (1969) report a case with typical appearances of pseudosarcoma but malignant spread of the sarcomatous element leading to death. HUGHES and CRUICKSHANK argue that wide rather than purely local excision is the wiser course for such tumors. RAZZUK et al. (1971) describe such a tumor excised quite locally but they provide no follow-up information of the outcome.

Carcinosarcoma, also usually pedunculated when presenting in the esophagus, contrasts with pseudosarcoma in the intimate admixture of carcinomatous and sarcomatous elements. It occurs especially in males, over the age of 45, and in the lower esophagus (GOWING, 1961). Cure by resection is quite possible, and when metastases occur, they are usually sarcomatous, although individual cases giving rise to both sarcomatous and carcinomatous metastases have been described. The importance of this type of tumor seems to be that it metastizes relatively late and apparent cures have been reported (STEINER et al., 1967). Such tumors are very difficult to distinguish from pleomorphic carcinoma on histological examination, but the pedunculation, sharp demarcation of carcinomatous and sarcomatous elements, and relative localization of the growth are characteristic (MOORE et al., 1963; LICHTER et al., 1968).

Such pedunculated tumors as pseudosarcoma and carcinosarcoma cannot be certainly diagnosed by endoscopic biopsy alone. Such a small specimen may provide a highly unrepresentative picture, possibly suggesting a highly malignant undifferentiated tumor for what is in reality a relatively curable lesion.

4. Malignant Melanoma

Malignant melanoma very rarely occurs as a primary esophageal tumor. Only rarely does normal melanotic tissue occur in the esophagus. Piccone et al. (1970) report a case of malignant melanoma occurring in a patient with melanosis of the esophagus. They were able to trace fewer than 30 cases in a review of the literature, 14 treated surgically, death nearly always occurring within a year.

5. Metastatic Tumors

The esophagus is an uncommon site to find blood-borne metastases but rare instances have been reported from a variety of primary tumors without any striking common features (Gowing, 1961).

Direct invasion of the esophagus by bronchial or thyroid carcinoma, or from metastatic paraesophageal lymph nodes secondarily invaded from nearby primary sites, is not uncommon.

6. Other Rare Malignant Tumors of the Esophagus

6.1. Carcinoid Tumor

Brenner et al. (1969) recently described a carcinoid tumor of the esophagus. There was no evidence of functional activity of this tumor.

6.2. Paget's Disease

Paget's disease may involve the esophageal mucosa in association with a carcinoma of the esophagus (Yates and Koss, 1968). As in Paget's disease of the breast, the epithelial changes characteristic of this disease were associated with a primary cancer close by. The epithelial lesion stretched over a considerable distance without any evidence of invasion of the submucosa by the Paget cells. In addition to involving the epithelium, the Paget cells also permeated the submucosal ducts of the esophagus. This seems to be a very rare lesion as the authors examined another 146 cases of squamous cell carcinoma and adenocarcinoma of the esophagus and were unable to find similar changes.

6.3. Hodgkin's Disease

Involvement of the esophagus by Hodgkin's disease is rare. According to Surks and Guttman (1966) only 30 cases of esophageal Hodgkin's disease have been reported. Such involvement usually does not occur as a primary event, but rather as an invasion from adjacent lymph nodes. In about 50 per cent of the reported cases the disease was discovered at postmortem examination. As in other types of esophageal tumors dysphagia is the most important symptom. Esophagoscopy may show nothing but a narrowing of extraesophageal origin and biopsy may be unrevealing as long as the esophageal mucosa is uninvolved (Hambly and Blundell, 1968).

The treatment of esophageal Hodgkin's disease is not different from the treatment of Hodgkin's disease involving other organs.

6.4. Granular Cell Myoblastoma

Some 10 cases of granular cell myoblastoma of the esophagus have been reported (FLEGE and EDMONDS, 1969). These tumors show groups of cells whose cytoplasm is filled with fine eosinophilic granules and which extend throughout the full thickness of the muscle layer. It is unknown whether these tumors arise from muscle cells, Schwann-cells, histiocytes, fibroblasts or paraganglionic cells. All but one of the reported cases have been in women between the ages of 19 and 48 years. The tumor may be small and localized to the esophagus, but in three of the reported cases it was associated with separate lesions in other parts of the body. Of the 10 patients only one had metastases. The tumors are radio-resistant. Treatment of the localized tumor has been by local excision and no recurrences have been reported, although follow-up information is incomplete.

6.5. Verrucous Squamous Cell Carcinoma

Verrucous squamous cell carcinoma is a rare variant of squamous cell carcinoma and may occur on any stratified squamous mucosa or modified skin (KRAUS and PEREZ-MESA, 1966). Five cases of esophageal involvement have been reported (MINIELLY et al., 1967). Verrucous squamous cell carcinoma is an exophytic, papillary or warty, slowly growing, often extensive neoplasm, that relentlessly invades local structures, but rarely metastasizes. It is frequently associated with surrounding leukoplakia. In four of the five reported cases the tumor occurred in patients with a previously diagnosed non-malignant esophageal lesion (two with achalasia and two with a pulsion diverticulum). The discrepancy between the clinical appearance of a large invading tumor and the well-differentiated nature of the growth on microscopic examination may create diagnostic difficulties. Therefore diagnosis is more likely when the pathologist is aware of the clinical nature of the lesion and when there is an adequate biopsy specimen to show the characteristic infiltrative growth pattern. The tumor has a definite tendency for recurrence and the prognosis of verrucous carcinoma of the esophagus is poorer than elsewhere in the body. For verrucous carcinoma surgical therapy, either diathermy or en-bloc resection, is much preferable to radiation therapy.

Acknowledgements

For the photomicrographs reproduced in Figs. 215–222 we are grateful to Professor G. O. BAIN of the Department of Pathology of the University of Alberta.

References

ADAMS, W. E.: The future outlook of surgical therapy for carcinoma of the esophagus. Surg. Gynec. Obstet. **100**, 366–368 (1955).

ADAMS, W. E., PHEMISTER, D. B.: Carcinoma of the lower thoracic esophagus. Report of a successful resection and esophagogastrostomy. J. thorac. Surg. **7**, 612–632 (1938).

AHLBOM, H. E.: Simple achlorhydric anemia. Plummer-Vinson syndrome, and carcinoma of the mouth, pharynx and oesophagus in women; observations at Radiumhemmet, Stockholm. Brit. med. J. **1936 II**, 331–333.

AHLBOM, H. E.: Prädisponierende Faktoren für Plattenepithelkarzinom in Mund, Hals und Speiseröhre. Eine statistische Untersuchung am Material des Radiumhemmets, Stockholm. Acta radiol. (Stockh.) **18**, 163–185 (1937).

AHMED, N., COOK, R.: The incidence of cancer of the oesophagus in West Kenya. Brit. J. Cancer **23**, 302–312 (1969).

AKAKURA, I., NAKAMURA, Y., KAGEGAWA, T., NAKAYAMA, R., WATANABE, H., YAMASHITA, H.: Surgery of carcinoma of the esophagus with preoperative radiation. Chest **57**, 47–57 (1970).

Akovbiantz, A., Aeberhard, P., Linder, E., Senning, Å.: Die Bedeutung der Mediastino-skopie für die Beurteilung der Operabilität des Oesophaguscarcinoms. Langenbecks Arch. klin. Chir. **313**, 360–363 (1965).

Allison, P. R., Borrie, J.: The treatment of malignant obstruction of the cardia. Brit. J. Surg. **37**, 1–21 (1949).

Allison, P. R., Johnstone, A. S.: The oesophagus lined with gastric mucous membrane. Thorax **8**, 87–101 (1953).

Ashbaugh, D. G.: Mediastinoscopy. Arch. Surg. **100**, 568–573 (1970).

Azzopardi, J. G., Menzies, T.: Primary oesophageal adenocarcinoma: confirmation of its existence by the finding of mucous gland tumours. Brit. J. Surg. **49**, 497–506 (1962).

Barrett, N. R.: Lower oesophagus lined by columnar epithelium. In: Modern trends in gastro-enterology, 2nd series. London: Butterworth 1958.

Beck, C.: Demonstrations of specimens illustrating a method of formation of a prethoracic esophagus. Illinois med. J. **7**, 463 (1905).

Belsey, R.: Reconstruction of the esophagus with left colon. J. thorac. cardiovasc. Surg. **49**, 33–55 (1965).

Bergman, F.: Cancer of the oesophagus: histological study of development and local spread of 10 cases of squamous cell carcinoma in the lower third of oesophagus. Acta chir. scand. **117**, 356–365 (1959).

Bigger, I. A., Vinson, P. P.: Carcinoma secondary to burn of the esophagus from ingestion of lye: report of a case. Surgery **28**, 887–889 (1950).

Bradshaw, E., Schonland, M.: Oesophageal and lung cancers in Natal African males in relation to certain socio-economic factors: an analysis of 484 interviews. Brit. J. Cancer **23**, 275–284 (1969).

Brenner, S., Heimlich, H., Widman, M.: Carcinoid of esophagus. N.Y. J. Med. **69**, 1337–1339 (1969).

Burgess, H. M., Baggenstoss, A. H., Moersch, H. J., Clagett, O. T.: Carcinoma of the esophagus: a clinicopathologic study. Surg. Clin. N. Amer. **31**, 965–976 (1951).

Burrell, R. J. W.: Distribution maps of esophageal cancer among Bantu in the Transkei. J. nat. Cancer Inst. **43**, 877–889 (1969).

Buschke, F.: Surgical and radiological results in treatment of esophageal carcinoma. Amer. J. Roentgenol. **71**, 9–24 (1954).

Buschke, F., Cantril, S. T.: Supervoltage roentgen therapy of oesophageal carcinoma. Radiology **42**, 480–492 (1944).

Camishion, R. C., Gibbon, J. H., Jr., Templeton, J. Y., III: Leiomyosarcoma of the esophagus: review of the literature and report of two cases. Ann. Surg. **153**, 951–956 (1961).

Case, R. A. M.: Mortality from cancer of the oesophagus in England and Wales. In: Neoplastic disease at various sites. Vol. IV. Tumours of the oesophagus, ed. N. C. Tanner and D. W. Smithers, p. 11–25. Edinburgh-London: Livingstone 1961 a.

Case, R. A. M.: Comparison of mortality from carcinoma of the oesophagus in selected countries. In: Neoplastic disease at various sites. Vol. IV. Tumours of the oesophagus, ed. N. C. Tanner and D. W. Smithers, p. 26–34. Edinburgh-London: Livingstone 1961 b.

Celestin, L. R.: Permanent intubation in inoperable cancer of the oesophagus and cardia. A new tube. Ann. roy. Coll. Surg. **25**, 165–170 (1959).

Churchill, E. D., Sweet, R. H.: Transthoracic resection of tumors of the stomach and esophagus. Ann. Surg. **115**, 897–920 (1942).

Clarke, C. A., Howel-Evans, A. W., McConnell, R. B.: Carcinoma of oesophagus associated with tylosis. (Correspondence.) Brit. med. J. **1957 I**, 945.

Cline, M. S.: Major problems in internal medicine. Vol. I. Cancer chemotherapy. Philadelphia-London-Toronto: Saunders 1971.

Cohen, N. N., Flowers, W.: Diagnosis of stenosing lesions of the esophagus using brush cytology. Gastrointest. Endoscopy **15**, 213–214 (1969).

Collis, J. L.: Carcinoma of the oesophagus: the case for surgical excision. Lancet **1957 II**, 613–616.

Collis, J. L.: Surgical treatment of carcinoma of the esophagus and cardia. Brit. J. Surg. **58**, 801–804 (1971).

Cox, R.: The management of dysphagia due to malignant disease of the thoracic and abdominal oesophagus. Ann. roy. Coll. Surg. **21**, 133–176 (1957).

Cummack, D. H.: Gastro-intestinal x-ray diagnosis; a descriptive atlas. Edinburgh-London: Livingstone 1969.

De Marco, A. R., Leon, W., Coleman, W. O., Welsh, R. A., Strug, L. H.: Pseudosarcoma of the esophagus. J. thorac. cardiovasc. Surg. **49**, 188–193 (1965).

Dodge, O. G.: The surgical pathology of gastro-oesophageal carcinoma. Brit. J. Surg. **49**, 121–125 (1961).

DOLL, R.: The geographical distribution of cancer. Brit. J. Cancer **23**, 1–8 (1969).

DOLL, W. R. S.: Prevention of cancer: pointers from epidemiology. London: Nuffield Provincial Hospital Trust 1967.

DORMANNS, E.: Das Oesophaguscarcinom: Ergebnisse der unter Mitarbeit von 39 pathologischen Instituten Deutschlands durchgeführten Erhebung über das Oesophaguscarcinom (1925–1933). Z. Krebsforsch. **49**, 86–108 (1939).

DUNLOP, E. E.: Carcinoma of oesophagus with survival. Aust. N.Z. J. Surg. **30**, 81–91 (1960).

ELLIS, F. G.: The natural history of achalasia of the cardia. Proc. roy. Soc. Med. **53**, 663–666 (1960).

ELLIS, F. H., JR.: Treatment of carcinoma of the esophagus and cardia. Proc. Mayo Clin. **35**, 653–663 (1960).

ELLIS, F. H., JR., JACKSON, R. C., KREUGER, J. T., MOERSCH, H. J., CLAGETT, O. T., GAGE, R. P.: Carcinoma of the esophagus and cardia. Results of treatment, 1946 to 1956. New Engl. J. Med. **260**, 351–358 (1959).

ENNUYER, A., CALLE, R., ROUSSEAU, S., BERTOLUZZI, M.: Les localisations œsophagiennes de la maladie de Hodgkin. Paris méd. **40**, 164–167 (1950).

FLEGE, J. B., JR., EDMONDS, T. T.: Granular cell myoblastoma of the esophagus. J. thorac. cardiovasc. Surg. **58**, 217–220 (1969).

FLEMING, J. A. C.: Carcinoma of the thoracic oesophagus: some notes on its pathology and spread in relation to treatment. Brit. J. Radiol. **16**, 212–216 (1943).

FLEMING, J. A. C.: Radiotherapy in cancer of thoracic oesophagus. Thorax **2**, 206–215 (1947).

GARLOCK, J. H.: The surgical treatment of carcinoma of the thoracic esophagus, with a report of three successful cases. Surg. Gynec. Obstet. **66**, 534–548 (1938).

GOODNER, J. T., MILLER, T. R., WATSON, W. L.: Sarcoma of the esophagus. Amer. J. Roentgenol. **89**, 132–139 (1963).

GOODNER, J. T., TURNBULL, A. D. M.: Bone metastases in cancer of the esophagus. Amer. J. Roentgenol. **111**, 365–367 (1971).

GOOLDEN, A. W. G.: Radiation cancer. A review with special reference to radiation tumours in the pharynx, larynx and thyroid. Brit. J. Radiol. **30**, 626–640 (1957).

GOWING, N. F. C.: The pathology of oesophageal tumours. In: Neoplastic disease at various sites. Vol. IV. Tumours of the oesophagus, ed. N. C. TANNER and D. W. SMITHERS, p. 91–135. Edinburgh-London: Livingstone 1961.

GUISEZ, J.: Malignant tumours of oesophagus. J. Laryng. Otol. **40**, 213–232 (1925).

GUISEZ, J., BARCAT, P.: Essais de traitement de quelques cas d'épithélioma de l'œsophage par les applications locales directes de radium. Bull. Soc. méd. Hôp. Paris **26**, 712–722 (1909).

HAMBLY, C. K., BLUNDELL, J. E.: Hodgkin's disease of the oesophagus. Aust. Radiol. **12**, 43–48 (1968).

HARTZ, P. H.: The incidence of carcinoma of the oesophagus in the Caribbean region and in Venezuela, compared with that of gastric cancer. Acta Un. int. Cancr. **14**, 548–553 (1958).

HOLUB, E., SIMECEK, C.: Pneumomediastinography in carcinoma of the esophagus. Thorax **23**, 77–82 (1968).

HUGHES, J. H., CRUICKSHANK, A. H.: Pseudosarcoma of the oesophagus. Brit. J. Surg. **56** 72–76 (1969).

HURST, E. E.: Malignant tumors in Alaskan Eskimos: unique predominance of carcinoma of the esophagus in Alaskan Eskimo women. Cancer **17**, 1187–1196 (1964).

ICHIKAWA, T.: The clinical effect of bleomycin against squamous cell carcinoma and further developments. Progress in antimicrobiol. and anticancer chemotherapy. Proceedings of the 6th Internat. Congr. of Chemotherapy, p. 1–3. Tokyo: University of Tokyo Press 1969.

JACKSON, C.: Carcinoma and sarcoma of esophagus. Sth. Surg. **4**, 1–11 (1935).

JACOBSSON, F.: The Paterson-Kelly (Plummer-Vinson) syndrome and carcinoma of the cervical oesophagus. In: Neoplastic disease at various sites. Vol. IV. Tumours of the oesophagus, ed. N. C. TANNER and D. W. SMITHERS, p. 53–60. Edinburgh-London: Livingstone 1961.

JOHNSTON, J. B., CLAGETT, O. T., McDONALD, J. R.: Smooth muscle tumors of the esophagus. Thorax **8**, 251–265 (1953).

KAY, S.: Mucoepidermoid carcinoma of the esophagus. Report of two cases. Cancer (Philad.) **22**, 1053–1059 (1968).

KELLEY, M. L., JR.: Intraluminal manometry in the evaluation of malignant disease of the esophagus. Cancer (Philad.) **21**, 1011–1018 (1968).

KELLING, G. E.: Oesophagoplastik mit Hilfe des Querkolon. Zbl. Chir. **38**, 1209 (1911).

KIVIRANTÁ, U. K.: Corrosion carcinoma of the esophagus; 381 cases of corrosion and nine cases of corrosion carcinoma. Acta oto-laryng. (Stockh.) **42**, 89–95 (1952).

KRAUS, F. T., PEREZ-MESA, C.: Verrucous carcinoma. Clinical and pathologic study of 105 cases involving oral cavity, larynx and genitalia. Cancer (Philad.) **19**, 26–38 (1966).

Lancet (N.A.): Annotation: oesophageal cancer in Africa. Lancet **1969**II, 1178.

Lane, N.: Pseudosarcoma (polypoid sarcoma-like masses) associated with squamous cell carcinoma of the mouth, fauces and larynx. Cancer (Philad.) 10, 19–41 (1957).

Leborgne, R., Leborgne, F., Jr., Barlocci, L.: Cancer of the esophagus: results of radiotherapy. Brit. J. Radiol. 36, 806–811 (1963).

Le Roux, B. T.: An analysis of seven hundred cases of carcinoma of the hypopharynx, the oesophagus and the proximal stomach. Thorax 16, 226–255 (1961a).

Le Roux, B. T.: Aortic erosion complicating oesophago-gastrectomy. Brit. J. Surg. 49, 271–277 (1961b).

Le Roux, B. T.: The influence of resection on the natural history of carcinoma of the hypopharynx, esophagus and proximal stomach. Surg. Gynec. Obstet. 115, 162–170 (1962).

Le Roux, B. T., Knothe, W.: The complications of oesophagogastrectomy for carcinoma. J. roy. Coll. Surg. Edinb. 7, 132–137 (1962).

Levy, J. I.: The diagnosis of carcinoma of the oesophagus in the plain chest radiograph. S. Afr. J. Radiol. 4, 1–5 (1966).

Li, K. H., Kao, J. C., Wu, Y. K.: A survey of the prevalence of carcinoma of the oesophagus in North China. Selected papers on cancer research. Shanghai, China: Shanghai scientific and technical publishers 1962.

Lichter, I., Smith, E. R., Gwynne, J. F.: Carcinosarcoma of the oesophagus. Thorax 23, 663–669 (1968).

Logan, A.: Gastro-oesophageal resection for carcinoma between the aortic arch and coeliac axis. J. roy. Coll. Surg. Edinb. 7, 223–227 (1962).

Logan, A.: The surgical treatment of carcinoma of the oesophagus and cardia. J. thorac. cardiovasc. Surg. 46, 150–161 (1963).

Lortat-Jacob, J. L., Maillard, J. N., Richard, C. A., Fekete, F., Huguier, M., Conte-Marti, J.: Primary esophageal adenocarcinoma: Report of 16 cases. Surgery 64, 535–543 (1968).

Lortat-Jacob, J. L., Maillard, J. N., Richard, C. A., Fekete, F., Launois, B.: Surgical treatment of cancer of the oesophagus. Brit. J. clin. Pract. 24, 13–16 (1970).

Lott, J. S., Smith, I. H.: Cobalt-60 beam therapy in carcinoma of the esophagus. Radiology 71, 321–326 (1958).

Luna, R., Ernst, R. W.: Colon interposition for treatment of benign and malignant constricting esophageal lesions. J. Amer. med. Ass. 184, 114 (1963).

MacPherson, I.: Carcinoma of lower end of oesophagus, with some comments on the possible role of tissue immunity. Brit. J. Surg. 53, 21–23 (1966).

Mahoney, E. B., Sherman, C. D.: Treatment of early carcinoma of midesophagus by resection with interposition reconstruction. Curr. surgical management, vol. III, p. 16. Philadelphia: Saunders 1965.

Marcial, V. A., Tomé, J. M., Ubiñas, J., Bosch, A., Correa, J. N.: Role of radiation therapy in esophageal cancer. Radiology 87, 231–239 (1966).

Martini, N., Goodner, J. T., D'Angio, G. J., Beattie, E. J.: Tracheoesophageal fistula due to cancer. J. thorac. cardiovasc. Surg. 59, 319–324 (1970).

McCort, J. J.: Radiographic identification of lymph node metastases from carcinoma of the esophagus. Radiology 59, 694–711 (1952).

McGlashan, N. D.: Oesophageal cancer and alcoholic spirits in central Africa. Gut 10, 643–650 (1969).

McPeak, E., Warren, S.: Histologic features of carcinoma of the cardio-esophageal junction and cardia. Amer. J. Path. 24, 971–991 (1948).

Menguy, R.: The role of bougienage in the palliative management of esophageal cancer. Surg. Gynec. Obstet. 119, 849 (1964).

Miller, C.: Carcinoma of the thoracic oesophagus and cardia: a review of 405 cases. Brit. J. Surg. 49, 507–522 (1962).

Minielly, J. A., Harrison, E. C., Jr., Fontana, R. S.: Verrucous squamous cell carcinoma of the esophagus. Cancer (Philad.) 20, 2078–2087 (1967).

Moore, T. C., Battersby, J. S., Vellios, F., Loehr, W. M.: Carcinosarcoma of the esophagus. J. thorac. cardiovasc. Surg. 45, 281–288 (1963).

Morson, B. C.: Spread of carcinoma of oesophagus. In: Neoplastic disease at various sites. Vol. IV. Tumours of the oesophagus, edit. by N. C. Tanner and D. W. Smithers, p. 136–145. Edinburgh-London: Livingstone 1961.

Morton, J. F.: Plants associated with esophageal cancer cases in Curaçao. Cancer Res. 28, 2268–2271 (1968).

Mousseau, M. M., Le Forestier, J., Barbin, J., Hardy, M.: Place de l'intubation à demeure dans le traitement palliatif du cancer de l'œsophage. Arch. Mal. Appar. dig. 45, 208–214 (1956).

Mustard, R. A.: Selection of therapy for esophageal cancer. Arch. Surg. 75, 674–677 (1957).

MUSTARD, R. A., IBBERSON, O.: Carcinoma of the esophagus. A review of 381 cases admitted to Toronto General Hospital 1937–1953 inclusive. Ann. Surg. **144**, 927–940 (1956).

NAKAYAMA, K.: Statistical review of five-year survivals after surgery for carcinoma of the esophagus and cardiac portion of the stomach. Surgery **45**, 883–889 (1959).

NAKAYAMA, K., ORIHATA, H., YAMAGUCHI, K.: Surgical treatment combined with preoperative concentrated irradiation for esophageal cancer. Cancer (Philad.) **20**, 778–788 (1967).

NELSON, R. S., LANZA, F. L.: The clinical value of radioactive phosphorus (32 p) in the diagnosis of esophageal cancer. Amer. J. dig. Dis. **14**, 538–544 (1969).

NIELSEN, J.: Clinical results with rotation therapy in cancer of the oesophagus; preliminary report based on 174 cases. Acta radiol. (Stockh.) **26**, 361–389 (1945).

OETTLÉ, A. G.: Cancer in Africa, especially in regions south of the Sahara. J. nat. Cancer Inst. **33**, 383–439 (1964).

OETTLÉ, A. G.: Cancer research in Africa, illustrated by a recent epidemic of cancer of the gullet. Raymond Dart Lectures, No. 3. Johannesburg: Witwatersrand University Press 1967.

OHSAWA, T.: The surgery of the oesophagus. Arch. jap. Chir. **10**, 605–695 (1933).

ONG, G. B., KWONG, K. H.: Management of malignant oesophagobronchial fistula. Surgery **67**, 293–301 (1970).

Pan-American Health Organization: Epidemiological research on cancer in Latin America. Report of advisory committee on medical research. Res. 2/7 Washington, D.C. (Regional office of the World Health Organization) 1963.

PARKER, E. F., BROCKINGTON, W. S.: Esophageal resection with end-to-end anastomosis. Experimental and clinical observations. Ann. Surg. **129**, 588 (1949).

PEARSON, J. G.: Radiotherapy of carcinoma of the oesophagus and post-cricoid region in South East Scotland. Clin. Radiol. **17**, 242–257 (1966).

PEARSON, J. G.: The value of radiotherapy in the management of esophageal cancer. Amer. J. Roentgenol. **105**, 500–513 (1969).

PEARSON, J. G.: The value of radiotherapy in the management of squamous oesophageal cancer. Brit. J. Surg. **58**, 794–797 (1971).

PICCONE, V. A., KLOPSTOCK, R., LE VEEN, H. H., SIKA, J.: Primary malignant melanoma of the esophagus associated with melanosis of the entire esophagus. J. thorac. cardiovasc. Surg. **59**, 864–870 (1970).

PIERCE, W. S., MACVAUGH, H., JOHNSON, J.: Carcinoma of the esophagus arising in patients with achalasia of the cardia. J. thorac. cardiovasc. Surg. **59**, 335–339 (1970).

PIERQUIN, B., TUBIANA, M., DUTREIX, J.: Étude de 54 cas de cancers de l'œsophage thoracique traités par le betatron (22 MeV). J. Radiol. Électrol. **39**, 725–736 (1958).

PIERQUIN, B., WAMBERSIE, A., TUBIANA, M.: Cancer of the thoracic oesophagus: two series of patients treated by 22 MeV betatron. Brit. J. Radiol. **39**, 189–192 (1966).

PLESTED, W. G., TILDON, T. T., HUGHES, R. K.: A philosophy of treatment of esophageal carcinoma. Amer. Surg. **34**, 650–656 (1968).

PROCTOR, D. S. C.: Carcinoma of the oesophagus: a review of 523 cases. S. Afr. J. Surg. **6**, 137–159 (1968).

RAPHAEL, H. A., ELLIS, F. H., JR., DOCKERTY, M. B.: Primary adenocarcinoma of the esophagus: 18 year review of literature. Ann. Surg. **164**, 785–796 (1966).

RAZZUK, M. A., URSCHEL, H. C., JR., RACE, G. J., NATHAN, M. J., PAULSON, D. L.: Pseudo-sarcoma of the esophagus. J. thorac. cardiovasc. Surg. **61**, 650–653 (1971).

RIDER, W. D., MENDOZA, R. D.: Some opinions on treatment of cancer of the esophagus. Amer. J. Roentgenol. **105**, 514–517 (1969).

SCANLON, E. F., MORTON, D. R., WALKER, J. M., WATSON, W. L.: The case against segmental resection for esophageal carcinoma. Surg. Gynec. Obstet. **101**, 290–296 (1955).

SEO, S.: Esophageal surgery. J. Jap. surg. Soc. (Japan) **33**, 1461 (1933).

SHEARMAN, D. J. C., FINLAYSON, N. D. C., ARNOTT, S. J., PEARSON, J. G.: Carcinoma of the oesophagus after gastric surgery. Lancet **1970 I**, 581–582.

SHINE, I., ALLISON, P. R.: Carcinoma of the oesophagus with tylosis. Lancet **1966 I**, 951–953.

SKINNER, M. E. G.: Malignant disease of the gastro-intestinal tract in the Rhodesian African, with special reference to the urban population of Bulawayo. A preliminary report. Nat. Cancer Inst. Monogr. **25**, 57–71 (1967).

SMITH, C. C. K., TANNER, N. C.: The complications of gastroscopy and oesophagoscopy. Brit. J. Surg. **43**, 396–403 (1955–56).

SMITHERS, D. W.: Adenocarcinoma of the oesophagus. Thorax **11**, 257–267 (1956).

SMITHERS, D. W.: The treatment of carcinoma of the oesophagus. Ann. roy. Coll. Surg. **20**, 36–49 (1957).

SMITHERS, D. W.: Radiotherapy of carcinoma of the oesophagus. In: Neoplastic disease at various sites. Vol. IV. Tumours of the oesophagus, ed. N. C .TANNER and D. W. SMITHERS, p. 258–271. Edinburgh-London: Livingstone 1961.

Smithers, D. W., Payne, P. M.: Analysis of the patients with carcinoma of the oesophagus seen at the Royal Marsden Hospital, 1936–1954. In: Neoplastic disease at various sites. Vol. IV. Tumours of the esophagus, ed. by N. C. Tanner and D. W. Smithers, p. 310–328. Edinburgh-London: Livingstone 1961.

Souttar, H. S.: A method of intubating the oesophagus for malignant stricture. Brit. med. J. 1924 I, 782–783.

Steiner, P. E.: The etiology and histogenesis of carcinoma of the esophagus. Cancer (Philad.) 9, 436–452 (1956).

Stener, B., Kock, N. G., Petterson, S., Zetterlund, B.: Carcinosarcoma of the esophagus. J. thorac. cardiovasc. Surg. 54, 746–750 (1967).

Stephen, S. J., Uragoda, C. G.: Some observations of oesophageal carcinoma in Ceylon, including its relationship to betel chewing. Brit. J. Cancer 24, 11–15 (1970).

Storey, C. F.: Acquired surgical lesions of the esophagus (II). Springfield, Ill.: Thomas 1962.

Stout, A. P., Lattes, R.: Tumors of the esophagus, sect. 5, fasc. 20. In: Atlas of tumor pathology. Washington, D.C.: Armed Forces Institute of Pathology 1957.

Surks, M. I., Guttman, A. B.: Esophageal involvement in Hodgkin's disease. Amer. J. dig. Dis. 11, 814–818 (1966).

Sweet, R. H.: Late results of surgical treatment of carcinoma of the esophagus. J. Amer. med. Ass. 155, 422–425 (1954).

Symonds, C. J.: A case of malignant stricture of the oesophagus illustrating the use of the new form of oesophageal catheter. Trans. clin. Soc. Lond. 18, 155–158 (1885).

Tanner, N. C.: Exfoliative cytological methods in the diagnosis of oesophageal tumours. In: Neoplastic disease at various sites. Vol. IV. Tumours of the oesophagus, ed. by N. C. Tanner and D. W. Smithers, p. 163–167. Edinburgh-London: Livingstone 1961.

Tanner, N. C., Smithers, D. W.: Neoplastic disease at various sites, 1st ed., vol. IV. Tumours of the oesophagus. Edinburgh-London: Livingstone 1961.

Turnbull, A. D. M., Goodner, J. T.: Primary adenocarcinoma of the esophagus. Cancer (Philad.) 22, 915–918 (1970).

Turner, G. G.: Some experiences in the surgery of the oesophagus. New Engl. J. Med. 205, 657–674 (1931).

Tuyns, A. J.: Cancer of the oesophagus: further evidence of the relation to drinking habits in France. Int. J. Cancer 5, 152–156 (1970).

Voutilainen, A., Koulumies, M.: Results of radiation therapy of cancer of the oesophagus. Ann. Chir. Gynaec. Fenn. 54, 40–51 (1965).

Wada, T., Matsumoto, Y., Amano, T.: Chemotherapy of esophageal cancer with bleomycin. Progress in antimicrobiol. and anticancer chemotherapy. Proceedings of the 6th Internat. Congr. of Chemotherapy, p. 41–46. Tokyo: University of Tokyo Press 1969.

Watson, T. A.: Radiation treatment of cancer of the oesophagus. Surg. Gynec. Obstet. 117, 346–354 (1963).

Watson, T. A.: Radiotherapy in the treatment of cancer of the oesophagus. Radiol. clin. (Basel) 36, 1–14 (1967).

Watson, T. A., Brown, E. M.: X-ray therapy in carcinoma of the esophagus. J. thorac. Surg. 22, 216–218 (1951).

Watson, W. L., Goodner, J. T., Miller, T. P., Pack, G. T.: Torek esophagectomy: case against segmental resection for esophageal cancer. J. thorac. Surg. 32, 347–359 (1956).

Wight, J. T., Richardson, P. C.: Squamous carcinoma of the thoracic oesophagus in malabsorption syndrome. Brit. med. J. 1967 I, 540–542.

Wookey, H.: The surgical treatment of carcinoma of the hypopharynx and the esophagus. Brit. J. Surg. 35, 249 (1948).

Wynder, E. L., Bross, I. J.: A study of etiological factors in cancer of the esophagus. Cancer (Philad.) 14, 389–413 (1961).

Yates, D. R., Koss, L. G.: Paget's disease of the esophageal epithelium. Arch. Path. 86, 447–452 (1968).

Younghusband, J. D., Aluwihare, A. P. R.: Carcinoma of the oesophagus: factors influencing survival. Brit. J. Surg. 57, 422–430 (1970).

Chapter 5

Inflammatory Lesions of the Esophagus

Reflux Esophagitis

B. S. Wolf and H. P. Lazar

With 12 Figures

1. Introduction

Since the original pathological (Hamperl, 1934) and clinical (Winkelstein, 1935) descriptions of "peptic esophagitis", a voluminous literature has appeared because of wide-spread interest by gastroenterologists, surgeons and radiologists. The designation of this condition as "peptic esophagitis" was based on the belief that peptic digestion of the esophageal mucosa was the etiological agent. The term "reflux esophagitis" is more suitable since identical pathological and clinical findings may result not only from reflux of gastric contents but also reflux of bile and pancreatic secretions, for example, after total gastrectomy. This chapter will attempt to indicate current concepts related to pathogenesis, diagnosis and therapy.

2. General Considerations

Reflux esophagitis refers to inflammatory changes in the distal esophagus due to the chemical action of gastric (or intestinal) contents which enter the esophagus as the result of retrograde flow. In a broad sense, it includes esophagitis associated with esophageal intubation, persistent vomiting, pregnancy, a severe illness or as a terminal event. Such circumstances, however, represent special cases. The bulk of this discussion will be directed to the common type of esophagitis resulting from insufficiency of the esophagogastric antireflux mechanism related to hiatal herniation. The term hiatal herniation is used in a general sense to include both congenital and acquired abnormalities in fixation of the distal esophagus to the crura of the diaphragm. The nature of the esophagogastric sphincteric or antireflux mechanism has been discussed in detail on p. 51. For the present purpose, it is assumed that this mechanism involves both intrinsic (Fyke et al., 1956) and extrinsic (Wolf, 1960; Vantrappen, 1960) factors.

The basic concept of reflux esophagitis is quite simple. If the antireflux mechanism becomes ineffective, usually as a result of a hiatal hernia, reflux of gastric contents into the terminal esophagus occurs. Acid peptic contents, usually confined to the stomach, act chemically on the squamous epithelium of the distal esophagus to produce inflammation, ulceration, and eventually scarring with stricture formation and fibrous shortening of the esophagus. However, this hypothesis must be a marked over-simplification since hernias and reflux are common conditions while esophagitis of significant severity is unusual. While minimal microscopic inflammatory changes may be common, progressive changes leading to a fibrous stricture are rare and usually occur in young children, in the postpartum period, or in elderly, frequently female, individuals. It is therefore necessary to examine in some detail the features of patients who do not, as well as those who do, develop significant esophagitis in association with herniation. In order to do this, a more precise understanding of herniation, reflux, and esophagitis is required.

2.1. Hiatal Hernia

Hiatal hernias are most suitably classified on the basis of their roentgen appearances. Two main types may be identified. The first may be designated as the concentric variety because the esophagus joins the stomach in axial or linear fashion, that is, at or immediately adjacent to the apex of the stomach. The shortening of the esophagus in the vast majority of such cases is functional and acquired as a result of loosening of the attachments of the lower esophagus and upper stomach to the diaphragm and neighboring structures. Some authors appear to limit the term "sliding" hiatal hernia or "short esophagus" type of hiatal hernia to this variety. In the second or eccentric variety, the esophagus joins the lateral aspect of the herniated portion of the stomach at an angle which is usually more acute and deeper than the normal angulation at the cardiac incisura. In this type, a portion of the hernial sac lies at a level above the esophagogastric junction, adjacent and parallel to the terminal esophagus which frequently appears to be displaced backward and somewhat compressed by the sac of stomach. When the esophagogastric junction is located above the hiatus, this type of hernia is referred to as a "rolling" hernia. When the squamocolumnar junction remains in its normal location, the term "paraesophageal" hernia is used. Both the rolling and paraesophageal variations may eventually lead to a so-called upside-down stomach. In the concentric variety, there may be some eccentric pouching of the hernial sac but the entrance of the esophagus into the hernial sac is direct and straight. The reasons for these two main types of hiatal hernia are not clear. The pathogenesis is discussed in Chapter 11, p. 743.

The important practical point is that significant esophagitis is practically confined to the concentric type (Skinner, 1966). The reason for this is that a relatively straight pathway between stomach and esophagus is required, even in the absence of any intrinsic sphincteric mechanism, if retrograde flow is to be free and easy. The size of the hernia is of little importance in this regard.

The concentric type of herniation (Fig. 235), when minimal, may be very difficult to identify since, in truth, no hernial sac is present above the hiatus of the diaphragm (Wolf, 1956; Stein and Finkelstein, 1960). Only the abdominal segment of the esophagus—a tubular segment which should be at least 2 cm in length with a caliber less than the tubular portion of the esophagus— is absent or effaced. Although the hiatus is wide anatomically, the width of the barium column traversing it, as seen radiologically, may be normal, increased, or show an inverted triangular or funnel appearance as it enters the fundus of the stomach. In newborn infants, this appearance when associated with reflux has been designated as "chalasia". However, a similar configuration can be recognized in adults at any stage. In such instances, it is not possible to determine whether the abdominal segment of esophagus was ever present or whether it has been displaced into or above the hiatus. At any rate, it is reasonable to refer to this appearance as hiatal herniation without a sac since its clinical and

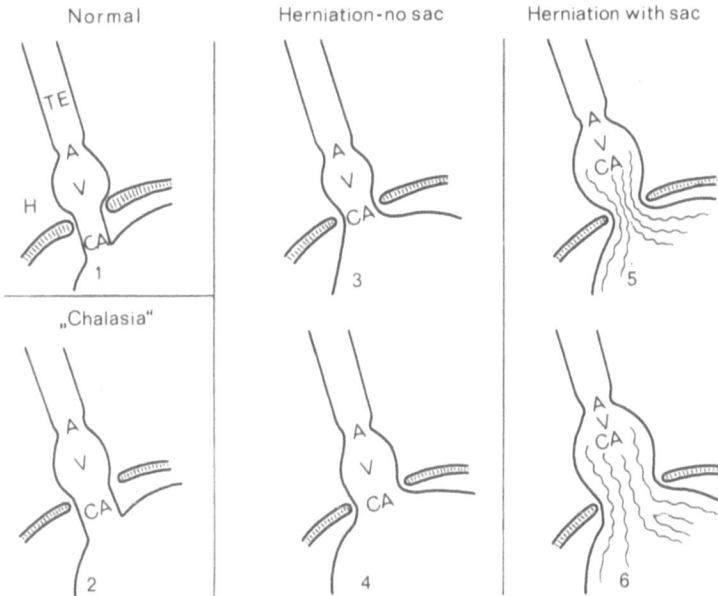

Fig. 235. Diagrammatic representation of types of concentric hiatal herniation. Panel 1 shows normal components of the esophagogastric region. The "A" level or "A ring" indicates the junction between the tubular esophagus (TE) and the phrenic ampulla or vestibule (V). The short tubular portion, in and below the hiatus (H), is the "submerged" or abdominal segment of the esophagus, also designated the cardiac antrum (CA). The squamocolumnar mucosal junction is not seen but is located within the submerged segment, probably close to its upper margin. Panel 2 shows an unusual configuration in which the submerged segment maintains a tubular configuration but, beginning at the level of the hiatus, is unusually distensible. This appearance of "chalasia" (hiatal and sphincteric incompetence) is seen rarely because the cardiac antrum is usually displaced into or above the hiatus or absorbed within the fundus of the stomach. Panels 3 and 4 show "herniation without a sac" as a result of widening of the hiatus and increased distensibility of the cardiac antrum. In Panel 3, widening of the hiatus is not obvious, presumably because adjacent soft tissue occupies the opening in addition to the cardiac antrum. A funnel-shaped configuration between the vestibule and the fundus of the stomach is present without any distinct cardiac orifice. In Panel 4, widening of the hiatus and absence of the normal submerged segment are indicated by the short, broad communication between the vestibule and the stomach. Herniation with a sac, Panel 5, usually shows a compressed slit-like sleeve of stomach within the hiatus. In other instances, however, Panel 6, a uniformly patulous hiatal communication is present. When, in addition, there is no discrete functional (sphincteric) activity related to the A or the V regions, reflux is likely to be free and easy

therapeutic significance is the same as any other type of concentric hernia (WOLF, 1970). Failure to include this variety in the concept of hiatal herniation has led to descriptions of "reflux without herniation" (HIEBERT and BELSEY, 1961; SKINNER, 1966; SKINNER et al., 1972) as if this were a separate syndrome. Under unusual circumstances, the abdominal segment appears to persist as a short but abnormally distensible tube. This appearance of an abnormally wide abdominal segment of the esophagus which is nevertheless normally located, "true chalasia", is seen in early scleroderma, after excessively forceful dilatation or bilateral myotomy for achalasia, or after hiatal hernia repair which has been successful in reducing the hernial sac but has failed to reconstruct a normal abdominal segment.

Minimal concentric hiatal herniation or herniation without a sac is significant because it forms the basis for further herniation. Moreover, when the hiatal channel is wide and patulous, free and easy reflux as well as severe symptoms of heartburn due to an incompetent sphincter are likely to be present. However, as further herniation of the fundus of the stomach into the hiatus occurs, the thicker wall of the stomach as well as adjacent fat and peritoneal attachments become trapped within the hiatus, creating a tubular sleeve of stomach which is compressed and narrowed and unable to distend (Sandmark, 1963b). This sleeve of stomach is not only tubular but also often slit-like and barium traversing it fills only the spaces between the rugae. The "width of the hiatus" in patients with a hernia is difficult to define since it is not a rigid region, and the hiatal opening is also occupied by soft tissue. With hernias of the same size, the amount of soft tissue surrounding the stomach in the hiatus varies from patient to patient. The width of the hiatus when exposed at operation or at necropsy after dissection and manipulation does not represent the anatomic relationships "in vivo". This distinction is of importance since a compressed sleeve of stomach within the hiatus serves as an antireflux mechanism. It is as if the extrinsic and intrinsic contributions to the normal antireflux mechanism in the esophagogastric region have become dissociated. As a result, in contrast to patients described as having herniation without a sac, two potential barriers to reflux are present, one at the level of the hiatus and the second more proximally in the region of the original sphincteric zone. The effectiveness of the hiatal mechanism depends on the degree of compression and the length of the gastric sleeve trapped in the deformed hiatus. These features can often been determined by careful roentgen observations of the barium column traversing the hiatus during swallowing or during reflux. From the functional point of view, the more proximal original sphincteric area may or may not be a more potent barrier to reflux than the hiatal mechanism, but reflux of substantial amounts of gastric contents into the esophagus can occur only if both are ineffective.

In the majority of patients with a concentric hernia, residual sphincteric activity in the displaced esophagogastric region can usually be recognized both radiologically and manometrically. A typical pull-through pressure curve as part of an esophageal motility study in an uncomplicated hiatal hernia shows a plateau of pressure related to the size of the hernial sac with peaks at its upper and lower ends (Code et al., 1962). The lower end corresponds to the hiatal mechanism described above while the upper end represents functional activity related to the original sphincteric zone. Radiologically, a contractile ring ("A ring") or ring-like segment ("vestibule") or both can usually be recognized between the end of the tubular esophagus and the true hernial sac. The contractile ring appears as a discrete intramural type of circumferential defect, a centimeter or less in length, which changes rapidly in width as it opens. This ring often delays the passage of a barium column both in a forward and retrograde direction until relaxation is induced by a voluntary swallow. Functional rings are considerably longer than the rings seen more distally at the squamocolumnar mucosal junction, which have no functional significance. As seen in profile, an "A ring" appears as a broad-based hemispherical defect rather than a notch. When it is completely relaxed, there is frequently no evidence of the ring although occasionally a short swallow circumferential indentation persists. Squamous epithelium is present for a short distance distal to this ring, within the so-called vestibule. The region of the A ring may be included in a more diffuse contraction of the vestibule as a whole giving rise to a contracted or sphincteric segment 2 to 3 cm in length. In the empty or contracted state, an A ring cannot be distinguished from the vestibule. However, an A ring may persist or open more slowly than the vestibule during filling and may contract prematurely while the vestibule remains filled. In some patients an A ring is unusually constant and opens only to a limited degree. Less commonly, the vestibule is prominent as an independent contractile segment. In other patients, there may be no evidence of any discrete contractile ring or segment. In this last group, the distal portion of the body of the esophagus (the portion above the site of an A ring) sometimes seems to act as a weak "sphincteric" region. These functional characteristics of the displaced esophagogastric region are best studied with cineradiography. The quantitative aspects, namely resting pressures and responses to various stimuli such as increased abdominal pressure, can be documented by intraluminal pressure measurements. For investigative purposes, cineradiography on film or television tape and manometry may be combined and performed simultaneously (HEITMANN et al., 1966; LONGHI and JORDAN, 1969; CLARK et al., 1970).

2.2. Esophagitis

The earliest changes indicative of reflux esophagitis are not visible grossly since they consist of relative widening of the basal cell portion of the epithelium and increase in height of the papillae so that their apices reach closer to the surface (ISMAIL-BEIGI et al., 1970). These changes suggest a more rapid turnover of the epithelial cells which might be expected as the result of chemical irritation. These changes are not specific and may be seen, for example, adjacent to a carcinoma (KANEKO). Leukocytic infiltration into the tunica propria is a less sensitive histological indicator of reflux esophagitis. More severe changes, grossly visible, consist of epithelial erosions, epithelial sloughing with membrane formation, edema, congestion and finally ulceration with marked cellular exudation and eventually scar formation.

Acute esophagitis is characterized by erosions of varying degrees. Later tissue destruction extends to all layers of the esophageal wall and fibrosis develops. In chronic superficial esophagitis the deeper lesions may be covered by a regenerated "intact" mucosa (PETERS, 1955; SANDRY, 1962). The process, however, is by no means smoothly progressive either circumferentially or longitudinally. The inflammatory changes are most severe, not immediately adjacent to the squamo-columnar mucosal junction, but a short distance above it. From the gross point of view, several varieties can be recognized which do not necessarily represent stages in the same process (MOERSCH et al., 1959; SANDRY, 1962; COLLIS, 1965). In the first variety, the changes remain histological. The patients may have typical heartburn of varying severity and frequency but, except for the presence of a hernia, no changes are visible radiologically or on endoscopy. In a second variety, the process is grossly evident but of moderate severity and remains superficial and chronic with periods of exacerbation and remission. The distal esophagus may be involved over a distance of 2 to 10 cm. The process may be confluent but is often spotty. There is no localized stricture but there may be a variable degree of diffuse narrowing as a result of the active inflammatory process as well as thickening of the muscle, presumably the result of failure of complete relaxation. This form of reflux esophagitis may be designated as chronic superficial diffuse esophagitis, which is rarely severe unless there is also a history of duodenal ulcer or intubation. A third type represents as a definite stricture resulting from scarring as well as intramural exudate and muscular hypertrophy. The stricture is located a short distance above the squamocolumnar mucosal junction and varies from $^1/_2$ to 2 cm in length. Active mucosal inflammatory changes may also be present but are usually relatively mild and extend for only a short distance on each side of the stricture. In a fourth variety, there is a discrete penetrating ulcer at the squamocolumnar mucosal junction which has many of the characteristics of a chronic peptic ulcer as seen in the duodenum or stomach (Wolf et al., 1953). There is always gastric epithelium of the cardiac type at the distal margin of such an ulcer and squamous epithelium along its proximal border. The ulceration penetrates into the muscularis propria and is associated with intramural exudate, fibrosis and stricture formation. There is usually a more superficial mucosal inflammatory process extending from the ulcer proximally for a distance of 2 to 4 cm. Squamocolumnar marginal peptic ulcer of this type is not related to peptic ulcer occurring in an esophagus lined with columnar epithelium as described by Barrett. Some confusion has arisen on this point since these marginal ulcers show a short collar or tubular segment distal to the ulcer, lined by columnar epithelium. This segment, however, is the normally columnar cell-lined portion of the abdominal esophagus or the "cardiac antrum" and does not represent heterotopic or ectopic gastric epithelium. A peptic ulcer as part of the Barrett anomaly usually occurs at the proximal margin of the "gastric-lined" segment, well above the esophagogastric or tube-sac junction. During the healing of a diffuse esophagitis, islands of metaplastic columnar epithelium may replace the squamous epithelium and simulate the Barrett anomaly. A fifth type of reflux esophagitis would include those patients with severe diffuse esophagitis and marked intramural fibrosis both circumferentially and longitudinally—an "ascending" fibrosis. This type is rare and appears to be almost confined to children or those with an originally "gastric-lined" esophagus who in addition develop a sliding hernia and reflux. A stenotic diaphragm-like ring at the squamocolumnar mucosal junction with no grossly evident inflammatory changes, that is, a Schatzki ring, is not included in this discussion of reflux esophagitis since its etiology is unknown.

One pathological feature that is difficult to study is decrease in length of the esophagus. In the absence of esophagitis, this appears to be reversible and the normal length of the esophagus can be restored at operation without great difficulty. When irreducible, it is often attributed to extensive longitudinal fibrosis but this is rarely evident pathologically. The muscle layer often appears thick and may be in a permanent state of "contracture". It is obviously difficult to exclude some degree of congenital shortening which originally may have been of minimal degree. A marked degree of periesophagitis, sometimes with perigastritis involving the hernial sac, may be present at operation and also interferes with reduction. It is difficult by any method currently available to determine preoperatively whether the esophageal shortening is reversible. If a fibrous stricture or penetrating ulcer is present which is fixed in position in relation to mediastinal landmarks, the possibility that simple hernia reduction at the time of operation will not be feasible must be anticipated.

Knowledge of the gross pathological types of esophagitis described above may be incorporated into a clinical classification (Table 20). Such a classification would include: (1) Patients with reflux and resulting heartburn, presumably with histological evidence of esophagitis, but no gross abnormality. (2) A diffuse chronic superficial esophagitis with mild mucosal changes on endoscopy and no significant roentgen findings except for a hernia. (3) Chronic superficial diffuse esophagitis evident both on endoscopy and on roentgen examination. The mucosal changes are obvious and there are often functional abnormalities such as limited distensibility of the distal esophagus. Significant stricture formation of a localized

Table 20. Clinical classification of peptic esophagitis

Histological lesions	Endoscopic signs	Roentgen features
1. Widening of basal cell portion heightening of papillae	Normal	Normal
2. Chronic superficial diffuse inflammation	Mild changes: hyperemia, friability, exudate, epithelial erosions	Normal
3. Chronic superficial diffuse inflammation	Similar as in "2"+ superficial ulceration, slight narrowing	Limited distensibility, finely serrated borders, distorted mucosal pattern, tapering configuration
4. Fibrotic stricture just above squamocolumnar junction	Stricture with or without chronic superficial inflammation in adjacent areas	Stricture 0.5 to 2 cm in length with or without signs of esophagitis similar to "3"
5. Marginal ulcer Stricture	Ulcer may not be visible due to stricture Chronic superficial inflammation proximal to stricture may be present	Ulcer niche or persistent patch of barium. Stricture. With or without signs of diffuse esophagitis
6. Diffuse inflammation and narrowing of long segment	Severe inflammatory changes Narrowing may preclude satisfactory esophagoscopy	Narrowing, irregularity and ulceration of long segment

nature, however, is not present. (4) The most prominent feature is a short, constant, at least partially fibrotic stricture located just above the squamocolumnar mucosal junction with or without evidence of superficial esophagitis immediately adjacent to the stricture. (5) The prominent feature is a discrete penetrating marginal ulcer at the squamocolumnar junction usually associated with localized stricture formation. There may be evidence of a more superficial inflammatory process proximal to the ulcer for a short distance. (6) Severe, diffuse narrowing of a long segment of the distal esophagus with marked mucosal changes and usually a history of intubation or some other superimposed inciting factor. A concentric hernia is present in all types except for unusual instances in the last category.

2.3. Reflux

It is possible, in any individual, to force gastric contents into the esophagus by progressively increasing intraabdominal and intragastric pressure, for example, by an encircling pressure cuff—if the patient will permit pressures of 100 mm of mercury or so. At some point, the normal antireflux mechanism will be overcome. Such maneuvers simply overpower the normal esophagogastric sphincter. However, if gastric contents flow into the esophagus simply on assuming the supine or Trendelenburg position, such reflux is clearly pathological. If reflux occurs in the Trendelenburg position only when the individual swallows (DE CARVALHO, 1951), that is, only when the intrinsic sphincteric mechanism is reflexly overcome, its possible clinical significance must be evaluated in the light of other factors (LINSMAN, 1965; CRUMMY, 1966). It is therefore clear that a simple statement, that reflux is present or absent, is not sufficient. Reflux may be observed in "normal" individuals on occasion and may be considered physiological (Venkatachalam, 1972; Winans, 1972). As pointed out above, during the course of a barium meal examination or on manometry, the antireflux mechanisms potentially present in the region of the hiatus and in the esophagogastric region may be observed and tested by a variety of maneuvers (Vanderwelde and Carlson, 1964; Brombart, 1967). Maneuvers which are designed to increase the difference in pressure between the abdomen and the thorax include direct compression of the abdomen, straight-leg raising, stooping over to touch the toes, the Valsalva maneuver and sniffing or the Mueller maneuver. Such maneuvers may be combined with a dry or a wet swallow. The water swallowing or siphonage test is usually most effective. The most common radiological finding is that maneuvers which increase intraabdominal pressure will displace barium into the hernial sac but that retrograde flow into the esophagus does not occur until a swallow is taken. To a limited degree, the roentgen observations can be quantitated by specifying not only the ease with which reflux occurs but also the width and height of the barium column that enters the body of the esophagus and the length of time that significant amounts of barium remain in the esophagus despite repeated swallows. A squirt of a small amount of barium into the terminal esophagus at the onset of a wet swallow which is then promptly returned with the swallowed fluid is probably harmless. However, if on swallowing a broad column of barium ascends into the mid-esophagus and, as a result of poor peristaltic or non-propulsive contractions, is not promptly returned to the stomach, such reflux is pathological. It should be noted that maneuvers designed to demonstrate reflux by increasing intraabdominal pressure may be self-defeating if additional herniation is induced and, as a result, compression on the sleeve of stomach within the hiatus increased. A deep inspiration may serve to increase abdominal pressure and increase reflux but it may have the opposite effect due to pinchcock action on the portion of the stomach located within the hiatus.

Other methods for the detection or study of esophageal reflux have been proposed (Benz, 1972). The most useful of these appears to be the determination of the pH by a suitable probe positioned at a point about 4 cm above the sphincteric zone after the instillation of 300 milliliters of 0.1 N hydrochloric acid into the body of the stomach (Tuttle and Grossman, 1958; Sandmark, 1963a; Piccone et al., 1965; Lockwood and Borgeskov, 1969; Hootkin et al., 1970). If the pH of the esophagus is persistently less than 4, independently of swallowing or belching, the test is considered positive for reflux. Several investigators believe that this test gives the best correlation with symptoms indicative of reflux and with the presence of esophagitis, for example, on suction biopsy. In comparison, roentgen tests for reflux are said to underestimate its incidence in symptomatic patients (Kantrowitz et al., 1969). Abnormally low resting pressures within the sphincteric region may be correlated with symptoms of reflux (Pope, 1967; Cohen and Harris, 1970; Haddad, 1970) but this does not appear to be a very selective test because of considerable overlapping of the measured values. In one study using a perfused catheter system (Bombeck et al., 1970a). no patient with a resting maximal inspiratory pressure greater than 15 cm of water exhibited reflux while all patients with values below 4 cm of water showed evidence of esophagitis on endoscopy. When maximal expiratory pressures were correlated, no patient with a pressure above 21 cm of water showed reflux and all patients with resting pressures below 12 cm of water had esophagitis endoscopically. Simultaneous manometric observations of pressure within the stomach, the sphincteric region, and the body of the esophagus while gradual compression is applied to the abdomen will demonstrate whether "a common cavity" is present (BUTTERFIELD et al., 1970). If pressures above and below the hiatus are measured during such compression, the effectiveness of the hiatal barrier can also be tested.

The acid perfusion test of BERNSTEIN (BERNSTEIN, 1958; BOMBECK et al., 1970a; HOOTKIN et al., 1970), that is, the instillation of 0.1 N hydrochloric acid within the body of the esophagus in an effort to reproduce the patient's symptoms, shows a high correlation with symptoms of reflux but, in effect, tests the reactivity or the sensitivity of the esophagus to acid rather than demonstrating actual reflux, although the two usually go together. In one study (SVOBODA et al., 1967), a positive acid perfusion test showed an 87% correlation with histological changes of esophagitis. In another study (ISMAIL-BEIGI, 1970), the acid perfusion test was performed in 21 patients with heartburn and objective evidence of reflux as indicated by intraesophageal pH measurements. It was found to be positive in 100% of these patients. Eighty three percent of the patients with reflux showed signs of esophagitis on histological examinations. Therefore a positive acid perfusion test suggests not only the presence of gastroesophageal reflux but also that of esophagitis. The Bernstein test is particularly useful when the symptoms of the patient are atypical. An acid clearing test in which, after the instillation of 0.1 N hydrochloric acid into the body of the esophagus, the patient is directed to take multiple swallows and the rate of disappearance of the acid is measured by means of a pH probe, has also been utilized. A clever modification of the acid perfusion test of BERNSTEIN has been devised for use in the course of roentgen examination (DONNER et al., 1966). A barium mixture, acidified with hydrochloric acid to pH of 1.7, is used. When this acid barium produces obvious abnormalities in the motility of the esophagus with irregular contractions and delay in emptying, the test is said to be positive provided peristaltic activity was normal with neutral barium and returns to normal after alkalinization. This test is less reliable than the conventional Bernstein test and usually does not reproduce the patient's symptoms.

2.4. Heartburn

Most people have, at one time or another, experienced heartburn and there is obviously a wide spectrum in its frequency and severity (TUTTLE et al., 1961). It is defined as a substernal burning sensation which typically radiates upward toward the neck, occurs usually after meals, is often induced by stooping, bending over or assuming the recumbent position, and comes in waves traveling upward and downward behind the sternum in repetitive fashion. It may or may not be accompanied by regurgitation of bitter or sour fluid into the mouth without coincident nausea. "Pure" heartburn should not be painful although marked discomfort may be present. When a patient gives a history of frequent heartburn exaggerated by the postures noted above, there is rarely any difficulty in demonstrating reflux. It is said that "burning" sensations which remain fixed in the substernal or epigastric region unrelated to posture may be due to a hiatal hernia without reflux or may be of "functional" origin. Moreover, typical heartburn as defined above may also be present without the ability to demonstrate reflux, at least on a single examination. The pressure barrier in the esophagogastric region or sphincteric zone is susceptible to a variety of stimuli, mechanical, (VAN DERSTAPPEN and TEXTER, 1964), hormonal (CASTELL and HARRIS, 1970) and pharmacological (SKINNER and CAMP, 1968; HOOKMAN and FLEISCHER, 1969), both excitatory and inhibitory. It is therefore not surprising that reflux may be demonstrable on one occasion and not on another. Severe heartburn and reflux may be present for many years without evident esophagitis. Although patients with significant esophagitis usually give a history of heartburn, stricture formation in patients with a hiatal hernia has been observed in the absence of previous heartburn (EDMUNDS, 1957). If dysphagia supervenes, heartburn ordinarily regresses or disappears.

2.5. Pathogenesis

Additional comments on the pathogenesis of reflux esophagitis must be made since the mechanism described above—herniation, reflux of acid gastric contents, a chemical esophagitis—has not been accepted by all (PALMER, 1968; JOHNSON, 1969). It has been suggested that reflux may be the primary phenomenon, followed by esophagitis, shortening of the esophagus and a traction type of hiatal hernia. Spontaneous reflux, however, is rare if the anatomical relationships of the esophagogastric region to the diaphragmatic crura are normal. If these are abnormal and the intrinsic sphincter incompetent, reflux may occur but "herniation without a sac" is usually present and can be identified. It is possible for an acute episode of esophagitis, for example, due to intubation or hyperemesis gravidarum, in a patient without a hernia, to heal with fibrosis and the production of a small "traction" hernia. The hernia may then increase slowly in size over a period of years and become in effect a traction-pulsion type of hernia, eventually with reflux esophagitis. It is also possible for certain individuals to learn to induce reflux voluntarily, for example, in merycism, by reproducing the physiological changes which permit vomiting—"physiological herniation". Such individuals tolerate reflux without developing esophagitis but may develop permanent herniation. A patient with reflux and herniation without a sac may develop esophagitis and the herniation may become more obvious as a result of traction by the inflamed esophagus. As pointed out above, however, it is more likely for such patients to develop a more obvious hernia with a sac above the hiatus and, at the same time, to show diminished reflux and heartburn. This last observation is confirmed by the fact that the incidence of herniation with a sac increases with age while the incidence of reflux without an obvious sac appears to decrease up to the sixth decade (STILSON et al., 1969).

The suggestion has also been made that the condition described above as herniation without a sac is a congenital anomaly related to a low attachment of the phrenicoesophageal membrane to the gastric region. It is postulated that, as a result, a distracting force is applied to the intrinsic sphincter which eventually makes it ineffective (BOMBECK et al., 1966; DILLARD and ANDERSON, 1966). Evidence has been presented to indicate that patients with esophagitis frequently have such low attachments. However, these observations do not change the basic fact that some variety of herniation precedes reflux and esophagitis. Incidentally, if this theory is correct, operative procedures which utilize the site of attachment of the phrenicoesophageal membrane as a landmark for hernia reduction would have to be modified to produce overcorrection. A relatively recent suggestion is that heartburn and significant esophagitis is more likely the result of reflux of duodenal contents into the stomach and then into the esophagus than reflux of acid gastric contents into the esophagus (GILLISON et al., 1969). In one investigation, a fairly good correlation between pyloric regurgitation and heartburn with a hernia was found. These observations, if confirmed, are of importance since many authors have recommended pyloroplasty as part of the treatment of a hiatal hernia with or without esophagitis. Moreover, the rationale for pyloroplasty as well as vagotomy or subtotal gastrectomy in the treatment of hiatal hernia and esophagitis is based on the thesis that refluxing, highly acid gastric contents, with or without gastric retention, are the important etiological agents in the induction of esophagitis. It has been suggested that patients with duodenal ulcer are under an increased risk of a severe stenosing esophagitis and that the effects of acid and pepsin must be predominant in such instances (WINKELSTEIN et al., 1954). It should be noted, however, that the bulk of the cases of esophagitis do not show obviously elevated acid levels and therefore should not require acid suppressing operations (SILBER, 1969). There is also no doubt that operative procedures which permit the entrance of duodenal or high jejunal contents into the esophagus also show a high incidence of reflux esophagitis (LEVRAT et al., 1962; MOFFAT, 1965). It therefore must be assumed at present that reflux esophagitis may be either acid or alkaline, "peptic" or "biliary", depending on specific circumstances. At any rate, esophagitis is rare if achlorhydria is present (PALMER, 1960).

Another argument against the reflux etiology points to the lack of perfect correlation between esophagitis and reflux. In one investigation during the course of selecting 43 patients with typical heartburn (ISMAIL-BEIGI and POPE, 1970), reflux was not demonstrated in 10. Despite this, however, 7 of the 10 showed microscopic evidence on suction biopsy of esophagitis. It is, however, difficult to deny that reflux would have been demonstrable at a second examination. In the same investigation, 33 of 42 patients with reflux showed histological evidence of esophagitis and this incidence might have been greater if additional biopsies had been done. This is a surprisingly good correlation of the incidence of heartburn with histological evidence of esophagitis.

The esophageal stimulus leading to the sensation of heartburn is assumed by some to be the direct action of the refluxed material on chemoreceptors or unmyelinated nerve fibers in the tunica propria. The histological finding that the apices of the papillae are closer to the surface of the epithelium in patients with typical heartburn is consistent with this hypothesis. During a Bernstein test, it takes some time for acid within the esophagus to produce heartburn. This time presumably is required for the acid to permeate the epithelium. Instillation of pontocaine may cause immediate cessation of induced heartburn or pain (COHEN, 1970). Another school of thought believes that refluxed material induces motility changes and the burning sensation is the result of abnormal contractions (SIEGEL and HENDRIX, 1963; SILBER, 1968). Manometric studies in patients who complain of heartburn or pain during the course of acid perfusion often, but not invariably, show repetitive contractions of high amplitude.

Intravenous probanthine during acid infusion may inhibit motor activity while symptoms persist (ATKINSON and BENNETT, 1968). Moreover, patients with scleroderma and reflux complain of heartburn despite the fact that the body of the esophagus has little motor activity. It must be realized, however, that some motor disturbances, e.g. changes in tone, may not be detectable by intraluminal pressure measurements. There may be better correlation of pain, rather than heartburn, with high amplitude repetitive contractions. It is obviously, however, not always easy for a patient to clearly distinguish between heartburn and pain in the course of acid perfusion, particularly when both may be present.

One factor which may not have received sufficient attention as a contributing factor to severe types of esophagitis, is the possibility of ischemia, particularly in elderly individuals. Experience with "ischemic colitis" and segmental infarction of the small bowel indicates that infarction of the mucosa may occur without obvious large vessel disease and lead to stricture. It is conceivable that a similar process may act in the distal esophagus in individuals so predisposed because of reflux. Spontaneous strictures, with a short history of dysphagia in elderly individuals ("geriatric" strictures), might be explained on this basis. However, an acute episode with bleeding as seen in ischemic colitis is not part of the history of such patients.

As a cause of reflux esophagitis, reflux of gastric contents at night has been emphasized in the belief that refluxed material may remain in the esophagus for long periods of time without swallowing of neutralizing saliva. Some evidence for this is the frequent occurrence of regurgitation at night which awakens the patient because of laryngeal aspiration. It is suspected that aspiration may occur without awakening the patient and induce bronchial and pulmonary inflammation (URSCHEL and PAULSON, 1967). It is not clear, however, how esophageal contents leak through the cricopharyngeal sphincter. Esophageal contents may enter the pharynx briefly at the onset of a swallow but rarely enter the larynx if pharyngeal deglutition is normal.

3. Clinical Features

Reports of the incidence of hiatal hernia with or without reflux vary considerably depending upon the criteria and methods used in making the diagnosis. There is no question, however, that a hernia is a frequent finding over the age of 50 and occurs perhaps in 30 to 50% of such individuals. A fraction of these patients, perhaps 20%, show easy reflux. The majority of these patients have mild symptoms, easily controlled by simple measures. Those patients who present for treatment are a selected group with more severe symptoms, which include persistent heartburn, post-prandial discomfort or pain, flatulence, dysphagia or bleeding. Typical heartburn usually indicates the presence of a concentric type of hernia while discomfort or bloating after meals, relieved by belching, suggests an eccentric hernia. Heartburn due to reflux is characteristically aggravated by bending, stooping, coughing, pregnancy, ascites, straining at stool and wearing tight garments or corsets. Sleepless nights due to regurgitation may be particularly bothersome. Heartburn usually follows a large meal or the intake of coffee, tea, alcohol or spicy foods. It often occurs, not immediately after eating, but sometime later when the acidity of the gastric contents is higher. The frequency of heartburn often depends on the emotional state of the patient as well. Characteristically, heartburn is promptly relieved by the intake of adequate amounts of antacids. When heartburn is the only complaint, it can be treated symptomatically without fear of any serious underlying disease. While there is insufficient information on the life history of such patients, the available evidence indicates that relatively few, certainly less than 5% will develop any serious complication (FLOOD et al., 1967; PALMER, 1968; SILBER, 1968). In children, heartburn is not a complaint but vomiting, regurgitation and failure to thrive are serious presenting symptoms.

In contrast to heartburn, the complaint of dysphagia requires determined study to identify its cause. A concentric hiatal hernia per se does not cause dysphagia. In the eccentric type of hiatal hernia the herniated sac may compress and narrow the lower esophagus, thereby causing dysphagia. In patients with only an occasional sticking sensation behind the sternum, promptly relieved by furhter swallowing, motility disturbances are likely to be the cause of the dysphagia. In patients with constant and persistent dysphagia to solid foods, some type of constant narrowing less than 12.5 mm in diameter should be demonstrated. Solids may become impacted at the stenosed segment, thereby giving rise to sudden episodes of pain and complete dysphagia, relieved only when the offending morsel of solid food lodged at the stricture is expelled or passes on. As the dysphagia increases or as a result of progressive narrowing, heartburn usually decreases in frequency and severity. With such a history of chronic or episodic dysphagia, there is usually little difficulty in demonstrating a stricture. Benign strictures due to reflux esophagitis are usually short, rarely more than 4 mm in length. Therefore, chronic dysphagia for liquids is unusual. These patients can drink at a normal speed. If the stricture becomes narrower or if the stenosed segment is relatively long, dysphagia for liquids may occur. As the result of the dysphagia, there may be some weight loss but this is rarely marked if the stricture is benign. Such patients usually maintain satisfactory nutrition on semi-solid foods for a surprisingly long period of time.

Pain of a spontaneous nature or during the course of swallowing is only rarely a prominent complaint in reflux esophagitis. When present, it is usually induced by an attempt to swallow too large a bolus or hot or cold foods, alcoholic drinks or even fruit juices. Patients with esophageal pain simulating angina pectoris may not show any evidence of esophagitis or free reflux in spite of the fact that a sliding hernia may be present. Most of these patients suffer from symptomatic diffuse spasm, a functional rather than inflammatory disease. If patients with reflux esophagitis do have persistent retrosternal pain, particularly if pain radiates to the back, it is likely that a penetrating marginal ulcer will be found or that a considerable degree of periesophagitis is present.

Bleeding of significant degree as a result of reflux esophagitis is uncommon. A penetrating marginal ulcer may bleed massively but similar bleeding from erosions in the diffuse superficial variety of esophagitis is unlikely. Patients with severe anemia due to a hernia usually show large hernias of the eccentric type with no evidence of esophagitis. In fact, the sleeve of stomach within the hiatus in such patients is almost always compressed rather than patulous. However, bleeding in association with reflux esophagitis is not uncommon in children and may result in chronic anemia in this age group.

There are no specific physical findings indicative of the presence of reflux esophagitis. Many of the patients are overweight but this is by no means invariable. It is nevertheless of importance to perform a careful physical examination to detect coincident disease. Any local tenderness of the upper abdomen, for example, cannot be attributed to esophagitis.

4. Roentgen Features

Prior to the performance of the roentgen examination of any patient in whom the suspicion of reflux esophagitis exists, the radiologist should be alerted to the specific symptomatology, namely the presence of heartburn, dysphagia, bleeding or pain. A complete examination of the esophagus utilizing all possible maneuvers, positions, projections, thicknesses of barium, double contrast, cineradiography etc., is a time-consuming procedure requiring considerable effort, not only on the part of the radiologist but of the patient as well. Such an examination is not indicated in routine gastrointestinal examinations. For example, there is little to be gained by heroic efforts to demonstrate reflux if the patient has no complaints referable to the esophagogastric region. If dysphagia is present and nothing is seen with the ordinary barium mixtures, the patient should be given a compressed barium tablet, 12.5 mm in diameter, to determine if a minimal stricture can be discovered. If the patient has pain, motor activity in the body of the esophagus must be carefully scrutinized and preferably recorded with movies. Tests for reflux must be done in such a fashion as to permit an evaluation

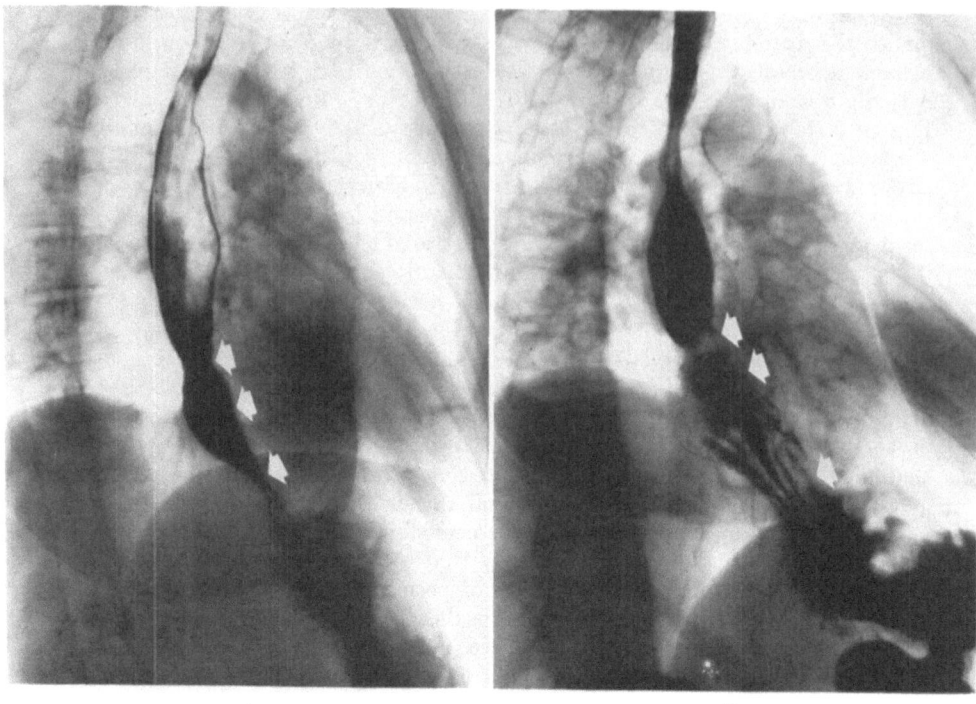

A   B

Fig. 236. Minimal reflux esophagitis. A In the erect position, a short funnel-shaped region (upper arrow) is noted at the distal end of the tubular esophagus. The barium-filled segment distal to this (middle arrow) has a tubular configuration but nevertheless represents a hiatal hernia. The barium column traversing the hiatus (lower arrow) is deceptively narrow. B Same patient in the prone position with a radiolucent bolster under the abdomen shows minimal persistent narrowing (upper arrow) at the end of the tubular esophagus. The sac is larger and appears to be composed of two components—a proximal portion (middle arrow) without gastric rugae (vestibule) and a distal portion with normal gastric rugae. The region of the hiatus (lower arrow) is obviously much wider than its apparent size in the erect position

of its significance. The detection of a hiatal hernia in patients with esophagitis is ordinarily not difficult since substantial shortening of the esophagus is practically always present. It is, however, necessary to examine the patient in the prone position, preferably with a bolster under the abdomen, to demonstrate the sac-like nature of the segment above the hiatus since it is often difficult to distend the hernial sac in the erect position. This is particularly true when a stricture is present since the hernial sac distal to the stricture will often maintain a tubular configuration. If one fails to recognize the presence of a hernia and assumes that the stricture is located, not at the end, but in the middle of the esophagus, the diagnosis of carcinoma must be made. Similarly, if a strictured segment occupies the region of the hiatus, it is unlikely to be benign. The hernia associated with stenosing esophagitis is concentric in nature and rarely despite the fact that it may not be evident in the erect position. The "width of the hiatus", that is, the potential maximum diameter of the barium column traversing the portion of the stomach within the hiatus, cannot be determined with the patient erect since it always appears narrow in this position. The width of the hiatus must be studied in the prone or supine positions while observing multiple

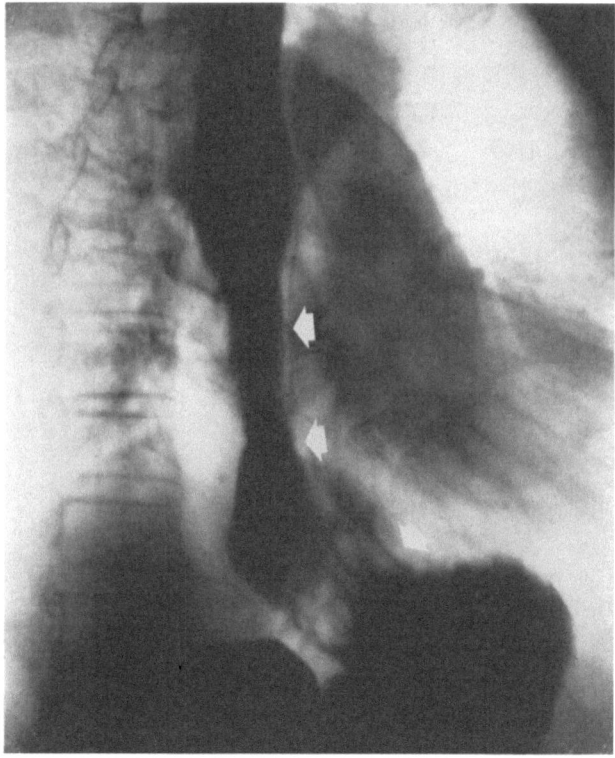

Fig. 237. Moderately severe reflux esophagitis. The distal esophagus (upper arrow) over a distance of about 7 cm is straight with limited distensibility and vertical parallel contours. The patient swallowed a considerable amount of air with the barium. The involved portion of the esophagus showed no typical stripping peristaltic wave. A fairly large concentric type of hiatal hernia is present. There is no evidence of any functional or sphincteric activity between the esophagus and the hernial sac (middle arrow). The barium column traversing the hiatus is unusually wide (lower arrow). This patient complained of rather severe heartburn, aggravated in the supine position, for about 10 years

phases during the course of filling. For this purpose, no bolster should be used under the abdomen and no compression applied. Even in patients with sizable hernias and reflux, a deep inspiration will narrow or obliterate the barium column traversing the hiatus. This maneuver is of use in distending the sac above the hiatus but misleading in attempts to determine the width of the hiatus. The diameter of the barium tablet noted above, that is, 12.5 mm, is approximately the minimum caliber of the gullet which will permit normal swallowing of solid boluses. When a narrowed segment smaller than the tablet is present, it becomes obstructed proximal to the stricture and fails to pass despite multiple additional wet swallows. The tablet is harmless because it disintegrates within a period of half an hour or so.

A chronic superficial diffuse esophagitis of mild degree may be present endoscopically in the absence of any remarkable roentgen features. In general, there is little reason to over-interpret minimal changes in motility of the distal esophagus or in the mucosal pattern in an effort to make the roentgen findings correlate with endoscopy since such changes have no special clinical significance.

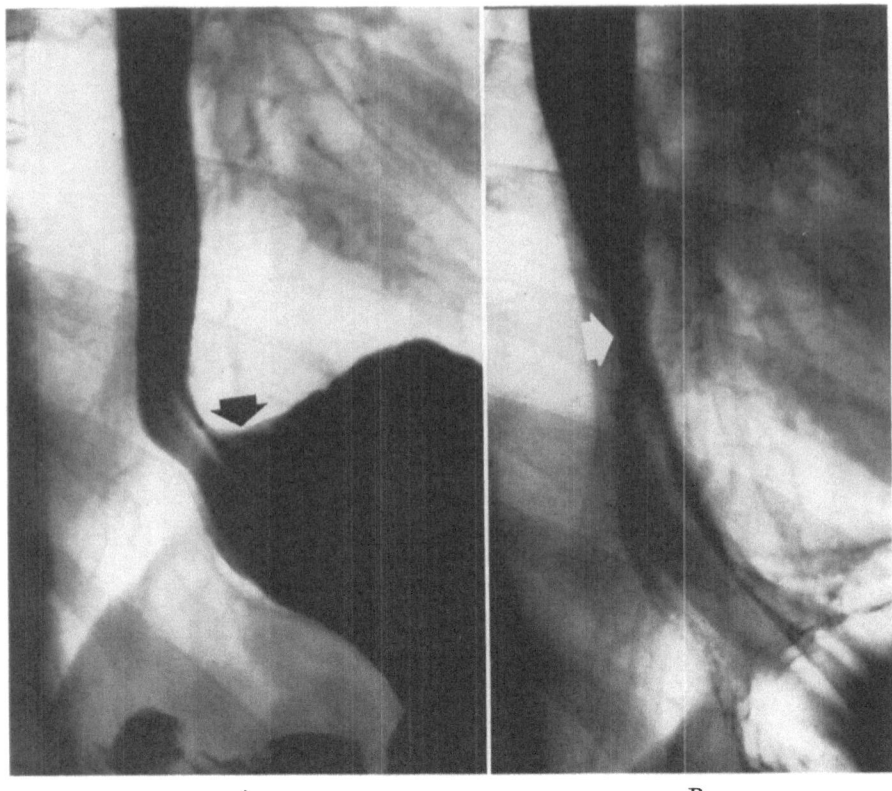

A   B

Fig. 238. Development of moderately severe reflux esophagitis. A Barium meal examination in 1955 was considered within normal limits. However, the esophagogastric region in and below the hiatus has a funnel configuration (arrow) and enters the fundus of the stomach through a wide communication. The abdominal segment of the esophagus or the "submerged" segment is absent; the "cardiac incisura" is effaced. This film was taken with the patient prone but without a bolster under the abdomen. B 12 years later, re-examination because of heartburn and occasional dysphagia shows distinct limited distensibility of the distal 2 inches of the tubular esophagus (arrow) with ragged contours. Note the stretched appearance of the concentric hiatal hernia and the broad communication through the hiatus between the sac and the stomach. This patient has been treated medically for 3 years since this examination with little change in his symptoms. The narrowing of the distal esophagus is somewhat more marked. The esophagogastric region on this and subsequent examinations was fixed in position in relationship to other mediastinal structures and was located at the same height above the hiatus in both the erect and recumbent positions. The fixed stretched appearance suggests that reduction of the hernia at operation is likely to be difficult

When esophagitis is more severe, roentgen features ranging from rather subtle to obvious findings may be detected. With the first swallow of fluid barium in the erect position (Fig. 236), the distal esophagus over a distance of 3 to 8 cm fails to open promptly or to distend normally. The normal slight curvature of the distal esophagus, backward toward the right, is absent and this portion of the esophagus appears unusually straight with vertical parallel margins (Fig. 237). When distensibility is only slightly limited, fine serrations may be seen along the borders. When the narrowing is marked, the borders appear more irregular or coarsely scalloped (Fig. 238). The most marked changes are

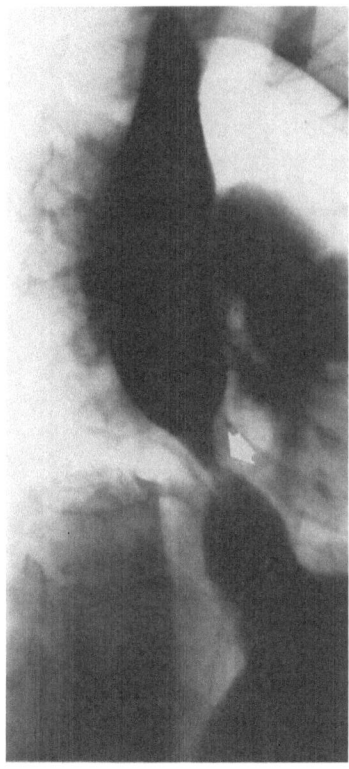 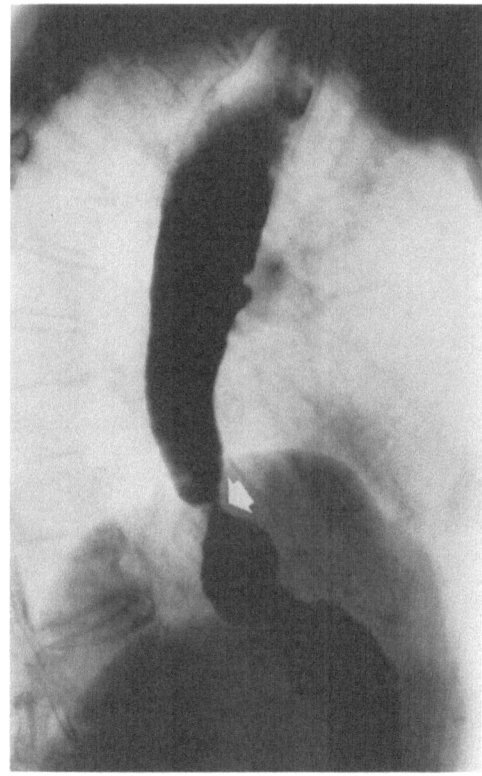

Fig. 239   Fig. 240

Fig. 239. Esophagitis with stricture. This patient complained of heartburn for about 15 years and then dysphagia for 6 months. There is a smooth narrow funnel-shaped segment about 2 cm in length involving the distal esophagus with the most marked narrowing just above the hernial sac (arrow). The stricture flares out proximally. The body of the esophagus is unusually distensible. The concentric hernia has a patulous communication through the hiatus with the stomach below. The funnel configuration suggests that there is some degree of functional component to the stricture with localized superficial inflammatory changes

Fig. 240. A 75 year old female with dysphagia for 2 years shows a short, marked stricture (arrow) between the esophagus and the hernial sac. The esophagus above is dilated with no forceful peristaltic wave. There is no evidence of esophagitis above the stricture. The stricture has smooth contours and funnels distally although proximally it widens abruptly. This woman had no history of previous heartburn that could be obtained. However, sometime before the onset of dysphagia, a left lumbar sympathectomy was performed because of impending gangrene of the big toe. Esophagoscopy after this barium meal examination showed a smooth white stricture. Biopsy of grossly normal mucosa proximal to the stricture showed squamous epithelium with thickening of its basal layer. A repeat blind biopsy distal to the stricture showed inflamed squamous epithelium. Clinically, there was also a question of scleroderma

present distally so that a somewhat tapering configuration is often seen. Emptying of the involved segment is usually abnormal also and a typical peristaltic stripping wave may not be evident. The involved segment seems to empty by a more diffuse contraction, maintaining a stretched appearance as it contracts. The esophagus above the involved segment may be somewhat dilated and show tertiary contractions although such contractions in the involved area are less frequent. These patients often swallow considerable amounts of air with the

Fig. 241 A—D. Patient with localized reflux esophagitis and stricture formation. Reproduction of 70 mm spot films

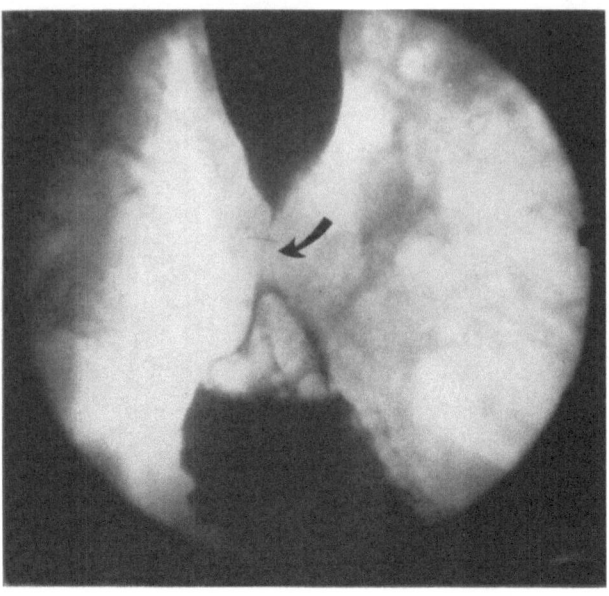

A. Erect position. There is a segment (arrow) about 3 cm in length between the esophagus and the hernial sac which fails to open promptly. The apex of the hernial sac has a triangular configuration, as does the distal end of the esophagus

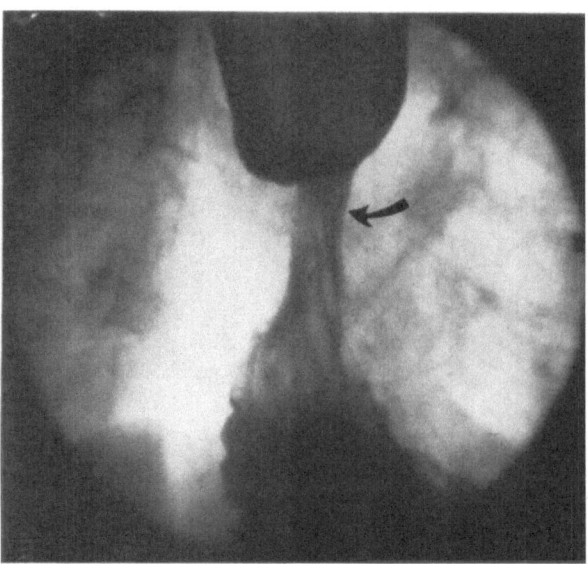

B. On repeated swallowing in the erect position, the strictured area opens and a waterfall effect (arrow) of barium entering the hernial sac is seen

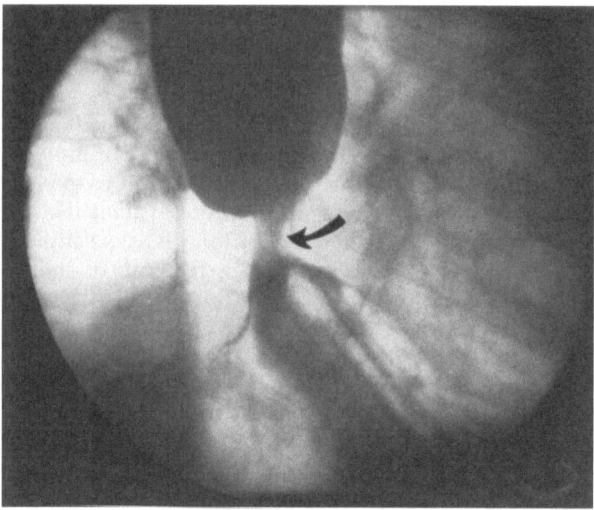

C. Same patient in the prone position with repeated swallowing shows the true length and width of the stricture (arrow). The proximal portion of the hernial sac maintains a triangular configuration and is flattened posteriorly

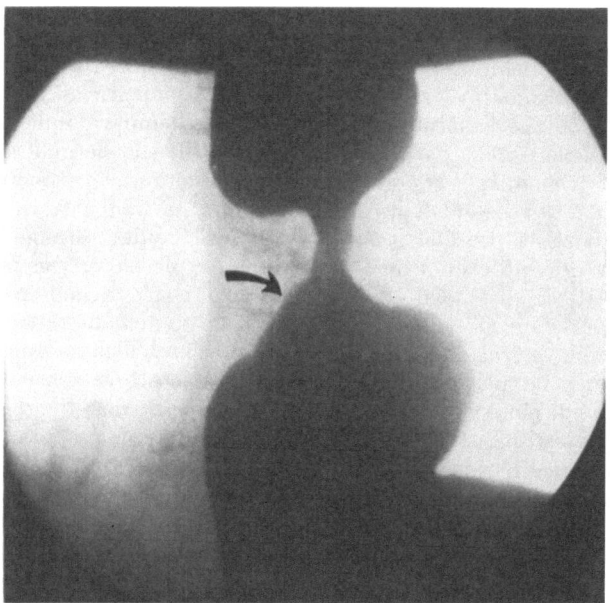

D. In the supine position after a swallow, free reflux of barium from the hernial sac into the esophagus through the stricture is demonstrated. Note the triangular cap (arrow) distal to the stricture. Esophagoscopy and biopsy showed a stricture with superficial inflammatory changes and no evidence of neoplasm

fluid barium and often a spontaneous double contrast is the best demonstration of limited distensibility. To demonstrate the mucosal pattern, a small amount of barium paste is administered. The normal longitudinal fold pattern is disorganized and distorted with irregular and discontinuous barium streaks. Transverse striations may be present but are more characteristic of a healing stage. It is worthy of note that, despite substantial healing of esophagitis as demonstrated by endoscopy and clinical improvement, it is rare to see a complete return to normal of the distal esophagus radiologically. Some lack of distensibility and a flattened mucosal pattern persist apparently indefinitely.

In the variety of esophagitis with a stricture in the esophagogastric region (Figs. 239, 240), the strictured site will usually be identified promptly with the first swallow of barium in the erect position. This position is particularly useful when the stricture is marked since it is possible to build up a column of barium above it in an attempt to force barium to pass through. The details of the stricture and its proximal margin can then be demonstrated. In order to delineate the distal margin of the strictured segment, distension of the hernial sac is required. This is normally best accomplished in the recumbent position, either prone or supine, with retained barium and swallowed air. Pressure on the abdomen, for example with a bolster, may be very helpful. Careful study of the margins of a stricture is essential in order to exclude a carcinoma. The majority of benign strictures, even though marked, have some functional component (Fig. 241). They close completely. When they open, they usually open fairly promptly to the same diameter and show the same configuration. The short transitional areas between the stricture and the esophagus above and the stomach below also show variable delay in opening as well as limitation of distensibility. They, however, change in configuration depending upon the degree of filling that can be induced. The esophagus for a distance of 2 cm or so above the stricture may, however, maintain a funnel shape toward the stricture despite efforts to distend it, presumably because of associated superficial esophagitis. The segment distal to the stricture may also show a similar funnel configuration with limited distensibility despite all efforts to fill the hernial sac. This may create a short triangular segment with straight contours between the stricture and the globular sac below. This segment shows no fold pattern although the sac distal to it shows normal gastric rugae. Free reflux through the stricture is usually not present even when the patient is placed in the prone position and the hernial sac distended. Barium does not wash to and fro through the stricture. However, in most instances, reflux can be demonstrated with relative ease, for example, by asking the patient to swallow. This is true even though the stricture may be marked. A typical benign stricture is concentric but many are eccentric, and, moreover, may be ovoid in shape so that the diameter differs in different projections. It is often essential to obtain an optimal projection of the involved area in order to avoid overlapping of the stricture by the adjacent distended esophagus or stomach. This is particularly true when the strictured segment is very short. The strictured segment, when somewhat longer, may be irregular and angulated in its course. This feature is therefore not useful in distinguishing benign from malignant strictures. The mucosal pattern within the benign stricture, as within a carcinoma, is absent. In general, a benign stricture associated with reflux esophagitis does not have the diaphragm or membranous character of a stenotic Schatzki ring. A similar appearance, however, can be seen after the inflammatory process becomes quiescent. Strictures with the characteristics described above have some fixed fibrous component but it is not possible to determine how much of the narrowing is due to active reversible exudate or muscular hypertrophy. The suggestion has been made that it might be possible to distinguish fixed from functional components by the use of relaxing drugs but this has not been sufficiently investigated.

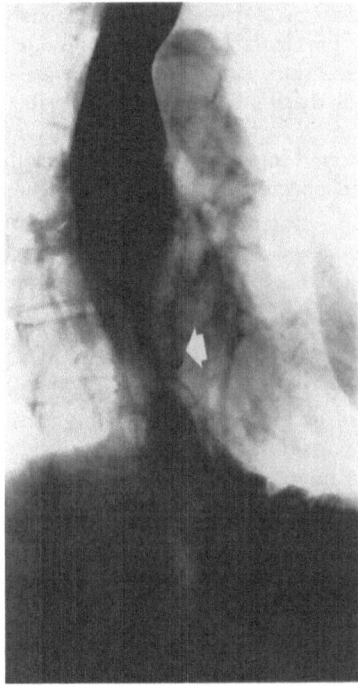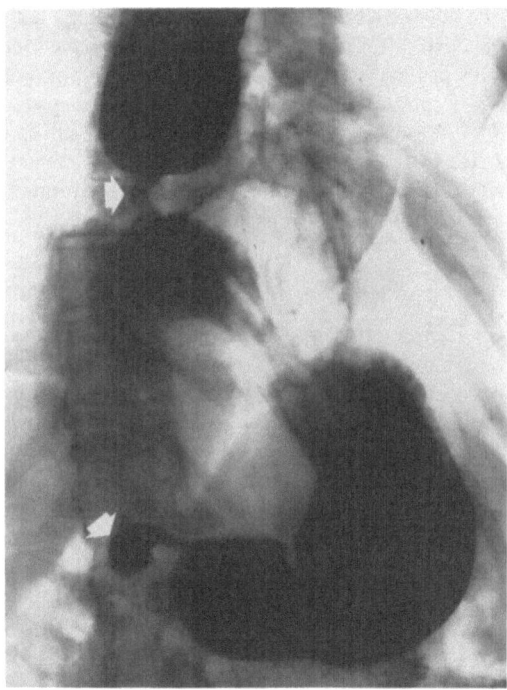

Fig. 242   Fig. 243

Fig. 242. Penetrating marginal esophagogastric ulcer. A middle-aged female complained of heartburn for some time, which decreased with the onset of dysphagia and occasional chest pain. Barium meal examination shows a persistent pocket of barium (arrow) located in the esophagogastric region, which has the appearance of an ulcer crater. The ulcer was best seen on this spontaneous "double-contrast" view. The esophagus at the site of the ulcer is narrowed and the body of the esophagus is dilated. A concentric hernia with a patulous hiatal region is present. There was free reflux

Fig. 243. Another patient, age 70, with a history of dysphagia for about a year shows a large hiatal hernia and a marked stricture almost 2 cm in length between the dilated esophagus and the hernial sac. Within the stricture, there is a discrete ulceration (upper arrow). This patient gave a history of a chronic duodenal ulcer. The duodenal bulb (lower arrow) was deformed but an active crater was not seen

A penetrating esophagogastric marginal ulcer (Figs. 242, 243) can usually be identified on careful roentgen examination as a projecting niche as well as a persistent patch of barium. It is frequently located within a stricture with many of the characteristics described above. The ulcer pocket may, however, not be easily demonstrated, presumably because of associated spasm and difficulty in filling and maintaining complete filling of the involved area. A spontaneous or intentional double contrast examination of the area is often most effective in demonstrating a crater when a suitable projection is obtained.

Despite special attention to the esophagogastric region, careful examination of the stomach and duodenum is required in order to exclude other lesions, specifically peptic ulceration, or other abnormalities which may be associated with gastric retention. As noted above, there is currently interest in the possibility that reflux of duodenal contents into the stomach may play a role in the induction of esophagitis. It is difficult to identify such reflux in the course of a conventional barium meal examination since barium is present simultaneously in both stomach and duodenum. Occasionally, particularly when the pyloric ring is patulous, streaming of barium in both directions can be identified, especially on cineradiography. A test for pyloric insufficiency has been described (Capper et al., 1966). In this test, barium is deposited in the duodenum by tube. After the removal of the tube, the patient is positioned in such a way as to permit reflux from the duodenum into the stomach which occurs quite promptly when pyloric insufficiency is present.

5. Endoscopy

Esophagoscopy is an invaluable method for the evaluation of the presence and severity of reflux esophagitis and in differential diagnosis. It should be preceded and guided by roentgen examination. In the absence of dysphagia and a stricture, esophagoscopy is ordinarily not essential unless a diagnostic problem exists or operative intervention is under consideration. Biopsy of normal appearing mucosa may nevertheless demonstrate microscopic evidence of esophagitis. In a recent study (Ismail-Beigi et al., 1970) esophagoscopy was performed in 34 subjects with heartburn. In 25 subjects the diagnosis of esophagitis was made endoscopically; in 22 of them, or 88%, biopsy also was abnormal. In 9 subjects the esophageal mucosa appeared normal endoscopically; in 7 of these subjects however, histological features of esophagitis were found to be present (i.e. relative widening of the basal cell portion of the epithelium and increase in height of the papillae). Therefore it would appear that biopsy is a more sensitive method for evaluation of the esophageal mucosa than endoscopy. The earliest gross changes are difficult to evaluate. The earliest endoscopic signs of reflux esophagitis usually appear on the dorsal wall of the esophagus, 1 or 2 cm proximal to the squamocolumnar mucosal junction. The central dorsal fold becomes erythematous and covered by a pseudomembranous exudate. Later the other folds become affected, the lesions spread upward and to the anterior wall and the patchy lesions become confluent. The mucosa is diffusely red, edematous, covered with exudate and friable. In more severe cases of esophagitis, longitudinal erosions appear, first on the dorsal wall, later more anteriorly and more proximally. If the entire circumference of the lower esophagus is affected, the lesions tend to become stenosing. In some cases a marginal ulcer can be observed at the squamocolumnar mucosal junction. Efforts to quantitate these endoscopic observations, are subjective. An estimate of the severity of the process on esophagoscopy correlates only in a rough fashion with roentgen changes since intramural changes causing limitation of distensibility are difficult to visualize. The utilization of fiber optic instruments has improved the ability of the endoscopist to study functional changes and color photography has contributed greatly to documentation and serial comparisons of the findings.

Esophagoscopy is not as reliable as roentgen examination in the detection of small sliding hiatal hernias. However, the presence of reflux can easily be recognized and the acidity of the gastric contents tested. When a stricture is anticipated, endoscopy can be performed with a rigid scope and an effort made to dilate the stricture. It is possible also to dilate the stricture with the aid of olive-tipped bougies, passed over a previously swallowed string, until the caliber of the stenosed segment is sufficiently wide to permit the passage of the esophagoscope. Such dilatations are necessary if observations distal to the stricture are to be made. Demonstration of a penetrating marginal ulcer is not difficult if the stricture can be passed. A "blind" biopsy distal to the stricture may be necessary to exclude carcinoma. An experienced endoscopist can also draw tentative conclusions as to the rigidity of the stricture and fixation of the area when operation and attempted reduction are anticipated.

6. Manometry

Manometric observations have contributed greatly to an understanding of the mechanism of reflux, and have also been used for diagnostic purposes. The manometric diagnosis of hiatal hernia is not very reliable, due to the high incidence of false positive and false negative results as compared to the X-ray techniques (COHEN, 1970). Quantitative measurements of the pressure relationships during resting, swallowing and a variety of maneuvers (application of pneumatic cuff, straight leg raising, manual compression) can be used as manometric tests of reflux. For example, free transmittal of modestly increased intraabdominal pressure into the body of the esophagus, resulting in an equalization of intragastric and intraesophageal pressure, is usually associated with a simultaneous fall in intraesophageal pH, indicating that free reflux is present (SANDMARK, 1963).

Measurements of intrasphincteric pressure with a perfused catheter system can be used as an estimate of sphincter competence. Sphincteric pressures obviously below the normal range show a good correlation with symptoms of reflux or esophagitis. Sphincteric pressures within the normal range do not necessarily signify absence of reflux or a competent sphincter since the sphincter pressures in patients with a hiatal hernia tend to decrease when the hernia is present and to rise when the hernia is reduced (HADDAD, 1970). Patients with esophagitis frequently show interference with the normal peristaltic pattern such as low amplitude or absent peristaltic waves (OLSEN and SCHLEGEL, 1965) but these features are not specific. In the presence of severe esophagitis or a stricture, intraluminal measurements may not be feasible or informative. Intraluminal pressure studies are of considerable importance in distinguishing reflux esophagitis from other abnormalities which are functional in nature, such as diffuse spasm and achalasia, as well as to document esophageal involvement in scleroderma and similar conditions. The combination of manometry and pH studies permits correct positioning of the exploring probe.

A thorough evaluation of a patient with reflux esophagitis includes a manometric study of the esophagus. The information obtained by manometric techniques may be used as a guide to therapy (AFFOLTER, 1967). Motor weakness of the lower esophagus and a weak or absent esophageal sphincter are arguments in favor of surgical intervention.

7. Diagnosis and Differential Diagnosis

Since the incidence of hiatal hernia is so high, the most common problem in differential diagnosis is a patient with indefinite gastrointestinal symptoms and a demonstrable hernia. If a hernia were not present and other diagnostic investigations were negative, such symptoms would be ordinarily attributed to some "functional" abnormality. It is therefore not possible to assume, because a hernia is present, that it is the cause of the patient's symptoms (RUDOLPH et al., 1971). If the patient's symptoms are atypical, even the demonstration of reflux must be evaluated carefully.

Severe heartburn or pain of esophageal distribution related to posture, and hypersensitivity to hot or alcoholic drinks suggest reflux esophagitis. A long history of heartburn followed by the development of dysphagia usually indicates a stenosing esophagitis. Peptic stenosis of the esophagus causes slowly progressive dysphagia for solids with occasional food impaction, but rarely dysphagia for fluids. By contrast, the dysphagia of malignant lesions is rapidly progressive, resulting after weeks or a few months in complete dysphagia for solids and fluids.

If the clinical features suggest reflux esophagitis, an acid perfusion test may be performed to confirm this clinical impression. This test is also helpful to distinguish esophageal pain from pain of other origin (e.g. myocardial ischemia, peptic ulcer, "functional" disturbances) since this test may reproduce the patient's symptoms. When esophagitis is severe, careful search for a peptic ulcer, particularly in the duodenum, which need not be active at the time of the examination, must be made. When other disease such as cholecystitis and cholelithiasis is discovered, a careful evaluation of the symptoms and objective findings is required to judge the contributions of each. In the presence of dysphagia, an abnormality in the swallowing mechanism must be present but all of the modalities of investigation may be required before a specific diagnosis can be made. A search for reflux is desirable if a chronic cough, "asthma" or recurrent pneumonitis without apparent etiology are a clinical problem. Esophagoscopy and/or biopsy are usually required to make a definite diagnosis of early reflux esophagitis. Clinical judgment will determine whether or not these rather unpleasant examinations are to be used. Radiological examinations are most helpful in the more advanced stages of the disease, when typical features are to be expected and esophagoscopy may be impossible due to the stenosis.

The most important radiological differential diagnosis is obviously carcinoma. When esophagitis is diffuse and non-stenotic, this problem rarely arises although there are instances of superficial spreading carcinoma, lymphoma or leukemia which may simulate esophagitis. When a strictured segment with or without ulceration is present, differential diagnosis becomes more difficult. Whenever there is any fixed soft tissue intrusion into the lumen above or below the stricture or any contour on either side of the stricture which remains straight or convex toward the lumen, the suspicion of carcinoma must be raised. Any evidence suggesting a mass, such as distinct or abrupt borders or an overhanging edge at either margin of the stricture, requires a working diagnosis of carcinoma until excluded by endoscopy and tissue biopsy, repeated if negative the first time. Ulceration within such carcinomas is usually present although difficult to discern because it is often superficial. Any irregular patch of barium suggesting "destroyed" mucosa which is repeatedly visualized, even if it does not remain filled, should suggest carcinoma. Thickening of the wall of the esophagus, when evident as a grey "stripe" against adjacent aerated lung, is present in benign strictures but should not form a discrete or globular mass. It should be emphasized that carcinoma of the esophagogastric region in association with a hiatal hernia is not rare and is frequently overlooked in the early stages.

It is also necessary to distinguish achalasia in association with a hernia from a benign stricture and reflux esophagitis. This may be very difficult since the hernia is concentric and the non-relaxing sphincter closely simulates a benign stricture. The body of the esophagus is ordinarily more markedly dilated in achalasia with no normal peristaltic activity. In patients with benign strictures of long standing, however, the esophagus may also be dilated with little evidence of peristalsis. Although a patient with achalasia and hernia is not likely to give a history of heartburn, endoscopy and manometric observations will generally be required to make this differential diagnosis.

Moniliasis of the esophagus shows characteristic diffuse superficial changes in the mucosal pattern, rarely with any stricture, which are usually promptly clarified by the clinical picture of an underlying disease, as well as the presence of similar changes in the mouth. Other types of specific diffuse esophagitis such as tuberculosis are relatively uncommon.

8. Therapy

In the absence of dysphagia and a stricture, patients with reflux esophagitis are treated medically—at least for a time. Since the esophagitis in the majority of instances is mild, simple medical measures usually produce prompt and lasting relief. Medical methods include avoidance of postures and activities which induce reflux and the use of non-absorbable antacids. Dietary measurements such as small meals, the avoidance of coffee, alcohol, tea, and other foods which aggravate symptoms are usually effective. Elevation of the head of the bed during sleep is necessary if heartburn or regurgitation at night is a problem. The avoidance of eating before going to bed, reduction in weight, and abandoning tight garments are other important measures. Anticholinergic drugs appear contraindicated because they decrease sphincteric pressure, retard gastric emptying and decrease esophageal peristalsis (SIEGEL, 1964). Cholinergic drugs can be used to increase the tone of the lower esophageal sphincter and to combat gastroesophageal reflux (FARRELL et al., 1973). When the esophagitis is more severe, a bland diet with 6 to 8 meals or even hourly feedings of milk or milk preparations should be given, together with adequate amounts of antacids in between the meals. In some cases it may be necessary to use an intraesophageal milk or antacid drip for periods of about two weeks. Intensive therapy of this type ordinarily will produce regression in the severity of the inflammatory process and improvement in the patient's symptoms which can frequently be maintained for considerable periods of time. It is obvious, however, that patients vary a great deal in their abilities to follow a strict regimen. The decision to operate will depend on the "intractability" of the patient's complaints—a matter of judgment for both the patient and the physician. Operation should also be considered when bleeding is recurrent. The results of surgical treatment for hernia and esophagitis without a stricture are said to be excellent with current techniques (SKINNER and BELSEY, 1967; URSCHEL and PAULSON, 1967). It should be realized, however, that reported successful results of surgical therapy of hiatal hernia and esophagitis may, in part, be due to the natural history of the disease. Moreover, in most studies the success is measured in terms of patient satisfaction rather than on the basis of objective criteria such as pH-electrode measurement, gastroesophageal reflux and radiological search for anatomical recurrence of the hernia. A small number of medically treated patients may at some future time develop a stricture but it is not possible to predict this in any specific case. However, such patients are at risk, for example if operative intervention of some type is required or if some episode associated with vomiting or periods of unconsciousness should supervene. Esophageal intubation should be avoided in these patients.

The treatment of esophagitis associated with a stricture is a difficult problem (ELLIS and PAYNE, 1965; BOMBECK et al., 1967; MENGUY, 1970). In many of these patients, the active inflammatory process is relatively quiescent and, fortunately, does not appear to be significantly aggravated by forceful dilatation of the stricture. It is therefore usually possible to dilate such strictures with esophageal bougies, often passed over a string or, in less severe cases or later

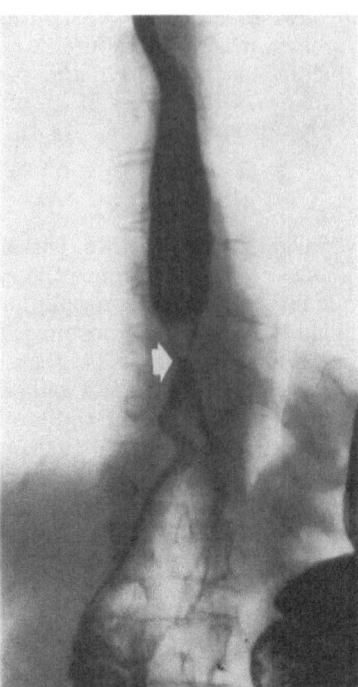

Fig. 244. An elderly female patient who, 10 years before this examination, underwent total gastrectomy for carcinoma of the stomach. An esophagoduodenostomy was performed without difficulty. Postoperatively, the patient did very well except for the prompt appearance and persistence of heartburn. One year before this examination, dysphagia appeared. Roentgen examination shows a tight short stricture (arrow) at the site of the anastomosis between the esophagus and the duodenum. Esophagoscopy showed the stricture and minimal superficial inflammatory changes. In view of the findings and history, this was assumed to be the result of reflux of duodenal contents

during treatment, by mercury-weighted tubes (Benedict, 1966). Such treatment has to be repeated at intervals, which, however, may be as long as a year or more. The technique of these dilatations is discussed on p. 800. After multiple dilatations, further efforts may become ineffective and operative intervention necessary. Operation will also be advised when bougienage has to be carried out too frequently. A variety of operations have been recommended in the treatment of strictures, suggesting that none is entirely satisfactory. Many of these are major procedures since it is unlikely that the shortened esophagus will permit reduction of the hernia. Recommended operations include esophagogastrectomy with excision of varying amounts of the esophagus and stomach, transplantation of the esophagogastric region to the dome of the diaphragm, esophagogastrectomy with interposition of jejunum or colon, formation of a gastric tube, and resection of the stricture plus a variety of procedures designed to suppress acid formation and produce prompt gastric emptying. Local resection or plastic procedures have regularly failed. To be effective, any procedure requires the correction of reflux. At the present time, the most popular operative procedure appears to be the Thal operation (Thal et al., 1965; Clarke et al., 1969), in which the strictured area is incised, the esophageal lumen widened, and the defect in the esophagus covered by the fundus of the stomach as a peritonealized patch. This is combined

with a plication procedure of the fundus around the esophagus in order to create
an antireflux mechanism. The patch becomes reepithelialized and, if reflux has
been controlled, the stricture should not recur. Other procedures which do not
directly attack the stricture but reconstruct an antireflux mechanism may be
successful if the structure can be forcibly dilated. Reflux esophagitis in children
may be rapidly progressive and unfortunately in this group operative procedures
appear less successful than in adults (SKINNER and BELSEY, 1967; McNAMARA
et al., 1969). They therefore form a special group and each case must be individualized.

There is a substantial danger of reflux esophagitis after any operative procedure
which excises, damages or bypasses the esophagogastric region due to the probability of inducing reflux of gastric or intestinal contents. Esophagoduodenostomy
is particularly likely to lead to reflux esophagitis of the alkaline or biliary type
(Fig. 244). Efforts to introduce a valvular antireflux mechanism, for example,
after esophagogastrectomy, are therefore desirable (BOMBECK and NYHUS, 1970b).
An interposed segment of jejunum or colon may act as an antireflux mechanism
if a portion of the segment is located below the hiatus. In the course of any
operative procedure for peptic ulcer, a careful examination of the hiatal region
is required. If herniation is present, a repair is necessary to prevent reflux despite
the fact that the operation is designed to produce achlorhydria. Repair may be
necessary if the performance of a vagotomy has compromised the hiatal region.
It must be emphasized that the reconstruction of an antireflux mechanism,
for example, by fundoplication or other maneuver, is the essential feature of
any operation for the repair of a hiatal hernia (LIND et al., 1965; POLK, 1969;
MUSTARD, 1970). This is obvious when the operation is performed because of
reflux. It is equally true, however, if the operation is done for any other reason
such as anemia since, if neglected, reflux esophagitis may follow hernia repair.

9. Other Types of Reflux Esophagitis

On the assumption that a predisposition to reflux esophagitis is present,
e.g. minimal herniation with or without a sac, a variety of factors may act as a
triggering mechanism to produce a severe esophagitis. The most common of
these (Fig. 245) is nasogastric intubation used after some type of operative
procedure, not primarily on the esophagus. Other contributing factors, however,
include persistent vomiting such as hyperemesis gravidarum, episodes of vomiting
associated with alcoholism, or the onset of duodenal ulceration or some systemic
disease such as scleroderma. Previous esophageal insults such as a lye burn
may also serve as a predisposing factor (IMRE and WOOLER, 1969).

The etiology of esophagitis after intubation is not entirely clear (DOUGLAS,
1956; NAGLER et al., 1960). Not all of these patients appear to have a hiatal
hernia or a previous history of reflux. It is sometimes evident when the tube
is inserted that reflux and spasm are occurring because the patient complains
of heartburn and pain. This, however, is not the usual story, perhaps because
many of these patients have other more serious problems in the postoperative
period. It does not seem possible to predict which of the many patients who are
intubated will present a week or a month after intubation with dysphagia and
a severe esophagitis. In such patients, a stricture usually appears surprisingly
rapidly and the further course is often comparable to that of a lye esophagitis.
The period of intubation, while usually several days, may be surprisingly short
and still create difficulty. There is probably a combination of etiological factors

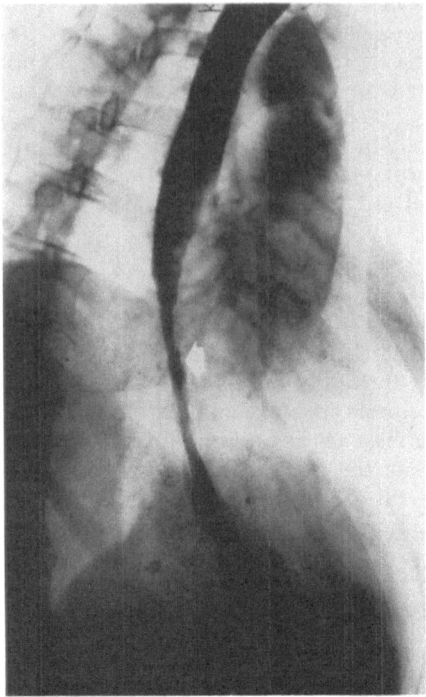
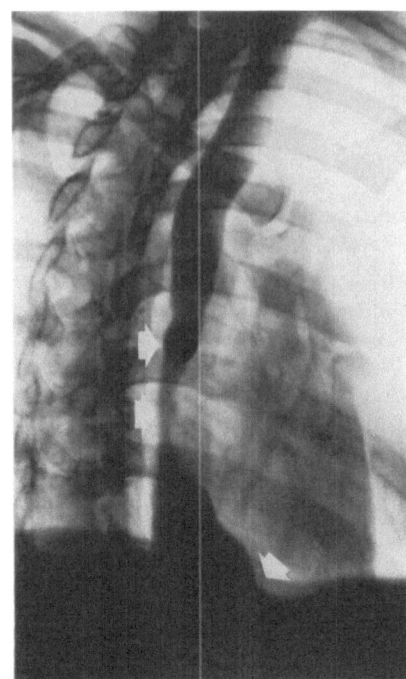

Fig. 245   Fig. 246

Fig. 245. Three months before this film was taken, this patient had undergone a hiatal hernia repair and was intubated for several days postoperatively. Dysphagia appeared promptly after the operation. Roentgen examination shows diffuse marked narrowing and mucosal irregularities of the distal esophagus (arrow) over a distance of 3 or 4 inches with no definite evidence of a hernia and no reflux. Esophagoscopy showed severe inflammatory changes. Narrowing progressed over a period of a year despite multiple dilatations. A second operation was performed and a severe periesophagitis was found. The esophagus was freed of adhesions and a second hernia repair performed. Dysphagia improved postoperatively with subsidence of active inflammatory changes, but the caliber of the esophagus is still distinctly limited

Fig. 246. A woman of 25 who vomited persistently during an episode of alcoholism. Dysphagia appeared shortly after this. Roentgen examination shows diffuse narrowing and irregularity of the distal portion of the tubular esophagus (middle arrow) with a concentric type of hernia and an unusually wide hiatal channel (lower arrow). A 12.5 mm compressed barium tablet (upper arrow) failed to pass. Esophagoscopy demonstrated severe inflammatory changes. Biopsy showed—unexpectedly—inflamed columnar type of epithelium

including prior herniation in some, reflux aggravated by the presence of the tube, mucosal ischemia because of compression of the esophageal mucosa between the tube within the lumen and spastic muscle, and the stress associated with the operation. Roentgen examination usually shows extensive involvement which is most severe often in the mid- rather than terminal esophagus. It is of interest that a hernia need not be present in such patients although the phrenic ampulla may simulate a small hernia. The inflammatory process seems to spare the phrenic ampulla as well as the abdominal segment of the esophagus. This is also true of the occasional case of severe esophagitis associated with a duodenal ulcer without a hernia, although a history of diagnostic intubation is often obtained in such substances. Treatment of intubation esophagitis is difficult and follows along the lines described above for severe esophagitis with a stricture.

Heartburn during the course of pregnancy is a common feature and may or may not be associated with a demonstrable sliding hernia or reflux esophagitis (DePaula Castro, 1967; Lind et al., 1968). Periodic incompetence of the anti-reflux mechanism is presumably the result of increased intraabdominal pressure with stretching of the phrenicoesophageal membrane as well as hormonal effects leading to relaxation of both the intrinsic sphincter and adjacent soft tissues. In general, such changes are reversible but some subtle permanent damage may have occurred. This is more likely in patients who during the course of pregnancy develop severe vomiting (Abbey Smith and Nelson, 1965). It has been stated that transient dysphagia of some degree is not an uncommon finding in the postpartum period. In a few cases, however, severe dysphagia appears promptly postpartum and a stricture is evident on roentgen examination. The findings in this group of patients are similar to those with intubation esophagitis and the prognosis and the therapy are comparable.

Persistent vomiting during an intercurrent illness from which the patient recovers appears to cause irreversible esophagitis only rarely. If vomiting is associated with markedly acid gastric contents, e.g., during a bout of alcoholism (Fig. 246) or diabetic ketosis, a fairly severe esophagitis may supervene, which ordinarily responds well to therapy. The incidence or the coincidence of vomiting and reflux esophagitis appears greater in children, although in such cases, cause and effect may be difficult to distinguish. When vomiting is treated by intubation, the possibility that a subsequent esophagitis is related to the intubation as well as the vomiting appears likely.

References

Abbey Smith, R., Nelson, C. S.: Oesophageal obstruction following hyperemesis gravidarum. Thorax 20, 528–531 (1965).

Affolter, H.: Pressure characteristics of reflux esophagitis. Helv. med. Acta 33, 395–402 (1967).

Atkinson, M., Bennett, J. R.: Relationship between motor changes and pain during esophageal acid perfusion. Amer. J. dig. Dis. 13, 346–350 (1968).

Benedict, E. B.: Peptic stenosis of the esophagus. A study of 233 patients treated with bougienage, surgery or both. Amer. J. dig. Dis. 11, 761–770 (1966).

Bernstein, L. M., Baker, L. A.: A clinical test for esophagitis. Gastroenterology 34, 760–781 (1958).

Benz, L. S., Hootkin, L. A., Margulies, S., Donner, M. W., Cauthorne, R. T., Hendrix, T. R.: A comparison of clinical measurements of gastroesophageal reflux. Gastroenterology 62, 1–5 (1972).

Bombeck, C. T., Aoki, T., Nyhus, L. M.: Anatomic etiology and operative treatment of peptic esophagitis. Ann. Surg. 165, 752–764 (1967).

Bombeck, C. T., Dillard, D. H., Nyhus, L. M.: Muscular anatomy of the gastroesophageal junction and the role of phrenoesophageal ligament. Ann. Surg. 164, 643–652 (1966).

Bombeck, C. T., Helfrich, G. B., Nyhus, L. M.: Planning surgery for reflux esophagitis and hiatus hernia. Surg. Clin. N. Amer. 50, 29–44 (1970a).

Bombeck, C. T., Nyhus, L. M.: Prevention of gastroesophageal reflux after resection of the lower esophagus. Surg. Gynec. Obstet. 130, 1035–1043 (1970b).

Brombart, M.: Roentgenology of the esophagus. In: Alimentary tract radiology, vol. 2, ed. A. R. Margulies and H. J. Burhenne, p. 337–352. St. Louis: C. V. Mosby 1967.

Butterfield, D. G., Struthers, J. E., Jr., Showalter, J. P.: A test of gastroesophageal sphincter competence: the common cavity test (abstract). Gastroenterology 58, 932 (1970).

Capper, W. M., Airth, G. R., Kilby, J. O.: A test for pyloric regurgitation. Lancet 1966 II, 621–623.

Castell, D. O., Harris, L. D.: Hormonal control of gastroesophageal sphincter strength. New Engl. J. Med. 282, 886–889 (1970).

CLARK, M. D., RINALDO, J. A., JR., EYLER, W. R.: Correlation of manometric and radiologic data from the esophagogastric area. Radiology **94**, 261–270 (1970).

CLARKE, J. M., RAYL, J. E., WOODWARD, E. R.: Experience with the Thal and Nissen operations in the treatment of reflux esophagitis with stricture: A preliminary report. Amer. Surg. **35**, 89–94 (1969).

CODE, C. F., KELLY, M. L., SCHLEGEL, J. F., OLSEN, A. M.: Detection of hiatal hernia during esophageal motility tests. Gastroenterology **43**, 521–531 (1962).

COHEN, B. R.: Manometry and related techniques in hiatal hernia and its complications. In: Progress in gastroenterology, vol. II, p.149–161, ed. G. B. J. GLASS. New York and London: Grune and Stratton 1970.

COHEN, S., HARRIS, L. D.: Lower esophageal sphincter strength. Gastroenterology **58**, 157–162 (1970).

COLLIS, J. L.: Benign stricture of the esophagus. In: Clinical surgery, No. 5. Thorax, ed. C. ROB and R. SMITH, p. 281–309. London: Butterworth & Co. 1965.

CRUMMY, A. B.: The water test in the evaluation of gastroesophageal reflux. Its correlation with pyrosis. Radiology **78**, 501–504 (1966).

DE CARVALHO, M.: Chirurgie du syndrome hiato-œsophagien (Communications prealable). Arch. Mal. Appar. dig. **40**, 280–293 (1951).

DE PAULA CASTRO, L.: Reflux esophagitis as the cause of heartburn in pregnancy. Obstet. and Gynec. **98**, 1–10 (1967).

DERSTAPPEN, G. VAN, TEXTER, E. C., JR.: Response of the physiologic and gastroesophageal sphincter to increased intra-abdominal pressure. J. clin. Invest. **43**, 1856–1868 (1964).

DILLARD, D. H., ANDERSON, H. N.: A new concept of the mechanism of sphincter failure in sliding esophageal hiatal hernia. Surg. Gynec. Obstet. **122**, 1030 (1960).

DONNER, M. W., SILBRIGER, M. L., HOOKMAN, P., HENDRIX, T. R.: Acid barium swallows in radiographic evaluation of clinical esophagitis. Radiology 87, 220–225 (1966).

DOUGLAS, W. K.: Oesophageal stricture associated with gastroduodenal intubation. Brit. J. Surg. **43**, 404–409 (1956).

EDMUNDS, V.: Hiatal hernia. A clinical study of 200 cases. Quart. J. Med. **26**, 445–465 (1957).

ELLIS, F. H., JR., PAYNE, W. S.: Motility disturbances of the esophagus and its inferior sphincter. In: Advances in surgery, ed. C. E. WELCH. Vol. I, p. 179–246. Chicago: Year Book Publishers 1965.

FARRELL, R. L., ROLING, G. T., CASTELL, D. O.: Cholinergic therapy of chronic heartburn: a controlled trial. Gastroenterology **64**, 726 (1973).

FLOOD, C. A., SEAMAN, W. B., BAKER, D. C., JR.: Development of esophagitis in hiatus hernia. In: The stomach; The Thirteenth Hahnemann Symposium, p. 72–83. New York: Grune and Stratton 1967.

FYKE, F. E., JR., CODE, C. F., SCHLEGEL, J. F.: The gastroesophageal sphincter in healthy human beings. Gastroenterologia (Basel) **86**, 135–150 (1956).

GILLISON, E. W., CAPPER, W. M., AIRTH, G. R., GIBSON, M. J., BRADFORD, I.: Hiatus hernia and heartburn. Gut **10**, 609–613 (1969).

HADDAD, J.: Relation of gastroesophageal reflux to yield sphincter pressures. Gastroenterology **58**, 175–184 (1970).

HAMPERL, H.: Peptische Oesophagitis. Verh. dtsch. path. Ges. **27**, 208–215 (1934).

HEITMANN, P., WOLF, B. S., SOKOL, E. M., COHEN, B. R.: Simultaneous cineradiographic—manometric study of the distal esophagus: Small hiatal hernias and rings. Gastroenterology **50**, 735–753 (1966).

HIEBERT, C. A., BELSEY, R.: Incompetency of the gastric cardia without radiologic evidence of hiatal hernia. J. thorac. cardiovasc. Surg. **42**, 352–362 (1961).

HOOKMAN, P., FLEISCHER, J.: Cholinergic alteration of lower esophageal sphincter pressure. Gastroenterology **56**, 1169 (1969).

HOOTKIN, L. A., BENZ, L. J., MARGULIS, S., CAUTHORNE, R. F., HENDRIX, T. R.: A comparison of clinical measurements of gastroesophageal reflux (abstract). Gastroenterology **58**, 1044 (1970).

IMRE, J., WOOLER, G.: Peptic ulceration of the oesophagus following corrosive burns. Thorax **24**, 762–764 (1969).

ISMAIL-BEIGI, F., HORTON, P. F., POPE, C. E., II: Histological consequences of gastroesophageal reflux in man. Gastroenterology **58**, 163–174 (1970).

JOHNSON, H. D.: The cardia and hiatus hernia. Springfield (Ill.): Charles C. Thomas 1968.

KANEKO, M.: Personal communication.

KANTROWITZ, P. A., CARSON, J. G., FLEISCHLI, D. J., SKINNER, D. B.: Measurements of gastroesophageal reflux. Gastroenterology **56**, 666–674 (1969).

LEVRAT, M., LAMBERT, R., KIRSHBAUM, G.: Esophagitis produced by reflux of duodenal contents in rats. Amer. J. dig. Dis. **7**, 564–573 (1962).

LIND, J. F., BURNS, C. M., MACDOUGALL, J. T.: "Physiological" repair for hiatus hernia—manometric study. Arch. Surg. **91**, 233–236 (1965).

LIND, J. F., SMITH, A. M., MCIVER, D. K., COOPLAND, A. T., CRISPIN, J. S.: Heartburn in pregnancy: Manometric study. Canad. med. Ass. J. **98**, 571–574 (1968).

LINSMAN, J. F.: Gastroesophageal reflux elicited while drinking water (water siphonage test); its clinical correlation with pyrosis. Amer. J. Roentgenol. **94**, 325–332 (1965).

LOCKWOOD, K., BORGESKOV, S.: Simultaneous measurement of intraluminal pressure and pH in the stomach and esophagus. Thorax **24**, 589–594 (1969).

LONGHI, E. H., JORDAN, P. H.: Pressure relationships responsible for reflux in patients with hiatal hernia. Surg. Gynec. Obstet. **129**, 734–748 (1969).

MCNAMARA, J. J., PAULSON, D. L., URSCHEL, H. C., JR.: Hiatal hernia and gastroesophageal reflux in children. Pediatrics,**43**, 527–532 (1969).

MENGUY, R.: Acquired short esophagus with stricture. Surg. Clinc. N. Amer. **50**, 45–55 (1970).

MOERSCH, R. N., ELLIS, F. H., JR., MCDONALD, J. R.: Pathologic changes occurring in severe reflux esophagitis. Surg. Gynec. Obstet. **108**, 476–484 (1959).

MOFFAT, R. C., BERKAS, E. M.: Bile esophagitis. Arch. Surg. **91**, 963–966 (1965).

MUSTARD, R. A.: A survey of techniques and results of hiatus hernia repair. Surg. Gynec. Obstet. **130**, 130–136 (1970).

NAGLER, R., WOLFSON, A. W., LOWMAN, R. M., SPIRO, H. M.: Effect of gastric intubation on the normal mechanisms preventing gastroesophageal reflux. New Engl. J. Med. **262**, 1325–1327 (1960).

OLSEN, A. M., SCHLEGEL, J. F.: Motility disturbances caused by esophagitis. J. thorac. cardiovasc. Surg. **50**, 607–612 (1965).

PALMER, E. D.: Subacute erosive "Peptic" esophagitis associated with achlorhydria. New Engl. J. Med. **262**, 927–929 (1960).

PALMER, E. D.: Hiatus hernia—esophagitis—esophageal stricture complex: Twenty-year prospective study. Amer. J. Med. **44**, 566–579 (1968).

PETERS, P.: The pathology of severe digestion oesophagitis. Thorax **10**, 269–286 (1955).

PICCONE, V. A., GUTELIUS, J. R., MCCORRISTON, J. R.: A multiphased esophageal pH test for gastroesophageal reflux. Surgery **57**, 638–646 (1965).

POLK, H. C., JR.: Fundoplication for complicated hiatal hernia: Rationale and results. Ann. thorac. Surg. **7**, 202–211 (1969).

POPE, C. E., II: A dynamic test of sphincter strength: its application to the lower esophageal sphincter. Gastroenterology **52**, 779–786 (1967).

RUDOLPH, I., HERRARA, A. F., STEIN, G. N., ROTH, J. L. A.: Mechanism of pyrosis. A clinical study. Amer. J. dig. Dis. **16**, 577–588 (1971).

SANDMARK, S.: Intraluminal pressures and pH in hiatus hernia and gastroesophageal reflux. Acta otolaryng. (Stockh.) **56**, 1–16 (1963a).

SANDMARK, S.: Hiatal incompetence: Studies on mechanics and principles of examination for hiatus hernia and gastroesophageal reflux. Acta radiol. (Stockh.) Suppl. **219**, 5–46 (1963b).

SANDRY, R. J.: Pathology of chronic esophagitis. Gut **3**, 189–200 (1962).

SIEGEL, C. I.: Heartburn. Gastroenterology **47**, 545–548 (1964).

SIEGEL, C. I., HENDRIX, T. R.: Esophageal motor abnormalities induced by acid perfusion in patients with heartburn. J. clin. Invest. **42**, 686–695 (1963).

SILBER, W.: Late results of the treatment of hiatal hernia. Amer. J. dig. Dis. **13**, 252–259 (1968).

SILBER, W.: Augmented histamine test in the treatment of symptomatic hiatal hernia. Gut **10**, 614–616 (1969).

SKINNER, D. B.: Symptomatic esophageal reflux. Amer. J. dig. Dis. **11**, 771–779 (1966).

SKINNER, D. B., BELSEY, R. H. R.: Surgical management of esophageal reflux and hiatus hernia. J. thorac. cardiovasc. Surg. **53**, 33–54 (1967).

SKINNER, D. B., BELSEY, R. H. R., HENDRIX, T. R., ZUIDEMA, G. D.: Gastroesophageal reflux and hiatal hernia. Boston: Little Brown & Co. 1972.

SKINNER, D. B., CAMP, T. F.: Relation of esophageal reflux to lower esophageal sphincter pressure decreased by atropine. Gastroenterology **54**, 543–551 (1968).

STEIN, G. N., FINKELSTEIN, A.: Hiatal hernia incidence and diagnosis. Amer. J. dig. Dis. **5**, 77–87 (1960).

STILSON, W. L., SANDERS, I., GARDINER, G. A., GORMAN, H. D., LODGE, D. F.: Hiatal hernia and gastroesophageal reflux. Radiology **93**, 1323–1327 (1969).

SVOBODA, A. C., KRAMER, C. M., GAMBLE, C. M., SOMMERS, S. C., MONROE, L. S.: Problems in the early diagnosis of peptic esophagitis. Gastrointest. Endosc. **13**, 14–17 (1967).

THAL, A. P., HATAFUKU, T., KURTZMAN, R.: New operation for distal esophageal stricture. Arch. Surg. **90**, 464–472 (1965).

TUTTLE, S. G., GROSSMAN, M. I.: Detection of gastroesophageal reflux by simultaneous measurement of intraluminal pressure and pH. Proc. Soc. exp. Biol. (N.Y.) **98**, 225–227 (1958).

Tuttle, S. G., Rufin, F., Bettarello, A.: The physiology of heartburn. Ann. intern. Med.
55, 292–300 (1961).

Urschel, H. C., Jr., Paulson, D. L.: Gastroesophageal reflux and hiatal hernia. J. thorac.
cardiovasc. Surg. 53, 21–32 (1967).

Vanderwelde, G. N., Carlson, H. C.: Esophageal reflux. Amer. J. Roentgenol. 92, 989–993
(1964).

Vantrappen, G., Texter, E. C., Jr., Barborka, C. J., Vandenbroucke, J.: The closing
mechanism at the gastroesophageal junction. Amer. J. Med. 28, 564–577 (1960).

Venkatachalam, B., Dacosta, L. R., Ip, S. K. L., Beck, I. T.: What is a normal esophagogastric junction? Gastroenterology 62, 521–527 (1972).

Winans, C. S.: Testing the normal gastroesophageal junction. Gastroenterology 62, 668–670
(1972).

Winkelstein, A.: Peptic esophagitis: A new clinical entity. J. Amer. med. Ass. 104, 906–908
(1935).

Winkelstein, A., Wolf, B. S., Som, M. L., Marshak, R. H.: Peptic esophagitis with duodenal or gastric ulcer. J. Amer. med. Ass. 154, 885–889 (1954).

Wolf, B. S.: The roentgen diagnosis of minimal hiatal herniation. J. Mt Sinai Hosp. 23, 90–
109 (1956).

Wolf, B. S.: The esophagogastric closing mechanism. J. Mt Sinai Hosp. 27, 404–416 (1960).

Wolf, B. S.: Roentgen features of the normal and herniated esophagogastric region. Clinical
correlations. In: Progress in gastroenterology, vol. II, ed. G. B. J. Glass, p. 288–315.
New York and London: Grune & Stratton 1970.

Wolf, B. S., Som, M., Marshak, R. H.: Short esophagus with esophagogastric or marginal
ulceration. Radiology 61, 473–495 (1953).

Lower Esophagus Lined with Columnar Epithelium

P. Heitmann

With 12 Figures

1. Historical Aspects, Definition, Incidence and Distribution

Over a long time, peptic stenoses and ulcers of the middle third of the esophagus (Fig. 247) have been considered to be the result of inflammatory shortening of this organ with ensuing displacement of a considerable portion of the stomach into the mediastinum. In 1950, Barrett pointed out that discrete ulcers of the esophagus were always surrounded by a gastric-like epithelium and thus reinforced this interpretation. In 1951, Bosher and Taylor described the presence of deep esophageal glands in the submucosa of the intrathoracic segment located below a stricture high in the esophagus. The radiological and anatomical observations of Allison and Johnstone in 1953 opened the way towards a correct

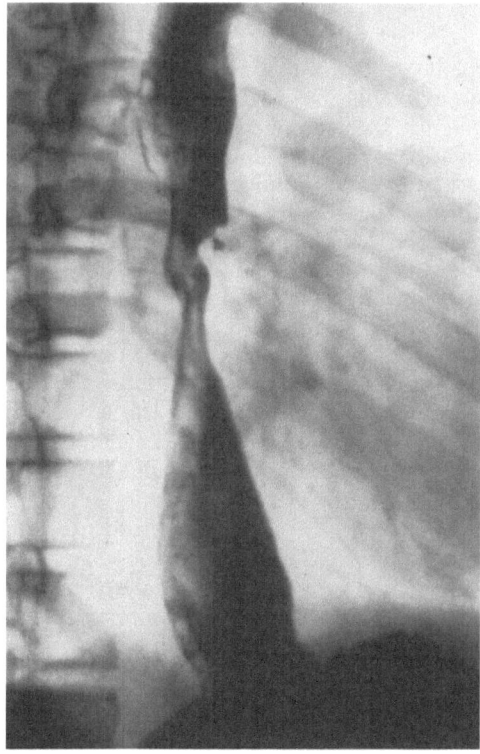

Fig. 247. Longitudinal stricture and penetrating ulcer in the middle third of the esophagus. Up to the level of the stenosis the esophagus is lined with fundic-like mucosa

interpretation of this disease. They noted that high peptic strictures and ulcers of the esophagus were always associated with a small hiatal hernia, but that the segment between the stricture and the hernia, although lined by columnar epithelium, had the vascular supply and the radiological and anatomical features of the esophagus. BARRETT agreed with this interpretation in 1957. In the same year, LORTAT-JACOB coined the term *endobrachyœsophagus* for this condition. In 1963, COHEN et al. reported on a simultaneous radiologic and intraluminal manometric study performed on a patient with this disease and they showed that the segment of esophagus lined with heterotopic columnar epithelium has the same motor behavior as the esophagus lined with squamous epithelium. HERSHFIELD et al. reported in 1965 that acid can be locally produced in the distal esophagus when this organ is lined with a fundic-like heterotopic mucosa. The pathogenesis of this interesting disease is still uncertain.

The exact incidence of this condition is unknown, but it seems to be relatively infrequent when compared with other inflammatory diseases of the esophagus. Thoroughly examined patients have been published as single case reports or in small series. However, our current knowledge about this disease lends support to the assumption that the overwhelming majority of the benign, high lying esophageal strictures of unknown etiology, as well as all the discrete, deep ulcers of the middle third of the gullet occur when this organ is lined with heterotopic columnar epithelium. The disease occurs with the same frequency in both sexes. In the majority of the patients, the first symptoms appear between the fourth and the seventh decade of life.

2. Pathologic Anatomy

The main morphologic feature is the presence of a continuous sheath of columnar epithelium extending from the stomach up to the distal or the middle third of the esophagus. The submucosa and the esophageal muscular coats show a normal structure. Blood is supplied via segmental arteries originating directly from the aorta (ALLISON and JOHNSTONE, 1953; WRIGHT, 1965). This has to be sharply differentiated from congenital ectopic gastric mucosal islands in the esophagus, which have no known relationship to this disease. These islands are frequently found in newborns and adults at the level of the pharyngo-esophageal junction. Their incidence in the middle and lower esophagus is smaller. They are always completely surrounded by squamous epithelium and have no continuity with the mucosa of the stomach (SCHRIDDE, 1904; RECTOR and CON-NERLEY, 1941; JOHNS, 1952; DE LA PAVA, PICKREN et al., 1964).

The single-layered cylindric epithelium in the esophagus shows no uniform structure. The surface is mainly formed by tall cells provided with glycoprotein inclusions and a brush border and arranged in flat villous-like structures. In the depth of the mucosa they form gland-like crypts (Fig. 248). In spite of their similarity with intestinal cells, they have no absorptive function. Some typical goblet cells are usually present. The structure is closely similar to the cardial epithelium of the stomach. However, electron microscopic studies performed by TRIER (1970) have shown that this epithelium is so typical that it can be distinguished morphologically from other epithelia of the gastrointestinal tract. Close to the cardia, the epithelium is frequently fundic-like and the mucosal glands are provided with peptic and parietal cells (Fig. 249). A true fundic mucosa occasionally lines the middle and the upper esophagus (WRIGHT, 1965; HERSH-FIELD et al., 1965; USTACH et al., 1969; HEITMANN et al., 1971; BURGESS et al., 1971). Rarely, a flat intestinal type of mucosa can be seen (DAVIDSON, 1964).

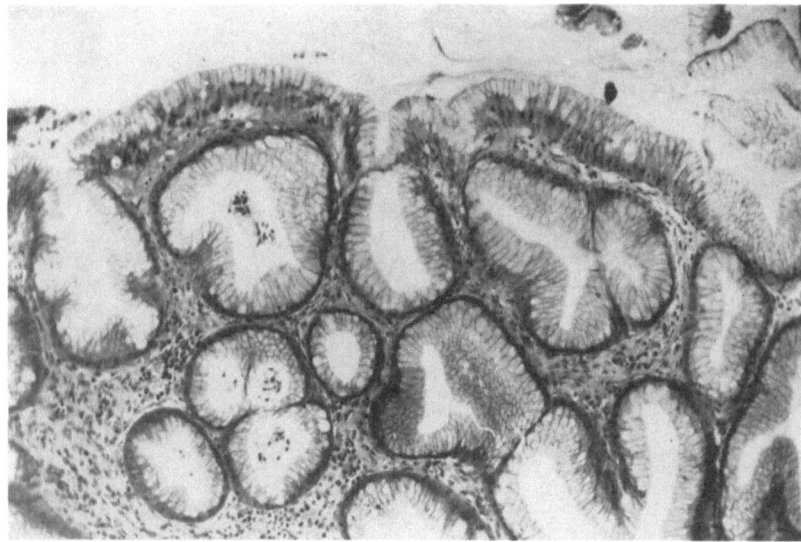

Fig. 248. Mucosal biopsy obtained immediately below a high esophageal stricture. Both the superficial layer and the glands have a structure similar to that of the cardial mucosa of the stomach

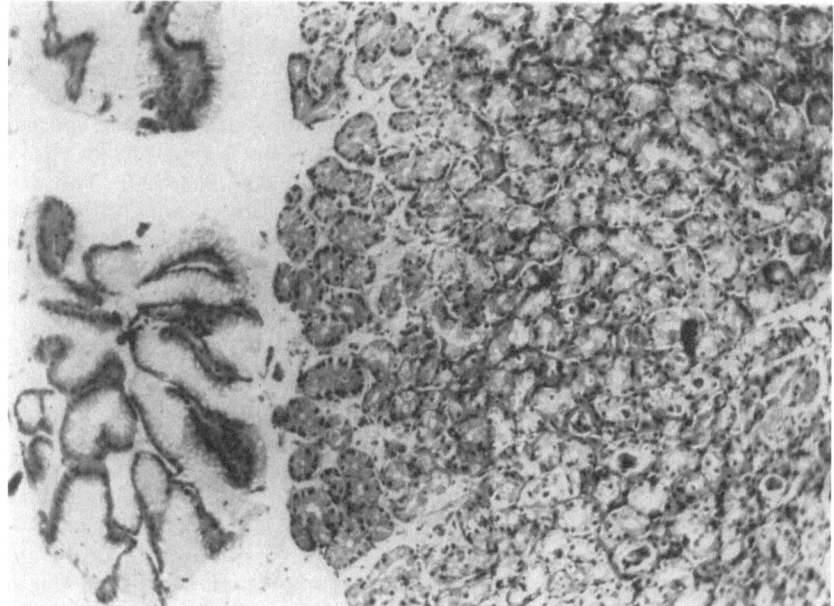

Fig. 249. Mucosal biopsy from the middle third of the esophagus of a patient with a high stricture and an esophageal ulcer. The structure is similar to that of the gastric fundus

Different types of mucosa are sometimes present along the esophagus without macroscopic transition (ABRAMS and HEATH, 1965; CORRIN et al., 1970; HEITMANN et al., 1971). The lamina propria in the distal segments of an ephagusos lined with columnar epithelium is usually normal and shows no inflammatory reaction.

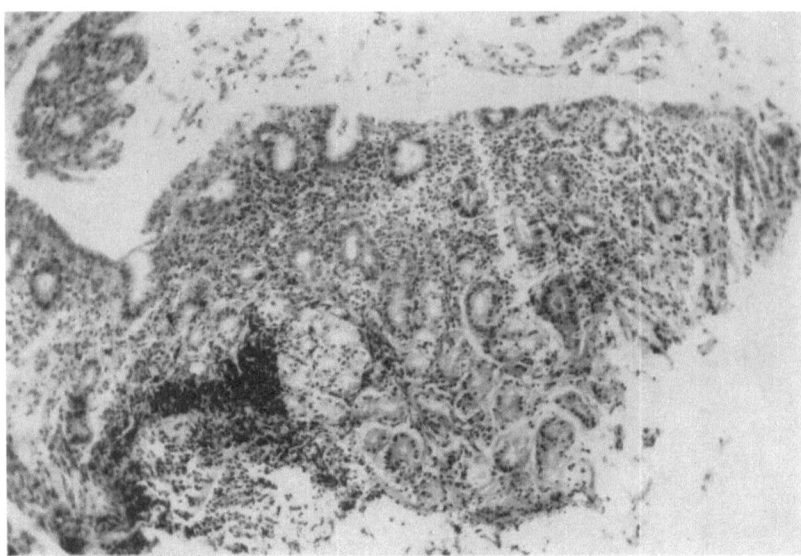

Fig. 250. Mucosal biopsy from the zone of a high esophageal stricture. The surface is ulcerated, there is an inflammatory infiltration and gland-like structures are visible in the depth

In the overwhelming majority of the patients with this disease, a peptic stricture develops in the proximal area of the columnar mucosa. This stricture is usually longitudinal and extends over a length of 1 to 4 cm. Sometimes it is short and ring-like. The transition between squamous and cylindric epithelium is proximal to it. At the level of the stenosis the mucosa is superficially ulcerated and gland-like structures remain visible in the depth (Fig. 250). The deeper layers and the periesophageal tissue are densely infiltrated with inflammatory cells; interstitial edema and vascular changes are present. The submucosa and the muscularis can be widely replaced by connective tissue and the stenotic zone usually adheres to the surrounding mediastinal structures. The adjacent lymphatic nodes are increased in size and show an inflammatory reaction. On extremely rare occasions, mainly when the esophagus is lined exclusively with cardial-like epithelium, a thin, membrane-like, stenotic ring without any inflammatory reaction originates at the level of the transition between cylindric and squamous epithelium (Heitmann et al., 1967).

One third or less of all patients develop a discrete, rounded, penetrating ulcer in the esophagus lined with columnar epithelium. It is usually located in the vicinity of the stenosis, but occasionally it may appear more distally. Its morphological features are similar to those of gastric and duodenal ulcers. It can erode greater vessels, perforate into the aorta or the mediastinum or heal with fibrous retraction.

The intensity of the inflammatory component may change in the course of time, but usually it remains unchanged for many years. However, in single cases the heterotopic epithelium has been seen to invade progressively more proximal areas of the esophagus (Goldman and Beckman, 1960; Mossberg, 1966). As it has been pointed out by Wright (1965) and by Rossetti (1966), adenocarcinomas originating in the heterotopic mucosa sometimes complicate this disease.

3. Pathophysiology

The function of the gastroesophageal junctional zone and of the esophagus lined with columnar epithelium has become better known since it has been explored by means of cineradiography, intraluminal manometry and secretory studies. Simultaneous radiographic and manometric studies have shown that the segment lined with columnar mucosa and located distally to a peptic stricture in the upper or middle third of the adult esophagus has the typical motility features of the esophagus and not those of a hiatal hernia (COHEN et al., 1963;

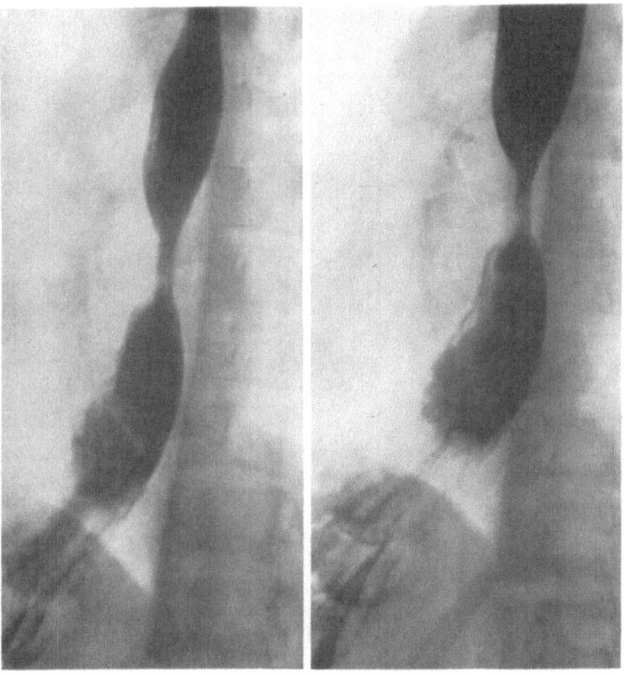

Fig. 251. Longitudinal stricture in the middle third of the esophagus. There is cardial and fundic-like mucosa at the level of the stricture and below it

HEITMANN et al., 1967; JORDAN and LONGHI, 1969; HEITMANN et al., 1971; BURGESS et al., 1971). The stricture is not located at the cardia, but in the tubular esophagus. The true gastroesophageal junction is situated as far as 12 cm below the stricture. This muscular gastroesophageal junction is displaced into the thorax due to the constant presence of a small hiatal hernia, which usually is 2 to 5 cm in length (Figs. 251–253).

It is still debated whether this constantly present hiatal hernia is important in the pathogenesis of this disease, or whether it is the consequence of some degree of longitudinal shortening of the esophagus. Gastroesophageal reflux is the distinguishing feature of some hiatal hernias. Reflux, however, is not due to the presence of a hiatal hernia, but depends mainly on the force of closure of the displaced gastroesophageal sphincter. This force of closure can be quantitated by means of intraluminal manometric studies performed with continuously infused catheters (WANKLING et al., 1965; HEITMANN et al., 1966; POPE, 1967; HEITMANN, 1969, 1970; KRAMER, 1969; COHEN and HARRIS, 1970, 1971; HADDAD,

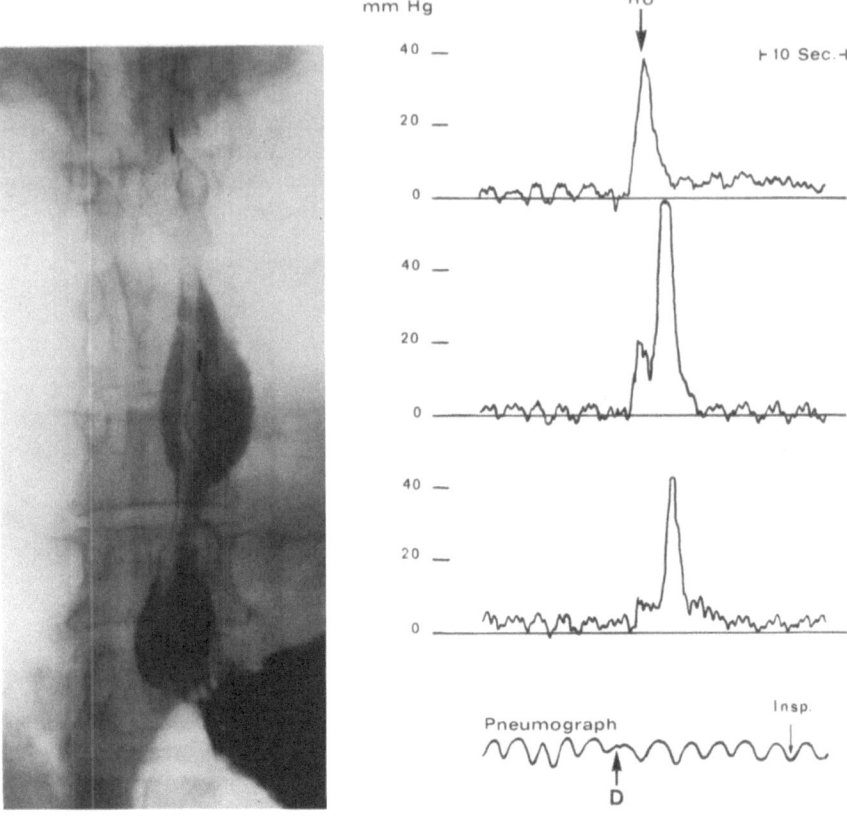

Fig. 252. Simultaneous radiographic and manometric study of a patient with findings similar to those shown in Fig. 251. Radiopaque marks indicate the points where intraluminal pressures were measured. After a swallow, a typical monophasic contraction wave, propagated downwards, appears in the body of the esophagus. The infrastenotic segment (lower mark, lower pressure tracing) exhibits a sequential contraction in spite of a fundic-like mucosal lining. (From Wienbeck et al., 1973)

1970). This type of measurements has shown that the majority of patients with strictures on top of an esophageal segment lined with columnar epithelium have a weak and incompetent gastroesophageal sphincter (Heitmann et al., 1971; Csendes and Larrain, 1972). This fact, which had been suspected earlier (Pierce and Creamer, 1963), has led to the assumption that peptic esophagitis may eventually induce a mucosal metaplasia in the distal esophagus. This has not been definitively proven. In most cases of severe, long-lasting reflux esophagitis there is no tendency for a transformation of an inflamed squamous epithelium into a cylindric type of epithelium. So far, experimental attempts to induce such a metaplasia have been unsuccessfull (van de Kerckhof and Gahagan, 1963; Hennessy et al., 1968), unless extreme and radical damage is inflicted to the junctional mucosa (Bremner et al., 1970). On the other hand it has been shown that some of these patients with heterotopic esophageal mucosa have a normal competent sphincter between the hernia and the esophagus and no radiological or manometric signs of reflux (Heitmann et al., 1967, 1970). If the lower esoph-

Histology   Motility

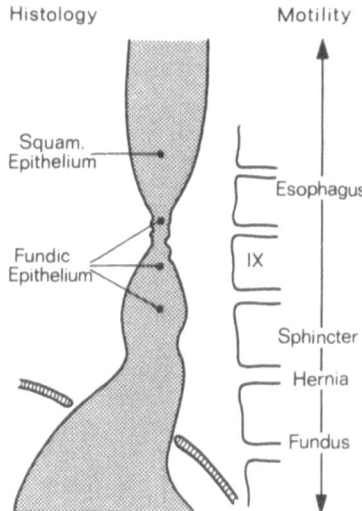

Fig. 253. Diagrammatic representation of important histologic, radiologic and manometric findings in patients with longitudinal esophageal strictures as shown on Figs. 251 and 252

agus of such patients is lined with cardial-like, non-acid-producing epithelium, there are no histological signs of esophagitis. A congenital anomaly and not an acquired metaplasia can be assumed to be present in these patients. When there is a fundic-like heterotopic mucosa in the distal esophagus, inflammatory changes which may lead to stricture formation and ulceration may develop in the absence of any detectable reflux. Local production of gastric juice (HERSHFIELD et al., 1965; USTACH et al., 1969) may be responsible for the development of these complications. Gastric secretion is normal in the majority of these patients; exceptionally it is markedly elevated. The important role of reflux for the development of strictures in the esophagus lined with columnar epithelium is suggested by the high rate of symptomatic relief and the objective improvement achieved by effective anti-reflux operative procedures (HILL et al., 1970; CSENDES and LARRAIN, 1972).

4. Symptomatology

In the absence of complications, the lower esophagus lined with columnar epithelium may be an asymptomatic condition, discovered by chance. Such cases are rare.

Symptoms are due to esophagitis and stricture formation. They appear predominantly after the fourth or fifth decade of life.

Dysphagia is the principal symptom. The sensation of food sticking behind the sternum increases in intensity in the course of months or years and then usually becomes stable. Solid foods such as meat, bread or certain fruits are most likely to cause it. The dysphagia is independent of emotional or external situations and is frequently accompanied by a painful sensation, which disappears when the retained food reaches the stomach or when it is regurgitated. Since peristaltic activity above the stricture is normal, there is no marked stasis. In the course of time, patients learn the optimal amount and consistence of food that can be swallowed with minimal difficulty and they are able to maintain an adequate nutrition. Extreme emaciation is exceptional; a complicating malignancy should be suspected in these cases. Complete dysphagia due to meat impaction can occur. Such an episode has been the first symptom in a few patients.

Heartburn is the second most frequent symptom. Usually, but not regularly, it precedes the onset of dysphagia for months or years. It is generally elicited by certain positions. Continuous heartburn with incomplete or brief relief after ingestion of antacids suggests the presence of widespread erosions or an esophageal ulcer.

Continuous gnawing, retrosternal or epigastric pain radiating into the back or the jaws which is not significantly relieved by antacids suggests the presence of a penetrating esophageal ulcer. A true periodicity or rhythmicity is not the rule. Ingestion of food exaggerates the pain, which is extremely refractory to therapy. Perforation into the mediastinum is infrequent since fibrous adhesions tend to seal the rent. The erosion of a greater vessel or of the aorta is characterized by massive brisk bleeding and regurgitation of fresh blood. Acute exsanguination may ensue. Superficial erosions of the mucosa in the region of the stricture can induce persistent occult bleeding and iron deficiency anemia.

As a whole, this is a severe and invalidating disease. Some partial spontaneous remissions may occur, but they are always short and never complete.

5. Diagnosis

The clinical history and the radiologic examination suggest the diagnosis, which is confirmed by the histologic examination of mucosal biopsy specimens taken at the level of the stricture and in the infrastenotic esophagus.

The most frequent radiologic finding in symptomatic patients is an organic stricture in the middle third of the esophagus. Usually it is 1 to 4 cm in length, the internal diameter varies between 3 and 9 mm and the normal mucosal pattern is destroyed and irregular (Figs. 247, 251). In about one third of the patients the stricture is shorter than 1 cm and looks like a broad, smooth, somewhat asymmetrical, ring-like narrowing (Fig. 254). Exceptionally, the stricture is membrane-like; in these cases it looks like a Schatzki ring in the middle or in the upper esophagus (Figs. 255, 256). The esophagus above the stenosis looks normal or slightly dilated and shows a normal peristaltic emptying. Below the stricture there is always a 2 to 12 cm long tubular segment; its wall is distensible and smooth and its mucosal pattern is similar to that of the normal esophagus in spite of the presence of columnar epithelium at this level. This segment empties itself in a peristaltic fashion. 2 to 5 cm above the hiatus it ends in a sliding hiatal hernia, which is characterized by broad mucosal folds and a passive and incomplete emptying. The transition is marked by a broad, dynamic narrowing, which represents the displaced gastroesophageal sphincteric zone (Figs. 253, 256). In some patients, this zone remains closed between swallows and prevents reflux. The majority of the patients show free reflux of barium from the stomach through the hernia into the distal esophagus. In some a discrete, deep ulcer can be seen in the region of the stricture or somewhat distal to it. The wall of the ulcer crater is smooth or only slightly irregular; a collar is usually visible (Figs. 247, 254). Endoscopically, the upper esophagus shows a normal or slightly reddened mucosa. A concentric, smooth narrowing of the lumen appears in the middle third of the esophagus, where the mucosa is swollen and bleeds easily. As far as the stenosis can be seen diffuse inflammatory changes and erosions are present. Usually the instrument cannot be passed beyond the stricture, unless the stenosis

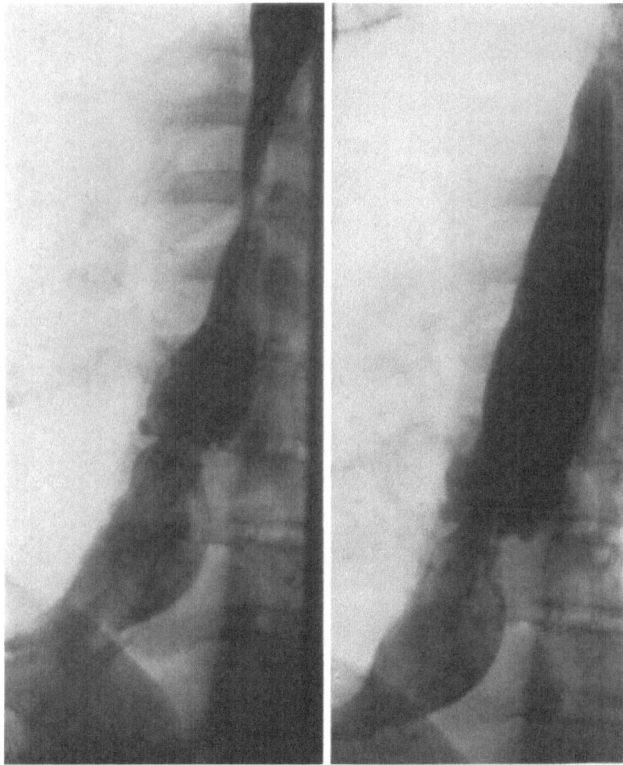

Fig. 254. Ring-like stricture and esophageal ulcer in a lower esophagus lined with fundic-like epithelium

has been dilated by bougienage. The mucosa of the substenotic segment has a normal appearance. If an ulcer is within the reach of the esophagoscope, a crater with smooth or somewhat irregular borders and a yellowish, granulating base is seen.

Biopsies of the mucosa of the upper esophagus show a normal squamous epithelium. At the level of the stricture and in its vicinity the mucosa is superficially ulcerated and gland-like structures are present in the densely infiltrated lamina propria. Biopsies from the mucosa of the infrastenotic segment can be made during esophagoscopy by means of a thin, flexible biopsy forceps or else through a suction biopsy device introduced under radioscopic control. The characteristics of the columnar epithelium at this level have been described in the chapter "Pathologic Anatomy". Multiple biopsies as well as cytologic examinations are necessary in order to exclude the presence of a carcinoma.

Intraluminal pressure measurements have contributed to a better understanding of this disease. From the diagnostic point of view, they can give information on the competence of the gastroesophageal sphincteric mechanism and manometric studies have shown that the esophageal segment lined with columnar epithelium has the typical motor behavior of the tubular esophagus. A carefully performed radiologic examination should be sufficient to provide the clinician with this information.

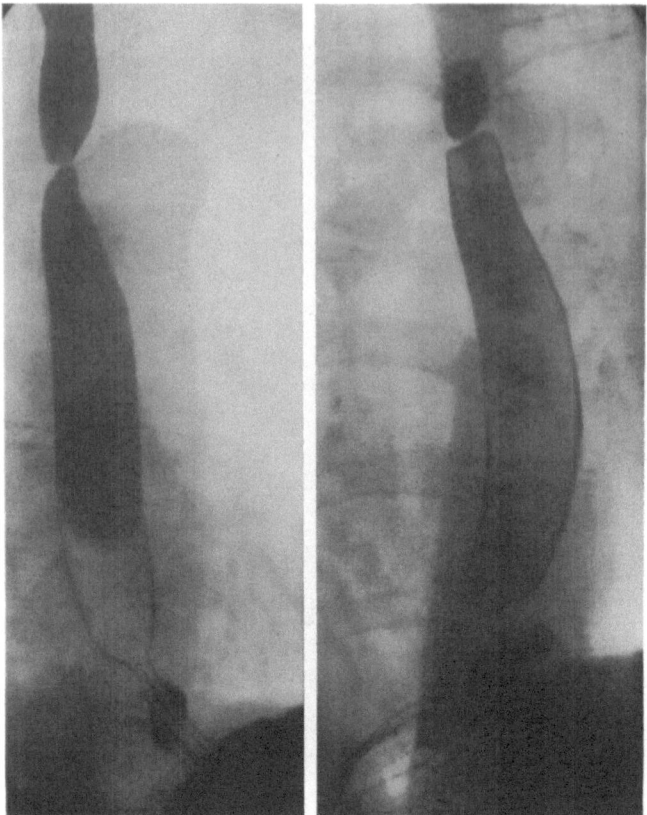

Fig. 255. Diaphragm-like narrowing of the lumen of the upper esophagus. Small hiatal hernia without reflux. The esophagus is lined with cardial-like mucosa up to the level of the ring. (From Heitmann et al., 1967)

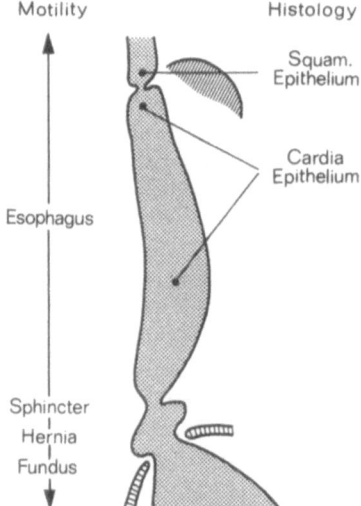

Fig. 256. Diagrammatic representation of manometric, radiologic and histologic findings in the patient's esophagus shown on Fig. 255

6. Differential Diagnosis

Esophageal strictures complicating a lower esophagus lined with columnar epithelium must be differentiated from conventional peptic stenoses complicating reflux esophagitis. The latter are located at the level of the displaced cardia. There is no tubular contractile segment between the stenosis and the hiatal

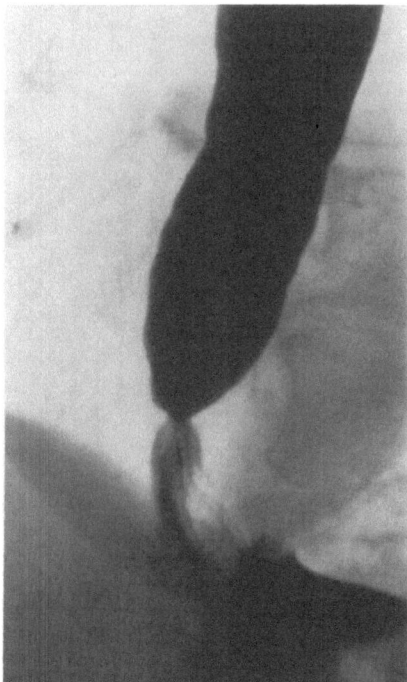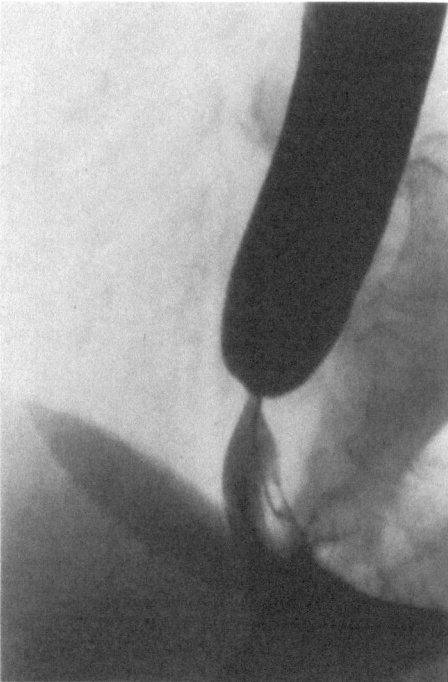

Fig. 257. Peptic stricture due to reflux esophagitis. The esophagus and the stenosis are lined with squamous epithelium. Immediately below the stricture there is a hiatal hernia with large mucosal folds

hernia. Broad gastric folds are visible immediately distal to the stenosis (Fig. 257). The stricture is lined with inflamed and superficially eroded squamous epithelium. Deep ulcers are rarely found and, when present, are at the level of the epithelial transition (WINKELSTEIN, 1935; WOLF et al., 1958; PAULSON, 1967). Esophageal stenosis following gastric resection or esophagoenterostomy as well as those complicating scleroderma of the esophagus can extend into the middle third of the gullet and give rise to difficult diagnostic problems. The differentiation of benign strictures in the middle third of the esophagus from esophageal carcinoma is of the utmost importance. Repeated biopsies and cytological examinations and in some cases even an exploratory thoracotomy have to be performed. The possibility of a complicating malignancy in the area lined with heterotopic mucosa makes repeated controls necessary. Caustic esophageal strictures rarely create differential diagnostic problems. However, esophageal strictures due to persistent vomiting or prolonged gastric intubation may present with similar radiologic features as strictures complicating heterotopic mucosal lining of the lower esophagus (Fig. 258). Important diagnostic features are that a hiatal

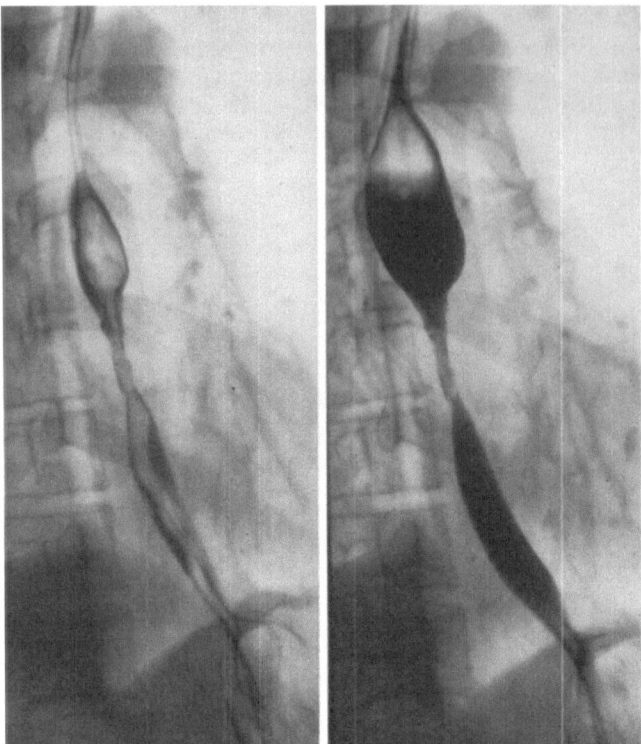

Fig. 258. Longitudinal stricture of the middle third of the esophagus, which developed after prolonged postoperative gastric intubation. The esophagus distal to the ulcerated and stenotic area is lined with squamous epithelium

hernia is not always present and that the infrastenotic esophagus is lined with squamous epithelium. Esophageal stenoses have been described which were thought to be due to Crohn's disease of the esophagus (GELFAND and KRONE, 1968; DYER et al., 1969; MADDEN et al., 1969). The histologic picture as well as the presence of typical intestinal lesions should lead to the diagnosis. Specific inflammations, extrinsic compressions and benign tumors can be recognized radiologically and endoscopically.

7. Treatment

Medical treatment appears justified in old patients, in those with mild dysphagia and in the absence of disabling complications. Symptoms can be alleviated by the intake of a soft diet, the avoidance of the horizontal position and the administration of antacids and local anesthetics or a continuous milk-alkali drip. Metoclopramide can aid in promoting gastric emptying. Anticholinergic drugs are to be avoided. This type of treatment has to be permanent. Bougienage of the stricture is often satisfactory but the result is transitory. Membrane-like rings can be mechanically dilated or ruptured.

Only surgical treatment offers permanent relief. Since gastroesophageal reflux appears to be important, an attempt should be made to effectively repair the hiatal hernia and to create a competent closing mechanism at the cardia along with pre- or peroperative bougienage (HILL et al., 1970; CSENDES and LARRAIN, 1972). A vagotomy and pyloroplasty can be performed if gastric secretion is increased. It has been repeatedly observed that after these relatively minor procedures inflammation and ulcerations heal and strictures become wider. However, if local production of acid impairs healing, or if the stricture is entirely fibrous, a resection and interposition operation has to be performed. These operations still carry a considerable morbidity and mortality.

References

ABRAMS, L., HEATH, D.: Lower oesophagus lined with intestinal and gastric epithelia. Thorax **20**, 66–72 (1965).

ALLISON, P. R., JOHNSTONE, A. S.: The oesophagus lined with gastric mucous membrane. Thorax **8**, 87–101 (1953).

BARRETT, N. R.: Chronic peptic ulcer of the oesophagus and oesophagitis. Brit. J. Surg. **38**, 175–182 (1950).

BARRETT, N. R.: The lower esophagus lined by columnar epithelium. Surgery **41**, 881–894 (1957).

BOSHER, L. H., TAYLOR, F. H.: Heterotopic gastric mucosa in the esophagus with ulceration and stricture formation. J. thorac. cardiovasc. Surg. **21**, 306–312 (1951).

BREMNER, C. G., LYNCH, V. P., ELLIS, F. H., JR.: Barrett's esophagus: congenital or acquired? An experimental study of esophageal mucosal regeneration in the dog. Surgery **68**, 209–216 (1970).

BURGESS, J. N., PAYNE, W. S., ANDERSEN, H. A., WEILAND, L. H., CARLSON, H. C.: Barrett esophagus. The columnar-epitheliallined lower esophagus. Mayo Clin. Proc. **46**, 728–734 (1971).

COHEN, B. R., WOLF, B. S., SOM, M., JANOWITZ, H. D.: Correlation of manometric, oesophagoscopic, and radiological findings in the columnar-lined gullet (Barrett syndrome). Gut **4**, 406–412 (1963).

COHEN, S., HARRIS, L. D.: Lower esophageal sphincter pressure as an index of lower esophageal sphincter strength. Gastroenterology **58**, 157–162 (1970).

COHEN, S., HARRIS, L. D.: Does hiatus hernia affect competence of the gastroesophageal sphincter? New Engl. J. Med. **284**, 1053–1056 (1971).

CORRIN, B., KENT HARRISON, G., JOHNSON, H. R. M.: High oesophageal stricture with hiatal hernia and a lower oesophagus lined by columnar epithelium. Thorax **25**, 89–90 (1970).

CSENDES, A., LARRAIN, A.: Effect of posterior gastropexy on gastroesophageal sphincter pressure and symptomatic reflux in patients with hiatal hernia. Gastroenterology **63**, 19–24 (1972).

DAVIDSON, J. S.: Ulceration of the esophagus in association with a tumor of the pancreas. J. thorac. cardiovasc. Surg. **48**, 200–204 (1964).

DE LA PAVA, S., PICKREN, J. W., ADLER, R. H.: Ectopic gastric mucosa of the esophagus. A study on histogenesis. N.Y. St. J. Med. **64**, 1831–1835 (1964).

DYER, N. H., COOK, P. L., KEMP HARPER, R. A.: Oesophageal stricture associated with Crohn's disease. Gut **10**, 549–554 (1969).

GELFAND, M. D., KRONE, C. L.: Dysphagia and esophageal ulceration in Crohn's disease. Gastroenterology **55**, 510–514 (1968).

GOLDMAN, M. C., BECKMAN, R. C.: Barrett syndrome. Case report with discussion about concepts of pathogenesis. Gastroenterology **39**, 104–110 (1960).

HADDAD, J. K.: Relation of gastroesophageal reflux to yield sphincter pressures. Gastroenterology **58**, 175–184 (1970).

HEITMANN, P.: Der gastrooesophageale Verschlußmechanismus bei Hiatusgleithernien. Internist (Berl.) **10**, 249–258 (1969).

HEITMANN, P.: Die Hiatusgleithernien mit einem hypertonischen gastro-ösophagealen Verschlußmechanismus. Dtsch. med. Wschr. **95**, 824–829 (1970).

HEITMANN, P., CSENDES, A., STRAUSZER, T.: Esophageal strictures and lower esophagus lined with columnar epithelium. Functional and morphologic studies. Amer. J. dig. Dis. **16**, 307–319 (1971).

HEITMANN, P., STRAUSZER, T., SAPUNAR, J., LARRAIN, A.: Lower esophagus lined with columnar epithelium: morphological and physiological correlation. Gastroenterology **53**, 611–624 (1967).

Heitmann, P., Wolf, B. S., Sokol, E. M., Cohen, B. R.: Simultaneous cineradiographic-manometric study of the distal esophagus: small hiatal hernias and rings. Gastroenterology 50, 737–753 (1966).

Hennessy, T. P. J., Edlich, R. F., Buchin, R. J., Tsung, M. S., Prevost, M., Wangensteen, O. H.: Influence of gastroesophageal incompetence on regeneration of esophageal mucosa. Arch. Surg. 97, 105–107 (1968).

Hershfield, N. B., Lind, J. F., Hildes, J. A., McMorris, L. S.: Secretory function of Barrett's epithelium. Gut 6, 535–539 (1965).

Hill, L. D., Gelfand, M., Bauermeister, D.: Simplified management of reflux esophagitis with stricture. Ann. Surg. 172, 638–646 (1970).

Johns, B. A. E.: Developmental changes in the oesophageal epithelium in man. J. Anat. (Lond.) 86, 431–442 (1952).

Jordan, P. H., Longhi, E. H.: Diagnosis and treatment of an esophageal stricture (ring) in a patient with Barrett's epithelium. Ann. Surg. 169, 355–363 (1969).

Kerckhof, J. van de, Gahagan, T.: Regeneration of the mucosal lining of the esophagus. Henry Ford Hosp. med. Bull. 11, 129–134 (1963).

Kramer, P.: Does a sliding hiatus hernia constitute a distinct clinical entity? Gastroenterology 57, 442–448 (1969).

Lortat-Jacob, J. L.: L'endobrachy-œsophage. Ann. Chir. 11, 1247 (1957).

Madden, J. L., Ravid, J. M., Haddad, J. R.: Regional esophagitis: a specific entity simulating Crohn's disease. Ann. Surg. 170, 351–367 (1969).

Mossberg, S. M.: The columnar-lined esophagus (Barrett syndrome)—an acquired condition? Gastroenterology 50, 671–676 (1966).

Paulson, D. L.: Benign stricture of the esophagus secondary to gastroesophageal reflux. Ann. Surg. 165, 765–776 (1967).

Pierce, J. W., Creamer, B.: The diagnosis of the columnar lined oesophagus. Clin. Radiol. 14, 64–69 (1963).

Pope, C. E., II: A dynamic test of sphincter strength: its application to the lower esophageal sphincter. Gastroenterology 52, 779–786 (1967).

Rector, L. W., Connerley, M. L.: Aberrant mucosa in the esophagus in infants and children. Arch. Path. (Chic.) 31, 285–294 (1941).

Rossetti, H.: Die Refluxkrankheit des Oesophagus. Stuttgart: Hippokrates 1966.

Schridde, H.: Über Magenschleimhautinseln vom Bau der Cardiadrüsenzone und Fundusdrüsenregion und den unteren Cardialdrüsen gleichende Drüsen im obersten Oesophagusabschnitt. Virchows Arch. path. Anat. 175, 1–16 (1904).

Trier, J. S.: Morphology of the epithelium of the distal esophagus in patients with mid-esophageal peptic strictures. Gastroenterology 58, 444–461 (1970).

Ustach, T. J., Tobon, F., Schuster, M. M.: Demonstration of acid secretion from esophageal mucosa in Barrett's ulcer. Gastrointest. Endosc. 16, 98–100 (1969).

Wankling, W. J., Warrian, W. G., Lind, J. F.: The gastroesophageal sphincter in hiatus hernia. Canad. J. Surg. 8, 61–67 (1965).

Wienbeck, M., Heitmann, P., Dombrowski, H., Schmitz-Moormann, P.: Das Barrett-Syndrom. Leber, Magen, Darm 3, 81–90 (1973).

Winkelstein, A.: Peptic esophagitis: a new clinical entity. J. Amer. med. Ass. 104, 906–909 (1935).

Wolf, B. S., Marshak, R. H., Som, M. L.: Peptic esophagitis and peptic ulceration of the esophagus. Amer. J. Roentgenol. 79, 741–759 (1958).

Wright, J. T.: Allison and Johnstone's anomaly. Amer. J. Roentgenol. 94, 308–320 (1965).

Caustic Lesions of the Esophagus

W. Pelemans and J. Hellemans

With 8 Figures

The swallowing of caustic substances causes a double therapeutical problem: the acute phase and its complications must be mastered, and care must be taken to prevent strictures and subsequent disturbances in swallowing. The way of achieving the latter is still debated although the introduction of early dilations (Salzer, 1920) and the use of antibiotics and steroids have improved the results of the preventive measures.

1. Incidence

Accidental caustic lesions occur mainly in children; in general rather small quantities are taken. At suicide attempts, which obviously occur mainly in adults or teen-agers, usually greater quantities of caustic substances are swallowed. Because strong acids immediately cause a burning pain in the mouth, acids are less frequently swallowed accidentally than alkalis, but they are used in suicide attempts.

2. Etiology

Various substances may cause caustic lesions of the esophagus: lye compounds, lysol, phenol, ammonium, potassium permanganate, acids (among others, concentrated acetic acid, sulfuric acid, hydrochloric acid), halogens, formaldehyde, clinitest tablets (NaOH), sodium hypochlorite (Clorox) and other products. Lye is the most common chemical agent implicated in chemical burns of the esophagus. Washing products, cleaners, polishers and detergents mostly contain very caustic substances. Many cleansing products used in the household incorporate sodium hydroxyde as their basic ingredient. Some products contain 8 to 50% sodium hydroxyde (Daly and Cardona, 1961) but in others the concentration may be as high as 90% (Borja et al., 1969).

3. Pathogenesis

Different factors determine the degree and the extent of the lesions: the nature of the caustic substance, its concentration, the quantity swallowed and finally the amount of time the product has come into contact with the tissues. Acids and alkalis influence tissue in a different way. Alkalis dissolve tissue and therefore penetrate more deeply. Acids cause a coagulative necrosis, a reaction which limits their penetration (Steigmann and Dolehide, 1956). In serious caustic burns from lyes it is mainly the esophagus which is affected. In burns from acids the most serious lesions may be found in the stomach (Steigmann and Dolehide, 1956). The squamous epithelium of the esophagus apparently offers more resistance to acids (Hodgson, 1959). According to Kinnman et al. (1969)

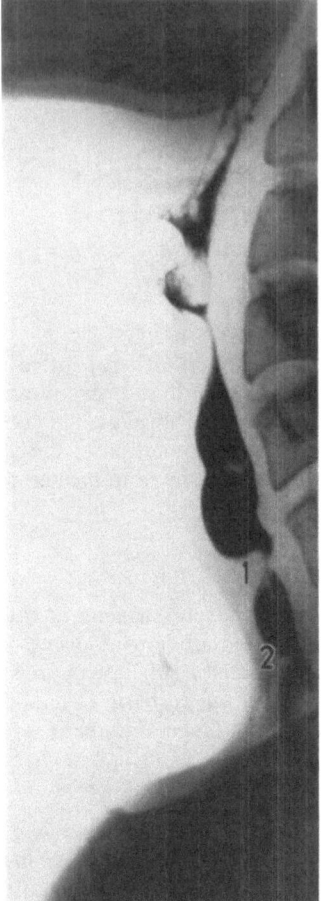 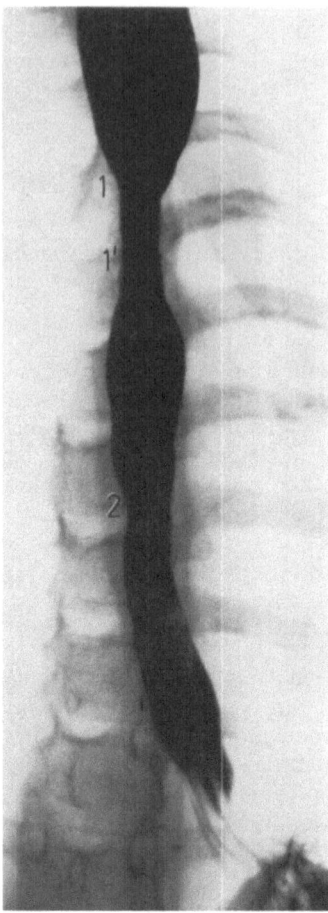

Fig. 259   Fig. 260

Fig. 259. Two short caustic stenoses in the pharyngoesophageal region (1–2). These stenoses developed after a symptom-free period of 4 months

Fig. 260. Caustic esophagitis. Moderate stenosis at the level of the left main bronchus (1—1'); a second slight narrowing (2) is seen more distally

the mortality rate of serious burns caused by acids is higher than that of burns caused by alkalis (30 and 9% resp.). In the acute stage of burns by strong acids renal damage and a serious systemic reaction must be feared.

Experiments on rats performed by Krey (1952) show that there is a clear correlation between the depth of the lesion and the concentration of the NaOH solution which was used. When a solution of 3.8% NaOH comes into contact with the esophagus for 10 sec, it causes a necrosis of the mucosa and of the submucosa which reaches the muscular layer. A concentration of 22.5% of NaOH pierces the whole esophageal wall and reaches the periesophageal tissues. The importance of these data is obvious if one remembers that cleansing products can contain up to 90% NaOH (Borja et al., 1969).

When greater quantities of caustic substances are swallowed, more extensive lesions occur and even the stomach and the duodenum are affected.

In certain parts the esophagus is narrower; passage in these parts is said to be somewhat slower so that the caustic substances are in longer contact with the underlying tissue. This would explain why the esophagus is preferentially and more heavily affected at the upper esophageal sphincter (Fig. 259), at the narrowing caused by aorta and left main bronchus (Fig. 260) and in the lower esophageal sphincter.

4. Pathology

The lesions caused by burns from lyes were studied experimentally by JOHNSON (1963). Schematically three phases must be distinguished.

4.1. The Acute Necrotic Phase

Coagulation of intracellular proteins results in cell necrosis. The living tissue surrounding the overlying area of necrosis develops intense inflammatory reactions. There is thrombosis of vessels and bacterial and hemorrhagic infiltration in the underlying layers. These lesions develop 1 to 4 days after the injury.

4.2. The Ulceration and Granulation Phase

The superficial necrotic tissue has sloughed three to five days after injury leaving an ulcerative, acutely inflamed base. Significant repair response occurs after 5 to 7 days. By the end of the first week inflammatory edema has infiltrated all layers of the esophagus and fresh granulation tissue appears at the surface. New blood vessels and fibroblasts originate during this stage. The granulation tissue fills in the defects left by sloughing, and collagenous connective tissue develops at days 10 to 12. Generally it is during this period that the esophagus is weakest.

4.3. The Phase of Cicatrization and Stricture Formation

From the beginning of the third week the collagenous connective tissue formation may begin to contract, and this results in narrowing of the esophagus. Adhesions between the granulating areas may occur with resultant pockets and bands. Muscle and nerve tissue degenerate. Ultimately the submucosa and muscular coats are replaced with a dense fibrous tissue layer. The inflammatory reaction stops after re-epithelization of the esophagus at 4 weeks to 3 months. This is the period when the most careful clinical vigilance must be maintained for signs of stricture formation. Since the epithelial and submucosal layers of severely burned areas have been sloughed off entirely there is no subsequent regeneration of the glandular and neurogenic contents of the submucosa. All these processes may permanently change the physiological behavior of the esophagus with a decrease in permeability, peristaltic movement and secretory activity.

5. Clinical Features

The clinical picture of an esophageal burn is determined by the degree and the extent of the lesions. In the initial phase the main complaints consist of pain in the mouth and in the substernal region (possibly irradiating into the epigastrium), hypersalivation, pain at swallowing and dysphagia. The presence or absence of fever seems to correlate best with the presence or absence of esophageal lesions after swallowing caustic substances (CANNON and CHANDLER, 1963). Bleeding can occur; frequently, the patient vomits. In severe cases there is shock, or the clinical picture is determined by the supervening complications.

This symptomatic phase is followed by a period of remission during which the complaints disappear. When after 2 or 3 weeks fibrosis and retraction have resulted in narrowing of the esophagus dysphagia reappears. It occurs within a month in 58% of esophageal burns leading to a stricture; after two months this number rises to 80%; if after 8 months no dysphagia occurs the development of dysphagia becomes very unlikely (1%) (Palmer, 1957).

Cho and Kinnman (1967) stress the serious systemic reaction that can occur in burns caused by strong acids. The intense stimulation by the acids can induce collapse and serious acidosis. Renal damage, especially involving the tubules, can be caused by shock and hypovolemia. The tubular function may be disturbed by resorption of toxic products from the lesions. A continuing shock can also provoke ischemic lesions in liver and heart. Important respiratory complications such as laryngospasm, larynxedema and eventually pulmonary edema may occur, especially when strong acids were aspirated into the airways.

6. Diagnosis

The history and the inspection of the oral cavity and pharynx can indicate that caustic substances were swallowed, but this does not mean that the esoph-

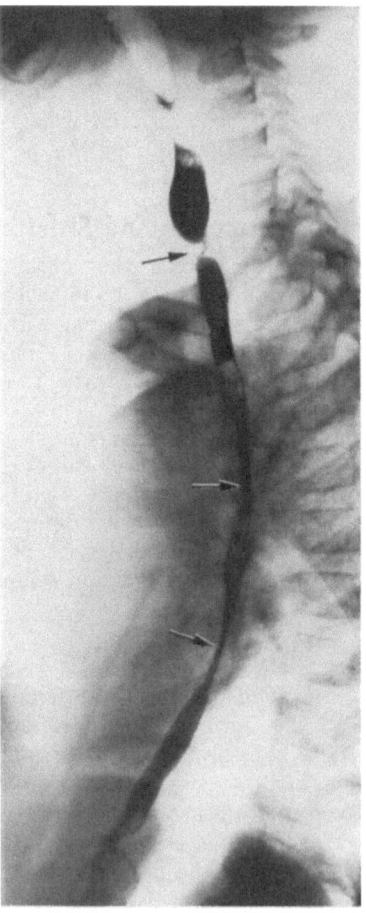

Fig. 261. Caustic esophagitis in a child, resulting in several stenotic segments (arrows)

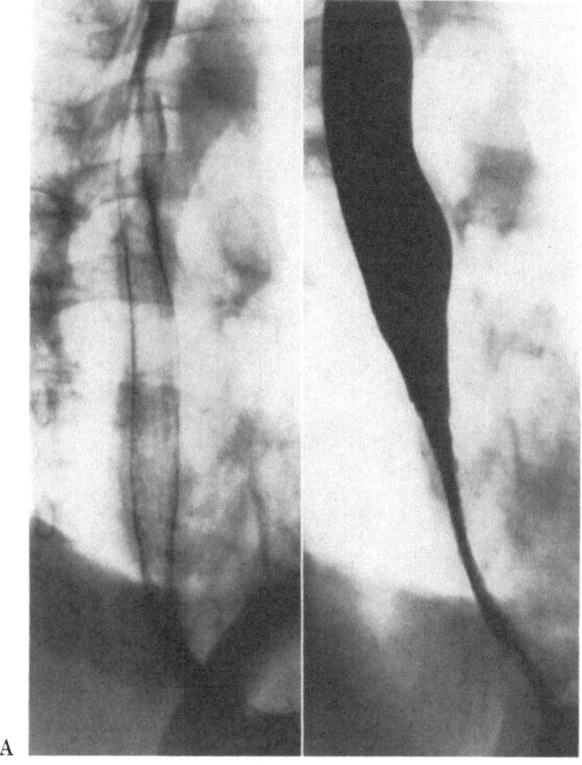

Fig. 262 A and B. Caustic esophagitis. A Abnormal mucosal pattern a few days after the burn (16/6/61). B Four months later (13/10/61) the distal esophagus is narrowed and there are still multiple ulcerations

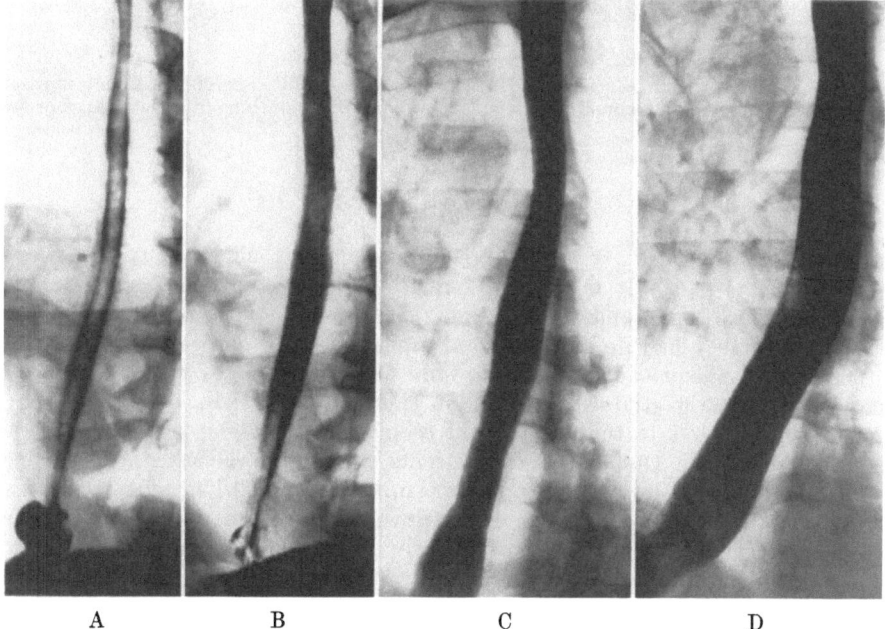

A   B   C   D

Fig. 263. A, B X-ray taken shortly after the burn. There is extensive narrowing and shortening of the esophagus with thickening of the folds. C The following day the narrowing is less severe but the borders are irregularly outlined. D Five months later the esophagus appears normal

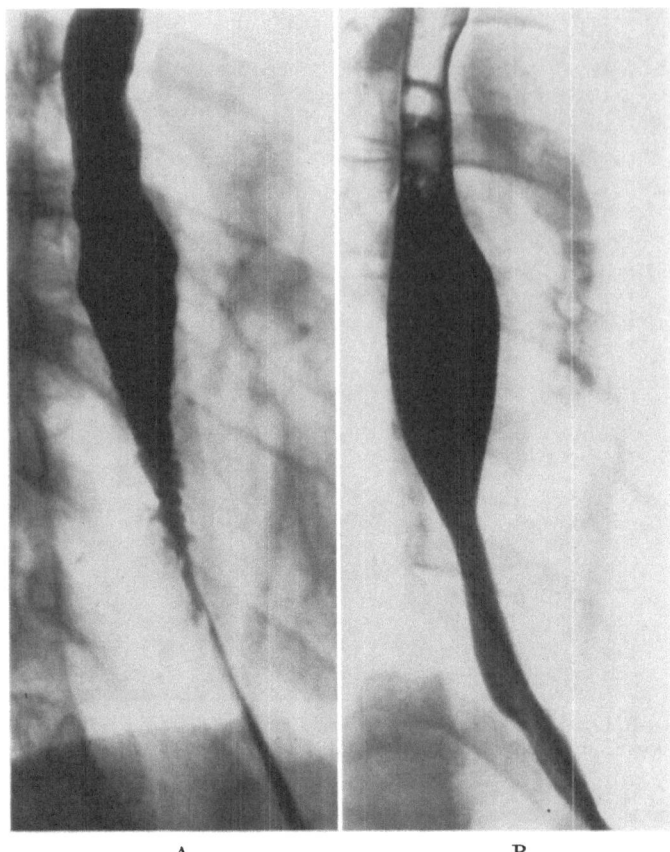

A   B

Fig. 264 A and B. Caustic stenosis in the lower esophagus. A 6/5/67: before treatment, multiple
ulcerations mimicking intramural diverticula. B 5/6/67: one month later, after treatment and
bougienage

agus has been burned. Webb et al. (1970) found in their study of 68 patients
that 26 (38%) had only burns of the mouth with no involvement of the esophagus. On the other hand, two patients had severe burns of the esophagus,
even though they had no apparent oral injuries. In the series of Bikhazi et al.
(1969) the esophagus was involved in only 56% of the cases with burns of the
oropharynx. In the study of Yarington et al. (1964) this incidence was about
25%. The latter state that in 15% of esophageal burns no lesions are found
in the oropharynx. Out of the 241 patients who swallowed caustic substances
and were evaluated by Cannon and Chandler (1963) 100 had burned only the
oropharynx. Because of the poor correlation between burns in oropharynx and
esophagus several authors advocate an early diagnostic esophagoscopy (Cannon
and Chandler, 1963; Yarington et al., 1964; Citron et al., 1968; Bikhazi
et al., 1969; Dafoe and Ross, 1969; Middelkamp et al., 1969), which allows
to establish with more certainty the presence of esophageal lesions. It also gives
some idea of the depth and the extent of the burn. Treatment can be adapted

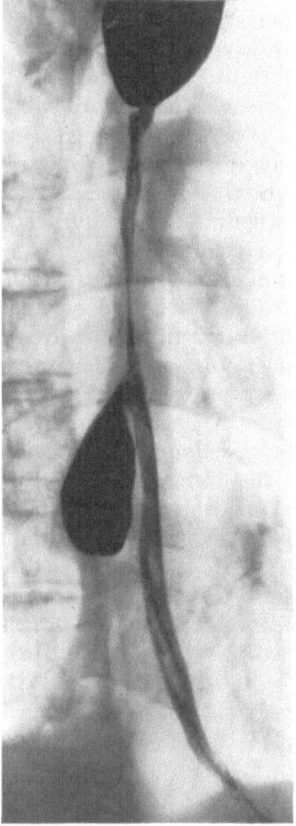

Fig. 265. Dilatation of the proximal esophagus above a narrow stenosis. In the middle third of the esophagus a large diverticular outpouching has developed

to these findings. Finally the evolution can be followed by serial esophagoscopies. The danger of this procedure, however, is instrumental perforation. Therefore it has been suggested not to introduce the endoscope beyond the proximal lesions in order to lessen the danger of perforation (CITRON et al., 1968; BIKHAZI et al., 1969; MIDDELKAMP et al., 1969). Even if esophagoscopy was negative, strictures may appear later (BIKHAZI et al., 1969) so that this method cannot be trusted blindly.

Radiographic examination, still very important for the follow-up of patients, is not suitable as a means of early diagnosis because it cannot establish with certainty the presence or absence of an esophageal burn. The early stages may be characterized by an abnormal mucosal pattern (Fig. 262A), by mucosal ulcerations or by extensive narrowing of the esophagus due to edema and "spasm" (Fig. 263A, B, C). These lesions may disappear completely (Fig. 263D) or lead to caustic stenoses which may assume different radiological appearances (Figs. 259, 260, 261, 262B). The stenosed segments frequently show signs of ulceration (Figs. 262B, 264A). Above the stenosis the esophagus may become markedly dilated: sometimes a diverticulum develops (Fig. 265).

7. Treatment

The treatment of caustic lesions of the esophagus attempts to cope both with the immediate and the late consequences of the injury. The therapeutic approach to the latter consequences has been changed markedly. Formerly one awaited the appearance of a stricture before treating it. In 1920 Salzer introduced the technique of early dilation, which was an important step toward preventive treatment. After Spain et al. had shown in 1950 that steroids have an important anti-inflammatory effect and inhibit fibrosis this medication was used in the treatment of esophageal burns.

The immediate treatment of esophageal burns consists of limiting the burning by neutralizing the swallowed products. To be effective this must be done as soon as possible, certainly within the first hour. Neutralizing lyes or other alkalis can be attempted with half-strength vinegar, lemon- or orange-juice. To neutralize acids, milk, white of egg or antacids can be used. Sodium bicarbonate is less indicated because it generates CO_2 which might increase the danger of perforation. Vomiting is potentially dangerous because it renews the contact of the caustic substance with the esophagus and can contribute to perforation if the vomiting movements are too forceful. Therefore the use of emetics is contraindicated. If necessary an urgent anti-shock treatment must be started, in which analgesia plays a very important role. A sufficient amount of fluid should be given. Broad spectrum antibiotics are immediately administered, in order to lessen the inflammatory reaction, to prevent infectious complications and to contribute to the healing of the burn. However, they do not prevent the formation of strictures (Johnson, 1963; McNeil and Welbourn, 1966). A thin non-irritating nasogastric tube is introduced from the very beginning. It allows the esophagus a partial rest. Although it does not prevent strictures to be formed, it keeps open a way for further dilations. Feeding via a nasogastric tube prevents that food particles remain in the esophagus and that these foreign bodies stimulate granulation. The tube has the disadvantage to irritate the esophagus continuously and to expose it to gastroesophageal reflux and peptic esophagitis. Some authors (Citron et al., 1968; Dafoe and Ross, 1969) prefer to leave the tube in the esophagus until complete re-epithelization has been reached; it seems better to remove it after a few days when the initial dysphagia has regressed and peroral feeding causes no more problems. If in later stages there is clinical or radiographic evidence for the development of a stricture, the patient is asked to swallow a thread to which a small latex bag, partially filled with mercury, is attached; this thread can be used as a guide for later dilations.

The prevention of stricture formation is important. Without preventive treatment 56 to 70% of the cases will develop strictures (68% according to Holinger and Johnston, 1950; 70% according to Finnerty, 1954; 56% according to Hardin, 1956).

The introduction of early dilation (Salzer, 1920) was a first steep toward the prevention of strictures. Dilation of the esophagus already from the first days after the injury aims at preserving an esophageal lumen by removing the adhesions that occur in the burned segments. When during further healing fibrosis and retraction occur the dilations attempt to prevent stricture formation and narrowing. Using this technique Daly and Cardona (1961) obtained healing with good esophageal function in 82% of their cases. In 1960 Appelberg published a series of 342 esophageal burnings treated with early dilations, complimented with intensive bougienage if stricture occurred. The results were evaluated in

250 patients and were found to be good in 236 of them. Follow-up studies of 111 cases showed that 96 patients had only minor radiological sequels, an observation which was confirmed endoscopically in 80 of them.

Several variants of this method are currently used. The type of dilator, the frequency of the dilations and the total duration of the treatment vary from one author to another. If one wants to use preventive dilations they are always started before any sign of stricture formation occurs. Some already start them the day after the injury, others wait until a week later, or until the patient is free from fever. The frequency of the dilations is progressively decreased.

Bougienage is not very comfortable for the patient and traumatizes the esophagus. APPELBERG (1960) reports 16 esophageal perforations, two of which were fatal, 1 gastric perforation and 4 esophageal bleedings. There are experimental data indicating that repeated dilations increase fibrosis because they always inflict new traumata (KNOX et al., 1967).

After SPAIN et al. (1950) showed experimentally that steroids inhibit inflammatory reaction and fibrosis in mice, this medication was used both experimentally and clinically for the treatment of esophageal burns. In experiments on dogs and rats steroids effectively limited fibrosis (ROSENBERG et al., 1951, 1953; JOHNSON, 1963; HALLER and BACHMAN, 1964; McNEIL and WELBOURN, 1966; KNOX et al., 1967). Only BYRNE et al. (1962) could not confirm this observation. Infectious complications occurred more frequently if steroids were used without antibiotics (ROSENBERG et al., 1951, 1953; HALLER and BACHMAN, 1964). If during treatment with steroids strictures did occur, they were less rigid (JOHNSON, 1963). This treatment had to be started as soon as possible in order to achieve the greatest effectiveness. The study of JOHNSON (1963), however, suggests that strictures can still be prevented, or at least be made less serious, if steroid treatment is started after 48 hours or even after 4 to 7 days. On stopping the administration of steroids further maturation of the cicatricial tissue and stricture formation may occur (JOHNSON, 1963).

No agreement has been reached as yet about dosage and duration of this treatment. In recent years (MIDDELKAMP et al., 1969; HALLER and ANDREWS, 1970; WEBB et al., 1970), very high initial doses have been used, from 100 mg of prednisone per day (or equivalent quantities of other steroids) up to 2–3 mg/kg/day. This dosage is then tapered off progressively. The total duration of this steroid treatment depends on the severity of the esophageal burns. Steroids are given until the re-epithelization stage has been reached (JOHNSON, 1963; DAFOE and ROSS, 1969). According to DAFOE and ROSS (1969), mild burns should be treated for one month, moderately severe burns for 6 to 8 weeks, and severe burns for 3 months. The general contraindications of steroids remain valid; perforation is an absolute contraindication.

A compilation of several studies (MILLER and WARREN, 1959; DALY and CARDONA, 1961; CANNON and CHANDLER, 1963; EGAN, 1969; BIKHAZI et al., 1969; BORJA et al., 1969; MIDDELKAMP et al., 1969; WEBB et al., 1970) indicates that 37 out of 233 cases developed strictures during treatment with antibiotics and steroids (16%). This figure agrees with the experience of HALLER et al. (1971); in a group of 69 children with esophageal burns proved by esophagoscopy 8 (12%) developed strictures under treatment with antibiotics and steroids. Although the therapeutic results have been improved by steroids, the studies of WEBB et al. (1970), of MIDDELKAMP et al. (1969) and the observations of CANNON and CHANDLER (1963) show that this preventive measure remains insufficient, especially in severe esophageal burns.

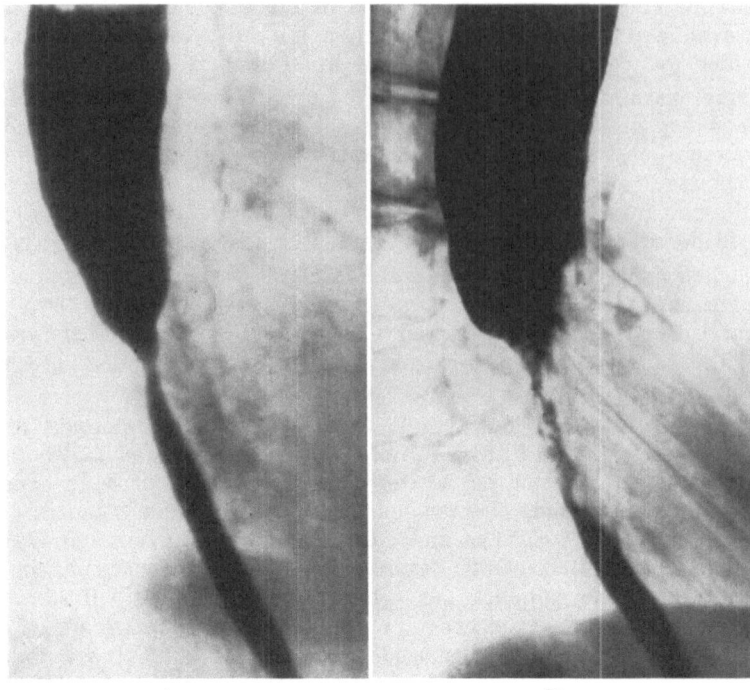

A   B

Fig. 266 A and B. Development of carcinoma in a case of caustic stricture. A 10/8/66: stenosis with benign aspect. B 10/3/72: Irregular filling defect in the stenosed segment due to squamous cell carcinoma

Finally the treatment with steroids can be combined with early dilations. The two approaches complement each other. The administration of steroids prevents fibrosis, while dilations model the esophagus by preventing or removing adhesions and by guiding the retraction of already existing fibrosis. However, the experimental and clinical data do not allow as yet definite conclusions. Knox et al. (1967) found that this combination was favorable in dogs: the evolution of the scarring was slower, dilations met with less resistance and did not have to be repeated as frequently. Haller and Bachman (1964), however, could not diminish the incidence of stricture formation in cats by adding early dilations to the treatment.

To summarize, the basic steps of the treatment are:

1. Immediate neutralization of the caustic substance.

2. Early esophagoscopy to confirm the existence of esophageal burns and to allow an estimate of the degree and the extent of the lesion.

3. Introduction of a stomach tube as soon as possible after the accident. The duration of the intubation varies from a few days to several weeks depending on the severity of the burn and the belief of the author in the effectiveness of this measure.

4. Immediate steroid and antibiotic therapy, eventually complimented by antishock therapy.

5. Especially during the initial period the patient must be watched carefully for the occurrence of disturbances in breathing and a tracheotomy may have to be performed.

6. Careful serial evaluation of the esophagus to detect early stricture formation.

7. Immediate and continuing dilation if stenosis begins.

In the later follow-up of patients with an esophageal burn one must keep in mind that a stricture can develop several months after the injury (Fig. 259). Many authors indicate that caustic lesions of the esophagus predispose to the later development of esophageal carcinoma (ALVAREZ and COLBERT, 1963; GROS-DIDIER et al., 1969; LANSING et al., 1969) (Fig. 266). Therefore, regular control of the patients remains indicated.

If in spite of preventive measures a stricture does occur or if a patient seeks medical advice with an already existing stricture, dilations should be preferred over surgical intervention if at all possible.

References

ALVAREZ, A. F., COLBERT, J. G.: Lye stricture of the esophagus complicated by carcinoma. Canad. J. Surg. 6, 470–476 (1963).

APPELBERG, H. R.: Corrosive burns of the esophagus and their treatment. Acta oto-laryng. (Stockh.) 158, 138–143 (1960).

BIKHAZI, H. B., THOMPSON, E. R., SHUMRICK, D. A.: Caustic ingestion: current status. A report of 105 cases. Arch. Otolaryng. (Chic.) 89, 770–773 (1969).

BORJA, A. R., RANSDELL, H. T., THOMAS, T. V., JOHNSON, W.: Lye injuries of the esophagus. Analysis of ninety cases of lye ingestion. J. thorac. cardiovasc. Surg. 57, 533–538 (1969).

BYRNE, W. D., SAMSON, P. C., DUGAN, D. J., NOEL, S. M., MAY, I. A.: Experimental lye burns of the esophagus in dogs: the effects of steroid administration. Surg. Forum 13, 254–256 (1962).

CANNON, S., CHANDLER, J. R.: Corrosive burns of the esophagus; analysis of one hundred patients. E.E.N.T. Monthly 42, 35–44 (1963).

CHO, K. J., KINNMAN, J. E. G.: Management of acid intoxication. J. Laryng. 81, 533–549 (1967).

CITRON, B. P., PINCUS, I. J., GEOKAS, M. C., HAVERBACK, B. J.: Chemical trauma of the esophagus and stomach. Surg. Clin. N. Amer. 48, 1303–1311 (1968).

DAFOE, C. S., ROSS, C. A.: Acute corrosive œsophagitis. Thorax 24, 291–294 (1969).

DALY, J. F., CARDONA, J. C.: Acute corrosive esophagitis. Arch. Otolaryng. (Chic.) 74, 629–634 (1961).

EGAN, R. S.: Corrosive esophagitis. A review of therapy. Northw. Med. (Seattle) 68, 1007–1009 (1969).

FINNERTY, J. J.: The late treatment of caustic strictures of the esophagus. Surg. Clin. N. Amer. 34, 353–361 (1954).

GROSDIDIER, J., ROBERT, D., WATELET, F., PARIETTI, R.: Cancer sur cicatrice de sténose caustique de l'œsophage datant de l'enfance. Sem. Hôp. Paris 41, 2512—2513 (1969).

HALLER, A., ANDREWS, H. G.: Pathophysiology and management of acute corrosive burns of the esophagus. Mod. Treatm. 7, 1182–1189 (1970).

HALLER, J. A., ANDREWS, H. G., WHITE, J. J., TAMER, M. A., CLEVELAND, W. W.: Patho-physiology and management of acute corrosive burns of the esophagus: results of treatment in 285 children. J. pediat. Surg. 6, 578–584 (1971).

HALLER, J. A., BACHMAN, K.: The comparative effect of current therapy on experimental caustic burns of the esophagus. Pediatrics 34, 236–245 (1964).

HARDIN, J. C.: Caustic burns of the esophagus. A ten-year analysis. Amer. J. Surg. 91, 742–748 (1956).

HODGSON, J. H.: Corrosive stricture of the stomach. Brit. J. Surg. 46, 358–361 (1959).

HOLINGER, P. H., JOHNSTON, K. C.: Caustic strictures of the esophagus. Illinois med. J. 98, 246–250 (1950).

JOHNSON, E. E.: A study of corrosive esophagitis. Laryngoscope (St. Louis) 73, 1651–1696 (1963).

KINNMAN, J. E. G., LEE, B. C., LEE, C. W., SHIN, H. I.: Management of severe lye corrosions of the oesophagus. J. Laryng. 83, 899–910 (1969).

Knox, W. G., Scott, J. R., Zintel, H. A., Guthrie, R., McCabe, R. E.: Bouginage and steroids used singly or in combination in experimental corrosive esophagitis. Ann. Surg. **166**, 930–941 (1967).

Krey, H.: On the treatment of corrosive lesions in the oesophagus. Acta oto-laryng. (Stockh.), Suppl. **102**, 1–49 (1952).

Lansing, P. B., Ferrante, W. A., Ochsner, J. L.: Carcinoma of the esophagus at the site of lye stricture. Amer. J. Surg. **118**, 108–111 (1969).

McNeil, R. A., and R. B. Welbourn: Prevention of corrosive stricture of the esophagus in the rat. J. Laryng. **80**, 346–358 (1966).

Middelkamp, J. N., Ferguson, T. B., Roper, C. L., Hoffman, F. D.: The management and problems of caustic burns in children. J. thorac. cardiovasc. Surg. **57**, 341–347 (1969).

Miller, C. L., Warren, R. O. Y.: Steroid treatment of lye burns of the esophagus. J. Amer. med. Ass. **170**, 1525–1527 (1959).

Palmer, E. D.: The esophagus and its diseases. New York: Paul B. Hoeber, Inc. 1957.

Rosenberg, N., Kunderman, P. J., Vroman, L., Moolten, S. E.: Prevention of experimental lye strictures of the esophagus by cortisone. Arch. Surg. **63**, 147–151 (1951).

Rosenberg, N., Kunderman, P. J., Vroman, L., Moolten, S. E.: Prevention of experimental esophageal stricture by cortisone. Arch. Surg. **66**, 593–598 (1953).

Salzer, H.: Frühbehandlung der Speiseröhrenverätzung. Wien. klin. Wschr. **33**, 307 (1920).

Spain, D. M., Molomut, N., Haber, A.: Biological studies on cortisone in mice. Science **112**, 335–337 (1950).

Steigmann, F., Dolehide, R. A.: Corrosive (acid) gastritis. New Engl. J. Med. **254**, 981–986 (1956).

Webb, W. R., Koutras, P., Ecker, R. R., Sugg, W. L.: An evaluation of steroids and antibiotics in caustic burns of the esophagus. Ann. thorac. Surg. **9**, 95–102 (1970).

Yarington, C. T., Bales, G. A., Frazer, J. P.: A study of the management of caustic esophageal trauma. Ann. Otol. (St. Louis) **73**, 1130–1135 (1964).

Acute Infectious Disease

W. Pelemans and G. Vantrappen

Acute infectious esophagitis can be divided in two distinct entities: primary suppurative esophagitis and esophagitis accompanying infectious diseases.

1. Suppurative Esophagitis

Suppurative esophagitis may develop as a complication of any condition interrupting the continuity of the esophageal mucosa and allowing pathogenic bacteria to penetrate into the esophageal wall. Traumatic lesions, produced by infected foreign bodies or instruments are probably an important cause of suppurative esophagitis (see also Foreign Bodies).

A suppurative infection of the esophagus may remain circumscribed and develop into one or, more rarely, into multiple submucosal abscesses, which tend to heal by draining into the lumen. However, the infection may also spread and lead to a phlegmon of the esophagus, involve the periesophageal tissue and the mediastinum, and form a fistula with adjacent cavities (TERRACOL, 1951).

Suppurative esophagitis produces rather severe symptoms including spontaneous substernal and/or cervical pain, dysphagia and pain on swallowing. If it is very extensive it will affect the general condition of the patient, with fever and general malaise.

Whereas the prognosis of an esophageal abscess is mostly favorable, as it often drains into the lumen, the phlegmonic involvement of the esophagus is often fatal. Adequate treatment of the esophageal trauma and antibiotics are the most important measures to prevent the development of suppurative complications. Indeed, the extensive use of antibiotics has made this complication of esophageal lesions exceptional. If necessary, an esophageal abscess may be drained endoscopically; an extensive suppurative esophagitis may require surgical drainage. Appropriate antibiotics are always indicated.

2. Esophagitis Secondary to Infectious Disease

Esophagitis may also be secondary to infectious diseases. Infections of the upper respiratory tract and influenza may involve the esophagus, and cause dysphagia. In an autopsy study of 601 cases of microscopic esophageal ulcerations, MOSES and CHEATHAM (1963) found indications of a viral etiology (intranuclear inclusions in the epithelial cells adjacent to the ulcerative lesions) in 2% of the cases. FINGERLAND et al. (1952) isolated the herpes virus from similar lesions. Herpetic esophagitis appears to be asymptomatic and frequently associated with malignancy (BERG, 1955; MOSES and CHEATHAM, 1963). It may occur even without other herpes localizations.

Exanthematous infectious diseases, such as measles and scarlet fever may involve the esophagus. In the course of scarlet fever a focal necrosis may develop in the esophagus, associated with ulcerations, edema and pseudomembranous

exudate. Phlegmonic esophagitis due to streptococcic infection is more exceptional, but may lead to esophageal perforation (Palmer, 1963). Necrotic ulcerations in pharynx and esophagus associated with measles have been described
by Rusza (1963).

Diphtheria may spread into the esophagus with lesions identical to those
in the throat (Palmer, 1963). However, the swallowing difficulties which occur
not infrequently in the course of diphtheria are more often caused by paralysis
of the pharyngeal muscles than by this form of esophagitis.

Together with the skin lesions of smallpox, an enanthema may develop in
the mucosa of the eyes and of the respiratory, gastrointestinal and genitourinaty
tract. The mucosa is edematous and shows erythematous spots; later blisters
develop which ulcerate rapidly. These mucosal lesions are the cause of the dysphagia and the dysphonia which sometimes are associated with smallpox (Bonnenfant, 1965).

Esophagitis accompanies typhoid fever (Varay, 1966) and severe infections
such as peritonitis, pneumonia and pyelonephritis in rare cases.

References

Berg, J. W.: Esophageal herpes; a complication of cancer therapy. Cancer (Philad.) 8, 731–
740 (1955).
Bonnenfant, F.: La variole. In: Maladies infectieuses, ed. P. Milliez, and F. Bonnenfant,
p. 807–826. Paris: Editions Médicales Flammarion 1966.
Fingerland, A., Vortel, V., Endrys, J.: Oesophagitis herpetica. Čas. Lék. česk. 91, 473–475
(1952). Cit. from author's English abstract.
Moses, H. L., Cheatham, W. J.: The frequency and significance of human herpetic esophagitis.
An autopsy study. Lab. Invest. 12, 663–669 (1963).
Palmer, E. D.: Clinical gastroenterology, second ed. New York: Hoeber 1963.
Ruzsa, G.: Gangrenous ulcerations in the pharynx and esophagus associated with measles.
Gyermekgyogyaszat 14, 374–376 (1963).
Terracol, J.: Les maladies de l'œsophage, 2⁰ éd. Paris: Masson & Cie. 1951.
Varay, A.: Précis de gastro-entérologie. Paris: Masson & Cie. 1966.

Tuberculosis of the Esophagus

W. Pelemans and J. Hellemans

1. Incidence

Tuberculosis of the esophagus is a rare disease. In autopsy series of patients dying from tuberculosis, the incidence varies from 0.04 to 0.2% (Lockard, 1913; Hlavacek, 1960). Calvet et al. (1961) observed one case among 36000 patients with pulmonary tuberculosis. Wexels (1954), in a review of the literature, encountered reports on 125 cases and Chung-Seh-Tung (1962) collected 150 cases of esophageal tuberculosis from the literature.

2. Pathogenesis

Although Audouin and Poulain (1950), Baron et al. (1961) and Fahmy et al. (1969) each reported a case of apparently primary esophageal involvement, tuberculosis of the esophagus is almost always secondary to other localizations. In cases of secondary esophageal involvement, the infection can reach the esophagus by several routes. In a patient with pulmonary tuberculosis it can be transferred via swallowed sputum, especially when he is undernourished, when there is stasis of food in the gullet, or when pre-existing esophageal lesions have destroyed the integrity of the esophageal mucous membrane. A tuberculous pharyngitis may descend into the gullet. Tuberculosis of the lung and of mediastinal lymph nodes and Pott's disease of the spine may lead to direct secondary invasion of the esophagus (Maillet, 1960; Roget et al., 1960; Lunel et al., 1963; Montandon, 1964; Hötter, 1965; Flabeau et al., 1968; Dieu and Adenis-Lamarre, 1971). Retrograde lymphatic spread from the lymph nodes around trachea, carina and bronchi has also been reported (Fahmy et al., 1969). Finally, hematogenous dissemination can occur in miliary tuberculosis but usually goes undetected.

3. Pathology

Tuberculosis of the esophagus, as of other parts of the gastrointestinal tract, can assume 3 different forms. The hypertrophic form is comparable with hypertrophic ileocecal tuberculosis, and appears as a stenosing tumor. The ulcerative type is characterized by the presence of solitary or multiple ulcers, which do not differ from tuberculous ulcerations elsewhere in the body. In the rare, granular form, the lesion is greyish in color and has a velvety appearance.

Tuberculosis of mediastinal lymph nodes may lead to esophageal fistula formation or to the development of traction diverticula in the middle third of the esophagus.

4. Clinical Features

Esophageal tuberculosis may remain asymptomatic; autopsy of patients with pulmonary tuberculosis occasionally reveals an unsuspected esophageal involvement. Traction diverticula also usually do not give rise to complaints. When esophageal symptoms occur, they are generally preceded by symptoms of other tuberculous localizations. Progressive dysphagia in a patient with pulmonary tuberculosis may be due to tuberculosis of the gullet. Ulcerative tuberculosis is frequently associated with pain in the throat and behind the sternum. This pain is mostly continuous and increases during swallowing. Coughing spells while eating or drinking suggest spill-over into the trachea or a tracheo(broncho)-esophageal fistula. An esophageal fistula can occasionally cause hematemesis (Montandon, 1964; Flabeau et al., 1968). Recurrent nerve paralysis is rare (Calvet et al., 1961).

5. Diagnosis

The development of painful dysphagia in a patient with established tuberculosis suggests the diagnosis. Radiological examination may reveal a narrowing of the esophageal lumen, ulcerations, an irregular outline of the esophagus due to periesophageal adhesions or compression by mediastinal lymph nodes. These signs, however, are all atypical (Lüdin, 1947). Although esophagoscopy can reveal an ulcerative or tumorous process or the orifice of an esophageal fistula, biopsy is necessary to establish the diagnosis. Finally, an attempt should be made to confirm the diagnosis by means of a culture, and to determine sensitivity to antibiotics.

6. Complications

Esophageal tuberculosis may entail several complications, such as traction diverticula, esophageal obstruction, recurrent nerve paralysis (Calvet et al., 1961) and fistulas between esophagus and bronchi (Montandon, 1964), esophagus and pleural cavity (Warembourg et al., 1959), esophagus and vena cava superior and between esophagus and aorta (Lahl, 1964; Lim Cheng Hong and Sugai, 1965).

7. Prognosis

The prognosis of esophageal tuberculosis is determined by the extent of the tuberculous infection and by the patient's response to treatment with tuberculostatics. In case of pulmonary tuberculosis with several cavities, invasion of the esophagus may be a fatal complication. With adequate treatment less extensive lesions can heal completely. Certain lesions, such as ganglioesophageal tuberculosis, can even heal spontaneously and leave only a small traction diverticulum.

8. Treatment

Treatment with tuberculostatics is indicated in all cases of esophageal tuberculosis. The ulcerative type usually will heal rapidly and completely. In cases of hypertrophic tuberculosis this therapy may not be sufficient because the esophageal obstruction may necessitate surgical intervention (Fahmy et al., 1969; Eckmann, 1969) especially if no other localizations are present. Dilatations may be necessary when stenosis develops. A fistula between esophagus and airways is usually an indication for surgical treatment.

References

AUDOUIN, J., POULAIN, J.: Tuberculose sténosante de l'œsophage, d'apparence primitive, guérie par l'œsophagectomie. Arch. franç. Mal. Appar. dig. **39**, 231–236 (1950).

BARON, F., VENISSE, C., LEGAL, G.: A propos d'un cas de tuberculose primitive de l'œsophage. Ann. Oto-laryng. (Paris) **78**, 142–145 (1961).

CALVET, J., COLL, J., SON-QUI: Tuberculose de l'œsophage révélée par une paralysie récurentielle droite. Ann. Oto-laryng. (Paris) **78**, 154–157 (1961).

CHUNG-SEH-TUNG, R. C.: Contribution à l'étude de la tuberculose de l'œsophage. Thése, Paris: Ed. Germain, 1962.

DIEU, J.-C., ADENIS-LAMARRE, F.: Les complications œsophagiennes de la tuberculose initiale. A propos de 20 cas. Pédiatrie **26**, 783–784 (1971).

ECKMANN, L.: Intramurales stenosierendes Tuberkulom des Ösophagus. Schweiz. med. Wschr. **99**, 538–539 (1969).

FAHMY, A. R., GUINDI, R., FARID, A.: Tuberculosis of the oesophagus. Thorax **24**, 254–256 (1969).

FLABEAU, F., LEPERCHEY, F., TERQUEM, J., SCEMAMA, P., ALNOT, J. Y.: Fistule tuberculeuse ganglio-œsophagienne révélée par des hématémèses. Mém. Acad. Chir. (Paris) **94**, 448–451 (1968).

HLAVACEK, V.: Deux cas de tuberculose de l'œsophage. Ann. Oto-laryng. (Paris) **77**, 196–202 (1960).

HÖTTER, G. J.: Tuberkulöse Ösophagus-Halslymphknotenfistel. Prax. Pneumol. **19**, 344–346 (1965).

LAHL, R.: Aortenbronchialfistel als tödliche Komplikation einer Lymphknotentuberkulose. Prax. Pneumol. **18**, 738–746 (1964).

LIM CHENG HONG, SUGAI, K.: Tuberculous aortic-oesophageal fistula. Report of a case. Singapore med. J. **6**, 164–167 (1965).

LOCKARD, L. B.: Esophageal tuberculosis: a critical review. Laryngoscope (St. Louis) **23**, 561–584 (1913).

LÜDIN, M.: Röntgenbefunde bei Oesophagustuberkulose. Schweiz. Z. Tuberk. **4**, 267–272 (1947).

LUNEL, J., NATALI, R., CHUNG-SEH-TUNG, R. C.: Tuberculose de l'œsophage d'allure primitive par fistule ganglio-œsophagienne. Genése des diverticules œophagiens épibronchiques. Arch. franç. Mal. Appar. dig. **52**, 530–538 (1963).

MAILLET, P.: Sténose œsophagienne consécutive au mal de Pott. Lyon chir. **56**, 924–926 (1960).

MONTANDON, A.: A propos de la tuberculose de l'œsophage. Fistule ganglio-broncho-œsophagienne. Ann. Oto-laryng. (Paris) **81**, 177–180 (1964).

ROGET, J., JAUDEL, J., BEAUDOING, A., VALOIS, J., GILBERT, Y.: Hématémèse révélatrice d'un diverticule ,,aortico-bronchique'' de l'œsophage chez un enfant de 11 ans. Rôle probable d'une fistulisation ganglionnaire tuberculeuse. Pédiatrie **15**, 190–192 (1960).

WAREMBOURG, H., DELACROIX, R., PAUCHANT, M., SERGENT, Y. H.: Fistule œsophagopleurale après pneumectomie pour tuberculose; guérison par plastie préthoracique. Arch. franç Mal. Appar. dig. **48**, 1772–1773 (1959).

WEXELS, P.: Tuberculosis of the esophagus. Acta tuberc. scand. **29**, 211–213 (1954).

Syphilis of the Esophagus

W. PELEMANS and G. VANTRAPPEN

1. Incidence

Syphilis of the esophagus is a rare condition. GUYOT (1931), reviewing the literature from 1717 to 1930, found only 55 cases and added two of his own. HUDSON and HEAD (1950) collected another 17 cases from the literature between 1930 and 1950, and reported one themselves. In recent years no cases have been reported. These data relate to the involvement of the esophagus by tertiary syphilis. Esophageal involvement during the other stages of the disease seems to be even more exceptional. According to PALMER (1963) congenital syphilitic ulcers have been described.

Chancres of the esophagus have not been found thus far. It is assumed that the esophagus can be involved during secondary syphilis, as can the skin and other mucous membranes. WILE (1914) offered the interesting speculation that the dysphagia that occasionally occurs in secondary syphilis may be due to involvement of the esophagus by syphilitic lesions. However, esophageal lesions during this stage have never been observed.

2. Pathology

From beginning to end syphilis is essentially a vascular disease, with the exception of the gumma, which is probably the result of a hypersensitivity phenomenon. Aside from gummas, the lesions of late syphilis are produced by obliterative endarteritis of terminal arterioles and small arteries and by the resulting inflammatory and necrotic changes. In general, the gross structure of the lesion of tertiary syphilis may assume one of two general forms, a sub-mucous gumma, or a diffuse inflammatory reaction with destruction of tissue and resultant scarring and stenosis. Either form may display erosions and ulcerations (HUDSON and HEAD, 1950). Usually the lesions occur in the upper end of the esophagus.

3. Clinical Features

Painless dysphagia is the most common symptom and is produced by obstructive lesions. The long duration of the dysphagia and its slowly progressive or non-progressive nature can be useful to differentiate tertiary syphilis from cancer (HUDSON and HEAD, 1950). When a gumma has led to the formation of a tracheoesophageal or a bronchoesophageal fistula, swallowing food or liquid will often elicit coughing (swallow-cough) (NOSNY et al., 1961).

4. Technical Examination

X-ray examination can reveal a stenosing or a rigid area, or it may suggest a tumor. At esophagoscopy the picture is rather variable, and depends upon the duration and severity of the involvement.

Generally the esophageal mucosa is edematous and engorged, and presents erosions or ulcers. Sometimes plaques of leucoplakia are observed. In other instances the mucosa is more granular and friable. The esophageal lumen may be slightly narrowed or stenosed to such a degree as to prevent the passage of the esophagoscope. A biopsy should be taken to exclude the possibility of other lesions, particularly cancer. The diagnosis of syphilis is suggested by the presence of perivascular round-cell infiltration and endarteritis phenomena.

5. Diagnosis

Tertiary syphilis of the esophagus is so rare that it is rarely considered in the differential diagnosis. However, chronic obstructive lesions of the esophagus in a patient with known syphilis and positive serological tests for syphilis should suggest the diagnosis. In view of the infrequency of this specific esophageal lesion, other more common diseases must be excluded first. The diagnosis is confirmed when the patient's condition improves under antiluetic therapy.

6. Complications

Tertiary syphilis of the gullet can lead to esophageal stenosis due to fibrosis. A tracheo(broncho)esophageal fistula occurs less frequently (NOSNY et al., 1961). Rupture of the esophagus has been described in two patients with neurosyphilis (GLASS and FREEMAN, 1935). As the esophagus ruptured during paretic seizures accompanied by retching and vomiting, it is not clear whether the rupture was due to syphilitic esophagitis itself or to the retching and vomiting movements. Finally it must be mentioned that extrinsic syphilitic lesions may be responsible for esophageal disorders. Thus KAMPMEIER and JONES (1941) reported on three cases in which gummas of the diaphragm around the hiatus were responsible for esophageal obstruction.

7. Treatment

Antibiotics, preferably penicillin, will generally lead to rapid improvement of esophageal lesions. If complications in the lungs can be avoided, a tracheo-(broncho)esophageal fistula may even heal under this medication (NOSNY et al., 1961). In case of esophageal stenosis, dilatation may be necessary. The further evolution can be followed radiologically and endoscopically; regression of the lesions under treatment confirms the diagnosis.

References

GLASS, W. E., FREEMAN, W.: Spontaneous rupture of the esophagus in syphilis. Amer. J. med. Sci. 189, 80–86 (1935).

GUYOT, R.: La syphilis de l'œsophage en particulier au point de vue anatomo-pathologique. Ann. Oto-laryng. (Paris) 1, 505–526 (1931).

HUDSON, T. R., HEAD, J. R.: Syphilis of the esophagus. J. thorac. Surg. 20, 216–221 (1950).

KAMPMEIER, R. H., JONES, E.: Esophageal obstruction due to gummata of esophagus and diaphragm. Amer. J. med. Sci. 201, 539–546 (1941).

NOSNY, P., LALUQUE, P., PLESSIS, J. L.: A propos d'une complication exceptionnelle de la syphilis: la fistule œsophago-aérienne. Med. Trop. (Marseille) 21, 435–439 (1961).

PALMER, E. D.: Syphilis. Clinical gastroenterology, second ed., p. 42. New York: Hoeber 1963.

WILE, U. I.: Syphilis of the esophagus. Amer. J. med. Sci. 148, 180–186 (1914).

Esophageal Mycoses

W. Pelemans and G. Vantrappen

With 2 Figures

1. Monilial Esophagitis

Monilial esophagitis or esophagitis candidosa caused by the yeast-like fungi of the genus Candida, is the most frequent mycotic infection of the esophagus.

1.1. History

Oral thrush was first described in 1764 by Rosen von Rosenstein, who mentions a disease of the mouth, which becomes severe if it spreads into the lungs. Thrush infections were later described by Langenbeck (1839), Berg (1841) and Robin (1953). Already in 1854 Virchow observed fungi which had penetrated into the esophageal wall down to the level of the submucosa; this may be the oldest description of esophagitis candidosa (Gemeinhardt and Deicke, 1967). But only since the introduction of antibiotics and corticosteroids into therapy has the literature paid more attention to this type of esophagitis. In 1956 Andren and Theander described for the first time the radiological appearance of monilial esophagitis.

1.2. Incidence

This infection of the esophagus remains a rare disease though its frequency has increased since the use of antibiotics and steroids. In 1964 Grieve published a review of the literature and collected 13 cases of monilial esophagitis. Since that time, however, many more cases have been described. Over a period of 10 years only 13 adults with esophageal mycoses were treated in Oxford (Holt, 1968). Out of 684 patients admitted into the Cancer Hospital in Jutland 98 (14%) suffered from moniliasis in the oral cavity or elsewhere and 35 patients (5%) had moniliasis of the esophagus (Jensen et al., 1964).

Autopsy studies on the incidence of esophagitis were performed by Gemeinhardt and Deicke (1967). Whenever macroscopic lesions were present the esophagus was studied histologically and cultures were made. In a series of 565 unselected autopsies they found 10 cases of esophageal mycoses; in the 103 children below the age of 1, the incidence was 5.8%, whereas in the 462 older patients it was only 0.87%. Vanbreuseghem (1970) did autopsy studies on the incidence of mycotic infections in 100 cancer patients. In this selected group he found in 67.4% of the cases fungi in the esophagus, mostly Candida albicans. The post mortem studies of Sherlock et al. (1970) revealed an incidence of gastrointestinal moniliasis ranging from 4% in patients with chronic leukemia, to 27% in patients with lymphosarcoma. In acute leukemias, the incidence was 15%. The esophagus was the most common site of gastrointestinal involvement.

1.3. Etiology

The yeast-like organisms of the genus Candida appear as septate branching mycelia 2 to 4 microns in diameter, and as ovoid yeast forms of slightly greater diameter. Although poorly stained with hematoxylin and eosin, the fungi can be visualized by P.A.S. and Gram stains and by phase microscopy (Louria et al., 1962). Esophageal mycotic lesions can be caused not only by Candida albicans, but also by Candida kruzei (Jensen et al., 1964; Delahunty, 1967), by Candida tropicalis (Jensen et al., 1964; Gemeinhardt and Deicke, 1967) and by Torulopsis glabrata (Jensen et al., 1964).

Several species of Candida are found in rotting vegetables and fruits, and also in dairy products, especially cheese, but Candida albicans is only very exceptionally found outside of humans and animals (Drouhet, 1957).

Candida is a normal sapropyhte of the mucosa and of the skin. According to Drouhet (1957) 6 to 30% of normal human subjects contain Candida in the mouth flora, and 15% have 'it in their stools. Candida is present in the vagina of non-pregnant women in 5 to 15% of the cases; in the last months of pregnancy this incidence increases to about 36%. Candida can also be found on the bronchial mucosa of normal subjects. The presence of Candida albicans on the skin, however, is abnormal, although other species of Candida can be found there. It should be noted, however, that the Candida found in the throat, the vagina, in the stools and on the bronchial mucosa of normal subjects are few in number and can be detected only by means of cultures.

1.4. Pathogenesis

Although this fungus can behave as a saprophyte and normal subjects can be carriers of Candida without having any complaints, Candida invasions of tissues are not a rare phenomenon (Seelig, 1966a). Serological studies show that the titer of Candida-inhibiting antibodies and of agglutinating antibodies increases with age.

Clinical studies show that Candida can become pathogenic under a wide variety of circumstances. Acute monilial esophagitis may occur without apparent underlying diseases (Brown and McKee, 1972). Infants are quite susceptible to oral thrush. The infection can occur at birth during the passage through an infected vagina, or the neonati may acquire it from other persons. Gemeinhardt and Deicke (1967) suggest that the use of gastric tubes may play a role in the pathogenesis of moniliasis of the esophagus. Diabetes and pregnancy, malignancy, blood diseases and a poor general condition also favor the development of monilial infections. Antibiotics and/or steroids significantly increase the risk of candidiasis. Thrush of the esophagus has also been described in association with a series of other diseases such as systemic lupus erythematodes (Hogewind-De Nijs and Hogewind, 1957; Goldberg and Dodds, 1968), caustic lesions of the esophagus (Gonzales-Crussi and Iung, 1965), ulcerative colitis (Buckle and Nichol, 1964; Guyer et al., 1971), achalasia (Guyer et al., 1971), hypoparathyroidism (Kenny and Holliday, 1964; Kantrowitz et al., 1969) and hemoglobin SC disease (Sanders et al., 1962).

The reason why the equilibrium between host and saprophyte is disturbed in these persons is not always clear. Often there is a combination of several pathogenetic factors such as a poor general condition, treatment with antibiotics and/or steroids. The mechanism by which antibiotics increase the hazards of candidiasis includes: overgrowth of Candida in the absence of competing organisms, local tissue damage and increased invasion by the candida, either as a consequence of the local tissue damage, or possibly due to the conversion of the candida to a more invasive mycelial form (Seelig, 1966a). Whether broad spectrum antibiotics directly stimulate the growth of Candida is a moot point, on which contradictory evidence has been presented. Antibiotics have been shown to inhibit both antibody synthesis and phagocytic activity, and thus may reduce the host resistance to invasions by Candida (Seelig, 1966a). The degree to which antibiotics depress host factors probably constitutes a serious problem only for patients with already poor immunological defenses. It is possible that impairment of phagocytic activity may be responsible for the increased susceptibility to Candida caused by corticosteroids. Some experiments (Louria and Browne, 1960) suggest that enhanced susceptibility due to cortisone is related primarily to the delayed appearance of phagocytes in parasitized tissues. Others (O'Grady et al., 1964) suggest that cortisone may interfere with the intracellular destruction of the engulfed organism. Evidence that impaired phagocytosis may play a part in the increased susceptibility of patients to Candida is provided by the reports of low phagocytic activity of polymorphonuclear leucocytes in patients with diabetes mellitus, hepatic disease and reticulo-endothelial neoplasms, all diseases characterized by a propensity towards Candida infections (Seelig, 1966a). Craig and Farber (1953) and later Baker (1962) drew attention to the profound neutropenia that is often present at the onset of mycotic infection in leukemia and aplastic anemia. In these diseases decreased phagocytosis may favor the development of moniliasis.

1.5. Clinical Features

Besides the associated pathology and its symptoms moniliasis of the esophagus can produce its own symptoms. Pain on swallowing is the most frequent complaint (Jensen, 1964; Holt, 1968). An acute onset of painful dysphagia for solids, hot or cold liquids and sometimes saliva suggests an infection with Candida. Continuous substernal pain, sometimes radiating into the back and obstruction of food passage frequently occur. Regurgitation and vomiting are also observed and in little children may cause attacks of cyanosis due to aspiration into the airways (Wagner and Kessel, 1958). In a retrospective study of autopsy data, Sherlock et al. (1970) found that out of a series of 70 patients with esophageal moniliasis, 20 had suffered from gastrointestinal bleeding. The authors do not mention, however, whether the bleeding was acute or chronic, and whether or not it was of esophageal origin. Moniliasis of the esophagus is often found in combination with oral thrush. Involvement of the mouth manifests itself by a great number of small round white specks, which can become larger, merge, and form a greyish coating. This may cover the tongue and spread to the cheeks, the palate and the pharynx, while the surrounding mucosa is erythematous. As a matter of fact the mucosa may show this red, smooth and varnished aspect before the white spots appear (Drouhet, 1957) or preserve it after they have disappeared.

Oral thrush can easily be recognized but it is not necessary part of the clinical picture. The possibility of moniliasis of the esophagus without clinical involvement of the mouth has often been stressed. Two of the 13 cases of esophageal candidiasis described by Holt (1968) did not show oral thrush. Of 13 cases of esophageal moniliasis collected from the literature by Grieve (1964) only 6 had oral involvement. Buckle and Nichol (1964) described two cases of esophageal involvement without a clear infection of Candida elsewhere; Greenbaum and Olmstead (1962) also report a case of esophageal moniliasis without thrush.

1.6. Technical Examination

The diagnosis of esophageal moniliasis can be confirmed by radiographic and endoscopic examinations, complimented by cultures of esophageal swabs and by biopsy.

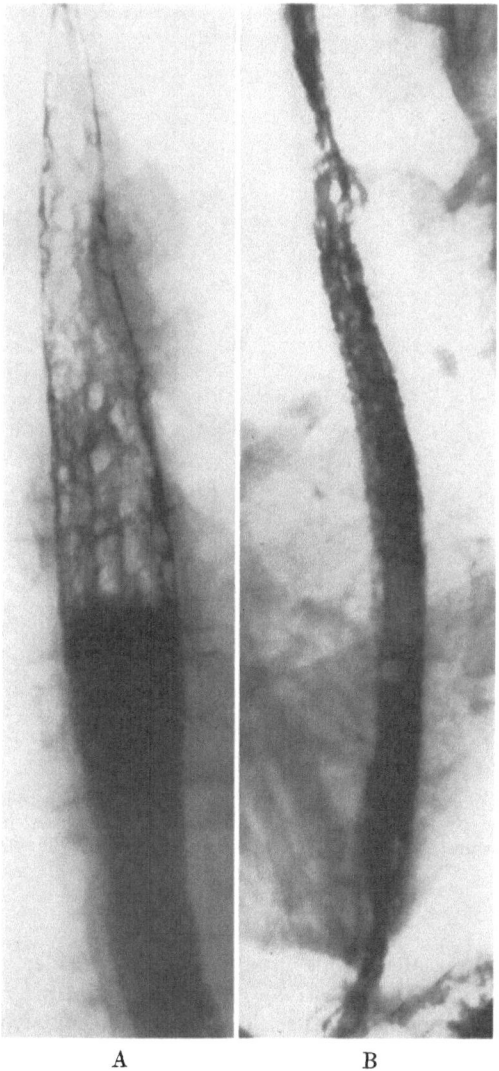

A   B

Fig. 267 A and B. Diffuse involvement of the esophagus by moniliasis in a patient with leukemia. Nodular filling defects (cobblestone pattern) on double contrast films (A) and shaggy outline (B)

The radiological features of esophageal moniliasis have been summarized by GUYER et al. (1971). The changes particularly affect the middle and lower thirds of the thoracic esophagus. A shaggy outline, due to mucosal ulcerations or slough within the lumen of the esophagus, is the most common abnormality

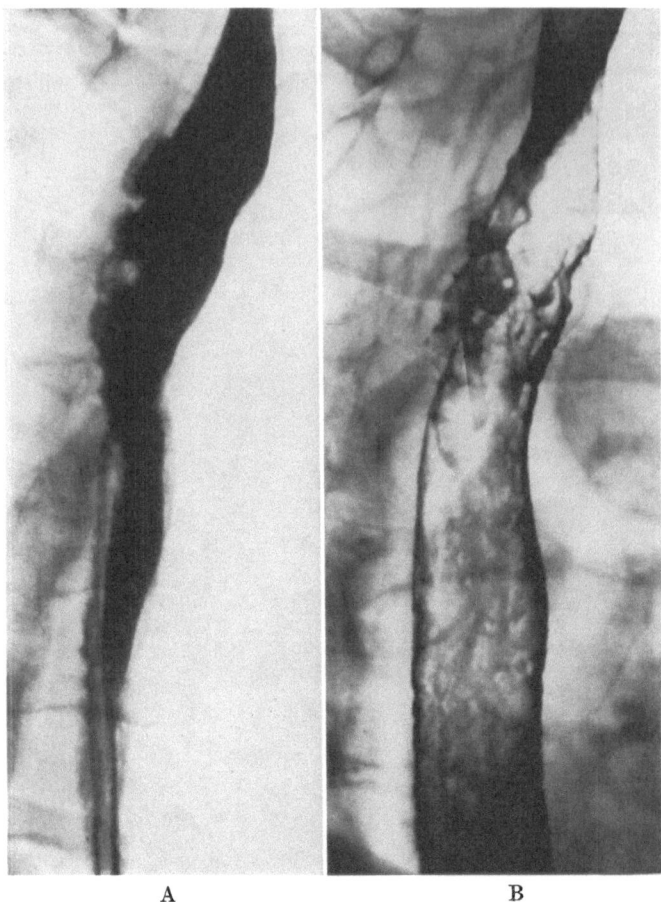

A   B

Fig. 268 A and B. Esophageal moniliasis in a 36-year old patient with reticulosarcoma. Lesions predominate in the upper third of the esophagus; abnormal mucosal pattern and marginal irregularities due to necrotic material adhere to the wall (slough) and to ulcerations

(Figs. 267 B, 268). Deep ulcerations give rise to typical ulcer craters. Nodular filling defects may occur (Fig. 267 A) and are ascribed to mucosal edema and ulceration, to pseudomembranes, or to actual colonies of Candida on the surface of the esophageal mucosa. Spasm of the esophagus may be sufficiently severe, particularly in children, to prevent the entrance of contrast material into the esophagus, and may lead to aspiration of the material into the trachea (WAGNER and KESSEL, 1958). Diminished esophageal peristalsis has been described by KAUFMAN et al. (1950), GRIEVE (1964), GUYER et al. (1971) and also by GOLDBERG and DODDS (1968), although the latter authors attribute this motor abnormality to the systemic lupus from which their patient was suffering. The contrast material may be so adherent to the mucosa that it remains visible for several hours. Finally, segmental narrowing has also been described in some patients. KANTROWITZ et al. (1969) point out that the radiographic appearance of the esophagus in chronic esophageal moniliasis does not resemble that seen in acute monilial infection. The cineradiographic examination of their case revealed a persistently narrowed but pliable segment of the esophagus extending from the thoracic inlet to approximately 4 cm above the aortic arch. Although the mucosal pattern was normal, peristaltic stripping was incomplete throughout the esophagus.

WOLF et al. (1955) noted severe dysphagia in small infants due to incoordination of the pharynx.

Normal radiological findings do not exclude moniliasis of the esophagus. The lesions apparent on endoscopy may not show up in the radiographies of up to 25% of the patients (JENSEN et al., 1964). Esophagoscopy therefore may be an extremely useful diagnostic tool. The esophagus appears edematous, reddened and friable, with erosions and ulcerations. Whitish spots of varying dimensions can fuse and form pseudomembranes. In other cases the lesions appear as pseudotumorous formations. At esophagoscopy swabs can be made for cultures and the fungus can be found in biopsy specimens.

1.7. Diagnosis and Differential Diagnosis

The history of the patient may reveal several elements suggestive of the diagnosis. When a patient is in poor general condition, when his defense mechanisms have been weakened, or when he has been treated with antibiotics and/or corticosteroids, the fairly acute development of painful dysphagia suggests the diagnosis, especially when oral thrush is present. A stool smear demonstrating the presence of monilial mycelia is highly suggestive of gastrointestinal fungal infection (SHERLOCK et al., 1970). The radiological examination will often provide the diagnosis. The radiological image must be differentiated from esophageal varices, peptic esophagitis, intramural diverticulosis, and other conditions associated with esophageal ulceration. On occasion the differential diagnosis with carcinoma of the esophagus can be difficult (GIBSON and HARRIS, 1967). Esophagoscopy with histological and bacteriological examinations may be necessary to confirm the diagnosis.

1.8. Complications

Esophagitis candidosa can lead to several complications. Bleedings, sometimes fatal, have been described in hemorrhagic necrotizing forms of infection (GEMEIN-HARDT and DEICKE, 1968). Monilial esophagitis can lead to organic stenosis (GIBSON and HARRIS, 1967), for which dilatations may be required (BECK, 1962; HAMMELBURG, 1967). Esophageal stenosis due to chronic candidiasis has been seen to regress under prolonged treatment with fungistatics (KANTROWITZ et al., 1969). There are reports of perforation due to acute infections (GONZALES-CRUSSI and IUNG, 1965), of fistulization (WEISS and EPSTEIN, 1962), and even of an esophagoaortic fistula (DELAHUNTY, 1967). The infection may spread to the lower gastrointestinal tract. When a Candida sepsis occurs the point of origin is to be found frequently in the gastrointestinal tract. In small children aspiration pneumonia is a common complication (GEMEINHARDT and DEICKE, 1967). TROU-PIN (1968) suggests the possibility of a causal relation between moniliasis of the esophagus and intramural esophageal diverticulosis; further evidence is needed to confirm this hypothesis.

1.9. Prognosis

Monilial esophagitis is mostly a concomitant disease of more serious and even life-threatening affections, which determine the prognosis of the patient. However, moniliasis itself can be the immediate cause of death due to bleeding and perforation. It also results in a higher morbidity for the patient and may lead to esophageal stenosis.

1.10. Treatment

Good results have been obtained with fungistatics. The drug of choice is nystatin, though intravenously administered amphotericin B has also been used successfully (JENSEN et al., 1964). Because of its toxicity (UTZ et al., 1964) the latter product is used for generalized moniliasis or deep seated infections (HOLT, 1968).

Nystatin should be given as a combined mouthwash, gargle and swallow, in a dose of a few million units, devided throughout the day. Higher doses can be given, if necessary, because the product is not absorbed. It seems to be more effective, however, to increase the viscosity of the suspension than to augment the dose because in this way nystatin can remain in contact with the lesions for a sufficiently long period of time to be absorbed by the fungi. To achieve the required degree of viscosity KANTROWITZ et al. (1969) added a concentration of 0.5% of methylcellulose to the suspension of nystatin. The mode of administering amphotericin B intravenously is to mix the drug with 5% dextrose in water and to infuse it over a period of several hours. To avoid local irritation and phlebitis the concentration should not exceed 1 mg of amphotericin/10 ml glucoses 5%. The dose should be increased progressively over a period of several days until it reaches $^1/_2$ mg/kg/day and this dose is maintained for about 14 days. Higher doses up to 1 mg/kg/day are usually administered only in cases of generalized moniliasis.

Amphotericin B has many undesirable effects, including the idiosyncratic reactions which occur in an isolated patient after only a small dose of the drug has been administered, and the side-effects which are dose-dependent and can occur in almost every patient (UTZ et al., 1964). The idiosyncratic reactions include anaphylactic shock, thrombocytopenia, acute liver failure, flushing, vertigo, generalized pain, grand mal convulsion, cardiac arrest and ventricular fibrillation. The side-effects of intravenous administration are phlebitis, fever, chills, nausea, vomiting, headache, anorexia, hypopotassemia, abnormal renal function, and anemia. It is clear therefore that patients undergoing this treatment need strict observation. The dose must be diminished and treatment may have to be interrupted temporarily, if the blood urea nitrogen or the serum creatinine increase. Antipyretic and antihistaminic drugs, chlorpromazine and hydrocortisone have been proposed to diminish the intensity of the side effects. Trauma to the veins can be markedly reduced by using pediatric scalp vein needles and by diluting the amphotericin B. It may even be advisable to add heparin to the infusion.

New products for the treatment of moniliasis are being studied (5-fluorocytosine-clotrimazole), but further experience is necessary to evaluate these drugs.

2. Other Mycotic Infections of the Esophagus

A limited number of mycotic diseases, other than moniliasis, may affect the esophagus in very rare instances.

2.1. Actinomycosis

Mediastinal lymph nodes, draining a pulmonary focus of infection, may produce caseating necrosis with secondary rupture into the esophagus, resulting in an esophagobronchial fistula (ANDERSON and SABISTON, 1965; WESSELHOEFT and KESHISHIAN, 1968; SEBASTIAN et al., 1969). Primary infection of the esophagus occurs rarely; ingestion of infected material has been proposed as a possible cause (AUBIN, 1951). A contiguous lesion may spread to the esophagus and this can be another way of esophageal infection. Esophageal involvement is mostly located in the upper third or at the bronchoaortic narrowing of the gullet. Dysphagia, hypersalivation, a burning sensation and retrosternal pain are possible complaints. Diagnosis is established by microscopic examination of the pus and by culture (AUBIN, 1951).

2.2. Mucormycosis

Fungi of the genus Mucor and Rhizopus occasionally proliferate in debilitated hosts, and may affect any organ of the body. In a series of 22 cases of gastrointestinal mucormycosis (NEAME and RAGNER, 1960) two patients showed esophageal involvement. Small ulcers, 1 cm in diameter, were found in one case; larger ulcers, 3 to 4 cm in diameter with a black necrotic centre and an edematous grayish border in the other. Rhizopus stolonifer (Rhizopus nigricans) was isolated in the last patient. KAHN (1963) described another case of esophageal mucormycosis discovered at post-mortem examination in a diabetic patient.

2.3. Histoplasmosis

Histoplasmosis is a localized or disseminated mycotic infection, primarily involving the reticuloendothelial system in various tissues and organs (MOSS and MCQUOWN, 1960). The disease is caused by Histoplasma capsulatum, a member of the group of the fungi imperfecti. It is probable that the infestation occurs via the respiratory tract. It is often asymptomatic and the disease may regress spontaneously. Hematogenous or lymphatic spread develops in a small minority of infected individuals. It may be generalized or limited to relatively few tissues.

Mediastinal lymph node involvement may be responsible for the formation of fistulas with the esophagus (HUTCHIN and LINDSKOG, 1964; SEBASTIAN et al., 1969). A cyst due to Histoplasma capsulatum is a rare cause of compression of the esophagus. HINSHAW and GUILFOIL (1964) described a man with vague complaints of epigastric discomfort. Radiologically a clearly delineated mass was found in the mediastinum causing compression of the gullet. At surgery a cyst was found between mucosa and muscularis mucosae, caused by Histoplasma capsulatum. Disseminated histoplasmosis, a rapidly fatal form if untreated (83% mortality), can occur in debilitated patients. Acute ulcerations in the esophagus, the stomach, the duodenum, the jejunum, the ileum and colon were found at post mortem examination of a 53 year old patient who died of severe gastrointestinal hemorrhage (STURIM et al., 1965).

2.4. Blastomycosis

Blastomyces brasiliensis is a yeast-like fungus which causes South-American blastomycosis. This chronic progressive granulomatous disease, which is found almost exclusively in Brazil, occasionally involves the esophagus (DE ABREU et al., 1966).

References

ABREU, M. DE, CUNHA, R. DA, PEREIRA, A. A., GOUVEIA, O. F. DE, LUNA, J. R. DE, SAAD, M., TEIXEIRA, D., MIGAHIRA, A. R.: Contribution à l'étude radiologique de la blastomycose sud-américaine de l'appareil digestif. Hospital **69**, 169–174 (1966).

ANDERSON, R. P., SABISTON, D. C.: Acquired bronchoesophageal fistula of benign origin. Surg. Gynec. Obstet. **121**, 261–266 (1965).

ANDREN, L., THEANDER, G.: Roentgenographic appearances of esophageal moniliasis. Acta radiol. (Stockh.) **46**, 571–574 (1956).

AUBIN, A.: Actynomycose. Encyclop. médico chirurgicale, oto-rhino-laryng. Paris: Editions Techniques 1951.

BAKER, R. D.: Leukopenia and therapy in leukemia as factors predisposing to fatal mycoses. Amer. J. clin. Path. **37**, 358–373 (1962).

BECK, L. K. L.: Über die Soorerkrankung und ihre Komplikation einer hochgradigen Ösophagusstenose. Z. Laryng. Rhinol. **41**, 348–353 (1962).

BROWN, J. W., MCKEE, W. M.: Acute monilial esophagitis occurring without underlying disease in a young male. Amer. J. dig. Dis. **17**, 85–88 (1972).

BUCKLE, R. M., NICHOL, W. D.: Painful dysphagia due to monilial oesophagitis. Brit. med. J. **1964 I**, 821–822.

CRAIG, J. M., FARBER, S.: The development of disseminated visceral mycosis during therapy for acute leucemia. Amer. J. Path. **29**, 601 (1953).

DELAHUNTY, J. E.: Oesophageal candidiasis and its radiological diagnosis. J. Laryng. **81**, 809–813 (1967).

DROUHET, E.: Biologie des infections à candida. Sur les manifestations pathologiques et les conditions étiologiques et pathogéniques de 175 cas de candidose. Sem. Hôp. (Paris) **33**, 807–828 (1957).

GEMEINHARDT, H., DEICKE, P.: Zur Kenntnis der Ösophagusmykose (Oesophagitis candidosa) durch Candida albicans. Dtsch. Gesundh.-Wes. **22**, 1897–1905 (1967).

GEMEINHARDT, H., DEICKE, P.: Tödliche Ösophagusmykose durch Candida albicans im Erwachsenenalter. Dtsch. Gesundh.-Wes. **23**, 1703–1707 (1968).

GIBSON, M. J., HARRIS, M.: An unusual case of monilial oesophagitis. Brit. J. Radiol. **40**, 391–392 (1967).

GOLDBERG, H. I., DODDS, W. J.: Cobblestone esophagus due to monilial infection. Amer. J. Roentgenol. **104**, 608–612 (1968).

GONZALES-CRUSSI, I. F., IUNG, O. S.: Oesophageal moniliasis as a cause of death. Amer. J. Surg. **109**, 634–638 (1965).

GREENBAUM, D. S., OLMSTEAD, E. V.: Esophageal moniliasis without thrush. J. med. Soc. N. J. **59**, 511–513 (1962).

GRIEVE, N. W. T.: Monilial œsophagitis. Brit. J. Radiol. **37**, 551–554 (1964).

GUYER, P. B., BRUNTON, F. J., ROOKE, H. W. P.: Candidiasis of the œsophagus. Brit. J. Radiol. **44**, 131–136 (1971).

HAMMELBURG, E.: L'œsophagite sténosante par moniliase. Ann. Oto-laryng. (Paris) **84**, 239–243 (1967).

HINSHAW, R. J., GUILFOIL, P. H.: Roentgenogram of the month. Intramural cystic lesion of the esophagus due to histoplasma capsulatum. Dis. Chest **47**, 555–556 (1965).

HOGEWIND-DE NIJS, J. J., HOGEWIND, F.: Röntgenologische afwijkingen van de slokdarm, veroorzaakt door candida albicans. Ned. T. Geneesk. **101**, 1325–1326 (1957).

HOLT, J. M.: Candida infection of the œsophagus. Gut **9**, 227–231 (1968).

HUTCHIN, P., LINDSKOG, G. E.: Acquired esophagobronchial fistula of infectious origin J. thorac. cardiovasc. Surg. **48**, 1–12 (1964).

JENSEN, K. B., STENDERUP, A., THOMSEN, J. B., BICHEL, J.: Oesophageal moniliasis in malignant neoplastic disease. Acta med. scand. **175**, 455–459 (1964).

KAHN, L. B.: Gastric mucormycosis: report of a case with review of the literature. S. Afr. med. J. **38**, 1265–1269 (1963).

KANTROWITZ, P. A., FLEISCHLI, D. J., BUTLER, W. T.: Successful treatment of chronic esophageal moniliasis with a viscous suspension of nystatin. Gastroenterology **57**, 424–430 (1969).

KAUFMAN, S. A., SCHEFF, S., LEVENE, G.: Esophageal moniliasis. Radiology **75**, 726–732 (1960).

KENNY, F. M., HOLLIDAY, M. A.: Hypoparathyroidism, moniliasis, Addison's and Hashimoto's disease. Hypercalcemia treated with intravenously administered sodium sulfate. New Engl. J. Med. **271**, 708–713 (1964).

LOURIA, D. B., BROWNE, H. G.: The effects of cortisone on experimental fungus infections. Ann. N.Y. Acad. Sci. **89**, 39–46 (1960).

LOURIA, D. B., STIFF, D. P., BENNETT, B.: Disseminated moniliasis in the adult. Medicine (Baltimore) **41**, 307–337 (1962).

MOSS, E. S., McQUOWN, A. L.: Atlas of medical mycology, second ed. Baltimore: Williams & Wilkins Co. 1960.

NEAME, P., RAGNER, D.: Mucormycosis: a report of twenty-two cases. Arch. Path. **70**, 261–268 (1960).

O'GRADY, F., COTTON, R. E., THOMPSON, R. E. M.: Morphology of cortisone-induced changes in mouse thigh candidiasis. Brit. J. exp. Path. **45**, 656–665 (1964).

SANDERS, E., LEVINTHAL, C., DONNER, M. W.: Monilial esophagitis in a patient with hemoglobin SC disease. Demonstration of esophageal motor abnormality by cine-radiofluorography. Ann. intern. Med. **57**, 650–654 (1962).

SEBASTIAN, S., PARKER, J. O., LYNN, R. B.: Acquired esophagobronchial fistulas in adults. Canad. med. Ass. J. **101**, 517–519 (1969).

SEELIG, M. S.: Mechanisms by which antibiotics increase the incidence and severity of candidiasis and alter the immunological defenses. Bact. Rev. **30**, 442–459 (1966a).

SEELIG, M. S.: The role of antibiotics in the pathogenesis of candida infections. Amer. J. Med. **40**, 887–917 (1966b).

SHERLOCK, P., GOLDSTEIN, M. J., ERAS, P.: Esophageal moniliasis. Mod. Treatm. **7**, 1250–1260 (1970).

SMITH, J. M. B.: Mycosis of the alimentary tract. Gut **10**, 1035–1040 (1969).

STURIM, H. S., KOUCHOUKOS, N. T., AHLVIN, R. C.: Gastrointestinal manifestations of disseminated histoplasmosis. Amer. J. Surg. **110**, 435–440 (1965).

TROUPIN, R. H.: Intramural esophageal diverticulosis and moniliasis. A possible association. Amer. J. Roentgenol. **104**, 613–616 (1968).

UTZ, J. P., BENNETT, J. E., BRANDRISS, M. W., BUTLER, W. T., HILL, G. J.: Amphotericin B toxicity. Ann. intern. Med. **61**, 334–354 (1964).

VANBREUSEGHEM, R.: Analyse mycologique du cadavre de malades morts du cancer. Brux.-méd. **11**, 1019–1025 (1970).

WAGNER, J. M., KESSEL, I.: Complications of candida albicans infection in infancy. Brit. med. J. **1958 II**, 362–366.

WEISS, J., EPSTEIN, B. S.: Esophageal moniliasis. Amer. J. Roentgenol. **88**, 718–720 (1962).

WESSELHOEFT, C. W., KESHISHIAN, J. M.: Acquired nonmalignant esophagotracheal and esophagobronchial fistulas. Ann. thorac. Surg. **6**, 187–195 (1968).

WOLFF, O. H., PETTY, B. W., ASTLEY, R., SMELLIE, J. M.: Trush esophagitis with pharyngeal incoordination treated with hydroxystilbamidine. Lancet **1955 I**, 991–994.

Granulomatous Esophagitis

W. Pelemans and G. Vantrappen

1. Crohn's Disease of the Esophagus

When in 1932, Crohn, Ginzburg and Oppenheimer described a disease they called regional enteritis, it was generally believed that this clinical and pathological entity was limited to the terminal ileum. It soon became apparent that the lesions may also be found elsewhere in the gut, and it is now realized that almost any part of the gastrointestinal tract may be affected.

Since 1950 a small number of case-reports have been published describing esophageal lesions which resemble those found in Crohn's disease. In some cases the esophagus was the only organ to be affected by the disease (Franklin and Taylor, 1950; Turina et al., 1968; Madden et al., 1969; Vogt-Moykopf and Wanke, 1970). In others a typical Crohn's disease of the small bowel or colon was associated with clinically important esophageal lesions (Gelfand and Krone, 1968; Dyer et al., 1969). Although no absolutely diagnostic features were found, the authors felt that the esophageal inflammation represented involvement of this organ by Crohn's disease. Heffernon and Kepkay (1954) described a man with "segmental esophagitis, gastritis and enteritis", but this case probably does not represent a true regional enteritis. Indeed, the clinical evolution was rather unusual for Crohn's disease and the pathological changes were non-specific at all sites. Achenbach et al. (1956) reported the case of a 25-year old man with ulcerating esophagitis, perianal fistulae, erythema nodosum, arthritis, pyoderma gangrenosum, splenomegaly and liver dysfunction. At operation several peri-esophageal fistulae were found to be present and at histological examination of the resected specimen foreign body giant cells were observed in a para-esophageal sinus tract.

The involvement of the esophagus by Crohn's disease is difficult to prove. The finding of esophageal lesions in a patient with Crohn's disease of the lower intestinal tract does not by itself indicate that the esophageal and intestinal lesions are of the same nature. An esophagoscopic biopsy is necessarily superficial and cannot establish the presence of the typical deeper lesions such as transmural lympho-plasma-cellular infiltration and deep fissurations. As long as more specific tests are not available the diagnosis must necessarily be based upon the presence of epithelioid granulomata in the lamina propria or submucosa. When the esophagus is the only organ affected by inflammatory lesions, the diagnosis of Crohn's disease is even more difficult. In the literature only two cases have been reported in whom more specific esophageal lesions seemed to be present. Turina et al. (1968) found at preoperative histological examination of the esophagus an epitheloid granulomatosis; examination of the resected specimen, however, could not confirm the presence of granulomas. The second case is that reported by Achenbach et al. (1956). Although the authors describe their case as ulcerative esophagitis, because in their opinion it was in many ways reminiscent of ulcerative colitis, the presence of chronic non-specific inflammation with fibrosis, and of foreign body giant cells in a paraesophageal sinus tract, suggest Crohn's disease rather than ulcerative esophagitis.

2. Sarcoidosis of the Esophagus

Sarcoidosis rarely affects the gastrointestinal tract. An analysis of 1254 cases of histologically proven sarcoidosis in the U.S.A. and in the United Kingdom allowed MAYOCK et al. (1953) to find only two cases of gastrointestinal involvement. In their comment on the occurrence of sarcoidosis in the gastrointestinal tract, POLACHEK and MATRE (1964) mention 25 cases of sarcoidosis of the stomach, 5 cases involving the small intestine, and 5 localized in the colon. Cases of sarcoidosis with esophageal symptoms but without histologically proven granulomatous involvement have been reported (LONGCOPE and FREIMAN, 1952; COWDELL, 1954; McKUSICK, 1953; COOK et al., 1970). Histological proof of such involvement has been given in only a few instances. KERLEY (1948) described a patient who had pulmonary involvement followed by extensive fibrosis, but no tubercle bacilli were isolated. The patient developed dysphagia, due to a stenosing lesion of the middle third of the esophagus. Biopsy of the gullet was reported as tuberculosis. In view of his good recovery and of the lack of tubercle bacilli, the patient was regarded as a cause of sarcoidosis of the lungs and the esophagus. SIEGEL et al. (1961) reported on a patient who complained about dysphagia; surgery revealed granulomas in the cricopharyngeal muscle. POLACHEK and MATRE (1964) described a patient with disseminated sarcoidosis of lungs, lymph nodes, liver, spleen and probably heart, with involvement of the esophagus proven by peroral biopsy. A patient of HARDY et al. (1967) complained mainly about dysphagia and dysphonia. Sarcoidosis of the lungs was established, with involvement of the cranial nerves and of the esophagus. WIESNER et al. (1971) observed a patient with dysphagia due to esophageal stenosis, with splenomegaly, paratracheal adenopathy and iron deficiency anemia. Histologic study of the tissue obtained at operation revealed a markedly thickened esophagus which contained many non-caseating granulomas with giant cells. The Kveim-test was positive. This is probably a case of sarcoidosis with primarily esophageal involvement. WIESNER et al. (1971) consider the case report of TURINA et al. (1968) as the fifth case of histologically proven esophageal granuloma with findings suggestive of sarcoidosis, but TURINA and his coworkers themselves report on it under the title "Crohn'sche Krankheit des Ösophagus".

In cases of non-caseating granulomatous esophagitis one should look for other more usual localizations of either Crohn's disease or sarcoidosis. If the esophagus is the only site of granulomatous involvement, the diagnosis is exceedingly difficult, because both diseases have similar histological and immunologic characteristics and their main difference is constituted by their divergent localization preference.

References

ACHENBACH, H., LYNCH, J. P., DWIGHT, R. W.: Idiopathic ulcerative esophagitis. Report of a case. New Engl. J. Med. **255**, 456–459 (1956).

COOK, D. M., DINES, D. E., DYCUS, D. E.: Sarcoidosis: report of a case presenting as dysphagia. Dis. Chest **57**, 84–86 (1970).

COWDELL, R. H.: Sarcoidosis: with special reference to diagnosis and prognosis. Quart. J. Med. **23**, 29–55 (1954).

Crohn, B. B., Ginzburg, L., Oppenheimer, G. D.: Regional ileitis: a pathologic and clinical entity. J. Amer. med. Ass. **99**, 1323–1329 (1932).

Dyer, N. H., Cook, P. L., Kemp Harper, R. A.: Oesophageal stricture associated with Crohn's disease. Gut **10**, 549–554 (1969).

Franklin, R. H., Taylor, S.: Nonspecific granulomatous (regional) esophagitis. J. Surg. **19**, 292–297 (1950).

Gelfand, M. D., Krone, C. L.: Dysphagia and esophageal ulceration in Crohn's disease. Gastroenterology **55**, 510–514 (1968).

Hardy, W. E., Tulgan, H., Haidak, G., Budnitz, J.: Sarcoidosis: A case presenting with dysphagia and dysphonia. Ann. intern. Med. **66**, 353–357 (1967).

Heffernon, E. W., Kepkay, P. H.: Segmental esophagitis, gastritis and enteritis. Gastroenterology **26**, 83–88 (1954).

Kerley, P.: Sarcoidosis. In: Modern trends in diagnostic radiology (first series), ed. McLaren, p. 150. New York: J. W. Hoeber 1948.

Longcope, W. T., Freiman, D. G.: A study of sarcoidosis. Based on a combined investigation of 160 cases including 30 autopsies from the Johns Hopkins Hospital and Massachusetts General Hospital. Medicine (Baltimore) **31**, 1–132 (1952).

Madden, J. L., Ravid, J. M., Haddad, J. R.: Regional esophagitis: a specific entity simulating Crohn's disease. Ann. Surg. **170**, 351–368 (1969).

Mayock, R. L., Bertrand, P., Morrison, C. E., Scott, J. H.: Manifestations of sarcoidosis. Analysis of 145 patients, with a review of nine series selected from the literature. Amer. J. Med. **35**, 67–89 (1963).

McKusick, V. A.: Boeck's sarcoid of the stomach with comments on the etiology of regional enteritis. Gastroenterology **23**, 103–113 (1953).

Polachek, A. A., Matre, W. J.: Gastrointestinal sarcoidosis. Report of a case involving the esophagus. Amer. J. dig. Dis. **9**, 429–433 (1964).

Siegel, C. I., Honda, M., Salik, J., Mendeloff, A. I.: Dysphagia due to granulomatous myositis of the cricopharyngeus muscle: physiological and cineradiographic studies prior to and following successful surgical therapy. Trans. Ass. Amer. Physiol. **74**, 342–352 (1961).

Turina, M., Schamaun, M., Waldvogel, W.: Crohnsche Krankheit des Ösophagus. Dtsch. med. Wschr. **93**, 2097–2099 (1968).

Vogt-Moykopf, I., Wanke, M.: Morbus Crohn des terminalen Ösophagus. Z. Gastroenterol. **8**, 163–167 (1970).

Wiesner, P. J., Kleiman, M. S., Condemi, J. I., Resnicoff, S. A., Schwartz, S. I.: Sarcoidosis of the esophagus. Amer. J. dig. Dis. **16**, 943–951 (1971).

Chapter 6

Esophageal Webs and Rings

J. A. RINALDO

With 5 Figures

1. Introduction

Web implies a thin, fragile diaphragm interrupting the esophageal lumen. *Ring* suggests a thicker, stronger diaphragm. However, both of these terms are often used to describe lesions that have a similar radiographic appearance. They are also used loosely to describe certain types of muscular contractions and stenoses. For these reasons, somewhat arbitrary but useful definitions have been coined to classify webs and rings (SHAMMA'A and BENEDICT, 1958; HILLE-MAND, 1968).

Evaluation of webs and rings should include a study of symptoms, signs, radiographic and manometric findings and, whenever possible, biopsy under direct vision (RINALDO and GAHAGAN, 1966). In the past only one or the other of these features has been used in an attempt to prove the nature of a web or ring. As will be noted in the text to follow, these features tend to be quite characteristic for the different webs and rings.

There are certain peculiarities about the radiographic findings of webs and rings that make some general remarks pertinent. The *web* and *ring* have sharp margins (Figs. 269–271) and vary in thickness from 0.1 to 0.3 cm. *Stenoses and muscle contractions* have more or less tapered margins and are 0.5 to over 1.0 cm thick (Fig. 272). The dynamic behavior of the lesions varies. *Web* and *ring* change not at all over a period of years or only slowly (WALDENSTRÖM and KJELL-BERG, 1939; SCHATZKI, 1963). *Muscle contractions* vary in rapidity of change (Fig. 273). The narrow types that are likely to be confused with webs and rings change quickly from moment to moment and can be distinguished by multiple spot films or cineradiography (Fig. 273). Muscle contractions of the type seen in achalasia are much thicker and taper smoothly. They change very little over a period of years. They are not a source of confusion. Contrarily, *stenoses* may decrease in size slowly over a period of weeks or months.

There are three other important points for clinicians to know in relation to the radiographic examination. First, the clinician should fully inform the radiologist concerning the suspected diagnosis. Second, the radiologist should use thick barium with the consistency of very thick cream or thin paste. A compressed barium tablet, 12.5 mm in diameter, may also be used. Third, the esophagus and stomach above and below a ring should be fully distended and in profile in order to delineate the ring properly (WIGGINS, 1967).

The upper limit of the esophagus is at the level of the cricoid muscle. This is usually taken as the dividing line between the pharynx and the esophagus. The lower limit is subject to considerable discussion (INGELFINGER, 1960). Fortunately, this problem can be avoided in patients with a lower esophageal ring.

Evidence is accumulating from both physiologic (HEITMAN et al., 1966; RINALDO and GAHAGAN, 1966) and autopsy studies (BAUER et al., 1970; GOYAL et al., 1970, 1971) that in these patients the narrow ring at the squamocolumnar junction is located at, or very close to, the junction of the esophageal and gastric muscle. Between these limits, it is usual to think of the esophagus as being divided into thirds, each segment being approximately 8 cm long. For reasons that will become apparent, it seems more appropriate to divide the esophagus into an upper segment 2 to 4 cm distal to the cricoid muscle, a middle segment, 20 to 22 cm long and a lower segment 2 to 4 cm long. The following classification of esophageal webs or rings is suggested to coincide with this division:

1. Upper esophageal web—The Paterson-Kelly or Plummer-Vinson syndrome.
2. Middle esophageal web.
3. Lower esophageal web.
4. Squamocolumnar or lower esophageal ring—the Schatzki ring.

Upper esophageal or postcricoid webs can be grouped together because these lesions have a peculiar anatomical and sex distribution and are frequently associated with buccal or esophageal carcinoma. All the rings that have been reported as lower esophageal webs or rings, but that are located in what is described here as middle esophageal segment, would be classified as middle esophageal webs (SALZMAN, 1965; MENDL and EVANS, 1962). This is appropriate since most of the webs classified as lower resemble middle esophageal webs in every way. Only webs in the lower 2 to 4 cm of the esophagus will be classified as lower esophageal webs primarily because they differ in radiographic appearance from the middle esophageal webs. The separation of the lower esophageal webs from the lower esophageal rings is justified because of their histological and radiographical differences. The reader should note that *web* will be used for all diaphragms in the upper, middle and lower segments and *ring* will be used only for the lesion at the squamocolumnar mucosal junction.

This division of webs and rings has many advantages. First it recognizes the proven differences in the epithelium overlying the web or ring—squamous epithelium over the lower esophageal web and squamous and columnar epithelium over the squamocolumnar rings. Second, it assists in defining the anatomy and its relation to function at the esophagogastric junction. For example, the surgeon who resects or biopsies a lower esophageal web should, when possible, identify the squamocolumnar junction and its relation to the web or ring in question. These should in turn be related to the radiographic anatomy using one of the more modern studies for reference (WOLF et al., 1968; BERRIDGE et al., 1966; CLARK et al., 1970). Third, this multivariate classification should help to determine the most appropriate modes of therapy in middle and lower esophageal webs as well as squamocolumnar rings.

2. Upper Esophageal Web
2.1. Definition

This is a narrowing in the postcricoid area of the esophagus due to a diaphragm formed by apparently normal mucosa (Fig. 269). (The reader should review the *Introduction* before proceeding further with this section.) The patient is usually a woman and often complains of dysphagia. There may be signs and laboratory evidence of an iron deficiency anemia. When there are, the eponyms Kelly-Paterson Syndrome or Plummer-Vinson Syndrome are used (KELLY, 1919; PATERSON, 1919; VINSON, 1922). Radiographically, there is a thin, eccentric lesion projecting into the barium column from the anterior wall of the esophagus at the level of the fifth to seventh cervical vertebrae.

2.2. Incidence

The prevalence of this web in patients undergoing routine radiographic examination of the upper gastroesophageal tract in a private hospital in Chicago was 0.36% (MILLER and LEWIS, 1963). However, in patients aged 40 to 75 years who complained of at least two years of dysphagia located between the hyoid bone and the suprasternal notch, 15.4% had one or more webs (ELWOOD et al., 1964). Strangely, only 12.5% of these patients had a web narrow enough to cause stenosis. This lesion has a peculiar geographic distribution; it occurs predominantly in the more northerly countries (Sweden, Scotland, Minnesota, etc.) and seems to be very rare in Africa.

Although this web has been reported in infants and adolescents, it is most common over the age of 30 (HOLINGER et al., 1951; ELWOOD et al., 1964; CRAWFURD et al., 1965; ENTWISTLE and JACOBS, 1965). The sex incidence is difficult to assess. Approximately 93% of patients with the Kelly-Paterson Syndrome are women (KELLY, 1919; PATERSON, 1919; MOERSCH and CONNER, 1926; SOTGIU and LABO, 1956; WYNDER and FRYER, 1958; JONES, 1961; ENTWISTLE and JACOBS, 1965). But when one considers asymptomatic upper webs, the relative incidence in women and men is uncertain, varying from 0 to 100% in two separated series (MILLER and LEWIS, 1963; ELWOOD et al., 1964).

2.3. Etiology and Pathogenesis

The etiology is unknown. The most strongly held theory is that iron deficiency causes alterations in the epithelial layer, which in turn cause dysphagia (WYNDER and FRYER, 1958; JONES, 1961). The frequently reported association of iron deficiency or anemia with upper esophageal webs, the fact that anemia or iron deficiency may be a precursor of dysphagia and the disappearance of dysphagia after iron therapy, all are in favor of this theory. However, in a careful epidemiological community study ELWOOD et al. (1964) found no evidence of a significantly increased prevalence of anemia or of latent iron deficiency in subjects with postcricoid dysphagia or in females with upper esophageal webs. Therefore, it seemed also possible that the web causes dysphagia and a decreased intake of iron-containing solid food. This nutritional deficiency along with the monthly loss of iron in females would in turn result in iron deficiency states. In addition, thyroid disease, Sjögren's Syndrome and riboflavin deficiency have all been mentioned as causing dysphagia (JONES, 1961; BLENDIS and KREEL, 1965). However, no authors suggest that these factors cause the upper web (ENTWISTLE and JACOBS, 1965). This problem has been studied again by CHISHOLM et al. (1971a, b) in a series of 168 individuals, who were chosen merely on the basis of iron deficiency anemia and who were compared to 98 age- and sex-matched controls. An upper esophageal web could be demonstrated by cinefluorography in 10% of the unselected iron-deficient patients, whereas no webs were found in the control subjects. When patients with webs were compared to subjects with iron deficiency but no webs (CHISHOLM et al., 1971a, b) it was found that tissue changes of iron deficiency such as angular stomatitis and glossitis were more common in the web patients. Moreover, patients with webs were more likely to be edentulous and to have an associated thyroid disease than the iron-deficient patient without webs. These observations seem to indicate that iron deficiency is a prerequisite for the development of upper esophageal webs, that thyroid disease is more common in this condition and that there is an increased incidence of tissue changes such as edentula and glossitis in patients with webs. The web has also been observed in infants, and it seems likely that in infants it is congenital in origin (HOLINGER et al., 1951).

2.4. Pathology

There is surprisingly little change in the normal histology of the esophageal mucosa in the upper web (ENTWISTLE and JACOBS, 1965). The squamous epithelium is intact but for some minor irregularities in the basal cell areas. There may be an increase in the number of mononuclear cells in the lamina propria and minimal fibrosis. There have also been some degenerative changes in striated muscle and nerves in the few cases where muscle has been studied. Interestingly, there has been no documented case to show a change from a web to a stricture, nor documented cases which show a reduction in lumen size over a period of months or years (ENTWISTLE and JACOBS, 1965). Thus, this appears to be a relatively static lesion with little or no evidence of inflammation. Little is known about the pathologic anatomy of the esophagus proper in this condition. Atrophy and hyperkeratinization of the esophageal epithelium with areas of desquamation and of degenerative changes in striated muscle and nerves have been described (SAVILAHTI, 1946).

2.5. Clinical Features

In adults, the symptoms may vary. In some, the web is discovered accidentally at the time of radiographic examination (MILLER and LEWIS, 1963). In others, dysphagia is the presenting complaint. In still others, there may be weakness, lassitude and loss of weight in addition to dysphagia (JACOBS and KILPATRICK, 1964; ELWOOD et al., 1964). The loss of weight is not sudden but occurs over a period of years. Dysphagia occurs with solids such as meat and bread, and not with liquids. The patient indicates that the passage of food is delayed or that food sticks between the hyoid bone and the suprasternal notch. Frequently the dysphagia has a sudden onset, when a particle of food, especially meat, becomes lodged in the throat. This gives rise to a sensation of choking but the patient has no pain.

In infants, there is usually no difficulty in swallowing until solids are added to the diet anywhere from five to 11 months. Then the child will frequently spit up his food. As he becomes a little older, solid particles of food will lodge in the web and may need to be removed at esophagoscopy. These children are considered "poor eaters". There may be repeated radiographic studies of the esophagus before the lesion is discovered (HOLINGER et al., 1951).

The signs vary from none at all in the patient who is discovered incidentally, to many in those with evidences of deficiency states (SOTGIU and LABO, 1956; WYNDER and FRYER, 1958; JONES, 1961). Pallor, a red smooth tongue with atrophic papillae, cracking at the angles of the mouth (cheilosis), depression of the nail beds (koilonychia), and brittle nails are results of iron deficiency. The signs of iron deficiency are not pathognomonic, since in one series matched controls had a significant incidence of these signs (WYNDER and FRYER, 1958). Moreover, manifestations of iron deficiency are not obligatory, since upper esophageal webs and postcricoid dysphagia may occur in patients who have no evidence of past or present iron deficiency (ELWOOD et al., 1964). Edentula is said to occur with greater frequency than usual in patients with upper esophageal web. Forty-six percent of the patients in one group had lost their teeth prior to the age of 39 as compared to 20% among the control group (WYNDER and FRYER, 1958). Splenomegaly was reported in the older literature but not recently (CAMERON, 1928).

2.6. Technical Features

Signs of iron deficiency should be looked for. Laboratory tests include the hemoglobin which is reduced disproportionately in relation to the red cell count. The red blood cells are microcytic. There is a reduction in mean corpuscular hemoglobin, mean corpuscular volume and mean corpuscular hemoglobin content. The level of serum iron is low with a normal or elevated iron binding capacity. Serum vitamin B_{12} and pyridoxine levels may be reduced (JACOBS and KILPATRICK, 1964; JACOBS and CAVELL, 1968). Achlorhydria is more common than in the normal population. Macrocytic anemia is sometimes seen.

Radiologic examination requires attention to the postcricoid area, if this lesion is to be discovered. Spot films of the barium-filled and distended upper esophagus or fluorocinematography must be obtained in the lateral position in order to visualize postcricoid webs. The clinician must indicate to the radiologist the diagnosis he is concerned about (see *Introduction* for other points). The web is a very thin projection into the barium column from the anterior wall of the esophagus just distal to the cricoid area. Usually it is less than 2 mm in width, (Fig. 269) and is best seen in the lateral view at the level of the fifth

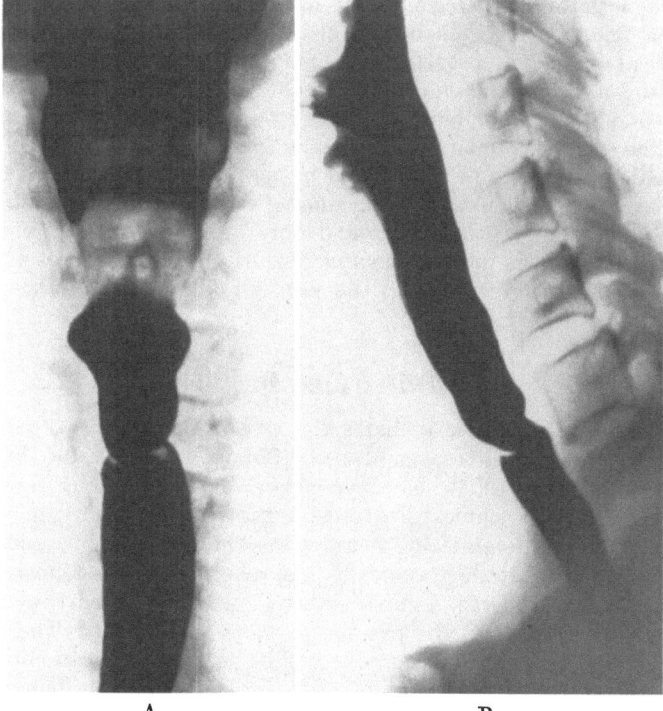

A   B

Fig. 269 A and B. Upper esophageal web. Anteroposterior and lateral view

to the seventh cervical vertebrae. It may be seen in the anteroposterior view if the web extends to the lateral walls of the esophagus (MILLER and LEWIS, 1963; PITMAN and FRASER, 1965). Some artifacts may be mistaken for the web (PITMAN and FRASER, 1965). It is felt that these postcricoid impressions are due to the ventral venous plexus. These impressions do not cause dysphagia. They can be best differentiated from the web by multiple spot films or cinematography because the ventral venous plexus changes its shape during the course of the examination and the web does not (BENEDICT, 1965) (Fig. 58). Rarely multiple webs are present in the upper esophagus or in the postcricoid region and the pharynx.

The endoscopic appearance of these webs varies from a transparent diaphragm with tiny vascular channels running in it to a thicker diaphragm that appears quite substantial (SHAMMA'A and BENEDICT, 1958). The web is usually eccentric, occluding only part of the lumen, but rarely it is concentric and occludes most of it. Sometimes a radiographically demonstrated web is not found on esophagoscopy, most likely because it is ruptured during endoscopy. The latter was always true when the Eder-Hufford esophagoscope was used because the obturator was used to pass the instrument. With the newer fiber-optic esophagoscope, it is important to start viewing as soon as one enters the esophagus.

There is only one manometric study of a patient with an upper esophageal web (KELLEY and FRAZER, 1966). This study was normal. Cytologic examinations have not been reported but one would anticipate that they will be normal.

2.7. Diagnosis

The diagnosis of upper esophageal web should be suspected if a patient, especially a middle-aged women, complains of intermittent dysphagia located in the cervical region and a sensation of choking. The presence of iron deficiency anemia is suggested by the clinical symptoms and signs. It is confirmed by red cell counts and hemoglobin determinations as well as serum iron and iron binding capacity. The presence of macrocytic anemia is determined by the usual methods. Pyridoxine deficiency can be established by serum determinations. The diagnosis may be discovered incidentally at the time of radiological examination for other reasons, but frequently it will be found only after careful examination of the postcricoid region in the active stage of deglutition. The diagnosis can be confirmed by esophagoscopy provided the web is not ruptured by the instrument or the preceding intubation.

2.8. Differential Diagnosis

The differential diagnosis includes the *postcricoid impression, inflammatory stenosis* and *postcricoid carcinoma* (JONES, 1961; ENTWISTLE and JACOBS, 1965; PITMAN and FRASER, 1965). The *postcricoid impression* was described in a preceding paragraph (Technical Features). *Inflammatory stenosis* may mimic the web clinically. The differentiating features are the radiographic, endoscopic and histologic appearance. Radiographically, the margins of the stenosis are thicker and the edges more tapered. Endoscopically, the lumen is narrowed and there is considerable resistance to the passage of the esophagoscope. The mucosa will be friable and eroded in acute lesions. It will be pale and firm in chronic lesions. Histologically, one finds evidence of acute and/or chronic inflammation with fibrosis. *Postcricoid carcinoma* is often associated with inflammatory strictures (JONES, 1961). It also may resemble upper esophageal web because it may be preceded by years of dysphagia and iron deficiency anemia. It is important that postcricoid carcinoma happens in women five times as frequently as in men. The reverse is true in carcinomas of the oropharynx, larynx and esophagus (JONES, 1961). The radiographic appearance has the characteristics of neoplasms elsewhere in the gastrointestinal tract. The lumen is irregular and mucosal markings are effaced. There are sharp margins at one or both ends of the lesions. Frequently the patient experiences difficulty in forcing the barium past the upper end of the esophagus, which results in retention of barium in the valleculae and pyriform sinuses. Endoscopically, postcricoid carcinoma shows friable, irregular, multicolored mucosa that projects into the lumen. Biopsies should be obtained when one suspects inflammatory strictures or postcricoid carcinoma.

2.9. Complications and Prognosis

Occasionally a bolus of meat will lodge in the stricture. The prognosis of the dysphagia associated with the upper esophageal web is excellent, if appropriate treatment is instituted. It must be emphasized, however, that carcinoma of the mouth, pharynx or upper esophagus has been observed in patients with upper esophageal webs, with sufficient frequency to consider this web as a precancerous lesion. About 70% of patients with carcinoma of the cricopharyngeal region give a long history of the Plummer-Vinson Syndrome (AHLBOM, 1936). Sixteen percent of the 58 patients with esophageal webs observed by SHAMMA'A and BENEDICT (1958) developed carcinoma in the mouth or esophagus. The malignancy tends to occur above the area of web formation, rather than in the web or below it. Three of the six patients of this series with carcinoma of the mouth had two webs.

2.10. Treatment

Treatment of upper esophageal web varies according to the clinical problem. In the asymptomatic web no treatment is indicated. In the patient with iron deficiency anemia, vigorous treatment with oral iron is needed. Preferably, this should be a liquid preparation. Where dysphagia is present the web is often fractured during the endoscopy (SHAMMA'A and BENEDICT, 1958). Where it is not, it is possible to remove portions of the web at esophagoscopy. Dilation with soft, mercury-filled bougies is seldom necessary. Surprisingly, simple treatment with iron may lead to disappearance of the web and of symptoms even if nothing is done to the ring (WALDENSTRÖM and KJELLBERG, 1939; JONES, 1961).

3. Middle Esophageal Web

This is a narrowing in the middle segment of the esophagus due to a mucosal diaphragm containing varying numbers of inflammatory cells (Fig. 270) (see *Introduction* before proceeding with this section). When present, dysphagia is the only symptom. Radiographically, there is a thin concentric or sometimes eccentric lesion projecting into the barium column.

3.1. Incidence

There are no precise figures on the incidence of this lesion. However, in one series of middle esophageal webs in which the patients were seen because of dysphagia, the incidence of middle esophageal web was only 4% of that of upper

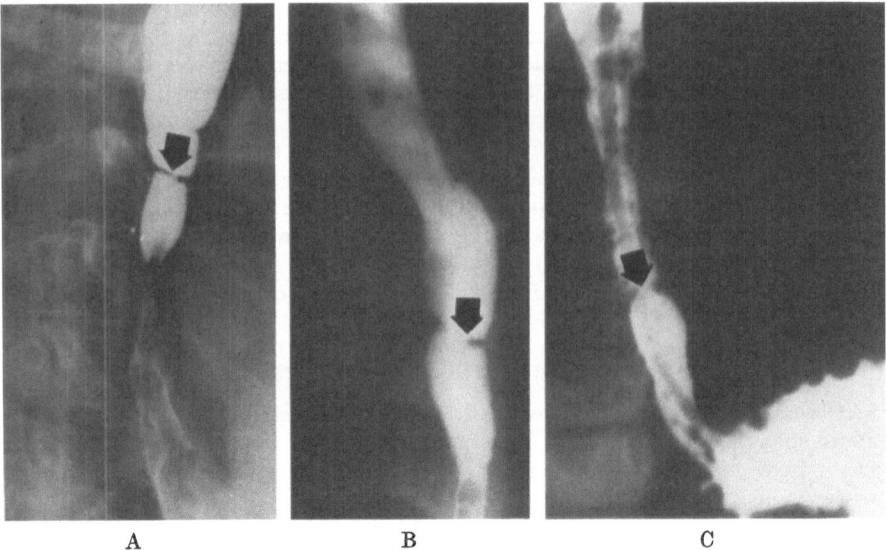

A   B   C

Fig. 270 A–C. Middle esophageal webs with slightly different configurations (arrows). A Upper part, very thin and symmetrical. B Middle part, thicker and slightly asymmetrical. C Lower part, still thicker but symmetrical. (Courtesy of LEO FIEGEL, M.D., Dept. Radiology, Grace Hospital, Detroit, Mich.)

esophageal web (SHAMMA'A and BENEDICT, 1958). The web occurs with equal frequency in men and women. It may occur in infants but is more common in adults.

3.2. Etiology

Some webs that occur in infants are most certainly congenital in orgin (HOLINGER et al., 1951). However, those in adults are of undetermined cause. Where an inflammatory reaction is present, it seems likely that the web is a result of the inflammation. However, the cause of the inflammation is unknown. Most often the web is composed of normal mucosa with normal epithelium. Sometimes there are more than the usual number of mononuclear cells. On occasion, minimal fibrosis is present in the lamina propria.

3.3. Clinical Features

In adults the web may be completely asymptomatic and may be found incidentally during radiographic examination. The only symptom, if any, is dysphagia for solids but not for liquids. The dysphagia is intermittent. Usually the patient indicates that food stops at midsternum, but sometimes the food is said to stop at the level of the suprasternal notch or the xiphoid. This may be associated with pain in the substernal area.

In infants, there are usually no symptoms until 5 or 11 months of age when the child is given solids to eat. Then the child begins to spit up food. Sometimes solids will occlude the narrow lumen and need to be removed at esophagoscopy. Once established the symptoms in adults and children vary little over a period of years. There are no physical findings related to the middle esophageal web.

3.4. Technical Features

Radiologically, this web is in the middle segment of the esophagus. It is 0.1 to 0.3 cm thick and may be eccentric or concentric. Other important features for the clinician will be found in the *Introduction*.

Endoscopic examination reveals a mucosal diaphragm without evidence of inflammation (SHAMMA'A and BENEDICT, 1958). Manometric examination has been reported on one occasion to be normal (KELLEY and FRAZER, 1966). Cytological examination has never been reported, but one would expect it to be normal.

3.5. Diagnosis

The diagnosis is suspected in infants from the history of normal eating habits until 5 months of age when the infant begins to spit up or has a sudden onset of esophageal obstruction (HOLINGER et al., 1951). In adults, the diagnosis is suggested by the occurrence of intermittent dysphagia when eating solids. Sometimes, when a morsel of food becomes impacted in the web, there is pain with the dysphagia. This is referred to the midsternum or sometimes to the suprasternal notch or the xiphoid. The differential diagnosis includes *inflammatory stenosis, muscle contraction* and *carcinoma*. *Inflammatory stenosis* is usually thicker and has gently tapering margins on radiographic examination. Endoscopically, there is friability of the mucosa with erosions, if the lesion is acute, or pale and tough mucosa if the lesion is older. A biopsy will show signs of acute or chronic inflammation, depending on the age of the stenosis. The type of *muscle contraction* that is confused with the middle esophageal web is very transient so that either multiple spot films, repeat films or cineradiography will make differentiation easy. *Carcinoma* of the esophagus is never manifested as a thin web with the sharp regular indentation in the barium column on radiographic examination.

3.6. Prognosis and Treatment

The only complication is occlusion of the esophageal lumen at the level of the web by a piece of solid food. This may necessitate removal at endoscopy. The prognosis is excellent. No treatment is necessary when the web is discovered incidentally during a routine radiographic examination. If dysphagia is present, dilation with bougies should be tried first. On occasion, it is necessary to resect pieces of the web through the esophagoscope. Rarely, it is necessary to resect the ring surgically, using a transthoracic approach.

4. Lower Esophageal Web

This lesion occurs in the 2 cm of the esophagus adjacent to the squamocolumnar junction (Fig. 271) (see *Introduction* before completing this section). It is a diaphragm formed by mucosa that contains only squamous epithelium and often has inflammatory cells in the lamina propria and submucosa. The symptoms are entirely similar to those of the squamocolumnar (Schatzki) ring. The radiographic appearance is not as unique as that of the squamocolumnar ring, but there are some radiographic patterns that suggest this diagnosis.

4.1. Incidence and Etiology

The incidence is unknown since the term "lower esophageal web" is used to describe lesions that on the one hand resemble middle esophageal webs and

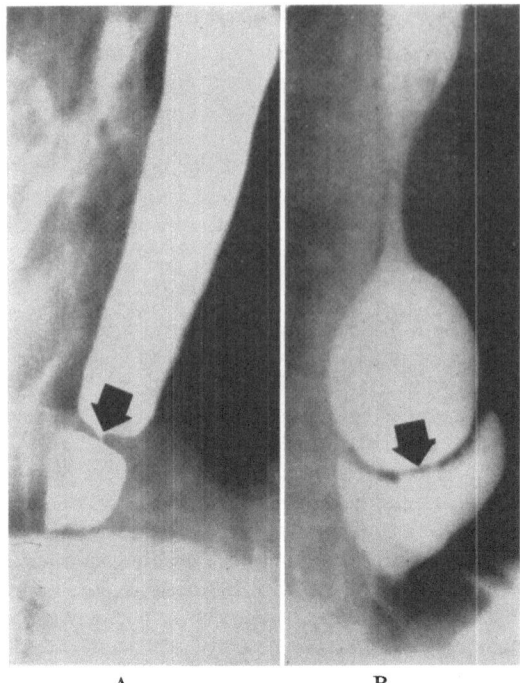

A   B

Fig. 271 A and B. A lower esophageal web (arrows). Two views in the same patient. Open biopsy of the web revealed squamous epithelium. A Web with esophagus above and below distended to the same extent. Web is at biconcave part of sphincter (see Fig. 272 for nomenclature). B Considerable distension of the esophagus above, and of the vestibular part of the sphincter below, giving the "beaked" appearance. [From Holyoake, Y.: Clin. Radiol. 14, 158 (1963)]

on the other hand resemble the squamocolumnar (Schatzki) ring (Figs. 270, 272) (Bugden and Delmonico, 1956; Mendl and Evans, 1962; Holyoake, 1963; Salzman, 1965). This appears to be a disease of adults within the age range from 40 to 70. The cause is unknown. The presence of submucosal inflammation suggests that it is an inflammatory lesion. The stimulus to this inflammation is uncertain. Progressive changes are slow, occurring over a period of many years.

This web is covered by squamous epithelium, which may show some hyperkeratosis. There is a chronic inflammatory infiltration in the submucosa (Bugden and Delmonico, 1956; Holyoake, 1963; Bjork and Charonis, 1967). The muscularis mucosa may be disrupted.

4.2. Clinical and Technical Features

The clinical features are entirely similar to those observed in lesions classified in the next section of this chapter as squamocolumnar ring. Radiologically, all of the techniques described in the *Introduction* should be followed. The lower esophageal web is 1–2 mm thick, or about the same thickness as the middle esophageal web and the squamocolumnar ring. In other respects, the radiographic appearance differs from that of the middle esophageal web and the squamocolumnar ring. First, the middle esophageal web has the same degree of distension of the esophagus above and below the web. Second, the squamocolumnar ring has a characteristic appearance that is described in the next section of this paper with biconcave and vestibular areas proximal to the squamo-columnar ring and asymmetrical stomach distal to it. The lower esophageal web has a symmetrical bulging proximal to the ring and an irregular distended area distal to it. There is disagreement on the interpretation of the radiographic anatomy of the lower esophageal web. Some interpret the distension of the esophagus proximal to this web as a gastroesophageal vestibule (HOLYOAKE, 1963). On the other hand, we feel that this web is at the level of the biconcave area of the inferior sphincter, not at the squamocolumnar junction, and the vestibular area of the sphincter is distal to the web (CLARK et al., 1970). The vestibular area may take on a wing-like appearance (see Fig. 271 b), which characterizes several of the reported cases (BUGDEN and DELMONICO, 1956; HOLYOAKE, 1963).

Endoscopic examination has the same shortcomings for this web as it does for the squamocolumnar ring.

4.3. Diagnosis

The diagnosis is suspected when a middle-aged man or woman complains of intermittent dysphagia. The symptom pattern is indistinguishable from that of the squamocolumnar ring. The differential diagnosis includes all those mentioned in the next section of this chapter entitled *squamocolumnar ring*. The chief difficulty is distinguishing this lesion from the squamocolumnar ring. The only means of separating the two is by radiographic appearance and by biopsy under direct vision. The radiographic characteristics have been discussed above. Treatment is the same as that of the squamocolumnar ring.

4.4. Comment

The reasons for separating this web from the squamocolumnar ring are discussed in the *Introduction*. The two seem to have the same inflammatory origin. The major difference between the two is a modest difference in location. The lower esophageal web appears to be up to 2 cm orad to the squamocolumnar ring. The grouping of the lower esophageal webs and squamocolumnar rings together has led to confusion concerning interpretation of the anatomy and function of the terminal esophagus.

5. Squamocolumnar Ring

5.1. Definition

This is a narrowing of the lumen at the squamocolumnar junction due to a diaphragm of mucosa which has varying degrees of acute and chronic inflammation (Fig. 272). More details of the classification of webs and rings will be found in the *Introduction*. Dysphagia occurs intermittently in those in whom the lumen at the level of the ring is less than 20 mm in diameter (SCHATZKI, 1963). The characteristic radiographic appearance consists of a symmetrical lesion 2 mm thick projecting into the lumen, and proximal to this ring a biconcave and vestibular area (Fig. 272) (RINALDO and GAHAGAN, 1966; CLARK et al., 1970).

5.2. Incidence

The incidence of this ring is 3.6% of routine radiographic examinations in the second decade, 8.5% in the third decade, and approximately 15% from

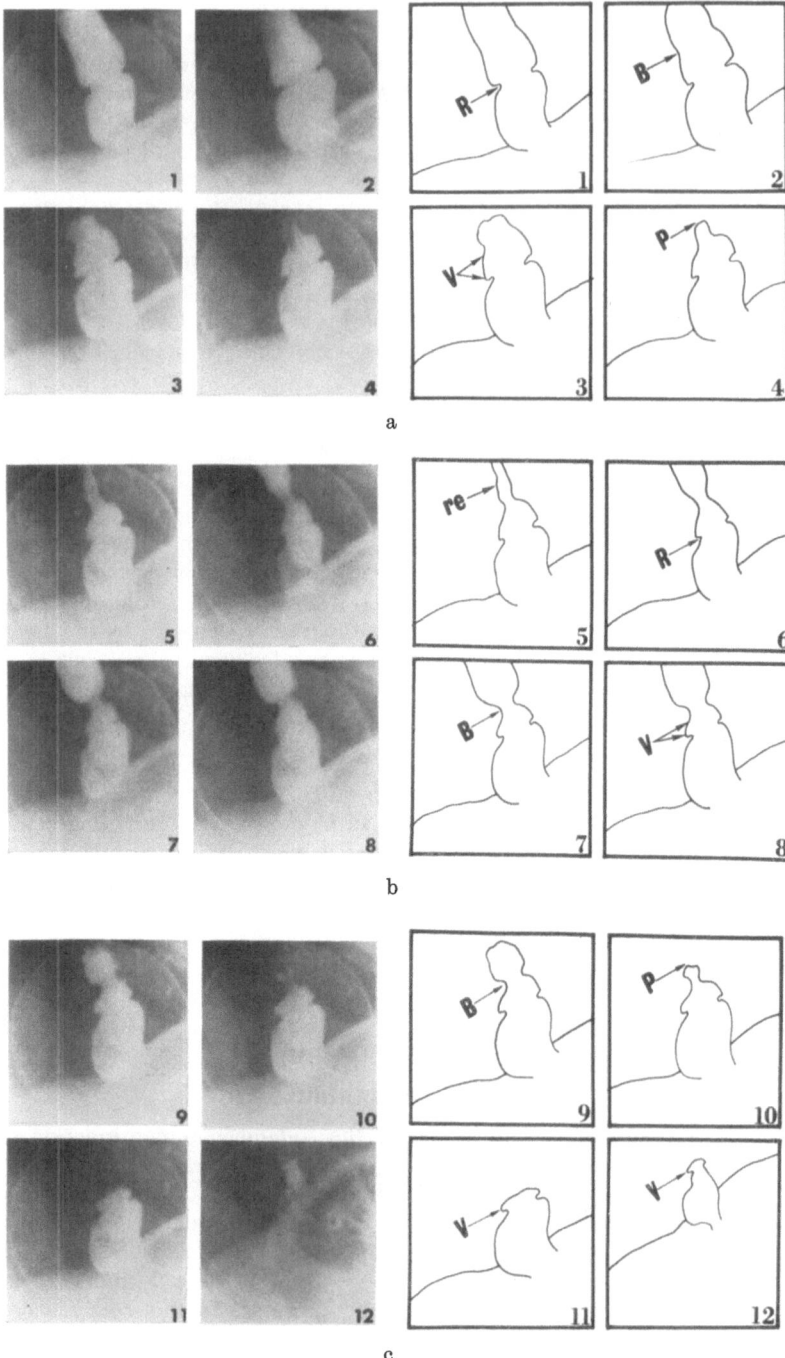

Fig. 272a–c. Muscular contraction and the squamocolumnar ring. This sequence of 70 mm spots shows the muscular contraction in various shapes during different phases of contractions but the constant shape of the ring. This is the radiographic appearance of the lower esophageal sphincter in the vast majority of patients who do not have a ring. Here one sees its relation to a squamocolumnar ring. a Relation of muscular ring to peristaltic wave and

the fourth decade on (KEYTING et al., 1960). Not all of these patients have dysphagia. Dysphagia is present only if the lumen at the level of the ring is narrow (see *Clinical Features*). In those who have persistent dysphagia, 75% are men (INGELFINGER and KRAMER, 1953; WILKINS and BARTLETT, 1963; RINALDO, 1966). The relation between men and women without symptoms has not been tabulated. Symptomatic squamocolumnar ring is rare under the age of 40. The mean age of the patients in two larger series was 53 and 56 years (WILKINS and BARTLETT, 1963; RINALDO and GAHAGAN, 1966).

5.3. Etiology and Pathogenesis

In those instances that fit the criteria of the definition, the ring is at the squamocolumnar junction. Three causes of this ring have been suggested; a transmucosal fold, a muscular ring, a fibrotic ring and a mucosal ring (INGEL-FINGER and KRAMER, 1953; POSTLETHWAIT and MUSSER, 1965; FRIEDLAND et al., 1966; GOYAL et al., 1970, 1971). The transmucosal fold theory was suggested by an autopsy study of patients who had had radiographic studies (FRIEDLAND et al., 1966). It ignores the large number of patients who have been operated upon and in whom the ring was found to be a firm narrowing at the squamo-columnar junction (WILKINS and BARTLETT, 1963; MONGES et al., 1964; POST-LETHWAIT and MUSSER, 1965; RINALDO and GAHAGAN, 1966; GROSDIDIER and BORRELLY, 1968). We suspect that the transmucosal fold accounts for many indentations at the junction of the esophagus and stomach but not the squamo-columnar ring. The original proponent of the theory that the ring is a muscular structure has since changed his point of view (INGELFINGER, 1960).

Surgical biopsy specimens of the squamocolumnar ring have shown greater or lesser degrees of inflammation and fibrosis. For this reason, it has been sug-gested that the ring results from inflammation leading to fibrosis and is a *forme fruste* of peptic esophagitis with stricture (WILKINS and BARTLETT, 1963; POST-LETHWAIT and MUSSER, 1965; RINALDO, 1966). The ring is very static in nature, changing in size over a period of five years in only 36% of symptomatic rings and 25% of asymptomatic rings. In those in whom change occurs, it is usually relatively slight but sometimes considerable (SCHATZKI, 1963). Thus, whatever the cause of the inflammatory process, it tends to be self-limiting and very slow in its progress. In a recent autopsy study it was felt that there is no inflammation (GOYAL et al., 1970, 1971). This would not account for decreases in size with

squamocolumnar ring. *1* A swallow has occurred and a bolus is approaching the lower segment. *R* Squamocolumnar ring. Area beyond *R* is stomach. *2* Leading edge of peristaltic wave just making its appearance at the top of this frame. *B* Biconcave part of the lower esophageal sphincter becoming more distinct. *3* Leading edge of peristaltic wave is now distinct. Biconcave part of sphincter closing. *V* Vestibular part of lower esophageal sphincter. *4* Same but more advanced. *P* Leading edge of peristaltic wave. b Independent contraction of biconvave area, *B*, but constant shape of squamocolumnar ring, *R*. *5* The patient swallowed some more barium as peristaltic wave completed travel at biconcave part of sphincter. *re* Reflux through biconcave part of sphincter before second bolus arrived. Supports concept that biconcave part, *B*, is upper part of sphincter. *6, 7, 8* Second bolus has arrived. Note biconcave part of sphincter closed in absence of peristaltic wave. c Closure of sphincter but constant shape of squamocolumnar ring until sphincter is empty. *9* Leading edge of peristaltic wave almost arrived at sphincter. *10* Leading edge of peristaltic wave has arrived and biconcave part has almost closed. *11* Biconcave part closed and vestibular part almost closed. *12* Entire sphincter now closed including biconcave and vestibular parts and stomach segment col-lapsing and traveling caudally

time (SCHATZKI, 1963). It may be that the inflammation disappears with time or it is conceivable that some patients have limitations in distensibility of the mucosa for unknown reasons.

5.4. Pathology

The upper surface of the ring is covered by squamous epithelium and the under surface by columnar epithelium. It has been said that this is not possible because the squamocolumnar junction is irregular (FRIEDLAND et al., 1966; SAVARY, 1970). This is true, but at endoscopy it has been possible for us to straighten the squamocolumnar line considerably by distending the esophagus with air. This point and the fact that such a large percentage of patients in whom the ring has been resected have the squamocolumnar junction in the specimen suggests that there are instances when this junction can be straight (WILKINS and BARTLETT, 1963; POSTLETHWAIT and MUSSER, 1965; RINALDO and GAHAGAN, 1966; GOYAL et al., 1970, 1971). Acanthosis and some degree of hyperkeratosis are noted in the squamous epithelium. An increase in the connective tissue and in the number of lymphocytes and plasma cells is present in the lamina propria. The muscularis mucosae has been found to be fragmented and arranged in bundles of varying size. The submucosa has proliferating connective tissue and numerous lymphocytes and plasma cells. No acute inflammatory cells are noted. These findings are all consistent with a chronic inflammatory reaction (POSTLETHWAIT and MUSSER, 1965).

5.5. Clinical Features

Many patients with lower esophageal rings experience no symptoms related to the ring. If present, the primary symptom is intermittent dysphagia. Attacks of dysphagia occur when the patient eats hurriedly and swallows solids, particularly chunks of meat, apple or bread. In some patients the ring is so narrow that they are unable to eat any solids. They will note that food is held up at the level of the xiphoid. Many patients first complain of dysphagia after removal of their teeth. Of 224 patients studied by SCHATZKI, 104 patients had repeated episodes of dysphagia (SCHATZKI, 1963). There were only two of these whose esophageal lumen at the level of the rings was greater than 20 mm wide. All patients with rings smaller than 13 mm had dysphagia. Forty percent of those with rings between 12 and 20 mm had repeated episodes of dysphagia. From these observations it is apparent that the occurrence and frequency of the attacks of dysphagia depend upon the bore of the ring. Pain with swallowing is common, particularly if the bolus lodges in the ring. The attacks of dysphagia last from about half an hour to several hours and end only when the patient can regurgitate or force the bolus past the narrow ring. Weight loss is rare because of the intermittent nature of symptoms. Heartburn is usually absent. There are no other systemic symptoms unless the patient has an associated disease such as systemic sclerosis. There are no signs associated with this ring.

5.6. Technical Features

Radiologic examination requires careful attention to some details to demonstrate the ring. These are set forth in the *Introduction*. It is important to emphasize that this ring of limited distensibility cannot be demonstrated unless the lower esophagus is distended beyond the maximal diameter of the ring. To detect

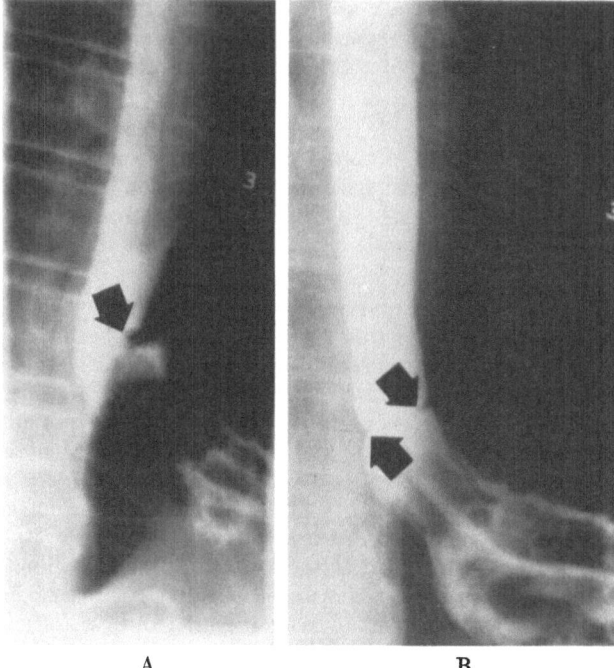

A   B

Fig. 273 A and B. Unusual appearances of a muscular contraction in the same position as
the biconcave area in Fig. 272. Same patient on both spot films. A Appears to be an asymmetrical ring (arrow). B Suggests a classical squamocolumnar ring with indentations on
both sides of the esophagus (arrows). The key to the diagnosis is the rapidly changing shape
as well as the overall appearance of this lower segment of the esophagus and upper segment
of the stomach

this lesion the patient should be placed in the prone horizontal position, partially
turned on the right side, and spot films should be taken at the moment a bolus
of thick barium reaches the lower esophagus which has been maximally dilated
by a deep breath. This ring is 0.2 to 0.3 cm thick. The diameter of the lumen
at the level of the esophagogastric junction varies from 0.5 to 3.0 cm in different
patients. In the individual patient the maximal diameter of the ring is remarkably
constant. The relation between the size of the lumen and the presence of dysphagia was discussed under *Clinical Features*.

In addition to the ring, there is a characteristic appearance proximal to it.
A narrow area about 1 to 2 cm orad to the ring is almost invariably present
(Fig. 273). This has been called the sphincter, the A-ring and the biconcave
area of the sphincter (BERRIDGE et al., 1966; WOLF et al., 1968; CLARK et al.,
1970). Between the narrow area and the squamocolumnar ring, a more distensible
area is present. This has been called the vestibule or the vestibular area of the
sphincter (BERRIDGE et al., 1966; WOLF et al., 1968; CLARK et al., 1970). Some
authors believe the narrow area and the distensible area together comprise the
inferior esophageal sphincter (BERRIDGE et al., 1966; CLARK et al., 1970). Other
authors believe the narrow area (A-ring) is a muscular contraction of unknown
cause in the distal esophagus (WOLF et al., 1968). Finally, some feel that this
characteristic appearance has nothing to do with the sphincter (HARRIS et al.,
1960; CAUTHORNE et al., 1965). In the view of these latter authors, the sphincter

is distal to the ring. A recent study would seem to finally dispel this point of view (GOYAL et al., 1970, 1971). But regardless of the interpretation, the radiographic appearance of the area proximal to the ring is characteristic and is important in the diagnosis.

Endoscopy has yielded variable results. If the ring has a bore of 10 to 12 mm, it is not seen with the standard round rigid 9 mm esophagoscope. It is some-times seen with the larger oval instruments. The new fiberscopes that allow distension with air while viewing the esophagus have given better results. With these instruments it is often possible to identify the ring and the squamocolumnar junction.

Manometry has yielded controversial results. In one study the inferior sphinc-ter pressure of those with rings was compared to normal controls and patients with hiatus hernias. The inferior sphincter pressure in patients with rings was equal to that of patients with hernias and lower than that of normals (RINALDO and GAHAGAN, 1966). In another study, the pressure in patients with rings was equal to that of controls. There was no difference between those with and those without dysphagia (CAUTHORNE et al., 1965). Thus, there is still no agree-ment concerning the manometrics of patients with lower esophageal ring. The main controversy from combined manometric and radiologic studies bears on the location of the ring with regard to the lower esophageal sphincter. According to HARRIS et al. (1960) and CAUTHORNE et al. (1965) the area below the ring has the manometric characteristics of a sphincter. However, others (HEITMANN et al., 1966; RINALDO, 1966; CLARK et al., 1970) believe that the lower esophageal sphincter lies just proximal to the lower esophageal ring. The latter view is strongly supported by a recent autopsy study (BAUER et al., 1970; GOYAL et al., 1970, 1971).

5.7. Diagnosis

The diagnosis is suggested by the presence of intermittent attacks of dys-phagia with meat in a patient, particularly a man over the age of 40, who has had his teeth pulled recently. The diagnosis is confirmed by radiographic examina-tion. However, the majority of such rings will be discovered incidentally at the time of routine radiographic examination for other reasons.

5.8. Differential Diagnosis

This includes the *transmucosal fold, muscular contraction, stenosis* and *neoplasm*. The *transmucosal fold* is an indentation in some patients at or near the cardiac incisura (FRIEDLAND et al., 1966). It is never associated with dysphagia, sub-sternal pain or weight loss. Radiographically, it does not have the characteristic ring-like appearance of the squamocolumnar ring. Endoscopically, the mucosa appears normal. *Muscular contraction* may be associated with dysphagia and pain. Radiographically, it is thicker and has more tapered margins than the ring. It also changes in diameter very quickly in a matter of fractions of a second (Fig. 273). On occasion this muscular contraction can resemble the ring very closely (Fig. 273 b) (BROMBART and HINS, 1965; WIGGINS, 1967). However, serial films or cineradiographic examination will allow differentiation of the ring and muscular contraction (Fig. 273). Endoscopically, the esophagus appears normal. *Stenosis* caused by reflux esophagitis is often preceded and accompanied by a history of heartburn. Dysphagia is more persistent and tends to become worse in the course of a year. Radiographically, it is thicker than the ring and the margins are more tapered. Stenosis is usually concentric. Endoscopically, one notes erythema and friability of the mucosa with erosions and narrowing of the lumen at the level of the stenosis. Biopsy reveals signs of acute and chronic inflammation. *Carconima* is associated with progressively more difficulty in swallowing over a period of weeks or months, almost always less than one year. Radiographically, the margins of the lesion are irregular and often the lumen is eccentric. Endoscopically, one finds friable mucosa which is multicolored and irregular. The diagnosis should be confirmed by biopsy.

5.9. Complications and Prognosis

There are no major complications of the ring. If the patient has a hiatal hernia, there may be the usual complications of the hernia. The prognosis is excellent with appropriate treatment.

5.10. Treatment

Some care in chewing food will often relieve the patient completely. Poorly fitting dentures may be provoking symptoms and should be remedied if possible. In the event that more aggressive treatment is needed, the use of mercury-filled bougies may afford some relief. Olive bougies passed over a metal wire which itself has been passed over a previously swallowed string also may improve the dysphagia. In both instances the diameter of the dilating instrument is progressively increased over a period of several days. The dilatations may have to be repeated after some time. Recently, pneumatic dilation has been suggested on the mistaken premise that this lesion is due to a muscular contraction. Nevertheless, it seems to give prompt and complete relief in many instances and is worth trying (BENEDICT, 1965; MOSSBERG, 1965; RIEGEL, 1967). If the patient has an incompetent inferior esophageal sphincter, dilation of the squamocolumnar ring may lead to gastroesophageal reflux. In this rare instance, hiatal hernia repair with a procedure to improve the function of the inferior sphincter may be necessary.

Another equally rare indication for surgery is the patient who has not been sufficiently improved by dilation. Repair of the hiatal hernia by abdominal approach should be combined with finger dilation and rupture of the ring through a gastrostomy. If the transthoracic approach is used the ring should be excsied through a longitudinal incision in the esophagus.

5.11. Comment

It is our belief that the squamocolumnar ring results from an unusual inflammatory reaction that seems to be self-limiting in most instances. The smaller the ring the more likely the patient will have dysphagia. This is not a functional lesion. It restricts the expansion of the wall of the esophagus at its junction with the stomach. A narrow ring should not be ignored. Appropriate treatment should be instituted.

We do not feel that the presence of the ring *per se* has any significance *vis-à-vis* the diagnosis of hiatal hernia because we feel the distal esophagus moves with swallowing (RINALDO, 1967; CLARK et al., 1970). Normal persons will have the squamocolumnar junction in the thorax as the peristaltic wave traverses the esophagus. The diagnosis of clinically significant hiatal hernia will depend on the size and asymmetry of the gastric pouch in the thorax correlated with the patient's symptoms as well as the endoscopic findings. Manometry may be a useful tool to evaluate the strength and competence of the lower esophageal sphincter.

The reason for separating the lower esophageal web from the squamocolumnar ring was explained in the *Introduction*. Briefly, the radiographic appearance of the two is distinctive, and the lower esophageal web has only squamous epithelium overlying it, whereas the lower esophageal ring is at the squamocolumnar junction.

References

AHLBOM, H. E.: Simple achlorhydric anaemia, Plummer-Vinson syndrome, and carcinoma of the mouth, pharynx and oesophagus in women. Brit. med. J. **1936 II**, 331–333.

BAUER, J. L., GOYAL, R. K., SPIRO, H. M.: The nature and location of the lower esophageal ring. Clin. Res. **118**, 376 (1970).

BENEDICT, E. B.: Forceful dilatation of the esophagus in the treatment of achalasia and lower esophageal ring. New Engl. J. Med. **272**, 1337–1338 (1965).

BERRIDGE, F. R., FRIEDLAND, G. W., TAGART, R. E. B.: Radiological landmarks at the oesophagogastric junction. Thorax **21**, 499–510 (1966).

BJORK, V. O., CHARONIS, C. G.: Lower esophageal web. Thorax **22**, 156–164 (1967).

BLENDIS, L. M., KREEL, L.: The aetiology of "sideropenic" web. Brit. J. Radiol. **38**, 112–115 (1965).

BROMBART, M., HINS, C.: L'anneau œsophagogastrique ou syndrome de Schatzki. Arch. Mal. Appar. dig. **54**, 1049–1061 (1965).

BUGDEN, W. F., DELMONICO, J. R., JR.: Lower esophageal web. J. thorac. cardiovasc. Surg. **31**, 1–18 (1956).

CAMERON, J. A. M.: Dysphagia and anemia. Quart. J. Med. **22**, 43–49 (1928).

CAUTHORNE, R. T., VAN HOUTTE, J. J., DONNER, M. W., HENDRIX, T. R.: Study of patients with lower esophageal ring by simultaneous cineradiography and manometry. Gastroenterology **49**, 632–640 (1965).

CHISHOLM, M., ARDRAN, G. M., CALLENDER, S. T., WRIGHT, R.: A follow-up study of patients with post-cricoid webs. Quart. J. Med. **40**, 409–420 (1971 a).

CHISHOLM, M., ARDRAN, G. M., CALLENDER, S. T., WRIGHT, R.: Iron deficiency and autoimmunity in post-cricoid webs. Quart. J. Med. **40**, 421–433 (1971 b).

CLARK, M. D., RINALDO, J. A., EYLER, W. R.: Correlation of manometric and radiologic data from the esophagogastric area. Radiology **94**, 261–270 (1970).

CRAWFURD, M. D., JACOBS, A., MURPHY, B., PETERS, D. K.: Paterson-Kelly syndrome in adolescence: a report of five cases. Brit. med. J. **1965 I**, 693–695.

ELWOOD, P. C., JACOBS, A., PITMAN, R. G., ENTWISTLE, C. C.: Epidemiology of the Paterson-Kelly syndrome. Lancet **1964 II**, 716–720.

ENTWISTLE, C. C., JACOBS, A.: Histological findings in the Paterson-Kelly syndrome. J. clin. Path. **18**, 408–413 (1965).

FRIEDLAND, G. W., MELCHER, D. M., BERRIDGE, F. R., GRESHAM, G. A.: Debatable points in the anatomy of the lower esophagus. Thorax **21**, 487–498 (1966).

GOYAL, R. K., BAUER, J. L., SPIRO, H. M.: The nature and location of the lower esophageal ring. New Engl. J. Med. **284**, 1175–1180 (1971).

GOYAL, R. K., GLANCY, J. J., SPIRO, H. M.: Lower esophageal ring. New Engl. J. Med. **282**, 1298–1305, 1355–1361 (1970).

GROSDIDIER, J., BORRELLY, J.: Cure chirurgicale de l'anneau de Schatzki. Arch. Mal. Appar. dig. **57**, 1041–1048 (1968).

HARRIS, L. D., KELLY, J. E., JR., KRAMER, P.: Relation of the lower esophageal ring to the esophagogastric junction. New Engl. J. Med. **263**, 1232–1235 (1960).

HEITMAN, P., WOLF, B. S., SOKOL, E. M., COHEN, B. R.: Simultaneous cineradiographic manometry study of the distal esophagus. Small hiatal hernia and rings. Gastroenterology **50**, 737–753 (1966).

HILLEMAND, P.: L'anneau de Schatzki. Bull. Soc. Med. Hôp. Paris **119**, 667–669 (1968).

HOLINGER, R. H., JOHNSTON, K. C., POTTS, W. J.: Congenital anomalies of the esophagus. Ann. Otol. (St. Louis) **60**, 707–717 (1951).

HOLYOAKE, Y.: Dysphagia due to lower oesophageal ring. Clin. Radiol. **14**, 158–162 (1963).

INGELFINGER, F. J.: The physiological background of heartburn, esophagitis and cardiospasm. Arch. intern. Med. **105**, 770–778 (1960).

INGELFINGER, F. J., KRAMER, P.: Dysphagia produced by a contractile ring in the lower esophagus. Gastroenterology **23**, 419–430 (1953).

JACOBS, A., CAVELL, I. A. J.: Pyridoxine and riboflavin status in the Paterson-Kelly syndrome. Brit. H. Haemat. **14**, 153–160 (1968).

JACOBS, A., KILPATRICK, G. S.: The Paterson-Kelly syndrome. Brit. med. J. **1964** II, 79–82.

JONES, R. F. M.: The Paterson-Brown-Kelly syndrome. Its relationship to iron deficiency anemia and postcricoid carcinoma. J. Laryng. **75**, 529–561 (1961).

KELLEY, M. L., FRAZER, J. P.: Symptomatic mid-esophageal webs. J. Amer. med. Ass. **197**, 143–146 (1966).

KELLY, A.: Spasm at the entrance to the esophagus. J. Laryng. **34**, 285–289 (1919).

KEYTING, W. S., BAKER, G. M., McCARVER, R. R., DAYWITT, A. L.: The lower esophagus. Amer. J. Roentgenol. **84**, 1070–1075 (1960).

MENDL, K., EVANS, C. J.: Incomplete lower esophageal diaphragm. Brit. J. Radiol. **35**, 165–171 (1962).

MILLER, J. D. R., LEWIS, R. B.: Esophageal webs in man. Radiology **81**, 498–501 (1963).

MOERSCH, H. J., CONNER, H. M.: Hysterical dysphagia. Arch. Otolaryng. **4**, 112–119 (1926).

MONGES, H., DOR, J., PAYAN, H., MONGES, A., HANEY, A.: Considérations sur l'image radiologique d'anneau de l'œsophage inférieur (lower esophageal ring) et son interpretation. Arch. Mal. Appar. dig. **53**, 1291–1302 (1964).

MOSSBERG, S. M.: Lower esophageal ring treated by pneumatic dilation. Gastroenterology **48**, 118–121 (1865).

PATERSON, D. R.: A clinical type of dysphagia. J. Laryng. **34**, 289–291 (1919).

PITMAN, R. G., FRASER, G. M.: The post-cricoid impression on the esophagus. Clin. Radiol. **16**, 34–39 (1965).

POSTLETHWAIT, R. W., MUSSER, A. W.: Pathology of lower esophageal web. Surg. Gynec. Obstet. **120**, 571–575 (1965).

RIEGEL, N.: Pneumatic dilatation in lower esophageal ring. N.Y. J. Med. **67**, 1081–1084 (1967).

RINALDO, J. A., JR.: The lower esophageal ring. Gastroenterology **51**, 1093–1094 (1966).

RINALDO, J. A., JR.: Movement of the distal esophagus during swallowing; a clue to cineradiographic and manometric examination. In: The esophagus and stomach, ed. E. POLISH, p. 47–53. New York: Grune and Stratton 1967.

RINALDO, J. A., JR., GAHAGAN, T.: The narrow lower esophageal ring: Pathogenesis and physiology. Amer. J. dig. Dis. **11**, 257–265 (1966).

SALZMAN, A. J.: Lower esophageal web associated with achalasia of the esophagus. N.Y. J. Med. **65**, 1922–1925 (1965).

SAVARY, M.: La jonction muqueuse gastro-œsophagienne: Aspect endoscopique normal et pathologique. Rev. méd. Suisse rom. **90**, 25–36 (1970).

SAVILAHTI, M.: On pathologic anatomy of Plummer-Vinson syndrome. Acta med. scand. **125**, 40–45 (1946).

SCHATZKI, R.: The lower esophageal ring. Long term follow-up of symptomatic and asymptomatic rings. Amer. J. Roentgenol. **90**, 805–810 (1963).

SHAMMA'A, M. H., BENEDICT, E. B.: Esophageal webs. New Engl. J. Med. **259**, 378–384 (1958).

SOTGIU, G., LABO, G.: Syndrome de Kelly-Paterson (formes frustes). Gastroenterologia (Basel) **86**, 167–173 (1956).

VINSON, P. P.: Hysterical dysphagia. Minn. Med. **5**, 107–108 (1922).

WALDENSTRÖM, J., KJELLBERG, S. R.: The roentgenological diagnosis of sideropenic dysphagia (Plummer-Vinson's syndrome). Acta radiol. (Stockh.) **20**, 618–638 (1939).

WIGGINS, C. A.: The lower esophageal ring. Austr. Radiol. **11**, 140–149 (1967).

WILKINS, E. W., JR., BARTLETT, M. K.: Surgical treatment of the lower esophageal ring. New Engl. J. Med. **268**, 461–464 (1963).

WOLF, B. S., HEITMAN, P., COHEN, B. R.: The inferior esophageal sphincter, the manometric high pressure zone and hiatal incompetence. Amer. J. Roentgenol. **103**, 251–276 (1968).

WYNDER, E. L., FRYER, J. H.: Etiologic considerations of Plummer-Vinson (Paterson-Kelly) syndrome. Ann. intern. Med. **49**, 1106–1128 (1958).

Chapter 7

Esophageal Diverticula

G. Vantrappen and W. Deloof

With 12 Figures

Esophageal diverticula are localized projections of the lumen of the gullet. They are distinguished from pseudo- or functional diverticula by the fact that the sacculation of the wall has a constant localization and is limited to a relatively small part of the esophageal circumference. Pseudodiverticula, however, are more or less circular protrusions of the esophageal wall, which are localized between two contraction rings and have a variable location.

Frequently a distinction is made between true and false diverticula, based upon the composition of the diverticular wall. According to some authors, the wall of a true diverticulum comprises all layers of the esophagus whereas that of a false diverticulum comprises only mucosa and submucosa (Jones et al., 1969; Spiro, 1970). Others have taken the opposite view (Terracol and Sweet, 1958). Therefore, it is better not to use this confusing distinction any more.

Diverticula can be congenital or acquired. Those of congenital origin contain all layers of the esophageal wall, whereas some acquired diverticula have a "complete" and others an "incomplete" wall. Hypotheses about the pathogenesis of diverticula have led to a classification in pulsion and traction diverticula. When the mucosa herniates through the muscle layers under the influence of an abnormal intraluminal pressure gradient, the diverticulum is called a pulsion diverticulum, whereas traction diverticula originate when the esophageal wall is attracted by adhesions (Rokitansky, 1840). When both factors seem to play a role in the pathogenesis the term *traction-pulsion diverticulum* is used.

The former classifications into congenital and acquired, pulsion and traction, false and true diverticula will be replaced by a classification based mainly on the localization of the diverticulum.

1. Lateral Pharyngeal Diverticula and Pouches

Protrusions of the lateral wall of the hypopharynx have variously been termed pharyngocoele (Kaufman, 1956), lateral pharyngeal pouch (Zaino et al., 1970) or lateral pharyngeal diverticulum (Ardran and Kemp, 1961; Templeton, 1964). Bachman et al. (1968) proposed to use the term pharyngeal diverticulum only for those outpouchings which are connected with the pharyngeal lumen via a narrow neck; if the connection of the outpouching with the pharyngeal lumen is wide they prefer the term pouch. Diverticula and pouches usually occur in the lateral wall of the pharynx, between the hyoid and the upper border of the thyroid cartilage (Fig. 274). More rarely diverticula can be located at the lowermost portion of the pyriform sinuses (Fig. 275).

Lateral pharyngeal pouches appear only during swallowing or during a modified Valsalva maneuver. These pouches are usually bilateral (Fig. 274), but

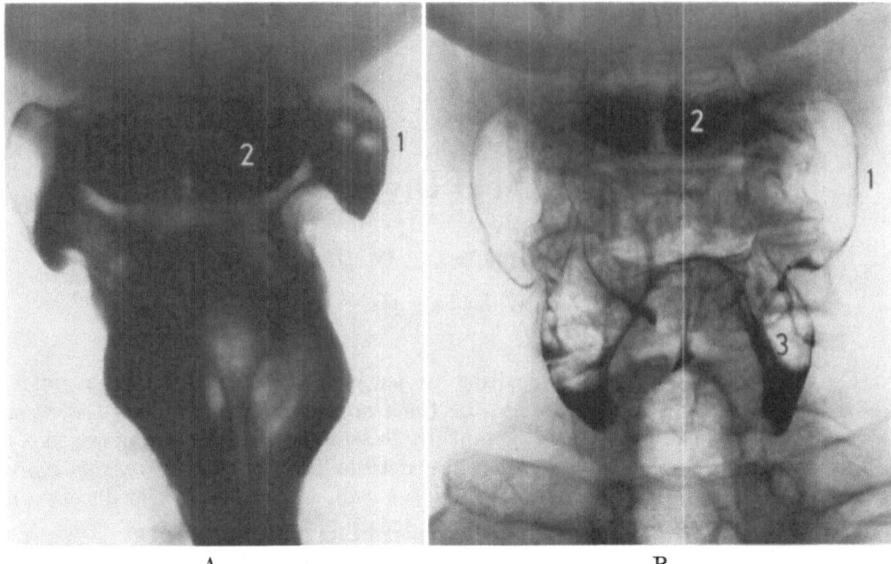

A   B

Fig. 274 A and B. Bilateral pharyngeal pouches. Ear-like outpouchings (*1*) appear during the swallowing act and during a modified Valsalva maneuver. Valleculae (*2*) and pyriform sinuses (*3*) are clearly visible

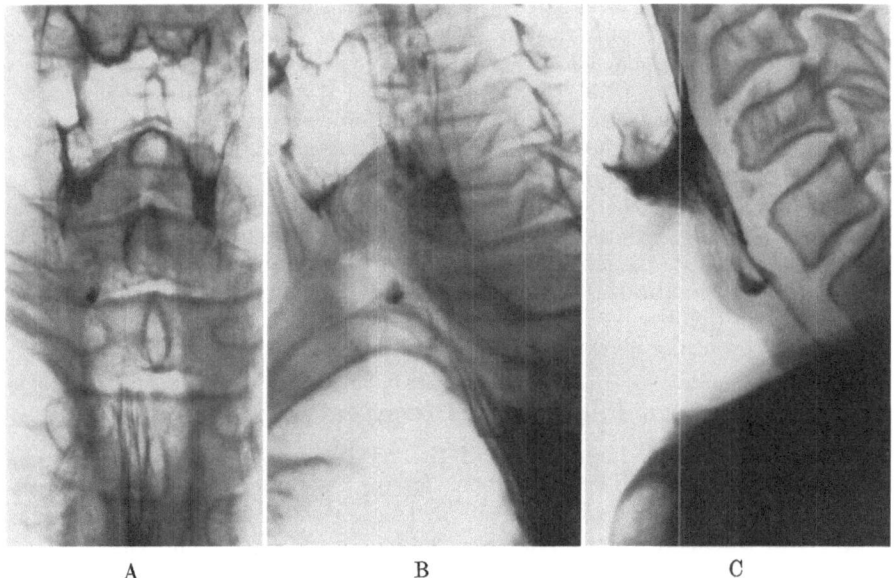

A   B   C

Fig. 275 A—C. Small lateral diverticulum of the lower border of right pyriform sinus demonstrated on post-deglutition films in anteroposterior (A), oblique (B) and lateral (C) position

they may be more pronounced on one side, or even confined to one side. As the connection with the pharyngeal lumen is broad there is no retention of swallowed material and usually no symptoms. Symptoms may occur when the pouch is so large as to hinder deglutition, but this is exceptional. The anomaly is mostly found in older subjects (ARDRAN and KEMP, 1961), and in glass blowers and trumpet players (KAUFMAN, 1956). It can be developed manually and is then used to store coins or other small objects. This has been observed in criminals (TEMPLETON, 1964) and in inhabitants of some regions of India (KAUFMAN, 1956).

Lateral pharyngeal diverticula can be congenital or acquired (KAUFMAN, 1956; BACHMAN et al., 1968). They can be visualized radiologically during swallowing or during a modified Valsalva maneuver. On frontal films they appear as a barium-filled sac of varying size, connected to the bulging portion of the hypopharynx by a short neck. On lateral films the filled diverticulum appears below the level of the valleculae and behind the plane of the epiglottis. These diverticula are often unilateral. There may be retention of barium which is cleared only after repeated dry swallows. Congenital diverticula, which are considered to be remnants of the third or fourth branchial cleft, are rare. The neck of these diverticula is often so narrow that they can be opacified only by a modified Valsalva maneuver, and that there is retention of barium for some time (BUCKSTEIN and REICH, 1950; FOWLER, 1962). Sometimes they cannot be opacified. In other cases the diverticulum is filled with air and is visible on plain films of the neck. Pharyngeal diverticula causing retention of swallowed material are likely to produce swallowing difficulties. In some cases it may even be necessary to resect such diverticular sacs. The small diverticula located at the lateral wall of the lowermost portion of the pyriform sinuses can best be demonstrated during the contraction phase of the pharynx and disappear when the pharynx is distended during the passage of a bolus or a modified Valsalva maneuver (BROMBART, 1961; ZAINO et al., 1970). The clinical significance of this type of diverticulum has not been established.

2. The Hypopharyngeal Diverticulum (Zenker's Diverticulum)

The hypopharyngeal diverticulum or Zenker's diverticulum is, strictly speaking, not an esophageal diverticulum, for it originates from the lower pharynx or hypopharynx. A variety of names have been given to these extrusions: pharyngoesophageal pouches, esophageal diverticula or pouches, pharyngocoeles, pharyngeal pouches, and retrocricoid diverticula. As a typical example of a pulsion diverticulum, it is formed by a protrusion of mucosa and submucosa through the muscle layers of the posterior pharyngoesophageal wall, usually at the level of the upper part of the cricopharyngeus (PERROTT, 1962). Abnormal intrapharyngeal pressure changes developing during swallowing are generally accepted to be the cause of this protrusion.

2.1. Incidence

In his series of 20000 routine radiographic examinations of the esophagus, WHEELER (1947) found 22 cases of hypopharyngeal diverticulum (0.11%). In a hospital population of 1400 patients SHALLOW and CLERF (1948) found a Zenker's diverticulum in 0.07%. In patients with dysphagia Zenker's diverticulum was observed in 1.8% (MACMILLAN, 1935), and in 308 cases with esophageal pathology the incidence was 4% (HARDY and CONN, 1962). The average age of patients with hypopharyngeal diverticulum is more than 50 years, and in many series even more than 60 years. The incidence is always higher in males than in females, the relation being about 3:1 (HARRINGTON, 1949).

2.2. Pathophysiology and Pathogenesis

The pathogenesis of Zenker's diverticulum is still not completely understood. It is generally believed that the protrusion of the mucosa is caused by a combination of two factors, i.e., an anatomically weak area in the posterior wall of the pharynx and disturbances in intrapharyngeal pressure. Standard descriptions of the anatomy of the pharynx in relation to the pathogenesis of Zenker's diverticula indicate that there are two weak areas in the posterior wall of the pharyngoesophageal junctional segment, which are known in the literature as the triangle of Killian (pharyngeal dimple) and the triangle of Laimer.

Cranially the triangle of Killian is bordered by the oblique fibers of the lower pharyngeal constrictor muscles and caudally by the horizontal fibers of the cricopharyngeal muscle. The latter muscle bundle forms the cranial border of the triangle of Laimer. The lower border of Laimer's triangle is formed by the circular and longitudinal fibers of the esophagus.

A careful dissection study of the hypopharynx in 40 cadavers (PERROTT, 1962) showed a considerable variation in the arrangement of the muscle fibers in this region. Weak spots in the muscular wall through which hypopharyngeal diverticula could be extruded were found in at least five different areas (Fig. 276 A): between the upper fibers of the cricopharyngeus and the lower fibers of the hypopharyngeus, in the upper part of the cricopharyngeus consisting of oblique fibers, between the lower oblique and circular fibers of the cricopharyngeus, at the junction of pharyngeal and esophageal muscles, and finally in the circular fibers at the upper end of the esophagus. On anatomical findings the commonest site of the commencement of a hypopharyngeal diverticulum appeared to be

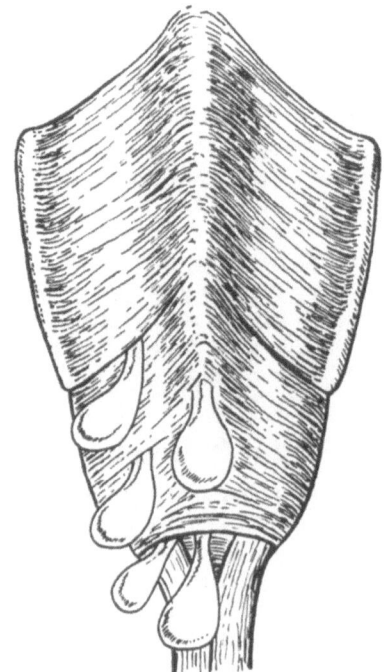

Fig. 276. A Different sites of diverticulum formation in the pharyngoesophageal region.
[From Perrot, J. W.: Aust. N. Z. J. Surg. **31**, 307 (1962)]

in the upper part of the cricopharyngeus, where the oblique fibers showed their highest incidence and greatest degree of divarication.

Weak spots in the musculature of the pharyngoesophageal region are present in all people but only a few develop a pouch. The reason why the mucosa extrudes in only a few people is not yet clear. According to BJÖRK (1960) predisposed individuals have such a weak anatomical structure of the posterior pharyngeal wall that normal physiological intrapharyngeal pressure suffices to cause herniation. Other authors also (COBURN, 1951) attach great importance to congenital predisposition and base this belief on the fact that Zenker's diverticulum may occur in several members of the same family (DUNHILL, 1950), and that it can be present at birth (RUSH and STINGILY, 1929). It should be stressed, however, that this diverticulum occurs mainly at an advanced age, which could point to a weakening of the pharyngeal wall secondary to senile atrophy (TEMPLETON, 1964).

In recent years attention has been drawn to a possible obstructive role of the cricopharyngeal muscle or pharyngoesophageal sphincter in the formation of these pouches. Different hypotheses have been proposed. The term cricopharyngeal achalasia, introduced by ASHERSON (1950) and revived by SUTHERLAND (1962) implies that the pharyngoesophageal sphincter fails to relax during the second stage of deglutition. This term, however, was applied to various neuromuscular disorders affecting the cricopharyngeal muscle without clear documentation of the failure of relaxation. Other disorders of the sphincter have also been implicated including delayed relaxation (CROSS, 1968), premature contraction (ARDRAN, 1961; LUND, 1968) and spasm (NEGUS, 1957; BELSEY, 1966). Few motility studies are available, however, to demonstrate these hypothetical disorders. KODICEK and CREAMER (1961) performed intraluminal pressure measurements with a non-perfused catheter system in 5 patients with a hypopharyngeal diverticulum. They failed to identify any abnormality of pharyngoesophageal sphincter function. The resting pressure in the sphincter was normal, suggesting absence of spasm; there was a normal fall in pressure in the high pressure zone on swallowing and the timing and amplitude of the fall were within the normal range, indicating a normal sphincteric relaxation. ELLIS et al. (1969) used a similar method to study 11 patients with Zenker's diverticula. They confirmed that the cricopharyngeal sphincters relaxed promptly and normally after every recorded swallow, that there was no "spasm" of the sphincter in these patients,

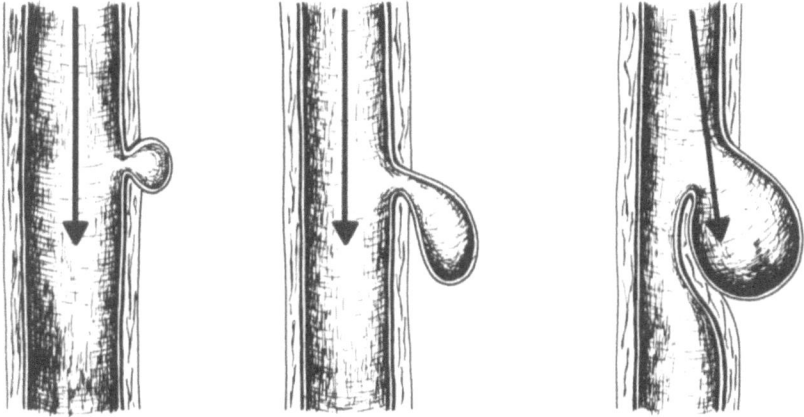

Fig. 276. B Different stages of Zenker's diverticulum

and that the sphincteric contractions were not excessive. But often the temporal relationship between the movements of pharynx and sphincter was abnormal, and this was the case in all patients at least some of the time. This intermittent abnormality was characterized by the occurrence of sphincteric contraction prior to completion of pharyngeal contraction. These studies confirm the cineradiographic observations of LUND (1965, 1968) and of ARDRAN and KEMP (1961), who noted premature contractions of the pharyngoesophageal sphincter in such patients. Indeed, the cricopharyngeus closed partly or completely before the whole of the bolus had been displaced from the pharynx. The contraction of the pharyngeal musculature upon the body of the bolus appeared to cause the protrusion of the diverticulum. Whether this incoordination of pharynx and pharyngoesophageal sphincter indeed plays a role in the genesis of the diverticulum remains an open question.

2.3. Pathology

At first the herniated mucosa forms a small pouch, which is always situated at or near the midline. Later it gradually increases in size. LAHEY and WARREN (1954) distinguish three stages in this development (Fig. 276B). In the first stage there is only a small protrusion of mucosa and submucosa in the form of a bulge; usually this stage is not associated with symptoms. In the second stage the diverticulum is bigger but the orifice of the pouch still lies in the plane of the normally oriented posterior wall of the pharynx. As it enlarges, the esophagus becomes displaced until finally, in the third stage, the diverticular orifice lies in a plane perpendicular to the original longitudinal axis of the pharyngoesophageal junctional segment, whereas the orifice of the esophagus lies parallel to this longitudinal axis (Fig. 276B). Food tends to enter the pouch and only spills over into the esophagus when the pouch is full. Because the diverticulum contains almost no muscular tissue it cannot contract and empties either by external compression or by changes in position. In this stage the diverticulum is a big atonic sac, which tends to descend into the mediastinum, usually on the left side of the esophagus. Eventually it can push aside and compress the gullet.

2.4. Symptoms

The hypopharyngeal diverticulum is the only esophageal diverticulum which is almost always associated with symptoms. In its initial stage, however, it can develop quite insidiously without causing symptoms. The most frequent first complaint is a sensation of dryness or scratching in the throat, which makes the patient clear his throat frequently and, therefore, may lead to a wrong diagnosis of chronic pharyngitis. Later the patient has a sensation of a foreign body in the throat after meals. Sooner or later he experiences some difficulty of swallowing for both liquids and solids. As the diverticulum enlarges the dysphagia increases and regurgitation of food and mucus ensues. When the pouch has become very large and causes an almost complete obstruction, the food can reach the esophagus only via an overflow from the diverticulum into the gullet. Then the dysphagia is so severe that a marked loss of weight and sometimes inanition occur. As in achalasia of the cardia dysphagia is often more marked when the patient is tense or when he has to eat in public places. Pain is rather rare in an uncomplicated diverticulum. Hoarseness due to compression of the recurrent laryngeal nerve has been reported in a few cases (BECKER and UNGEHEUER, 1970). The most typical symptom of a hypopharyngeal diverticulum is regurgitation of both food and liquid immediately after swallowing. This food is mostly undigested and smells and tastes as it was ingested. The regurgitated food can also have been ingested several hours or even a few days before; then it will smell and taste bad. The stagnating food can also be the cause of a bad taste in the mouth and a smelling breath. Another frequent complaint is the occurrence of gurgling noises during deglutition, usually of liquids. In some instances this symptom becomes so noticeable that the patient is embarrassed and gives up eating in the presence of others. Most patients learn that by assuming certain positions or by massaging the neck, they can free the sticking food. Sometimes regurgitation of food and mucus occurs at night. This may cause laryngeal irritation and cough. The regurgitation can also go unnoticed and lead to aspiration pneumonia and, if it occurs frequently, to chronic bronchopulmonary infection. Recurrent pulmonary symptoms are sometimes the first and only symptom which leads the patient to seek medical advice.

The clinical examination is mostly not very relevant. Gurgling noises may be heard during drinking or such noises may be provoked by massage of the neck in patients with large pouches. In less than one third of the cases a swelling can be observed in the left side of the neck, just anterior to the sternomastoid. This swelling increases after a meal and it can be emptied by pressing this region.

2.5. Diagnosis

The most characteristic clinical symptom of a hypopharyngeal diverticulum is that sometimes both liquids and food return into the mouth immediately after they have been swallowed. The diagnosis is suggested by regurgitation of unaltered food, minutes or hours after a meal and particularly while the patient lies down or bends the head to the left. It is also suggested by the production of a gurgling noise or the emptying of a swelling in the neck on pushing the finger upwards along the medial wall of the sternomastoid muscle.

The diverticulum is best demonstrated by radiographic examination. Antero-posterior, lateral and oblique projections are necessary to show small diverticula, to determine the site of origin and the neck of the diverticulum and to distinguish a pouch from an esophageal dilation above an esophageal web. When the diverticulum empties itself quickly it can sometimes be visualized only in the recumbent position. The image can change under the influence of swallowing and of a Valsalva maneuver. Undeep diverticula may disappear on X-rays taken when the pharynx is distended by contrastmedium, to reappear as soon as the bolus has passed.

The size of the diverticula varies from a few millimeters to several centimeters. In the initial stage the diverticulum looks like a thorn and is located on the proximal part of the semilunar impression, at or near the midline of the posterior pharyngeal wall (Fig. 277). Gradually the protrusion assumes a more globular shape but it remains perpendicular to the longitudinal axis of the pharynx (Fig. 278). Later the diverticulum takes on the form of a pouch (Fig. 279). By then it is usually more than 1 cm long and it begins its descent into the mediastinum so that the longitudinal axis of the diverticulum becomes parallel to the axis of the pharynx. In this stage the diverticulum does not compress the esophagus and it fills at the same time as the esophagus. Finally the diverticulum becomes very large and the esophagus is filled with barium mainly by overflow from the diverticulum. In this stage the esophagus is markedly compressed (Fig. 280) and may even become obstructed (Fig. 281). The contour of the diverticulum is smooth but in greater pouches retention of food may cause filling

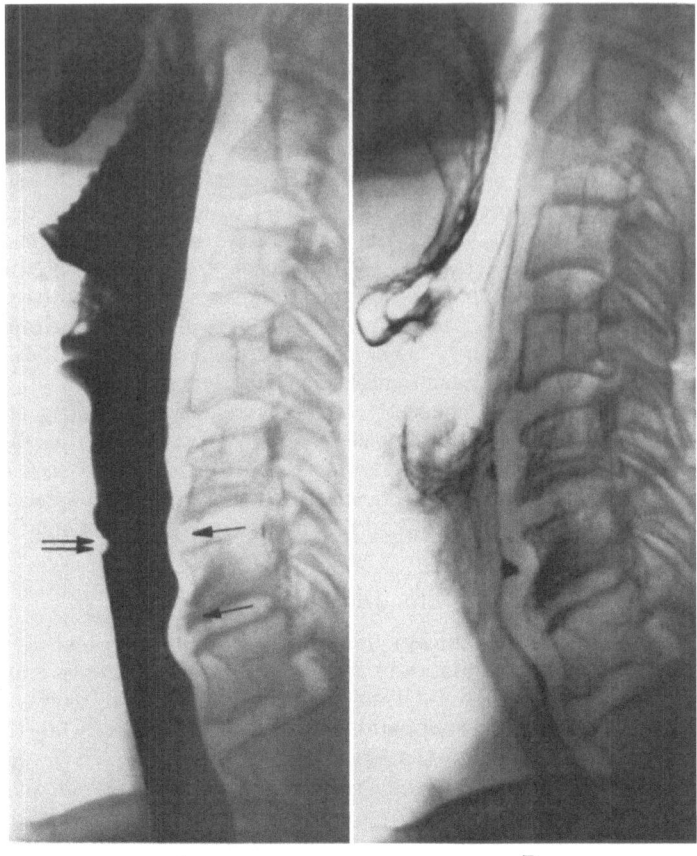

A   B

Fig. 277 A and B. Pharyngoesophageal region during (A) and after (B) swallowing. A small triangular outpouching of the posterior wall appears during the contractive phase (B) and disappears on filling (A). Note also the impression on the posterior wall caused by osteophytes (←) and the small defect of the anterior wall caused by the venous plexus (⇉)

defects, which must be differentiated from carcinoma in the bottom of the diverticulum.

Endoscopic examination can be useful to exclude other lesions such as carcinoma and to judge the condition of the esophageal mucosa. This examination is not without danger, because the esophagoscope tends to penetrate the larger diverticula and may lead to perforation of the diverticular wall. Intraluminal pressure measurements are of limited diagnostic importance, but they can indicate the presence of pharyngoesophageal incoordination.

2.6. Complications of Untreated Diverticula

Aspiration of food into the airways may result in bronchopulmonary complications. Pressure on the recurrent laryngeal nerve can cause hoarseness, and pressure on sympathetic nerves a Claude Bernard-Horner syndrome. Diverticulitis with ulceration, perforation and eventually bronchoesophageal fistula is rare. Spontaneous perforation does not occur, unless a sharp object has pene-

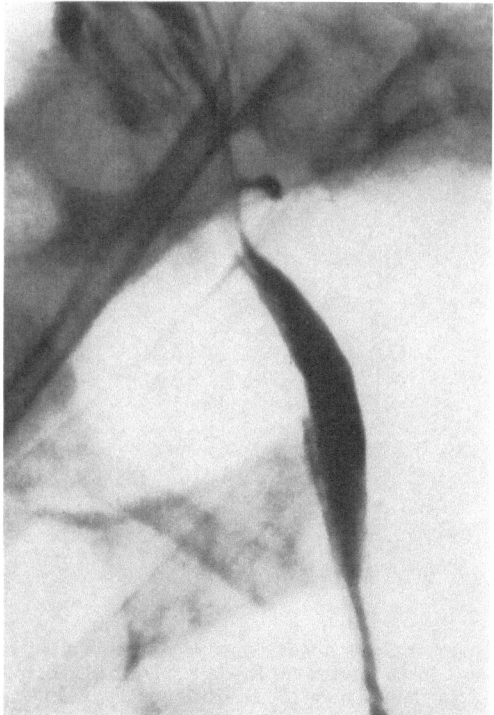

Fig. 278. Small hypopharyngeal (Zenker's) diverticulum

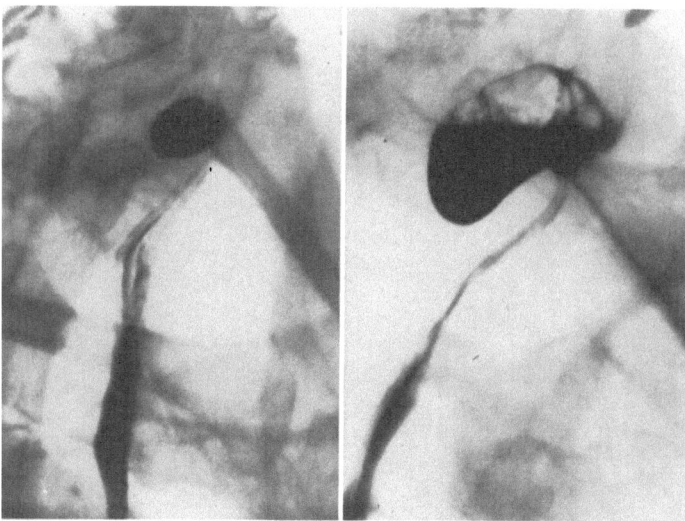

Fig. 279. Hypopharyngeal diverticulum. Evolution over a 10-year period

trated the pouch. Bleeding is very rare and should always suggest the possibility of a carcinoma in the diverticulum. SOM and DEITEL (1967) described such a case and collected from the literature 15 other cases of a malignant tumor developing

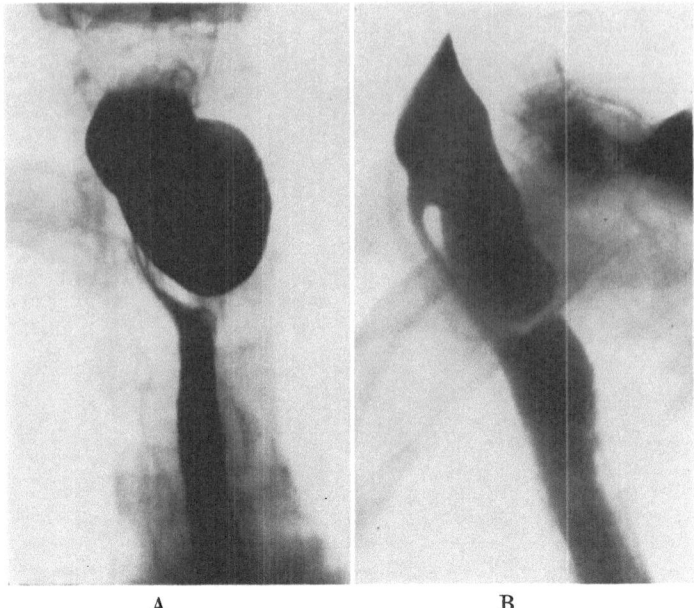

A   B

Fig. 280 A and B. Hypopharyngeal diverticulum of moderate size. On the frontal view (A) the diverticulum is seen to be located on the left side of the cervical esophagus, which is displaced to the right. The lateral view (B) shows the pouch behind the compressed cervical esophagus

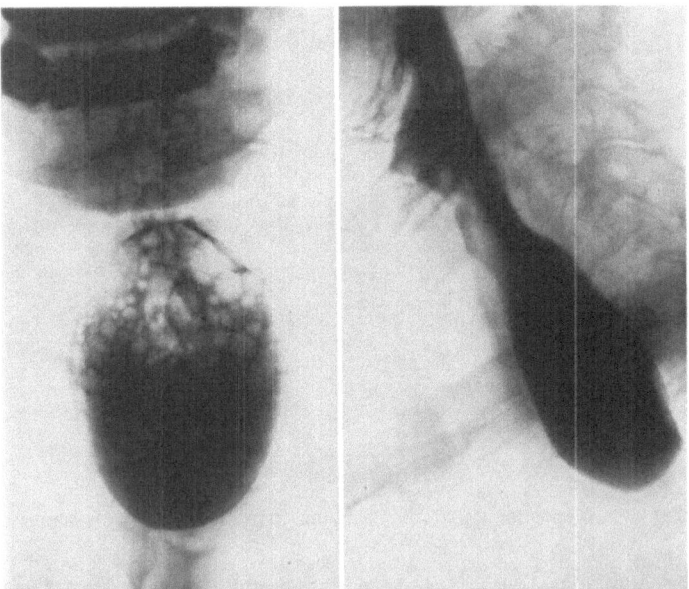

Fig. 281. Huge hypopharyngeal diverticulum. The barium fills the pouch and does not enter the esophagus

in a Zenker's diverticulum. Change in symptomatology, recent weight loss and the appearance of blood in the regurgitated material are often seen with an associated carcinoma (PIERCE and JOHNSON, 1969).

2.7. Evolution and Prognosis

A hypopharyngeal diverticulum usually increases in size very slowly so that it takes many years before the pouch is so big as to cause a serious displacement of the esophagus. The size and symptoms of smaller diverticula, however, can remain unchanged for many years (EINARSSON and HALLEN, 1967). The prognosis of the hypopharyngeal diverticulum is good, provided the patient has not yet incurred chronic pulmonary lesions.

2.8. Treatment

Small asymptomatic diverticula which are found incidentally during a radiological examination require no treatment. Small symptomatic diverticula can be treated by dilatation of the upper esophageal sphincteric segment. According to NEGUS (1950) a wide dilatation is required, which can be done with a hydrostatic or pneumatic bag. Depending on the evolution of the symptoms and of the radiological signs a new series of dilatations may be necessary after a few months. One must be certain, however, that no cicatricial scarring with stenosis exists because in these cases hydrostatic or pneumatic dilatation could easily provoke perforation. Dilatations by means of bougies or olives of progressively increasing diameter are indicated in these fibrotic stenoses. For such small diverticula an operation is not indicated, because the pouch will not necessarily increase in size; dilatations are even capable to arrest the evolution of the pouch.

As a general rule patients with bigger pouches, i.e. those who are in stage II or III of the LAHEY and WARREN classification (1954), should be treated surgically. Their pouches tend to become progressively larger; dysphagia and regurgitation are frequent and there is a real risk of aspiration pneumonia and of malnutrition.

A number of surgical procedures have been advocated. Surgical excision was first attempted in the later part of the nineteenth century. The earlier operations were associated with high mortality and morbidity rates. In the early years of the twentieth century a two-stage operation was developed and it greatly reduced the complications and hazards of operation for this lesion (LAHEY, 1953; LAHEY and WARREN, 1954). As a first step the pouch was isolated and sewed under the skin incision in the neck in an inverted position; about a week later the sac was removed. However, this technique requires two surgical procedures and a rather long period of hospitalization. Extirpation of the diverticulum today is performed almost always as a one-step operation. A stapling device has been used in resection of these diverticula (HOELM and PAYNE, 1969). The fact that the primary mortality of this operation is brought down to below 1% (CLAGETT and PAYNE, 1960; BOYD, 1961) is a good reason why most surgeons use this type of operation almost exclusively. The present status of the one-stage pharyngoesophageal diverticulectomy is discussed by WELSH and PAYNE (1973).

The technique of the operation has been described by several authors (CLAGETT and PAYNE, 1960; BOYD, 1964). The diverticulum should be dissected free down to the neck of the sac at its site of origin. Care should be taken to avoid injury to the recurrent laryngeal nerve. Care should be taken also to accomplish complete removal of the sac. When a small pouch is left it predisposes to the development of a recurrent diverticulum. Too broad a resection on the other hand can lead to stenosis. Many surgeons use a nasoesophageal tube as a guide to localize the esophagus and to help in the determination of the extent of the resection. Before the operation the pouch should be emptied by continuous suction with a catheter for one or more days. The pouch may also be washed out by taking effervescent drinks after meals and bending down the head between the knees to induce regurgitation.

Negus (1950) has strongly stressed the importance of the preoperative wide dilatation of the pharyngoesophageal sphincter. Also, Clagett and Payne (1960) used preoperative dilatation, with a previously swallowed silk thread as a guide for the dilating bougie if there is evidence of marked angulation or obstruction of the esophagus.

The results of the one-stage diverticulectomy were described by several authors (Clagett and Payne, 1960; Sweet, 1956; Warren, 1960). Immediate postoperative results are good and complaints mostly disappear completely. The operative mortality rate is low and varies from 0 to 0.8%. Mediastinitis has become an extremely rare complication. The most frequent complication is lesion of the recurrent laryngeal nerve (2.8 to 10.7% of the cases). Vocal cord paralysis and hoarseness always recuperate completely. Fistulas occur in 0.7 to 3.5% of all cases, but they close spontaneously. The incidence of postoperative dysphagia and serious stricture, which requires dilatation, decreases with increasing technical experience of the surgeon. Recurrence of the diverticulum in the first weeks after the operation is found in 1.2 to 3.0% of the cases. Long term follow-up studies on sizable series of patients are not available. In a number of smaller series, in which the patients were followed for a period of up to 12 years after surgery (Gammelgaard, 1955; Nicholson, 1962; Einarsson and Hallen, 1967), systematic radiographic examination revealed recurrence of diverticula in 65 to 85%. In many cases the radiological recurrence was not associated with clinical symptoms. To diminish the danger of recurrence Negus (1950) proposes postoperative dilatation of the cricopharyngeal region in addition to the preoperative dilatations.

The importance attached in recent years to motility disturbances of the pharynx and upper esophageal sphincter in the pathogenesis of these diverticula has led many surgeons to perform a myotomy of the cricopharyngeal muscle in the treatment of this disorder. Some combine the myotomy with a classical diverticulectomy during the same procedure (Cross et al., 1961; Wilkins, 1964; Smith and Buchtel, 1968; Rosetti, 1971). Others perform a myotomy without resection of the diverticulum (Harrison, 1958; Sutherland, 1962; Belsey, 1966; Davis et al., 1966; Blakeley et al., 1968; Lund, 1968). Ellis et al. (1969) performed this myotomy in 18 patients with hypopharyngeal diverticula. Of the 14 patients subjected to myotomy alone or combined with diverticulopexy, 9 were asymptomatic, 4 had occasional symptoms and only 1 was not improved by the operation. This and other studies show that myotomy can be a valuable therapeutic measure. It has not been decided as yet whether the adding of the diverticulectomy will improve the long term results.

Apart from diverticulectomy with or without myotomy other surgical procedures were and are used. Diverticulopexy consists of the fixation of the isolated pouch to the prevertebral muscles or to the pharynx in an inverted position.

This operation has been abandoned except in combination with myotomy. Invagination, too, is practically no longer performed. In this procedure the pouch was isolated and inverted into the esophagus and the defect in the wall of the pharynx was closed. Probably the only indication is a large diverticulum in a poor risk patient (COBURN, 1951).

The endoscopic treatment of Zenker's diverticulum was described for the first time in 1917 by MOSHER. Later the procedure was given up to be revived by DOHLMAN and MATTSSON (1960) and by LEWIS and EDWARDS (1962). The technique consists in cutting the wall between the diverticulum and the esophagus via a modified esophagoscope. By dividing this wall, diverticulum and esophagus form a single lumen. Moreover the procedure automatically includes a myotomy of the cricopharyngeal muscle. The cutting of this wall does not seem to involve undue risks because the long evolution of the pouch usually results in firm adhesions between the diverticulum and the esophagus. Although the procedure is said to be relatively simple and short, most authors use this method only for elderly or poor risk patients, for cases in which abnormalities of the neck make an external incision undesirable and for patients who refuse an operation but allow an endoscopic procedure. The procedure is less safe for small diverticula, and is contraindicated in cases of thyroid enlargement, after strumectomy or after a previous external operation because of the danger that certain blood vessels will have an abnormal course.

3. Esophageal Diverticula

Most authors agree that diverticula of the thoracic esophagus occur less frequently than pharyngoesophageal diverticula. SHIELDS and ANDERSON (1959) estimate their incidence to be about 10% of all esophageal diverticula. BROM-

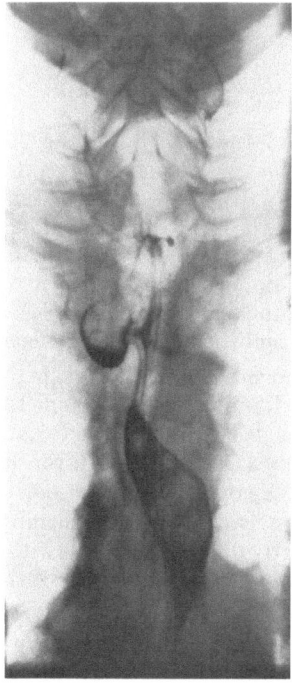

Fig. 282. Pulsion diverticulum in the upper third of the esophagus. The neck of the diverticular outpouching is well visualized. Note also the barium residue in a small lateral diverticulum of the left pyriform sinus

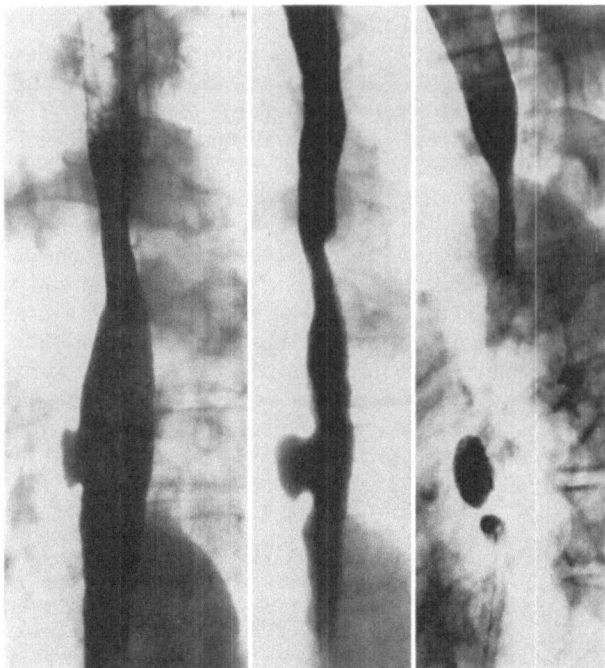

Fig. 283. Midesophageal traction-pulsion diverticula. The outpouchings increase in size or appear during esophageal contraction

BART (1961), however, found that 76.8% of the 350 esophageal diverticula he observed were located in the supra-aortic segment and in the middle third of the esophagus, whereas only 10.8% were situated in the pharyngoesophageal region. This discrepancy he ascribes to the technique of radiological examination and he stresses the importance of taking X-ray pictures of the esophagus in the left oblique position to detect the majority of the thoracic diverticula. The relative frequency of epibronchial diverticula was already stressed by KRAGH (1922–1923) who found 51 epibronchial diverticula in a series of 556 autopsies.

According to their pathogenesis the esophageal diverticula can be classified into congenital and acquired anomalies. Although the congenital origin of diverticula is hard to prove, it is generally accepted that they do occur. Based upon embryological studies RAVEN (1933) describes the following types of congenital esophageal diverticula: (1) the diverticulum associated with a tracheoesophageal fistula; (2) the diverticulum caused by an incomplete separation of esophagus and trachea; (3) the diverticulum associated with multiple diverticula of the colon; and (4) diverticula of the posterior wall of the esophagus which originate from epithelial inclusions.

The acquired diverticula can be divided, according to their pathogenesis, into traction, pulsion and pulsion-traction diverticula. The most suitable classification is that based on the anatomical localization and distinguishes between midesophageal and epiphrenic diverticula, although diverticula may occur in other segments of the esophagus as well (Figs. 282, 283).

3.1. Midesophageal Diverticula

Diverticula of the thoracic esophagus are usually situated in the middle third of the gullet at the level of the lunghilus (Fig. 283). According to BROM-BART (1956), diverticula situated in the triangular space limited by the aortic arch, the descending aorta and the left main bronchus constitute a separate group; they originate from the left anterior lateral wall and are pulsion diverticula. As long ago as 1915 LE COUNT described in this segment pulsion diverticula which were unattached to lymph nodes and which were considered hernias of the mucosa through the muscular layers of the esophagus.

3.1.1. Pathogenesis and Pathology

Traction diverticula are caused by an extrinsic process producing traction on the esophageal wall. Such a diverticulum thus contains all layers of the normal esophageal wall. The extrinsic processes are mostly inflamed lymph nodes which lie very close to the gullet wall in the region of the trachea and bronchi. Tuberculosis is the most frequent cause of this lymphadenopathy, but mycotic infection may also be the cause. DIEU and ADENIS-LAMARRE (1971) observed 20 cases of midesophageal diverticula among 2000 children with tuberculosis of mediastinal lymph nodes. Traction diverticula have also been ascribed to lesions of the vertebral column (STEWART, 1931; HOYNE and ROGERS, 1951; CORNELL, 1956; BOCKUS, 1963) and to benign intramural tumors of the esophagus. CROSS et al. (1961) suggested that congenital attachment to the trachea or periesophageal structures, akin to the more common tracheoesophageal anomalies, might be the cause of the traction diverticulum.

The traction diverticulum is more or less triangular in shape and is usually small, measuring less than 2 cm. It originates from the anterior or anterolateral wall of the gullet with its long axis directed anteriorly and upward, so that the apex lies higher than the mouth of the diverticulum. Unlike the pharyngo-esophageal diverticulum the traction diverticulum does not have a neck but opens into the esophageal lumen through a wide stoma. Due to this anatomical disposition and to the muscular elements in the wall of the diverticulum it retains food only rarely. If a parietal obstruction in the distal esophagus supervenes, pulsion may contribute to the further development of the sac, thus giving rise to a pulsion-traction diverticulum.

3.1.2. Symptoms

Midesophageal traction diverticula are mostly asymptomatic and discovered only as incidental findings on routine barium study of the esophagus or at autopsy examination. MACMILLAN (1935) examined 1000 patients with dysphagia and ascribed this symptom only 4 times to the presence of a traction diverticulum. There is general agreement that the esophageal symptoms of a patient with a traction diverticulum are due to complications or to associated lesions. When a patient with an uncomplicated midesophageal diverticulum complains of substernal pain or heartburn, dysphagia, heaviness in the chest, regurgitations or respiratory symptoms, other causes should be carefully excluded before attributing these symptoms to the diverticulum. A large pulsion or pulsion-traction diverticulum, however, may be a rare cause of these symptoms, particularly of dysphagia and regurgitation of retained food.

3.1.3. Complications

Complications of the traction diverticulum are rare, but do occur. These include diverticulitis, occasionally leading to abscess formation and even to perforation with localized mediastinitis (PALMER, 1955; GUILLON et al., 1955; WEBSTER, 1957). Instances have been reported of fistula formation between the esophagus and a variety of mediastinal structures, i.e., the trachea, the bronchi, the pericardium, the pleural cavity and even the superior vena cava and the aorta. There has also been a report on phlebitis of the vena anonyma and the left subclavian vein secondary to a localized mediastinitis caused by diverticulitis. Formation of a fistula with large mediastinal blood vessels results in exsanguination (POWELL, 1957; CHEITLIN et al., 1961). Hemorrhage may also be caused by ulceration of the diverticular mucosa. The bleeding may be massive or chronic and occult and lead to iron deficiency anemia or to frequent regurgitation of small amounts of blood. Perforation into the airways, though the most frequent complication, remains rare. COLEMAN and BUNCH (1950) estimate that 15% of the nonmalignant esophageal fistulas are caused by complicated traction diverticula. According to NASH and PALMER (1947) 5% of all fistulas between esophagus and bronchi are secondary to these diverticula. Up to 1961, 22 such cases were reported.

3.1.4. Diagnosis

Most traction diverticula are discovered incidentally on barium examination of the esophagus. The radiological picture is typical. The diverticulum is cone- or tent-shaped and does not assume a dependent position. Calcified lymph nodes may be noticed close to the pouch. As these diverticula frequently originate from the right anterior lateral wall, pictures in the left oblique position may be required to visualize the pouch. On rare occasions an ulcer niche is demonstrable in the diverticular wall.

Esophagoscopy is indicated in symptomatic patients in order to recognize associated lesions.

3.1.5. Treatment

Uncomplicated traction diverticula do not require any treatment. When complicated by esophagitis conservative measures, such as a bland diet and antacids, may alleviate the complaints. Stenosing lesions should be dilated. Conservative treatment, including antibiotics, is indicated in cases of acute diverticulitis. However, when peridiverticulitis has led to perforation and to abscess or fistula formation, surgery is required. When there is a communication between the esophagus and a small bronchus, closure of the fistula is usually sufficient. In some cases, particularly when there are bronchiectasies in the communicating pulmonary segment, segmental resection of the lung may be required.

3.2. Epiphrenic Diverticula
3.2.1. Incidence

The epiphrenic diverticulum is an uncommon entity. GOODMAN and PARNES (1952) found only 126 cases in the literature up to 1952. Since that time, additional reports have appeared, a.o. by HABEIN et al. (1956a, b), who described 121 epiphrenic pulsion diverticula seen at the Mayo Clinic during the 10 year period from 1944 through 1953. Basing himself upon a number of papers published between 1926 and 1960 EERLAND (1962) calculated the relative incidence of different types of esophageal pouches and found 1 421 pharyngoesophageal, 436 midesophageal and 177 epiphrenic diverticula. HARRINGTON (1949) had only seen 8 patients with epiphrenic diverticula, whereas he operated on 216 patients with Zenker's diverticulum. LAHEY and WARREN (1954) had 9 and 365 patients respectively, and SWEET (1965) 10 and 67. The experience of WHEELER (1947) probably reflects the frequency of natural occurrence in that only 3 examples were encountered during 20 000 radiological examinations of the esophagus, an incidence of 0.015%.

Epiphrenic diverticula have been observed in infants and children (MEADOWS, 1970), but usually they are found in middle aged men. The age of the 97 patients reported by HABEIN et al. (1956) ranged from 34 to 81, with an average of 59. The ratio of men to women was a little more than 2:1. In 15 of these 97 cases there were multiple esophageal diverticula, with as many as 3 lesions in some patients. HIRD and HORTENSTINE (1959) reported the occurrence of multiple epiphrenic diverticula in various members of different generations of the same family. HEBESTREIT and LÜTGEMEIER (1971) reported a case with two large epiphrenic diverticula associated with achalasia. Eight of the 80 patients observed by BRUGGEMAN and SEAMAN (1973) had multiple diverticula.

3.2.2. Pathology

These diverticula are generally considered to be of the pulsion type, and occur in the lower 5 to 10 cm of the esophagus. The opening of the pouch is usually located in the posterior wall of the gullet, and is, in almost two thirds of the cases, directed toward the right thoracic cavity. The wall is composed of mucosa, submucosa, muscularis mucosae and an outer fibrous layer of varying density. The size of these diverticula varies within relatively large limits from less than 1 cm to more than 9 cm. Of the 103 epiphrenic diverticula, occurring in 97 patients, HABEIN et al. (1956) found 62 to measure between 1 and 3 cm, and 22 between 3 and 5 cm. As the sacculation increases in size, it tends to assume a more dependent position in relation to the esophagus, with distortion, angulation and partial obstruction of the esophagus distal to the opening of the pouch. The neck of the diverticulum is usually short, measuring only 0.5 cm or less.

3.2.3. Etiology

The etiology and pathogenesis are not known. Several mechanisms have been postulated, including a congenitally weak wall associated with a distal esophageal obstruction and/or motility disorders of the distal esophagus. Abnormally high or long-lasting intraluminal pressures would result in a progressive outpouching of the inner esophageal layer through the weak spot in the wall. In favor of this hypothesis is the observation that epiphrenic diverticula are frequently associated with other lesions of the distal part of the esophagus and diaphragm.

ALLEN and CLAGETT (1965) observed in a series of 160 patients with epiphrenic diverticula that 34% had a hiatal hernia, 24% had diffuse esophageal spasm, 10% achalasia and 9% esophagitis. The vast majority of patients with any of these distal esophageal diseases, however, never develops an epiphrenic diverticulum. As the presence of a congenital or acquired weak spot in the esophageal wall is difficult to prove in a particular case, the relation between the diverticulum and the distal esophageal diseases remains hypothetical.

3.2.4. Symptoms

The symptoms of patients with epiphrenic diverticula are extremely variable. Approximately one third of the patients have no clinical symptoms that can in any way be regarded as related to the diverticulum. When symptoms are present it is often difficult to determine whether they are generated by the diverticulum itself or are related to other lower esophageal and diaphragmatic lesions, which are so frequently associated with these diverticula. The epiphrenic diverticulum thus seems to be completely asymptomatic in one third of the patients; another third have aspecific esophageal complaints, which could be due to either the diverticulum or the associated lesion; in 15 to 20% of the patients the symptoms are clearly related to the associated disease and in only 15 to 20% do the symptoms seem to be directly caused by the diverticulum itself. Habein et al. (1956) reported on a series of 24 operated and 97 non-operated epiphrenic diverticula and found that 42% of these patients had dysphagia, 32% of their non-operated patients had dysphagia but it could be attributed to the diverticulum in only 13%. The dysphagia was usually described as a sensation of food sticking in the lower esophagus. Regurgitation of undigested food was observed in 38% of the cases and was favored by changes in position. In some patients regurgitation occurred only on lying down. These patients are particularly liable to present a chronic cough and choking spells and to develop pulmonary complications.

Julian (1953) described a patient with anginal pain radiating into the left arm and associated with electrocardiographic changes of coronary insufficiency, both of which disappeared on resection of the diverticulum. Rarely hematemesis melena or iron deficiency anemia is the first sign. Exceptionally the patient notices a gurgling noise in the lower substernal region on swallowing or on changes of position. Trempe (1955) described the symptom of delayed drunkenness and Nylander (1952) observed a patient who was relieved of both his dysphagia and asthma on resection of an epiphrenic diverticulum.

The symptoms do not correlate well with the size of the pouch, but pouches with a short and broad neck tend to cause less difficulty. The duration of symptoms prior to diagnosis varies from a few months to several years. The evolution is not necessarily characterized by a progressively deteriorating symptomatology. Habein et al. (1956) found that no more than 5 out of 25 patients developed more serious symptoms in the course of a 5 year follow-up period.

3.2.5. Diagnosis

On chest X-ray a round or oval shadow or an air-fluid level in the right or left paracardial region may suggest the presence of a diverticulum. The diagnosis is made by radiographic examination of the esophagus with contrast medium. Characteristically the epiphrenic pulsion diverticulum has a globular shape and a discernible neck or stalk which connects the body of the pouch with the esophagus (Figs. 284, 285). The shape and size of the pouch can change quickly during the passage of the bolus. Filling defects, due to the presence of food remnants in the diverticulum, are frequently observed. Large diverticula may compress and displace the esophagus, but the mucosal pattern remains normal. In some cases it may be difficult to differentiate it from a large penetrating peptic ulcer of the distal esophagus or it may be masked by an associated hiatal hernia. Whenever an epiphrenic diverticulum is found the esophagus should be thoroughly examined, because this pouch is frequently associated with other

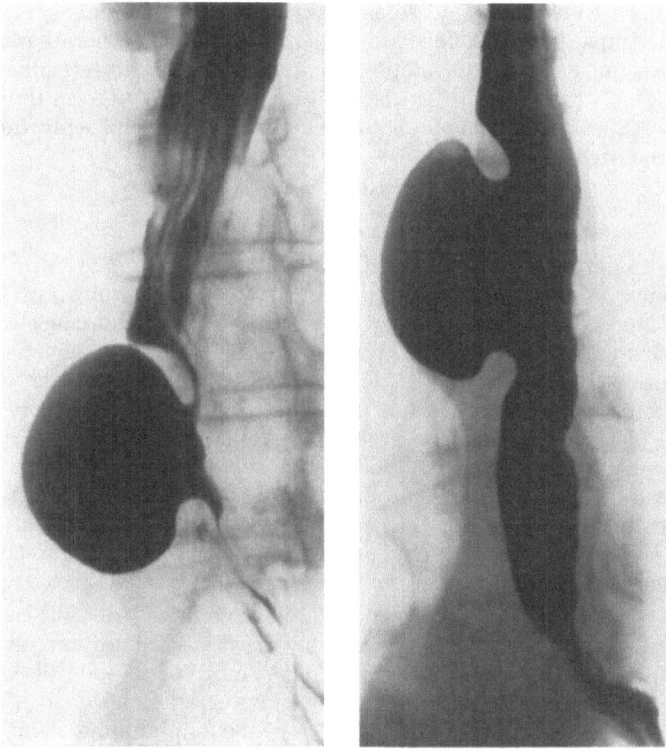

Fig. 284   Fig. 285

Fig. 284. Typical epiphrenic diverticulum

Fig. 285. Epiphrenic pulsion diverticulum located about 10 cm above the cardia

lesions of the esophagus. Failing to recognize and treat these associated diseases may be the cause of persisting symptoms after diverticulectomy. As most of these associated diseases result in motility disorders of the esophagus, intra-luminal pressure measurements and other motility studies may be useful.

Esophagoscopy with a flexible fiberscope may disclose or confirm the presence of some associated lesions but should always be done with the greatest care. According to PALMER (1951) and EFFLER (1964) esophagoscopy is contraindicated, because the endoscope tends to penetrate the pouch rather than the lumen of the distal esophagus and may thus cause a perforation of the diverticulum.

3.2.6. Complications

Complications of an epiphrenic pulsion diverticulum are exceptional. Diver-ticulitis may develop and this may give rise to ulceration or to perforation with mediastinitis, empyema or fistula formation with mediastinal structures. Aspira-tion of regurgitated material into the airways may result in bronchopulmonary infections. Hemorrhages have also been reported. Esophageal strictures are more likely to result from associated anomalies such as hiatal hernia than from the diverticulum itself. SADASIVAN and UMAPATHY (1962) reported on a patient with an epiphrenic diverticulum, in whom the dysphagia suddenly worsened as a result of the impaction of a bone fragment in the pouch. There have also been a few reports on a tumor developing in an epiphrenic diverticulum (Putney and Clerf, 1953; Allen and Clagett, 1965; Hodge, 1970). According to Hodge (1970) only 12 cases of leiomyoma developing in an epiphrenic diverticulum have been reported.

3.2.7. Treatment

The treatment of an epiphrenic diverticulum depends on the seriousness of the symptoms. A small asymptomatic pouch does not require any treatment. But even a larger diverticulum may go untreated if it does not cause compression of the esophagus or regurgitation. When symptoms develop, such as dysphagia or regurgitations, one should try to determine whether the symptoms are related to the pouch or to associated lesions. If there is doubt whether the diverticulum is the cause of the symptoms conservative therapeutic measures will be directed toward the relief of the associated conditions, such as hiatal hernia, esophagitis, achalasia or diffuse spasm of the esophagus. Measures will also be taken to keep the diverticulum empty as much as possible, especially by advising the patient to sleep in a position that promotes emptying of the sac. A sufficient amount of liquid should be used to wash out the sac and the esophagus.

The selection of patients for operative treatment will depend primarily on the magnitude of the symptoms, the size of the diverticulum and, if associated lesions are present, the persistence of serious symptoms in spite of conservative treatment. Since 50 to 70% of patients with lower esophageal diverticula have other lesions of the distal part of the gullet or of the diaphragm, careful evaluation of the distal esophagus in all epiphrenic diverticula is important. Habein et al. (1956) suggested that surgical treatment of the diverticulum should not be undertaken if correction of the associated lesions cannot be accomplished. Allen and Clagett (1965) found an unsatisfactory incidence of complications, suture line leaks, bronchoesophageal fistulas, lesions of the vagal nerves, and hemorrhages when only excision of the pouch was done. They compared their experience in 24 patients treated between 1944–1953 by excision alone with 17 managed between 1954–1963 by excision of the sac, long esophagomyotomy, and correction of hiatal hernia. Complications were significantly diminished in the latter group. Therefore, there is general agreement that resection of the epiphrenic diverticulum should be complemented with correction of the associated lesions of the lower esophagus or diaphragm.

The long-term results of 24 patients treated by resection of the diverticulum alone are not particularly good (Habein et al., 1956). Almost 50% of these patients had either moderate or severe symptoms following the operation. Long-term results of sizable series patients, treated by diverticulectomy and correction of the associated lesion, have not yet been published.

3.3. Subphrenic Diverticula

Subphrenic diverticula are very rare. According to Coburn et al. (1971) only two cases have been reported. In both instances the pouch was demonstrated to be anterior in location. The diverticulum may intermittently herniate upward through the diaphragmatic hiatus and cause symptoms and signs of gastroesophageal reflux.

References

ALLEN, T. H., CLAGETT, O. T.: Changing concepts in the surgical treatment of pulsion diverticula of the lower esophagus. J. thorac. cardiovasc. Surg. 50, 455–462 (1965).

ARDRAN, G. M., KEMP, F. H.: The radiography of the lower lateral food channels. J. Laryng. 75, 358–370 (1961).

ARDRAN, G. M., KEMP, F. H., LUND, W. S.: The aetiology of the posterior pharyngeal diverticulum; a cineradiographic study. J. Laryng. 78, 333—349 (1964).

ASHERSON, N.: Achalasia of the cricopharyngeal sphincter: A record of cases, with profile pharyngograms. J. Laryng. 64, 747–758 (1950).

BACHMAN, A. L., SEAMAN, W. B., MACKEN, K. L.: Lateral pharyngeal diverticula. Radiology 91, 774–782 (1968).

BECKER, H., UNGEHEUER, E.: Zur Klinik und Therapie des Ösophagusdivertikels. Med. Klin. 65, 589–594 (1970).

BELSEY, R.: Functional disease of the esophagus. J. thorac. cardiovasc. Surg. 52, 164–188 (1966).

BJÖRK, H.: Some pathological conditions of the esophagus. Acta oto-laryng. (Stockh.), Suppl. 158, 126 (1960).

BLAKELEY, W. R., GARETY, E. J., SMITH, D. E.: Section of the cricopharyngeus muscle for dysphagia. Arch. Surg. 96, 745–762 (1968).

BOCKUS, H. L.: Gastroenterology. Philadelphia: W. B. Saunders Co. 1963.

BOYD, D. P.: Diverticula of the esophagus. Surg. Clin. N. Amer. 41, 769–772 (1961).

BOYD, D. P.: Esophageal diverticulum. Surg. Clin. N. Amer. 44, 589–595 (1964).

BROMBART, M.: À propos des diverticules de l'œsophage: Définition, distribution, aspects radiologiques. J. belg. Radiol. 39, 362–374 (1956).

BROMBART, M.: Clinical radiology of the oesophagus. Bristol: John Wright and Sons 1961.

BRUGGEMAN, L. L., SEAMAN, W. B.: Epiphrenic diverticula. An analysis of 80 cases. Amer. J. Roentgenol. Radium Ther. Nucl. Med. 119, 266–276 (1973).

BUCKSTEIN, J., REICH, S.: Lateral pharyngeal diverticula, as a cause of dysphagia. J. Amer. med. Ass. 144, 1154–1155 (1950).

CHEITLIN, M. D., KAMIN, E. J., WILKES, D. J.: Midesophageal diverticulum: Report of a case with fistulous connection with the superior vena cava. Arch. intern. Med. 107, 252–259 (1961).

CLAGETT, O. T., PAYNE, W. S.: Surgical treatment of pulsion diverticula of the hypopharynx: One-stage resection in 478 cases. Dis. Chest 37, 257–261 (1960).

COBURN, D. E.: The treatment of esophageal diverticulum by inversion. New Engl. J. Med. 244, 791–795 (1951).

COBURN, W. M., DANA, E. R., GAYLE, B. W.: Subphrenic esophageal diverticulum in a case studied by cinemanometry. Johns Hopk. med. J. 128, 41–44 (1971).

COLEMAN, F. P., BUNCH, G. H., JR.: Acquired non-malignant esophago-tracheobronchial communications. Dis. Chest 18, 31–48 (1950).

CORNELL, A.: Diverticula of the esophagus. J. Mt. Sinai Hosp. 23, 40—55 (1956).

CROSS, F. S.: Esophageal diverticula related neuromuscular problems. Ann. Otol. (St. Louis) 77, 914–926 (1968).

CROSS, F. S., JOHNSON, G. F., GEREIN, A. N.: Esophageal diverticula: Associated neuromuscular changes in the esophagus. Arch. Surg. 83, 525–533 (1961).

DAVIS, M. V., MITCHEL, B. F., ADAM, M.: Cricopharyngeal achalasia: Variant of hypopharyngeal diverticulum syndrome. Texas Med. 62, 47 (1966).

DIEU, J. C., ADENIS-LAMARRE, F.: 20 cas de diverticules œsophagiens parabronchiques décelés parmis 2000 enfants atteints de tuberculose ganglio-bronchique. Rev. Tuberc. (Paris) 35, 103–109 (1971).

DOHLMAN, G., MATTSSON, O.: The endoscopic operation for hypopharyngeal diverticula. Arch. Otolaryng. 71, 744–752 (1960).

DUNHILL, T.: Pharyngeal diverticulum. Brit. J. Surg. 37, 404–415 (1950).

EERLAND, L. D.: Slokdarmdivertikels. Ned. T. Geneesk. 106, 357–364 (1962).

EFFLER, D. B.: Benign esophageal lesions. Read at the postgraduate course in thoracic surgery. Clinical Congress, American College of Surgeons, Oct. 5 to 9, 1964, Chicago, Ill.

EINARSSON, S., HALLEN, O.: On the treatment of esophageal diverticula. Acta oto-laryng. (Stockh.) 64, 30–36 (1967).

ELLIS, F. H., JR., SCHLEGEL, J. F., LYNCH, V. P., PAYNE, W. S.: Cricopharyngeal myotomy for pharyngo-esophageal diverticulum. Ann. Surg. 170, 340–349 (1969).

FOWLER, W. G.: Lateral pharyngeal diverticula. Ann. Surg. 155, 161–165 (1962).

GAMMELGAARD, A.: Esophageal diverticula. Results of operative treatment in one stage. Acta chir. scand. 109, 181–183 (1955).

Goodman, H. I., Parnes, I. H.: Epiphrenic diverticula of the esophagus. J. thorac. Surg. **23**, 145 (1952).

Guillon, H., Batisse, R., Jacques, A.: Diverticulum of the lower esophagus fistulizing into the mediastinum. Ann. Oto-laryng. **72**, 440 (1950).

Habein, H. C., Jr., Kirklin, J. W., Clagett, O. T., Moersch, H. J.: Surgical treatment of lower esophageal pulsion diverticula. Arch. Surg. **72**, 1018–1024 (1956).

Habein, H. C., Jr., Moersch, H. J., Kirklin, J. W.: Diverticula of the lower part of the esophagus. A clinical study of one hundred forty-nine non-surgical cases. Arch. intern. med. **97**, 768–777 (1956).

Hardy, J. D., Conn, J. H.: Diseases of the esophagus. An analysis of 308 consecutive cases. Ann. Surg. **155**, 971–990 (1962).

Harrington, S. W.: The surgical treatment of pulsion diverticula of the thoracic esophagus. Ann. Surg. **129**, 606–618 (1949).

Harrison, M. S.: The aetiology, diagnosis and surgical treatment of pharyngeal diverticula. J. Laryng. **72**, 523–534 (1958).

Hebestreit, H. P., Lütgemeier, J.: Zwei ungewöhnliche Divertikel des epiphrenischen Ösophagus. Fortschr. Roentgenstr. **115**, 540–541 (1971).

Hird, W. E., Hortenstine, C. B.: Familial esophageal epiphrenal diverticula. J. Amer. med. Ass. **171**, 1924–1927 (1959).

Hodge, G. B.: Esophageal leiomyoma associated with an epiphrenic diverticulum and hiatus hernia. Amer. Surg. **36**, 538–543 (1970).

Hoelm, J. G., Payne, W. S.: Resection of pharyngoesophageal diverticulum using stapling device. Mayo Clin. Proc. **44**, 738–741 (1969).

Hoyne, R. M., Rogers, J. C. T.: Esophageal fibromyoma associated with diverticulum. Amer. J. Surg. **81**, 592–594 (1951).

Jones Avery, F., Gummer, J. W. P., Lennard-Jones, J. E.: Clinical gastroenterology. Oxford and Edinburgh: Blackwell Scientific Publications 1969.

Julian, D. G.: Epiphrenic oesophageal diverticulum with cardiac pain. Lancet **1953 II**, 915.

Kaufman, S. A.: Lateral pharyngeal diverticula. Amer. J. Roentgenol. **75**, 238–241 (1956).

Kodicek, J., Creamer, B.: A study of pharyngeal pouches. J. Laryng. **75**, 406–411 (1961).

Kragh, J.: Tuberculous diverticula of the oesophagus (so-called traction diverticula). Acta oto-laryng. (Stockh.) **4**, 49 (1922–1923).

Lahey, F. H.: Esophageal diverticula. Surg. Clin. N. Amer. **33**, 813–826 (1953).

Lahey, F. H., Warren, K. W.: Esophageal diverticula. Surg. Gynec. Obstet. **98**, 1–28 (1954).

Le Count, E. P.: Epibronchial pulsion diverticula of the esophagus. Chicago Path. Soc. **10**, 35 (1915).

Lewis, R. S., Edwards, W. G.: The treatment of pharyngeal diverticula. Brit. J. Surg. **50**, 1—5 (1962).

Lund, W. S.: A study of the cricopharyngeal sphincter in man and in the dog. Ann. roy. Coll. Surg. Engl. **37**, 225–246 (1965).

Lund, W. S.: The cricopharyngeal sphincter: Its relationship to the relief of pharyngeal paralysis and the surgical treatment of the early pharyngeal pouch. J. Laryng. **82**, 353–367 (1968).

MacMillan, A. S.: Statistical study of diseases of the esophagus. Surg. Gynec. Obstet. **60**, 394 (1935).

Meadows, J. A., Jr.: Esophageal diverticula in infants and children. Sth. med. J. (Bgham, Ala.) **63**, 691–694 (1970).

Nash, E. C., Palmer, W. L.: The clinical significance of diverticulosis including diverticulitis of the gastrointestinal tract. Ann. intern. Med. **27**, 41–63 (1947).

Negus, V. E.: Pharyngeal diverticula. Observations on their evolution and treatment. Brit. J. Surg. **38**, 129–146 (1950).

Negus, V. E.: The etiology of pharyngeal diverticula. Bull. Johns Hopk. Hosp. **101**, 209 (1957).

Nicholson, W. F.: The late results of operations for pharyngeal pouch. Brit. J. Surg. **49**, 548–552 (1962).

Nylander, P. E. A.: Diverticulum of thoracic esophagus. Two cases of special interest. Acta chir. scand. **103**, 473–480 (1952).

Palmer, E. D.: The esophagus and its diseases. New York: Paul B. Hoeber, Inc. 1951.

Palmer, E. D.: Clinical problems associated with esophageal diverticula. Amer. J. med. Sci. **229**, 16–21 (1955).

Perrott, J. W.: Anatomical aspects of hypopharyngeal diverticula. Aust. N.Z. J. Surg. **31**, 307–317 (1962).

Pierce, W. S., Johnson, J.: Squamous cell carcinoma arising in a pharyngoesophageal diverticulum. Cancer **24**, 1068–1070 (1969).

Powell, M. E. A.: A case of aortic esophageal fistula. Brit. J. Surg. **45**, 55–57 (1957).

PUTNEY, F. J., CLERF, L. H.: Epiphrenic esophageal diverticulum. Trans. Amer. broncho-esoph. Ass. **34**, 30 (1953).

RAVEN, R. W.: Pouches of the pharynx and oesophagus with special reference to the embryo-logical and morphological aspects. Brit. J. Surg. **21**, 235–256 (1933).

ROKITANSKY, C.: Med. Jb. d. K. k. Österr. Staates **21**, 219f. (1840) (Lehrbuch Path. Anat., W. Barumuller).

ROSETTI, M.: Zur Operationstechnik des zervikalen Ösophagusdivertikels. Helv. chir. Acta **38**, 237–239 (1971).

RUSH, L. V., STINGILY, C. R.: Congenital diverticulum of esophagus; case report. Sth. med. J. (Bgham, Ala.) **22**, 546–548 (1929).

SADASIVAN, C. S., UMAPATHY, A.: Epiphrenic diverticulum of the oesophagus complicated by the impaction of a foreign body. Thorax **17**, 267–270 (1962).

SHALLOW, T. A., CLERF, L. H.: One stage pharyngeal diverticulectomy: Improved technique and analysis of 186 cases. Surg. Gynec. Obstet. **86**, 317–322 (1948).

SHIELDS, T. W., ANDERSON, M. C.: Thoracic esophageal diverticula. Report of three cases. Amer. J. dig. Dis. **4**, 522–533 (1959).

SMITH, S., BUCHTEL, B. C.: Pharyngo-esophageal diverticula and dysfunction of the crico-pharyngeus muscle. Sth. med. J. (Bgham, Ala.) **61**, 826 (1968).

SOM, M. L., DEITEL, M.: Carcinoma in a large pharyngoesophageal diverticulum. Arch. Surg. **94**, 35–38 (1967).

SPIRO, H. M.: Clinical gastroenterology. London: The McMillan Company, Collier-MacMillan Limited 1970.

STEWART, J. D., JR.: Myoma of the esophagus with associated diverticula. Arch. Path. **12**, 77–84 (1931).

SUTHERLAND, H. D.: Cricopharyngeal achalasia. J. thorac. cardiovasc. Surg. **43**, 114–126 (1962).

SWEET, R. H.: Excision of diverticulum of the pharyngo-esophageal junction and lower esophagus by means of the one stage procedure. A subsequent report. Ann. Surg. **143**, 433–438 (1956).

TEMPLETON, F. E.: X-Ray examination of the stomach. Revised ed. Chicago-London: The University of Chicago Press 1964.

TERRACOL, J., SWEET, R. H.: Diseases of the esophagus. Philadelphia: W. B. Saunders Co. 1958.

TREMPE, F.: Large pulsion diverticulum of middle third of thoracic oesophagus. Canad. med. Ass. J. **73**, 38–39 (1955).

WARREN, K. W.: Some technical considerations in the management of pharyngo-esophageal diverticulum. Surg. Clin. N. Amer. **40**, 633–643 (1960).

WEBSTER, B. H.: Spontaneous perforation of an oesophageal diverticulum. Report of a case with survival. Dis. Chest **31**, 345–348 (1957).

WELSH, S. F., PAYNE, W. S.: Present status of one-stage pharyngo-esophageal diverticul-ectomy. Rev. Surg. **30**, 370–371 (1973).

WHEELER, D.: Diverticula of the foregut. Radiology **49**, 476–481 (1947).

WILKINS, S. A., JR.: Indications for section of the cricopharyngeus muscle. Amer. J. Surg. **108**, 533–538 (1964).

ZAINO, C., JACOBSON, H. G., LEPOW, H., OZTURK, C. H.: The pharyngo-esophageal sphincter. Springfield, Ill.: Ch. C. Thomas 1970.

Chapter 8

Congenital Anomalies of the Esophagus

Esophageal Atresia

G. Fransen and A. Lacquet

With 5 Figures

1. History

The earliest description of a case of esophageal atresia, associated with the typical form of tracheoesophageal fistula, was presented in 1697 by Thomas Gibson in his then popular work "The anatomy of human bodies epitomized". Already in 1670 William Durston had reported a simple type of esophageal atresia without associated tracheoesophageal fistula in an embryo of a monster-type thoracopagus. In 1861, Hirschsprung was able to publish a remarkable series of 14 cases of the anomaly, including 4 cases which had come under his own notice. Although the anomaly thereafter was well known and described many times, attempts to correct the lesion were sporadic: the first gastrostomy for esophageal atresia was performed by Hoffman in 1898. In 1913 Richter substantially altered the surgical approach to the anomaly by the first transpleural ligation of a tracheoesophageal fistula. The first primary esophageal anastomosis through a right extrapleural approach was done by Langman in 1936. The deformity was uniformly fatal until 1935, when the first child born with atresia without fistula survived thanks to treatment by gastrostomy and many years later by esophageal substitution. In 1939 the first surviving patients having the common type of esophageal atresia with tracheoesophageal fistula were operated upon independently by Leven and Ladd, who used multiple stages in the therapeutic approach (gastrostomy—extrapleural division of the fistula—cervical esophagostomy and much later esophageal substitution). In 1941 Cameron Haight performed the first successful primary end-to-end anastomosis, which has become the generally accepted technique. In Europe reports of successes with this method came not earlier than 1947, when Ten Kate of Holland, Franklin of England and Sandblom of Sweden reported their initial successes.

2. Incidence

Considerable variation in the incidence of atresia of the esophagus is found in the articles which refer to its frequency. Numbers as high as 1 in 800 and as low as 1 in 10000 live births are given (Bettex and Crivelli, 1960). Scott and Wilson (1957) and Cuendet (1968) give an incidence of about 1/2000 and Freeman (1969) found the lesion in 1/3000 live births; the majority of authors agree that these numbers reflect the real incidence. There is a slight preponderance for males (60%) (Pellerin et al., 1963; Wayson et al., 1965; Rohmsdahl et al.,

1966; Koop and Hamilton, 1968; Holden and Wooler, 1970). This sex predilection cannot be explained. The incidence of esophageal atresia in more than
one child of the same parents has rarely been described. Haight (1957) and
Koop and Hamilton (1968) found in their series of 208 and 249 cases that
the anomaly occurred in two siblings in only one family. In a review of this
subject, Sloan and Haight (1956) were able to find only 5 proven instances
of esophageal atresia in siblings. Hausmann et al. (1957) described the occurrence
of esophageal atresia with and without fistula in three consecutive siblings.
In 1924 Ysander described an esophageal atresia with tracheoesophageal fistula
in both components of an 8 mm embryo of the monster type thoracopagus tetra-
brachius. Woolley et al. (1961) reported the only known instance in which
twins were affected. The finding of an esophageal atresia in only one of the twins,
however, is more frequent (Ingalls and Prindle, 1949; Brown and Brown,
1950; Leven et al., 1952; Haight, 1957; Freeman, 1969). Blank et al. (1967)
reported the presence of the anomaly in each of a pair of identical twins, but
in the pairs of identical twins in the series of Haight (1957) the anomaly occurred
only in one of the twins. These data indicate that genetic factors are not important in the etiology of esophageal atresia.

3. Embryology

It has been suggested that anomalous vessels such as an aberrant right
subclavian artery, anomalous aortic arches, fourth aortic arch remnants and
vascular rings, can produce esophageal atresia by local pressure (Fluss and
Poppen, 1951). Langman (1952) and Roe and Nobis (1963) even postulated
that, if no trace of a primitive right aorta is found at the time of operation, it
may still have persisted several weeks too long during embryonal life and have
caused the lesion. Most authors, however, think it is improbable that direct
compression by aberrant vessels plays an important role in the formation of
esophageal anomalies, since no consistent relation can be found between abnormalities in the cardiovascular system and esophageal atresia, although they
are frequently associated. Since the development of the various organs after
the 4th week of gestation, when the fetal heart starts beating, depends on a
normal blood supply, it has been suggested that esophageal atresia is due to a
deficient blood supply (Lister, 1963), possibly caused by the vascular anomalies
(Ingalls et al., 1952). Louw (1959) has shown experimentally that small bowel
atresia can be produced by surgical interference with the blood supply to the
gut of puppies in utero.

The "epithelial occlusion theory" (based on the work of Tandler, 1902),
which explains the atresia by an arrest of revacuolization and recanalization
after the phase of solid development of the esophagus, has received much attention. This theory, however, cannot explain fistula formation and conclusive
evidence of a solid stage in esophageal development is still lacking. Although
the pathogenetic mechanisms of esophageal atresia and/or tracheoesophageal
fistula are not yet fully understood, there is no doubt that these anomalies
originate during the differentiation of the esophagus and trachea between the
end of the third and the sixth week of gestation. In normal embryos of 21 to
23 days (4 mm) the primordial respiratory tract anlage appears from the ventral
side of the primitive foregut. This outgrowth separates from the future esophagus
by lateral growth ridges which fuse to form a tracheoesophageal septum, which
is complete at 27 to 32 days (8 mm). The completion of the system first takes
place in the caudal end of the pouch and extends subsequently in a cephalad

direction up to the top of the larynx. From this one can infer that a local non-fusion of the lateral tracheoesophageal grooves results in a tracheoesophageal fistula, and furthermore, that incompleteness, dorsal or ventral displacement, or twisting of the lateral infoldings can account for the atresia.

4. Pathological Anatomy

An almost infinite number of types of atresia can be encountered, as is evident from the numerous case reports (DAUM, 1970). It is generally agreed that there are 5 basic anomalies, including 4 types of esophageal atresia with and without fistula and the H-type tracheoesophageal fistula without atresia. Some authors have arbitrarily suggested and applied different alphabetical and numerical schemes to these anomalies, which are summarized in Table 21. Other authors, however, prefer to use an entirely descriptive or diagrammatic classification, in order to avoid confusion (HOLDER and ASHCRAFT, 1966; CUENDET, 1968; KOOP and HAMILTON, 1968; MILLER and MOYNIHAN, 1970). The relative incidence of the various anomalies, observed in some of the larger series of patients, is presented in Table 22. Esophageal atresia with a fistula from the trachea to the lower segment of the esophagus is the most common variety. Esophageal atresia without fistula was found in about 8% of the cases. Other anatomical varieties are rare but are important to look for, inasmuch as the mortality is highest in these rarer varieties. The frequency of atresia combined with both upper and lower fistulas is stated to be between 1 and 2%, but the real number is probably higher because the existence of the upper fistula may easily be over-looked (either pre-, per-, or postoperatively) (HAYS et al., 1966b; COZZI, 1967; HASSE, 1968).

The blind upper pouch is usually dilated to a diameter of 10 mm and hyper-trophied, so that the mucosal layer can easily be distinguished from the sub-mucosa and the muscularis; this pouch gets a rich blood supply from the inferior thyroid artery. The distal segment is always hypoplastic with a poor blood supply, especially in its most proximal portion. The fistulous traject from the trachea to the distal segment may extend toward the cardia over varying distances,

Table 21. Classification of different types of tracheoesophageal fistula and esophageal atresia with a survey of the most frequently used symbols

Descriptive nomenclature	Atresia without fistula	Atresia with upper segment tracheoesophageal fistula	Atresia with lower segment tracheoesophageal fistula	Atresia with upper and lower segment tracheoesophageal fistula	Tracheo-esophageal fistula without atresia
VOGT (1929)	2	3a	3b	3c	—
LADD (1944)	I	II	III–IV	V	—
SWENSON (1948)	2	4	1	5	3
GROSS (1953)	A	B	C	D	E
STEPHENS (1956)	B	E	A	D	C

Table 22. Incidence of different types of tracheoesophageal fistula and esophageal atresia. (N = number of patients)

	Atresia without fistula		Atresia with upper segment tracheoesophageal fistula		Atresia with lower segment tracheoesophageal fistula		Atresia with upper and lower segment tracheosophageal fistula		Tracheoesophageal fistula without atresia		Total number of patients
	N	%	N	%	N	%	N	%	N	%	
Surgical section of the American Academy of Pediatrics 1964	82	7.7	9	0.8	916	86.5	7	0.7	44	4.2	1058
Haight 1957	20	10	0	0	165	82.5	2	1	7	3.5	207
Waterston 1962	19	8.7	2	1	190	87.2	3	1.3	4	1.8	218
Desjardins 1964		8		1		87		1		3	264
Humpreys 1964	17	16.2	3	2.9	81	77.1	0	0			105
Mellins 1964	12	6.6	2	1.1	164	89.6	2	1.1	3	1.6	183
Rehbein 1964	8	3.4	1	0.4	220	92.4	5	2.1	4	1.7	238
Holinger 1965	10				123	84.2	1		12		146
Martin 1965	8	8	0	0	79	81.4	1	1	8	8	97
Wayson 1965	3	3.5	0	0	80	93	0	0	3	3.5	86
Hays 1966		10.2		3		70.8		5		11	108
Cozzi 1967	6	6.4	4	4.3	76	81.7	2	2.1	5	5.3	98
Ferguson 1970	4	5.8	0	0	64	92.8	0	0	1	1.4	69
Holden 1970		2		2		86		1		1	116

but the terminal esophagus has in most instances a quite normal caliber; sometimes, however, the distal segment is so narrow that it does not even allow the passage of air into the stomach (SWENSON et al., 1962).

Marked variations are found in the distance between the upper and lower esophageal pouches, from overlapping up to 6 cm, but the gap between the two segments is usually greatest in the cases of atresia without fistula. In the usual type of atresia with lower tracheoesophageal fistula, the proximal pouch mostly ends blindly at a depth of 10 to 12 cm from the upper alveolar ridge. The distal esophageal pouch has a greater variability in length. The distal fistula enters the trachea in an end-to-side manner at or just above the tracheal bifurcation in a majority of cases, whereas a proximal pouch fistula enters the trachea most commonly at its midportion or slightly below. In atresias with unusually long and dilated upper pouches extending below the carina, as described by DAFOE and ROSS (1960), MINNIS et al. (1962), YAHR et al. (1962), LISTER (1963), ROE and NOBIS (1963), WOLF et al. (1965) and HOLCOMB and DANIEL (1966), the fistulous communication with the distal esophageal segment is usually long and enters the trachea at the level of the thoracic inlet. According to the observations of REHBEIN (1964a) an upper fistula is frequently found if the distal segment communicates with the trachea high up and if this lower fistula is overlapped by the upper pouch. A case with two fistulas in the lower segment is reported by DEVENS and RITZ (1965) and a case with an upper fistula ending in a lower fistula by DAUM and VAN KAICK (1970).

5. Pathophysiology
5.1. Hydramnios

There is a definite interrelationship between hydramnios in the mother and those fetal lesions which interfere with normal swallowing and alimentation (LLOYD and CLATWORTHY, 1958). The fetus participates in the turnover of the amniotic fluid by intermittent swallowing; the ingested fluid is then absorbed by the gastrointestinal tract and transferred to the maternal circulation via the placenta. Any obstructive lesion in the proximal portion of the gastrointestinal tract or inability of the fetus to swallow leads to an excessive accumulation of amniotic fluid.

Of the 13 cases of esophageal atresia observed by SCOTT and WILSON (1957) hydramnios was present in 12; its absence in the remaining case was due to a double communication between both segments of the esophagus and trachea, so that swallowed liquid could pass into the lower absorptive segments of the alimentary tract. It is estimated that one out of 10 to 12 cases of hydramnios is due to esophageal atresia (SCOTT and WILSON, 1957; MOYA et al., 1960); hydramnios is therefore an important aid in early diagnosis. The occurrence of polyhydramnios and esophageal atresia without a fistula was as high as 57% in the series of KOOP and HAMILTON (1968) and as high as 85% in the series of WATERSTON et al. (1963). In cases of atresia with a fistula polyhydramnios was reported in 17% of KOOP's (1968) and in 32% of WATERSTON's (1963) cases. A similar correlation was also recognized by HAIGHT (1961) and CUENDET (1968), but the real incidence is thought to be very much higher because good obstetrical histories were often unavailable to the authors.

5.2. Prematurity

Some 25 to 40% of infants with esophageal atresia are premature (weight at birth less than 2500 g) (SWENSON et al., 1962; HOLDER et al., 1964; HERTZLER, 1965; MARTIN, 1965; HECKER et al., 1966; COZZI and WILKINSON, 1969; FERGUSON, 1970; SLIM and BICKERS, 1970); this may be related to overdistension of the pregnant uterus with amniotic fluid, since there is a high incidence of hydramnios in cases of esophageal atresia. According to HAIGHT (1957), HOLDER et al. (1964) and HAYS et al. (1966b), the incidence of prematurity is considerably higher in patients without a patent lower segment fistula (56 to 75%) than in those with patent fistulas (25 to 49%). With the exception of imperforate anus, which occurs with about the same frequency in full-term and premature infants, all other anomalies associated with esophageal atresia occur with greater frequency in the premature ones. When there is an additional anomaly of the cardiovascular system the incidence of prematurity is 52% (Mellins and Blumenthal, 1964) and probably much higher when the anomaly interferes with a reasonable life expectancy. When there is an associated intestinal atresia the incidence of prematurity is 80% (Holder et al., 1964); when there are associated anorectal anomalies, 64% (Cozzi and Wilkinson, 1969).

5.3. Pneumonia

At the time the diagnosis is established pneumonia is a concomitant finding in most patients with esophageal atresia and tracheoesophageal fistula. It is caused by the aspiration or overflow of nasopharyngeal mucus and saliva from the upper blind pouch immediately after birth and the regurgitation of gastric contents through a patent fistula.

Circumstances which increase the frequency of pulmonary complications are prematurity (Cozzi, 1967), delay of diagnosis and appropriate treatment (Scott and Wilson, 1957; Hertzler, 1965; Koop and Hamilton, 1968), number of feedings attempted before diagnosis (Pellerin and Nihoul-Fekete, 1967), pre-operative radiological examination with contrast material (Koop and Hamilton, 1968; Ingelrans et al., 1969) and certain anatomical types (Rehbein, 1964a; Cozzi, 1967). The onset of the pulmonary lesions is usually situated in the right upper lobe (Hertzler, 1965; Cozzi, 1967; Thomas and Chrispin, 1969). Severe bilateral pneumonia soon after birth suggests the presence of an upper fistula (Rehbein, 1964a).

A significantly increased prevalence of pneumonia in infants with a patent fistula (Waterston et al., 1963; Cozzi, 1967) suggests that regurgitated gastric contents are a greater irritant to the lungs than inhaled saliva or feedings from the upper pouch. While crying the glottis of the newborn infant closes, the intra-thoracic pressure increases, and forces air from the lungs through the tracheo-esophageal fistula and the lower esophageal segment into the stomach. The consequent overdistension of the stomach and elevation of the diaphragm periodically result in regurgitation of gastric juice into the lungs (Martin, 1965), because gastroesophageal reflux is facilitated by the poor function of the lower esophageal sphincter mechanism during the first days of life (Gryboski et al., 1963). It is known that the contents of the stomach in the first hours of life are distinctly acid. The damage caused by this reflux in the fistulous traject and the lungs was histologically proven by Pellerin and Nihoul-Fekete (1967), and by Cuen-det (1968). As the newborn is a primarily diaphragmatic breather the elevation of the diaphragm itself also causes respiratory embarrassement by preventing full expansion of the lungs and adequate cough. Pneumatic gastric rupture resulting from massive distension of the stomach as a result of tracheoesophageal fistula has been described by Othersen and Gregorie (1963).

6. Associated Anomalies

(Table 23)

Forty-eight percent of 1058 infants with tracheoesophageal anomalies reviewed by the surgical section of the American Academy of Pediatrics had other con-

Table 23. Incidence of different anomalies associated with esophageal atresia

Author	Number of patients	Number of patients with anomalies	Number of cardiovasc. anomalies	Number of gastroint. anomalies	Genito-urinary anomalies	Musculo-skeletal anomalies +face	Central nervous anomalies	Mongolism
HAIGHT 1957	200		47	37	29	26	9[b]	
HAYS[a] 1962	141	46	28	25	20	3	2	4
SWENSON 1962	61		17	19	21	13	2	6
WATERSTON 1962	218	117	59	54	35		6	
MARTIN 1965	97	31	11	11	5	13	3	
HERTZLER 1965	143	65	43	55	20	10		
HOLDER 1964	1058	505	222	233	109	144	35	28
WAYSON[a] 1965	80		21	12	5	6		3
ROHMSDAHL 1965	38	20	23	6	5	16	1	3
COZZI 1970	93		21	28	10			

[a] Only major anomalies.
[b] Including mongolism.

genital malformations (a total of 849 anomalies). Esophageal atresia without tracheoesophageal fistula is most frequently associated with another anomaly (58%) whereas tracheoesophageal fistula without atresia has the lowest incidence of associated malformations (27%). The common type of atresia with lower segment fistula is associated with other congenital defects in 48% of the patients (HOLDER et al., 1964; HUMPHREYS and FERRER, 1964). The percentage of patients with significant anomalies increases with decreasing birth weight. Multiplicity of anomalies is not rare and patients with particularly significant complexes of anomalies are described by HAYS (1962), KOLB (1963), MELLINS and BLUMEN-THAL (1964), REHBEIN and HOFFMAN (1964b), KIRKPATRICK et al. (1965), WILLICH (1965), FRANKEN and SALDINO (1969) and AHMED (1970). Evaluation of infants combining two or more associated anomalies is very difficult, so that few generalizations can be made regarding the way of management. Although some of these anomalies are considered surgically correctable, they are of life-threatening significance.

In large series 20 to 30% of the patients have one or more cardiovascular anomalies (HAIGHT, 1957; HOLDER et al., 1964; MELLINS and BLUMENTHAL, 1964; HERTZLER, 1965). Atrial septal defects, ventricular septal defects and patent ductus arteriosi are the most common associated cardiac anomalies (MELLINS and BLUMENTHAL, 1964; WAYSON et al., 1965). Other malformations, in decreasing order of frequency, are anomalous pulmonary and aortic valves, anomalous right subclavian artery, persistent left superior vena cava, coarctation of the aorta, right aortic arch, tetralogy of Fallot, transposition of the great vessels, Ebstein's anomaly and dextrocardia. In the series of Mellins and Blumenthal (1964) 97 cardiovascular anomalies occurred in 48 patients.

Gastrointestinal anomalies form the second major group of malformations associated with atresia. Imperforate anus is by far the most frequent of these, followed in decreasing frequency by intestinal atresia, malrotations, Meckel's diverticulum, hypertrophic pyloric stenosis, perforations of the intestinal tract, strictures of the lower esophagus, annular pancreas and various intestinal duplications. Any distal obstruction, but particularly upper intestinal obstructions, will contribute to the pulmonary complications encountered with tracheoesophageal fistula because of gastric distension and vomiting into the trachea. For this reason and because of the difficulties to detect and manage such lesions, they have been studied carefully (Rehbein and Hoffman, 1964b; Franken and Saldino, 1969; Raffensperger, 1970). Especially the coexistence of a separate distal esophageal stenosis may seriously change the outcome of surgical treatment of esophageal atresia, because it is very difficult to demonstrate these lower strictures prior to the operative correction (Mahour et al., 1961; Tuquan, 1962). Calibration of the distal esophagus at the time of operation usually demonstrates these lower esophageal stenoses, but Overton and Creech (1958) reported a case with a weblike membrane in the distal segment of such an elasticity that it could be stretched as far as the stomach, and thus gave an erroneous impression of patency. In cases with an open lower tracheoesophageal fistula and no air in the gastrointestinal tract a distal esophageal stenosis must be highly suspected. The incidence of pyloric stenosis in cases of esophageal atresia ranges from 1 to 10% indicating that there is an association of the two anomalies (Holder et al., 1964; Franken and Saldino, 1969), although this association may be coincidental (Raffensperger, 1970). The presence of hypertrophic pyloric stenosis is often obscured because the symptoms of vomiting secondary to pyloric stenosis are delayed until the third to sixth week of life and thus may be attributed to a postoperative complication.

The associated genitourinary anomalies include horseshoe kidney, congenital absence of kidney, polycystic disease, stricture of PUJ, patent urachus, atresia of ureter, hypospadias, crossed renal ectopia and fusion, and rectourogenital fistulas. These genitourinary anomalies also have a poor prognosis. The chance of survival for infants with associated major urogenital defects can be expected to be as small as or smaller than that of infants with cardiovascular abnormalities (Holder et al., 1964; Mellins and Blumenthal, 1964; Wayson et al., 1965). Osseous anomalies that are most frequent are absence or hypoplasia of portions of bones in the extremities, although the spine and the ribs can also be involved. The occurrence of esophageal atresia in cretins was noted by Hays (1962), Swenson et al. (1962), Mellins and Blumenthal (1964), Holder et al. (1964), Rehbein and Hoffman (1964b), Rohmsdahl et al. (1966), Krishinger and Woolley (1969), and Lister (1969).

7. Diagnostic Procedures

7.1. Nasogastric Intubation

Any infant born of a mother with unexplained hydramnios should have nasogastric intubation in the immediate newborn period (delivery room). This should also be done in any infant who seems to have an excess of mucus in the nose or mouth or who has episodes of coughing, choking, apnea, cyanosis or

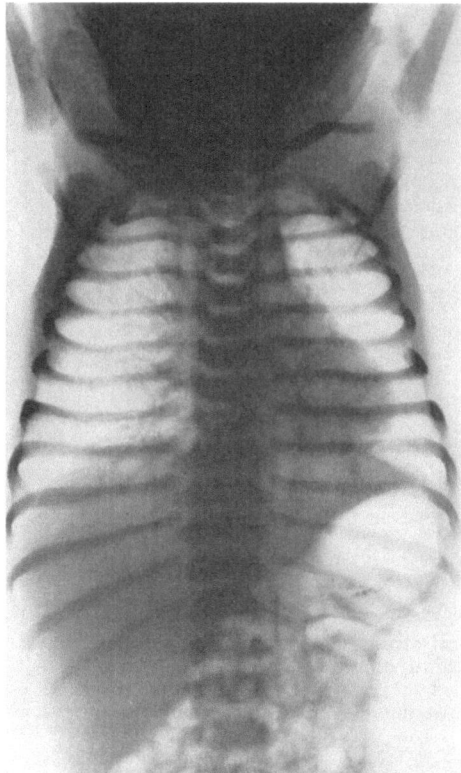

Fig. 286. Esophageal atresia with tracheoesophageal fistula. The plain thoraco-abdominal film suggests the diagnosis: the upper pouch is distended with air and produces a radiolucent area in the upper mediastinum; the right wall of the pouch is clearly outlined; the pressure of air in stomach and intestine indicates the existence of a tracheoesophageal fistula

other signs of respiratory distress in the first few hours of life. The recognition of these symptoms calls for an immediate catheterisation of the esophagus; if a moderately stiff, radiopaque catheter introduced in the esophagus encounters a resistance at a quite constant distance of approximately 11 cm from the upper alveolar ridge, the diagnosis of atresia is established (Fig. 110). To rule out false negative results due to coiling of the catheter in a blind upper pouch, confirmatory roentgenograms in frontal and lateral view are to be made. The simple determination of the pH of the fluid aspirated through the catheter also can easily and with certainty indicate whether the catheter tip has reached the stomach or not (JOHNSONBAUGH, 1968). This prompt catheterization can be an important contribution to making an early diagnosis.

7.2. Radiological Examinations

A plain film of the thorax may show an air-filled upper pouch (Fig. 286) and should also be made to visualize the inserted catheter and to assess the state of the lungs (Fig. 287). The presence of air in the stomach and intestines with a completely obstructed upper pouch is a proof of a patent fistula between the lower esophageal segment and the tracheobronchial tree, but the presence

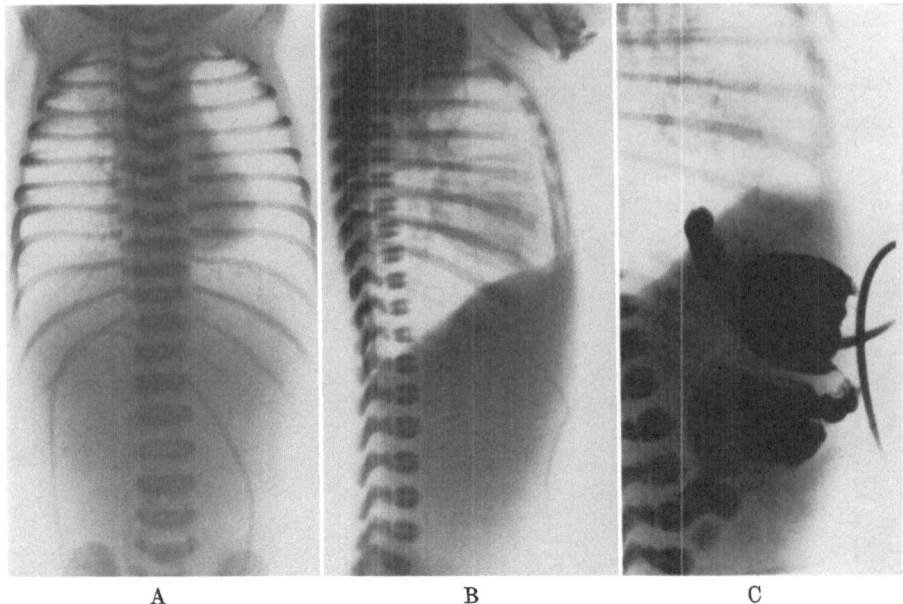

Fig. 287 A—C. Esophageal atresia without tracheoesophageal fistula. A The upper pouch is distended and filled with air; there is no air in the abdomen. B A catheter introduced into the esophagus was coiled in the upper air-containing pouch. C Retrograde opacification through a gastrostomy demonstrates the short post-atretic distal esophagus

or absence of air in the abdomen does not help in the diagnosis of an upper pouch fistula and can even be misleading in cases with a non-patent lower pouch fistula (about 1.5% appears to be non-patent) or with an associated structure in the lower esophageal segment. Further detailed information on the upper pouch (size, presence of a fistula, abnormal configurations) can be obtained by means of contrast material (Fig. 288), although some surgeons found it too dangerous or inadvisable (Kafka et al., 1966; Cuendet, 1968; Koop and Hamilton, 1968; Jaubert de Beaujeu and Mollard, 1970). Most radiologists feel that the use of small amounts of contrast material is safe, provided all precautions are taken to prevent overflow or aspiration of contrast material into the tracheobronchial tree. For this purpose all secretions are aspirated, a catheter with an opening only at its tip is inserted into the upper pouch and a limited amount (0.5 cc) of aqueous Dionosil (a contrast material used for bronchography) is instilled with the infant held in the upright position; after the roentgenograms are taken, the contrast material has to be aspirated immediately with the syringe, which is left attached to the catheter during the whole procedure.

FRITZ and SCHOBER (1969) advocate the double contrast method after the insufflation of a few ml of air (Fig. 288), while KAFKA et al. (1966), CUENDET (1968), INGELRANS et al. (1969), and JAUBERT DE BEAUJEU and MOLLARD (1970) favor pneumoesophagography, because this technique eliminates the use of possibly harmful contrast materials.

COHEN (1965), ALTMAN et al. (1966) and SWISCHUK (1968) suggest that the delineation of the distal esophageal pouch in cases of esophageal atresia without fistula should become a routine procedure in the preoperative assessment. This

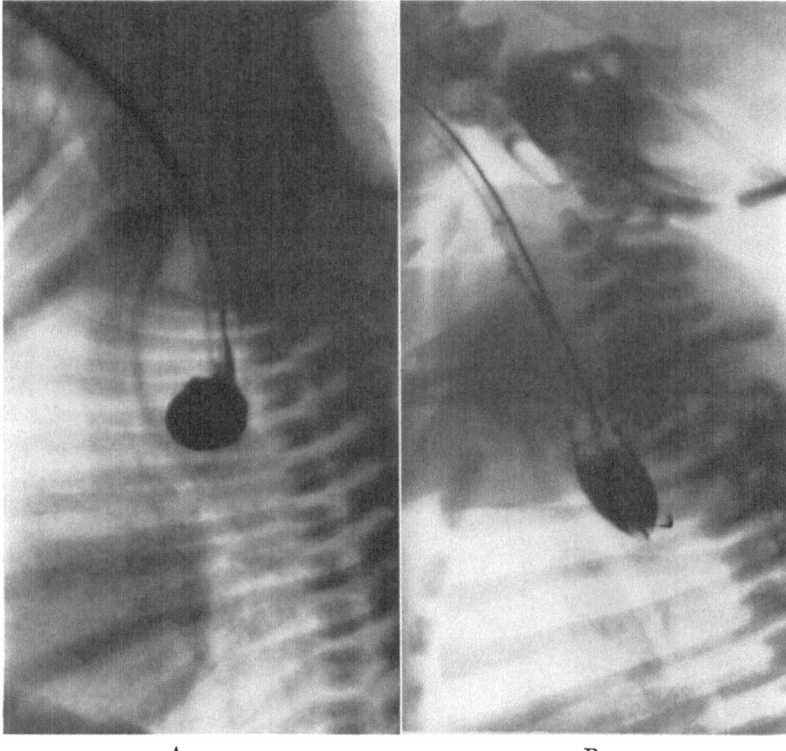

A   B

Fig. 288 A and B. Esophageal atresia. Opacification of the upper pouch with (A) and without (B) injection of air

can be achieved by performing a gastrostomy and inducing reflux of contrast material from the stomach into the esophagus (Fig. 287, 289).

8. Treatment

8.1. Principles of Management

1. The operative correction of esophageal atresia is not strictly an emergency procedure and all adequate measures should first be taken to correct—or with increasingly prompt diagnosis to prevent—the pulmonary insult and to maintain the infants in a satisfactory condition. In all cases the level of general care and nursing afforded these children (pre- and postoperatively) is the most important factor in the survival rate, and the role played by especially trained nursing personnel cannot be overemphasized.

2. In full-term infants in a good general condition with uncomplicated esophageal atresia and distal tracheoesophageal fistula the treatment of choice is an undelayed thoracotomy with division and closure of the fistula and primary esophageal anastomosis.

3. In all other infants definitive surgical repair must be delayed until the patient's condition and size allow it. The chance of successful treatment by primary repair is extremely small in premature and critically ill infants. In infants

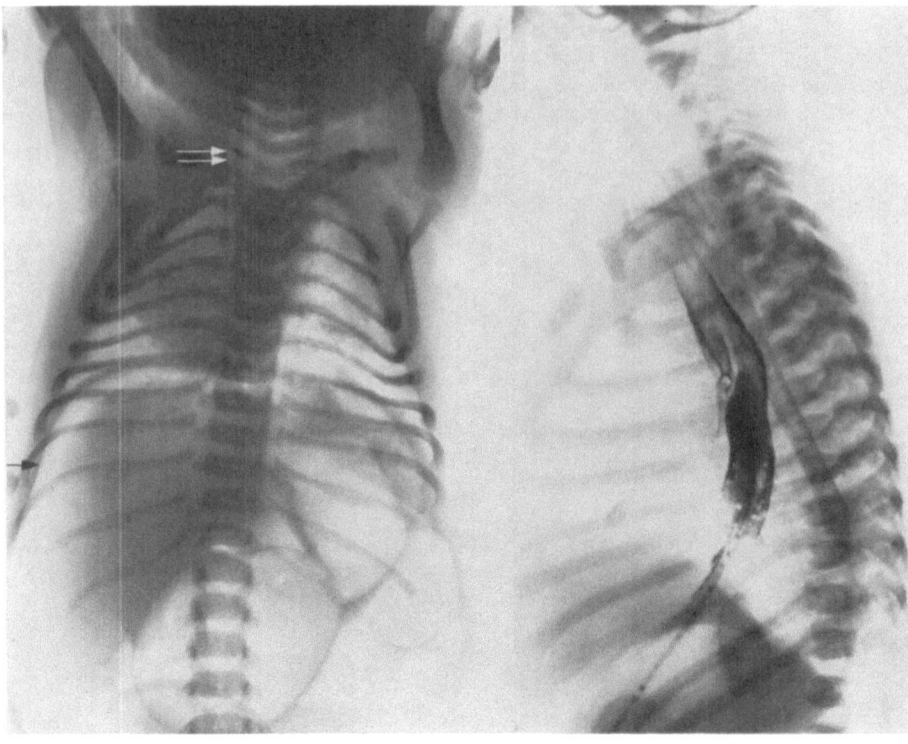

A   B

Fig. 289 A and B. Esophageal atresia with inferior tracheoesophageal fistula and associated duodenal atresia. On the plain film (A) the stomach is seen to be enormously dilated. Over-filling with air has led to free air in the abdomen (→). Note also the radiolucent area in the region of the upper mediastinum (⇒) due to air in the upper esophagus. A catheter intro-duced as far as possible into the upper esophagus was halted at the lower end of the air-filled pouch (B). A laparotomy was performed because of the free air in the abdomen. Through a gastrostomy a catheter was introduced into the distal esophagus and contrast material was injected, which clearly outlined the tracheoesophageal fistula

whose only complicating factor is aspiration pneumonia, esophageal reconstruc-tion with division and closure of the fistula usually must be delayed for only a short time, i.e. until there is clearing of the pulmonary problems. In high risk patients, however, (extreme prematurity by weight, severe resistent pneumonia, additional major anomalies, unusual types of atresia with a wide gap between the esophageal segments), only a staging program of management can contribute to a higher survival rate. In these instances staged operative techniques, during a period of prolonged intensive conservative therapy, can include gastrostomy, division and closure of a fistula, cervical esophagostomy, bougienage of an upper pouch, esophageal reconstruction and other procedures.

8.2. Preoperative Management

The pharynx and upper esophageal pouch should be aspirated every fifteen minutes regardless of apparent need, so that the pouch is empty at all times. Immediate replacement of the aspiration catheter is imperative when its lumen becomes occluded by secretions. REPLOGLE (1963) was the first to obtain satisfying results by employing a sump catheter especially designed for this purpose[1]. This double-lumen tube has been used since effectively by many surgeons for prolonged drainage, even in premature and poor risk infants, sometimes via a right-sided pharyngostomy (TALBERT and HALLER, 1965). Irrigation of the upper pouch with a mucolytic agent to liquefy tenacious secretions can be done under continuous suction, but the greatest care should be taken to avoid overflow in the tracheobronchial tree.

Elevation of head and thorax is important prior to establishment of a gastrostomy and perhaps until definitive operation. The infant's position should be changed from side to side at least each hour but never without prior aspiration of the proximal pouch.

For maintenance of a normal body temperature—which is of the utmost importance—the infants are placed in a warm Isolette. A humidified atmosphere offers valuable benefits in liquefying secretions. Oxygen therapy should be available to those who require it.

Antibiotic therapy is started routinely at the time of admission to the hospital and is subsequently adapted to the results of sensitivity studies on culture specimens obtained from the nasopharynx and the upper esophageal pouch.

The parenteral administration of fluids will assure a good nutritional state, an adequate intake of calories and a positive nitrogen balance. Any method of staging treatment ought to include some means of feeding the baby with milk from an early stage (HUGHES et al., 1965).

Atelectasis or evidence of retained secretions call for prompt tracheobronchial aspiration by direct laryngoscopy and the aspiration should be repeated until there is substantial improvement, i.e. until the lungfields are clear on roentgen examination.

In all cases when definitive surgery cannot be done without delay, a gastrostomy should be performed as an emergency procedure to maintain gastric decompression, to avoid acid reflux, and to permit feeding after the tracheoesophageal fistula has been divided.

8.3. Operative Management

The first aim of all types of operative management (primary repair or staged procedures) is division and closure of the fistulous communication between the trachea and esophageal pouch. Single or multiple ligation of the fistula without section is unsatisfactory and frequently leads to recanalization (WOOLLEY et al., 1961; PELLERIN et al., 1963; KOOP and HAMILTON, 1965; HOLDER and ASHCRAFT, 1966; MAHOUR et al., 1971). In infants who are unable to withstand any but a minimal procedure, simple division of the fistula can easily be done under local anesthesia with an extrapleural approach. In order to eliminate any thoracic procedure in compromised infants, RANDOLPH et al. (1968) performed a complete gastric division with gastrostomies in the proximal and distal gastric pouches (for suction and feeding respectively) as an alternative to the transthoracic division of the fistula. Partition of the gastric lumen with a single "pull-out" plication suture seems to be a superior alternative to complete gastric division (TOULOUKIAN and STINSON, 1970).

When the gap between the esophageal segments is short enough an esophagoesophagostomy is carried out. There are three basic types of anastomosis. (1) The

---

[1] Replogle sump tube. Aloe Medical, 1831 Olive St., St. Louis, Mo.

single layer end-to-end anastomosis is the most popular procedure and unquestionably the easiest to perform. The incidence of leaks and the mortality of these leaks are higher than with other procedures but the risk of stricture formation is lower. (2) The Haight telescopic end-to-end anastomosis has the lowest incidence of leaks but the highest incidence of strictures. (3) The two layer end-to-end anastomosis is the most difficult to perform and can be used only when both ends of the esophagus are well developed; as to the anastomotic complications it takes an intermediate position.

In cases where the ends of the esophagus are found to be in contact or in close approximation Ty et al. (1967) and Leix and Schwab (1969) carried out the Duhamel end-to-side anastomosis; this technique seems to be safe and successful in their hands. The best method of approaching the site of anastomosis is still controversial and there are many proponents of both the transpleural and the extrapleural approach. Those who approach the lesion transpleurally believe that the better exposure, the easier dissection and the shorter operating time compensate for the added risks of pleural empyema in the event of a leaking anastomosis. The use of an extrapleural drain after suturing the mediastinal pleura can probably avoid this complication almost completely (Koop and Hamilton, 1968). The retropleural approach permits only a limited exposure and is often complicated by opening of the pleural cavity. In spite of these drawbacks this method causes less of a trauma to the lungs and results in a lower postoperative mortality if a leak develops. Statistical data on comparable series indicate that the best survival rates are obtained by this extrapleural approach (Holder et al., 1964; Hays, 1966 a, b).

In 15% of the infants born with atresia (including most of the cases with isolated atresia without fistula) the gap between the upper and lower segments is too long for a safe end-to-end anastomosis. In such cases therapy consists of cervical esophagostomy, division of the fistula if present, a feeding gastrostomy and, only much later, esophageal replacement. Various types of esophageal substitutes have been tried but most surgeons now use some portion of the colon, with satisfactory results in many cases (Martin and Flege, 1964; Hanna et al., 1967; Othersen and Clatworthy, 1967; Rehbein et al., 1968). Although Koop and Verhagen (1961), Petterson (1962), Rehbein and Hoffman (1964 b) and Bentley (1965) have used primary one stage colonic substitution in newborn infants, in whom direct esophagoesophagostomy was not possible, the colonic substitution is usullay delayed until the child has reached the age of 6 to 24 months.

When there are associated colonic or anal malformations and when the blood supply to the colon is unsuitable for support of a transplant, Burrington and Stephens (1968) perform esophagoplasties with tubes made of the stomach.

In 1965, Howard and Myers published their remarkable paper on elongation of the upper blind pouch by daily bougienage: they demonstrated in a case with a wide gap between the two esophageal segments that the upper pouch could be elongated greatly by repeated daily stretching with a mercury bougie over a period of several weeks, so that a direct esophageal anastomosis could be accomplished subsequently. To estimate the distance between the ends of the esophageal pouches during the elongation procedure Hamilton (1966) placed silver clips on the distal esophagus at the time of division of the fistula. Other successes described by Johnston (1965), Hays et al. (1966 a, b), Köllermann and Gall (1966), Young (1967 a, b), Woolley et al. (1969), Ferguson (1970) and Jaubert de Beaujeu and Mollard (1970) support the idea of many surgeons that probably a great number of infants can successfully be treated by this technique, which eliminates the necessity for a colon graft in the majority of cases. The ultimate esophageal function in such cases is thought to be superior to that obtained by means of colon interposition. Stretching the lower pouch in a retrograde fashion through the gastrostomy opening can also be done (LAFER and BOLEY, 1966; HAYS et al., 1966a; WOOLLEY et al., 1969) but seems more difficult and even more risky. A new method of elongating both the upper and lower segment has been developed (REHBEIN and SCHWEDER, 1972). At surgery a nylon thread is passed from the upper to the lower esophageal segment and exteriorized through the gastrostomy. Over this thread silver olives are passed to elongate simultaneously both segments. In this way colon transplantation becomes unnecessary. During the elongation procedure, however, the danger of aspiration pneumonia remains and this can only be obviated by careful attention in keeping the upper pouch free from saliva, so that excellent and intensive nursing care must be available night and day for a period of several weeks. Although no complications directly related to introduction of the dilatators into the upper pouch have been encountered, this procedure can also stretch an upper tracheo-esophageal fistula, making its recognition at the time of operation very difficult (HAYS et al., 1966a, b; WOOLLEY et al., 1969), so that division of such a fistula sometimes has to be done as a separate procedure. An upper esophageal pouch, which at operation is found to expand synchronously with breathing suggests the existence of an upper fistula (REHBEIN, 1964a).

9. Anastomotic Complications

9.1. Leaks

Anastomotic leaks, pulmonary complications and associated congenital anomalies are the three most important causes of postoperative death. The incidence of an anastomotic leak after primary esophageal anastomosis ranges from 10 to 25%, with a mortality of 40 to 60% (SWENSON et al., 1962; HOLDER et al., 1964; MARTIN, 1965; HERTZLER, 1965; WAYSON et al., 1965; ERAKLIS and GROSS, 1966; KOOP and HAMILTON, 1968; LIVADITIS et al., 1969). This complication usually develops between the second and seventh postoperative day. In general, the earlier the leak occurs the larger it tends to be. The surgical approach and the type of anastomosis are important factors in the pathogenesis of leaks.

Other factors which contribute to the development of this complication are tension on the suture line, dimensional and structural disproportion between the esophageal segments, damage to the blood supply of the distal segment and severe respiratory distress.

A significant increase in the infant's respiratory rate, dyspnoe, signs of toxicity and deterioration of the general condition suggest an anastomotic leak. In this case some degree of mediastinitis will invariably be present and if the anastomosis was done extrapleurally, a mediastinal abscess can occur. If the approach was transpleural, an early leak will result in empyema. However, a fluid collection in the pleural cavity is often a late finding, whereas a pneumothorax soon after surgery is strongly indicative and sometimes the first indication of an ·(impending) anastomotic leak (LIVADITIS et al., 1969). The size of the leak is important to determine the type of treatment; if small it can often be handled by an adequate drainage while ceasing oral feedings; but if it is large, only continuous esophageal suction or a cervical esophagostomy, a gastrostomy for constant evacuation of the stomach, and feeding via a duodenal catheter can reduce the mortality (Eraklis and Gross, 1966). Reoperation of the inflamed region for closure of the leak is not advisable and accounts for many deaths. Those who survive the complication develop almost invariably a stricture at the anastomotic site which later requires dilations or even operative resection or esophagoplasty.

9.2. Strictures

The most common complication in infants who survive esophageal anastomosis is stricture formation. Significant difficulties due to postanastomotic strictures were observed in at least 25% of the patients (Schultz and Clatworthy, 1963; Holinger et al., 1965; Martin, 1965; Hertzler, 1965; Chrispin et al., 1966; Koop and Hamilton, 1968; Holder and Ashcraft, 1970) and most of them require some further procedure for dysphagia (Fritz and Schober, 1969; Ferguson, 1970; Holden and Wooler, 1970; El Shafie and Rickham, 1971). On routine roentgenographic re-examination about 80% of the patients had varying degrees of stricture (Desjardins et al., 1964), but no consistent relation could be found between the severity of the radiologically demonstrated stricture and the patient's clinical state.

The factors which appear to contribute to postoperative stricture formation following esophageal anastomosis have been outlined by Schultz and Clatworthy (1963). Tension on the suture line and/or too extensive mobilization of the esophagus seem to be the most important factors (Holder and Ashcraft, 1966). The type of anastomosis also plays an important role; the single layer end-to-end anastomosis is the procedure which is least likely, and the Haight anastomosis the one which is most likely to be followed by strictures (Holder et al., 1964); in cases where an end-to-side anastomosis was possible no stenosis was found (Leix and Schwab, 1969). Leakage at the site of anastomosis and infection cause some degree of stricture formation in almost all instances. Experimental studies show a high stricture tendency when chromic catgut or silk were used.

A typical stricture becomes symptomatic in the first ten weeks following surgery when solid foods are added to the diet, but in a number of patients the symptoms appear only later during infancy. Dysphagia with chronic cough, choking and even cyanosis during feedings is the dominant symptom, but recurrent aspiration pneumonia is also commonly observed. At least 15% of the patients have to be hospitalized for removal of foreign bodies lodged at the anastomotic site (Hertzler, 1965; Holinger et al., 1965; Livaditis et al., 1968; El Shafie and Rickham, 1971). The radiological appearance of these strictures is rather variable. In some cases it is a ring-like narrowing only a few millimeters long, at the level of the anastomosis; in other cases it appears as a slight decrease in esophageal diameter over several centimeters. Contour irregularities and axial deviations are not uncommon. The oral segment of the esophagus may reveal varying degrees of dilatation, sometimes causing tracheal dislocation and compression.

The mortality associated with tight and persistent strictures is high and usually due to aspiration pneumonia. The unexpected sudden deaths which have also been noted (Haight, 1963; Schultz and Clatworthy, 1963) are probably due to respiratory obstructions caused by compression of the soft posterior tracheal wall by the distended proximal segment of the esophagus.

In view of the high frequency of stricture formation and because experience has demonstrated that it is easier to treat a beginning constriction while the site of anastomosis is still soft rather than fibrotic, surgeons now recommend a more liberal use of dilatations in the early postoperative period, or even try to prevent the development of strictures by routine dilatations of all cases post-operatively. Dilatations should be the initial treatment in all patients with an established stenosis. Resection with reanastomosis or esophagoplasty is indicated only for tight strictures which are resistent to prolonged treatment by bougie-nage. The injection of triamcinolone into the stricture site at endoscopy (HOLDER et al., 1969) has been reported to be a successful means of preventing recurrence after dilatations.

9.3. Recurrent Tracheoesophageal Fistula

In reviewing the literature KAFROUNI et al. (1970) found 64 cases of recurrent tracheoesophageal fistulas out of 578 cases in which primary repair of such a fistula was done; this means that the incidence of this complication (11%) is higher than usually suspected. The main factor leading to the re-establishment of a fistula seems to be the extension from a leaking esophageal suture line (even through the capillarity of the suture material only) into the site of the tracheal closure (MOSKOVITZ et al., 1960; COWLEY, 1967; KOOP and HAMILTON, 1968). Recurrent fistulas can occur soon after the initial repair and should be suspected in patients who have persistent upper respiratory infections or re-current pneumonia, and coughing, choking or cyanosis following drinking or eating.

The diagnosis, even when strongly suspected, is difficult and often defies the most thorough examination. Of the 51 cases of recurrent tracheoesophageal fistulas whose outcome is known, 21 recurrences were found just prior to death or at autopsy (KAFROUNI et al., 1970). KÖLLERMANN and GALL (1966) stated that the presence of marked air bubbles in the esophagus filled with opaque medium is a radiological sign of this complication.

The overall mortality rate of this complication is approximately 50 to 60% and even after operation for recurrent fistula the fatality rate is high (SWENSON et al., 1962; KOOP and HAMILTON, 1968; KAFROUNI et al., 1970). Treatment will be the division of the recurrent fistula with interposition of some neutral tissue between the closed ends of the fistula. Satisfactory repair is unlikely if the operation is undertaken less than two or three months following the initial operation.

9.4. Neurogenic Dysfunction

In addition to stenosis, a functional disturbance in motor activity of the primarily repaired esophagus may be responsible for causing dysphagia in some cases. Several authors used cinefluoroscopy to study esophageal function after repair of esophageal atresia (HAIGHT, 1957; KIRKPATRICK et al., 1961; DES-JARDINS et al., 1964; CHRISPIN et al., 1966; SHEPARD et al., 1966; TY et al., 1967; BURGESS et al., 1968; CUENDET, 1968; HOLDER and ASHCRAFT, 1970). They found that the primary peristaltic wave invariably died out below the line of anastomosis and that below this level a lack of peristalsis occurred over a distance of at least 3 to 5 cm; in this aperistaltic segment secondary contractions could be observed, resulting in both anterograde and retrograde flow with some-times a considerable delay in the emptying time of this segment; the function of the inferior esophageal sphincter was considered normal. Intraluminal pres-sure recordings showed somewhat conflicting results: in contrast to LIND et al.

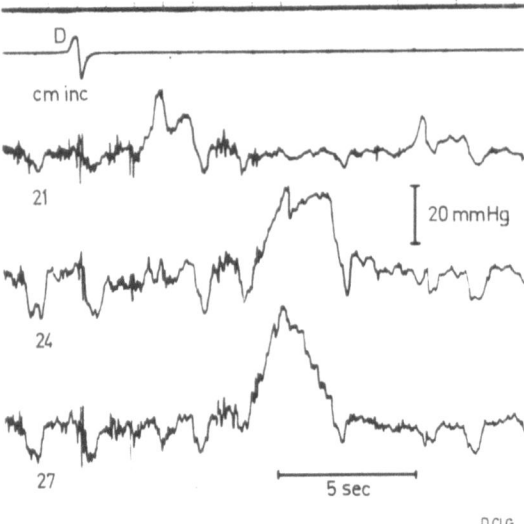

Fig. 290. Manometry after repair of esophageal atresia. The peristaltic contraction stops below the level of 21 cm from the incisors, probably above the level of the anastomosis. More distally, from 24 to 27 cm, simultaneous contractions appear, after a delay of 2 to 3 sec. In the lowest segment of the esophagus the contractions are normal again. Although no stenosis could be demonstrated on roentgen examination, the patient complained of dysphagia

(1966), who found a disordered motility pattern in the entire esophagus, indistinguishable from that of achalasia in adults, SHEPARD et al. (1966) and BURGESS et al. (1968) noted an aperistaltic segment of only 6 to 15 cm near the anastomotic site and a completely normal lower esophageal sphincter; in the aperistaltic segment no reaction on deglutition or only aperistaltic simultaneous and often repetitive contractions occurred (Fig. 290).

There is no uniformity of opinion as to whether this motor dysfunction results from a congenital defect in the vagal innervation or musculature, or whether it is the result of trauma at the time of operation causing interruption of the esophageal branches of the vagal nerves or extensive periesophageal fibrosis. Although the possibility of a congenital etiologic factor cannot be excluded, an acquired lesion seems the most likely explanation for the motor disorder. HOLDER and ASHCRAFT (1970) reported that the cases with non-motile segments in the reconstructed esophagus all had extensive mobilization of the esophageal segments in order to attempt to gain more length when preparing the anastomosis, and TY et al. (1967) showed good esophageal motility patterns in cases in which an end-to-side anastomosis had not necessitated extensive periesophageal dissection. These observations, however, are not confirmed by CHRISPIN et al. (1966), who found no relationship between surgical technique and postoperative motor disorders. BURGESS et al. (1968) postoperatively tested the integrity of the vagal trunks with a Hollander insulin test and found it to be normal. In an infant that could be studied before repair of the atresia KIRKPATRICK et al. (1961) found an abnormal motility in the distal segment of the esophagus and CHRISPIN et al. (1966) preoperatively could not find stripping waves in the esophagus of two patients with a tracheoesophageal fistula. KRISHINGER and WOOLLEY (1969) reported the case of a boy who developed achalasia at the age of six and who had previously been treated for atresia and tracheoesophageal fistula.

The dysfunction usually causes only minor symptoms but careful questioning always reveals some degree of dysphagia (usually for solids) even when no stricture can be demonstrated. Most children chew their foods longer and more carefully than their siblings and have some difficulties with large boluses poorly masticated. Impaction and intermittent regurgitation sometimes occur, and the patient's preference for an upright position while eating is usually clear. There seems to be a correlation between the abnormalities observed by motility studies and the symptomatology (SHEPARD et al., 1966; LIND et al., 1966; CHRISPIN et al., 1966; TY et al., 1967; BURGESS et al., 1968), although some degree of deficiency in the peristalsis can also be demonstrated in children who have no difficulties with a normal diet several years after the operation.

10. Trends in Survival

In 1960, survival after primary repair of uncomplicated esophageal atresia of the usual type approached 95% in good pediatric centers throughout the world. At the same time, however, the overall mortality ranged from 40 to 60%; thus a significant mortality was found when the atresia was of the less common anatomical type or was complicated by associated anomalies or pneumonia and when the infants were premature by weight. This group constituted a majority of the infants. The rigorous use of the Waterston's classification of risks (WATERSTON et al., 1963) (Table 24) has done much to clarify the prognosis of the individual baby at the time of admission to the hospital. Since that time there has been a consistent gradual fall in the mortality associated with the treatment of esophageal atresia both among mature and premature infants; this improvement has accompanied the trend toward increased use of delayed surgical management, but has also been associated with many other concurrent advances in clinical management.

There is a trend today to investigate the mortality in function of the type of management used: (1) Undelayed primary anastomosis. (2) Primary anastomosis after a short delay of less than 2 weeks. This type of treatment is indicated in patients with pneumonia, prematurity, respiratory distress syndrome or hyperbilirubinemia. (3) Staged "long" delays. Extreme prematurity, additional major anomalies, resistent pneumonia and atresia with a wide gap between the segments make this type of treatment unavoidable.

The overall survival has now reached 80%. The delayed cases undoubtedly represent a less favorable group. When undelayed primary anastomosis can be performed (about 40% of all infants) survival is the rule.

Table 24. Progression of esophageal atresia based on Waterston's classification of risks (WATERSTON et al., 1962)

Risk group A	Birthweight over 2500 g and well
Risk group B₁	Birthweight 2000 to 2500 g and well
B₂	Higher birthweight, moderate pneumonia and congenital anomaly
Risk group C₁	Birthweight under 2000 g
C₂	Higher birthweight and severe pneumonia and severe congenital anomaly
Survival	A: >90%; B: 60 to 70%; C: <10%

References

Ahmed, S.: Right-sided Bochdalek hernia associated with esophageal atresia and tracheo-esophageal fistula. J. Pediat. Surg. 5, 256 (1970).

Altman, D. H., Mencia, L. F., Litt, R. E., Gilbert, M. G.: Esophageal atresia. A simple radiological technic to facilitate surgical management. Radiology 86, 1112–1114 (1966).

Ashcraft, K. W., Holder, T. M.: The story of esophageal atresia and tracheoesophageal fistula. Pediat. Surg. 65, 332–340 (1969).

Bentley, J. F. R.: Primary colonic substitution for atresia of the esophagus. Surgery 58, 731–736 (1965).

Bettex, M., Crivelli, T.: Der heutige Stand der Chirurgie der Oesophagusatresie. Schweiz. med. Wschr. 90, 671–677 (1960).

Blank, R. H., Prillaman, P. E., Minor, G. R.: Congenital esophageal atresia with tracheo-esophageal fistula occurring in identical twins. J. thorac. cardiovasc. Surg. 53, 192–196 (1967).

Bluestone, C. D., Kerry, R., Sieber, W. K.: Congenital esophageal stenosis. Laryngo-scope (St. Louis) 79, 1095–1104 (1969).

Brown, R. K., Brown, E. C.: Congenital esophageal anomalies: Review of twenty-four cases and report of three. Surg. Gynec. Obstet. 91, 545–550 (1950).

Burgess, J. N., Carlson, H. C., Ellis, F. H., Jr.: Esophageal function after successful repair of esophageal atresia and tracheoesophageal fistula. J. thorac. cardiovasc. Surg. 56, 667–673 (1968).

Burrington, J. D., Stephens, C. A.: Esophageal replacement with a gastric tube in infants and children. J. Pediat. Surg. 3, 246–252 (1968).

Chrispin, A. R., Friedland, G. W., Waterston, D. J.: Aspiration pneumonia and dys-phagia after technically successful repair of esophageal atresia. Thorax 21, 104–110 (1966).

Cloud, D. T.: Anastomotic technic in esophageal atresia. J. Pediat. Surg. 3, 561–564 (1968).

Cohen, S. J.: Unusual types of esophageal atresia and tracheoesophageal fistulae. Diagnostic aids and procedures. Clin. Pediat. 4, 271–275 (1965).

Cowley, L. L.: Congenital tracheo-esophageal fistula: recurrence after repair. Amer. Surg. 33, 409–410 (1967).

Cozzi, F.: Oesophageal atresia. Lancet 1967 II, 1222–1225.

Cozzi, F., Wilkinson, A. W.: Intrauterine growth rate in relation to anorectal and oesoph-ageal anomalies. Arch. Dis. Childh. 44, 59–62 (1969).

Cuendet, A.: Le traitement des atrésies de l'œsophage. Helv. chir. Acta 35, 338–367 (1968).

Dafoe, C. S., Ross, C. A.: Tracheo-esophageal fistula and esophageal atresia. Dis. Chest 37, 42–51 (1960).

Daum, R.: Formen der Oesophagusfehlbildungen. Z. Kinderchir. 8, 39–44 (1970).

Daum, R., Kaick, G. van: Seltene Variante einer Ösophagusatresie. Fortschr. Röntgenstr. 113, 112–113 (1970).

Desjardins, J. G., Stephens, C. A., Moes, C. A. F.: Results of surgical treatment of con-genital tracheo-esophageal fistula, with a note on cine-fluorographic findings. Ann. Surg. 160, 141–145 (1964).

Devens, K., Ritz, O.: Eine bisher unbekannte Form der Ösophagusatresie. Z. Kinderchir. 2, 484–486 (1965).

El Shafie, M., Rickham, P. P.: Long-term results after primary repair of oesophageal atresia and tracheo-oesophageal fistula. Z. Kinderchir. 9, 309–316 (1971).

Eraklis, A. J., Gross, R. E.: Esophageal atresia — Management following an anastomotic leak. Surgery 60, 919–923 (1966).

Ferguson, C. C.: Management of infants with esophageal atresia and tracheoesophageal fistula. Ann. Surg. 172, 750–754 (1970).

Fluss, Z., Poppen, K. J.: Embryogenesis of tracheoesophageal fistula and esophageal atresia. Arch. Path. 52, 168–181 (1951).

Franken, E. A., Saldino, R. M.: Hypertrophic pyloric stenosis complicating esophageal atresia with tracheoesophageal fistula. Amer. J. Surg. 117, 647–649 (1969).

Freeman, N. V., Rickham, P. P., Johnston, J. H.: In: Neonatal Surgery, p. 198–223. London: Butterworths 1969.

Fritz, W., Schober, K. L.: Ein Beitrag zur Therapie der kongenitalen Ösophagusatresie. Zbl. Chir. 94, 1637–1646 (1969).

Gans, S. L., Lackey, D. A., Zuckerbraun, L.: Duplications of the cervical esophagus in infants and children. Surgery 63, 849–852 (1968).

Giedon, A.: Angeborene hohe Ösophagotrachealfistel von H-Typus. Helv. paediat. Acta 15, 155–162 (1960).

Greenough, W. G.: Congenital esophageal strictures. Amer. J. Roentgenol. 92, 994–999 (1964).

GROSS, R. E.: An atlas of children's surgery, p. 2–7. Philadelphia-London-Toronto: W. D. Saunders Company 1970.

GRYBOSKI, J. D., THAYER, W. R., SPIRO, H. M.: Esophageal motility in infants and children. Pediatrics **31**, 382–395 (1963).

HAIGHT, C.: Some observations on esophageal atresias and tracheo-esophageal fistulas of congenital origin. J. thorac. Surg. **34**, 141–172 (1957).

HAIGHT, C.: The management of congenital esophageal atresia and tracheoesophageal fistula. Surg. Clin. N. Amer. **41**, 1281–1293 (1961).

HAIGHT, C.: In: Discussion of SCHULTZ, L. R., CLATWORTHY, H. W.: "Esophageal strictures after anastomosis in esophageal atresia" Arch. Surg. **87**, 120–124 (1963).

HAMILTON, J. P.: Esophageal atresia. Technical points in the staged procedures leading to esophageal anostomosis. J. pediat. Surg. **1**, 253–255 (1966).

HANNA, E. A., HARRISON, A. W., DERRICK, J. R.: Long-term results of visceral esophageal substitutes. Ann. thorac. Surg. **3**, 111–118 (1967).

HASSE, W.: Ösophagusatresie. Thoraxchirurgie **16**, 432–438 (1968).

HAUSMANN, P. F., CLOSE, A. S., WILLIAMS, L. P.: Occurrence of tracheoesophageal fistula in three consecutive siblings. Surgery **41**, 542–543 (1957).

HAYS, D. M.: An analysis of the mortality in esophageal atresia. Amer. J. Dis. Child. **103**, 765–770 (1962).

HAYS, D. M., WOOLLEY, M. M., SNYDER, W. H.: Changing techniques in the management of esophageal atresia. Arch. Surg. **92**, 611–616 (1966a).

HAYS, D. M., WOOLLEY, M. M., SNYDER, W. H.: Esophageal atresia and tracheoesophageal fistula: management of the uncommon types. J. pediat. Surg. **1**, 240–252 (1966b).

HECKER, W. C.: Ösophagusstenosen im Kindesalter und ihre Therapie. Münch. med. Wschr. **36**, 2026–2033 (1968).

HECKER, W. C., DAUM, R., RÜTER, E.: Bedeutsame prognostische Faktoren in der Behandlung der Oesophagusmißbildungen. Mschr. Kinderheilk. **114**, 225—227 (1966).

HERTZLER, J. H.: Congenital esophageal atresia. Problems and management. Amer. J. Surg. **109**, 780–787 (1965).

HOLCOMB, G. W., DANIEL, R. A.: Unusual tracheoesophageal fistulas with membranous atresia of the middle or distal esophagus. Surgery **59**, 1112–1119 (1966).

HOLDEN, M. P., WOOLER, G. H.: Tracheo-esophageal fistula and oesophageal atresia: results of 30 years' experience. Thorax **25**, 406–412 (1970).

HOLDER, T. M., ASHCRAFT, K. W.: Esophageal atresia and tracheoesophageal fistula. Curr. Probl. Surg. 3–68, August, 1966.

HOLDER, T. M., ASHCRAFT, K. W.: Esophageal atresia and tracheoesophageal fistula. Ann. thorac. Surg. **9**, 445–467 (1970).

HOLDER, T. M., ASHCRAFT, K. W., LEAPE, L.: The treatment of patients with esophageal strictures by local steroid injection. J. pediat. Surg. **4**, 646–653 (1969).

HOLDER, T. M., CLOUD, D. T., LEWIS, J. E., PILLING, G. P.: Esophageal atresia and tracheoesophageal fistula. A survey of Its members by the Surgical Section of the American Academy of Pediatrics. Pediatrics **34**, 542–549 (1964).

HOLDER, T. M., McDONALD, V. G., WOOLLEY, M. M.: The premature or critically ill infant with esophageal atresia: increased succes with a staged approach. J. thorac. cardiovasc. Surg. **44**, 344–358 (1962).

HOLINGER, P. H., BROWN, W. T., MAURIZI, D. G.: Endoscopic aspects of post-surgical management of congenital esophageal atresia and tracheoesophageal fistula. J. thorac. cardiovasc. Surg. **49**, 22–32 (1965).

HOLINGER, P. H., JOHNSTON, K. C.: Postsurgical endoscopic problems of congenital esophageal atresia. Ann. Otol. **72**, 1035–1049 (1963).

HOPKINS, W. A., ZWIREN, G. T.: Colon replacement of the esophagus in children. J. thorac. cardiovasc. Surg. **46**, 346–358 (1963).

HOWARD, R., MYERS, N. A.: Esophageal atresia: a technique for elongating the upper pouch. Surgery **58**, 725–727 (1965).

HUGHES, E. A., STEVENS, L. H., TOMS, D. A., WILKINSON, A. W.: Oesophageal atresia: metabolic effects of operation. Brit. J. Surg. **52**, 403–410 (1965).

HUMPHREYS, G. H., FERRER, J. M.: Management of esophageal atresia. Amer. J. Surg. **107**, 406–411 (1964).

INGALLS, T. H., PRINDLE, R. A.: Esophageal atresia with tracheo-esophageal fistula. Epidemiologic and teratologic implications. New Engl. J. Med. **240**, 987–995 (1949).

INGALLS, T. H., CURLEY, F. J., PRINDLE, R. A.: Experimental production of congenital anomalies. Timing and degree of anoxia as factors causing fatal deaths and congenital anomalies in the mouse. New Engl. J. Med. **247**, 758–768 (1952).

INGELRANS, P., LACHERETZ, M., DEBEUGNY, P., FIEVEZ, E.: Le facteur respiratoire dans l'atrésie congénitale de l'œsophage. Importance pronostique et problèmes thérapeutiques. Lille méd. **14**, 693–697 (1969).

Ishida, M., Tsuchida, Y., Saito, S., Tsunoda, A.: Congenital esophageal stenosis due to tracheobronchial remnants. J. pediat. Surg. 4, 339–345 (1969).

Jaubert de Beaujeu, M., Mollard, P.: Diagnostic et traitement de l'atrésie de l'œsophage. Rev. Prat. 20, 1099–1110 (1970).

Jaubert de Beaujeu, M., Mollard, P., Campo-Paysaa, A., Bochu, A.: Traitement des atrésies de l'œsophage avec impossibilité d'anastomose d'emblée. Ann. Chir. infant. 9, 289–296 (1968).

Johnsonbaugh, R. E.: A new diagnostic procedure for evaluating esophageal atresia. Amer. J. Dis. Child. 116, 175–178 (1968).

Johnston, P. W.: Elongation of the upper segment in esophageal atresia: report of a case. Surgery 58, 741–744 (1965).

Kafka, V., Hucin, B., Koutecky, J., Kolihova, E.: Ösophagusatresie. Bemerkungen zur Diagnostik und prä- und postoperativen Behandlung. Z. Kinderchir. 3, 460–472 (1966).

Kafrouni, G., Baick, C. H., Woolley, M. M.: Recurrent tracheoesophageal fistula: a diagnostic problem. Surgery 68, 889–894 (1970).

Kelley, M. L., Murtagh, J., McCarty, W. C.: Reduplication of the esophagus. J. Amer. med. Ass. 204, 73–75 (1968).

Keshishian, J. M., Cox, P. A.: Esophageal stricture at anastomotic site following repair of tracheoesophageal fistula. J. thorac. cardiovasc. Surg. 53, 754–756 (1967).

Kirkpatrick, J. A., Cresson, S. L., Pilling, G. P.: The motor activity of the esophagus in association with esophageal atresia and tracheoesophageal fistula. Amer. J. Roentgenol. 86, 884–887 (1961).

Kirkpatrick, J. A., Wagner, M. L., Pilling, G. P.: A complex of anomalies associated with tracheoesophageal fistula and esophageal atresia. Amer. J. Roentgenol. 95, 208–211 (1965).

Köllermann, M. W., Gall, F.: Ein Beitrag zur Behandlung der Oesophagusatresie. Z. Kinderchir. 3, 472–478 (1966).

Kolb, E.: Kombination von Oesophagusatresie, Duodenalstenose, Anusatresie mit multicystischer Niere. Helv. paediat. Acta 18, 240–245 (1963).

Koop, C. E.: Atresia of the esophagus: Technical considerations in surgical management. Surg. Clin. N. Amer. 42, 1387–1395 (1962).

Koop, C. E., Hamilton, J. P.: Atresia of the esophagus: increased survival with staged procedures in the poor-risk infant. Ann. Surg. 162, 389–401 (1965).

Koop, C. E., Hamilton, J. P.: Atresia of the esophagus: Factors affecting survival in 249 cases. Z. Kinderchir. 5, 319–333 (1968).

Koop, C. E., Verhagen, A. D.: Early management of atresia of the esophagus. Surg. Gynec. Obstet. 113, 103–112 (1961).

Krishinger, G. L., Woolley, M. M.: Esophageal atresia and tracheo-esophageal fistula. 25 years' experience and current management. Calif. Med. 111, 165–168 (1969).

Ladd, W. E.: The surgical treatment of esophageal atresia and tracheoesophageal fistula. New Engl. J. Med. 230, 625–637 (1944).

Ladd, W. E.: Congenital anomalies of the esophagus. Pediatrics 6, 9–19 (1950).

Lafer, D. J., Boley, S. J.: Primary repair in esophageal atresia with elongation of the lower segment. J. pediat. Surg. 1, 585–587 (1966).

Langman, J.: Oesophageal atresia accompanied by a remarkable vessel anomaly. Arch. chir. neerl. 4, 39–42 (1952).

Leix, F., Schwab, C. E.: End to side operative technic for esophageal atresia with tracheoesophageal fistula. Amer. J. Surg. 118, 225–235 (1969).

Leven, N. L., Varco, R. L., Lannin, B. G., Tongen, L. A.: The surgical management of congenital atresia of the esophagus and tracheoesophageal fistula. Ann. Surg. 136, 701–719 (1952).

Lind, J. F., Blanchard, R. J., Guyda, H.: Esophageal motility in tracheoesophageal fistula and esophageal atresia. Surg. Gynec. Obstet. 123, 557–564 (1966).

Lister, J.: An unusual variation of oesophageal atresia. Arch. Dis. Childh. 38, 176–179 (1963).

Lister, J.: The blood supply of the oesophagus in relation to oesophageal atresia. Arch. Dis. Childh. 39, 131–137 (1964).

Lister, J.: Oesophageal atresia in a cretin. Proc. roy. Soc. Med. 62, 1094–1095 (1969).

Livaditis, A., Okmian, L., Eklöf, O.: Esophageal atresia. Anastomotic strictures following primary surgical management. Scand. J. thorac. cardiovasc. Surg. 2, 151–158 (1968).

Livaditis, A., Okmian, L., Eklöf, O.: Esophageal atresia. Anastomotic disruption following primary surgical management. Scand. J. thorac. cardiovasc. Surg. 3, 39–43 (1969).

Lloyd, J. R., Clatworthy, H. W.: Hydramnios as an aid to the early diagnosis of congenital obstruction of the alimentary tract: a study of the maternal and fetal factors. Pediatrics 21, 903–909 (1958).

Lorimier, A. A. de: Treatment of esophageal atresia with a short proximal esophageal segment. J. Amer. med. Ass. 195, 697–698 (1966).

Louw, J. H.: Congenital intestinal atresia and stenosis in the newborn. Observations on its pathogenesis and treatment. Ann. roy. Coll. Surg. Engl. **25**, 209–234 (1959).

Mahour, G. H., Johnston, P. W., Gwinn, J. L., Hays, D. M.: Congenital esophageal stenosis distal to esophageal atresia. Surgery **69**, 936–939 (1971).

Martin, L. W.: Management of esophageal anomalies. Pediatrics **36**, 342–350 (1965).

Martin, L. W., Flege, J. B.: Use of colon as a substitute for the esophagus in children. Amer. J. Surg. **108**, 69–74 (1964).

Mellins, R. B., Blumenthal, S.: Cardiovascular anomalies and esophageal atresia. Amer. J. Dis. Child. **107**, 160–164 (1964).

Miller, R. C., Moynihan, P. C.: Esophageal atresia. Sth. med. J. (Bgham, Ala.) **63**, 939–945 (1970).

Minnis, J. F., Burko, H., Brevetti, G.: Segmental duplication of the esophagus associated with esophageal atresia and tracheo-esophageal fistula. Ann. Surg. **156**, 271–275 (1962).

Moskovitz, W. S., Hughes, C. W., Bowers, W. F.: Recurrent tracheoesophageal fistula. Amer. J. Surg. **100**, 110–112 (1960).

Moya, F., Apgar, V., James, L. S., Berrien, C.: Hydramnios and congenital anomalies. J. Amer. med. Ass. **173**, 1552–1556 (1960).

Othersen, H. B., Clatworthy, H. W.: Functional evaluation of esophageal replacement in children. J. thorac. cardiovasc. Surg. **53**, 55–63 (1967).

Othersen, H. B., Gregorie, H. B.: Pneumatic rupture of the stomach in a newborn infant with esophageal atresia and tracheoesophageal fistula. Surgery **53**, 362–367 (1963).

Overton, R. C., Creech, O.: Unusual esophageal atresia with distant membranous obstruction of the esophagus. J. thorac. cardiovasc. Surg. **35**, 674–677 (1958).

Pellerin, D., Bienayme, J., Aicardi, J., Dolsa, E.: Traitement de l'atrésie de l'œsophage et résultats. Arch. franç. Pédiat. **20**, 821–837 (1963).

Pellerin, D., Nihoul-Fekete, C.: Atrésie de l'œsophage, succes et échecs. Arch. franç. Pédiat. **24**, 319–328 (1967).

Petterson, G.: Experiences in oesophageal reconstruction. Arch. Dis. Childh. **37**, 184–189 (1962).

Polk, H. C., Burford, T. H.: Disorders of the distal esophagus in infancy and childhood. Amer. J. Dis. Child. **108**, 243–251 (1964).

Raffensperger, J.: Gastrointestinal-tract defects associated with esophageal atresia and tracheo-esophageal fistula. Arch. Surg. **101**, 241–244 (1970).

Randolph, J. G., Tunell, W. P., Lilly, J. R.: Gastric division in the critically ill infant with esophageal atresia and tracheoesophageal fistula. Surgery **63**, 496–502 (1968).

Rehbein, F.: Oesophageal atresia with double tracheo-oesophageal fistula. Arch. Dis. Childh. **39**, 138–142 (1964a).

Rehbein, F., Hofmann, S.: Ösophagusatresie mit Duodenalverschluß und Analatresie, zugleich ein Beitrag zur primären Kolonersatzplastik. Z. Kinderchir. **1**, 57–74 (1964b).

Rehbein, F., Schweder, N.: Neue Wege in der Rekonstruktion der kindlichen Speiseröhre. Dtsch. med. Wschr. **97**, 757–770 (1972).

Rehbein, F., Schweder, N., Willich, E.: Rekonstruktion der kindlichen Speiseröhre durch Colon. Dtsch. med. Wschr. **93**, 720–727 (1968).

Replogle, R. L.: Esophageal atresia: plastic sump catheter for drainage of the proximal pouch. Surgery **54**, 296–297 (1963).

Roe, B. B., Nobis, P. D.: Congenital tracheo-esophageal fistula. Amer. J. Dis. Child. **106**, 489–491 (1963).

Römer, K. H.: Nouveaux aspects de la chirurgie des atrésies de l'œsophage. Bronches **18**, 286–289 (1968).

Rohmsdahl, M. M., Hunter, J. A., Grove, W. J.: Tracheoesophageal fistula and esophageal atresia. J. thorac. cardiovasc. Surg. **52**, 571–578 (1966).

Schultz, L. R., Clatworthy, H. W.: Esophageal strictures after anastomosis in esophageal atresia. Arch. Surg. **87**, 120–124 (1963).

Scott, J. S., Wilson, J. K.: Hydramnios as an early sign of oesophageal atresia. Lancet **1957 II**, 569–572.

Shepard, R., Fenn, S., Sieber, W. K.: Evaluation of esophageal function in postoperative esophageal atresia and tracheoesophageal fistula. Surgery **58**, 608–617 (1966).

Slim, M. S., Bickers, W. M.: Esophageal atresia with tracheo-esophageal fistula. Arch. Surg. **100**, 577–581 (1970).

Sloan, H., Haight, C.: Congenital atresia of the esophagus in brothers. J. thorac. Surg. **32**, 209–215 (1956).

Stephens, H. B.: H-type tracheoesophageal fistula complicated by esophageal stenosis. J. thorac. cardiovasc. Surg. **59**, 325—329 (1970).

Swenson, O., Lipman, R., Fisher, J. H., Duluca, F. G.: Repair and complications of esophageal atresia and tracheoesophageal fistula. New Engl. J. Med. **267**, 960–963 (1962).

Swischuk, L. E.: Demonstration of the distal esophageal pouch in esophageal atresia without fistula. Amer. J. Roentgenol. **103**, 277–280 (1968).

Talbert, J. L., Haller, J. A.: Temporary tube pharyngostomy in the staged repair of congenital tracheoesophageal fistula. Surgery **58**, 737–740 (1965).

Thomas, P. S., Chrispin, A. R.: Congenital tracheo-oesophageal fistula without oesophageal atresia. Clin. Radiol. **20**, 371–374 (1969)

Touloukian, R. J., Stinson, K. K.: Temporary gastric partition: a model for staged repair of esophageal atresia with fistula. Ann. Surg. **171**, 184–188 (1970).

Tuquan, N. A.: Annular stricture of the esophagus distal to congenital tracheoesophageal fistula. Surgery **52**, 394–395 (1962).

Ty, T. C., Brunet, C., Beardmore, H. E.: A variation in the operative technic for the treatment of esophageal atresia with tracheo-esophageal fistula. J. pediat. Surg. **2**, 118–126 (1967).

Vidne, B., Levy, M. J.: Use of pericardium for esophagoplasty in congenital esophageal stenosis. Surgery **68**, 389–392 (1970).

Waterston, D. J., Bonham-Carter, R. E., Aberdeen, E.: Oesophageal atresia: tracheo-oesophageal fistula. A study of survival in 218 infants. Lancet **1962 I**, 819–822.

Waterston, D. J., Bonham-Carter, R. E., Aberdeen, E.: Congenital tracheo-oesophageal fistula in association with oesophageal atresia. Lancet **1963 II**, 55–57.

Wayson, E. E., Garnjobst, W., Chandler, J. J., Peterson, C. G.: Esophageal atresia with tracheoesophageal fistula. Amer. J. Surg. **110**, 162–167 (1965).

Willich, F.: Lungenaplasie rechts mit Situs Inversus totalis, Ösophagusatresie und Abgang des unteren Ösophagussegmentes aus dem re. Hauptbronchus. Z. Kinderchir. **2**, 120–121 (1965).

Wolf, R. Y., Duncan, L., Pate, J. W.: Tracheoesophageal fistula associated with esophageal duplication. Surgery **58**, 728–730 (1965).

Woolley, M. M., Chinnock, R. F., Paul, R. H.: Premature twins with esophageal atresia and tracheo-esophageal fistula. Acta paediat. **50**, 423–430 (1961).

Woolley, M. M., Leix, F., Johnston, P. W., Hays, D. M.: Esophageal atresia types A and B: Upper pouch elongation and delayed anatomic reconstruction. J. pediat. Surg. **4**, 148–153 (1969).

Yahr, W. Z., Azzoni, A. A., Santulli, T. V.: Congenital atresia of the esophagus with tracheoesophageal fistula: an unusual variant. Surgery **52**, 937–941 (1962).

Young, D. G.: Successful primary anastomosis in esophageal atresia after reduction of a long gap between the blind ends by bouginage of the upper pouch. Brit. J. Surg. **54**, 321–324 (1967a).

Young, D. G.: Dilatation and elongation of the proximal pouch in oesophageal atresia. Z. Kinderchir. **4**, 11–16 (1967b).

Isolated Tracheoesophageal Fistula

A. Lacquet and G. Fransen

The first report of a tracheoesophageal fistula without atresia appears to be Lamb's paper in 1873; the lesion was diagnosed at autopsy in a 7-week old infant. The first successful closure of a fistula appears to have been performed by Imperatori in 1939 via a transtracheal route, in a 6-year old child. The first transthoracic repair was apparently that reported by Haight in 1948; and Miller used the first transcervical aproach in 1958 for a fistula which was situated at the lower pole of the thyroid.

Isolated tracheoesophageal fistula is a rarely diagnosed malformation and seems to account for only 4% of the congenital esophageal anomalies. The rarity of the anomaly is more apparent than real and the more frequent detection of cases in recent years tends to confirm the opinion that the lesion is more common than is generally believed (Giedion, 1960; Lynn and Davis, 1961; Cohen, 1965; Thomas and Chrispin, 1969). About 60% of the patients are males (Killen and Greenlee, 1965). The most plausible pathogenetic theory postulates the failure of the lateral cell masses to separate completely the primitive foregut into anterior and posterior components (trachea and esophagus). In about 65% of the cases the fistulas are located at the level of the second thoracic vertebra or above (Schneider and Becker, 1962; Thomas and Chrispin, 1969). Of the 41 cases of isolated tracheoesophageal fistula collected by Lynn and Davis (1961), ten were cervical, 22 were high thoracic and only nine were in the region of the carina. Johnston and Hastings (1966), in reviewing all cases in the English medical literature, found that the fistulas most commonly occurred at the level of C_7 and T_1. Cleland (1968) found the fistulas in his twelve cases high up in the trachea, always attainable by a cervical approach. Cases with two fistulous communications between trachea and esophagus are described by Rabbitt (1957), Goldenberg (1960) and Hays (1966b) and the occurrence of three fistulas is reported by Eckstein and Somasundaram (1966) in a boy of twelve. In these cases the upper fistula ended invariably high into the trachea so that it could not be found by thoracic exploration. Although the position of the fistula may change slightly with crying and coughing, usually the fistula has an oblique course running cephalad from the esophagus into the trachea. Autopsy reports emphasize that the esophageal apertures of these fistulas are often slitlike and covered by mucosal folds, so that they may easily be missed when a tracheoesophageal fistula is looked for from the esophageal lumen; on autopsy, examination of the posterior surface of the trachea greatly enhances the likelihood of finding a fistula.

Patients with isolated tracheoesophageal fistulas can be classified in three distinct clinical groups: (1) Those with acute pulmonary symptoms soon after birth: severe pneumonia with respiratory distress and episodes of choking and cyanosis associated with feedings. (2) Those with a delayed onset of symptoms, primarily of gastrointestinal nature: abdominal distension caused by the passage of large volumes of air, especially when crying, frothy stools, coughing and occasional choking spells after taking liquids and preference for semisolid food and for eating in the supine position. Respiratory symptoms may appear later but are less overwhelming. (3) Those in whom the diagnosis is delayed for a long time (Lansden and Falor, 1960; Haas, 1961; Tenta and Ford, 1967; Zack and Owens, 1967; Gelissen and Persijn, 1968). The patients complain of severe long-standing pneumonia treated on innumerable occasions, chronic cough, hemoptysis and postural drainage of copious quantities of sputum. Throughout these reports it is striking how often the correct diagnosis is suspected early by the clinician, to be discarded later as a result of negative diagnostic procedures so that many cases have masqueraded under the diagnosis of faulty deglutition and recurrent pneumonia of unknown origin.

Simple auscultation of the thorax before and after the infant has attempted to swallow liquids may give strong evidence of a tracheoesophageal communication if dramatic increase in rales and ronchi is noted (Luomanen, 1962; Johnston and Hastings, 1966; Cleland, 1968; Grob, 1968; Thomas and Chrispin, 1969). A simple method of diagnosing and locating the fistula has been suggested by Cohen (1965) and Johnston and Hastings (1966), but its ultimate value has not yet been determined: a firm catheter with its free end immersed in water is slowly passed into the esophagus; when the fistula is approached, air escapes from the tube and bubbles are seen in the water, especially when the patient is crying and straining. Esophageal atresia is quickly ruled out by the passage of the catheter down the esophagus into the stomach.

No type of roentgenographic examination or endoscopic maneuver is infallible in making the diagnosis. Endoscopic procedures have met with more failures than successes, even when the diagnosis had already been established by other methods (Stephens, 1970). Esophagoscopy offers little aid by itself to establish the diagnosis but its use has been recommended in conjunction with other procedures. The instillation of methylene blue through an endotracheal tube frequently makes it possible to observe the dye as it appears in the esophagus, if the instillation of dye is done sufficiently high in the trachea and if positive pressure is applied (Herweg and Ogura, 1955; Kafrouni et al., 1970). Cohen (1965) and Johnston and Hastings (1966) increased the usefulness of endoscopy by auscultation through the esophagoscope, while pressing air into the trachea with positive pressure breathing.

Tracheoscopy offers a more immediate chance of identifying a fistula, the lining mucosa being less likely to obscure the opening of the fistula. A forward viewing telescopic lens system seems to be ideal for examination of the posterior wall of the trachea and sometimes an ureteral catheter can be passed across the fistula (Killen and Greenlee, 1965; Winslow et al., 1966; Putney, 1967). Routine esophagograms usually fail to visualize the lesion itself but the absence of an esophageal stripping wave, together with air in the esophagus on lateral radiographs and gaseous distention of the gut are highly suggestive (Johnston and Hastings, 1966; Tenta and Ford, 1967; Zack and Owens, 1967; Thomas and Chrispin, 1969). There is little doubt that cineradiography, taken in the prone or prone oblique position by a high speed camera, is by far the most useful diagnostic tool; it can be done safely and with confidence in its reliability. But since the filling and emptying of the fistula are almost instantaneous, the site of the fistula can only be seen on a few frames and a frame-by-frame analysis is needed (Thomas and Chrispin, 1969). This technique was used very effectively by Kappelman et al. (1969) who filled the esophagus with contrast material in a retrograde fashion.

The precise localization of the fistula is important to determine the choice of the operative approach. A right thoracic incision used to be the classical approach but most of the recently reported cases have been approached by a cervical incision, which is always used when the level of the fistula is above T_2. The cervical approach has even been successfully employed in fistula division as low as the carina and HAYS (1966a, b) defends this procedure irrespective of the level of the fistula. The fistula should be severed and the esophagus and trachea closed with interrupted sutures. SCHNEIDER and BECKER (1962), HAYS (1966a, b), COZZI (1967), CLELAND (1968), and THOMAS and CHRISPIN (1969) had no deaths in their series when the fistulas could be closed at the time of operation, despite a high complication rate. Because of the difficulties in establishing a clear diagnosis, however, the presence of a fistula is proven only at autopsy in about 20% of the cases.

References

BABBITT, D. P.: Double tracheoesophageal fistula without atresia. New Engl. J. Med. **257**, 713–717 (1957).

CLELAND, W. P.: Fistules trachéo-œsophagiennes (sans atrésie de l'œsophage). Bronches 18, 175–179 (1968).

CLOUD, D. T.: Anastomotic technic in esophageal atresia. J. pediat. Surg. **3**, 561–564 (1968).

COHEN, S. J.: Unusual types of esophageal atresia and tracheoesophageal fistulae. Diagnostic aids and procedures. Clin. Pediat. **4**, 271–275 (1965).

COZZI, F.: Oesophageal atresia. Lancet **1967 II**, 1222–1225.

COZZI, F., WILKINSON, A. W.: Intrauterine growth rate in relation to anorectal and oesophageal anomalies. Arch. Dis. Childh. **44**, 59–62 (1969).

ECKSTEIN, H. B., SOMASUNDARAM, K.: Multiple tracheoesophageal fistulas without atresia. Report of a case. J. pediat. Surg. **1**, 381–383 (1966).

GANS, S. L., LACKEY, D. A., ZUCKERBRAUN, L.: Duplications of the cervical esophagus in infants and children. Surgery **63**, 849–852 (1968).

GELISSEN, H. J., PERSIJN, N.: Fistules œsophago-tracheobronchiques. Bronches 18, 180–195 (1968).

GIEDON, A.: Angeborene hohe Ösophagotrachealfistel von H-Typus. Helv. paediat. Acta **15**, 155–162 (1960).

GOLDENBERG, I. S.: An unusual variation of congenital tracheoesophageal fistula. J. thorac. cardiovasc. Surg. **40**, 114–116 (1960).

GREENOUGH, W. G.: Congenital esophageal strictures. Amer. J. Roentgenol. **92**, 994–999 (1964).

GROB, M.: Les fistules œsophago-trachéo-bronchiques d'origine congénitale. Bronches 18, 161–174 (1968).

HAAS, L.: Congenital tracheo-esophageal fistula. Proc. roy. Soc. Med. **54**, 329–330 (1961).

HAYS, D. M., WOOLLEY, M. M., SNYDER, W. H.: Changing techniques in the management of esophageal atresia. Arch. Surg. **92**, 611–616 (1966a).

HAYS, D. M., WOOLLEY, M. M., SNYDER, W. H.: Esophageal atresia and tracheoesophageal fistula: management of the uncommon types. J. pediat. Surg. **1**, 240–252 (1966b).

HECKER, W. C.: Ösophagusstenosen im Kindesalter und ihre Therapie. Münch. med. Wschr. **36**, 2026–2033 (1968).

HECKER, W. C., DAUM, R., RÜTER, E.: Bedeutsame prognostische Faktoren in der Behandlung der Oesophagusmißbildungen. Mschr. Kinderheilk. **114**, 225–227 (1966).

HERWEG, J. C., OGURA, J. H.: Congenital tracheo-esophageal fistula without esophageal atresia. An endoscopic diagnostic technique. J. Pediat. **47**, 293–299 (1955).

HOPKINS, W. A., ZWIREN, G. T.: Colon replacement of the esophagus in children. J. thorac. cardiovasc. Surg. **46**, 346–358 (1963).

ISHIDA, M., TSUCHIDA, Y., SAITO, S., TSUNODA, A.: Congenital esophageal stenosis due to tracheobronchial remnants. J. pediat. Surg. **4**, 339–345 (1969).

JOHNSTON, P. W., HASTINGS, N.: Congenital tracheoesophageal fistula without esophageal atresia. Amer. J. Surg. **112**, 233–240 (1966).

KAFROUNI, G., BAICK, C. H., WOOLLEY, M. M.: Recurrent tracheoesophageal fistula: a diagnostic problem. Surgery **68**, 889–894 (1970).

KAPPELMAN, M. M., DORST, J., HALLER, A., STAMBLER, A.: H type tracheo-esophageal fistula. Diagnostic and operative management. Amer. J. Dis. Child. **118**, 568–575 (1969).

KILLEN, D. A., GREENLEE, H. B.: Transcervical repair of H-type congenital tracheo-esophageal fistula. Ann. Surg. **162** 145–150 (1965).

Lansden, F. T., Falor, W. H.: Congenital esophagorespiratory fistula in the adult. J. thorac. cardiovasc. Surg. **39**, 246–251 (1960).

Luomanen, R. J. K.: Tracheoesophageal fistula without atresia of the esophagus. N.Y. St. J. Med. **62**, 3987–3990 (1962).

Lynn, H. B., Davis, L. A.: Tracheo-esophageal fistula without atresia of the esophagus. Surg. Clin. N. Amer. **41**, 871–882 (1961).

Polk, H. C., Burford, T. H.: Disorders of the distal esophagus in infancy and childhood. Amer. J. Dis. Child. **108**, 243–251 (1964).

Putney, F. J.: Bronchoesophagology. Arch. Otolaryng. **86**, 117–121 (1967).

Römer, K. H.: Nouveaux aspects de la chirurgie des atrésies de l'œsophage. Bronches **18**, 286–289 (1968).

Schneider, K. M., Becker, J. M.: The "H type" tracheoesophageal fistula in infants and children. Surgery **51**, 677–686 (1962).

Stephens, H. B.: H-type tracheoesophageal fistula complicated by esophageal stenosis. J. thorac. cardiovasc. Surg. **59**, 325–329 (1970).

Tenta, L. T., Ford, L. H.: Congenital H type TE fistula in a young adult. Arch. Otolaryng. **85**, 675–679 (1967).

Thomas, P. S., Chrispin, A. R.: Congenital tracheo-oesophageal fistula without oesophageal atresia. Clin. Radiol. **20**, 371–374 (1969).

Vidne, B., Levy, M. J.: Use of pericardium for esophagoplasty in congenital esophageal stenosis. Surgery **68**, 389–392 (1970).

Waterston, D. J., Bonham-Carter, R. E., Aberdeen, E.: Oesophageal atresia: tracheo-oesophageal fistula. A study of survival in 218 infants. Lancet **1962I**, 819–822.

Winslow, P. R., Bryant, L. R., Hasbrouck, J. D.: Cystoscope endoscopy in the H-type tracheoesophageal fistula. Arch. Surg. **93**, 520–522 (1966).

Zack, B. J., Owens, M. P.: Congenital tracheoesophageal fistula in the adult. Arch. Surg. **95**, 674–677 (1967).

Bronchoesophageal Fistula

G. Fransen and A. Lacquet

Accumulation of case reports of bronchoesophageal fistula in recent years suggests that this lesion occurs more frequently than was once thought. The embryological explanation lies in an incomplete separation of the tracheobronchial tree from the esophagus, the low site of the fistula being due to an early caudad elongation of the trachea and esophagus.

Braimbridge and Keith (1965) described four different types of congenital bronchoesophageal fistula. Type I is formed by a wide-necked esophageal diverticulum which penetrates into the lung. Although there is a congenital background these fistulas themselves are acquired. In type II a short, straight track runs directly from the esophagus to a lobar or segmental bronchus (Frater and Dowdle, 1964; Braimbridge and Keith, 1965; John et al., 1965; Le Brigand et al., 1967; Hivet and Dorf, 1970; Nelson and Benfield, 1970; Smith, 1970). Type III is characterized by a lung cyst which communicates directly with the bronchus and via a fistulous tract with the esophagus (Braimbridge and Keith, 1965; Galey et al., 1968). In type IV the fistula communicates with a sequestrated segment or lobe of the lung which receives an independent blood supply directly from the aorta (Das et al., 1959; Boyden et al., 1962; Louw and Cywes, 1962; Ashley and Evans, 1966; Arcomano and Azzoni, 1967; Gerle et al., 1968; Lewis and Murray, 1968; Moscarella and Wylie, 1968).

In studying the problem of pulmonary sequestration with gastrointestinal communication Halasz et al. (1962) and Gerle et al. (1968) postulated that all forms of pulmonary sequestration or foregut duplications (either intralobular or extralobular, with or without associated diaphragmatic hernia, with or without abnormal blood supply have a common embryogenesis and are only developmental stages of the same disorder. Previously the observations of Beskin (1961), who found enteric tissue within an intralobular sequestration which communicated with a duplication of the esophagus, also suggest that pulmonary sequestration is an anomaly of foregut development. Gerle et al. (1968) proposed a classification of all possible variants of pulmonary sequestrations based on the presence or absence of a connection with the gastrointestinal tract, whether this connection was patent or not.

The congenital nature of these fistulas is difficult to prove, because they usually reveal themselves only in adolescent or early adult life. However, the absence of past or present surrounding inflammations, the lack of adherent lymphnodes and the presence of a definite mucosa and muscularis are generally accepted as sufficient evidence of their congenital origin. The bronchoesophageal fistulas are usually lined by stratified squamous epithelium (Halasz et al., 1962; Frater and Dowle, 1964; Braimbridge and Keith, 1965; John et al., 1965; Ashley and Evans, 1966; Le Roux and Williams, 1968; Hivet and Dorf, 1970; Nelson and Benfield, 1970; Smith, 1970) but columnar or transitional epithelial linings have also been noticed (Das et al., 1959; Braimbridge and Keith, 1965; Gerle et al., 1968; Lewis and Murray, 1968). Symptoms sometimes begin in childhood but seldom at birth as might be expected from their congenital origin. They usually begin only in adult life and are often intermittent. This late onset of symptoms is variously attributed to the presence of a membrane which subsequently ruptures, to a fold of esophageal mucosa which initially overlaps the orifice but later becomes a less effective operculum, and to the fact that the fistula runs in a rostral direction from the esophagus to the bronchus and may close during swallowing. Esophagobronchial fistulas are usually insidious in their onset. The symptoms are those of bronchopulmonary suppuration and may be associated with systemic evidence of such an infection, especially finger clubbing (Das et al., 1959; Frater and Dowdle, 1964; Le Roux and Williams, 1968; Nelson and Benfield, 1970). The main complaint is chronic productive cough; hemoptysis is usually moderate and intermittent, but massive hemoptysis has also been reported (Halasz et al., 1962; Ashley and Evans, 1966; Gerle et al., 1968; Kinley and Lang, 1969). Choking and coughing on swallowing liquids or with a change in posture, and the appearance of food in the sputum are recorded in about half the reported cases, but these symptoms, when present, often can be so mild that they are only elicited in retrospect after the diagnosis has been made by other means. The stomach may fill with air on expiration and this may cause gastroesophageal reflux (Braimbridge and Keith, 1965; Hivet and Dorf, 1970). The duration of symptoms varies from six months to 50 years with a mean of 17 years (Braimbridge and Keith, 1965), the usual history being one of recurrent episodes of pneumonia of obscure origin.

The most reliable investigation for demonstrating an esophagobronchial fistula is the esophagogram with thin contrast material while the patient assumes the position in which he finds his symptoms most marked; false negative results, however, are not uncommon.

A bronchogram serves to demonstrate the extent and degree of bronchial damage (bronchiectasis is frequent) but outlines the fistulous tract only exceptionally.

Endoscopy, although often not helpful, may demonstrate the opening of the fistula into the bronchus or more rarely into the esophagus, but usually the orifices are recognized only when the exact sites are already known. The endobronchial instillation of methylene blue has also been successful in establishing the diagnosis (Le Brigand et al., 1967; Galey et al., 1968). In about a third of the patients the congenital communication is found only during surgery, in spite of extensive preoperative investigation.

The treatment advocated today is surgical excision of the fistulous tract with closure of both its ends. If the associated segment or lobe of lung is too severely damaged by infection, it also must be removed. The results of surgical treatment are eminently sactisfactory. Obliteration of the fistula with silvernitrate cauterization is an unreliable technique, which should be reserved for those patients who cannot withstand an operation (Le Brigand et al., 1967).

References

Arcomano, J. P., Azzoni, A. A.: Intralobar pulmonary sequestration and intralobar enteric sequestration associated with vertebral anomalies. J. thorac. cardiovasc. Surg. 53, 470–476 (1967).

Ashley, D. J. B., Evans, C. J.: Oesophago-pulmonary fistula. Brit. J. Surg. 53, 739–740 (1966).

Beskin, C. A.: Intralobar enteric sequestration of the lung containing aberrant pancreas. J. thorac. cardiovasc. Surg. 41, 314–317 (1961).

BOYDEN, E. A., BILL, A. H., CREIGHTON, S. A.: Presumptive origin of a left lower accessory lung from an esophageal diverticulum. Surgery 52, 323–329 (1962).

BRAIMBRIDGE, M. V., KEITH, H. I.: Oesophago-bronchial fistula in the adult. Thorax 20, 226–233 (1965).

DAS, J. B., DODGE, O. G., FAWCETT, A. W.: Intralobar sequestration of lung, associated with foregut diverticulum (oesophagobronchial fistula) and an aberrant artery. Brit. J. Surg. 46, 582–586 (1959).

FRATER, R. W. M., DOWDLE, E. B.: Congenital esophagobronchial fistula. Arch. Surg. 89, 949–954 (1964).

GALEY, J. J., VANETTI, A., NEVEUX, J. Y.: Les fistules œsophago-aériennes de l'adulte. Bronches 18, 196–217 (1968).

GERLE, R. D., JARETZKI, A., ASHLEY, C. A., BERNE, A. S.: Congenital bronchopulmonary-foregut malformation. Pulmonary sequestration communicating with the gastrointestinal tract. New Engl. J. Med. 278, 1413–1419 (1968).

HALASZ, N. A., LINDSKOG, G. E., LIEBOW, A. A.: Esophagobronchial fistula and broncho-pulmonary sequestration. Ann. Surg. 155, 215–220 (1962).

HIVET, M., DORF, G.: Fistule œso-bronchique sans doute congénitale chez un adulte. Sem. Hôp. 41, 2563–2566 (1970).

JOHN, S., GOPINATH, N., McPHAIL, J. L.: Congenital oesophagobronchial fistula. Brit. J. Surg. 52, 941–943 (1965).

KINLEY, C. E., LANG, H. B.: Congenital bronchoesophageal fistula in an adult: a case presenting with massive hemoptysis. Canad. med. Ass. J. 100, 390–392 (1969).

LE BRIGAND, H., WAPLER, C., LUIZY, J., ROCHAINZAMIR, A., TESTARD, J.: Neuf cas de fistules œsophago-bronchiques bénignes et non traumatiques de l'adulte. Mém. Acad. Chir. 93, 233–246 (1967).

LE ROUX, B. T., WILLIAMS, M. A.: Congenital oesophagobronchial fistula with presentation in adult life. Brit. J. Surg. 55, 306–308 (1968).

LEWIS, J. E., MURRAY, R. E.: Pulmonary sequestration with bronchoesophageal fistula. J. pediat. Surg. 3, 575–579 (1968).

LOUW, J. H., CYWES, S.: Extralobar pulmonary sequestration communicating with the oesophagus and associated with a strangulated congenital diaphragmatic hernia. Brit. J. Surg. 50, 102–105 (1962).

MOSCARELLA, A. A., WYLIE, R. H.: Congenital communication between the esophagus and isolated ectopic pulmonary tissue. J. thorac. cardiovasc. Surg. 55, 672–676 (1968).

NELSON, R. J., BENFIELD, J. R.: Benign esophagobronchial fistula. Arch. Surg. 100, 685–688 (1970).

SMITH, D. C.: A congenital broncho-oesophageal fistula presenting in adult life without pulmonary infection. Brit. J. Surg. 57, 398–400 (1970).

Cleft Larynx
Laryngotracheoesophageal Cleft
Persistent Esophagotrachea

A. LACQUET and G. FRANSEN

RICHTER is credited with the first diagnosis of cleft larynx in 1792 when he inserted his finger in the throat of an infant and found the gullet and larynx to be a common cavity. Since then, reports of about 40 proven cases of laryngotracheo-esophageal cleft have been published, the majority dating from the last years. The apparent rarity of this anomaly may be due in part to a general una-wareness of its existence and to the difficulties in making the correct diagnosis. HAIGHT and WILLIAMS (1962) found the lesion in four patients out of approximately 2000 autopsies. Because of the small number of reported cases it is virtually impossible to establish positive conclusions with respect to incidence, clinical pattern or associated anomalies. As with other congenital anomalies of the esophagus, there seems to be a relation with both immaturity and hydramnios (ZACHARY and EMERY, 1961; HAIGHT and WILLIAMS, 1962; BLUMBERG et al., 1965; FRATES, 1967; FISHER, 1969). The sex distribution is approximately equal and a familial tendency has been described (CROOKS, 1954; ZACHARY and EMERY, 1961).

The associated anomalies include esophageal atresia with fistula (WELCH and HUSAIN, 1958; HAIGHT and WILLIAMS, 1962; DAUM et al., 1965; DELAHUNTY and CHERRY, 1969), Meckel's diverticulum (BLUMBERG et al., 1965; FISHER, 1969; DELAHUNTY and CHERRY, 1969), absence of a kidney (WELCH and HUSAIN, 1958; DELAHUNTY and CHERRY, 1969), extrophy of the bladder (GRISCOM, 1966), hiatus hernia (JAHRSDOERFER et al., 1967), severe cleft palate and persistence of a left vena cava (HAIGHT and WILLIAMS, 1962), incomplete iris (FISHER, 1969), ventricle septal defect (DAUM et al., 1965), bifid spleen, imperforate anus, annular pancreas, patent ductus arteriosus, coarctation of the aorta, urethrorectal fistula (DELA-HUNTY and CHERRY, 1969).

The respiratory tract is first recognizable as a pouch arising from the anterior aspect of the primitive foregut. As the gut elongates the pouch also progresses caudad but it becomes separated from the developing esophagus by the union, from below upward, of infoldings of mesodermal origin from each side of the common tube; this separation of esophagus and trachea up to the level of the larynx is completed in the embryo of 9 to 10 mm ($\pm$ 33 days). The cricoid cartilage, coming from the fifth or sixth branchial arch, develops as two lateral centers of cartilage that fuse first ventrally and then dorsally at about the forty-fifth gestational day. The development and functioning of the vocal cords and the ability of the epiglottis to cover the glottis depend on the dorsal fusion of the cricoid cartilages. The pathogenesis of a laryngotracheoesophageal cleft seems to be due to an arrest in the rostral development of the tracheoesophageal septum which in turn prevents the dorsal fusion of the cricoid cartilages. The defect apparently begins to appear arround the thirty-fifth gestational day (this is approximately 10 days before the normal fusion of the cricoid cartilage). The severity of the cleft will vary with the stage of development reached by the embryo at the time the growth of the tracheoesophageal septum was arrested. It may involve only the cricoarytenoid area (FINLAY, 1949; CROOKS, 1954; DAUM et al., 1965; HARRISON et al., 1965; SHAPIRO et al., 1966; JAHRSDOERFER et al., 1967; IMBRIE and DOYLE, 1969; DELAHUNTY and CHERRY, 1969; FISHER, 1969); it may extend downward beyond the cricoid cartilage into the trachea (PETTERSON, 1955; ZACHARY and EMERY, 1961; BLUMBERG et al., 1965; GEIGER et al., 1970); or it may be so extensive that the septum is completely absent, resulting in a persistent esophagotrachea (WELCH and HUSAIN, 1958; TRIBOLETTI, 1958; ZACHARY and EMERY, 1961; GRISCOM, 1966; FISHER, 1969).

The clinical picture chiefly includes respiratory distress, sometimes with pronounced mucous secretions and marked episodes of cyanosis, and feeding difficulties (with incoordination of swallowing and aspiration of food). There is also a high incidence of laryngeal stridor and vocal changes in the form of a weakness of voice or frank aphonia, due to an air leak through the cleft and the inability to approximate the vocal cords. The symptoms develop immediately after birth and, if no stridor occurs, may be indistinguishable from esophageal atresia with tracheoesophageal fistula. Untreated the infants will almost always succumb to aspiration pneumonia or sudden respiratory death. The more extensive the communication between airway and gullet, the freer the aspiration and the sooner the death of the infant may be expected. Except for the case described by JAHRSDOERFER (1967), which is exceptional in that the infant lived 46 months in the hospital before a proper diagnosis was made and surgery undertaken, all other cases without successful surgical correction have been fatal in early infancy.

Diagnosis is extremely difficult. This can be attributed in some cases to intermittent opening and closure of the posterior margins of the larynx and trachea during respiration and in other cases to a lack of knowledge of the condition. Routine chest films show only the secondary changes of aspiration pneumonia, although the shadows of the air contained in trachea and esophagus may arouse suspicion. Esophagograms show spillage of contrast material into the trachea but by themselves do not allow a correct diagnosis. In cases of persistent esophagotrachea cineradiography during swallowing can lead to a correct preoperative diagnosis if a persistent fusion of the tracheal and esophageal lumen is found (FRATES, 1967). Endoscopic procedures (laryngoscopy, tracheoscopy, esophagoscopy) might be expected to reveal a greater percentage of cases but frequently the larynx will appear surprisingly normal. Neither roentgenographic evaluation, nor endoscopy, nor surgical exploration have been uniformly successful in reaching a correct diagnosis. All patients in whom the diagnosis was made preoperatively had undergone intensive investigation, including X-ray examinations, endoscopic explorations and even surgical procedures. Often a right diagnosis could only be made at the time of surgical exploration (BLUMBERG et al., 1965; GRISCOM, 1966; DELAHUNTY and CHERRY, 1969; FISHER, 1969; GEIGER et al., 1970) or at postmortem examination (WELCH and HUSAIN, 1958; TRIBOLETTI, 1958; HAIGHT and WILLIAMS, 1962; DAUM et al., 1965; HARRISON et al., 1965; FISHER, 1969).

The surgical approach depends on the size of the cleft. If it extends downward for a few tracheal rings only, repair of the defect can be attempted by an anterior (JAHRSDOERFER et al., 1967; DELAHUNTY and CHERRY, 1969) or a lateral pharyngeal (SHAPIRO et al., 1966) approach. Large defects extending down to the carina require a combined thoracic-cervical approach. Although a prolonged delay in total correction of the lesion does not seem advisable, a short waiting period to clear an eventual pneumonic process and to improve the nutritional state will increase the chances of survival. In such cases tracheostomy, feeding gastrostomy and full-time nursing are required as temporary measures. At the operation meticulous anatomical repair of the entire cleft with fine atraumatic sutures should be performed in two layers and extend proximally to the interarytenoid area. Interposition of a viable muscle pedicle to separate the suture lines can aid in preventing recurrence. Firm anchorage of the dorsal arch of the cricoid will assure restoration of a normal alimentary function and vocal cord alignment.

Almost 50% of all cases of laryngotracheoesophageal cleft found in the literature have had definitive surgery. Only PETTERSON (1955), SHAPIRO et al. (1966), DELAHUNTY and CHERRY (1969) and GEIGER et al. (1970) have described successful surgical procedures. A partially successful cleft larynx repair was done by JAHRSDOERFER et al. (1967). Attempts at surgical repair of persistent esophagotrachea, the most severe degree of laryngotracheoesophageal cleft, has until now been invariably lethal (ZACHARY and EMERY, 1961; GRISCOM, 1966; FISHER, 1969).

References

BLUMBERG, J. B., STEVENSON, J. K., LEMIRE, R. J., BOYDEN, E. A.: Laryngotracheoesophageal cleft, the embryologic implications: Review of the literature. Surgery 57, 559–566 (1965).

CROOKS, J.: Non-inflammatory laryngeal stridor in infants. Arch. Dis. Childh. 29, 12–17 (1954).

DAUM, R., HECKER, W. C., ROSSNER, J. A., WENZ, W.: Kongenitale oesophago-laryngotracheale Kommunikationen, ein Beitrag zur Differentialdiagnose der oberen Oesophagotrachealfisteln. Z. Kinderchir. 2, 314–325 (1965).

DELAHUNTY, J. E., CHERRY, J.: Congenital laryngeal cleft. Ann. Otol. 78, 96–106 (1969).

FINLAY, H. V. L.: Familial congenital stridor. Arch. Dis. Childh. 24, 219–223 (1949).

FISHER, J. H.: Extensive tracheoesophageal communication. Bronches 19, 105–109 (1969).

FRATES, R. E.: Roentgen signs in laryngotracheoesophageal cleft. Radiology 88, 484–486 (1967).

GEIGER, J. P., O'CONNELL, T. J., CARTER, S. C., GOMEZ, A. C., ARONSTAM, E. M.: Laryngotracheal-esophageal cleft. J. thorac. cardiovasc. Surg. 59, 330–334 (1970).

GRISCOM, N. T.: Persistent esophagotrachea. Amer. J. Roentgenol. 97, 211–215 (1966).

HAIGHT, C. A., WILLIAMS, T. C.: Cleft larynx: a cause of laryngeal obstruction and incompetence. J. Laryng. 76, 381–387 (1962).

HARRISON, H. S., FUQUA, W. B., GIFFIN, R. B.: Congenital laryngeal cleft: report of a case. Amer. J. Dis. Child. 110, 556–558 (1965).

IMBRIE, J. D., DOYLE, P. J.: Laryngotracheoesophageal cleft. Laryngoscope (St. Louis) 79, 1252–1274 (1969).

JAHRSDOERFER, R. A., KIRCHNER, J. A., THALER, S. U.: Cleft larynx. Arch. Otolaryng. 86, 82–87 (1967).

PETTERSON, G.: Inhibited separation of larynx and the upper part of trachea from oesophagus in a newborn. Acta chir. scand. 110, 250–254 (1955).

SHAPIRO, M. J., FALLA, A., IRVINGTON, N. J.: Congenital posterior cleft larynx. Ann. Otol. (St. Louis) 75, 961–967 (1966).

TRIBOLETTI, E.: Unusual congenital anomaly involving the larynx, trachea and esophagus. New Engl. J. Med. 258, 1002–1003 (1958).

WELCH, R. G., HUSAIN, O. A. N.: Atresia of the esophagus with common tracheo-oesophageal tube. Arch. Dis. Childh. 33, 367–370 (1958).

ZACHARY, R. B., EMERY, J. L.: Failure of separation of larynx and trachea from the esophagus: persistent esophagotrachea. Surgery 49, 525–529 (1961).

Vascular Rings

G. FRANSEN and W. PELEMANS

With 7 Figures

Vascular Anomalies Causing Tracheoesophageal Symptoms

1. Introduction

In this chapter only those vascular anomalies are discussed that cause symptoms of tracheal and/or esophageal compression. These vascular anomalies have all one common characteristic, i.e. they form a complete vascular ring around the trachea and/or the esophagus. For a more complete review the reader is referred to the excellent monograph "Esophagography in anomalies of the aortic arch system" (KLINKHAMER, 1969). The main feature of a congenital vascular ring is that the esophagus and trachea no longer occupy their normal retrovascular position but are encircled to a greater or lesser degree by anomalous vascular structures. The embryologic development of the aorta and its branches permits a great variety of possible anomalies (EDWARDS, 1948; BLAKE and MANION, 1962). These aberrant arteries in the upper mediastinum assume importance when they compress the trachea or the esophagus or both. The clinical signs of this compression are not characteristic of any particular type of anomaly; these malformations can all produce similar symptoms. In general they manifest themselves in two age groups: in the first years of life if the ring around the trachea and esophagus is so narrow that compression becomes apparent very soon, and in the elderly if the ring, which was initially too wide to cause compression, begins to narrow and becomes rigid as a result of arteriosclerotic changes and reduced elasticity of the vascular wall.

2. Clinical Picture

In general, the clinical picture of tracheoesophageal compression depends on the age of the patient: in infants and children the compression will give rise mainly to respiratory symptoms and in adults dysphagia and feeding problems are more apt to be the principal complaints (MATHEY et al., 1959; SCHMIDT-HABELMANN et al., 1968; KLINKHAMER, 1969). However, the vast majority of vascular rings which are serious enough to cause symptoms will come to the attention of the clinicians in the early years of life. In a critical review of the literature, LASHER (1958) noted that a minority of patients with a complete vascular ring live to adult life.

2.1. Respiratory Symptoms

The child usually exhibits a crowing type of respiration with a marked inspiratory and expiratory stridor. There may be a wheeze loud enough to be heard many feet away. A persistent, brassy cough is present in most cases and repeated attacks of "croup" are noted. The respiratory rate is increased and a marked air hunger is present in many cases. Cyanosis and attacks of "croup" can occur, particularly during exertion or feeding.

Deep respiratory retractions can be observed as accessory muscles of respiration are required to obtain an adequate exchange of air. A finding characteristic of compression of the trachea is the position of the head in extreme hyperextension, because in this position the trachea pushes away from its anterior surface any structure which is impinging upon it; hyperextension of the head can considerable diminish the respiratory distress.

Recurring episodes of respiratory infection are a common feature. The most severe forms are incompatible with life and the patients die in infancy of asphyxia or pneumonia. As already mentioned, in many of the young patients there are no problems with the digestive tract, but the respiratory symptoms can be exaggerated during feedings and attempts at swallowing. In many adults there are symptoms or signs of respiratory distress but some of these patients suffered from dyspnea, stridor and respiratory infection already in their first years of life.

2.2. Feeding Problems

Dysphagia is usually provoked by hurried swallowing or ingestion of bulky or very cold foods. A sensation of substernal fullness and an awareness of difficulty in getting ingesta past a point high up in the thorax may be noted. There is no pain other than the substernal discomfort. This dysphagia is a constant daily problem and makes the patient anxious and can even lead to emaciation and depression.

A vascular ring can usually be diagnosed accurately by radiological examination of the esophagus (Mathey et al., 1959; Hallman et al., 1966; Schmidt-Habelmann et al., 1968; Klinkhamer, 1969). Angiography can delineate the abnormal arterial patterns more precisely but is not essential for effective treatment. Surgical correction of vascular anomalies causing tracheoesophageal compression should be undertaken as soon as possible after the diagnosis has been established. Preliminary treatment of a respiratory tract infection may be necessary but if the general condition is good, surgical correction is urgent. The operation always has to include interruption of the vascular ring by division of a nonessential vessel, division of the ductus arteriosus (ligamentum) and dissection of all fascial bands and attachments to the trachea and esophagus (Mathey et al., 1959; Hallman et al., 1966; Schmidt-Habelmann et al., 1968). Clinical results of surgical interruption of the vascular rings are almost invariably gratifying, especially in children.

3. Different Types of Anomalies
3.1. Aberrant Right Subclavian Artery (A. lusoria)
(Fig. 291)

Clinical interest for this anomaly dates from 1946, when Gross performed the first successful operation for the relief of the symptoms resulting from an aberrant right subclavian artery. In most instances this aberrant vessel originates near the bend of the aortic arch, passes obliquely through the mediastinum behind the esophagus, from below and from the left upward and to the right, whereafter it continues its course to the upper limb in an anatomically normal way. Reports of a pre-esophageal or pretracheal course of the artery are more exceptional (Schmidt, 1957a; Klinkhamer, 1969). Embryologically an aberrant right subclavian artery represents the persisting portion of the right fourth aortic arch while the cranial

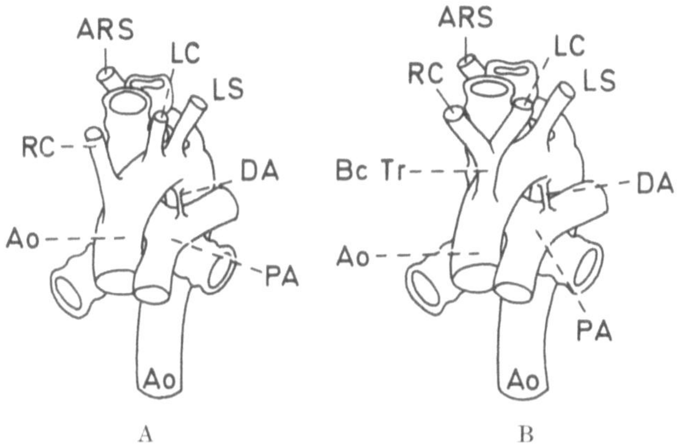

Fig. 291 A and B. Diagrammatic representation of the aberrant right subclavian artery. A Normal origin of the carotid arteries. Trachea and esophagus can shift forward by using the space between the two carotid arteries. B Common origin of the carotid arteries: bicarotid truncus. The V in front of the trachea prevents the trachea and the esophagus from bending forward. Both organs are hemmed in, dorsally by the aberrant right subclavian artery, and ventrally by the carotid fork. *Ao* aorta; *PA* pulmonary artery; *DA* ductus arteriosus; *RC* right carotid artery; *LC* left carotid artery; *LS* left subclavian artery; *ARS* aberrant right subclavian artery; *BcTr* bicarotid truncus. (From KLINKHAMER, A. C.: Esophagography in anomalies of the aortic arch system. Exc. Med. Found. Amsterdam, 1969)

portion of this arch is obliterated. The first segment of this "arteria lusoria" is often dilated at its origin (the so-called diverticulum of Kommerell).

An aberrant right subclavian artery without evidence of any other congenital abnormality of the vascular system occurs in about 0.5 to 1% of the population (SCHMIDT, 1957a; LASHER, 1958; STEWART et al., 1964; GRANT and BASMAJIAN, 1965); in cases with congenital heart diseases this incidence is higher. About 10% of the patients with aberrant right subclavian artery have symptoms of compression and, as already mentioned, respiratory symptoms are more frequent in childhood, dysphagia more commonly occurs in adults. Aberrant right subclavian artery, however, is the type of ring that is most likely to cause symptoms in later life (HALLMAN and COOLEY, 1964). The occurence of 11 adult patients in one physician's experience (PALMER, 1955) indicates that the lesion is not exceptional. An aberrant right subclavian artery gives rise to clinical manifestations only when the right and the left carotid arteries originate together from the aortic arch (bicarotid truncus) or close to each other (< 4 cm) so that the trachea and esophagus cannot escape compression because they cannot migrate forward between the two carotids (KLINKHAMER, 1966; NATHAN and GITLIN, 1968). KLINKHAMER (1966) in reviewing the literature found that in 29% of the reports an aberrant right subclavian artery was associated with truncus bicaroticus and in another 10% the two carotid vessels were situated closer to each other than normal. The diagnosis can be made by radiological examination of the esophagus (Fig. 292): the frontal esophagogram at the level of the aortic arch or just above it shows an oblique filling defect in the barium-filled esophagus, extending from below and from the left upward and to the right; the segments above and below the defect are displaced in the sense of a

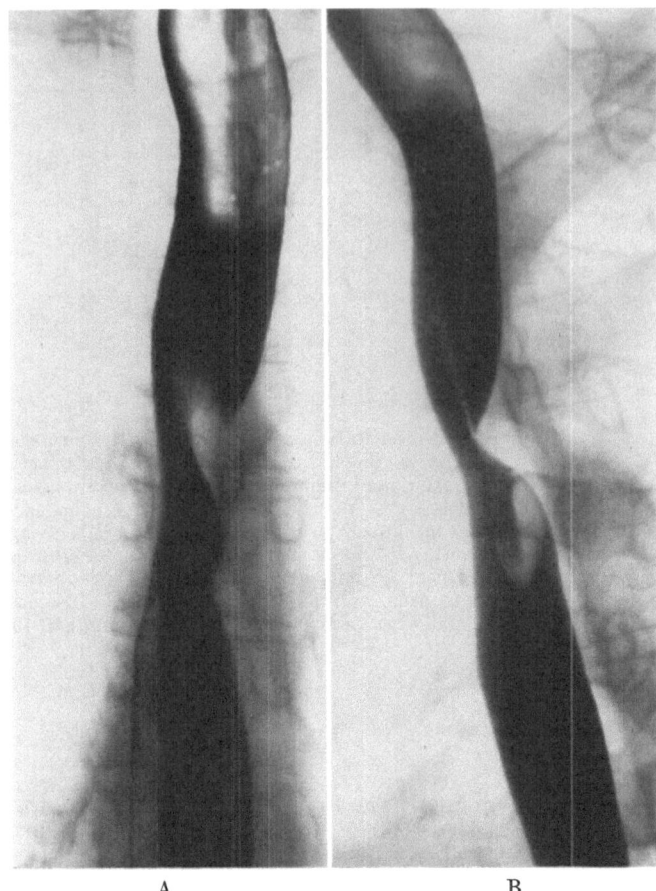

A   B

Fig. 292 A and B. Typical indentation on left and posterior border of the middle third of the esophagus due to an aberrant right subclavian artery. The anteroposterior view (A) shows the oblique ascending indentation on the left contour, the left oblique anterior view (B) shows the wedge-shaped appearance of the posterior contour

"dislocatio ad latidudinem" in a bone fracture. Sometimes, however, the aberrant artery produces only a small impression on the right margin of the esophagus. In the right anterior oblique position, the esophagus is seen to spiral upward just above the aortic arch. In the left anterior oblique projection and in the lateral view, a wedge-shaped impression on the dorsal aspect of the barium-filled esophagus can be noted.

In adults esophagoscopy serves to exclude extramucosal esophageal tumors; sometimes a pulsatile protrusion may be evident and compression of the aberrant artery by the tip of the esophagoscope may obliterate the right radial pulse (LICHTER, 1963). Bronchoscopic examination can also reveal the pulsatile nature of the constriction, while compression of the artery with the endoscope may cause obliteration of the right radial pulse (MUSTARD et al., 1962). A similar compression was previously done by FACQUET et al. (1955) by means of a mercury bougie.

The classic surgical treatment consists of ligating and dividing the anomalous artery (GROSS, 1955; MUSTARD et al., 1962; LICHTER, 1963). As a rule the operation is technically easy and therapeutically sactisfactory. However, technical difficulties are reported when a Kommerell's diverticulum is present (SHANNON, 1961). In older patients, it may be necessary to re-establish a good blood flow to the right arm. This can be accomplished by reanastomosing the aberrant subclavian artery to the ascending aorta (HALLMAN and COOLEY, 1964). The purpose of this procedure is to avoid the remote possibility of ischemic symptoms in the upper extremity due to an inadequate collateral circulation and to prevent the development of a subclavian steal syndrome in the subsequent years.

3.2. Double Aortic Arch

(Fig. 293)

A double aortic arch results from the persistence of the fourth branchial arches at both the right and left side. The double aortic arch forms, together with the ductus arteriosus (ligamentum) and the pulmonary artery, a ring around the trachea and the esophagus, which is usually too small to accomodate a trachea and an esophagus of normal size; pressure on these organs is likely to occur in almost all cases. In the majority of cases the left (or anterior) arch is the smaller of the two and the descending aorta is usually situated on the left side of the spinal column (NUBOER, 1951; GROSS, 1955; HALLMAN and COOLEY, 1964; SCHMIDT-HABELMANN et al., 1968). Although a double aortic arch is compatible with a long life and only minor symptoms, the difficulties are usually serious enough to be diagnosed during early infancy (NUBOER, 1951; STOREY and CRITTENDEN. 1951; GROSS, 1955; MATHEY et al., 1959; BRUNNER et al., 1960; MUSTARD et al., 1962; HALLMAN et al., 1966). There may be problems with swallowing but the alarming symptoms come from the tracheal narrowing. Variations in size and course of the arches can result in a variable picture of indentations on the esophagogram. On frontal esophagograms a bilateral impression in the barium-filled esophagus occurs when the two limbs of the arch are situated at the same level: if they are situated at different levels, a sinuous course of the esophagus between the two impressions can be noted. In this case the impression on the right aspect of the esophagus lies more cranially than the one on the left aspect. The typical radiological pattern of a double aortic arch can usually be recognized most easily on lateral views because of the anteroposterior compression of the esophagus.

A double aortic arch which gives no rise to symptoms requires no treatment, but only a few children with symptoms of compression survive more than two years without surgical intervention (EKSTRÖM and SANDBLOM, 1952); they usually die within the first months of life.

In cases with pronounced symptoms surgery is urgent. The only rational therapy consists of the division of the smaller of the two aortic arches. The suspension of the distal end of the transsected arch by suturing it, to the anterior endothoracic fascia if the left or anterior arch is divided, to the prevertebral fascia on the right of the vertebral column if the right or posterior arch is divided, can be helpful in lessening the likelihood of residual compression (HALLMAN and COOLEY, 1964; SCHMIDT-HABELMANN et al., 1968). The ligamentum or ductus arteriosus also should be divided in all instances to allow the pulmonary artery to slide forward and sideways. Of the 26 patients operated upon by GROSS (1955) 21 survived and had extraordinary relief of symptoms. Comparable results are reported by MUSTARD et al. (1962) and MATHEY et al. (1959). All the patients

654

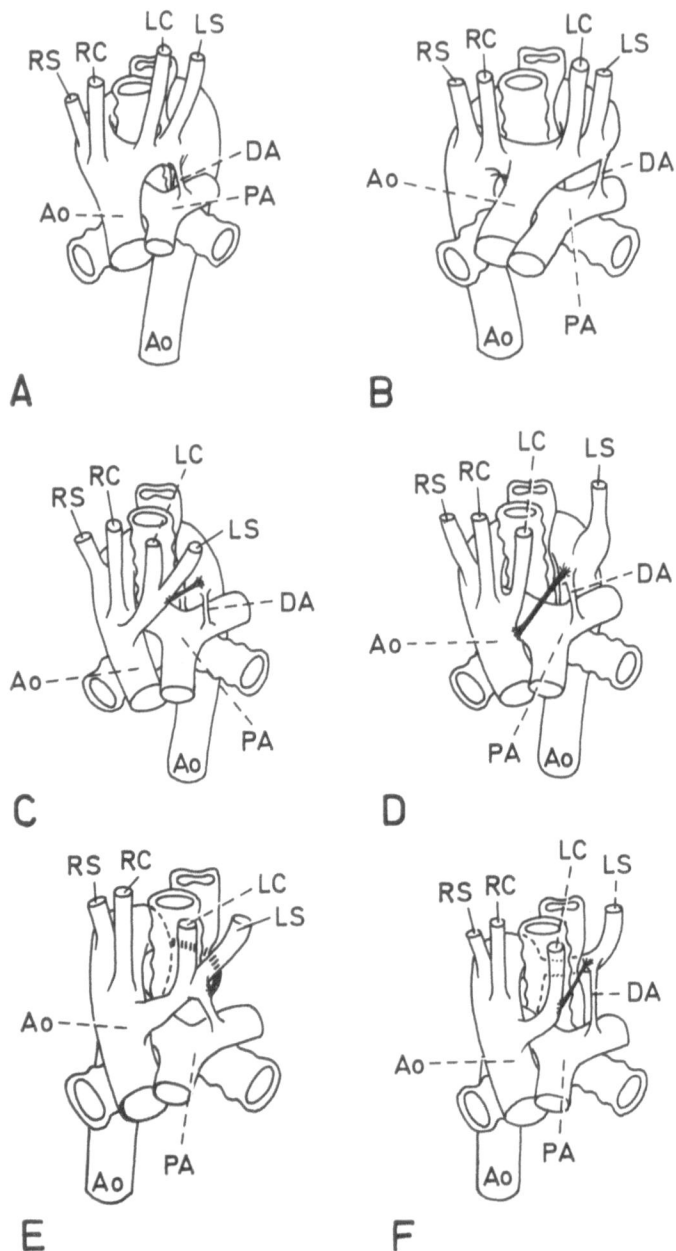

Fig. 293 A—F. Diagrammatic representation of different types of double aortic arch. A With a left-sided ductus arteriosus and a left-sided descending aorta. B With a left-sided ductus arteriosus and a right-sided descending aorta. C With a left-sided descending aorta. The left anterior arch between the origin of the left subclavian artery and the descending aorta is atretic. D With a left-sided descending aorta. The left anterior arch between the origin of the left carotid artery and that of the left subclavian artery is atretic. E With the right-sided descending aorta. The left posterior arch between the origin of the left subclavian artery and the descending aorta is atretic. F With a right-sided descending aorta. The left posterior arch between the origins of the left carotid artery and the left subclavian artery is atretic. *Ao* aorta; *RC* right carotid artery; *PA* pulmonary artery; *LC* left carotid artery; *DA* ductus arteriosus; *RS* right subclavian artery; *LS* left subclavian artery. (From KLINKHAMER, A. C.: Esophagography in anomalies of the aortic arch system. Exc. Med. Found. Amsterdam, 1969)

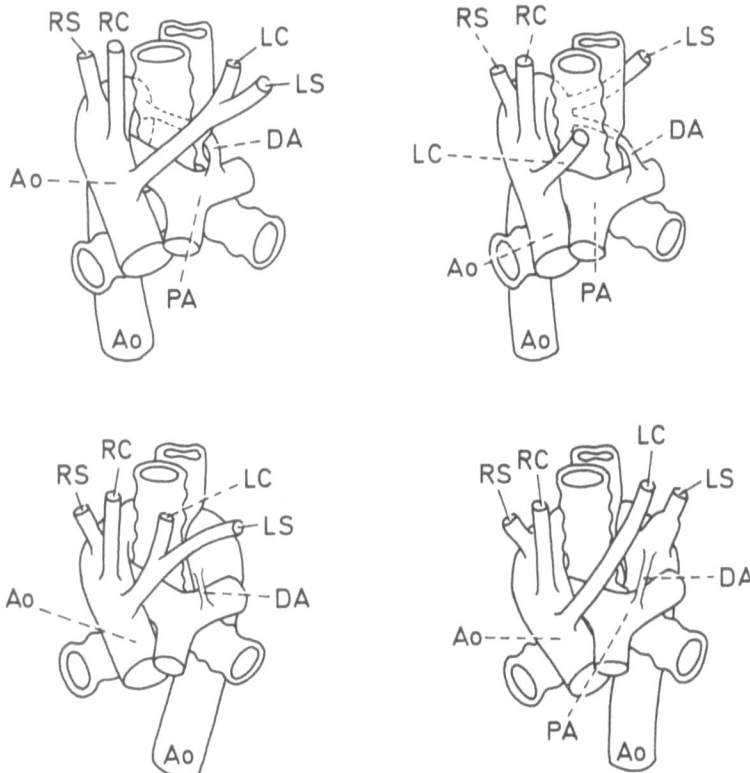

Fig. 294. Diagrammatic representation of different types of right-sided aorta with complete vascular ring. (From KLINKHAMER, A. C.: Esophagography in anomalies of the aortic arch system. Exc. Med. Found. Amsterdam, 1969)

reported on by HALLMAN and COOLEY (1964) and SCHMIDT-HABELMANN et al. (1968) survived and were free of complaints. A slight stridor may remain for some time, due to softening and distortion of the cartilage rings of the trachea since early embryonal life.

3.3. Right-sided Aortic Arch

(Fig. 294)

The incidence of a right-sided aortic arch is about 0.02 to 0.1% (SCHMIDT, 1957b; HASTREITER et al., 1966). Numerous anatomical variations of right-sided aortic arch are described (HOUBEN and LAMERS, 1964; D'CRUZ et al., 1966; KLINK-HAMER, 1969) according to the course of the descending aorta, the origin of the brachiocephalic vessels from the aortic arch and the course of the ductus arteriosus (ligamentum). Only these varieties which form a complete ring around the trachea and the esophagus are of clinical significance and in all these instances the ultimate cause of the tracheoesophageal constriction seems to be the ductus arteriosus (KEATS and MARTT, 1962; MUSTARD et al., 1962; HALLMAN and COOLEY, 1964; KLINKHAMER, 1969).

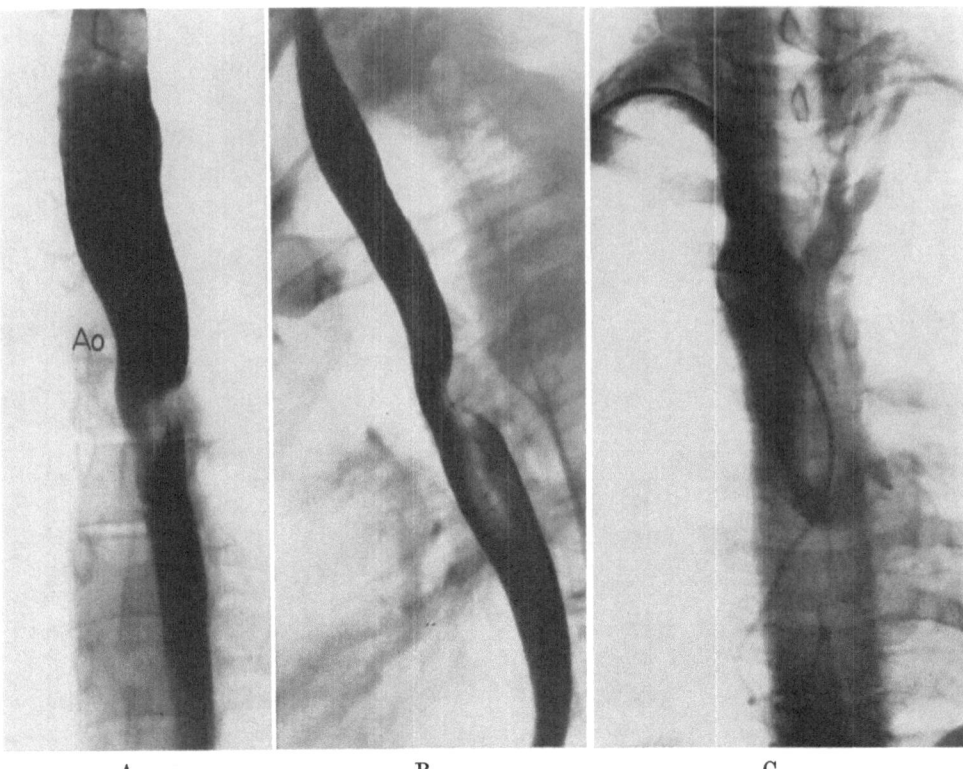

A   B   C

Fig. 295 A—C. Right-sided aortic arch, with right descending aorta and retroesophageal aortic diverticulum. A Esophagogram in frontal view shows a transversal radiolucency beneath the aortic knob (*Ao*). B The wedge-shaped appearance of the indentation is apparent in the left oblique view. C Aortogram showing the aortic arch with the left common trunk of carotid and subclavian artery and the right descending aorta

A right aortic arch, especially when associated with a right descending aorta, is very often associated with other congenital malformations as well (Blake and Manion, 1962; D'Cruz et al., 1966; Hastreiter et al., 1966; Schmidt-Habel-mann et al., 1968), especially with the tetralogy of Fallot.

Usually the symptoms begin a little later in childhood than those of a double aortic arch and they are not as severe (Gross, 1955). The anomaly has also been recognized in an adult from an episode of acute dysphagia, caused by ingestion of a big lump of food (Barbier, 1957).

The deformations of the barium-filled esophagus depend on the anatomical variations but usually a large indentation is seen at the level of the aortic arch on the right and posterior surface (Mustard et al., 1962; Hallman and Cooley, 1964) (Fig. 295).

Treatment of this condition consists of dividing the ductus arteriosus (ligamentum), thus breaking the constricting ring. Whenever a left subclavian artery is found behind the esophagus, it should be severed also (Gross, 1955; Mathey et al., 1959; Keats and Martt, 1962; Mustard et al., 1962; Hallman et al., 1966; Levine and Serfas, 1967). It is important to perform surgical therapy early

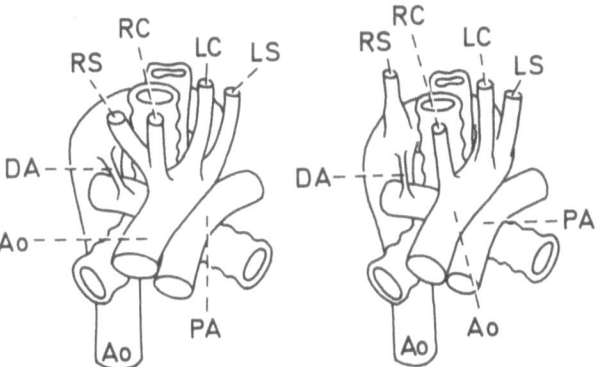

Fig. 296. Different types of left-sided aortic arch with right descending aorta and retro-esophageal course of the transverse portion of the arch. (From KLINKHAMMER, A. C.: Esopha-gography in anomalies of the aortic arch system. Exc. Med. Found. Amsterdam, 1969)

in life before the tracheal wall has become permanently deformed. The results of surgical intervention are eminently satisfactory.

3.4. Left-sided Aortic Arch with Right-sided Descending Aorta
(Fig. 296)

In this very rare anomaly the left-sided aortic arch joins a retroesophageal or a pretracheal transverse aorta which continues as a right-sided descending aorta. If part of the arch lies behind the esophagus, a ring is formed around the trachea and the esophagus and can produce symptoms of tracheoesophageal compression. The anomaly is described in children but the symptoms, if they are present at all, are far from constant in the few cases reported.

3.5. Cervical Aortic Arch

A few cases of cervical aortic arch have been described; in most of them the aortic arch is of the right-sided type (HARLEY, 1959; MASSUMI et al., 1963; MA-HONEY and MANNING, 1964; D'CRUZ et al., 1966; KLINKHAMER, 1969). This dis-order is due to the development of the aortic arch from the third instead of from the fourth branchial arch. The anatomic features of a right-sided cervical arch are similar to those of a right-sided aortic arch with left descending aorta. The left-sided cervical arch can be placed in the category of left-sided aortic arch with right descending aorta; the cervical position of the aortic arch, however, justifies a separate classification, particularly because the symptoms of this anomaly are different from those found in the intrathoracic vascular rings.

A true cervical aortic arch extends up to the lower cervical region and presents clinically as a pulsatile mass in this region; it resembles an aneurysm of the in-nominate, carotid or subclavian arteries. Half of the cases with right-sided cervical aortic arch reported in the literature had symptoms of tracheoesophageal com-pression, the ductus arteriosus being responsible for the constriction and the vascular ring being formed by (1) the right-sided segment of the aortic arch on the right, (2) the retroesophageal segment of the aortic arch dorsally, (3) the junction of the arch with the descending aorta and the ductus arteriosus on the left, and (4) the pulmonary artery ventrally.

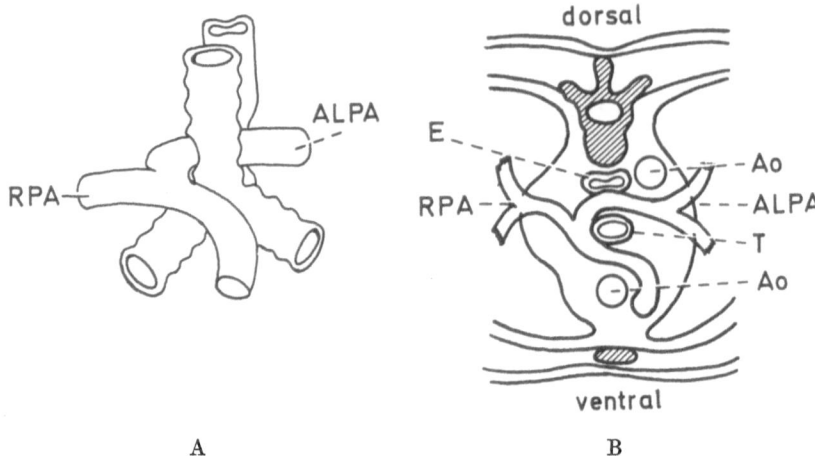

Fig. 297A and B. Aberrant left pulmonary artery. A Frontal view. B Transverse view. *T* Trachea; *E* esophagus; *RPA* right pulmonary artery; *ALPA* aberrant left pulmonary artery. (From KLINKHAMER, A. C.: Esophagography in anomalies of the aortic arch system. Exc. Med. Found. Amsterdam, 1969)

3.6. Aberrant Left Pulmonary Artery
(Fig. 297)

An aberrant left pulmonary artery arises from the right pulmonary artery, passes over the right main bronchus and behind the trachea and reaches the hilus of the left lung. Thus it may constrict the right main stem bronchus and, to a lesser degree, the trachea just above the carina. As the esophagus is not encircled by the vascular ring, dysphagia and other feeding problems are not associated with this anomaly, but the symptoms of respiratory obstruction are usually severe (in more than 90% of the cases) and already present at birth in 50% (CLARKSON et al., 1967). Autopsy studies reveal a high frequency of associated anomalies, and in almost half of the cases associated malformations in more than one body system are recorded (JUE et al., 1965).

On lateral esophagograms the aberrant left pulmonary artery is seen as an indentation in the anterior aspect of the esophagus at the level of the tracheal bifurcation. The trachea is displaced forward at this level (KLINKHAMER, 1969). Surgical therapy consists of altering the course of the aberrant vessel by dividing and reanostomosing it anterior to the trachea. MUSTARD et al. (1962) treated successfully a case of aberrant left pulmonary artery by simple division of the ligamentum arteriosum, which completed the vascular ring in this patient.

Failure to recognize a symptomatic aberrant left pulmonary artery results almost invariably in death, usually before the age of one (JUE et al., 1965).

References

BARBIER, F.: Dysphagie par arcus aortae dexter circumflexus. Acta gastro-ent. belg. **20**, 905–909 (1957).

BLAKE, H. A., MANION, W. C.: Thoracic arterial arch anomalies. Circulation **26**, 251–265 (1962).

BRUNNER, S., GAMMELGARD, A., PETERSEN, O., STORM, O.: Arterial malformation in the superior mediastinum. Acta radiol. (Stockh.) **53**, 105–112 (1960).

CLARKSON, P. M., RITTER, D. G., RAHIMTOOLA, S. H., HALLERMANN, F. J., McGOON, D. C.: Aberrant left pulmonary artery. Amer. J. Dis. Child. **113**, 373–377 (1967).

D'CRUZ, I. A., CANTEZ, T., NAMIN, E. P., LICATA, R., HASTREITER, A. R.: Right-sided aorta. Part II: Right aortic arch, right descending aorta, and associated anomalies. Brit. Heart J. **28**, 725–739 (1966).

EDWARDS, J. E.: Anomalies of the derivation of the aortic arch system. Proc. Mayo Clin. **32**, 925–949 (1948).

EKSTROM, G., SANDBLOM, P.: Double aortic arch. Acta chir. scand. **102**, 183–202 (1952).

FACQUET, J., WELTI, J. J., ALHOMME, P.: Dysphagie lusoria mortelle par anomalie de la sous-clavière droite. Nouveau procédé diagnostique. Arch. Mal. Cœur **48**, 582–596 (1955).

GRANT, J. C. B., BASMAJIAN, J. V.: Grant's method of anatomy, 7th ed. Baltimore: Williams and Wilkins 1965.

GROSS, R. E.: An atlas of children's surgery, p. 2–7. Philadelphia-London-Toronto: W. D. Saunders Company 1970.

GROSS, R. E.: Arterial malformations which cause compression of the trachea or esophagus. Circulation **11**, 124–134 (1955).

GROSS, R. E., HOLCOMB, G. W., FARBER, S.: Duplications of the alimentary tract. Pediatrics **9**, 449–468 (1952).

HALLMAN, G. L., COOLEY, D. A.: Congenital aortic vascular ring. Arch. Surg. **88**, 666–675 (1964).

HALLMAN, G. L., COOLEY, D. A., BLOODWELL, R. D.: Congenital vascular ring. Surg. Clin. N. Amer. **46**, 885–892 (1966).

HARLEY, H. R. S.: The development and anomalies of the aortic arch and its branches. With a report of a case of right cervical aortic arch and intrathoracic vascular ring. Brit. J. Surg. **46**, 561–573 (1959).

HASTREITER, A. R., D'CRUZ, I. A., CANTEZ, T.: Right-sided aorta. Part I: Occurrence of right aortic arch in various types of congenital heart disease. Brit. Heart J. **28**, 722–725 (1966).

HEIM DE BALSAC, R.: Left aortic arch (posterior or circumflex type) with right descending aorta. Amer. J. Cardiol. **5**, 546–550 (1960).

HOUBEN, M. L. M., LAMERS, J. J. H.: Twee patiënten met een rechter aortaboog en een aorta-divertikel als onderdeel van een vaatring. Mschr. Kindergeneesk. **32**, 434–439 (1964).

JUE, K. L., RAGHIB, G., AMPLATZ, K., ADAMS, P., EDWARDS, J. E.: Anomalous origin of the left pulmonary artery from the right pulmonary artery. Amer. J. Roentgenol. **95**, 598–610 (1965).

KEATS, T. E., MARTT, J. M.: Tracheoesophageal constriction produced by an unusual combination of anomalies of the great vessels. Amer. Heart J. **63**, 265–269 (1962).

KLINKHAMER, A.: Aberrant right subclavian artery. Clinical and roentgenologic aspects. Amer. J. Roentgenol. **97**, 438–446 (1966).

KLINKHAMER, A.: Esophagography in anomalies of the aortic arch system. Amsterdam: Excerpta Medica Foundation 1969.

LASHER, E. P.: Types of tracheal and esophageal constriction due to arterial anomalies of the aortic arch, with suggestions as to treatment. Amer. J. Surg. **26**, 228–233 (1958).

LEVINE, S., SERFAS, L. S.: Dysphagia lusoria secondary to complete vascular ring. Amer. J. Surg. **113**, 435–438 (1967).

LICHTER, I.: The treatment of dysphagia lusoria in the adult. Brit. J. Surg. **50**, 793–796 (1963).

LISTER, J.: The blood supply of the oesophagus in relation to oesophageal atresia. Arch. Dis. Childh. **39**, 131–137 (1964).

MAHONEY, E. B., MANNING, J. A.: Congenital abnormalities of the aortic arch. Surgery **55**, 1–14 (1964).

MASSUMI, R., WIENER, L., CHARIF, P.: The syndrome of cervical aorta. Amer. J. Cardiol. **11**, 678–685 (1963).

MATHEY, J., BINET, J. P., DENIS, B.: Anomalies de développement des arcs aortiques. J. Chir. **77**, 505–526 (1959).

MUSTARD, W. T., TRIMBLE, A. W., TRUSLER, G. A.: Mediastinal vascular anomalies causing tracheal and esophageal compression and obstruction in childhood. Canad. med. Ass. J. **87**, 1301–1305 (1962).

NATHAN, H., GITLIN, G.: Thoracic duct terminating on the right side associated with aberrant retro-oesophageal right subclavian artery and truncus bicaroticus. Thorax **23**, 266–270 (1968).

NUBOER, J. F.: Double aortic arch. J. thorac. Surg. **22**, 208–215 (1951).

PALMER, E. D.: Dysphagia lusoria: clinical aspects in the adult. Ann. intern. Med. **42**, 1173–1180 (1955).

Schlamowitz, S. T., Di Giorgi, S., Gensini, G. G.: Left aortic arch and right descending aorta. Amer. J. Cardiol. **10**, 132–137 (1962).

Schmidt, J.: Röntgendiagnostische Besonderheiten der Arteria Lusoria. Fortschr. Röntgenstr. **86**, 188–192 (1957a).

Schmidt, J.: Besonderheiten der Herzgefäßfigur im sagittalen Röntgenbild beim Rechtsaortenbogen. Fortschr. Röntgenstr. **87**, 597–604 (1957b).

Schmidt-Habelmann, P., Klinner, W., Meisner, H., Sebening, F., Struck, E.: Frühkindlicher Stridor und Dysphagie. Dtsch. med. Wschr. **93**, 335–344 (1968).

Shannon, J. M.: Aberrant right subclavian artery with Kommerell's diverticulum. J. thorac. cardiovasc. Surg. **4**, 408–411 (1961).

Stewart, J. R., Kincaid, O. W., Edwards, J. E.: An atlas of vascular rings and related malformations of the aortic arch system. Springfield (Ill.): Charles C. Thomas 1964.

Storey, C. F., Crittenden, J. W.: Double aortic arch. Dis. Chest **20**, 611–629 (1951).

Chapter 9

Mechanical Lesions of the Esophagus

Traumatic Lesions of the Esophagus

J. Janssens and P. Valembois

A great number of mechanical factors may cause esophageal lesions. They all have in common that they forcebly violate the integrity of the esophageal wall. In this section only those mechanical lesions of the esophagus which are due to external traumata will be discussed.

1. Pathogenesis

The first case of rupture of the esophagus due to traumatic injury described in the literature appears in the Smith Papyrus (1800 B.C.; cited by Breasted, 1930). Mechanical lesions of the esophagus due to external traumata are rare, because of the well protected location of the esophagus in the thorax; moreover, the gullet is elastic and very mobile, which also diminishes the chance of injury.

Mechanical esophageal lesions can be caused by blunt external trauma of the chest or by penetrating wounds (gunshot-wounds, knife-wounds, etc.).

1.1. Blunt Trauma

The first case of esophageal rupture due to blunt external trauma was described by Whipham in 1903. A man who fell from his horse sustained a depressed fracture of the skull. The fracture was repaired but after the procedure the patient's condition became progressively worse and he died 24 hours later. Autopsy showed rupture of the esophagus in the lower left part. Worman et al. (1962) published the first survey. They found 27 cases described in the English literature and added 3 of their own. Blair et al. (1968) found 8 additional cases in the other European literature and described one more of their own. Barrie et al. (1961) described the first case of rupture of the abdominal esophagus due to blunt external trauma. In this case the abdominal esophagus was completely transected. Miller (1968) reported on a similar case.

The incidence of esophageal lesions due to blunt external trauma has recently increased together with the number of car accidents; 7 of the 14 cases reported by Reichenecker (1963) and 13 of the 17 patients with a tracheoesophageal fistula resulting from nonpenetrating trauma of the chest, collected from the literature by Killen and Collins (1965), were due to a car accident. In most instances the esophageal lesion is due to the pressure of the steering-wheel on the driver's thorax; hence the name "steering-wheel injuries". The esophageal lesion is most likely caused by a sudden increase in intraluminal pressure and favored by associated regurgitation under pressure of gastric contents into the esophagus (Nelson, 1959). Another external blunt trauma which may cause esophageal lesions is external cardiac massage. Thus Lundbergh et al. (1967) found, on autopsy, esophageal tears of the Mallory-Weiss type in 10% the of patients who had undergone closed-chest cardiac massage.

The localization of the esophageal tear due to blunt trauma is largely determined by the site of impact (Nelson, 1959). If it hits the lower chest or the upper abdomen, the distal esophagus is injuried; if the crushing force hits higher,, the esophageal lesion also will be localized higher. In the latter case a tracheo-esophageal fistula may occur. The first case of a tracheoesophageal fistula following blunt trauma was described by Vinson (1936). Several analogous cases have been described since (Killen and Collins, 1965). The fistula has the form of a slit or of an ovoid, with its longitudinal axis in the cephalocaudal direction. The fistula itself is formed by apposition of longitudinal tears in the anterior wall of the esophagus and in the dorsal membraneous part of the trachea. These lesions are probably due to the compression of both organs between sternum and spinal column, followed by necrosis and fistulization. A relatively late manifestation of the fistula, a few days after the trauma, is fairly typical. Indeed in most cases a swallow-cough appears only 3 to 5 days after the trauma. This latent period occurs either because an incomplete tear needs some time to become a complete fistula, or because an extensive lesion needs some time to become necrotic and give rise to communications between both structures. In a few exceptional cases symptoms developed 3 to 6 months after the injury (Grimes, 1972). Actually, the formation of a tracheoesophageal fistula considerably improves the prognosis because it allows some drainage of the mediastinitis. Thus the survey of Worman et al. (1962) shows 10 survivors out of a series of 12 patients with a fistula, whereas only 3 out of 15 patients without fistula survived their trauma.

1.2. Penetrating Wounds

Esophageal lesions may also be due to penetrating wounds of the thorax, caused for instance, by bullets or knives. The degree and the nature of these penetrating wounds is obviously very heterogeneous. For instance, Malt et al. (1963) described a knife wound of the neck, with transection of the esophagus; Bliznak and Ramsey (1971) even described a case of atrioesophageal fistula after a gunshot wound.

1.3. Mechanical Agents Acting from Inside the Lumen

Mechanical agents can also cause lesions from inside the lumen of the esophagus; e.g., air under high pressure may accidentally enter the esophagus (Petren, 1908; Kerr et al., 1953; Cole and Burcher, 1961; Randolph et al., 1967). The mechanism causing esophageal lesions in such instances is similar to that responsible for the Mallory-Weiss syndrome.

2. Symptoms

The symptoms of esophageal lesions due to blunt external trauma are similar to those of spontaneous or iatrogenic perforations of the esophagus, and are described in the appropriate sections. However, the esophageal injuries produced by external trauma are mostly combined with lesions of other intrathoracic organs, and the symptoms of these lesions may dominate the clinical picture. Esophageal injury must always be suspected if an apparently moderate thoracic trauma produces unduly severe symptoms of cyanosis, dyspnea, shock and prostration. "Swallow-cough" is the typical symptom of a tracheo(broncho)esophageal fistula. As noted above, this symptom occurs only after a latent period of a few days.

3. Diagnosis

The diagnosis of an esophageal lesion due to external trauma is quite difficult, because the patient usually has several traumata and is frequently unconscious. Yet an early diagnosis is extremely important. Indeed, the extent of the mediastinitis will be the most important factor delimiting the possibilities of treatment. The technical examinations which aid the diagnosis are described in the sections on spontaneous or iatrogenic rupture of the esophagus.

4. Treatment

The treatment of esophageal lesions due to external trauma remains controversial. These injuries are rare and vary greatly in severity and extent; the concomitant lesions of other intrathoracic organs also are greatly variable. It is therefore difficult to evaluate the different treatments that have been proposed (MILLER, 1968). STEPHENS (1965) advocates immediate surgery if the diagnosis is established in the first few days. If it is established later, a gastrostomy is necessary before the lesion can be repaired in a second procedure. According to MILLER (1968) primary repair of the lesion is always contraindicated because of the usually extensive necrosis; he therefore advocates treatment by the exclusion principle (JOHNSON et al., 1956). Tracheoesophageal fistulas do not heal spontaneously; they always require surgical repair. Because the development of a fistula is a favorable factor in case of mediastinitis (WORMAN et al., 1962), an immediate operation is not usually required. The general condition of the patient and the extent of the mediastinitis and of the associated lesions will determine the timing of the operation.

References

BARRIE, J., SARRAZIN, R., BONNET-EYMARD, J.: Rupture traumatique de l'oesophage abdominal. Mém. Acad. Chir. (Paris) 87, 662–667 (1961).

BLAIR, D. W., HART, D. D., MACKAY, W. D., MILLS, K. L. G.: Rupture of the esophagus from blunt external trauma. J. roy. Coll. Surg. Edinb. 13, 46–48 (1968).

BLIZNAK, J., RAMSEY, J. D.: Atrio-esophageal fistula secondary to gunshot wound of the chest. Milit. Med. 136, 584–585 (1971).

BREASTED, J.: The Edwin Smith Papyrus. Chicago: Chicago Univ. Press 1930.

COLE, D. S., BURCHER, S. K.: Accidental pneumatic rupture of esophagus and stomach Lancet 1961 I, 24–25.

GRIMES, O. F.: Nonpenetrating injuries to the chest wall and esophagus. Surg. Clin. N. Amer. 52, 597–610 (1972).

JOHNSON, J., SCHWEGMAN, C. W., KIRBY, C. K.: Esophageal exclusion for persistent fistula following spontaneous rupture of the esophagus. J. thorac. Surg. 32, 827–832 (1956).

KERR, H. H., SLOAN, H., O'BRIEN, C. E.: Rupture of the esophagus by compressed air. Surgery 33, 417 (1953).

KILLEN, D. A., COLLINS, H. A.: Tracheoesophageal fistula resulting from nonpenetrating trauma to the chest. J. thorac. cardiovasc. Surg. 50, 104–110 (1965).

LUNDBERG, G. D., MATTEI, I. R., DAVIS, C. J., NELSON, D. E.: Hemorrhage from gastroesophageal lacerations following closed chest cardiac massage. J. Amer. med. Ass. 202, 123–126 (1967).

MALT, R. A., HEAD, J. H., SWEET, R. H.: Knife wound of the neck, with transection of the esophagus and contralateral hemopneumothorax. New Engl. J. Med. 268, 1353 (1963).

Miller, D. R.: Transection of the esophagus at the esophagogastric junction by blunt trauma. Report of a case. J. Trauma 8, 1105–1110 (1968).

Nelson, R. E.: Traumatic rupture of the esophagus. J. thorac. Surg. 37, 220–223 (1959).

Petren, G.: Ein Fall von traumatischer Oesophagus-Rupture, nebst Bemerkungen über die Entstellung der Oesophagus-Rupturen. Beitr. Klin. Chir. 61, 265 (1908).

Randolph, H., Melick, D. W., Grant, A. R.: Perforation of the esophagus from external trauma or blast injuries. Dis. Chest 51, 121–124 (1967).

Reichenecker: Thesis, Grenoble 1963, cit. by: Piaget, F., Jaudel, Reichenecker: A propos des ruptures traumatiques de l'œsophage thoracique par traumatismes fermés. Ann. Oto-laryng. (Paris) 82, 290–293 (1965).

Stephens, T. W.: Traumatic tracheo-oesophageal fistula following steering-wheel type of injury. Brit. J. Surg. 52, 370–372 (1965).

Vinson, P. P.: External trauma as a cause of lesions of the esophagus. Amer. J. Dig. Dis. 3, 457–459 (1936).

Whipham, T. R. C.: Lancet 1903 II, 749.

Worman, L. W., Hurley, J. D., Pemberton, A. H., Narodick, B. G.: Rupture of the esophagus from external blunt trauma. Arch. Surg. 85, 333–338 (1962).

Foreign Bodies in the Esophagus

J. Janssens and P. Valembois

With 5 Figures

1. Incidence

Small children frequently swallow foreign bodies during their games. Eating too fast without masticating sufficiently or the bad habit of drinking abundantly during meals increase the danger of swallowing foreign bodies. In some professions (tailor or carpenter) people have the habit of keeping in their mouth certain objects which can easily be swallowed. The risk of swallowing foreign bodies is increased in all situations which entail a diminished ability to distinguish a foreign body once it is in the mouth: after a cerebrovascular accident, wearing a dental prothesis with a palate etc. This accident occurs also in senile and psychotic persons.

All kinds of foreign bodies can be swallowed: non-traumatizing ones such as coins (Fig. 298), buttons, dental crowns, fruit stones or large lumps of meat (Fig. 84); more traumatizing objects also have been found in the esophagus, such as open safety pins (Fig. 299), nails (Fig. 300) and other metal objects (Fig. 301), pieces of glass, fish and meat bones (Fig. 302) and even small dental protheses (JACKSON, C., and JACKSON, C. L., 1936–1959; JACKSON, C. L., 1957; BOGAARS, 1962; BERENDES et al., 1963; BARBARY and BADRAWY, 1968; DONNELLY and DEVERALL, 1968; JACKSON, C., 1969; TUCKER, 1970).

Whenever a foreign object is swallowed it usually passes the entire gastrointestinal tract without any problems and is evacuated with the stools. Rarely do they get caught in the gullet. In a normal esophagus a foreign body is usually trapped at one of the naturally narrowed parts: just below the cricopharyngeal muscle, at the crossing of the aorta or left main bronchus, and at the gastroesophageal junction. Pathological narrowings caused by fibrosis, strictures, webs or carcinoma may cause impaction of relatively small objects. Stenosis has been observed with increasing frequency in recent years because the incidence of serious caustic lesions, caused by strong detergents, is increasing and because more patients with congenital or acquired esophageal diseases are treated surgically, resulting in an increased number of postoperative side effects (HOLINGER and JOHNSTON, 1963; FRIEDBERG and BLUESTONE, 1970; RICKHAM, 1971).

2. Pathogenesis and Pathology

An esophageal lesion caused by a foreign body can be as insignificant as a minimal mucosal tear but it can also be a serious esophageal perforation involving the mediastinal structures. The foreign object itself can directly cause the lesion; in other cases the lesion is secondary to impaction. In both instances secondary esophageal contractions and repeated swallowing attempts of the patient who tries to evacuate the foreign body will aggravate the lesion. Unless the foreign body has

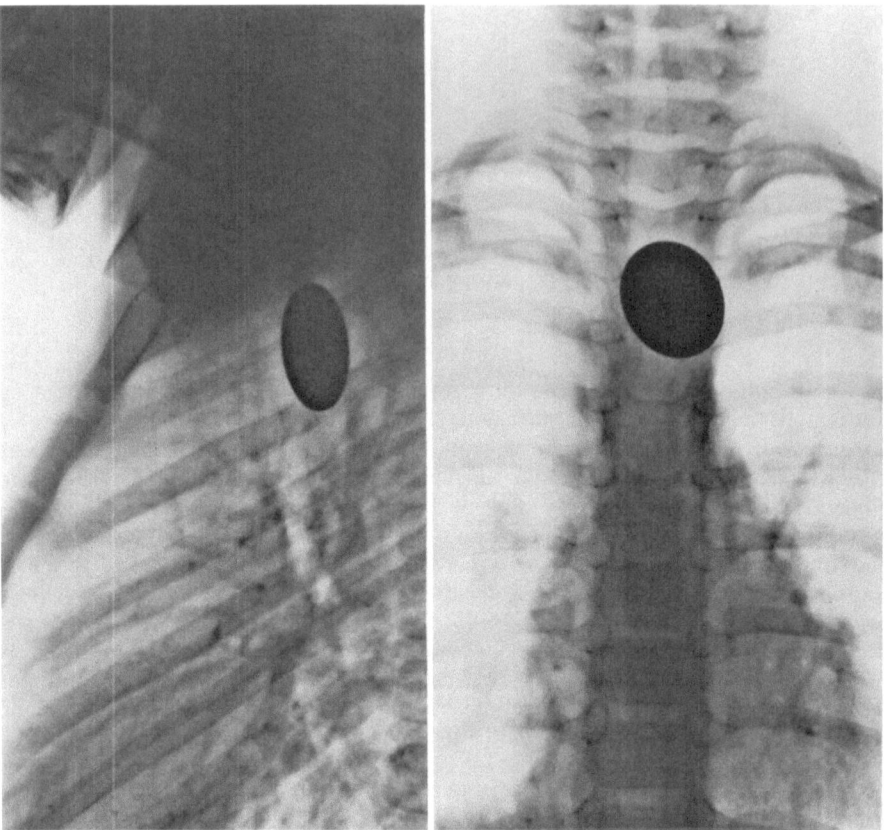

Fig. 298. Coin in the upper part of the thoracic esophagus, lying nearly in a frontal plane

sharp points, a free esophageal perforation will mostly not occur, not even if the foreign body remains trapped for a long time. Ulcerations may penetrate the esophageal wall but a barrier of inflammatory tissue usually prevents a free perforation. The great danger of a foreign body remaining impacted for a long time is fistula formation. Penetration of the ulceration into a bronchus results in a bronchoesophageal fistula. The ulceration may also perforate into a blood vessel, even the aorta, and cause an eventually fatal mediastinal bleeding (SLOOP and THOMPSON, 1967). Rarely sharp foreign bodies such as an open safety pin may erode the pericardium and may result in heart tamponade (NORMAN and CASS, 1971). The most important point is to find out whether an incomplete or a complete esophageal perforation is present (DONNELLY and DEVERALL, 1968). An incomplete perforation causes only superficial inflammation with edema, ulceration and sometimes intramural abscesses. A complete perforation, however, causes an extramural abscess, mediastinitis and involvement of the surrounding structures. The prognosis is determined in part by the localization of the perforation. A thoracic, and more rarely, a posteropharyngeal perforation causes mediastinitis, while the inflammatory reaction associated with a perforation of the anterior or lateral part of the cervical esophagus, mostly remains localized.

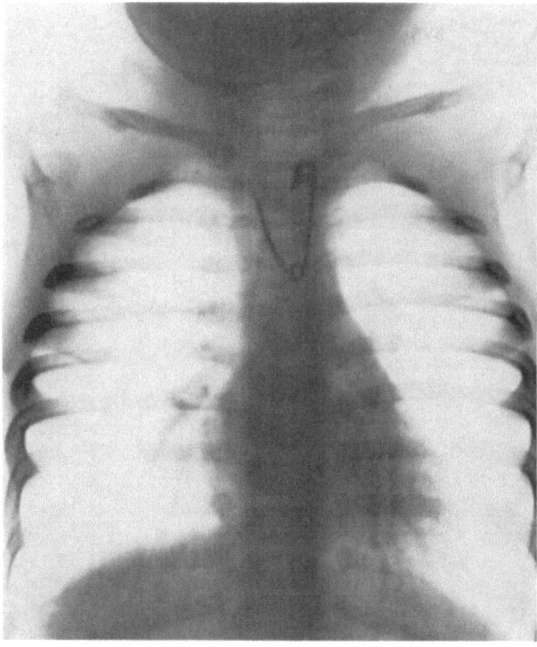

Fig. 299. Open safety pin in the upper part of the thoracic esophagus

3. Clinical Features

Mostly the patient is aware that he has swallowed the foreign body and often he himself has the impression that "something got stuck in the esophagus". In other cases the impaction occurs during the meal, even though the patient does not have the impression that he has swallowed an abnormally big bolus or an unusual object.

The most important symptoms of a foreign body in the esophagus are pain and dysphagia. In addition, an excessive amount of saliva may be produced and the patient feels a continuous need to swallow.

Spontaneous pain is a frequent symptom; typically the pain increases markedly during swallowing (odynophagia). The patient may be able to point to the exact location of the foreign body. It must be remembered, however, that the site at which an obstruction is localized by the patient is frequently incorrect. A foreign body in the hypopharynx usually causes discomfort above the level of the cricoid; a foreign object in the distal part of the esophagus may cause referred pain in the neck. A foreign body in the intraabdominal part of the esophagus usually results in epigastric discomfort. Pain radiating to the thorax or toward the back suggests the possibility of an esophageal perforation. When the patient claims he swallowed only a meat bolus but has intense pain, one must always take a radiograph to exclude the presence of a piece of bone in the bolus. An intraesophageal foreign body almost always causes dysphagia. Complete obstruction results in dysphagia for both liquids and solids. It the obstruction is located in the lower part of the esophagus the patient is still able to take a small amount of food or fluid which piles up in the esophagus and can eventually be regurgitated afterwards. An obstruction in the upper part of the gullet results in an overflow of all swallowed

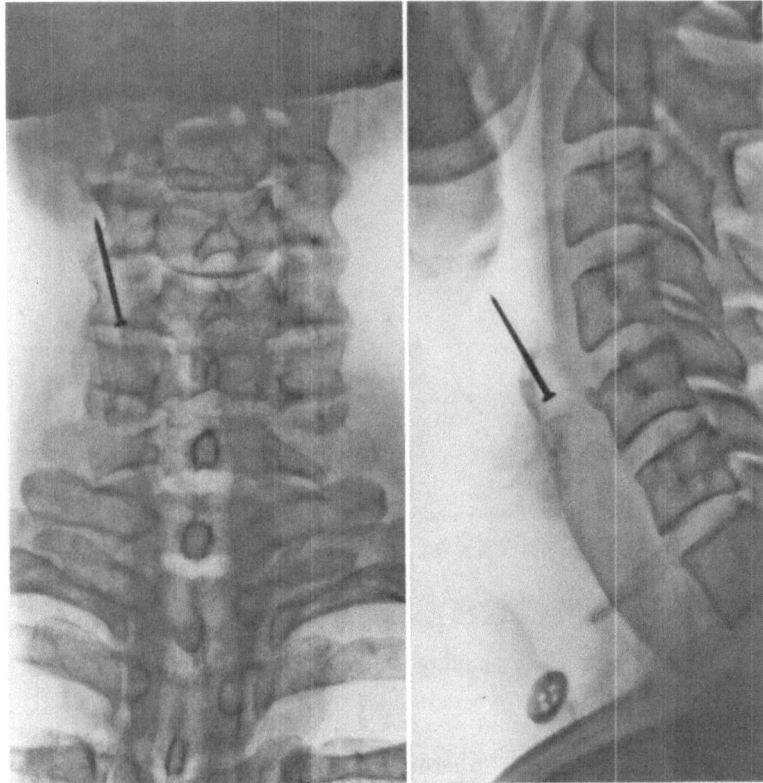

Fig. 300. Nail in right pyriform sinus

material into the larynx. When a patient with a known stenosing lesion of the esophagus experiences a sudden increase of his dysphagia, the possibility of a foreign body in the esophagus must always be considered. Children and psychotic patients may swallow objects which are sufficiently big to compress the trachea and cause difficulties in breathing (Bockus, 1963; Friedberg and Bluestone, 1970). When the foreign body or the ensuing ulceration ruptures the esophageal wall, the clinical picture of an esophageal perforation is found in addition to the already described symptoms.

Finally it must be stressed that the history is not always typical. Sometimes it will yield only few indications of the fact that the primary pathology is a foreign body in the esophagus (Lacomme and Lo, 1969). Baltzell (1968) reported the history of a 20 month old child described by his mother as "doing poorly"; radiographic examination of the thorax revealed a coin in the esophagus; esophagoscopy showed that it was completely overgrown with granulation tissue. Moure (1931) reports a case in which the diagnosis of foreign body was made 23 years after the patient had swallowed a dental prothesis. Especially in children respiratory complaints and continuous productive cough, caused by aspiration pneumonia, can be the dominating symptom after the swallowing of a foreign object that initially caused only slight or no discomfort at all (Glass and Goodman, 1966; Donnelly and Deverall, 1968; Friedberg and Bluestone, 1970).

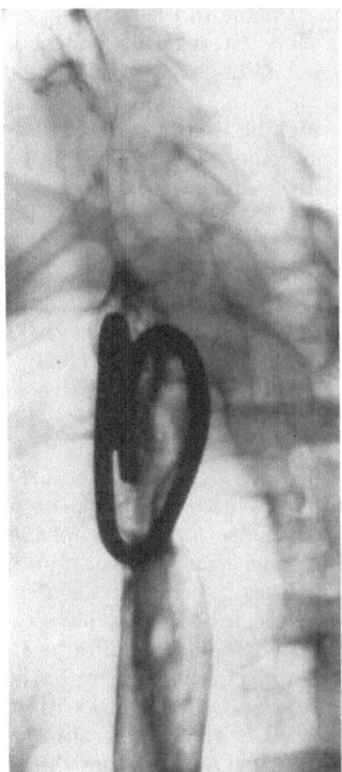 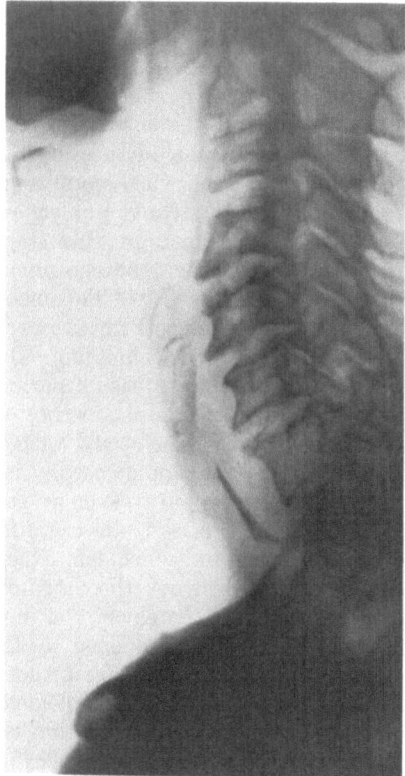

Fig. 301   Fig. 302

Fig. 301. Bent metal wire in the upper third of the thoracic esophagus

Fig. 302. Chicken bone in the cervical esophagus

4. Diagnosis

Whenever a patient seeks medical advice because he has swallowed a foreign object the situation should be taken seriously until the opposite has been proven. Often the patient's only complaint, compelling him to see the doctor, is fear. Many parents want an examination because they think their child swallowed something. One always starts with the examination of pharynx and hypopharynx by means of a laryngoscope, followed by a radiographical examination of neck and thorax, at first without contrast medium to recognize a radiopaque foreign body. To visualize foreign bodies of slight radiopacity high contrast pictures are needed; therefore a low voltage technique without a grid is used. A lateral and an anteroposterior X-ray of the neck is taken, as well as a lateral and an oblique chest radiograph. The radiological examination of pharynx and neck in lateral projection is very important, particularly to distinguish slightly opaque foreign bodies from the osseous structures of the cervical spine and from linear calcifications of the laryngeal tissues (GOLDMAN, 1951) (Fig. 302). It also permits to detect a non-radiopaque foreign object if it is surrounded by air or has caused a thickening of the prevertebral soft tissue space at the level of the hypopharyngeal outlet (WENZ, 1969). Special attention should be paid to the physiological narrowings of the esophagus. A swallowed coin lies in a frontal plane in the esophagus, and in anteroposterior direction in the trachea (Fig. 298). Even if the foreign body is not radiopaque, its presence can be established indirectly when a fluid level exists in the esophagus or when edema or abscess formation has caused swelling of periesophageal soft tissue, resulting in a widening of the prevertebral space. These routine radiographic pictures may also show signs of esophageal perforation, such as mediastinal or cervical emphysema, pleural effusion or pneumothorax.

If these examinations have not yet revealed a foreign object and if there are real symptoms, one must, at this stage of the examination, decide whether esophagoscopy or further radiographical examination with contrast medium should be performed. St. Clair Thompson and Negus (1955) advocate esophagoscopy at this stage whereas Pulvertaft and Stayte (1965) prefer a radiological examination with contrast medium. Donnelly and Deverall (1968) advise radiological examination in case a perforation or a mediastinal involvement are suspected, or in case the esophagoscopy would be too difficult. These radiological examinations should be performed with water-soluble contrast media.

As a matter of fact esophagoscopy is not only a diagnostic procedure but in the first place an attempt at treatment. It should be pointed out that an esophageal perforation in itself is not an absolute contraindication for esophagoscopy. However, an impaction which has existed for some time is a contraindication because impaction destroys the surrounding tissues, increasing the risk of an iatrogenic perforation. Moreover, the impacted foreign body may have caused a local abscess which can be opened by the esophagoscope. Even after esophagoscopy the possibility remains that a radiolucent object, covered by granulation tissue, is overlooked. Further radiological exploration is performed with a liquid barium suspension or, if a perforation is suspected, with Gastrografin, to check whether the outline of the esophageal lumen is normal and whether the contrast medium passes easily. Afterwards a less fluid barium mixture is administered, which may reveal a remnant of barium sticking to a foreign body. Eventually one can ask the patient to swallow a barium pill. The pill must be rather large (5 to 7 mm in diameter) and must be swallowed with as little water as possible. When this barium pill es held up at a certain level for a few minutes this part is mostly the place where a foreign body got caught. The use of a semisolid object like a cotton ball (Roth, 1963) or of a marshmallow soaked in barium is recommended by some authors to detect small foreign bodies, such as fish or chicken bones (Wenz, 1969). However, if these objects get impacted at the level of the foreign body they may compromise its endoscopic removal. Gastrografin has some advantages over barium as a contrast medium. It can be used even when a perforation is suspected and it is absorbed quickly by the tissues so that a subsequent esophagoscopy remains feasible (Donnelly and Deverall, 1968).

In spite of these various techniques of examination a firm diagnosis cannot always be made. Out of his series of 100 cases of foreign bodies in the esophagus, Bogaars (1962) was unable to visualize the foreign body in 10 of his patients, neither by radiology nor by esophagoscopy.

5. Treatment

A foreign body in the esophagus is only rarely a real emergency, and some measures, which are thought by the public mind to be urgent, must be carefully avoided (Tucker, 1970; Friedberg and Bluestone, 1970). One should never try to remove a foreign body by inserting a finger in the throat. A voluminous foreign body, which permitted adequate respiration when lying in the hypopharynx, may be pushed into the larynx and cause asphyxia. Turning the patient upside down usually has no effect on an intraesophageal object but can dislodge a foreign body from the lower trachea into the larynx, resulting in asphyxia. Emetics will never be administered because the vomiting movements may cause injury or even perforation of the esophagus if the foreign body has sharp edges.

When a patient seeks medical advice because he has swallowed a foreign body, one starts with an examination of the pharynx followed by X-rays of the neck and thorax, possibly complemented by radiological examination with contrast medium. If all these examinations are negative and if the complaints of the patient are not too serious one can await the development. Mostly the foreign body passes through the entire gastrointestinal tract without complications and is evacuated with the stools. Antacids and coating powders should be administered because the foreign body may always have caused an esophageal lesion. If the symptoms persist after 24 to 48 hours, an esophagoscopy is performed or a more complete radiological exploration, if that has not yet taken place. If these examinations reveal that the foreign object is trapped in the esophagus it must be removed either by esophagoscopy or by surgery. One shall never neglect to look for an organic narrowing of the esophagus which has favored the impaction. In many cases the foreign body can be removed at esophagoscopy (in 78,5% of the cases of BOGAARS, 1962). The technique of removal has been described by JACKSON and JACKSON (1934, 1936, 1948, 1957, 1959, 1969), and more recently by FRIEDBERG and BLUESTONE (1970) and by TUCKER (1970). Based on the radiographic data one should try to obtain a duplicate of the foreign body. An equivalent of this foreign body and a discussion of the difficulties which are to be expected with that particular object can usually be found in the tabulated data of the JACKSON collection (JACKSON and JACKSON, 1936). Consequently the extraction procedure will be imitated and exercised on a rubber tube with open manikin board. In this way it is possible to select the most suitable esophagoscope and extraction forceps. The endoscope should be sufficiently long because the foreign body may be pushed distally during the manipulations. A laryngoscope and a laryngeal grasping forceps must be available in case the foreign body is regurgitated and aspirated in the larynx.

Care should be taken to select the most suitable type of anesthesia (TUCKER, 1968–1970; TUCKER et al., 1969). Usually local anesthesia is sufficient. For children and subjects who are unable to collaborate, general anesthesia may be necessary. When the foreign body lies in the upper part of the esophagus the introduction of the tracheal tube may result in perforation of the esophagus if the tube is pushed too far dorsally. An adequate dose of atropine must be given to decrease esophageal secretion. Once the foreign body has been visualized endoscopically it will be grasped with the preselected forceps, pulled up as far as possible into the esophagoscope and so removed. If the foreign body is too voluminous it will be withdrawn together with the endoscope, but this may be a dangerous procedure for sharp objects.

More specific methods for the removal of special kinds of foreign bodies have been described in the literature. One of the most difficult problems is the endoscopic removal of an open safety pin, particularly if the top is directed orally (Fig. 299) (if the top is pointing downward the pin will close automatically when it is pulled up in the esophagoscope). JACKSON has described as many as 16 different methods, indicating that no one is entirely satisfactory in all cases. In the technique of BARLOW (1960) a ring, fixed obliquely on a shaft, is brought under the pin under esophagoscopic control. With a stiletto, the pin is pushed down through the ring, thus closing it. When it is dangerous to extract a foreign object with the esophagoscope because it has a sharp side pointed upward, one can push it down carefully into the stomach and perform a gastrotomy, which is always to be preferred above a thoracotomy (Donnelly and Deverall, 1968). The same can be done for a less sharp object which cannot be removed endoscopically. Once it has reached the stomach the foreign object often passes down the intestine without much trouble. Bigler (1966) and Symbas (1968) described a technique to extract a blunt foreign object from the esophagus by means of a *Foley catheter:* the balloon is inflated distally from the foreign object, which thereby leaves the wall if it had penetrated it slightly and falls on the top of the balloon; it can then easily be extracted. This technique should not be used for sharp objects or more than 24 hours after the incident in view of the perforation danger. Blind methods, which try to remove the object by grasping it with a hook or pushing it with a tube, are dangerous and should not be used.

Broad spectrum antibiotics and parenteral feeding must be used until the lesions are healed. A careful follow-up is necessary not to overlook a residual abscess; pain, persisting dysphagia and fever are signs of such an abscess.

Sometimes surgical extraction of the foreign body is preferred over endoscopic removal. According to Seed (1952) removal by external surgical approach is required if the foreign body is impacted, if it has produced periesophagitis after unsuccessful attempts at removal through the esophagoscope, or if it is lodged in a periesophageal abscess. If the foreign object has caused an esophageal perforation, which is discovered within the first 24 hours, surgery is indicated so that the tear may be closed at the same time. The presence of a mediastinal abscess, which has to be drained anyway, is also an indication for surgery (Donnelly and Deverall, 1968). Whenever a foreign body in pharynx or esophagus has been visualized on plain films, it is recommended to check its location in the operation room immediately before the anesthesia is performed.

6. Complications

The most serious complication is perforation of the esophagus. Although foreign objects with sharp sides are most likely to produce this complication, voluminous objects may slowly erode the esophageal wall and finally cause perforation. Inexpert attempts at endoscopic removal also may result in an iatrogenic perforation.

Another serious complication is the development of an intramural abscess, which may cause periesophagitis and eventually mediastinitis. The ulceration may penetrate into the trachea and result in a tracheoesophageal fistula, or perforate into a blood vessel and cause a serious mediastinal hemorrhage. Edwards et al. (1971) report the history of a 22 year old patient who, while being treated for bronchitis, had a chest X-ray which revealed a safety pin in what appeared to be the esophagus. On further examination the pin was found to have eroded the anterior wall of the esophagus and was lodged between esophagus and trachea.

Vogel (1921) collected from the literature 50 cases of hemorrhage secondary to erosion of mediastinal blood vessels and found that 30 of these were due to erosion of the aorta.

7. Esophageal Obstruction from Meat Impaction

Obstruction of the esophagus from meat impaction occurs mostly in persons with an organic esophageal narrowing [11 out of 17 in the series of Richardson

(1945)] and in persons with an upper dental prothesis which misleads the patient in judging the exact size of a meat bolus [12 out of 17 patients in the series of RICHARDSON (1945)]. A chest X-ray must always be taken not to overlook the presence of a bone fragment in the bolus. One shall attempt to relax the esophagus maximally by means of antispasmodics; this in itself is often sufficient to allow spontaneous evacuation of the bolus or to push it down into the stomach by means of a gastric tube. Eventually one can attempt to remove the bolus endoscopically.

DREW (1945) and after him RICHARDSON (1945) pointed to the possibility of removing the bolus enzymatically with Caroid, the most important part of which is papain (papayatin). This substance is a vegetable pepsin from the juice of the fruit and leaves of Carica papaya L. (papaw tree). The following products can be used for enzymatic digestion of a meat bolus (MILLER and GODFREY, 1955): (1) Trypsin (0.125 gm in 10 ml of Sörensen's phosphate buffer) appears to be the most active product in vivo and can be sterilized. (2) Caroid (papaya) (10 ml of a 10% suspension in isotonic salt solution) appears to be the most powerful preparation in vitro. (3) Proteinase A (30000 U. in 10 ml of isotonic salt solution) is very active. The patient takes about 10 ml of one of these solutions and tries to keep it in his esophagus as long as possible. Intermittently the pieces already digested are sucked up. When the bolus has become sufficiently small, it spontaneously slides down into the stomach or is regurgitated. The entire treatment lasts usually from 1 to 1.5 hours. This type of treatment has occasionally resulted in digestion of the esophageal wall and fatal perforation (ANDERSEN et al., 1959).

References

ANDERSEN, H. A., BERNATZ, P. E., GRINDLEY, J. H.: Perforation of the esophagus after use of a digestant agent. Ann. Otol. (St. Louis) 68, 890–896 (1959) and Trans Amer. bronchoesoph. Ass. 39, 80 (1959).

BALTZELL, W.: Unusual foreign bodies. Laryngoscope (St. Louis) 78, 479–486 (1968).

BARBARY, A. S., BADRAWY, R.: Foreign bodies in the oesophagus. (A record of 500 cases.) J. Egypt. med. Ass. 51, 325–336 (1968).

BARLOW, D.: Device for removing an open safety pin from oesophagus or bronchial tree. Lancet 1960 I, 208.

BERENDES, J., LINK, R., ZÖLLNER, F.: Fremdkörper des Ösophagus. Hals-Nasen-Ohrenheilkunde, p. 581–596. Stuttgart: Georg Thieme 1963.

BIGLER, F. C.: The use of Foley catheter for removal of blunt foreign bodies from the esophagus. J. thorac. cardiovasc. Surg. 51, 759–760 (1966).

BOCKUS, H. L.: Gastroenterology, vol. I, p. 225. Philadelphia-London: W. B. Saunders Co. 1963.

BOGAARS, A. H.: Survey of 100 cases of corpora aliena in the esophagus. Pract. oto-rhinolaryng. (Basel) 24, 125–127 (1962).

DONNELLY, R. J., DEVERALL, P. B.: The management of oesophageal foreign bodies and their complications. Postgrad. med. J. 44, 830–835 (1968).

DREW, F. P.: Cit. by RICHARDSON, J. R., New treatment for esophageal obstruction due to meat impaction. Ann. Otol. (St. Louis) 54, 328–348 (1945).

EDWARDS, H., JR., MCNICHOLS, W. A., SR., DIKMAN, S.: Esophageal perforation by a safety pin. J. Amer. med. Ass. 218, 740 (1971).

FRIEDBERG, S. A., BLUESTONE, C. D.: Foreign body accidents involving the air and food passages in children. Otolaryng. Clin. N. Amer. 3, 395–403 (1970).

GLASS, W. H., GOODMAN, M.: Unsuspected foreign bodies in the young child's oesophagus presenting with respiratory symptoms. Laryngoscope (St. Louis) 76, 605–615 (1966).

GOLDMAN, J. L.: Fish bones in the esophagus. Ann. Otol. (St. Louis) 60, 957–973 (1951).

HOLINGER, P. H., JOHNSTON, K. C.: Postsurgical endoscopic problems of congenital esophageal atresia. Ann. Otol. (St. Louis) 72, 1035–1049 (1963).

JACKSON, C. L.: Foreign bodies in the esophagus. Amer. J. Surg. 93, 308–312 (1957).

JACKSON, C.: Foreign bodies in the air and food passages. In: Otolaryngology, vol. 5 (COATES, H. P., SCHENK, M., MILLER, eds.), chap. 1. Hagerstown: Harper 1969.

Jackson, C., Jackson, C. L.: Foreign bodies in air and food passages. Ann. Roentgen. New York: Paul B. Hoeber 1934.

Jackson, C., Jackson, C. L.: Diseases of the air and food passages of foreign body origin. Philadelphia-London: W. B. Saunders Co. 1936.

Jackson, C., Jackson, C. L.: Foreign bodies in air and food passages. Postgrad. Med. 4, 281–290 (1948).

Jackson, C., Jackson, C. L.: Diseases of the nose, throat, and ear, 2nd ed. Philadelphia-London: W. B. Saunders Co 1959.

Lacomme, Y., Lo, R.: Troubles persistants de la déglutition chez un nourisson par volumineux corps étranger méconnu. J. franç. Oto-rhino-laryng. 18, 818–820 (1969).

Miller, J. H., Godfrey, G. C.: Treatment of impaction of cooked meat in the esophagus with trypsin. Arch. Otolaryng. 62, 202–203 (1955).

Moure, E. J.: Zahnprothese, zweieinhalb Jahre am Oesophaguseingang gelegen. Mschr. Ohrenheilk. 65, 1297–1300 (1931).

Norman, M. G., Cass, E.: Cardiac tamponade resulting from a swallowed safety pin. Pediatrics 48, 831–833 (1971).

Pulvertaft, C. N., Stayte, D. J.: Dangers of radiotranslucent dental plates. Brit. med. J. 1965 II, 420–421.

Richardson, J. R.: A new treatment for esophageal obstruction due to meat impaction. Ann. Otol. (St. Louis) 54, 328–348 (1945).

Rickham, P. P.: Ingested foreign bodies in childhood. Ann. roy. Coll. Surg. Engl. 48, 25 (1971).

Roth, J. L. A.: Esophagitis and peptic ulcer of the esophagus. In: H. L. Bockus, Gastroenterology. Philadelphia-London: W. B. Saunders Co. 1963.

Seed, G. S.: Diseases of the ear, nose and throat, ed. by W. G. Scott-Brown. London: Butterworth & Co., Ltd. 1952.

Sloop, R. D., Thompsom, J. C.: Aorto-esophageal fistula: report of a case and review of literature. Gastroenterology 53, 768–777 (1967).

St. Clair Thompson, Negus, V. E.: Disease of the nose and throat, p. 843. London: Cassell 1955.

Symbas, P. N.: Indirect method of extraction of foreign body from the esophagus. Ann. Surg. 167, 78–80 (1968).

Tucker, G. F., Jr.: Anesthesia in peroral endoscopy. Otolaryng. Clin. N. Amer. 1, 37 (1968).

Tucker, G. F., Jr.: Management of foreign bodies in the esophagus. In: Modern treatment, vol. 7, p. 1301–1319. New York: Harper and Row 1970.

Tucker, G. F., Jr., Adriani, J., Atkins, J.: Anesthesia in peroral endoscopy. Trans Amer. broncho-esoph. Ass. 49, 116 (1969).

Vogel, R.: Über Fremdkörper in der Speiseröhre. Langenbecks Arch. klin. Chir. 115, 910 (1921).

Wenz, W.: Oesophagus. In: Handbuch der medizinischen Radiologie, Bd. XI, Teil 1. Berlin-Heidelberg-New York: Springer 1969.

Spontaneous Rupture of the Esophagus

(Boerhaave's Syndrome)

J. Janssens and P. Valembois

With 1 Figure

1. Definition

Spontaneous rupture of the esophagus can be defined as a complete tear of all layers in an apparently normal gullet. A distinction must be made between perforation and rupture. A perforation results from a lesion, iatrogenic or not, or is a final stage of an esophageal disease. What is described as a spontaneous rupture is mostly caused by vomiting and is therefore called "primary pressure rupture of the esophagus" (Moynihan, 1954). The term "secondary pressure rupture of the esophagus" (Toghill et al., 1968) is used when other causes of increased intraabdominal pressure, such as a status asthmaticus (Raffle, 1958) or epilepsy (Klein and Grossman, 1943) produce the rupture. In some cases the rupture seems to be "really spontaneous"; Heroy (1952) described a case of spontaneous rupture of the esophagus which occurred during T.V. watching and Clark and Tankel (1964) described one that took place while the person was asleep.

2. History and Incidence

Boerhaave (1724) was the first to describe a spontaneous rupture of the esophagus in an autopsy report of his patient Baron von Wassenaer, Grand Admiral of the Dutch fleet. Meyer (1858) made the first pre-mortem diagnosis and already in 1877 Fitz published a review about the new syndrome. In 1944 Graham described two cases of rupture of the esophagus who survived after surgical drainage of the pleura, while Collis et al. (1944) described the first attempt at primary closure of the rent by open thoracotomy. But it was only in 1947 that Barrett performed the first successful thoracotomy with primary closure of the rupture. Although spontaneous rupture of the esophagus remains rare, more than 280 cases have already been described in the literature.

3. Pathogenesis

A rupture of the esophagus almost always occurs after a fairly sudden increase of the intraabdominal pressure by vomiting (75 to 80%), straining at defecation, childbirth or an attack of epilepsy. The speed of the increase in pressure is probably more important than the absolute value of the pressure (Burt, 1931). This sudden increase in pressure is more dangerous when the stomach is full, because the fundus of a full stomach is less able to handle the increase in pressure.

During a normal vomiting reflex the esophagus is opened completely so that the stomach contents can be evacuated. When incoordination of this mechanism occurs, the upper esophageal sphincter may not relax or a localized segment of the esophagus may contract; the intraesophageal pressure increases and may rupture the esophagus. This muscular incoordination occurs frequently after administration of heavy sedatives, after alcohol abusus, in diseases of the central nervous system (especially when midbrain or hypothalamus are affected), during changes of blood pH and shortly after a general anesthesia (MACKLER, 1952; MEAGHER et al., 1962; O'CONNELL, 1967). Frequently, however, an underlying pathology diminishing the resistance of the esophageal wall is found in cases of esophageal rupture, e.g. peptic esophagitis (BRACKNEY et al., 1955) and malnutrition with disturbances of protein metabolism (ANDERSON, 1952). In cases of acute esophagitis the esophageal wall is said to have such a low resistance that a forceful deglutition movement alone would already suffice to cause a rupture, particularly when there is a distal obstruction due to a web or a stenosing esophagitis (CONTE, 1966).

Experimental studies stress the importance of both the increase in abdominal pressure and of the pathology of the esophageal wall in the pathogenesis of spontaneous rupture. Already in 1884 McKENZIE showed that at an average intraluminal pressure of 7 lb/inch² a rupture occurs in the esophagus removed from adult cadavers; either all layers burst at the same time or first the muscle and only then the mucosa rupture. MACKLER (1952) found an average pressure at rupture of 5 lb/inch² in a preparation of esophagus and stomach of cadavers. TIDMAN and JOHN (1967) found an average value of 2.3 lb/inch² for an isolated preparation of esophagus and stomach and 4.6 lb/inch² for the esophagus in situ. These values are still within the physiological range since ATKINSON et al. (1961) measured intragastric pressure peaks up to 200 mm Hg ($=3.866$ lb/inch²) during provoked vomiting in volunteers. This pressure is transmitted into the esophagus if the cardia is open and the upper esophageal sphincter closed during vomiting. The importance of an intact esophageal mucosa was stressed by DERRICK et al. (1958), who showed that the bursting strength of the intact human esophagus in situ is much higher (3 to 7.5 lb/inch²) than that of an esophagus from which the mucosa had been removed (1 to 2.25 lb/inch²). When the cat esophagus is infused with acid pepsin under a constant pressure of 20 cm H_2O it ruptures more easily than when it is infused with 0.1 N HCl (FERGUSON et al., 1950). The experiments of BRACKNEY et al. (1955) show that regurgitation of acid gastric contents in dogs clearly increases the danger of perforation during vomiting. All these studies seem to indicate that a certain increase in intraabdominal pressure is the factor provoking rupture of the esophagus, but that the chances of rupture are greater if the esophageal mucosa has been affected by gastroesophageal reflux.

4. Pathology

The tear of a spontaneous esophageal rupture is linear with clear-cut edges, mostly longitudinal; it is 0.5 to 4 cm long, sometimes more. In 70 to 80% of the cases the tear is located in the left postero-lateral wall of the esophagus, 2.5 to 7.5 cm above the cardia (HOCHBERG and PARLAMIS, 1961; MEAGHER et al., 1962; O'CONNELL, 1967. This preferential localization remains in esophagi removed from cadavers (MACKLER, 1952), and is probably related to a splaying out of the muscle fibers and to the entrance of numerous blood vessels and nerves at that place.

Only a few cases have been described of spontaneous rupture in the middle third of the esophagus (FITZ, 1877; PRIVITERI and GAY, 1951; MOYNIHAN, 1954;

WACHTEL and GENKINS, 1955; ROSS, 1961; HAMILTON, 1967; BATES, 1969) or in its upper part (JORDAN, 1964; HAMILTON, 1967; RUSSELL and McDONALD, 1968). Microscopic examination of the tear shows only acute inflammatory lesions and no chronic inflammatory cell infiltration or fibrous reaction (MACKLER, 1952).

5. Clinical Features

Spontaneous rupture of the esophagus occurs mainly in males (85% of the cases). The peak incidence is between the ages of 50 and 60 (LAUSCHKE et al., 1970). It almost always starts with an episode of vomiting, followed by an abrupt tearing or burning pain in the low retrosternal or high epigastric region. The pain frequently radiates to the left hypochondrium, the back or the left shoulder and is so intense that often even morphine cannot stop it. Respiratory movements, reclining and moving about clearly increase it. There is also marked dysphagia. Sometimes the patient says he had the impression that something tore inside. Often he experiences a sensation of extreme thirst (ANDERSON, 1952). The condition of the patient may be dramatic from the very beginning because of shock from pain and hypoxia, and, more rarely, from blood loss; but mostly the situation turns critical only after some time.

Other symptoms can occur more rarely. SAMSON (1951) described a nasal tone of the voice few hours before the development of cervical emphysema. Sometimes the vomiting does not precede the acute attack of pain, but occurs later; or the patient may have a slight hematemesis (MACKLER, 1952).

BANGASH et al. (1968) described the history of a 73 year old woman, who suddenly became dyspneic without any clear cause. A few hours before, she had complained of a short attack of retrosternal pain not preceded by vomiting. Autopsy showed a transverse tear in the lower part of the esophagus, empyema and mediastinitis. In the initial phase the paucity of the clinical signs is in sharp contrast with the severity of the symptoms. Mostly one finds only tachypnea and slight abdominal tenderness. Initially, the esophageal tear produces only a slight mediastinitis and mediastinal emphysema, which obviously are rather insusceptible to clinical examination. A discrete and initially sterile effusion in the left pleural cavity may develop. More rarely a mediastinal "crunching" sound (the Hamman sound) can be heard on auscultation of the thorax (MEAGHER et al., 1962; O'CONNELL, 1967). Severe clinical signs appear only when involvement of the mediastinal pleura by the infectious process results in pleural effusion (mostly at the left side), pneumothorax, or hydro- or pyopneumothorax. Rarely even a tension pneumothorax may occur (TOGHILL et al., 1968). In case of a bilateral pleural effusion the exsudate in the right pleural cavity is often sterile and not connected with the left pleural effusion which is infected (SMEAD, 1931). After a few hours the mediastinal emphysema can rise into the neck, where in 65% of the cases typical snow crepitation can be felt (TESLER and EISENBERG, 1963). The triad described by BARRETT (1946–1947), i.e. tachypnea, abdominal muscle tenderness and subcutaneous emphysema in the neck, is almost pathognomonic for an esophageal rupture. In some cases the mediastinal emphysema can be so marked that it causes respiratory distress (ANDERSON, 1952). If the retropharyngeal space is involved in the infectious process stiffness of the neck can also be found. Rarely a purulent pericarditis can occur as a complication of esophageal rupture with mediastinitis (BOYD and WITTMANN, 1971). Without adequate treatment the general condition of the patient progressively deteriorates by the spreading mediastinitis, resulting in sepsis, shock, cyanosis and exitus.

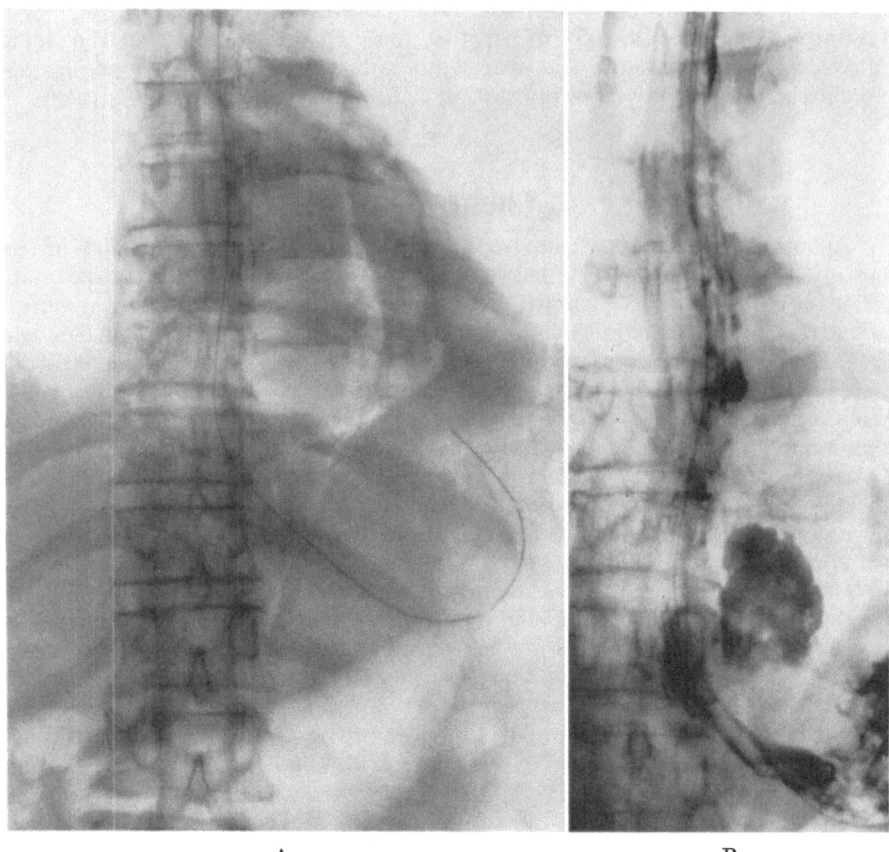

A B

Fig. 303. A Spontaneous perforation of the esophagus. Penetrated plain chest film showing pneumomediastinum with air along the descending aorta and left diaphragmatic dome. B Same case, showing the site of perforation and the extravasation of contrast medium

6. Technical Examinations

One of the earliest signs of an esophageal rupture is mediastinal emphysema, which can often be shown radiologically several hours before subcutaneous emphysema in the neck is found. In the most typical case the air in the mediastinum takes on the shape of a V (V-sign of Naclerio, 1957): the air rises along the left side of the aorta (vertical limb of the V) and spreads laterally over the left diaphragm (horizontal limb of the V) (Fig. 303). In view of the rather fast evolution of this phenomenon it is indicated to repeat an initially negative examination whenever a rupture is suspected on clinical grounds.

The chest X-ray usually shows a pleural effusion; in other cases one finds a pneumothorax or a hydropneumothorax, rarely even a tension pneumothorax. An over-exposed radiograph can sometimes provide useful supplementary information such as the presence of gastric contents behind the heart shadow or of a fluid level (O'Connell, 1967).

An attempt should always be made to localize radiologically the site of perforation by administering to the patient a water-soluble contrast medium. The rather intense pain the patient experiences on drinking it confirms the diagnosis. KERR (1962) described a technique to localize with more certainty the site of extravasation; through a soft catheter, introduced into the stomach, contrast medium is injected while the catheter is slowly withdrawn. This technique will also prevent the overlooking of a second tear (SEALY, 1963). However, these radiological techniques will not always offer an exact picture of the magnitude of the tear because the contrast medium sometimes leaks only from the lower part of the lesion (BATES, 1969).

7. Diagnosis

As is often the case in rare diseases, the most important step in making the diagnosis is to think of the possibility of a spontaneous rupture of the esophagus. Only rarely the diagnosis is made on admission of the patient (BRIGGS et al., 1961). The history, however, is often quite typical. The triad of BARRETT (1946–1947) is practically pathognomonic. The radiological demonstration of mediastinal emphysema, of extravasated contrast medium or of an esophagopleural fistula proves the diagnosis. If gastric contents or traces of swallowed dye (methylene blue) are found in the pleural cavity the diagnosis is equally certain (LEVINE and KELLEY, 1965).

Several conditions have to be considered in the differential diagnosis of esophageal rupture. A perforated gastric or duodenal ulcer can be recognized by the presence of free air under the diaphragm. Acute pancreatitis can also mimic a spontaneous esophageal rupture and cause a pleural effusion; but mostly this disease begins with abdominal pain which is later followed by vomiting. An esophageal rupture is often considered initially to be a myocardial infarction; the E.C.G. will help to exclude this diagnosis. In dissecting aneurysm of the aorta, the pain tends to diminish after a while, whereas it rather increases in case of esophageal rupture. A spontaneous pneumothorax usually does not cause the extremely intense pain of a rupture of the esophagus, and the general condition of the patient is less affected. The Mallory-Weiss syndrome will cause more bleeding and much less pain; also there are no signs of mediastinitis.

More rarely a spontaneous rupture of the esophagus is confused with mesenteric thrombosis, pulmonary embolism, bronchial rupture, volvulus or strangulation of a diaphragmatic hernia, perforation of a peptic ulcer of the esophagus, intestinal obstruction or strangulation, or rupture of the gallbladder (ANDERSEN, 1952; LEVINE and KELLEY, 1965; PANARO and LESLIE, 1965; MECKSTROTH and BROENNLE, 1968). Only in the very rare case of perforation of an intrathoracic stomach or intestinal segment can the differential diagnosis not be made; but this is not very important since both conditions require the same treatment (ANDERSON, 1952; CHAMBERLAIN and BYERLY, 1957).

8. Prognosis

Spontaneous rupture of the esophagus is always a very serious condition with considerable mortality. Even if the diagnosis is made early and the patient is treated by thoracotomy, closure of the tear and pleural drainage, the mortality is still around 25%. If the diagnosis is made late and if treatment must be limited to pleural drainage, the mortality is much higher. Without treatment the condition is almost always fatal.

9. Treatment

Since Graham's report in 1944 on the first two cases of esophageal rupture treated successfully by surgical drainage of the pleura and since Barrett's first successful closure of the tear in 1947, most authors agree on the necessity of immediate surgery. There is some discussion, however, whether treatment must only be pleural drainage by thoracotomy or pleural drainage with primary closure of the tear. Already in 1951 Samson published a series of 30 cases of spontaneous esophageal rupture, 15 of which were treated by pleural drainage and suture of the tear with a mortality of 33%; in the other cases, treated by pleural drainage via a thoracotomy without primary closure of the tear, the mortality was 47%. Later reviews have confirmed these results (Derbes and Mitchell, 1956; Anderson, 1957). Postlethwait and Sealy (1961) collected from the literature 117 cases; pleural drainage with suture of the tear resulted in an average mortality of 31% whereas the mortality of pleural drainage alone amounted to 54%. However, both groups are not entirely comparable since drainage without closure of the tear usually was performed only in those patients in whom the diagnosis had been made rather late. In these cases the prognosis was obviously less favorable.

The most logical attitude seems to be the following. If the diagnosis has been made early (i.e. within 24 hours) thoracotomy with suture of the tear and drainage of the pleural cavity yields the best results. Unless the radiological examination clearly shows that the tear is located at the right side, a left thoracotomy is performed. It is important to buttress the suture carefully with pleura to prevent postoperative fistula formation. This is a very frequent complication; in some series it occurred in 45% to 50% of the cases (Briggs et al., 1961; Derbes and Mitchell, 1965). It usually develops about 8 to 10 days after the operation; a careful pleural drainage will usually result in closure of the fistula in a few weeks. Recently a technique of transabdominal suture of the tear, complemented by a closed intercostal drainage, was proposed by Berne et al. (1969). If on the contrary the diagnosis is made after more than 24 hours, only a thoracotomy with pleural drainage must be performed because the edges of the tear are already infected to such an extent that a safe primary suture is no longer possible (Sanderson, 1965; Bradham et al., 1967; Hamilton, 1967).

General measures such as antibiotics and parenteral feeding are of course indicated. A few cases have been published in which the diagnosis was made very late, yet the general condition of the patient remained good without evidence of increasing mediastinitis or empyema; in such cases conservative treatment is acceptable (Movsas, 1966).

10. Esophageal Rupture in Children

Derbes and Mitchell (1956) showed that the esophagus of children is much more resistant than that of adults (13 times more resistant during the first year of life and 4 times at the age of 12). It is not to be wondered therefore that spontaneous rupture of the esophagus in children is very rare (only about 2% of all spontaneous esophageal ruptures).

Only a few cases in children have been described (Boyd, 1882; Menne and Moore, 1921; Derbes and Mitchell, 1956). The lesion can also occur in the neonatus (Dorsey et al., 1959; Wiseman et al., 1959; Hochberg and Parlamis, 1961; Le Brigand et al., 1961). Whereas in adults the tear is usually located in the left posterolateral aspect of the gullet, in young children it occurs rather at the right side and causes right pleural effusion. This is probably due to the fact that in young children the esophagus is located more to the right and is protected at its left side by the aorta (HOHF et al., 1962). Treatment is the same as in adults.

References

ANDERSON, R. L.: Rupture of the esophagus. J. thorac. Surg. 24, 369–388 (1952).

ANDERSON, R. L.: Spontaneous rupture of the esophagus. Amer. J. Surg. 93, 282–290 (1957).

ATKINSON, M., BOTTRILL, M. B., EDWARDS, A. T., MITCHELL, W. M., PEET, B. G., WILLIAMS, R. E.: Mucosal tears at the oesophagogastric junction (the Mallory-Weiss syndrome). Gut 2, 1–11 (1961).

BANGASH, M., DEMOS, N. J., TIMMES, J. J.: Spontaneous rupture of the esophagus. One transverse rupture. N.Y. J. Med. 68, 1857–1860 (1968).

BARRETT, N. R.: Spontaneous perforation of the oesophagus: review of the literature and report of three new cases. Thorax 1, 48–70 (1946).

BARRETT, N. R.: Report of case of spontaneous perforation of oesophagus successfully treated by operation. Brit. J. Surg. 35, 216–218 (1947).

BATES, M.: Pressure rupture of the mid-thoracic oesophagus. Brit. J. Surg. 56, 327–331 (1969).

BERNE, C. J., SHADER, A. E., DOTY, D. B.: Treatment of effort rupture of the esophagus by epigastric celiotomy. Surg. Gynec. Obstet. 129, 277–280 (1969).

BOERHAAVE, H.: Atrocis, nec descripti pirus, Morbi Historia, secundum medicae Artis Leges Conscripta. Lugdunum Batavorum (1724).

BOYD, D. P., WITTMANN, C. J., JR.: Some principles in treating perforation of esophagus. Surg. Clin. N. Amer. 51, 567–574 (1971).

BOYD, S.: Rupture of the oesophagus. Trans. path. Soc. Lond. 33, 125–129 (1882).

BRACKNEY, E. L., CAMPBELL, G. S., THAL, A. P., WANGENSTEEN, O. H.: Spontaneous perforation of the esophagus; experimental study. Proc. Soc. exp. Biol. (N.Y.) 88, 307–310 (1955).

BRADHAM, R. R., BRIDGMAN, A. H., SCOTT, S. M., BETTS, R. H.: Spontaneous esophageal perforation. Management of the "intermediate" phase. Ann. thorac. Surg. 3, 6–14 (1967).

BRIGGS, J. N., HAMEL, N. C., SCHULKINS, T. A.: Spontaneous rupture of the esophagus. West. J. Surg. Obstet. Gynec. 69, 351–354 (1961).

BURT, C. V. A.: Pneumatic rupture of intestinal canal. Arch. Surg. 22, 875–902 (1931).

CHAMBERLAIN, J. M., BYERLY, W. G.: Rupture of the esophagus. Amer. J. Surg. 93, 271–281 (1957).

CLARK, D. H., TANKEL, H. I.: Pressure rupture and spontaneous perforation of the esophagus. Gut 5, 86–89 (1964).

COLLIS, J. L., HUMPHREYS, D. R., BOND, W. H.: Spontaneous rupture of the esophagus. Lancet 1944 II, 179–180.

CONTE, B. A.: Esophageal rupture in absence of vomiting. J. thorac. cardiovasc. Surg. 51, 137–142 (1966).

DERBES, V. J., MITCHELL, R. E., JR.: Rupture of the esophagus. Surgery 39, 688–709 (1956).

DERRICK, J. R., HARRISON, W. H., HOWARD, J. M.: Factors predisposing to spontaneous perforation of the esophagus. The mechanical strength of the ulcerated esophagus. Surgery 43, 486–489 (1958).

DORSEY, J. H., HOHF, R. P., LYNN, T. E.: Relationship of peptic esophagitis to spontaneous rupture of the esophagus. Arch. Surg. 78, 878–888 (1959).

FERGUSON, D. J., SANCHEZ-PALOMERA, E., SAKO, Y., CLATWORTHY, H. W., TOON, R. W., WANGENSTEEN, O. H.: Studies on experimental esophagitis. Surgery 28, 1022–1039 (1950).

FITZ, R. H.: Rupture of the healthy esophagus. Amer. J. Med. Sci. 73, 17–36 (1877).

GRAHAM, E. A.: Editorial comment: Year book of General Surgery, p. 382 (1944).

HAMILTON, S. G. I.: Spontaneous rupture of the esophagus. Brit. J. Surg. 54, 304–306 (1967).

HEROY, W. W.: Discussion of ANDERSON, R. L., J. thorac. Surg. 24, 369–388 (1952).

HOCHBERG, L. A., PARLAMIS, N.: Spontaneous perforation and rupture of the esophagus with report of five cases. Amer. J. Surg. 102, 428–438 (1961).

HOHF, R. P., KIMBALL, E. R., BALLENGER, J. J.: Rupture of the esophagus in the neonate. J. Amer. med. Ass. 181, 939–943 (1962).

JORDAN, O.: Spontan ruptur of cervikale oesophagussegment. Ugeskr. Laeg. 126, 1170–1173 (1964).

KERR, I. M.: A method af demonstrating the site of perforation of the esophagus. Brit. J. Radiol. 35, 255–260 (1962).

KINSELLA, T. J., MORSE, R. W., HERTZOG, A. J.: Spontaneous rupture of the esophagus. J. thorac. Surg. 17, 613–631 (1948).

KLEIN, L., GROSSMAN, M.: Rupture of the esophagus. Med. Bull. Veterans' Adm. (Wash.) 19, 277–283 (1943).

Lauschke, H., Hau, T., Peiper, H. J.: Rupturen und Perforationen der Speiseröhre unter besonderer Berücksichtigung der pathologischen, klinischen und therapeutischen Unterschiede. Langenbecks Arch. Chir. **326**, 186–211 (1970).
Le Brigand, H., Bordes, J., David, G.: Spontaneous perforation of esophagus in newborn infant. Mem. Acad. Chir. **87**, 687–691 (1961).
Levine, P. H., Kelley, M. L., Jr.: Spontaneous perforation of esophagus simulating acute pancreatitis. J. Amer. med. Ass. **191**, 343–345 (1965).
Mackler, S. A.: Spontaneous rupture of the esophagus. An experimental and clinical study. Surg. Gynec. Obstet. **95**, 345–356 (1952).
McKenzie, M.: A manual of diseases of the nose and the throat, p. 160. New York: Wm. Wood & Co. 1880–1884.
Meagher, R. P., Lupien, J., Albert, S. N.: Postoperative rupture of the esophagus. Surg. Gynec. Obstet. **115**, 677–681 (1962).
Meckstroth, C. V., Broennle, A. M.: Post-emetic rupture of the esophagus. Case report. Ohio St. med. J. **64**, 69–72 (1968).
Menne, F. R., Moore, C. V.: Spontaneous rupture of esophagus in infant. Arch. Pediat. **38**, 672–676 (1921).
Meyer, J.: Ueber Zerreißung der Speiseroehre. Med. Ztg. Berl. **1**, 189 (1858).
Movsas, S.: Spontaneous rupture of the esophagus: Is conservative treatment ever justified? Thorax **21**, 111–114 (1966).
Moynihan, N. H.: Pressure perforation and rupture of the esophagus. Lancet **1954 II**, 728–732.
Naclerio, E. A.: The "V-sign" in the diagnosis of spontaneous rupture of the esophagus (an early roentgen clue). Amer. J. Surg. **93**, 291–298 (1957).
O'Connell, N. D.: Spontaneous rupture of the esophagus. Amer. J. Roentgenol. **99**, 186–203 (1967).
Panaro, V. A., Leslie, E. S.: Spontaneous rupture of the esophagus. Ann. Surg. **161**, 213–217 (1965).
Postlethwait, R. W., Sealy, W. C.: Surgery of the esophagus, p. 133–138. Springfield (Ill.): Thomas 1961.
Priviteri, C. A., Gay, B. B., Jr.: Spontaneous rupture of the esophagus with report of five cases. Radiology **57**, 48–57 (1951).
Raffle, E. J.: Spontaneous rupture of the esophagus and bronchial astma. Lancet **1958 I**, 938–940.
Ross, J. G.: Spontaneous rupture of the middle third of the oesophagus. Brit. J. Surg. **48**, 633–635 (1961).
Russell, J. Y. W., McDonald, N.: Spontaneous rupture of the oesophagus. Brit. J. Surg. **55**, 311–314 (1968).
Samson, P. C.: Post-emetic rupture of esophagus. Surg. Gynec. Obstet. **93**, 221–229 (1951).
Sanderson, R. G.: Spontaneous rupture of the esophagus; report of survival without surgical management. Amer. J. Surg. **109**, 506–508 (1965).
Sealy, W. C.: Rupture of the esophagus. Amer. J. Surg. **105**, 505–510 (1963).
Smead, L. F.: Spontaneous rupture of the esophagus following vomiting. Amer. J. Surg. **13**, 497–501 (1931).
Tesler, M. A., Eisenberg, M. M.: Collective review; spontaneous esophageal rupture. Int. Abstr. Surg. **117**, 1–10 (1963).
Tidman, M. K., John, H. T.: Spontaneous rupture of the esophagus. Brit. J. Surg. **54**, 286–292 (1967).
Toghill, P. J., MacGuire, C. F., Raut, P. S.: "Spontaneous" rupture of healthy esophagus. Postgrad. med. J. **44**, 504–508 (1968).
Wachtel, F. W., Genkins, G.: Spontaneous rupture of normal esophagus: report of case with unusual clinical course and pathologic findings. J. Mt. Sinai Hosp. **22**, 6–14 (1955).
Wiseman, H. J., Celano, E. R., Hester, F. C.: III. Spontaneous rupture of the esophagus in a newborn infant. J. Pediat. **55**, 207–210 (1959).

Iatrogenic Perforations of the Esophagus

J. Janssens and G. Vantrappen

1. Definition

When a perforation of the esophagus is due to diagnostic or therapeutic procedures, it is called iatrogenic.

2. Incidence

Although a wide variety of technical examinations and procedures can cause esophageal perforations, most are caused during endoscopy. The incidence of esophageal perforations due to endoscopic exploration has increased during the last few years, in spite of the advent of flexible instruments. This is probably related to the steadily increasing number of endoscopies, sometimes performed by less experienced endoscopists. When performed expertly, however, esophagoscopy carries a low risk of perforation, the reported figures since 1950 being between 0.06 and 0.10% of the examinations (Table 25). The risk of perforation at gastroscopy is considerably lower still.

Comparable data about the incidence of iatrogenic esophageal perforations due to other causes than endoscopy are not available. It appears that dilatations, particularly when performed without a guiding thread, are the second most frequent cause (Table 26).

Table 25: Incidence of esophageal perforations by endoscopy

Author	Number of examinations	Incidence of esophageal perforations in %
Jones et al., 1951	49 000 gastroscopies	0.1
Bell et al., 1956	35 000 endoscopies	0.71
Smith and Tanner, 1956	605 esophagoscopies 7 200 gastroscopies	1.5 0.3
Palmer and Wirts, 1957	40 540 esophagoscopies 267 175 gastroscopies	0.23 0.06
Brick, 1961	1 000 esophagoscopies	0.2
Elner and Dahlbäck, 1962	3 965 esophagoscopies	0.5
Steyn and Brunnen, 1962	1 978 esophagoscopies	0.4
Alford et al., 1963	2 156 esophagoscopies	0.3
Johnson and Schwegeman, 1967		0.8
Hegemann and Gall, 1967	978 esophagoscopies	0.6
Wychulis et al., 1969	8 038 endoscopies gastroscopies alone	0.4 0.06
Mark and Knauer, 1969	700 endoscopies	0.7

Table 26. Relative importance of several procedures in the pathogenesis of esophageal perforation
Number of perforations

	Groves, 1966	Zittel and Boden, 1966	Maillard, 1967	Hegemann and Gall 1967	Youngs and Nicoloff, 1969	Wichern, 1970	Total
Endoscopy with or without biopsy	10	91	11	9	12	66	199
Endoscopy with dilatation	2					21	23
Endoscopy with extraction of foreign body		23	4				27
Dilatation	4	54	7	9	3	25	102
Gastric or duodenal tube insertion		1	3	2	2	9	17
Endotracheal intubation	1	4				13	18
Surgery						19	19
Total	17	173	25	20	17	153	405

3. Etiology and Pathogenesis

Most endoscopic perforations are due to crushing of the posterior esophageal wall between the instrument and the cervical spine. Exaggerated hyperextension of the neck and the presence of cervical osteophytes increase the risk of perforation. The danger of crush injuries was decreased by the advent of fiber endoscopes. But even with the fiber endoscope, an instrument which was thought to be completely safe, 5 esophageal perforations were reported recently (Anselm et al., 1970). The practice of intubating the trachea whenever esophagoscopy is performed under general anesthesia has been abandoned as it increases the risk of crush injuries of the posterior wall of the esophagus (Wychulis et al., 1969).

Spasm of the cricopharyngeal muscle, which results in a deviation and kinking of the pharyngoesophageal lumen, increases the risk of perforation of the pyriform sinus. No wonder that, at the time of the rigid esophagoscope, this level was called "the gate of tears" of the inexperienced esophagoscopist. This complication is observed more frequently when the endoscopy is performed under local anesthesia than when it is carried out under general narcosis (Flavell, 1963). Firm closure of the mouth of the esophagus should not be forced by exerting pressure on the endoscope, but can be overcome by asking the patient to swallow.

An endoscopic perforation can also occur at the level of the esophageal body, generally when an organic lesion is present (diverticulum, achalasia, stricture, carcinoma). In a normal esophageal body, the perforation is almost always located at one of its 3 natural narrowings, i.e. at the level of the aortic arch, the left main bronchus or the pillars of the diaphragm. Exceptionally the endoscope may perforate the mucosa first, continue for a few centimeters intramurally, and then perforate the muscular layer (DUBOST and EVARD, 1964). In other instances the endoscope causes a mucosal trauma, resulting in an intramural abscess which perforates later (MOUNIER-KUHN et al., 1963; PIQUET et al., 1964). Endoscopic removal of foreign bodies carries a higher risk of perforation, especially if the object to be extracted is fairly large or has sharp edges.

Bougienage is the second most frequent cause of iatrogenic esophageal perforations (Table 26). Yet the risk of perforation is very small if a guiding thread is used. BILL et al. (1963) reported 10 perforations in a series of 300 dilatations without guiding thread, whereas no perforation occurred in the 120 cases where this guide was used. Pneumatic dilatations for achalasia of the cardia cause perforation in about 2% of the cases (OLSEN et al., 1959; VANTRAPPEN et al., 1971) (Fig. 183). Other causes of iatrogenic perforation of the esophagus are endotracheal intubation (ZITTEL and BODEN, 1966; WICHERN, 1970), insertion of a Mackler tube for inoperable carcinoma (YOUNGS and NICOLOFF, 1969), introduction of radium-containing sounds (STEPHENSON et al., 1968), and aspiration of mucus secretion in the newborn (ASTLEY and ROBERTS, 1970). A Sengstaken-Blakemore tube for tamponade of bleeding esophageal varices can also lead to perforation (ZITTEL and BODEN, 1966). The esophagus can be perforated accidentally during surgery in the proximity of the gullet, such as thyroid surgery (STEPHENSON et al., 1968), lung resection or excision of a bronchogenic cyst (BRIGGS and GERMANN, 1968), vagotomy (POSTLETHWAIT et al., 1969) or hiatal hernia repair (FOSTER et al., 1965). A more ingenious perforation occurred in a patient with an esophageal diverticulum, who had taken a hydrophilic laxative, part of which was retained in the pouch where it swelled and caused a rupture (WICHERN, 1970).

4. Symptoms and Diagnosis

The symptoms of an iatrogenic esophageal perforation are determined by the nature of the examination or the procedure which caused it. An accidental perforation during surgery in the proximity of the esophagus is generally noticed during the procedure and can be closed at once. By contrast, an esophageal perforation during aspiration of pharyngeal secretions in the newborn is likely to go unrecognized for some time. An endoscopic perforation in the body of the esophagus is usually noticed during the examination itself, but crush-injuries of the cervical esophagus and perforations of the piriform sinus are rarely diagnosed immediately. The only sign of perforation may be blood on the distal extremity of the endoscope after examination (SPIRO, 1970). Perforation should be suspected if the examination was technically difficult or accompanied by considerable bleeding, or if the patient suffers severe pain or unexplained fever after the examination.

Pain is a very telling symptom. Immediately after endoscopy a patient frequently has discomfort or mild pain in the throat. If it continues for more than 12 hours after the examination or if it is more pronounced and increases in the course of time, a traumatic lesion of the esophagus should be strongly suspected. Cervical lesions are associated with pain in the neck, which occurs mainly after deglutition and aggravates when an inflammatory reaction develops. Usually there is abundant secretion of saliva, which may be bloody. Thoracic lesions produce pain in the substernal region and in the back, increasing upon deglutition and respiration. If the perforation occurs in the abdominal segment of the esophagus, it produces epigastric pain radiating to the back and mimicking an acute abdomen. Soon dysphagia develops together with fever and leukocytosis. Hematemesis can occur but is seen only rarely (MAILLARD, 1967). The mediastinal emphysema associated with a thoracic esophageal perforation will ascend into the neck and cause the typical crepitation on palpation. A cervical perforation, when large, may also lead to emphysema. Respiratory difficulties due to pleural involvement occur late, unless the perforation is very large. In some cases the typical symptoms of an instrumental esophageal perforation may be delayed for hours, restlessness and tachycardia being the only symptoms (STEPHENSON et al., 1968).

The triad consisting of pain, dyspnea and fever is observed in about 50% of the instrumental esophageal perforations and should be considered pathognomonic unless the contrary is proven (GERARD et al., 1968; STEPHENSON et al., 1968). Subcutaneous emphysema in the neck establishes the diagnosis. If the perforation remains untreated, the infection spreads and, in the case of a high perforation, causes redness and induration in the supraclavicular and suprasternal regions. Thoracic perforations lead to mediastinitis and pleural effusion with hydro-(pneumo)thorax. Finally cyanosis, shock and death ensue.

The technical examinations to ascertain and localize an iatrogenic perforation have been described in the chapter on spontaneous esophageal rupture.

5. Treatment

The treatment of an iatrogenic perforation of the esophagus is determined in part by the presence or absence of underlying esophageal pathology. A distal obstruction, for instance, must be treated if leakage of the sutured perforation is to be avoided. If the perforation occurs in an apparently normal esophagus the treatment is determined by the localization of the perforation, its size and by the time interval since the accident. Some authors advocate conservative treatment. MENGOLI and KLASSEN (1965) reported on their series of 21 esophageal perforations due to esophagoscopy, 18 of whom were treated conservatively; the mortality rate was 5.5%. Yet most authors agree that the majority of iatrogenic esophageal perforations must be treated immediately with drainage and, if possible, closure of the rupture, whereas only the smaller cervical lesions can be treated conservatively. ZITTEL and BODEN (1966) collected from the literature 177 cases of iatrogenic esophageal perforation; 70 patients were treated conservatively, with a mortality rate of 37.1%; 58 were treated with drainage only, with a mortality of 22.4%, and in 49 cases the drainage was complemented by suturing of the rupture, which resulted in a mortality of only 10.2%. The mortality rate of cervical perforations after either conservative or surgical treatment was considerably lower ($\pm 15\%$) than that of thoracic perforations ($\pm 30\%$). Most authors seem to agree with the following therapeutical scheme (GROVES, 1966; ZITTEL and BODEN, 1966; BRIGGS and GERMANN, 1968; YOUNGS and NICOLOFF, 1969; BOYD and WITTMANN, 1971).

Conservative treatment is sufficient for pinpoint perforations of the cervical esophagus as well as for perforations due to dilatation of a caustic stricture which is often associated with extensive periesophageal fibrosis. Large cervical perforations with infection spreading to the mediastinum, however, generally require surgical drainage of neck and mediastinum. Thoracic perforations must always be treated surgically. If the treatment can be undertaken within 24 hours after the accident a pleural drainage and suture of the perforation are performed. The suture must be carefully protected with a pleural flap (DOOLING and ZICK, 1967). Treatment beginning at a later stage must be limited to pleural drainage via a thoracotomy. Perforations of the distal segment of the esophagus can be treated in the same manner and the suture can be protected with an onlay gastric patch (HATAFUKU and THAL, 1964; MARK and KNAUER, 1969). Perforations by pneumatic dilatations for achalasia can be treated conservatively if they are recognized immediately (VANTRAPPEN et al., 1971) (see Treatment of Achalasia).

A very aggressive treatment was proposed by JOHNSON et al. (1956, 1968) and consists of exteriorization of the cervical esophagus and ligation of the distal esophageal segment, to be followed in a later stage by the interposition of a colonic segment. This type of treatment should be carried out only if other measures are impossible or insufficient.

High doses of a broad spectrum antibiotic and parenteral feeding are indicated. Sometimes even a jejunostomy must be performed (BOYD and WITTMANN, 1971). In cases of cervical perforation, or of thoracic rupture which can be closed surgically, drinking can be resumed after 48 hours, but a normal diet should not be started until after the 7th or 8th day (GROVES, 1966; BRIGGS and GERMANN, 1968).

References

ALFORD, B. R., JOHNSON, R. L., HARRIS, H. H.: Penetrating and perforating injuries of the esophagus. Ann. Otol. 72, 995–1004 (1963).

ANSELM, K., SHARTSIS, J. M., CARANDANG, N. V., PRIEST, R. J.: Perforation of the esophagus with the gastrocamera fiberscope. Amer. J. dig. Dis. 15, 311–315 (1970).

ASTLEY, R., ROBERTS, K. D.: Intubation perforation of the oesophagus in the newborn baby. Brit. J. Radiol. 43, 219–222 (1970).

BELL, J. W., BESKIN, C. A., STARKEY, G. W. B.: Mediastinal abscess following instrumental perforation of the esophagus. Amer. J. Surg. 91, 999–1003 (1956).

BILL, A. H., JR., MEBUST, W. K., SAUVAGE, L. R.: Evaluation of techniques of esophageal dilatations in relation to the danger of perforation: A study of 441 dilatations of benign strictures in children. J. thorac. cardiovasc. Surg. 45, 510–514 (1963).

BOYD, D. P., WITTMANN, C. J., JR.: Some principles in treating perforation of the esophagus. Surg. Clin. N. Amer. 51, 567–574 (1971).

BRICK, I. B.: Esophagoscopy by and for the internist: A review of results in a thousand patients. Amer. J. med. Sci. 241, 289–295 (1961).

BRIGGS, J. N., GERMANN, T. D.: Traumatic perforations of the esophagus. Surg. Clin. N. Amer. 48, 1297–1302 (1968).

DOOLING, J. A., ZICK, H. R.: Closure of an esophagopleural fistula, using onlay intercostal pedicle graft. Ann. thorac. Surg. 3, 553–557 (1967).

DUBOST, C., EVARD, C.: A propos de deux accidents de la gastroscopie, reconnus tardivement et guéris. Ann. Chir. 18, 1556–1562 (1964).

ELNER, A., DAHLBÄCK, O.: Instrumental perforation of the esophagus. Acta oto-laryng. (Stockh.) 54, 279–286 (1962).

FLAVELL, G.: The oesophagus. London: Butterworths 1963.

FOSTER, J. H., JOLLY, P. C., SAWYERS, J. L., DANIEL, R. A.: Esophageal perforation: diagnosis and treatment. Ann. Surg. 161, 701–709 (1965).

GERARD, F. P., SABETY, A. M., TRILLO, R. A., FERNANDO, M. B.: Esophageal perforation. Arch. Surg. 96, 414–419 (1968).

GROVES, L. K.: Instrumental perforation of the esophagus. What is conservative management? J. thorac. cardiovasc. Surg. 52, 1–10 (1966).

HATAFUKU, T., THAL, A. P.: The use of the onlay gastric patch with experimental perforations of the distal esophagus. Surgery 56, 556–560 (1964).

HEGEMANN, G., GALL, F.: Diagnose und Behandlung instrumenteller Ösophagusverletzungen. Thoraxchirurgie 15, 233–240 (1967).

JOHNSON, J., SCHWEGMAN, C. W.: Iatrogenic and spontaneous perforation of the esophagus. Amer. J. Gastroent. 47, 365–372 (1967).

JOHNSON, J., SCHWEGMAN, C. W., KIRBY, C. K.: Esophageal exclusion for persistent fistula following spontaneous rupture of the esophagus. J. Thorac. Surg. 32, 827–832 (1956).

JOHNSON, J., SCHWEGMAN, C. W., McVAUGH, H.: Early esophagogastrostomy in the treatment of iatrogenic perforation of the distal esophagus. J. Thorac. Cardiovasc. Surg. 55, 24–29 (1968).

JONES, F. A., DOLL, R., FLETCHER, C., RODGERS, H. W.: The risk of gastroscopy: a survey of 49,000 examinations. Lancet 1951 I, 647.

MAILLARD, J. N.: Les plaies de l'oesophage. Acta chir. belg. 66, 725–746 (1967).

MARK, J. B. D., KNAUER, C. M.: Use of the onlay gastric patch in instrumental rupture of the esophagus. J. thorac. cardiovasc. Surg. 57, 813–816 (1969).

Mengoli, L. R., Klassen, K. P.: Conservative management of esophageal perforation. Arch. Surg. **91**, 238–240 (1965).

Mounier-Kuhn, P., Gaillard, J., Haguenauer, J. P., Charachon, P., Morgon, A., Charachon, D.: Les incidents et accidents de l'oesophagoscopie. J. franç. Oto-rhino-laryng. **17**, 473–474 (1963).

Olsen, A. M., Harrington, S. W., Moersch, H. J., Andersen, H. A.: The treatment of cardiospasm: analysis of a twelve-year experience. J. thorac. cardiovasc. Surg. **22**, 164–187 (1959).

Palmer, E. D., Wirts, W. C.: Survey of gastroscopic and esophagoscopic accidents. Report of committee on accidents of the American Gastroscopic Society. J. Amer. med. Ass. **164**, 2012–2015 (1957).

Piquet, J., Decroix, G., Piquet, J. J.: Les perforations de l'oesophage. Ann. Oto-laryng. (Paris) **81**, 119–127 (1964).

Postlethwait, R. W., Seuk, K. K., Dillon, M. L.: Esophageal complications of vagotomy. Surg. Gynec. Obstet. **128**, 481–488 (1969).

Smith, C. C. K., Tanner, N. C.: Complications of gastroscopy and oesophagoscopy. Brit. J. Surg. **43**, 396–403 (1956).

Spiro, H. M.: Clinical gastroenterology, p. 79. New Haven: Yale University School of Medicine 1970.

Stephenson, H. E., McLeod, R. A., McCraw, J. B., McKenzie, J. W., McDonald, W., English, M. T.: Perforation of the esophagus. A challenge to early diagnosis. Amer. J. Surg. **115**, 648–650 (1968).

Steyn, J. H., Brunnen, P. L.: Perforation of cervical esophagus at esophagoscopy. Scot. med. J. **7**, 494–497 (1962).

Vantrappen, G., Hellemans, J., Deloof, W., Valembois, P., Vandenbroucke, J.: Treatment of achalasia with pneumatic dilatations. Gut **12**, 268–275 (1971).

Wichern, W. A., Jr.: Perforation of the esophagus. Amer. J. Surg. **119**, 534–536 (1970).

Wychulis, A. R., Fontana, R. S., Payne, W. S.: Instrumental perforation of the esophagus. Dis. Chest **55**, 184–189 (1969).

Youngs, J., Nicoloff, D.: Management of esophageal perforation. Surgery **65**, 264–268 (1969).

Zittel, R. X., Boden, T.: Erkennung und Behandlung iatrogener Ösophagusperforationen. Med. Klin. **61**, 1111–1113 (1966).

Mallory-Weiss Syndrome

J. JANSSENS and P. VALEMBOIS

1. Definition

The syndrome of Mallory-Weiss can be defined as a gastrointestinal bleeding caused by mucosal laceration at the lower part of the esophagus and/or the cardiac portion of the stomach, elicited by a more or less sudden increase of the intragastric pressure.

2. History

In 1929 MALLORY and WEISS published 4 cases of acute upper gastrointestinal bleeding, which at autopsy were found to be due to mucosal tears at the cardia. In 1932 they added another 15 clinically analogue cases to the series; this time, however, without surgical or pathological proof. Actually, already in 1879 QUINCKE had described a similar case of gastrointestinal bleeding, but he had not noticed the connection with vomiting. WHITING and BARRON (1955) described the first ante-mortem diagnosis in a patient who underwent successful surgery afterwards. The first endoscopic diagnosis was made by HARDLY (1956). Until 1960 only a few case reports were published, but afterwards more attention was again paid to the syndrome as a possible cause of massive high gastrointestinal bleeding, and several series of more than 10 cases were published (ATKINSON et al., 1961; GRIMES, 1964; FREEARK et al., 1964; HOLMES, 1966; DAGRADI et al., 1966; NIELSEN and ZACHARIAE, 1970).

3. Incidence

The syndrome of Mallory-Weiss is considered to be the cause of between 1 and 15% of all massive upper gastrointestinal bleedings. BERKOWITZ (1963) published 200 autopsy cases of patients who died from the consequences of an upper gastrointestinal bleeding; in 2 cases he found mucosal tears. KATZ et al. (1965) examined endoscopically 297 hospitalized patients with gastrointestinal bleeding and made a diagnosis of Mallory-Weiss syndrome in 2.02% of them. PALMER (1961) found the syndrome to be the cause of upper gastrointestinal bleeding in 3.5% of 650 cases. In 1966 his series had increased to 2178 cases and the incidence of mucosal tears had increased to 4.9%. By endoscopy DAGRADI et al. (1966) found mucosal tears in 12% of all massive gastrointestinal bleedings, while WELLS (1967) observed by endoscopy an actively bleeding tear around the cardioesophageal junction in 25 cases out of 170 acute gastrointestinal bleedings (14%). Probably the latter number comes closest to the real incidence. If no early fiber esophagogastroscopy is performed, many gastrointestinal bleedings go undiagnosed [in the series of AVERY JONES (1956) 21%]; part of these are probably caused by mucosal tears.

The syndrome occurs more frequently in men than in women (DOBBINS, 1963; CLEMENZ and DAWSON, 1966). Although it may be observed at all ages the peak incidence lies between 40 and 50.

4. Pathogenesis

In their original article Mallory and Weiss (1929) described the syndrome as a massive hematemesis after prolonged alcoholic indulgence and preceded by bloodless vomiting. The causative lesion is a tear in the mucosa with bleeding from the submucosal lacerated arteries. The esophagogastric junction is rich in blood vessels, which explains why even a superficial tear can cause considerable loss of blood.

Although vomiting is frequently the cause of the mucosal tears Atkinson and Mitchell (1962) demonstrated that the provoking factor is an increase of the intraabdominal pressure, whatever its origin. In their series of 14 patients vomiting was found in only 6; other causes of mucosal tears were intense coughing-fits, an attack of epilepsy, a status asthmaticus or non-productive retching. By inflating the stomachs of cadavers in situ they demonstrated that mucosal tears could be caused from a pressure of 150 mm Hg. The localization of the tears at the esophagogastric junction is due to extragastric factors, because in an isolated stomach no specific localization is prominent. Atkinson et al. (1961) further demonstrated in volunteers that during provoked vomiting the intragastric pressure may rise for several seconds to levels of 120 to 160 mm Hg, whereas peak pressures up to 200 mm Hg also occur. Not the absolute intragastric pressure is important but the pressure difference across the gastric wall. Therefore, hiatus hernia is a predisposing factor. Since the intraesophageal pressure, which is a measure of the intrathoracic pressure, reaches only 50 mm Hg during vomiting (Atkinson et al., 1961), the pressure gradient across the wall of the herniated sac can reach up to 100 mm Hg at that moment. Already Fleischner (1956) pointed to the importance of a sliding hernia in the pathogenesis of the Mallory-Weiss syndrome. In the series of Atkinson et al. (1961) a hiatus hernia could be demonstrated radiologically in 4 out of 11 cases, while Dagradi et al. (1966) found a small sliding hernia in all of their 30 patients. Although a hiatus hernia cannot be clearly demonstrated radiologically in each patient with mucosal tears, it is not impossible that a temporary hernia occurs during the vomiting movements. Nauta (1956) demonstrated that this is indeed the case in dogs.

It is difficult to find out to what extent mucosal atrophy plays an important etiological role, because this lesion occurs so frequently. It is not impossible that the required pressure gradient is lower when the mucosa is atrophic. This would also explain why mucosal tears are found especially at a later age. Nielsen and Zachariae (1970) determined the gastric acid secretion after histamine stimulation in 8 of their patients with Mallory-Weiss syndrome and found very divergent values suggesting that extensive atrophic gastritis is not an obligatory factor.

Though Mallory and Weiss (1929–1932) cited chronic alcoholism as a constant finding in these patients, this was not confirmed in later series. On the other hand it is logical that rupture occurs more easily after copious meals, because a filled stomach can withstand an increase in pressure less easily.

The pathogenesis of mucosal tears and of spontaneous esophageal rupture is identical. Transitions between both lesions are known such as the intramural dissection of the esophagus (Thompson et al., 1967). As yet not a single case of a proven Mallory-Weiss syndrome which ruptured afterward has been described, except maybe the patient described by Zikria et al. (1965); in this patient the diagnosis of mucosal tears was established only on clinical data.

Why an increase in intragastric pressure results in a mucosal tear at the gastroesophageal junction or in a rupture of the esophagus has not been definitely determined. There is some evidence that in the stomach and in the most distal part of the esophagus the muscularis can be still further extended at the moment that the mucosa has been extended maximally: somewhat higher in the esophagus this difference in elasticity does not exist any more (LION-CACHET, 1963).

5. Clinical Features

The most typical history begins with retching or vomiting of normal stomach contents on one or more occasions, followed by vomiting of red blood. In contrast with the esophageal rupture the epigastric pain is much less pronounced and it is especially the bleeding that is prominent. Because it is an arterial bleeding it can be massive: in the series of FREEARK et al. (1964) (13 cases) a mean of 5.7 liters of blood was necessary; HOLMES (1966) gave to 8 patients who were operated upon an average of 5.2 liters each with an average of 3.5 liters preoperatively.

In other cases the bleeding is less pronounced and causes only melena, or a hematemesis after several hours (KELLEY, 1958). Sometimes bleeding is minimal with only a few traces of blood through the vomited material; it may be even totally absent as was described by ATKINSON et al. (1961) and KATZ et al. (1965).

As already indicated, vomiting is not obligatorily the provoking factor; all factors which cause an increase in intragastric pressure can provoke mucosal tears. In the literature we found 151 cases of Mallory-Weiss syndrome the etiology of which was indicated; in 138 cases (91%) the tear had occurred after vomiting; 65 patients (43%) had a history of vomiting after alcohol abusus. In other cases the cause was a severe coughing-fit, a status asthmaticus, an attack of epilepsy, a blunt abdominal trauma and squeezing during delivery. A few cases occurred in which the bleeding itself was the first symptom.

Clinical examination is not very relevant except for the symptoms of bleeding which can be more or less severe.

6. Diagnosis

The most important point in diagnosing mucosal tears is to think of the possibility, especially when hematemesis occurs after a period of vomiting. When mucosal tears happen without bleeding, and both ATKINSON et al. (1961) and KATZ et al. (1965) described such cases, clinical diagnosis is practically impossible.

Once the possibility of Mallory-Weiss syndrome has been taken into account, the diagnosis can usually be confirmed most easily by an esophagogastroscopy. For an experienced endoscopist the active bleeding is mostly not an insuperable obstacle to localize the site of bleeding (KATZ et al., 1965). On endoscopical examination one finds one or more longitudinal fissures with sharp edges and a base which is covered with blood or seropurulent exudate.

According to ATKINSON et al. (1961) the diagnosis can even be established retrospectively, when esophagoscopy is performed within 8 days after the bleeding has stopped. The healing tear appears as a linear greyish scar with red edges.

The radiological diagnosis of mucosal tears is very difficult. Only a few cases have been described in which the radiological diagnosis was suspected by the presence of contrast material in the wall of the stomach or the esophagus (DOBBINS, 1963; SPARBERG, 1968). Recently ANTONIO et al. (1970) described a proven case of Mallory-Weiss syndrome in which a persisting collection of contrast material could be seen radiologically in the upper left lateral aspect of a small hiatus hernia.

KOEHLER (1969) succeeded in confirming the diagnosis in three cases by selective arteriography of the celiac artery. The differential diagnosis must of course be made with all causes of upper gastrointestinal bleeding, especially with spontaneous rupture of the esophagus.

7. Pathology

The macroscopic lesion consists of one or more longitudinal fissures of the mucosa and submucosa in the lower part of the esophagus and/or the cardiac portion of the stomach. These tears are 3 to 20 mm long and 2 to 3 mm wide. Sometimes the lesions occur pear-shaped, with the sharp end turned towards the stomach. The basis is covered with blood or with yellow slough; the edges are sharp with some swelling of the surrounding mucosa. Microscopically it appears as an acute inflamed ulcer, which perforates the muscularis mucosa. Mostly these ulcers are not deeper than the submucosa, rarely they reach the musculosa. The craters contain blood and a fibrinopurulent exudate; the bottom is edematous and acutely inflamed. There is no fibrous reaction. Usually one finds a network of broad thin-walled blood vessels in the surrounding submucosa.

8. Treatment

The treatment is determined by the severity of the bleeding. In the beginning conservative treatment is indicated. Mostly the bleeding will stop spontaneously. The gastric contents will be evacuated by tube, as a full stomach is a contributing factor to the genesis of mucosal tears. Antiemetics must be administered to prevent further vomiting and new bleeding. When the bleeding has stopped, the nasogastric tube is removed after 24 hours and fluid feeding can be started (Holmes, 1966).

If the bleeding does not stop spontaneously or if it cannot be controlled by conservative means an urgent laparotomy is indicated; after ligating the bleeding points the tears are sewed with catgut. A Sengstaken-Blakemore tube will mostly not suffice because the bleeding is arterial and the pressure in the balloon is not sufficently high to compress the arteries. At any rate, a blind subtotal gastrectomy for a massive bleeding without known etiology must be rejected. In these cases the gastrotomy will be elongated to the upper side and the cardia can be explored eventually with a sterile endoscope in order not to miss the possibility of a mucosal tear at the cardia.

The prognosis is favourable when the diagnosis has been made in time by an early esophagogastroscopy or by an exploratory gastrotomy.

In the series of Wells (1967), consisting of 25 cases in which the diagnosis was made endoscopically during the phase of active bleeding, not a single death occurred; no more than 5 patients needed surgery with suture of the tear. Except for one case in the series of Wells (1967) and one in the series of Nielsen and Zachariae (1970) no recurrences have been reported.

References

Antonio, J. M. T., Hunter, C. H., Dobbins, W. O.: Mallory-Weiss syndrome: A radiologic diagnosis. Amer. J. dig. Dis. 15, 1043–1044 (1970).

Atkinson, M., Bottrill, M. B., Edwards, A. T., Mitchell, W. M., Peet, B. G., Williams, R. E.: Mucosal tears at the esophagogastric junction (the Mallory-Weiss syndrome). Gut 2, 1–11 (1961).

Atkinson, M., Mitchell, W. H.: The mechanism whereby Mallory-Weiss mucosal tears at the cardia are produced. Surgical physiology of the gastrointestinal tract. Proceedings of a symposium held in the Royal College of Surgeons of Edinburgh, p. 35–39. Edinburgh and London: Morrison and Gibb Ltd. 1962.

BERKOWITZ, D.: Fatal gastrointestinal hemorrhage: Diagnostic implications from a study of 200 cases. Amer. J. Gastroent. 40, 372–377 (1963).

CLEMENZ, F. W., DAWSON, R. G.: Esophageal dyskinesia and the Mallory-Weiss syndrome. Arch. Surg. 93, 614–615 (1955).

DAGRADI, A. E., BRODERICK, J. T., JULER, G., WOLINSKY, S., STEMPIEN, S. J.: The Mallory-Weiss syndrome and lesion. A study of 30 cases. Amer. J. dig. Dis. 11, 710–721 (1966).

DOBBINS, W. O.: Mallory-Weiss syndrome: a commonly overlooked cause of upper gastrointestinal bleeding. Report of three cases and review of the literature. Gastroenterology 44, 689–695 (1963).

FLEISCHNER, F. G.: Hiatus hernia complex. Hiatus hernia, peptic esophagitis, Mallory-Weiss syndrome, hemorrhage and anemia, and marginal esophagogastric ulcer. J. Amer. med. Ass. 162, 183–191 (1956).

FREEARK, R. J., NORCROSS, W. J., BAKER, R. J., STROHL, E. J.: The Mallory-Weiss syndrome. Arch. Surg. 88, 882–887 (1964).

GRIMES, O. F.: Surgical management of massive gastrointestinal hemorrhage from cardio-esophageal lacerations. Amer. J. Surg. 108, 285–296 (1964).

HARDLY, J. T.: Mallory-Weiss syndrome. Report of case diagnosed by gastroscopy. Gastroenterology 30, 681–685 (1956).

HOLMES, K. D.: Mallory-Weiss syndrome: review of 20 cases and literature review. Ann. Surg. 164, 810–820 (1966).

JONES, F. A.: Hematemesis and melena with special reference to causation and to the factors influencing the mortality from bleeding peptic ulcer. Gastroenterology 30, 166–190 (1956).

KATZ, D., FREUD, M., McKINNON, W. M. P.: The Mallory-Weiss syndrome: evaluation by early endoscopy of its clinical picture and its incidence in upper gastrointestinal hemorrhage. Amer. J. dig. Dis. 10, 314–323 (1965).

KELLEY, M. L., JR.: Massive hemorrhage following gastroscopy. Probable example of Mallory-Weiss syndrome. Amer. J. dig. Dis. 3, 454–463 (1958).

KOEHLER, P. R.: New approaches to the radiological diagnosis of Mallory-Weiss syndrome. Brit. J. Radiol. 42, 354–357 (1969).

LION-CACHET, J.: Gastric fundal mucosal tears. Brit. J. Surg. 50, 985–986 (1963).

MALLORY, G. K., WEISS, S.: Hemorrhages of the cardiac orifice of the stomach due to vomiting. Amer. J. med. Sci. 178, 506–515 (1929).

NAUTA, J.: The closing mechanism between the esophagus and the stomach. Gastroenterologia (Basel) 86, 219–232 (1956).

NIELSEN, P. E., ZACHARIAE, F.: The Mallory-Weiss syndrome. Acta path. microbiol. scand., Suppl. 212, 166–175 (1970).

PALMER, E. D.: Diagnosis of upper gastrointestinal hemorrhage. Springfield (Ill.): Charles C. Thomas 1961.

PALMER, E. D.: Seasonal incidence of upper gastrointestinal tract bleeding. J. Amer. med. Ass. 198, 184–185 (1966).

QUINCKE, H.: Ulcus oesophagi ex digestione. Dtsch. Arch. klin. Med. 24, 72 (1879).

SPARBERG, M.: Roentgenographic documentation of the Mallory-Weiss syndrome. J. Amer. med. Ass. 203, 151–152 (1968).

THOMPSON, N. W., CALVIN, B. E., FRY, W. J.: The spectrum of emetogemic injury to the esophagus and stomach. Amer. J. Surg. 113, 13–26 (1967).

WEISS, S., MALLORY, G. K.: Lesions of the cardiac orifice of the stomach produced by vomiting. J. Amer. med. Ass. 98, 1353–1355 (1932).

WELLS, R. F.: A common cause of upper gastrointestinal bleeding. The Mallory-Weiss syndrome. Sth. med. J. (Bgham, Ala.) 60, 1197–1201 (1967).

WHITING, E. G., BARRON, G.: Massive hemorrhage from a laceration, apparently caused by vomiting, in the cardiac region of the stomach, with recovery. Calif. Med. 82, 188–189 (1955).

ZIKRIA, B. A., ROSENTHAL, A. D., POTTER, R. T., FERRER, J. H.: Mallory-Weiss syndrome and emetogenic (spontaneous) rupture of the esophagus. Ann. Surg. 162, 151–155 (1965).

Intramural Rupture and Bleeding

J. Janssens and G. Vantrappen

1. Etiology

In some cases traumata of the esophagus are limited to part of the esophageal wall, without causing a complete perforation; they may then result in intramural dissection, intramural bleeding or intramural abscess formation. The intramural lesion may be caused by endoscopic exploration (Borrie, 1958; Lichter and Borrie, 1965) or by aspiration of the oropharynx of the neonate with a suction catheter (Eklöf et al., 1969). Sanborn (1960) mentioned foreign bodies as another cause of intramural esophageal perforations with abscess formation (Fig. 99). He suggested that the "esophageal phlegmons" that are described by endoscopists may in fact be due to intramural rupture by foreign bodies. The first case of "spontaneous" intramural esophageal dissection after vomiting was described by Thompson et al. (1967). Marks and Keet (1968) described an intramural esophageal perforation occurring during a rather hurriedly eaten meal. Borrie and Sheat (1970) reported on a patient who suffered an intramural perforation because "he stifled a sneeze in the very act of swallowing a portion of a sandwich lunch".

In other cases the intramural lesion is associated with an extensive intramural hematoma (Williams, 1957). An intramural hematoma may develop during the course of treatment with anticoagulants (Benjamin and Hanks, 1965), or as a complication of, for instance, vagotomy (Rabiah and Elliott, 1968).

2. Pathogenesis

The pathogenesis of an intramural lesion due to an esophageal trauma caused by a foreign body or by the insertion of instruments is clear enough. If the trauma does not penetrate beyond the mucosa into the muscle layer, infected material such as saliva and food accumulates between the mucosa and the muscle layer and may lead to a progressive dissection, eventually resulting in an intramural abscess. When the lesion is located in the upper part of the esophagus the dissection is usually arrested at the level of the aortic arch (Borrie and Sheat, 1970). The pathogenesis of the so-called spontaneous intramural perforations and hemorrhages is less obvious. As in the Boerhaave or the Mallory-Weiss syndrome, it could be due to a sudden increase in intraesophageal pressure (Thompson et al., 1967; Talley and Nicks, 1969). However, as the mucosa offers a greater resistance to tears than any other layer of the esophagus (McKenzie, 1884; Derrick et al., 1958), it must be assumed that the intramural perforation is favored by already existing minor lesions of the mucosa, due, for instance, to esophagitis (Talley and Nicks, 1969).

3. Symptoms

Intramural rupture is characterized by sudden severe retrosternal pain and dysphagia, usually occurring during a meal, and frequently by a small hematemesis

(TALLEY and NICKS, 1969). In contrast with complete esophageal rupture, there is no mediastinal or cervical subcutaneous emphysema, and the general condition of the patient is not nearly as bad. He may have some fever and a reactive pleural effusion is not infrequent. Whereas the Mallory-Weiss syndrome is characterized primarily by hematemesis, the prominent symptoms of intramural rupture are pain and dysphagia (MARKS and KEET, 1968).

In infants a traumatic submucosal perforation may mimic the symptoms of esophageal atresia: hypersalivation, choking, coughing and cyanosis during attempts at feeding.

4. Radiological Features and Diagnosis

Radiology is the main diagnostic tool. The examination should be started by plain chest X-rays to look for signs of complete perforation, such as air in the mediastinum. As it is difficult to exclude a complete perforation beforehand, water-soluble contrast media, such as Gastrografin, must be used. If the swallowed contrast medium penetrates into the intramural dissecting lesion, a narrow stripe of contrast medium is seen parallel to the esophagus. This has been described as "double barrelled esophagus" (LICHTER and BORRIE, 1965; THOMPSON et al., 1967; ALBOT et al., 1969; JOFFE and MILLAN, 1970) or as "mucosal stripe sign" (LOWMAN et al., 1969). It is important to have the patient drink some water during the examination, which will remove the intraluminal but not the extraluminal contrast medium. X-rays taken some time after the contrast swallow are very informative because they show persistent contrast medium in the esophageal wall, or, if the contrast medium has disappeared there, because they are an argument for the existence of a second opening (BORRIE and SHEAT, 1970). Sometimes filling of the false intramural channel can only be obtained on a second contrast swallow a few days later (JOFFE and MILLAN, 1970).

The contrast medium extravasated in intramural lesions remains in close approximation with the esophageal lumen. This is generally not the case in complete esophageal perforations and this may help to differentiate both conditions. In children, the image of a "double barrelled esophagus" may also be due to congenital duplication of the esophagus, but here the communication is generally located in the distal part of the gullet (GROSS, 1953; EKLÖF et al., 1969).

If the swallowed contrast medium does not penetrate into the dissecting space, filling defects are found instead of a "double barrelled esophagus". Healing sometimes results in esophageal stenosis (ALBOT et al., 1969).

The hematoma formation secondary to vagotomy may cause a narrowing of the distal esophagus, mimicking achalasia both radiologically and clinically (RABIAH and ELLIOTT, 1968). Endoscopy is contraindicated in view of the danger of complete perforation.

5. Treatment

Before treatment is started it is mandatory to establish the differential diagnosis between complete and partial esophageal perforation, because complete rupture generally requires surgery, whereas an intramural lesion can be managed by conservative means (MARKS and KEET, 1968; EKLÖF et al., 1969; LOWMAN et al., 1969; TALLEY and NICKS, 1969; ALBOT et al., 1969; BORRIE and SHEAT, 1970).

Peroral feeding is stopped, antibiotics are administered, and it may be useful to aspirate the stomach in order to prevent reflux. These conservative measures are generally sufficient for complete healing, but severe complications such as hemorrhage, complete perforation or abscess formation can always occur, so that surgical intervention may yet become necessary (Lichter and Borrie, 1965).

References

Albot, G., Autier, C., Libande, H.: Traumatisme instrumental mineur de l'œsophage inférieur chez un sujet porteur d'un brachy-œsophage. Actualités hépato-gastro-entérol. Hôtel-Dieu **5**, B 225–B 230 (1969).

Benjamin, B., Hanks, J. J.: Submucosal dissection of the oesophagus due to hemorrhage. A new radiographic finding. J. Laryng. **79**, 1032–1038 (1965).

Borrie, J.: The management of emergencies in thoracic surgery, p. 275. New York: Appleton-Century-Crofts 1958.

Borrie, J., Sheat, J.: Spontaneous intramural oesophageal perforation. Thorax **25**, 294–300 (1970).

Derrick, J. R., Harrison, W. H., Howard, J. M.: Factors predisposing to spontaneous perforation of the esophagus. The mechanical strength of the ulcerated esophagus. Surgery **43**, 486–489 (1958).

Eklöf, O., Löhr, G., Okmian, L.: Submucosal perforation of the esophagus in the neonate. Acta radiol. — Diagnosis (Stockh.) 8, 187–192 (1969).

Gross, R. E.: The surgery of infancy and childhood. Its principles and techniques. Philadelphia-London: W. B. Saunders Co. 1953.

Joffe, N., Millan, V. G.: Postemetic dissecting intramural hematoma of the esophagus. Radiology **95**, 372–380 (1970).

Lichter, I., Borrie, J.: Intramural oesophageal abscess. Brit. J. Surg. **52**, 185–188 (1965).

Lowman, R. M., Goldman, R., Stern, H.: The roentgen aspects of intramural dissection of the esophagus. Radiology **93**, 1329–1331 (1969).

Marks, I. N., Keet, A. D.: Intramural rupture of the esophagus. Brit. med. J. **1968 III**, 536–537.

McKenzie, M.: A manual of disease of the nose and the throat, p. 160. New York: Wm. Wood & Co. 1880–1884.

Rabiah, F. A., Elliott, H. B.: Intramural hematoma of the esophagus. An unusual complication of vagotomy. Amer. J. dig. Dis. **10**, 925–928 (1968).

Sanborn, E. B.: Intramural abscesses of the esophagus: a complication of foreign bodies. J. thorac. cardiovasc. Surg. **41**, 586–592 (1960).

Talley, N. A., Nicks, R.: Spontaneous submucosal haematoma of the oesophagus: Oesophageal apoplexy. Med. J. Aust. **2**, 146–150 (1969).

Thompson, N. W., Ernst, C. B., Fry, W. J.: The spectrum of emetogenic injury to the esophagus and stomach. Amer. J. Surg. **113**, 13-26 (1967).

Williams, B.: Oesophageal laceration following remote trauma. Brit. J. Radiol. **30**, 666–668 (1957).

Chapter 10

Esophageal Varices

J. Fevery and J. De Groote

With 8 Figures

1. Definition

Esophageal varices are dilated and tortuous veins in the esophageal wall, secondary to increased venous pressure in the splanchnic venous bed or in the superior vena cava. Dilated veins in the gastrointestinal organs are most common in the submucosal layer. However, in the distal few centimeters of the esophagus, the main veins, and consequently the varices, run right underneath the epithelium (Butler, 1951; De Carvalho, 1966; Stelzner and Lierse, 1968). The source of most hemorrhages from esophageal varices, therefore, is found in that area (Chiles et al., 1953, 84%; Orloff and Thomas, 1963, 75%; Burgmann, 1965, 80%; Dagradi et al., 1966, 86%).

2. Anatomy and Histopathology

The venous drainage of the esophagus constitutes an anastomosis between the systemic superior vena cava and the portal system. Schematically the distal third of the esophagus drains into the left gastric coronary vein and into the right gastro-epiploic vein. There is some drainage into phrenic veins and a minor part of the blood flows through the short gastric veins to the spleen. The gastric coronary and the inferior mesenteric vein usually drain into the splenic vein. Sometimes the inferior and superior mesenteric veins join each other. The short portal vein is formed by the confluent splenic and superior mesenteric veins (Ruzicka and Rossi, 1970; Fig. 304). The upper two thirds of the esophagus mainly drain into the azygos and hemiazygos system, whereas blood from the upper end flows into the subclavian, the thyroid, and the first intercostal veins. There is also some drainage into lower intercostal, bronchial and vertebral veins (Fig. 304).

The venous system of the esophagus itself (Butler, 1951) is composed of (1) The intrinsic veins, including a subepithelial plexus in the lamina propria, a submucosal plexus, and perforating veins, which join the two plexuses and drain into the extrinsic veins. (2) The veins accompanying the vagal nerves that run in the adventitial wall of the esophagus. (3) Some twenty extrinsic veins, formed by groups of perforating veins.

Most authors agree that both the subepithelial and submucosal plexus exist over the entire length of the esophagus, the subepithelial plexus being far more important in the distal portion of the esophagus where most veins run in the longitudinal axis of the gullet (Butler, 1951; De Carvalho, 1966; Stelzner and Lierse, 1968). These longitudinal veins end directly into the deeper subglandular veins of the gastric wall (Fig. 305). Submucosal and perforating veins are rather sparse in the distal 2 to 3 cm of the esophagus. The subepithelial localization of the veins favors easy bleeding in the distal esophagus when varices exist. However,

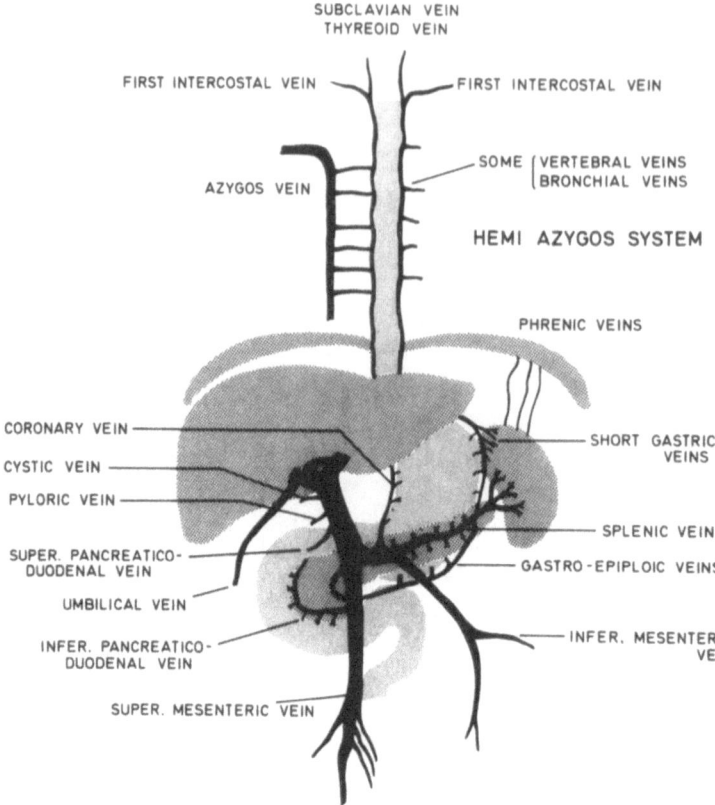

SUBCLAVIAN VEIN
THYREOID VEIN

FIRST INTERCOSTAL VEIN

FIRST INTERCOSTAL VEIN

SOME ⎰VERTEBRAL VEINS
      ⎱BRONCHIAL VEINS

AZYGOS VEIN

HEMI AZYGOS SYSTEM

PHRENIC VEINS

CORONARY VEIN

SHORT GASTRIC
VEINS

CYSTIC VEIN

PYLORIC VEIN

SPLENIC VEIN

SUPER. PANCREATICO-
DUODENAL VEIN

GASTRO-EPIPLOIC VEINS

UMBILICAL VEIN

INFER. PANCREATICO-
DUODENAL VEIN

INFER. MESENTERI
VEI

SUPER. MESENTERIC VEIN

Fig. 304. Portal venous system and venous drainage of the esophagus. (Modified from RU-ZICKA and ROSSI, and from BUTLER)

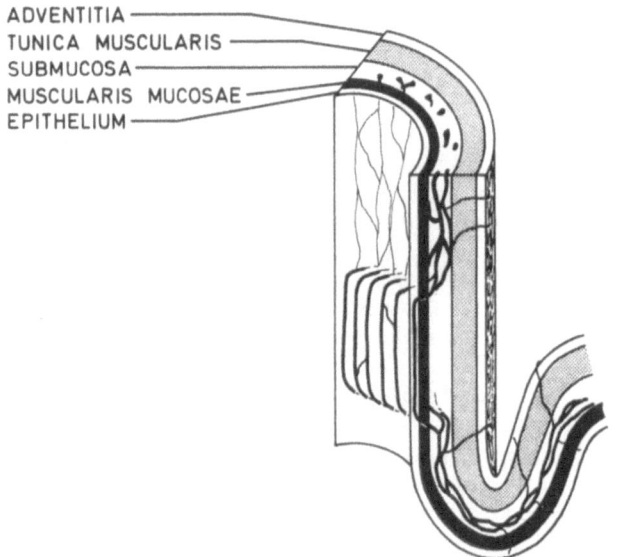

ADVENTITIA
TUNICA MUSCULARIS
SUBMUCOSA
MUSCULARIS MUCOSAE
EPITHELIUM

Fig. 305. The intrinsic venous plexuses of the esophagus and of the gastroesophageal junctional segment. (Modified from DE CARVALHO, and from STELZNER and LIERSE)

esophageal submucosal and gastric subglandular veins may also give rise to bleeding.

Although varices in surgical or autopsy specimens are usually spread over all layers of the esophageal wall, only one single bleeding point, located in the subepithelial plexus of the distal esophagus, is found in most instances (BURGMANN, 1965).

3. Incidence

Few reports are available on the overall incidence of esophageal varices. WEINBERG (1949) found them to be present in 8% of 1189 consecutive necropsy specimens. In cirrhotic patients esophageal varices are reported in 22.5 to 63% of the cases, depending on the type of patients studied and the method of detection used (PALMER and BRICK, 1953; PALMER et al., 1954). The incidence of cirrhosis varies from 1 to 6% in autopsy studies (TUMEN and COHN, 1965), and from 0.17 to 4.91% in clinical surveys (MÜTING et al., 1966; STONE et al., 1968; MÖRL and FEIGE, 1969).

4. Etiology and Pathogenesis
(see Table 27)

Esophageal varices are usually caused by increased pressure in the venous splanchnic bed, i.e. in the splenic, superior mesenteric, or portal veins. This increased venous pressure, which will be called "Portal Hypertension" opens up pre-existing collateral vessels that reach the esophageal veins via the gastric coronary, the gastroepiploic, and the short gastric veins (Fig. 304). Esophageal varices may also be due to obstruction of the superior vena cava by esophageal or bronchial cancer. As these varices result from an increased resistance in their own outflow tract they are called "downhill varices".

4.1. Esophageal Varices Secondary to "Portal Hypertension"

Portal hypertension may be of presinusoidal and/or postsinusoidal origin. In the first category the main lesion is presumed to be situated before the hepatic sinusoids, in the last behind the sinusoids. In both instances the lesion may be either intra- or extrahepatic (TUMEN and COHN, 1965; SHERLOCK, 1968; SCHMID, 1968). This classification corresponds to the experimental observation of increased splenic pulp pressure with normal wedged hepatic venous pressure in the presinusoidal type, whereas both pressures are increased in the postsinusoidal type. Although it may be very difficult to determine the exact location of the disorder within the liver lobule and although the lesion is frequently of a mixed nature, this classification is still useful.

4.1.1. Presinusoidal Causes
4.1.1.1. Prehepatic Pathology
4.1.1.1.1. Forward Flow Group

4.1.1.1.1.1. Banti-Syndrome and Tropical Splenomegaly. In the so-called *Banti-syndrome*, which has been frequently described in mediterranean countries, splenomegaly is supposed to be the primary defect. Portal hypertension and "minor" liver lesions are said to develop as secondary phenomena, but accurate descriptions of the liver lesions are sparse. The accent has been on the huge spleen with signs

Table 27. Etiology of Esophageal Varices

4.1. Secondary to Portal Hypertension
  4.1.1. Presinusoidal Causes
    4.1.1.1. Presinusoidal Prehepatic Causes
      4.1.1.1.1. Forward Flow Group
        4.1.1.1.1.1. Banti-syndrome and Tropical Splenomegaly
        4.1.1.1.1.2. Arteriovenous shunts in the Portal System
      4.1.1.1.2. Portal Vein Thrombosis and Compression
      4.1.1.1.3. Splenic Vein Thrombosis
    4.1.1.2. Presinusoidal Intrahepatic Causes
      4.1.1.2.1. Hepatic Schistosomiasis
      4.1.1.2.2. Myeloproliferative Diseases
      4.1.1.2.3. Granulomatous Diseases
      4.1.1.2.4. Congenital Hepatic Fibrosis (Fibroangioadenomatosis)
      4.1.1.2.5. Polycystic Liver Disease, Hydatid Cysts
      4.1.1.2.6. Liver Metastases
      4.1.1.2.7. Wilson's Disease
      4.1.1.2.8. Acute Hepatitis
  4.1.2. Sinusoidal Causes
    4.1.2.1. Acute Hepatitis
    4.1.2.2. Fatty Liver
    4.1.2.3. Early Stage of Chronic, Non-suppurative, Destructive Cholangitis (Primary Biliary Cirrhosis)
    4.1.2.4. Kupffer Cell Hypertrophy with Perisinusoidal Fibrosis
  4.1.3. Postsinusoidal Causes
    4.1.3.1. Postsinusoidal Intrahepatic Causes
      4.1.3.1.1. Liver Cirrhosis
        4.1.3.1.1.1. Alcoholic Liver Cirrhosis
        4.1.3.1.1.2. Post-necrotic Liver Cirrhosis
        4.1.3.1.1.3. Cryptogenic Liver Cirrhosis
        4.1.3.1.1.4. Primary Biliary Cirrhosis
        4.1.3.1.1.5. Secondary Biliary Cirrhosis
        4.1.3.1.1.6. Cardiac Cirrhosis
        4.1.3.1.1.7. Indian Type of Infantile Cirrhosis
        4.1.3.1.1.8. Miscellaneous
      4.1.3.1.2. Liver Cirrhosis Associated with Metabolic Disorders
        4.1.3.1.2.1. Hemochromatosis
        4.1.3.1.2.2. Wilson's Disease
        4.1.3.1.2.3. Galactosemia
        4.1.3.1.2.4. Cystic Fibrosis of Pancreas
        4.1.2.1.2.5. Fructose Intolerance
        4.1.3.1.2.6. Glycogenosis Type IV
        4.1.3.1.2.7. Tyrosinosis
        4.1.3.1.2.8. Deficiency of α1-antitrypsine
        4.1.3.1.2.9. Gaucher's Disease
        4.1.3.1.2.10. Hepatic Porphyria
        4.1.3.1.2.11. Sickle-Cell Disease
      4.1.3.1.3. Alcoholic Hepatitis
      4.1.3.1.4. Partial Nodular Transformation
      4.1.3.1.5. Veno-occlusive Disease
    4.1.3.2. Postsinusoidal Extrahepatic Causes
      4.1.3.2.1. Budd-Chiari Syndrome
      4.1.3.2.2. Congestive Heart Failure
      4.1.3.2.3. Obstruction of Inferior Vena Cava
4.2. Esophageal Varices without Portal Hypertension
  4.2.1. Obstruction of Vena Cava Superior (Downhill Varices)
  4.2.2. Carcinoma at the Gastroesophageal Junction
  4.2.3. "Idiopathic Esophageal Varices"
  4.2.4. Esophageal Varices in Patients with Liver Disease, but Normal Portal Pressure
4.3. Unclassified Miscellaneous Causes

of "hypersplenism". The Anglo-Saxon equivalent "Tropical, Fibrocongestive or Idiopathic Splenomegaly" has been more critically studied (BASU and AIKAT, 1963; BOYER et al., 1967). Intrasplenic pressures were found to be increased in 45% of the 83 patients with tropical splenomegaly studied by LEATHER (1961), MARSDEN et al. (1964) and WILLIAMS et al. (1966). The portal hypertension seemed to be caused by an increased portal blood flow, which itself was secondary to increased splenic flow or to hypervolemia with dilution anemia (see also 4.1.1.1.1.2. and 4.1.1.1.2.). However, very recently multiple small thrombi were found in intrahepatic portal vein branches (BOYER et al., 1974).

4.1.1.1.1.2. Arteriovenous Shunts in the Portal System. Arteriovenous shunts of the splenic vessels are said to produce portal hypertension and varices by increasing flow and pressure in the splenic vein (LINDER et al., 1968). The fistulas may be congenital but more frequently they are acquired by trauma (gunshot) (JOHNSTON and GIBSON, 1965), surgery (suturing together of the artery and the vein), or by spontaneous rupture of aneurysms of the splenic artery.

Esophageal varices caused by fistulas between the mesenteric artery and vein are very rare; only one documented case has been described (GRAFE and STEINBERG, 1966). Intrahepatic arteriovenous shunts, leading to portal hypertension and esophageal varices, may be caused by percutaneous suction biopsy of the liver (PREGER, 1967b), familial hereditary telangiectasia (GRAHAM et al., 1964) as well as by the above mentioned causes of intrasplenic fistulas (LINDER et al., 1968; DONOVAN et al., 1969; FULTON and WOLFEL, 1970). Shunts between the smaller hepatic and portal branches have been described as a cause of portal hypertension by POPPER et al. (1952). These arteriovenous fistulas cause bleeding from esophageal varices in 30% of the cases (LINDER et al., 1968). They can be suspected by a bruit and a thrill, and sometimes by calcifications of the original aneurysm, but angiography is required to confirm the diagnosis. Surgical therapy consists of ligation of the artery, resection of the splenic shunt, partial hepatectomy or simple closure of the fistula (MADDING et al., 1954; SHUMACKER and WALDHAUSEN, 1961).

The histological lesions include slight hepatic fibrosis, highly vascularized portal spaces and thickened walls of the intrahepatic portal venules (DONOVAN et al., 1969). This condition thus resembles the hepatoportal sclerosis described in tropical splenomegaly and in the so-called Banti-syndrome. It is not yet certain whether these minor abnormalities cause an increased presinusoidal resistance or whether they are secondary to an elevated portal flow.

Intrahepatic arteriovenous anastomoses, escaping detection by the now available "rough" methods, may be the cause of portal hypertension in some cases with patent portal vein and nearly normal liver histology (TISDALE et al., 1959).

4.1.1.1.2. Portal Vein Thrombosis or Compression

Portal vein thrombosis is the classical example of presinusoidal prehepatic portal hypertension, with highly increased splenic and portal pressure and normal wedged hepatic vein pressure. It was found in 12.5% of Hunt's 584 cases of portal hypertension (HUNT, 1965).

When occurring in childhood, the main cause is umbilical sepsis (CLATWORTHY and BOLES, 1959; SHALDON and SHERLOCK, 1962b; THOMPSON and SHERLOCK, 1964; VOORHEES et al., 1965; STATHERS and BLACKBURN, 1968; O'DONNELL and MOLONEY, 1968). Neonatal thrombosis is frequently followed by a fine recanalization, resulting in a cavernous transformation of the portal tract. The portal vein may also be congenitally absent. Portal pylephlebitis caused by infection and abcedation of the gallbladder, appendix or right colon, or secondary to osteo-myelitis and severe leg abscesses may also result in portal vein thrombosis (Stath-ers and Blackburn, 1968). Invasion or compression of the portal vein by primary malignant tumors of the liver, gall bladder, pancreas, stomach, and colon is an other cause of thrombosis (Albacete et al., 1967). Rarely acute pancreatitis (McDermott, 1960), pancreatic pseudocysts (Varriale et al., 1963) or adenop-athies in the hilus of the liver may cause such a compression. Thrombosis also occurs in blood diseases with increased coagulability, such as thrombocytemia, polycytemia and myelofibrosis (Shaldon and Sherlock, 1962a; Scherl and Klein, 1970) and as a complication of liver cirrhosis (Hunt and Whittard, 1954). An exhaustive list of causes of portal vein thrombosis and suppurative pyle-phlebitis is given by Jones (1965).

The hepatic lesions in this group are nearly always indistinguishable from those described as "hepatoportal sclerosis" (Mikkelsen et al., 1965) and from those found in cases with partial occlusions. Mikkelsen et al. (1965), therefore, suggest that they may be variants of the same underlying disease mechanism, whereby the occlusive process is sometimes restricted to small intrahepatic portal venules or is accompanied by partial or total occlusion of the large portal branches.

4.1.1.1.3. Splenic Vein Thrombosis

Thrombosis of the splenic vein causes left-sided extrahepatic "portal" hyper-tension. The ensuing collateral circulation runs over the stomach to the esophageal veins or to the coronary and portal veins (Paraf and Chalut, 1962; Basu and Aikat, 1963; Grünert et al., 1966; Rignault et al., 1968; Turrill and Mikkel-sen, 1969; Jenny, 1969; Sutton et al., 1970). Chronic alcoholic pancreatitis is the most frequent cause of the thrombosis. Therapy consist primarily in resection of the spleen and splenic vessels.

4.1.1.2. Presinusoidal Intrahepatic Disorders

4.1.1.2.1. Hepatic Schistosomiasis (Schistosoma Mansoni, Hematobium, Japonicum) (Mendes, 1965)

Involvement of the liver by Schistosomiasis, particularly of the Mansoni variety, is the most frequent cause of portal hypertension in Asia, Africa and South-America. The ova are put in or carried to mesenteric and portal venules where they may cause a mild granulomatous lesion or extensive fibrosis (the so-called "white clay-pipestem fibrosis") (Symmers, 1904). The endo- and peri-phlebitis of the portal venules causes a presinusoidal hypertension with normal wedged hepatic venous pressure, absence of cirrhosis and of regeneration nodules, and increased intrasplenic pressure (Aufses et al., 1959; Andrade, 1965; Cou-tinho, 1968; Sherlock, 1968). Diagnosis in the chronic forms is established by direct microscopical demonstration of the eggs in the stools or in a deep rectal biopsy, by complement fixation tests, by immunofluorescence techniques (Da Sil-va and Pontes, 1965), or by a liver biopsy with direct "squash" examination (Kubasta et al., 1965) or after Ziehl-staining (Scheuer, 1968).

The portal hypertension is treated by splenorenal (Da Silva and Pontes, 1965) or portocaval anastomosis and splenectomy. Recently, extracorporeal filtra-tion of the portal blood after injection of antimony preparations to mobilize the parasites has been advocated before a shunt operation is performed (Goldsmith et al., 1967; Kean and Goldsmith, 1969).

4.1.1.2.2. Myeloproliferative Diseases, Myelofibrosis

Infiltration around the portal venules by reticuloses, leukemia or Hodgkin's disease may cause a presinusoidal hypertension, due to "diminished distensibility with increased resistance" (LIMA et al., 1962; SHALDON and SHERLOCK, 1962a; ROSENBAUM et al., 1966). In addition, the hepatic blood flow was found to be inereased in some cases (SHALDON and SHERLOCK, 1962a; ROSENBAUM et al., 1966). Similarly portal hypertension was noted in a patient with osteopetrosis (DENISON et al., 1971), and in myelofibrosis (SULLIVAN et al., 1974). Increased splenic blood flow may play an additional role.

4.1.1.2.3. Granulomatous Diseases

Large and well-organized granulomas in or near the portal tracts are found in 60–80% of patients with sarcoidosis (ISRAEL and SONES, 1964; LEBACQ, 1964; SCHEUER, 1968). These lesions can produce presinusoidal portal hypertension and esophageal varices in the absence of cirrhosis (LEBACQ et al., 1957; CHEITLIN et al., 1960; PORTER, 1961; MISTILIS et al., 1964; IBER and MADDREY, 1965). Fifteen such cases have been documented: most of them had esophageal varices (VILINS-KAS et al., 1970). Similar lesions occur in Brucellosis but portal hypertension has not been documented.

4.1.1.2.4. Congenital Hepatic Fibrosis (Fibroangioadenomatosis)

This is a congenital and frequently familial disorder characterized by the presence of broad fibrous septa in the portal areas containing only a small number of small portal vein branches (SWEETHAM and SYKES, 1961; SCHEUER, 1968). Portal hypertension is thought to be caused by the lack of normal portal branches or by the compression of the branches within the fibrous septa and is therefore presinusoidal. The disease occurs in childhood or adolescence, usually with signs of portal hypertension and normal liver function (KERR et al., 1961; HERMANN and HAWK, 1967; ZEEGEN et al., 1970).

4.1.1.2.5. Polycystic Liver Disease

The cysts of polycystic liver disease have a typical bile duct epithelium and can be considered as dilated intralobular ducts (MELNICK, 1955). They rarely lead to portal hypertension, which is presumably caused by compression of the intra-hepatic veins or to fibrous reaction in the portal area (CAMPBELL et al., 1958; LATHROP, 1959; SEDACCA et al., 1961). Hydatid cysts causing presinusoidal portal hypertension were described by GILSANZ et al. (1961).

4.1.1.2.6. Liver Metastases

The importance of liver metastases as a cause of esophageal varices has probably been underestimated (HYUN et al., 1964). In a series of 1 189 consecutive post mortem studies WEINBERG (1949) found liver secondaries to be the cause of esophageal varices in 4 out of 95 cases. LUNA et al. (1968) examined the esophagus of 40 autopsy cases with liver secondaries and found esophageal varices in 5 of them.

Neoplastic infiltration with occlusion of portal venules was always present and thrombi in the centrolobular venules were frequently observed. Neoplastic emboli in the portal venules are assumed to be the initial hepatic lesion. Later, the intravenous tumor growth is said to invade the parenchyma and the centro-lobular vessels; this invasion will eventually result in the compression of liver tissue and of larger intrahepatic vessels (Ruprecht and Kinney, 1956; Hyun et al., 1964). Portal hypertension, therefore, seems to be of presinusoidal origin.

4.1.1.2.7. Wilson's Disease (see further sub 4.1.3.1.2.2.)

In the early precirrhotic stages of Wilson's disease, portal hypertension develops, with normal wedged hepatic venous pressure. The obstruction therefore seems to be located in the smaller intrahepatic radicles of the portal veins (Taylor et al., 1959).

4.1.1.2.8. Acute Hepatitis

Temporary esophageal varices, increased splenic pulp pressure, and increased pressure in esophageal varices have been observed in acute hepatitis (Palmer and Brick, 1954–1955; Reichman and Davis, 1957; Haerter and Palmer, 1959). This could be due partly to portal inflammation and edema, and would then be presinusoidal in nature (Preisig, 1967). However, as the main lesion is centro-lobular, it seems likely that a sinusoidal factor is involved as well.

4.1.2. Sinusoidal Causes
(Rappaport et al., 1970)

4.1.2.1. Acute Hepatitis
(cfr. supra 4.1.1.2.8.)

4.1.2.2. Fatty Liver

Fatty liver, secondary to alcoholism, diabetes, heart disease, and obesity, has been reported as the cause of varices in a few cases (Palmer and Brick, 1954, 1955; Leevy, 1962; Chiandussi et al., 1963; Madore, 1970; Rappaport et al., 1970).

4.1.2.3. Early Stage of Chronic, Non-Suppurative, Destructive Cholangitis (Primary Biliary Cirrhosis)

Portal hypertension seems to be more frequent in this disease than is generally thought and occurs from the early stages of the disease, prior to the full development of cirrhosis and even in the absence of regenerating noduli (Zeegen et al., 1969; Sicot and Benhamou, 1971). In the early phase the hypertension could well be due to sinusoidal lesions such as doubling of the cell-plates and slight mononuclear cell infiltration (Scheuer, 1968). If the lesions are more granulomatous in type the portal hypertension is probably presinusoidal. Later on, biliary cirrhosis develops with regenerating noduli, causing postsinusoidal hypertension (see 4.1.3.1., and Kew et al., 1971).

4.1.2.4. Kupffer Cell Hypertrophy with Perisinusoidal Fibrosis

Esophageal varices have been described in 2 patients, 7 and 21 years old, with a history of an acute abdominal infectious disease. Liver function was normal and no histologic lesions were found in the portal tracts on light microscopy. The increased portal system pressure seemed to be due to perisinusoidal fibrosis and grossly enlarged Kupffer cells which had caused narrowed sinusoidal lumina. Wedged hepatic venous pressure was measured in one case and was found to be normal (Kluge et al., 1970).

4.1.3. Postsinusoidal Portal Hypertension
4.1.3.1. Postsinusoidal Intrahepatic Causes

In adults, chronic liver disease accounts for 85–90% and liver cirrhosis for 80% of portal hypertensions (WELCH, 1960; STROHMEYER and DÖLLE, 1963). Extrahepatic obstruction of the portal vein is more important in children. It was observed in 58 of the 98 children with portal hypertension studied by VOORHEES et al. (1965).

4.1.3.1.1. Liver Cirrhosis

The portal vascular bed is reduced in the cirrhotic liver due to disappearance of portal venules and sinusoids by collapse, fibrosis and regenerating nodules (POPPER et al., 1952; SHERLOCK, 1965, 1968, and other authors). Dilated sinusoids shunting the portal blood to the centrolobular vein without contact with the regenerating nodules ("internal Eck fistulas") may also contribute to the development of portal hypertension (POPPER et al., 1952). Besides these changes, a postsinusoidal block has generally been accepted as the most important factor in causing portal hypertension in the cirrhotic patient. Centrolobular vein compression by the regenerating nodules was thought to increase post-sinusoidal pressure (as measured by wedged hepatic venous pressure) and, in a retrograde way, portal venous pressure (as measured by intrasplenic or omphaloportal pressure) (KELTY et al., 1950). Recent observations have cast some doubt on the importance of a post-sinusoidal block and regenerating nodules, since portal hypertension has been found in the absence of these nodules in early stages of primary biliary cirrhosis (ZEEGEN et al., 1969; SICOT and BENHAMOU, 1970), in subacute viral hepatitis (REICHMAN and DAVIS, 1957), steatosis (LEEVY, 1962), and in the early non-cirrhotic stages of alcoholic injury (REYNOLDS et al., 1969). Esophageal varices are found in 22 to 70% of the cirrhotics, depending upon the technique used for diagnosis (BRICK and PALMER, 1953; PALMER et al., 1954; GARCEAU et al., 1963; STONE et al., 1968). Different types of cirrhosis must be distinguished according to the etiology. (For a recent discussion see also REYNOLDS, 1973.)

4.1.3.1.1.1. Alcoholic Liver Cirrhosis. Alcohol is the outstanding cause of liver cirrhosis in the U.S.A. and in the larger cities of Western Europe (GARCEAU et al., 1963). A daily intake of 80 g of alcohol for more than 10 years gives 37% chance of developing cirrhosis; if the daily intake is 160 g for 10 years the risk is as high as 60% (CAROLI and PEQUINOT, 1959; LELBACH, 1967; PEQUINOT, 1970).

4.1.3.1.1.2. Post-Hepatitis or Post-Necrotic Liver Cirrhosis. It is difficult to prove a direct relationship between cirrhosis and a previous episode of acute hepatitis (SCHAEFER et al., 1967). In Europe about one third of the cirrhotics have a history of hepatitis. Recent investigations in Austria and Germany demonstrated the presence of Hepatitis-Associated-Antigen (Australian or SH-antigen) in about one third of the cirrhotics (KRASSNITZKY et al., 1970; KABOTH et al., 1970). Cirrhosis was found to develop in 1–3% of the patients with acute hepatitis (KALK and WILDHIRT, 1960). But chronic agressive hepatitis seems to be more directly related to cirrhosis. 15% of patients with this disease develop cirrhosis (DE GROOTE et al., 1968; SELMAIR et al., 1969).

4.1.3.1.1.3. Cryptogenic Cirrhosis. This group constitutes roughly the other third of the patients and may well be related to anicteric or undocumented hepatitis, to toxic liver injury (methyl dopa, oxyfenisatine, etc.) or to compensated alcoholic cirrhosis in people who stopped drinking.

4.1.3.1.1.4. Primary Biliary Cirrhosis. Varices can be found at all stages of the disease (see 4.1.1.2.3., 4.1.2.3.), and they are one of the main clinical problems in the late stage, where a typical cirrhosis has developed. Eight of the 22 patients described by Ahrens et al. (1950) had esophageal varices and 4 of them had a bleeding episode.

4.1.3.1.1.5. Secondary Biliary Cirrhosis. Cirrhosis is a relatively uncommon complication of biliary tract obstruction (Scheuer, 1968). Secondary biliary cirrhosis is usually caused by strictures of the bile tract, following complicated interventions for stones. It can also be caused directly by calculeous disease or obstructing neoplasm. 19–25% of the patients with biliary cirrhosis develop portal hypertension with bleeding varices (Scobie et al., 1965; Sedgwick et al., 1966; Adson and Wychulis, 1968). In childhood, biliary atresia is the most frequent cause of secondary biliary cirrhosis. Sclerosing cholangitis (frequently associated with chronic inflammatory diseases of the colon) is another cause in adults.

4.1.3.1.1.6. Cardiac Cirrhosis. Chronic congestive failure is another rare cause of cirrhosis. Mitral valve disease, especially when associated with tricuspid insufficiency, and constrictive pericarditis are the main etiological disorders. Esophageal varices are extremely rare.

4.1.3.1.1.7. Indian Type of Infantile Cirrhosis. This disease of unknown etiology is found in children of the higher economical classes in India. It may develop as an acute disease resembling sometimes alcoholic hepatitis without steatosis, or as a more chronic disorder with a fine macronodular cirrhosis, portal hypertension, and variceal bleeding (Smetana et al., 1961; Scheuer, 1968).

4.1.3.1.1.8. Miscellaneous. Cirrhosis and esophageal varices can develop late in the course of a variety of other diseases, such as ulcerative colitis, arsenicum poisoning, systemic lupus erythematodes, etc. There seems to be no direct relationship between syphilis and cirrhosis, but injections, alcoholism and arsenotherapy favor liver disease. In some series, 10–28% of the cirrhotics had syphilis (Karmi et al., 1969). Furthermore, tertiary syphilis with fibrous retractions may rarely produce portal hypertension (Shapiro and Weiner, 1951). Arsenotherapy itself can induce portal hypertension because of non-cirrhotic portal vein sclerosis (Morris et al., 1974) or real cirrhosis.

4.1.3.1.2. Liver Cirrhosis Associated with Metabolic Disorders

This group of diseases is discussed separately for several reasons. Its concerns mainly familial, genetic disorders, which are frequently associated with a number of extrahepatic symptoms and signs; cirrhosis with portal hypertension usually develops late in the course of the disease and may sometimes be prevented by dietary and drug therapy (Iber and Maddrey, 1965).

4.1.3.1.2.1. Hemochromatosis (Sheldon, 1935; Finch and Finch, 1955). Although some people still doubt the genetic nature of hemochromatosis (MacDonald, 1964) an increasing number of familial and of twin-incidences are being recorded. Iron absorption seems to be greatly enhanced; this causes near saturation of the iron binding capacity in the blood and gradual deposition of iron in liver, heart, pancreas, gastric chief cells and other tissues. Fibrosis develops, eventually resulting in cirrhosis with broad dense fibrous septa (Knoblauch and Hedinger, 1963). If treated by frequent phlebotomies from an early stage on, the process can be arrested. In our own series varices were found in 35% of the cases at the time of diagnosis and were the cause of death in 3 out of 10 deaths. Secondary hemochromatosis and hemosiderosis can develop in patients receiving multiple transfusions or massive iron therapy. Varices have been found in four hemosiderosis patients (Palmer and Brick, 1955).

4.1.3.1.2.2. Hepato-Lenticular Degeneration, Wilson's Disease. This recessive inborn error of copper metabolism may be related to a deficiency of ceruloplasmin, a copper-binding α_2-globulin in blood serum (SCHEINSBERG and GITLIN, 1952). Increased intestinal absorption of copper (CARTWRIGHT et al., 1955) together with the disturbance in copper-binding leads to tissue accumulation of this metal with Kayser-Fleisher corneal rings, lenticular lesions with neuro-psychiatric disturbances, liver cirrhosis and renal tubular changes (WALSHE and BRIGGS, 1962). Portal hypertension and esophageal varices seem to be very frequent. Massive hematemesis is observed in 5–10% of the patients (STERNLIEB et al., 1970). In advanced cirrhosis portal hypertension is presumably postsinusoidal in type; in the early stages some data suggest a presinusoidal origin, since the wedged hepatic venous pressure can be normal in contrast to the greatly enhanced intrasplenic pressure (TAYLOR et al., 1959). Portal-systemic shunt operations are frequently followed by severe and often fatal neurological deterioration (STERNLIEB et al., 1970). Prognosis is therefore worse than in the usual cirrhotic. Abnormally increased affinity for copper of hepatic metallothionein in Wilson's disease might be the primary defect (EVANS et al., 1973).

4.1.3.1.2.3. Galactosemia. The primary defect is a deficiency of galactose-1-phosphate-uridyl transferase in liver and red blood cells with accumulation of galactose-1-phosphate (ISSELBACHER, 1959). The clinical picture includes cataract, hepatosplenomegaly with macronodular cirrhosis and portal hypertension, malnutrition and mental disturbances (HSIA and WALKER, 1961). Diagnosis is made by finding in the urine a Benedict-positive, reducing hexose which is not glucose (negative glucose oxidase test). Therapy of this autosomal recessive disease is elimination of food containing galactose from the diet.

4.1.3.1.2.4. Cystic Fibrosis of the Pancreas, Mucoviscidosis. The liver disturbances which are frequently observed in cystic fibrosis of the pancreas result from partial obstruction of the bile canaliculi, with development of a focal biliary fibrosis (DI SANT'AGNESE and BLANC, 1956; DI SANT'AGNESE and TALAMO, 1967). Biliary cirrhosis is rare, occurring in about 2% of the cases (DI SANT'AGNESE, 1956; ROBERTS, 1962).

4.1.3.1.2.5. Fructose Intolerance. This autosomal, recessive deficiency in fructose-1-phosphate-aldolase causes fructosuria, hypoglycemic attacks and liver steatosis with intralobular and periportal fibrosis (LEVIN et al., 1968). Portal hypertension develops, if fructose is not banned from the diet.

4.1.3.1.2.6. Glycogenosis Type IV (Andersen's disease 1956). This rare disease is caused by deficiency of the branching enzyme (amylo-1, 4→1, 6-transglucosidase). Abnormal glycogen is formed and accumulates in the liver, leading to liver cirrhosis with "giant cells" and progressive portal hypertension (SIDBURY et al., 1962; SCHEUER and WILLIAMS, 1965; BROWN and BROW, 1966).

4.1.3.1.2.7. Tyrosinosis and Hypermethioninemia. Tyrosinosis was recently described as a rare cause of liver cirrhosis mainly in French-Canadian children (LAROCHELLE et al., 1967). Hypermethioninemia also can progress to liver cirrhosis (PERRY et al., 1965), but is mostly secondary to tyrosinosis.

4.1.3.1.2.8. Deficiency of α_1-Antitrypsine. This deficiency is mainly related to obstructive pulmonary disease, but may also result in liver cirrhosis (SHARP et al., 1969; BERG and ERIKSSON, 1972), and in neonatal cholestasis (AAGENAES et al., 1973).

4.1.3.1.2.9. Gaucher's Disease. This familial disease is characterized by accumulation of galactosidero- and glucosiderocerebrosides and of glycolipids in the histioreticular system, resulting in hepatosplenomegaly, enlarged lymph nodes, and bone marrow infiltration. In the chronic adult form, extensive liver infiltration with portal hypertension has been reported (Morrison and Lane, 1955).

4.1.3.1.2.10. Hepatic Porphyria. Acute intermittent porphyria (Swedish type), porphyria variegata, which is frequently encountered in South-Africa, and porphyria cutanea tarda with attacks related to alcohol intake may produce hepatic lesions. Cirrhosis was found in half of the adult patients of Brugsch et al. (1960).

4.1.3.1.2.11. Sickle-Cell Disease. This genetically dominant disorder of hemoglobin synthesis is associated with liver cirrhosis in about 25% of the cases (Green et al., 1953; Song, 1957). Cirrhosis seems to be due to multiple small ischemic infarcts of sickle cell erythrocytes, and to the increased release of thromboplastine. Hemosiderosis, secondary hemochromatosis, serum hepatitis, and gallstone disease are additional causes of liver injury in this disease (Jordan, 1957; Barrett-Connor, 1968).

4.1.3.1.3. Alcoholic Hepatitis

Acute or chronic alcoholic hepatitis may be associated with an increased portal vein pressure together with an increased wedged hepatic vein pressure and normal or reduced hepatic blood flow. Esophageal varices were found in 12 of the 28 patients described by Reynolds et al. (1969), although cirrhosis and regenerating nodules were absent. Alcoholic sclerosing hyaline necrosis seems to cause a sufficient disturbance of the hepatic venous blood flow to induce portal hypertension and varices.

4.1.3.1.4. Partial Nodular Transformation

Four cases of this rare disease were described by Sherlock et al. (1966) and a fifth was recently reported by Classen et al. (1970). All cases had marked portal hypertension with esophageal varices and hematemesis. The liver is not enlarged, but non-cirrhotic nodules, mainly in the perihilar region, replace and compress the remaining lobules. Diagnosis is usually made at autopsy, but should be suspected in the presence of significant portal hypertension, with nearly normal liver function tests and nearly normal liver punction biopsy.

4.1.3.1.5. Veno-Occlusive Disease

This disease is characterized by an acute, subacute or chronic obliteration of the small hepatic vein radicles, which is followed by centrolobular congestion, necrosis and fibrosis (Bras and Hill, 1956). The disease occurs mainly in Jamaica, Asia and Africa. It can be produced by monocrotaline (Hill et al., 1958). In Jamaica, Bush teas made from Crotalaria fulva extracts are thought to be responsible. Hepatomegaly, ascites and acute liver failure may follow or the disease may go into the chronic stage with marked portal hypertension (Sherlock, 1968). A similar syndrome can be caused by cytotoxic drugs or irradiation (Weinbren, 1966).

4.1.3.2. Extrahepatic Postsinusoidal Portal Hypertension

4.1.3.2.1. Budd-Chiari Syndrome

Although obstruction of the hepatic veins can be produced by a large number of intra- or extrahepatic disorders, the etiology in more than half of the cases of Budd-Chiari syndrome remains unknown (Parker, 1959). Hepatic tumors, primary or secondary, infiltration of the inferior vena cava by renal carcinoma, and polycythemia vera (Vaquez' disease) are listed as the most frequent causes.

Membraneous obliteration in the hepatic portion of the vena cava (KIRURA et al., 1963; SCHAFFNER et al., 1967), oral contraceptives causing thrombosis of the hepatic veins (ECKER et al., 1966; STERUP and MOSBECH, 1967), and massive involvement by Aspergillus resulting in thrombosis (YOUNG, 1969) have been added to this list. When the onset of the disease is acute the patients are severely ill and suddenly develop massive ascites, abdominal pain, hepatomegaly and mild jaundice. Liver coma and death may rapidly develop if the venous outflow block is total. In the more chronic cases, abdominal pain and ascites are the main features, with signs of portal hypertension gradually developing (CLAIN et al., 1967; SCHAFFNER et al., 1967; SHERLOCK, 1968).

An increased serum alkaline phosphatase and a high protein content in the ascitic fluid are the main laboratory findings. Liver biopsy shows centrolobular congestion and necrosis and marked sinusoidal dilation (SCHEUER, 1963). Hepatic venography may show narrowing or occlusion of some hepatic veins, while a spiderweb pattern is seen in adjacent vessels (CLAIN et al., 1967). Obstruction of the hepatic portion of the inferior vena cava causing a Budd-Chiari syndrome seems to be more frequent in Japan than in Western countries (NAKAMURA et al., 1968).

4.1.3.2.2. Congestive Heart Failure

According to LUNA et al. (1968) 8% of the esophageal varices in non-cirrhotic patients result from chronic congestive heart failure (see also PALMER and BRICK, 1954). The increased pressure in the inferior vena cava is transmitted to the hepatic veins and causes a postsinusoidal hypertension.

4.1.3.2.3. Obstruction of Inferior Vena Cava

See previous Section 4.1.3.2.1.

4.2. Esophageal Varices without Portal Hypertension
4.2.1. Obstruction of Vena Cava Superior (Downhill Varices)
(Fig. 306)

The venous outflow of all but the distal portion of the esophagus drains via intercostal and vertebral veins and especially via the azygos system into the superior vena cava. Obstruction of the superior vena cava results in a reversal of the flow direction. Esophageal veins drain part of the venous blood to intercostal or vertebral veins below the obstruction and probably to the portal system (SNODGRASS and MELLINKOFF, 1961; STOLZE, 1964; REX and RICHTER, 1967). Superior vena cava obstruction is usually caused by neoplastic disease; mediastinal fibrosis, gigantic thyroid struma, aortic aneurysms, and idiopathic thrombosis are other causes.

4.2.2. Carcinoma at the Gastroesophageal Junction

Varices in the distal esophagus have been observed in patients with carcinoma at the gastroesophageal junction, presumably due to blocking of the venous return to the gastric veins (TESCHENDORF, 1958; LEICHNER-WEIL, 1965).

4.2.3. Idiopathic Esophageal Varices

PALMER and BRICK (1955) reported 13 cases of varices in the distal esophagus without evident cause; in 4 of these normal venous pressures were documented with normal liver function and normal histology. SCHAEFER et al. (1964) reported 2 cases with normal splenic pulp and mesenteric vein pressures and normal splenic

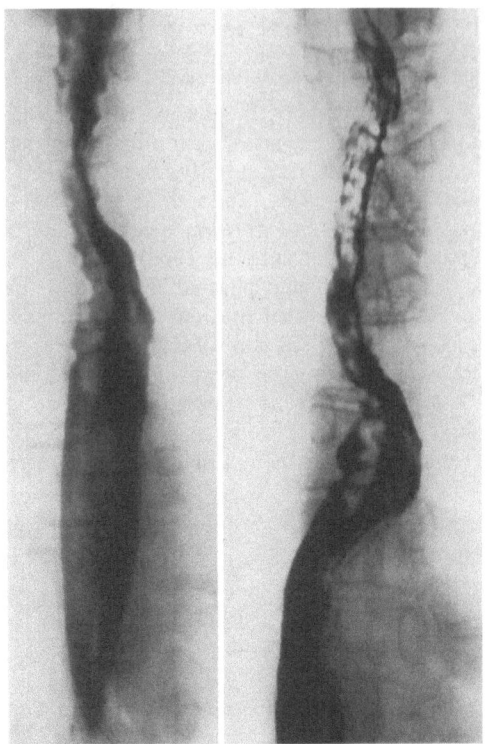

Fig. 306. Downhill varices in a 65-year old woman with recurrent goiter after thyroidectomy. The caval vein was not obstructed. Typical intraluminal defects are apparent in upper and middle third of the esophagus

venography; liver biopsy in both cases showed no lesions except for a moderate degree of fatty metamorphosis. The pathogenesis of these idiopathic esophageal varices is unknown.

4.2.4. Esophageal Varices in Patients with Liver Disease, but Normal Portal Pressure

Esophageal varices have been reported in patients with liver disease in the absence of portal hypertension (Homer et al., 1964; Greene et al., 1965). However, variations in portal pressure are known to occur and transient esophageal varices have been described (Bennett et al., 1953; Palmer, 1953). Reversible fatty liver changes have been observed in alcoholics who stop drinking (Bennett et al., 1953; Leevy et al., 1958).

4.3. Unclassified Miscellaneous Causes

Portal hypertension and esophageal varices have been reported in amyloidosis (Kapp, 1965; Brandt et al., 1968), hiatus hernia (Palmer, 1958; Dagradi and Stempien, 1962), normal pregnancy, achalasia, intrathoracic arteriovenous aneurysms, kala azar, fascioliasis and amebic hepatitis (Palmer and Brick, 1954, 1955).

Varices of the cervical esophagus have been found in 3 patients by PALMER (1952). They were located in the posterior wall and were believed to be due to venous congestion, produced by the cricopharyngeal muscle or to abnormal extensions of the posterior hypopharyngeal venous plexus.

5. Clinical Features : Bleeding
5.1. Incidence

Three to seven percent of massive upper gastrointestinal hemorrhages are due to esophageal varices (HISLOP et al., 1966; HALMAGYI, 1970). Bleeding occurred in 38% of 467 cirrhotic patients with known varices studied during a three year period (GARCEAU et al., 1963). The incidence of bleeding in other clinical reports ranges from 25–56% and in autopsy series from 30–70% of patients with esophageal varices (McCRAY et al., 1969). Hemorrhage was the cause of death in one third of such patients (BECK and CREUTZFELDT, 1962; GARCEAU et al., 1964).

5.2. Pathogenesis of the Bleeding

The mechanisms that trigger the actual bleeding episode are still controversial. Esophagitis with erosion, lesions by food substances and sudden increase in esophageal portal pressure (explosion theory) have all been suggested as the immediate cause of bleeding (HARTMANN, 1964). Autopsy studies showed evidence of esophagitis in about 50% of the cases who died from esophageal hemorrhage (CHILES et al., 1953; WAGENKNECHT et al., 1953). Mucosal alterations, however, may be due to circulatory failure in shock and preagonal stages, to irritation by nasogastric aspiration or balloon-tamponnade tubes and to postmortem changes (LIEBOWITZ, 1961; ORLOFF and THOMAS, 1963). Bleeding has been observed in patients with achlorhydria, total gastrectomy, or partial esophagogastrectomy with interposition of a jejunal segment (LIEBOWITZ, 1961; SMITH and EDWARDS, 1966). OSTROW et al. (1960) found achlorhydria in one third of their alcoholic cirrhotics, and decreased gastric acid secretion in all cirrhotics studied. Similar findings have been reported by BENDETT et al. (1963), but not by TABAQCHALI and DAWSON (1964), who found the acid secretion to be normal or even slightly increased in cirrhotic patients (mostly non-alcoholics). To settle the problem of esophagitis as a cause of bleeding varices, ORLOFF and THOMAS (1963) studied the esophagus in 20 cirrhotics (19 alcoholics) who were treated by varix ligation within 5 to 56 hours after the onset of bleeding; a solitary bleeding point was found within 1.5 cm of the gastroesophageal junction in 16 of them. The source of bleeding could not be determined in the remaining 4 patients. Macroscopic evidence of esophagitis was found in only one patient, who had been drinking heavily until just before the bleeding. In an endoscopic study, DAGRADI et al. (1966) found only one bleeding point in each of the 35 patients bleeding from esophageal varices; mild esophagitis was observed in only 2 patients. BRICK and PALMER (1964) examined by esophagoscopy 1000 cirrhotics. Among the 704 patients with varices (81% of them were alcoholics) they found subacute erosive esophagitis in 72 (10.2%), esophageal ulcer in 6 (0.9%) and erosive gastritis in 19 cases (2.7%).

Sudden changes in pressure within the varices can be related to local changes in the distal esophagus or to changes in portal pressure. Any maneuver that increases intraabdominal pressure will cause a rise in portal pressure (LEEVY et al., 1960a; LIEBOWITZ, 1961; SILVA et al., 1969). A five-minute period of vigorous exercise or administration of drugs containing epinephrine or Levophed have been shown to increase wedged hepatic pressure by up to 10 mm of Hg (Leevy et al., 1958). Plasma-volume expansion with dextran or albumin has been shown to produce a temporary increase in portal pressure in compensated cirrhosis ($2^1/_2$ h) and a long-lasting hypertension in patients with gross ascites (Boyer et al., 1966). Ascites itself may be associated with a significant elevation in portal pressure (Panke et al., 1959). Local pressure changes in the lower esophageal sphincter may also play a role, since at least 75% of the bleeding points are located within 1–5 cm of the gastroesophageal junction (Chiles et al., 1953; Orloff and Thomas, 1963; Burgmann, 1965; Dagradi et al., 1966).

5.3. Clinical Symptoms

In most instances the hemorrhage results in a sudden massive hematemesis. During meals or straining the patient feels blood welling up without nausea or sickness. These hemorrhages frequently cause shock and exsanguination, and may be followed by coma in patients with poor liver function. Sometimes the acute bleeding episode is followed by chronic loss of blood.

Immediate mortality is high (33%: Ratnoff and Patek, 1942; 44%: Sherlock and Alpert, 1965). Prognosis is even worse in patients with ascites, jaundice or coma, in whom mortality amounts to 97% as compared to 9% for those with reasonable liver function (Sherlock, 1964). Brick and Palmer (1964) reported that 44% of their patients died during the first bleeding episode and half of the survivors required more than 2.5 l of blood.

The time of the subsequent hemorrhages is unpredictable; in some patients the interval is as long as 13 years (Tumen and Cohn, 1965). One to two thirds of the survivors, however, die within the first year (Sherlock, 1964; Patek et al., 1948; Garceau et al., 1963).

It has been shown endoscopically that larger varices are associated with more severe degrees of bleeding (Dagradi et al., 1966). Furthermore, there is a clear correlation between high portal pressure and actual variceal hemorrhage (Turner et al., 1957; Jackson, 1963); but there is no correlation of portal pressure with variceal size (Brick and Palmer, 1964; Peternel et al., 1967).

6. Diagnosis
6.1. Diagnosis of Esophageal Varices

The diagnosis of esophageal varices can be established by radiography, esophagoscopy, splenoportography and arteriography of the celiac trunk. Umbilico-portography and ammonia tolerance tests can also be used.

6.1.1. Barium Swallow[1]

Varices detected by radiography are classically described as sigmoidal, tortuous, and nodular filling defects (Fig. 307), indenting the barium column of a slightly dilated esophagus. The presence of thickened longitudinal folds with variable rounded expansions, and scalloping of the inner border of a dilated lower esophagus are also valuable signs. Varices occur usually in the distal half of the esophagus and, as a rule, they are most prominent in the lower end of the gullet, where they may produce marked filling defects displacing the pleuroesophageal line (Fig. 308).

In cooperation with J. Pringot.

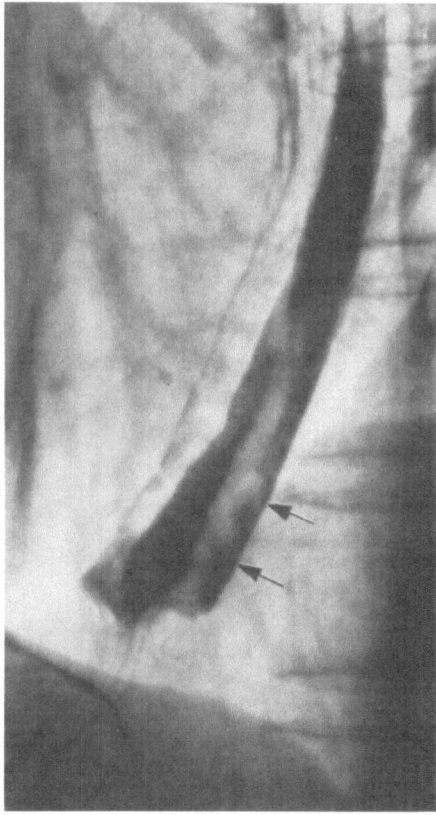

Fig. 307. Minute esophageal varices. The nodular thickening of the mucosal folds (arrow) were shown by esophagoscopy to be due to varices

As the esophageal peristaltic contractions usually result in the emptying of the varices, X-ray films should be made while the esophagus is relaxed, or ahead of a peristaltic contraction. Usually they are better visualized in the recumbent than in the upright position (Fig. 309, 310). Submucosal metastases may cause filling defects, which, when multiple, may mimic esophageal varices (Fig. 311).

Varices are detected by radiography in 27.5% (BRICK and PALMER, 1964) to 66% (PETERNEL et al., 1967) of the patients in whom the presence of varices is proven by another method. In different groups of cirrhotic patients, varices were demonstrated radiologically in 20–70%. However, these groups are not comparable.

Recently, cineradiography has been used to improve detection of varices. Positive results were reported in 88% of the patients examined by ADLER et al. (1964). A rapid dextran infusion (1 000 ml of 6% dextran in saline over 30–40 min) has been reported to enhance visualization of varices by increasing portal hypertension (PREGER, 1967a). Anticholinergic drugs will have the same effect (GHAHREMANI et al., 1972). A meal rich in proteins may also permit an easier radiological demonstration of varices, presumably by increasing portal venous pressures (CASTLEMAN et al., 1958; ORREGO et al., 1965; DEBAU et al., 1968).

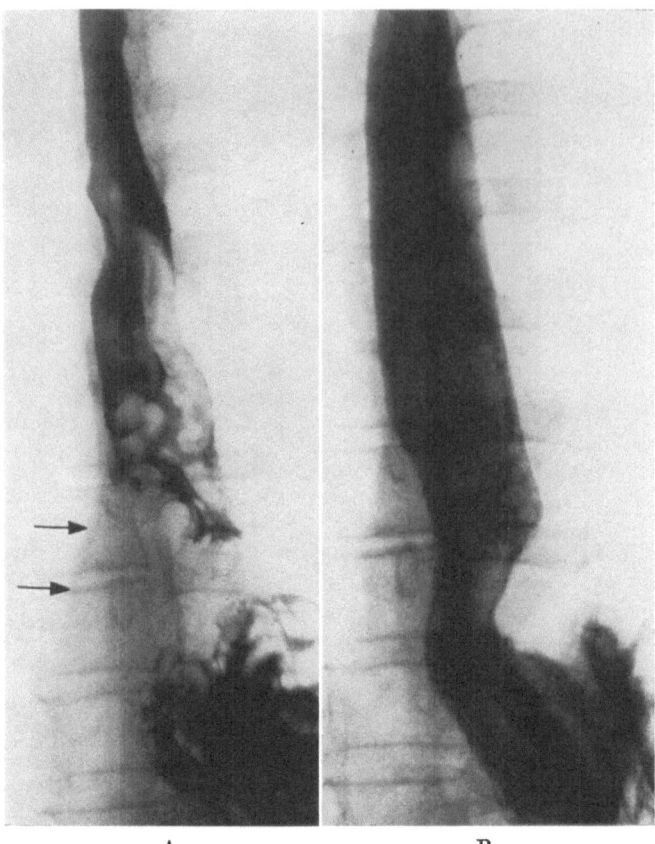

Fig. 308 A—C. Esophageal varices. A Intraluminal filling defects corresponding to sub-mucosal varices. Displacement to the right of the pleuroesophageal line (arrow). B When the esophagus has been filled the varicosities cannot be seen, but the segmental thickening of the right pleuroesophageal line is better distinguishable. C Splenoportography shows that the zone of thickening is due to voluminous periesophageal varices (double arrow). Note also the associated hiatus hernia

6.1.2. Esophagoscopy

This method allows direct visualization of the varices and, even more important, visualization of the bleeding point. Semi-rigid and fiberesophagoscopes give comparable detection rates (CONN et al., 1967a). Varices are seen as serpentine elevations of the mucosa, persisting during breathing and wrinkling in inspiration (Fig. 122). With the rigid or semi-rigid esophagoscope varices have a bluish color. This characteristic helps in the differentiation from mucosal folds if it is present, but its absence means little. Through the fiberscope the bluish color is less evident and one must rely more on the tortuous course and the persistence during respiration.

Varices have been graded as mild (less than 3 mm), moderate (3–6 mm) or severe (BRICK and PALMER, 1964) or as grade 1 (less than 2 mm in diameter), grade 2 (2–3 mm), grade 3 (3–4 mm), grade 4 (4–5 mm), grade 5 (more than 5 mm, occluding the lumen, grape-like or sometimes varices on top of varices) (DAGRADI

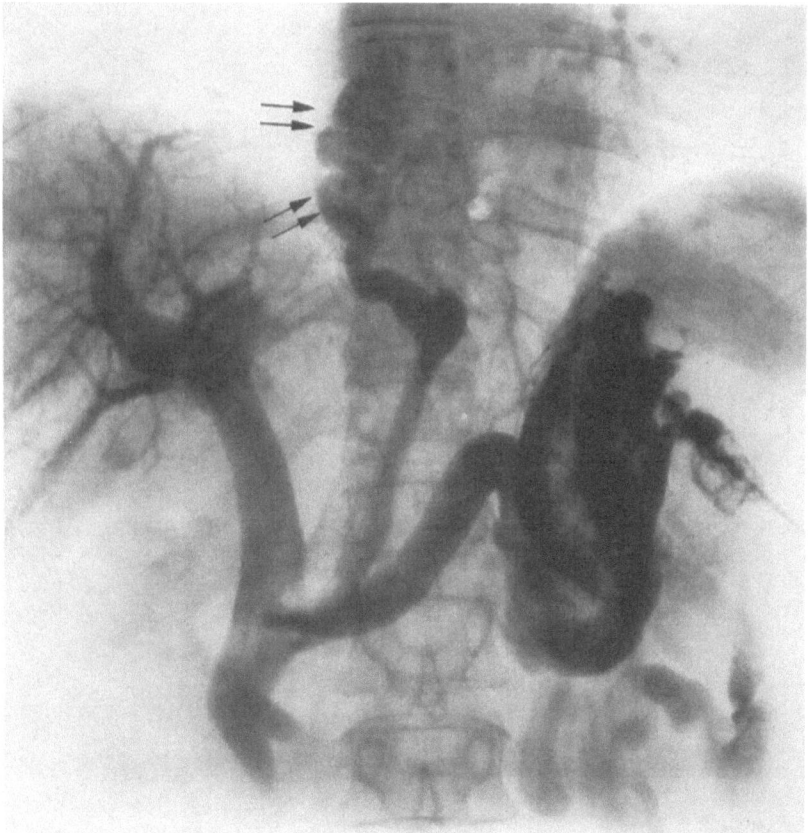

Fig. 308 C

et al., 1966). The extent of the esophagus involved in varix formation should also be noted. Endoscopy has the advantage of direct visualization, but observer variation in the same patient was found to be as high as 33% (CONN et al., 1965). Attempts have been made to improve differentiation from mucosal folds by using red filters (CONN et al., 1967 b) and by color photography. A more dubious advantage of esophagoscopy is the possibility to measure portal venous pressure by trans-esophagoscopic needling of the varix (ALLISON, 1951; BRICK and PALMER, 1964). The main advantage of esophagoscopy is that it makes a precise diagnosis of the bleeding cause possible. In a selected series of 27 patients with proven varices, liver disease, and hematemesis, only 5 were actually bleeding from ruptured varices, gastritis being the most frequent cause of the bleeding (McCRAY et al., 1969; DAGRADI et al., 1970).

6.1.3. Splenoportography

Opacification of the splenic and portal vein system by injecting contrast material into the splenic pulp is used to demonstrate the patency of the portal vein and the presence of gastric and esophageal varices (Fig. 308 C) (ABEATICI and CAMPI, 1951; BOULVIN et al., 1951; LEGER, 1951). The technique consists of a

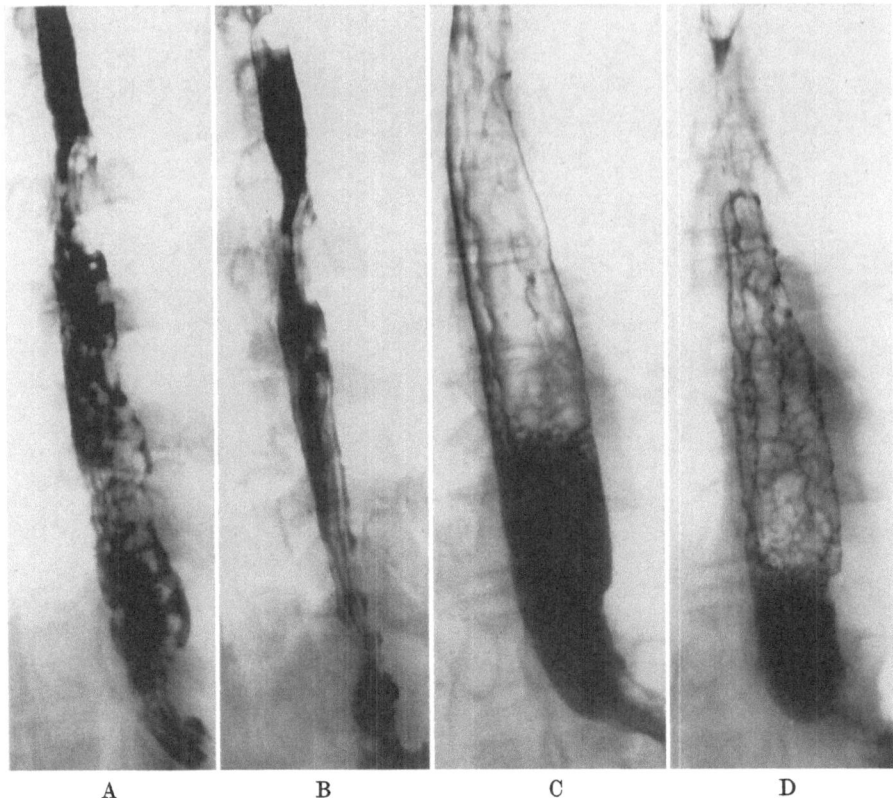

A   B   C   D

Fig. 309 A—D. Extensive esophageal varices in a 55-year old patient. A Supine position: the
visualization of varices is easier in the recumbent position and when the esophagus is relaxed.
B Esophageal contraction collapses the varices and makes visualization difficult. C In the
upright position the distension of the esophagus during drinking is frequently insufficient to
visualize the varices. D Varices are better visible in front of peristaltic contractions, even in
the upright position

percutaneous puncture of the spleen under local anesthesia, using a polyethylene
catheter over a 10 cm long needle or a needle with a stilletto. The needle is introduced in the mid-axillary line at the level of the 8th or 9th intercostal space
and moved in a slightly cranioposterior direction. When the appearance of a free
drip of blood has established that the needle is in the correct position, intrasplenic pressure is measured and a small test injection is made under fluoroscopic
control. There after, about 50 ml of water-soluble contrast material is injected
and X-ray films are made at a rate of 2 frames per second during the first 3 seconds
followed by 1 per second from the 4th to the 20th second. Ascites, marked jaundice,
and coagulation disorders are contraindications to the procedure (LEGER, 1966;
WARREN et al., 1967; KREEL, 1970). The only serious complication is bleeding
from the puncture site, which in 1–2% of the patients may be sufficiently severe
to require transfusion.

It has been attempted to improve the technique by using a multiperforated
needle, to inject larger doses (100 ml; McNULTY, 1968) and by using the prone
position (MOSKOWITZ et al., 1968). A patent portal vein and varices can be clearly

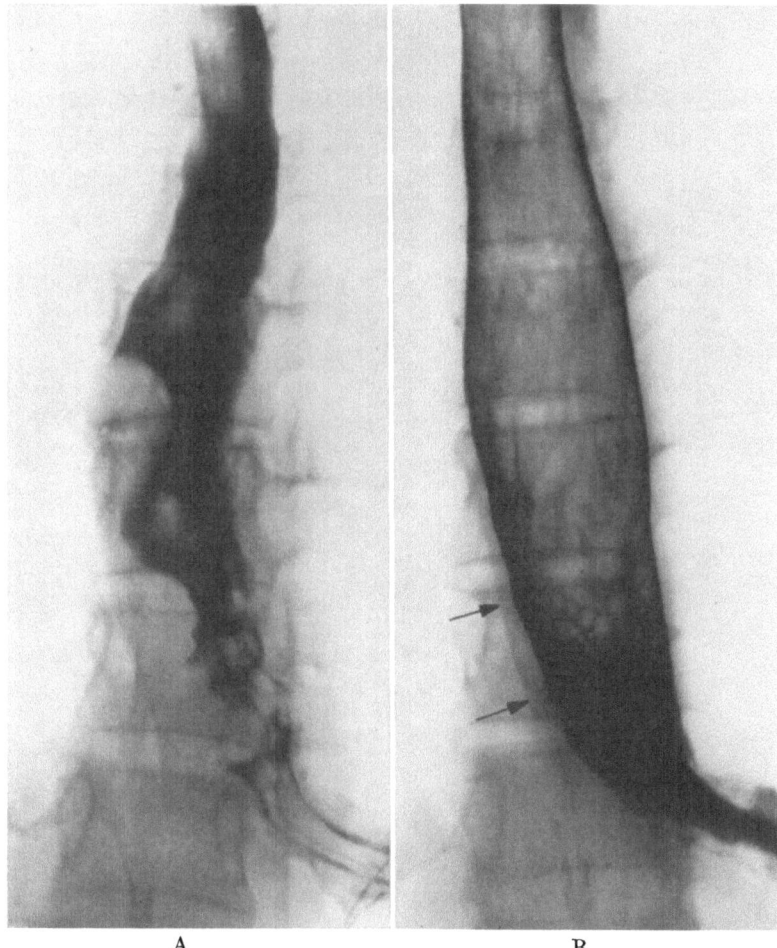

A
B

Fig. 310. A Extensive varices predominant on the right side of the lower third of the esophagus.
B In the upright position when the esophagus is distended, the scalloped contour disappears
whereas a slight enlargement of the right pleuroesophageal line persists (arrow)

visualized but the technique is too complicated to be used routinely. It is mainly
applied in relation to planned surgical intervention. Indirect splenoportography
is the result of the venous phase of an intraarterial injection in the splenic artery.
Great advances have recently been made in this field (VIAMONTE et al., 1970).

6.1.4. Umbilical Vein Portography

Injection of contrast material through a catheter put into the surgically reopened umbilical vein was first described by CARBALHAES (1959). In addition to
visualizing the venous patterns of liver, spleen and intestine, this technique
permits early detection of varices (BAYLY and CARBALHAES, 1964; KESSLER and
ZIMMON, 1967; LAVOIE et al., 1967; JOLY et al., 1968; RACHLIN et al., 1970).

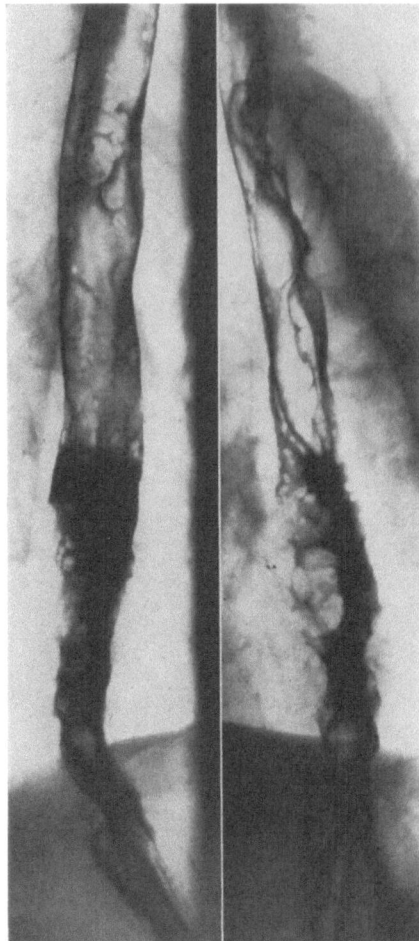

Fig. 311. Submucosal metastases of a gastric carcinoma, spread diffusely over the esophagus. The irregular confluence of the filling defects in the lower esophagus, and their persistence in the upright position as well as during peristalsis aid to distinguish it from varices (Dr. P. Dan- haive, Namur)

6.1.5. Ammonia Tolerance; Indirect Test for Esophageal Varices

High levels of ammonia in arterial and venous blood were found after oral intake of ammonium chloride in patients with cirrhosis (Van Caulaert and De- viller, 1932). This was related to intestinal blood shunting the liver (Kirk, 1936). Conn (1961) has used this test as an index of portosystemic shunting. Non enteric coated tablets of ammonium chloride (0.4 g per 10 kg body weight) are administered with 250 ml water to fasting subjects and after 45 min an arterial blood sample is taken. In compensated liver cirrhosis this test permits differentiation between pa- tients with and without portosystemic shunting; poor liver function, yielding in itself abnormal ammonia curves, precludes this differentiation (McDermott and Huston, 1963). Arterial blood levels over 250 µg/100 ml agreed in 70% with other methods used for the detection of varices in cirrhotic patients (Conn, 1967).

Table 28. Detection rates of esophageal varices by different diagnostic techniques

	X-ray (%)	Esoph-agos-copy (%)	Spleno-portog-raphy (%)	Ammonia tolerance test (%)	Patients
BRICK and PALMER, 1964	27.5	70.4			1000 "unselected" cirrhotics seen over 11 years who underwent both examinations
GREENE et al., 1965		90	50		60 "selected" cirrhotics
CONN, 1967	37	43		39	275 "unselected" cirrhotics undergoing the 3 examinations
CONN et al., 1967	26	39			54 unselected cirrhotics
PETERNEL et al., 1967	66	97.6	73		83 cirrhotics selected because of varices proven by one method

Nearly normal levels of ammonia were found in patients with schistosomiasis who had esophageal varices (WARREN and REBOUCAS, 1964); it looks therefore as if varices must be accompanied by some liver function disturbances to result in a positive ammonia test.

6.1.6. Evaluation of the Different Techniques Used

The techniques used to detect esophageal varices yield different results (Table 28). Although esophagoscopy gives the highest detection rates, radiography will mostly be used first because of its simplicity, safety, and convenience.

6.2. Diagnosis of Bleeding from Esophageal Varices

If variceal hemorrhage is suspected in a patient with upper gastrointestinal bleeding, attempts should be made first to demonstrate liver disease by history and by clinical examination for hepatosplenomegaly, collateral circulation, cutaneous manifestations, fetor hepaticus and flapping tremor. Laboratory tests include mainly serum levels of bilirubin, albumin, globulines, transaminases, coagulation proteins, and ammonia. If a normal ammonia level is found in venous blood 3 hours after a hematemesis, bleeding from esophageal varices is very unlikely (MARTINI and WIEBEL, 1964). Similarly a normal BSP-test makes variceal bleeding unlikely; the contrary is not true because BSP extraction may be decreased in acute bleeding, presumably as a result of a decreased liver blood flow (ENQUIST et al., 1964).

Varices should be demonstrated by the methods discussed in the previous paragraphs. The presence of esophageal varices in a patient with upper gastrointestinal bleeding does not mean that the varices are the source of the hemorrhage. Peptic ulcer and hemorrhagic gastritis are a frequent cause of bleeding in cirrhotics, especially in alcoholics (DAGRADI et al., 1970). Before diagnosing bleeding of variceal origin the bleeding point should be visualized endoscopically or by selective angiography. Endoscopy has many advantages over radiology because

it allows direct inspection of the bleeding site, whereas radiology can only demonstrate the presence of varices. Moreover, superficial lesions cannot be visualized
radiologically. Emergency endoscopy for bleeding requires a thorough lavage of
the stomach with ice water through a large gastric tube until the returns are clear,
as well as continuous instillation and suction in the esophagus during examination.
Recently selective angiography has been used as another means of demonstrating
the bleeding site. The escape of injected contrast material into the esophageal or
gastric lumen can be visualized if at least 2 ml of blood is lost each minute.

7. Therapy

Therapy of esophageal varices consists mainly in treatment of the underlying
disease. In some rare instances (fatty liver, hepatitis etc.) this treatment may
result in disappearance of the varices. Prophylactic shunt operations can also be
performed to treat portal hypertension. Therapy of bleeding varices is the major
problem and has to be divided into emergency medical and surgical care; both
may or may not have to be followed by "definitive" operations.

7.1. Medical Management of Bleeding Varices

(Sherlock, 1967; Schaffner, 1968; Williams and Dawson, 1968)

The aims of medical treatment are to prevent shock and liver anoxia by
restoring the blood volume, to prevent hepatic encephalopathy and to arrest
further bleeding.

7.1.1. Blood Transfusion

Adequate amounts of blood should be given as soon as possible to restore blood
volume. Fresh blood and Vitamin K (10 mg I.V.) will help to improve coagulation.
Large amounts of blood are necessary, for it has been found that at least 50% of
the patients require more than 2.5 l to survive (Brick and Palmer, 1964; Sherlock and Alpert, 1965). As recurrent bleeding is noted in almost 70% of the
patients close supervision of the patient is required (Sherlock and Alpert, 1965).

7.1.2. Prevention of Hepatic Encephalopathy (in Cirrhotics)

Encephalopathy is a common consequence of bleeding because of cerebral
anoxia, resorption of blood protein derivatives, hypopotassemia and sometimes
because of the administration of sedatives. Purging with magnesium sulphate or
other preparations and administration of enemas is indicated to remove swallowed
blood. Neomycine (4–6 g daily) should be given to depress bacterial breakdown of
blood and production of ammonia. Lactulose, an unabsorbable disaccharide, has
been proven to lower blood ammonia and to prevent hepatic coma (Rottiers
et al., 1968; Elkington et al., 1969). It can be given orally in a dose of 100 g a
day, or as an enema containing 300 g of lactulose in 1 l of fluid.

7.1.3. Arrest of Further Bleeding
7.1.3.1. Drugs

Vasopressine in a dose of 20 U administered intravenously over a period of
20 min lowers portal pressure to 30 to 40% of the control value, presumably by
vasoconstriction of the splanchnic arterioles (Shaldon et al., 1961; Tsakiris et al.,
1964; Silva et al., 1969). The effect lasts for about one hour. Octapressine (phenyl-
alanine-lysine-vasopressine) has the same effect but causes less systemic vaso-

constriction. The dose may be repeated after two hours, with diminishing effect, however. The maximal decrease of splanchnic blood flow in 5 normal subjects during and immediately after the administration of the drug reached 50% of the control value; it returned to 73% after 15 min and to 90% after 50 min (JACOBSEN et al., 1969; SILVA et al., 1969). The effects on wedged hepatic venous pressure and hepatic resistance are variable, mainly because of changes in cardiac output (Cocco et al., 1963). Arfonad, an autonomic ganglionic blocking agent, caused systemic hypotension with reduced cardiac output, and a decrease in hepatic blood flow, wedged hepatic vein pressure, and calculated vascular resistance (Cocco et al., 1963). An intravenous drip of a 0.1% solution of Arfonad R administered to bleeding cirrhotics at a rate sufficient to produce a controlled hypotension of 70–80 mm Hg for 1 h stopped the hemorrhage in the six patients of KUHN et al. (1967). Splenic portal pressure decreased by 31% (CINCOTTI and HUEMER, 1971).

7.1.3.2. Gastric Cooling

Gastric hypothermia, produced by circulation of a cooled 50% ethanol-water mixture (0° C) into a gastric balloon, was introduced by WANGENSTEEN et al. (1963) in the therapy of esophageal bleeding. After controlling the exact position of the gastric balloon, infusion of 700 ml of cooled fluid is started and circulation is maintained for 24 h at a rate of 1 l/min. Body temperature should be maintained by electrical blankets and physiotherapy. This method stops bleeding in 80% of the patients (WALKER et al., 1964; NAGEL et al., 1966; RODGERS et al., 1966). Recurrent bleeding shortly after removing the gastric balloon was seen in 6 out of 20 patients. The mechanism whereby bleeding stops seems to be local vasoconstriction, as no changes in portal pressure were observed (WALKER et al., 1964). The high cost of the machine, and the need for specialized staff prevent broader use of the technique. Furthermore, gastric rupture was a frequent complication in the early period but could be avoided by safety devices. Development of pneumonia is the most frequent complication.

7.1.3.3. Balloon Tamponade

The commonly used Sengstaken-Blakemore tube consists of a gastric balloon, filled with water and some water-soluble contrast material, and of an esophageal balloon, to be inflated with some air under gentle pressure. A third outlet allows continuous suction of gastric contents as well as washing and instillation of drugs (neomycine, lactulose etc.). Traction (with 750 g) has to be applied and the best system uses a pulley wheel to suspend the tube. The gastric balloon exerts compression on gastric varices and on the veins draining into the esophageal varices, while the esophageal balloon may compress the esophageal varices. The tube is highly effective for acute esophageal bleeding, but is unpleasant for the patient and recurrent bleeding is frequent (LIEDBERG, 1968). It should be deflated after 24 hours, in order to avoid erosive esophagitis (READ et al., 1960). Complications are not infrequent, occurring in 35% of the cases in one series (CONN and SIMPSON, 1967). They include bronchial aspiration of regurgitated material, rupture of the esophagus and airway obstruction.

7.1.3.4. Intraarterial Infusion

Recent investigations in dogs with portal hypertension (NUSBAUM et al., 1967) and in man (NUSBAUM et al., 1968) indicate that selective infusion in the superior mesenteric artery of vasopressin and derivatives causes a decrease of the superior mesenteric and portal flow, and results in a decrease of portal pressure. Epinephrine derivatives had no sustained portal hypotensive action. Murray-Lyon et al. (1973) used this method for the treatment of acute variceal bleeding, but did not see any advantage over the venous route and a rather high incidence of complications.

By using one of these methods bleeding can be stopped temporarily in 70 to 80% of the patients.

Usually treatment is started with vasopressine, transfusion, and drug therapy to prevent hepatic encephalopathy. When bleeding cannot be controlled a Sengstaken-Blakemore tube may be used and left for 24 hours. However, when a Sengstaken tube or gastric cooling is really needed the bleeding is likely to be so massive and the risk for recurrence so high that emergency surgery may be preferable. Esophageal transection, sometimes with polar gastric resection or emergency portocaval anastomosis is then performed.

7.2. Surgical Management of Bleeding Esophageal Varices

Surgery may be directed against the varices (transection and ligation procedures) or against the portal hypertension (shunt operation). It is nearly impossible to get exact figures of the mortality rate, complications, and survivals in the different types of surgery, because everything has been mixed up: emergency operations with elective and prophylactic interventions, extra- and intrahepatic causes of portal hypertension; even in the group of cirrhotics, the disease can be more or less advanced, the etiology may be different, and the alcoholic may or may not continue to drink (Grace et al., 1966; Powell and Klatskin, 1968). An attempt at unraveling some of the published data is presented in Table 29 and Table 30.

7.2.1. Emergency Surgical Treatment

Emergency surgery is indicated if massive bleeding with impending shock and encephalopathy cannot be controlled by medical treatment. Three different types of operations can be performed: an emergency shunt operation, esophageal or gastric resections, or the more simple ligation-transection procedures. The decision about the type of surgery will depend mainly on the patient's age and liver function (jaundice, ascites, albuminemia, etc.) because these factors determine his chance to survive a more definitive but troublesome operation, such as emergency portocaval anastomosis, esophagus transection with polar gastric resection, or replacement of the esophagus by a segment of jejunum or colon.

Splenoportography should always be performed prior to shunt operations to make sure that the portal vein is open and suitable for anastomosis. The skill and experience of the available surgeon is another important factor in deciding the type of operation. Ligation and transection procedures are probably the simplest surgical emergency procedures, but the mortality of these operations is not significantly lower than that of urgent shunt operations (see Table 29), mainly because the bleeding cirrhotic is "metabolically bankrupt" and has a poor tolerance for anesthesia, further transfusion, etc. (Sherlock, 1967). Liver failure is the most frequent cause of postoperative death if bleeding can be controlled. Mortality rates of ligation and transection procedures vary from 10 to 80% with a mean around 45%, whereas emergency shunt operations have a mean mortality rate of 31.8% (Grace et al., 1966). Similar results are reported by Orloff (1967),

Table 29. Results of surgical intervention and of conservative treatment of esophageal bleeding due to intrahepatic portal hypertension

Treatment	Authors	Operative mortality (within 1 month) %	Enceph-alopathy %	Thrombo-sis or re-bleeding %	Longterm survival % after X years	Number of pa-tients	Type studied
Conservative	LINTON and ELLIS, 1956	50 (mortality — related to acute bleeding)			38 (1 yr)	22	Cirr. (good risk)
	EDMUNDS and WEST, 1964	82			14 (3 yr)	45	
	ORLOFF, 1968 (M)	86			9.5 (5 yr)	14	
Emergency operations							
Transsesophageal suture	LINTON and ELLIS, 1956	10		75 received later definitive operation		20	Cirr.
	MILNES WALKER, 1964	80				5	Cirr. (poor risk)
	ORLOFF, 1967	46				15	Cirr.
	HUNT, 1967	35		31 later → P.C. shunt		51	mostly Cirr.
Subcardiac gastric transection	TANNER, 1961	36	18	27		11	Cirr.
Dissection ligature of cardia (Vossschulte)	GRUENAGEL and HANKE, 1968	70		14	14 (4 yr)	7	Cirr.
Ligation + splenectomy	JOHNSON et al., 1966	63				27	Cirr. (21 poor risk)
Portacaval shunt	AKOVBIANTZ et al., 1968 (M)	50				10	Cirr.
	HIVET and CHEVREL, 1968 (M)	36				33 Cirr.	Cirr.
	MÉGEVAND, 1968 (M)	29				24	Cirr. (50% ascites, jaund.)
	ORLOFF, 1968 (M)	47				40	Cirr. (50% poor risk)
	GÜTGEMANN and ESSER, 1968	51				15	Cirr. (20% alcohol)
	GRAHAM et al., 1972	15				7	Cirr. (moderate grade; 25% alcohol)
Splenorenal shunt	HEPP et al., 1967	25				4	Cirr. (alcohol)
	RENWICK et al., 1969	62				8	mostly Cirr.
All types of emergency shunts (review)	GRACE et al., 1966	32	19	2.1		173	

Table 29 (continued)

Treatment	Authors	Operative mortality (within 1 month) %	Enceph- alop- athy %	Thrombo- sis or re- bleeding %	Longterm survival % after X years	Number of pa- tients	Type studied
Elective therapy							
Ligation and esoph- ageal transection	Milnes Walker, 1964	18		11	36 (3 yr)	11	Cirr. (poor risk)
Ligation and gastric transection	Tanner, 1961	0	7	{14 major / 43 minor}		14	Cirr.
Ligation and splenec- tomy	Johnson et al., 1966	19		42	43 (5 yr)	26	Cirr. (good risk)
	Smith, 1970	21		34		19	Cirr. (17)
Splenectomy alone	Hallenbeck et al., 1963	—		66	55 (5 yr)	73	Cirr.
Portocaval shunt	Linton and Ellis, 1956	15	13	10	65 (5 yr)	33	Cirr.
	Mc Dermott et al., 1961	12	68	19	36 (5 yr)	71	Cirr. ($^2/_3$ good risk)
	Linton et al., 1961	15	25	24	50 (5 yr)	47	Cirr. ($^2/_2$ good risk)
	Hallenbeck et al., 1963	11.4			38 (5 yr)	51	Cirr. (good rask)
	Edmunds and West, 1964	9.5				22	Cirr. (good risk)
	Schreiber et al., 1964	7		4.7		134	
	Hivet and Chevrel, 1968 (M)	16			53 (1 yr)	20	Cirr.
	Mégevand, 1968 (M)	5				234	mostly Cirr.
	Gütgemann and Esser, 1968	14.5	26	1.4	23 (5 yr)	210	Cirr. (75% alc.; 31% fair; 7% poor risk)
	Panke et al., 1968	10					Cirr.
(controlled study)	Barnes et al., 1971	17	20	4	39 (5 yr)	103	Cirr. non-shunt. contr.
	Jackson et al., 1971	13		4.5	{38 (5$^1/_2$ yr) / 57 (5$^1/_2$ yr)}	51	Cirr. shunted
	Graham et al., 1972	0	30			67	
review	Grace et al., 1966	16.8	22	2.8	38 (5 yr)	26	Cirr. (20% poor risk)

				Survival	No.	Characteristics
Splenorenal shunt						
LINTON and ELLIS, 1956	13				70	Cirr.
LINTON et al., 1961	11	24	19	57 (5 yr)	122	Cirr. (2/3 good risk)
MC DERMOTT et al., 1961	17	7	18	73 (5 yr)	166	Cirr. (2/3 good risk)
HALLENBECK et al., 1963	6	5	25	62 (5 yr)	70	Cirr. (good risk)
HIVET and CHEVREL, 1968 (M)	19				37	Cirr.
HEPP et al., 1968 (M)	3.5	3.5	3.5		29	(mostly alc.) Cirr.
RENWICK et al., 1969	7.5	13.5 (mild)	23 major / 15 minor	56 (5 yr)	39	mostly Cirr.
BARNES et al., 1971	10	4	7	39 (5 yr)	70	Cirr.
review — GRACE et al., 1966	19.2	13.4	19			
Distal splenorenal shunt						
WARREN et al., 1969	52				15	Cirr.
SALAM et al., 1971	6				16	Cirr.
Portorenal shunt						
SIMEONE and HOPKINS, 1967	36				11	Cirr.
Combined shunt-operations						
AKOVBIANTZ et al., 1968 (M)	11				33	Cirr.
DALICHOU, 1968 (M)	16	16	7		30	Cirr.
LATASTE and ROBIN, 1968	16			66 (2 yr)	45	Cirr. (mostly alc.)
DAGHER et al., 1971	18	24		44 (5 yr)	50	Cirr. (90%)
review — GRACE et al., 1966	15.5	19	6.7	42 (5 yr)		
Prophylactic shunts						
JACKSON et al., 1968 — Shunts	13.5			48.7 (4 yr)	37	Cirr. 30% poor risk
Non-shunted				70.6 (4 yr)	17	
Conservative control				72.5 (4 yr)	58	
CONN and LINDENMUTH, 1969 — Shunts	25			90 (2 yr)	12	Cirr. with asc. +jaund. 50%
Controls	25			48 (2 yr)	16	Alc. Cirr.
RESNICK et al., 1969 — Shunts	52	2.1		53 (5 yr)	48	2/3 poor risk
Controls	37	27		51 (5 yr)	45	Alc. Cirr.
CONN and LINDENMUTH, 1968 (M) — Shunts				51 (4 yr)	25	50% jaundice 75% ascites
Controls				62 (5 yr)	31	

(M) refers to papers published in the book "The Therapy of Portal Hypertension" edited by MARKOFF, N.G.

Table 30. Treatment and prognosis in portal hypertension due to schistosomiasis or extrahepatic block

Treatment	Authors	Operative mortality (%)	Rebleeding or thrombosis (%)	Longterm survival	Number of patients
Schistosomiasis					
Gastroesophageal decongestion with splenectomy	Hassab, 1967	9.9	3		35
Extrahepatic block					
Esophageal transection	Milnes Walker, 1964	0	16 minor 33 major	88 (5 yr)	25
Gastric subcardiac transection	Tanner, 1961	0	20 minor 60 major		5
	Hamilton and Hunt, 1970	0	73		15
Proximal gastric resection	Rothwell-Jackson and Hunt, 1970	3.5	24.5 minor 10.5 major	86 (10 yr)	28
Splenectomy	Stathers and Blackburn, 1968	0	25 minor 75 major, requiring other surgery		12
	Fonkalsrud and Longmire, 1969				6
	Hamilton and Hunt, 1970	23	90		27
Portocaval shunt	Fonkalsrud and Longmire, 1969	0			7
Splenorenal shunt	Stathers and Blackburn, 1968		40		10
	Renwick et al., 1969		23	92 (5 yr)	14
	Hamilton and Hunt, 1970	0	65 { 36 if shunt >10 mm 100 if shunt <10 mm		21
Mesentericocaval shunt	Fonkalsrud and Longmire, 1969		0		3

who used both approaches in a group of cirrhotics, half of which were poor risk cases because of jaundice and ascites. In view of these discouraging results a conservative attitude is justified in old and poor risk cases. Different types of ligation and transection procedures have been described (Tanner, 1961; Milnes-Walker, 1964; Boerema et al., 1967; Gruenagel and Hanke, 1968; and others). Although they differ from simple oversewing to proximal gastric resection, operative mortality is not statistically different, indicating once more that survival is mainly determined by the general condition of the patient. In a carefully controlled therapeutical study Jackson et al. (1971) give evidence of a significantly prolonged survival (57% versus 36%) in cirrhotic patients with a portocaval shunt versus a randomized control group.

7.2.2. Elective Surgical Treatment in Liver Cirrhosis with Bleeding Varices

Conservative treatment, splenectomy with or without omentopexy and the various ligation-transection procedures yield a 40 to 60% chance of recurrent bleeding. Although survival with conservative therapy is reported to be lower than with surgery (EDMUNDS and WEST, 1964), it has not been proven that shunt operations prolong survival. In most studies the operated patients are compared with a group of poor risk patients, not undergoing surgery because of a poor general condition. All elective operations have about the same operative mortality. Recurrence of variceal bleeding is certainly more frequent in the ligation-transection procedures, and is somewhat more frequent in splenorenal anastomosis as compared to portocaval shunt. Recurrent bleeding after splenorenal shunt depends in part on the width of the anastomosis (a stoma smaller than 10 mm always thromboses; one that is larger than 10 mm occludes in only 36% of the cases) (HAMILTON and HUNT, 1970). Severe encephalopathy occurs more frequently after portocaval than after splenorenal anastomosis. The 5 year survival rate for the different types of surgery is about 50% (see Table 28). The result seems to depend more on the patient's liver function than on the type of surgery, if an operation prevents the patient from bleeding for a shorter or longer period of time, it gives him more chance of dying from liver failure. According to McDERMOTT et al. (1961) 70% of deaths occur in patients who do not meet the optimal criteria for shunt operation. However, what are these optimal criteria? Most authors refer to a serum bilirubin level of more than 2 mg/100 ml, a prothrombin time less than 50%; a serum albumin level of less than 3 g/100 ml, and the continuous presence of ascites as negative factors. Furthermore, age 50 or above, and precoma during bleeding are other negative factors. Certainly those patients do worse, but would they do better if they were not operated?

JACKSON et al. (1971) recently reported on a controlled study of therapeutic elective shunt operations in patients who had bled from varices. The shunted patients had a significantly better survival (57% after 5 years) than the controls (36%).

7.2.3. Prophylactic Shunt Operations in Liver Cirrhosis

The problem of prophylactic shunt operations has been studied by several groups of investigators (JACKSON et al., 1968; CONN and LINDENMUTH, 1968, 1969; RESNICK et al., 1969). The 5 year survival rate of cirrhotics who had not bled prior to the start of the trial was comparable in the non-shunted and shunted group. Nearly all these patients were alcoholics, and at least half of them had jaundice and/or ascites; encephalopathy was present in 39% in one study. Bleeding was far more frequent in the non-shunted group, and was the most important cause of death, whereas the shunted group presented more signs of hepatic failure and encephalopathy. In fact, in JACKSON et al. 's series non-operated patients did better. In a group of cirrhotics with ascites and jaundice, shunted patients did better after 2 years than the controls, but the group is small and the follow-up period too short to draw valid conclusions (CONN and LINDENMUTH, 1969).

7.2.4. Prophylactic Operations in Extrahepatic Block

Patients with portal hypertension of extrahepatic origin have a far better prognosis, because their liver function tends to be normal. Their first risk therefore is death from hemorrhage. Shunt operations, i.e., splenorenal and mesentericocaval anastomosis are the procedures of choice (ZUIDEMA and EBERT, 1967).

Ligation-transection operations, even with colonic or jejunal replacement of the esophagus, have also been performed (Perry et al., 1963; Koop and Kavanian, 1965). The 5 year survival rate after ligation-transection procedures is not bad, mainly because the general condition of these patients is good and because the incidence of recurrent bleeding tends to decrease with the increasing age of the patients.

7.3. Thoracic Duct Drainage

As the production of thoracic duct lymph was found to be increased in cirrhotic patients, thoracic duct drainage has been used in the treatment of intrahepatic portal hypertension (Dumont and Mulholland, 1965). Thoracic duct pressure, however, does not correlate with portal pressure (Warren et al., 1968). If the drained lymph is efficiently replaced by fluid, wedged hepatic vein pressure and ascites are not reduced (Yamamoto et al., 1964; Warren et al., 1968). In some patients lymph drainage could not control hemorrhage (Kessler et al., 1969).

Although this problem has not yet been settled (Dumont, 1969), the general feeling is that thoracic duct drainage is not the therapy of choice for bleeding varices.

7.4. Transumbilical Portal Decompression

The portal vein can be drained by extracorporeal catheters connecting the reopened umbilical vein with a systemic vein, usually the femoral or external jugular vein. These artificial shunts can be constructed as a temporary aid in lowering portal pressure to control hemorrhage or they can have a more permanent character. They usually result in a rapid drop of portal pressure (Piccone and Leveen, 1967; White et al., 1968).

7.5. Sclerosing Injections for Esophageal Varices

At esophagoscopy sclerosing material can be injected into the submucosa close to the varices (Wodak, 1965a, b), or directly into varices (Pinel et al., 1965, 1971; Hardcastle, 1969). Usually a 5% solution of sodium morrhyate, a 5% solution of quinine chlorhydrate and urea (Sclerana) or a linol-linolen mixture (Phlebocid) is used. This technique was mostly used in patients who could not be subjected to surgery; bleeding episodes seem to be reduced by this therapy.

References

Aagenaes, O., Matlary, A., Elgjo, K., Munthe, E., Fagerhol, M.: Neonatal cholestasis in Alpha$_1$-antitrypsin deficient children. Acta paediat. Scand. 61, 632–642 (1972).

Abeatici, S., Campi, L.: Sur les possibilités de l'angiographie hépatique. La visualisation du système portal. Acta radiol. (Stockh.) 36, 383–392 (1951).

Adler, D. C., Haverback, B. J., Meyers, H. I.: Cineradiography of esophageal varices. J. Amer. med. Ass. 189, 77–80 (1964).

Adson, M. A., Wychulis, A. R.: Portal hypertension in secondary biliary cirrhosis. West. Surg. Ass. 96, 604–612 (1968).

Ahrens, E. H., Jr., Payne, M. A., Kunkel, H. G., Eisenmenger, W. J., Blondheim, S. H.: Primary biliary cirrhosis. Medicine (Baltimore) 29, 299–364 (1950).

Akovbiantz, A., Hefti, M., Bircher, J., Ammann, R., Haemmerli, U. P., Schmid, M.: 44 Shuntoperationen bei portaler Hypertonie: Indikationen und Resultate. In: The therapy of portal hypertension, ed. N. G. Markoff, p. 5–7. Stuttgart: Georg Thieme 1968.

Albacete, R. A., Matthews, M. J., Saini, N.: Portal vein thromboses in malignant hepatoma. Ann. intern. Med. 67, 337–348 (1967).

ALLISON, P.: The measurement of blood pressure in oesophageal varices. Thorax 6, 325–327 (1951).

ANDERSEN, D. H.: Familial cirrhosis of the liver with storage of abnormal glycogen. Lab. Invest. 5, 11–20 (1956).

ANDRADE, Z. A.: Hepatic schistosomiasis. Progress in liver diseases, eds. H. POPPER and F. SCHAFFNER, vol. II, p. 228–242. New York: Grune and Stratton Co. 1965.

AUFSES, A. H., JR., SCHAFFNER, F., ROSENTHAL, W. S., HERMAN, B. H.: Portal venous pressure in "Pipestem" fibrosis of the liver due to schistosomiasis. Amer. J. Med. 27, 807–810 (1959).

BARNES, B. A., ACKROYD, F. W., BATTIT, G. E., KANTROWITZ, P. A., SCHAPIRO, R. H., STROLE, W. E., JR., TODD, D. P., McDERMOTT, W. V., JR.: Elective portasystemic shunts: morbidity and survival data. Ann. Surg. 174, 76–84 (1971).

BARRETT-CONNOR, E.: Cholelithiasis in sickle cell anemia. Amer. J. Med. 45, 889–898 (1968).

BASU, A. K., AIKAT, B. K.: Tropical splenomegaly. London: Butterworths Co. 1963.

BAYLY, J. H., CARBALHAES, O. G.: The umbilical vein in the adult: Diagnosis, treatment and research. Amer. Surg. 30, 56–60 (1964).

BECK, K., CREUTZFELDT, W.: Über die unmittelbaren Todesursachen bei der Leberzirrhose. Med. Klin. 57, 860–864 (1962).

BENDETT, R. Y., FRITZ, H. L., DONALDSON, R. M., JR.: Gastric acid secretion after parenterally and intragastrically administered histamine in patients with portacaval shunt. New Engl. J. Med. 268, 511–516 (1963).

BENHAMOU, J. P., GUILLEMOT, R., TRICOT, R., LÉGER, L., FAUVERT, R.: Hypertension portale essentielle. Presse méd. 70, 2397–2399 (1963).

BENNETT, H., LORENTZEN, C., BAKER, L.: Transient esophageal varices in hepatic cirrhosis. Arch. intern. Med. 92, 507–522 (1953).

BERG, N. O., ERIKSSON, S.: Liver disease in adults with Alpha-Antitrypsin deficiency. New Engl. J. Med. 287, 1264–1267 (1972).

BERTRAND, L., MICHEL, H.: Regenerative nodules are not responsible for portal hypertension in alcoholic cirrhosis, p. 20. Proceedings 4th Meeting I.A.S.L. Elsinore 1970.

BLENDIS, L. M., BANKS, D. C., RAMBOER, C., WILLIAMS, R.: Spleen blood flow and splanchnic haemodynamics in blood dyscrasia and other splenomegalies. Clin. Sci. 38, 73–84 (1970).

BOEREMA, I., KLOPPER, P. J., HOLSCHER, A. A.: Afbinding van de gehele slokdarm bij bloedende varices. Ned. T. Geneesk. 111, 1549–1554 (1967).

BOULVIN, R., CHEVALIER, M., GALLUS, P., NAGEL, M.: La portographie par voie splénique transpariétale. Acta chir. belg. 50, 534–544 (1951).

BOYER, J. L., CHATTERJEE, C., IBER, F. L., BASU, A. K.: Effect of plasma volume expansion on portal hypertension. New Engl. J. Med. 275, 750–755 (1966).

BOYER, J. L., GUPTA, K. P. S., BISWAS, S. K., PAL, N. C., MALLICK, K. C. B., IBER, F. L., BASU, A. K.: Idiopathic portal hypertension. Ann. intern. Med. 66, 41–68 (1967).

BRANDT, K., CATHCART, E. S., COHEN, A. S.: A clinical analysis of the course and prognosis of forty-two patients with amyloidosis. Amer. J. Med. 44, 955–969 (1968).

BRAS, G., HILL, K. R.: Veno-occlusive disease of the liver: essential pathology. Lancet 271, 161–163 (1956).

BRICK, I. B., PALMER, E. D.: Incidence and diagnosis of esophageal varices in cirrhosis of the liver: an esophagoscopic study. Gastroenterology 25, 378–384 (1953).

BRICK, I. B., PALMER, E. D.: One thousand cases of portal cirrhosis of the liver. Arch. intern. Med. 113, 501–511 (1964).

BROWN, B. I., BROW, D. M.: Lack of an X-1,4-glucan: α-1,4 glucan 6-glucosyltransferase in a case of Type IV glycogenosis. Proc. nat. Acad. Sci. (Wash.) 56, 725–729 (1966).

BRUGSCH, J., BRANDT, H. H., MUNCH, O.: Über Leberveränderungen bei Porphyrien des Erwachsenen. Acta hepato-splenol. (Stuttg.) 7, 333–360 (1960).

BURGMANN, W.: Die wechselnde Füllung der Ösophagusvarizen. Med. Welt 27, 1507–1512 (1965).

BUTLER, H.: The veins of the oesophagus. Thorax 6, 276–296 (1951).

CAMPBELL, G. S., BICK, H. D., PAULSEN, E. P., LOBER, P. H., WATSON, C. J., VARCO, R. L.: Bleeding esophageal varices with polycystic liver. New Engl. J. Med. 259, 901–910 (1958).

CARBALHAES, O. G.: Hepatoportografia por via umbilical. Rev. Sanid. milit. (Mex.) 12, 42 (1959).

CAROLI, J., PEQUINOT, G.: Enquête sur les circonstances diététiques de la cirrhose alcolique en France. World Congr. Gastroenterology, Washington 1958, vol. 1, p. 661–665. Baltimore: Williams and Wilkins Co. 1959.

CARTWRIGHT, G. E., BUSH, J. A., MARKOWITZ, H., MAHONEY, J. P., GUBLER, C. J.: Further studies on the abnormalities in the metabolism of copper in Wilson's disease. J. clin. Invest. 34, 925 (1955).

CASTLEMAN, L., BRANDT, J. L., RUSKIN, H.: The effect of oral feedings of meat and glucose on hepatic vein wedge pressure in normal and cirrhotic subjects. J. Lab. clin. Med. **51**, 897–903 (1958).

CAULAERT, C. VAN, DEVILLER, C.: Ammoniémie expérimentale après ingestion de chlorure d'ammonium chez l'homme à l'état normal et pathologique. C. R. Soc. Biol. (Paris) **111**, 50–52 (1932).

CINCOTTI, J., HUEMER, R.: Reduction of portal hypertension by ganglionic blockade. Amer. J. dig. Dis. **16**, 517–521 (1971).

CHEITLIN, M. D., SULLIVAN, B. H., JR., MYERS, J. E., JR., HENCH, R. F.: Portal hypertension in hepatic sarcoidosis. Gastroenterology **38**, 60–69 (1960).

CHIANDUSSI, L., GRECO, F., INDOVINA, D., CESANO, L., VACCARINO, A., MURATORI, F.: Hepatic steatosis and portal hypertension with presinusoidal obstruction. Gastroenterology **44**, 532–535 (1963).

CHILES, N. H., BAGGENSTOSS, A. H., BUTT, H. R., OLSEN, A. M.: Esophageal varices: comparative incidence of ulceration and spontaneous rupture as a cause of fatal hemorrhage. Gastroenterology **25**, 565–573 (1953).

CLAIN, D., FRESTON, J., KREEL, L., SHERLOCK, S.: Clinical diagnosis of the Budd-Chiari syndrome. Amer. J. Med. **43**, 544–554 (1967).

CLASSEN, M., ELSTER, K., PESCH, H. J., DEMLING, L.: Portal hypertension caused by partial nodular transformation of the liver. Gut **11**, 245–249 (1970).

CLATWORTHY, H. W., BOLES, T., JR.: Extrahepatic portal bed block in children: pathogenesis and treatment. Ann. Surg. **150**, 371–383 (1959).

COCCO, T. B., KENNETH, H. J., LEEVY, C. M.: Observations on intrahepatic vascular pressure regulation in portal hypertension. Ann. Surg. **158**, 109–116 (1963).

CONN, H. O.: Ammonia tolerance as an index of portal-systemic collateral circulation in cirrhosis. Gastroenterology **41**, 97–106 (1961).

CONN, H. O.: Ammonia tolerance in the diagnosis of esophageal varices. A comparison of endoscopic, radiologic and biochemical techniques. J. Lab. clin. Med. **70**, 442–451 (1967).

CONN, H. O., BINDER, H., BRODOFF, M.: Fiberoptic and conventional esophagoscopy in the diagnosis of esophageal varices. Gastroenterology **52**, 810–818 (1967a).

CONN, H. O., BRODOFF, M., GORDON, M. E.: Red filters in the esophagoscopic diagnosis of esophageal varices. Amer. J. dig. Dis. **12**, 1209–1215 (1967b).

CONN, H. O., LINDENMUTH, W. W.: Observations on prophylactic portacaval anastomosis in cirrhotic patients with esophageal varices. In: Therapy of portal hypertension, ed. N. C. MARKOFF, p. 78–86. Stuttgart: Georg Thieme 1968.

CONN, H. O., LINDENMUTH, W. W.: Prophylactic portacaval anastomosis in cirrhotic patients with esophageal varices and ascites. Amer. J. Surg. **117**, 656–661 (1969).

CONN, H. O., SIMPSON, J. A.: Excessive mortality associated with balloon tamponade of bleeding varices. A critical reappraisal. J. Amer. med. Ass. **202**, 587–591 (1967).

CONN, H. O., SMITH, H. W., BRODOFF, M.: Observer variation in the endoscopic diagnosis of esophageal varices. A prospective investigation of the diagnostic validity of esophagoscopy. New Engl. J. Med. **272**, 830–834 (1965).

COUTINHO, A.: Hemodynamic studies of portal hypertension in Schistosomiasis. Amer. J. Med. **44**, 547–556 (1968).

DAGHER, F. J., KHURI, S., DAGHER, I. K.: Surgical management of portal hypertension. A ten-year experience. Arch. Surg. **103**, 363–370 (1971).

DAGRADI, A. E., MEHLER, R., TAN, D. T. D., STEMPIEN, S. J.: Sources of upper gastrointestinal bleeding in patients with liver cirrhosis and large esophagogastric varices. Amer. J. Gastroent. **54**, 458–463 (1970).

DAGRADI, A. E., STEMPIEN, S. J.: Symptomatic esophageal hiatus sliding hernia. Clinical, radiologic and endoscopic study of 100 cases. Amer. J. dig. Dis. **7**, 613–633 (1962).

DAGRADI, A. E., STEMPIEN, S. J., OWENS, L. K.: Bleeding esophagogastric varices. Arch. Surg. **92**, 944–947 (1966).

DALICHAU, H., UNGEHEUER, E.: Das Schicksal des Patienten mit blutenden Oesophagusvarizen. In: The therapy of portal hypertension, ed. N. G. MARKOFF, p. 8–10. Stuttgart: Georg Thieme 1968.

DA SILVA, L. C., PONTES, J. F.: Clinical aspects of schistosomiasis mansoni. Progress in liver diseases, eds. H. POPPER and F. SCHAFFNER, vol. II, p. 243–252. New York: Grune and Stratton Co. 1965.

DEBAU, M., OPROIV, A., TACORIAN, S., DEBAU, M., HOANCA, O., RUSSU, M., IONESCO, M.: Une nouvelle méthode radiologique pour le diagnostic des varices œsophagiennes. Rev. int. Hépat. **18**, 515–522 (1968).

DE CARVALHO, C. A. F.: Zur Untersuchung der Beziehung zwischen Arterien und Venen der Übergangszone zwischen Magen und Oesophagus des Menschen. Anat. Anz. **118**, 261–280 (1966).

DE GROOTE, J., DESMET, V. J., GEDIGK, P., KORB, G., POPPER, H., POULSEN, H., SCHEUER, P. J., SCHMID, M., THALER, H., UEHLINGER, E., WEPLER, W.: A classification of chronic hepatitis. Lancet 1968 II, 626–628.

DENISON, E. K., PETERS, R. L., REYNOLDS, T. B.: Portal hypertension in a patient with osteopetrosis. Arch. intern. Med. 128, 279–283 (1971).

DI SANT'AGNESE, P. A.: Cystic fibrosis of the pancreas. Amer. J. Med. 21, 406–422 (1956).

DI SANT'AGNESE, P. A., BLANC, W. A.: A distinctive type of biliary cirrhosis of the liver associated with cystic fibrosis of the pancreas. Pediatrics 18, 387–409 (1956).

DI SANT'AGNESE, P. A., TALAMO, C.: Cystic fibrosis of the pancreas. New Engl. J. Med. 277, 1287–1344 (1967).

DONOVAN, A. J., REYNOLDS, T. B., MIKKELSEN, W. P., PETERS, R. L.: Systemic-portal arteriovenous fistulas: pathological and hemodynamic observations in two patients. Surgery 66, 474–482 (1969).

DUMONT, A. E.: Comments: On the effect of lymph drainage on portal pressure and bleeding esophageal varices. Gastroenterology 57, 232–234 (1969).

DUMONT, A. E., MULHOLLAND, J. H.: Hepatic lymph in cirrhosis. In: Progress in liver disease, eds. H. POPPER and F. SCHAFFNER, vol. II, p. 427–441. New York: Grune and Stratton Co. 1965.

ECKER, J. A., MCKITTRICH, J. E., FAILING, R. M.: Thrombosis of the hepatic veins. "The Budd-Chiari syndrome"—a possible link between oral contraceptives and thrombosis formation. Amer. J. Gastroent. 45, 429–443 (1966).

EDMUNDS, R., WEST, J. P.: Treatment of bleeding esophageal varices. Five-year comparison of medical and surgical procedures. J. Amer. med. Ass. 189, 854 (1964).

ELKINGTON, S. G., FLOCK, M. H., CONN, H. O.: Lactulose in the treatment of chronic portal systemic encephalopathy. New Engl. J. Med. 281, 408–412 (1969).

ENQUIST, I. F., DENNIS, C., FIERST, S. M., KARLSON, K. E.: Validity of the bromsulphalein test in patients with acute severe upper gastrointestinal hemorrhage. Amer. J. Surg. 107, 306–310 (1964).

EVANS, G. W., DUBOIS, R. S., HAMBRIDGE, K. M.: Wilson's disease: Identification of an abnormal copper-binding protein. Science 181, 1175–1176 (1973).

FINCH, S. C., FINCH, C. A.: Idiopathic hemochromatosis, an iron storage disease. Medicine (Baltimore) 34, 381–430 (1955).

FONKALSRUD, E. W., LONGMIRE, W. P.: Reassessment of operative procedures for portal hypertension in infants and children. Amer. J. Surg. 118, 148–157 (1969).

FULTON, R. L., WOLFEL, D. A.: Hepatic artery—portal vein arteriovenous fistula. Arch. Surg. 100, 307–309 (1970).

GARCEAU, A. J., CHALMERS, T. C., and the Boston Inter-Hospital Liver Group: The natural history of cirrhosis. I. Survival with esophageal varices. New Engl. J. Med. 268, 469–473 (1963).

GARCEAU, A. J., DONALDSON, R. M., JR., O'HARA, E. T., CALLOW, A. D., MUENCH, H., CHALMERS, T. C., and the Boston Inter-Hospital Liver Group: A controlled trial of prophylactic portocaval-shunt surgery. New Engl. J. Med. 270, 496–500 (1964).

GHAHREMANI, G. G., PORT, R. B., WINANS, C. S., WILLIAMS, J. R.: Esophageal varices. Enhanced radiologic visualization by anticholinergic drugs. Amer. J. dig. Dis. 17, 703–712 (1972).

GILSANZ, V., GALLEGO, M., YUSTE, P. C.: Portal circulation in hydatid cyst of the liver. Arch. intern. Med. 108, 540–547 (1961).

GITLIN, N., GRAHAME, G. R., KREEL, L., WILLIAMS, H. S., SHERLOCK, S.: Splenic blood flow and resistance in patients with cirrhosis before and after portacaval anastomoses. Gastroenterology 59, 208–213 (1970).

GOLDSMITH, E. I., CARVALHO LUZ, F. F., PRATA, A., KEAN, B. H.: Surgical recovery of schistosomes from the portal blood. J. Amer. med. Ass. 199, 235–240 (1967).

GRACE, N. D., MUENCH, H., CHALMERS, T. C.: The present status of shunts for portal hypertension in cirrhosis. Gastroenterology 50, 684–691 (1966).

GRAFE, W. R., STEINBERG, I.: Superior mesenteric arterio-venous fistula following small bowel resection. Gastroenterology 51, 231–235 (1966).

GRAHAM, K. J., BARRATT-BOYES, B. G., COLE, D. S.: The results of shunt operation for bleeding varices due to intrahepatic obstruction. Surg. Gynec. Obstet. 134, 47–50 (1972).

GRAHAM, W. P., EISEMAN, B., PRYOR, R.: Hepatic artery aneurysm with portal vein fistula in a patient with familial hereditary telangiectasia. Ann. Surg. 159, 362–367 (1964).

GREEN, T. W., CONLEY, C. L., BERTHRONG, M.: The liver in sickle cell anemia. Bull. Johns Hopk. Hosp. 92, 99–127 (1953).

GREENE, L., WEISBERG, H., ROSENTHAL, W. S., DOUVRES, P. A., KATZ, D.: Evaluation of esophageal varices in liver disease by splenic-pulp manometry, spleno-portography and esophagogastroscopy. Diagnostic discrepancies. Amer. J. dig. Dis. 10, 284–292 (1965).

Gruenagel, H. H., Hanke, M.: Die Dissektionsligatur nach Vossschulte zur Behandlung der Oesophagusvaricenblutung. Chirurg **39**, 270–273 (1968).

Grunert, R. D., Oeff, K., Gerstenberg, E., Schmidt, H.: Diagnosis of isolated splenic vein occlusion by radioportography. Surgery **59**, 364–367 (1966).

Gütgemann, A., Esser, G.: Portal hypertension, varicose vein bleeding and shunt operation. Minn. Med. **51**, 1517–1525 (1968).

Haerter, W., Palmer, E. D.: Portal hypertension with esophageal varices in acute infectious hepatitis: further observations. Amer. J. med. Sci. **237**, 596–599 (1959).

Hallenbeck, G. A., Wollaeger, E. E., Adson, M. A., Gage, R. P.: Results after portal systemic shunts in 120 patients with cirrhosis of the liver. Surg. Gynec. Obstet. **116**, 435–442 (1963).

Halmagyi, A.: A critical review of 425 patients with upper gastro-intestinal hemorrhage. Surg. Gynec. Obstet. **130**, 419–430 (1970).

Hamilton, D. W., Hunt, A. H.: Extrahepatic portal obstruction. Med. J. Aust. **1**, 493–499 (1970).

Hardcastle, B.: Sclerosing injections for esophageal varices. Eye, Ear, Nose Thr. Monthly **48**, 693–695 (1969).

Hartmann, G.: Diagnostik und Therapie der akuten Ösophagusvarizenblutung. Dtsch. med. Wschr. **89**, 125–131 (1964).

Hassab, M. A.: Gastroesophageal decongestion and splenectomy in the treatment of esophageal varices in bilharzial cirrhosis: Further studies with a report on 355 operations. Surgery **61**, 169–176 (1967).

Hepp, J., Moreaux, J., Bismuth, H.: Résultats des anastomoses spléno-rénales dans la cirrhose. Bull. Soc. Méd. Hôp. (Paris) **118**, 1101–1107 (1967).

Hermann, R. E., Hawk, W. A.: Congenital hepatic fibrosis as a cause of portal hypertension: report of two cases. Surgery **62**, 1095–1099 (1967).

Hill, K. R., Stephenson, C. F., Filshie, I.: Hepatic veno-occlusive disease produced experimentally in rats by the injection of monocrotaline. Lancet **1958I**, 623.

Hislop, I. G., Waters, T. E., Kellock, T. D., Swannerton, B.: The natural history of haemorrhage from oesophageal varices. Lancet **1966I**, 945–948.

Hivet, M., Chevrel, J. P.: Indications et résultats immédiats des dérivations porto-caves dans l'hypertension portale de l'adulte. In: The therapy of portal hypertension, ed. N. G. Markoff, p. 13–16. Stuttgart: Georg Thieme 1968.

Homer, S., Yanoff, M., Brooks, F. P.: Gastrointestinal bleeding in 3 patients with chronic liver disease, esophageal varices and normal portal pressure. Amer. J. dig. Dis. **9**, 406–415 (1964).

Hsia, D. Y., Walker, F. A.: Variability in the clinical manifestations of galactosemia. J. Pediat. **59**, 872–883 (1961).

Hunt, A. H.: An analysis of 584 cases of portal obstruction seen between 1947–1963, with particular reference to surgical treatment. St. Bart. Hosp. J., Clinical and research Suppl. **69**, 1–15 (1965).

Hunt, A. H.: Observations on treatment and prognosis of portal hypertension.. Colston Papers **19**, 371–374 (1967).

Hunt, A. H., Whittard, B. R.: Thrombosis of the portal vein in cirrhosis hepatis. Lancet **1954I**, 281–284.

Hyun, B. H., Singer, E. P., Sharrett, R. H.: Esophageal varices and metastatic carcinoma of liver. A report of three cases and review of the literature. Arch. Path. **77**, 292–298 (1964).

Iber, F. L., Maddrea, W. C.: Familial hepatic diseases with portal hypertension with or without cirrhosis. Progress in liver diseases, eds. H. Popper and F. Schaffner, vol. II, p. 290–302. New York: Grune and Stratton Co. 1965.

Israel, H. L., Sones, M.: Selection of biopsy procedures for sarcoidosis diagnosis. Arch. intern. Med. **113**, 255–260 (1964).

Isselbacher, K. J.: Galactose metabolism and galactosemia. Amer. J. Med. **26**, 715–723 (1959).

Jackson, F. C.: "Directional" flow patterns in portal hypertension. Arch. Surg. **87**, 307–319 (1963).

Jackson, F. C., Perrin, E. B., Felix, W. R., Smith, A. G.: A clinical investigation of the portacaval shunt: V. Survival analysis of the therapeutic operation. Ann. Surg. **174**, 672–701 (1971).

Jackson, F. C., Perrin, E. B., Smith, A. G., Dagradi, A. E., Nadal, H. M.: A clinical investigation of the portacaval shunt. II. Survival analysis of the prophylactic operation. Amer. J. Surg. **115**, 22–42 (1968).

Jacobsen, K. R., Ranek, L., Tygstrup, N.: Liver function and blood flow in normal man during infusion of vasopressin. Scand. J. clin. Lab. Invest. **24**, 279–284 (1969).

Jenna, M.: Die Milzvenenthrombose. Helv. chir. Acta **36**, 77–80 (1969).

JOHNSON, G., JR., DART, C. H., JR., PETERS, R. M., MACFIE, J. A.: Hemodynamic changes with cirrhosis of the liver: Control of arteriovenous shunts during operation for esophageal varices. Ann. Surg. **163**, 692–703 (1966).

JOHNSTON, G. W., GIBSON, J. B.: Portal hypertension resulting from splenic arteriovenous fistulae. Gut **6**, 500–502 (1965).

JOLY, J. G., BERNIER, J., LAVOIE, P., LEGARE, A., VIALLET, A.: Hemodynamic and radiological evaluation of patients with hepatic or pancreatic disease by combined umbilico-portal and systemic venous catheterization. Canad. med. Ass. J. **98**, 16–24 (1968).

JONES, C. A.: Diseases of the portal vein. In: Gastroenterology, ed. H. L. BOCKUS, vol. III, p. 441–452. Philadelphia-London: W. B. Saunders Co. 1965.

JORDAN, R. A.: Cholelithiasis in sickle cell disease. Gastroenterology **33**, 952–958 (1957).

KABOTH, U., SCHOBER, A., ARNDT, H. J., VIDO, I., SELMAIR, H., GALLASCH, E., VERMA, P., THOMSSEN, R., CREUTZFELDT, W.: Australia (S.H.)-Antigen-Befunde bei Leberkranken und Blutspendern. Dtsch. med. Wschr. **95**, 2157–2165 (1970).

KALK, H. E., WILDHIRT, E.: Probleme der chronischen Hepatitis. Internist (Berl.) **1**, 141–147 (1960).

KAPP, J. P.: Hepatic amyloidosis with portal hypertension. J. Amer. med. Ass. **191**, 497–499 (1965).

KARMI, G., THIRKETTLE, J. L., READ, A. E. A.: The association of syphilis with hepatic cirrhosis: a report of six cases and a review of the literature. Postgrad. med. J. **45**, 675–679 (1969).

KEAN, B. H., GOLDSMITH, E. I.: Schistosomiasis Japonica. Treatment by extracorporeal hemofiltration. Amer. J. Med. **47**, 546–552 (1969).

KELTY, R. H., BAGGENSTOSS, A. H., BUTT, H. R.: The relation of the regenerated liver nodule to the vascular bed in cirrhosis. Gastroenterology **15**, 285–295 (1950).

KERR, D. N. S., HARRISON, C. V., SHERLOCK, S., WALKER, R. M.: Congenital hepatic fibrosis. Quart. J. Med. **30**, 91–117 (1961).

KESSLER, R. E., SANTONI, E., TICE, D. A., ZIMMON, D. S.: Effect of lymph drainage on portal pressure and bleeding esophageal varices. Gastroenterology **56**, 538–547 (1969).

KESSLER, R. E., ZIMMON, D. S.: Umbilical vein catheterization in man. Surg. Gynec. Obstet. **124**, 594–597 (1967).

KEW, M. C., VARMA, R. R., DOS SANTOS, H. A., SCHEUER, P. J., SHERLOCK, S.: Portal hypertension in primary biliary cirrhosis. Gut **12**, 830–834 (1971).

KIMURA, C., SHIROTANI, H., HIROOKA, M., TERADA, M., IWAHASKI, K., MAETANI, S.: Membranous obliteration of the inferior vena cava in the hepatic portion. J. cardiovasc. Surg. **4**, 87–98 (1963).

KIRK, E.: Amino acid and ammonia metabolism in liver disease. Acta med. scand. (Suppl.) **77**, 1–147 (1936).

KLUGE, T., SOMMERSCHILD, H., FLATMARK, A.: Sinusoidal portal hypertension. Surgery **68**, 294–300 (1970).

KNOBLAUCH, M., HEDINGER, C.: Die Hämochromatoseleber. Virchows Arch. path. Anat. **337**, 205–214 (1963).

KOOP, C. E., KAVIANIAN, A.: Reappraisal of colonic replacement of distal esophagus and proximal stomach in the management of bleeding varices in children. Surgery **57**, 454–456 (1965).

KRASSNITZKY, O., PESENDORFER, F., WEWALKA, F.: Australia / S.H.-Antigen und Lebererkrankungen. Dtsch. med. Wschr. **95**, 249–253 (1970).

KREEL, L.: Radiology of the portal system. Gut **11**, 620–626 (1970).

KUBASTA, M., DUSEK, J., KUBASTOVA, B., KODOUSEK, R.: Needle biopsy of the liver in schistosomiasis mansoni. Gastroenterology **49**, 280–286 (1965).

KUHN, T., JOSEPH, W. L., CINCOTTI, J. J.: Ganglionic blocking agents as a method of avoiding emergency portal decompression. Surg. Forum **18**, 394–395 (1967).

LAROCHELLE, J., MORTEZAI, A., BELANGER, M., FREMBLEY, M., CLAVEAU, J. C., AUBIN, G.: Experience with 37 infants with Tyrosinemia. Canad. med. Ass. J. **97**, 1051–1056 (1967).

LATASTE, J., ROBIN, B.: Les hémorragies digestives hautes chez les cirrhotiques (139 cas). Presse méd. **76**, 307–309 (1968).

LATHROP, D. B.: Cystic disease of the liver and kidney. Pediatrics **24**, 215–224 (1959).

LAVOIE, P., LEGARE, A., VIALLET, A.: Portal catheterization via the round ligament of the liver. Amer. J. Surg. **114**, 822–830 (1967).

LEATHER, H. M.: Portal hypertension and gross splenomegaly in Uganda. Brit. med. J. **1961I**, 15–18.

LEBACQ, E.: Etudes cliniques et biologiques concernant la sarcoidose de Besnier-Boeck-Schaumann. Brussels: Ed. Arscia 1964.

LEBACQ, E., PLUYGERS, E., TIRZMALIS, A.: Les localisations hépato-spléniques de la sarcoidose de Besnier-Boeck-Schaumann. Diagnostic et traitement. Acta gastro-ent. belg. **20**, 534–554 (1957).

Leevy, C. M.: Fatty liver: a study of 270 patients with biopsy proven fatty liver and a review of the literature. Medicine (Baltimore) **41**, 249–276 (1962).

Leevy, C. M., Cherrick, G. R., Davidson, C. S.: Portal hypertension. New Engl. J. Med. **262**, 397–403 (1960a).

Leevy, C. M., Cherrick, G. R., Davidson, C. S.: Portal hypertension. New Engl. J. Med. **262**, 451–456 (1960b).

Leevy, C. M., Zinke, M., Barber, J., Chey, W. Y.: Observations on the influence of medical therapy on portal hypertension in hepatic cirrhosis. Ann. intern. Med. **49**, 837–851 (1958).

Léger, L.: Phlébographie portale par injection splénique intra-parenchymateuse. Mém. Acad. Chir. **77**, 712 (1951).

Léger, L.: Splenoportography: diagnostic phlebography of the portal venous system. Springfield (Ill.): Charles C. Thomas 1966.

Leichner-Weil, Z.: Venen- und Lymphgefäßerweiterungen im Oesophagus beim Tumor der Kardia. Fortschr. Röntgenstr. **102**, 102–103 (1965).

Lelbach, W. K.: Zur leberschädigenden Wirkung verschiedener Alkoholika. Dtsch. med. Wschr. **92**, 233–238 (1967).

Levin, B., Snodgrass, G. J., Oberholzer, V. G., Burgess, E. A., Dobbs, R. H.: Fructosaemia: observations on seven cases. Amer. J. Med. **45**, 826–838 (1968).

Liebowitz, H. R.: Pathogenesis of esophageal varix rupture. J. Amer. med. Ass. **175**, 874–879 (1961).

Liedberg, G.: Esophageal tamponage in the treatment of massive bleeding from esophageal varices, with special reference to volume and pressure in the balloons. Acta chir. scand. **134**, 249–253 (1968).

Lima, P. J., von Eye, G., Paranhos de Lima, C., Ludwig, O. K.: Portal venous pressure in Hodgkin's disease with hepatic involvement and esophageal varices. Amer. J. Med. **32**, 618–620 (1962).

Linder, F., Vollmar, J., Krumhaar, D.: Die arterio-venösen Fisteln des Pfortadergebietes. Langenbecks Arch. klin. Chir. **320**, 50–63 (1968).

Linton, R. R., Ellis, D. S.: Emergency and definitive treatment of bleeding esophageal varices. J. Amer. med. Ass. **160**, 1017–1023 (1956).

Linton, R. R., Ellis, D. S., Geary, J. E.: Critical comparative analysis of early and late results of splenorenal and direct portacaval shunts performed in 169 patients with portal cirrhosis. Ann. Surg. **154**, 446–459 (1961).

Luna, A., Meister, H. P., Szanto, P. B.: Esophageal varices in the absence of cirrhosis. Incidence and characteristics in congestive heart failure and neoplasm of the liver. Amer. J. clin. Path. **49**, 710–717 (1968).

MacDonald, R. A.: Hemochromatosis and hemosiderosis. Springfield: Charles C. Thomas 1964.

Madding, G. F., Smith, W. L., Hershberger, L. R.: Hepatoportal arteriovenous fistula. J. Amer. med. Ass. **156**, 593–596 (1954).

Madore, P.: Variceal hemorrhage in a case of hepatic steatosis. Amer. J. Gastroent. **54**, 267–271 (1970).

Markoff, N. G.: The therapy of portal hypertension. Proc. Int. Symposium. Stuttgart: Georg Thieme 1968.

Marsden, P. D., Hutt, M. S., Banwell, J. G.: Abnormal splenovenograms in non-cirrhotic patients with portal hypertension and marked splenomegaly. J. trop. Med. Hyg. **67**, 239–245 (1964).

Martini, G. A., Wiebel, J. P.: Die Ammoniakbestimmung im Blut zur Differentialdiagnose akuter Blutungen im oberen Verdauungskanal. Med. Klin. **59**, 618–621 (1964).

McCray, R. S., Martin, F., Amir-Ahmadi, H., Sheahan, D. G., Zamcheck, N.: Erroneous diagnosis of hemorrhage from esophageal varices. Amer. J. dig. Dis. **14**, 755–760 (1969).

McDermott, W. V., Jr.: Portal hypertension secondary to pancreatic disease. Ann. Surg. **152**, 147–150 (1960).

McDermott, W. V., Jr., Huston, C. J. W.: The oral ammonium tolerance test as aid in the investigation of suspected esophago-gastric varices. Ann. Surg. **158**, 820–826 (1963).

McDermott, W. V., Jr., Pallazi, H., Nardi, G. L., Mondet, A.: Elective portal systemic shunt. An analysis of 237 cases. New Engl. J. Med. **264**, 419–427 (1961).

McNulty, J. G.: High dose percutaneous transplenic portal venography. Brit. J. Radiol. **41**, 55–58 (1968).

Megevand, R. P.: Indications and results of porta-caval shunts. In: The therapy of portal hypertension, ed. N. G. Markoff, p. 11–13. Stuttgart: Georg Thieme 1968.

Melnick, P. J.: Polycystic liver. Arch. Path. **59**, 162–172 (1955).

Mendes, T. F.: The schistosomiases. In: Gastroenterology, ed. H. L. Bockus, vol. III, p. 52–84. Philadelphia-London: W. B. Saunders Co. 1965.

Mikkelsen, W. P., Edmondson, H. A., Peters, R. L., Redeker, A. G., Reynolds, T. B.: Extra- and intrahepatic portal hypertension without cirrhosis (hepatoportal sclerosis). Ann. Surg. **162**, 602–620 (1965).

MISTILIS, S. P., GREEN, J. R., SCHIFF, L.: Hepatic sarcoidosis with portal hypertension. Amer. J. Med. **36**, 470–475 (1964).

MÖRL, H., FEIGE, G.: Leberzirrhose nach Magenresektionen, bei Magen-Duodenalgeschwüren und Geschwürsnarben. Dtsch. med. Wschr. **94**, 2167–2170 (1969).

MORRIS, J. S., SCHMID, M., NEWMAN, S., SCHEUDER, P. J., SHERLOCK, S.: Arsenic and noncirrhotic portal hypertension. Gastroenterology **66**, 86–94 (1974).

MORRISON, A. N., LANE, M.: Gaucher's disease with ascites: a case report with autopsy findings. Ann. intern. Med. **42**, 1321–1329 (1955).

MOSKOWITZ, H., CHAIT, A., MARGULIES, M., MELLINS, H. Z.: Prone Splenoportography. Radiology **90**, 1132–1135 (1968).

MÜTING, D., LACKAS, N., REIKOWSKI, H., RICHMOND, S.: Leberzirrhose und Diabetes mellitus. Studie von 140 Kombinationsfällen. Dtsch. med. Wschr. **91**, 1433–1438 (1966).

MURRAY-LYON, I. M., PUGH, R. N. H., NUNNERLEY, H. B., LAWS, J. W., DAWSON, J. L., WILLIAMS, R.: Treatment of bleeding oesophageal varices by infusion of vasopressin into the superior mesenteric artery. Gut **14**, 59–63 (1973).

NAGEL, M., RAHMANZADEH, R., SCHIER, J.: Lokale Hypothermie des Magens zur Unterstützung der konservativen Behandlung massiver gastroösophagealer Blutungen. Münch. med. Wschr. **108**, 2005–2011 (1966).

NAKAMURA, T., NAKAMURA, S., AIKAWA, T.: Obstruction of the inferior vena cava in the hepatic portion and the hepatic veins. Angiology **19**, 479–498 (1968).

NUSBAUM, M., BAUM, S., KURODA, K., BLAKEMORE, W. S.: Control of portal hypertension by selective mesenteric arterial drug infusion. Arch. Surg. **97**, 1005–1012 (1968).

NUSBAUM, M., BAUM, S., SAKIYALAK, P., BLAKEMORE, W. S.: Pharmacologic control of portal hypertension. Surgery **62**, 299–310 (1967).

O'DONNELL, B., MOLONEY, M. A.: Development and course of extrahepatic portal obstruction in children. Lancet **1968 I**, 789–791.

ORLOFF, M. J.: Emergency portocaval shunt: A comparative study of shunt, varix ligation and nonsurgical treatment of bleeding esophageal varices in unselected patients with cirrhosis. Ann. Surg. **166**, 456–478 (1967).

ORLOFF, M. J., THOMAS, H. S.: Pathogenesis of esophageal varix rupture. Arch. Surg. **87**, 301–307 (1963).

ORREGO, H., MENA, I., BARAONA, E., PALMA, R.: Modifications in hepatic blood flow and portal pressure produced by different diets. Amer. J. dig. Dis. **10**, 239–248 (1965).

OSTROW, J. D., TIMMERMAN, R. J., GRAY, S. J.: Gastric secretion in human hepatic cirrhosis. Gastroenterology **38**, 303–313 (1960).

PALMER, E. D.: Primary varices of the cervical esophagus as a source of massive upper gastrointestinal hemorrhage. Amer. J. dig. Dis. **19**, 375–377 (1952).

PALMER, E. D.: On correlations between portal venous pressure and the size and extent of esophageal varices in portal cirrhosis. Ann. Surg. **138**, 741–744 (1953).

PALMER, E. D.: Esophageal varices associated with hiatus hernia in the absence of portal hypertension. Amer. J. med. Sci. **235**, 677–681 (1958).

PALMER, E. D., BRICK, I. B.: Sources of upper gastrointestinal bleeding in cirrhotic patients with esophageal varices. New Engl. J. Med. **248**, 1057–1058 (1953).

PALMER, E. D., BRICK, I. B.: Esophageal varices in non-cirrhotic patients. Esophagoscopic study. Amer. J. Med. **17**, 641–644 (1954).

PALMER, E. D., BRICK, I. B.: Varices of the distal esophagus in the apparent absence of portal and of superior caval hypertension. Amer. J. med. Sci. **230**, 515–519 (1955).

PALMER, E. D., BRICK, I. B., JAHNKE, E. J.: Esophageal varices without hemorrhage in cirrhosis; a proper indication for shunting procedures. New Engl. J. Med. **250**, 863–865 (1954).

PANKE, W. F., ROUSSELOT, L. M., MORENO, A. H.: Splenic pulp manometry as an emergency test in differential diagnosis of acute upper gastrointestinal bleeding. Surg. Gynec. Obstet. **109**, 270–278 (1959).

PANKE, W. F., ROUSSELOT, L. M., BURCHELL, A. R.: A sixteen-year experience with end-to-side portacaval shunt for varical hemorrhage: Analysis of data and comparison with other types of portasystemic anastomoses. Ann. Surg. **168**, 957–965 (1968).

PARAF, A., CHALUT, Y.: Les thromboses splénoportales. Paris: Expansion édit. 1962.

PARKER, R. G. F.: Occlusion of the hepatic veins in man. Medicine (Baltimore) **38**, 369–402 (1959).

PATEK, A. J., JR., POST, J., RATNOFF, O. D., MANKIN, H., HILLMAN, R. W.: Dietary treatment of cirrhosis of the liver; results in one hundred and twenty-four patients observed during a ten year period. J. Amer. med. Ass. **138**, 543–549 (1948).

PATRASSI, G., DAL PALU, C., RUOL, A.: La pletora portale, p. 331. Roma: Pozzi 1961.

PEQUINOT, G.: About the geographical aspects of cirrhosis. In: Alcohol and the liver, eds. GEROK, SICKINGER and HENNEKEUSER, p. 469–473. Stuttgart-New York: Schattauer 1970.

Perry, J. F., Jr., Root, H. D., Miller, F. A., Varlo, R. L.: Total removal of the intra-thoracic esophagus and antethoracic jejunal esophageal replacement for treatment of esophageal varices due to extrahepatic portal block. Ann. Surg. **158**, 126–128 (1963).

Perry, T. L., Hardwick, D. F., Dixon, G. H., Dolmar, C. L., Hansen, S.: Hypermethionin-emia: a metabolic disorder associated with cirrhosis, islet cell hyperplasia and renal tubular degeneration. Pediatrics **36**, 236–250 (1965).

Peternel, W. W., Dagradi, A. E., Rogers, A. I., Nadal, H. M., Perrin, E. B., Jackson, F. C.: Clinical investigation of the portacaval shunt. III. The diagnosis of esophageal varices. J. Amer. med. Ass. **202**, 1081–1084 (1967).

Piccone, V. A., Leveen, H. H.: Transumbilical portal decompression. Surg. Gynec. Obstet. **125**, 66–72 (1967).

Pinel, J., Richard, R., Dentan, Th., Trotoux, J., Léger, L.: Sclérose des varices œsopha-giennes. 66 malades traités et suivis. Presse méd. **79**, 1739–1741 (1971).

Pinel, J., Richard, R., Forest, H.: Les injections sclérosantes dans le traitement des varices œsophagiennes hémorrhagiques. Ann. Oto-laryng. (Paris) **82**, 966–969 (1965).

Popper, H., Elias, H., Petty, D.: Vascular pattern of the cirrhotic liver. Amer. J. clin. Path. **22**, 717–729 (1952).

Porter, G. H.: Hepatic sarcoidosis. A cause of portal hypertension and liver failure; Review. Arch. intern. Med. **108**, 483–495 (1961).

Powell, W. J., Klatskin, G.: Duration of survival in patients with Laennec's cirrhosis. Influence of alcohol withdrawal and possible effects of recent changes in general management of the disease. Amer. J. Med. **44**, 406–420 (1968).

Preger, L.: Enhanced visualization of esophageal varices by dextran infusion. A preliminary report. Amer. J. Roentgenol. **101**, 476–471 (1967a).

Preger, L.: Hepatic arteriovenous fistula after percutaneous liver biopsy. Amer. J. Roentgenol. **101**, 619–620 (1967b).

Preisig, R.: The pathogenesis of portal hypertension during human and canine viral hepatitis. In: The therapy of portal hypertension, ed. N. G. Markoff, p. 189. Stuttgart: Georg Thieme 1968.

Rachlin, L., Hansen, R. H., Carolan, J. J.: Umbilical vein catheterization and cirrhosis. Surg. Gynec. Obstet. **130**, 272–274 (1970).

Rappaport, A. M., Knoblauch, M., Black, R. G., Ohira, S.: Hepatic microcirculatory changes leading to portal hypertension. Ann. N.Y. Acad. Sci. **170**, 48–66 (1970).

Ratnoff, O. D., Patek, A. J., Jr.: The natural history of Laennec's cirrhosis of the liver. An analysis of 368 cases. Medicine (Baltimore) **21**, 207–268 (1942).

Read, A. E., Dawson, A. M., Kerr, D. N. S., Turner, M. D., Sherlock, S.: Bleeding oesophageal varices treated by oesophageal compression tube. Brit. med. J. **1960 I**, 227–231.

Reichman, S., Davis, W. D., Jr.: The splenic approach to the portal circulation. Intrasplenic and intrahepatic tissue pressure measurements in acute and convalescent hepatitis. Gastroenterology **33**, 609–615 (1957).

Renwick, S. B., Loewenthal, J., Mills, F. H.: Splenorenal anastomosis. Med. J. Aust. **1**, 755–760 (1969).

Resnick, R. H., Chalmers, T. C., Ishihara, A. M., Garceau, A. J., Callow, A. O., Schimmel, E. M., O'Hara, E. T., and the Boston Inter-Hospital Liver Group: A controlled study of the prophylactic portacaval shunt. A final report. Ann. intern. Med. **70**, 675–688 (1969).

Rex, J., Richter, K.: Ösophagusvarizen und Dilatation der Azygosvenen bei Obstruktion der Vena Cava Cranialis. Fortschr. Röntgenstr. **106**, 885–887 (1967).

Reynolds, T. B.: Portal hypertension in chronic liver disease. In: The Liver, eds. E. A. Gall and F. K. Mostofi, p. 370–383. Baltimore: Williams & Wilkins Co. 1973.

Reynolds, T. B., Hidemura, R., Michel, H., Peters, R.: Portal hypertension without cirrhosis in alcoholic liver disease. Ann. intern. Med. **70**, 497–506 (1969).

Rignault, D., Nine, J., Moine, D.: Splenoportographic changes in chronic pancreatitis. Surgery **63**, 571–575 (1968).

Roberts, W. C.: The hepatic cirrhosis of cystic fibrosis of the pancreas. Amer. J. Med. **32**, 324–328 (1962).

Rodgers, J. B., Older, T. N., Stabler, E. V.: Gastric hypothermia: A critical evaluation of its use in massive upper gastrointestinal bleeding. Ann. Surg. **163**, 367–372 (1966).

Rosenbaum, D. L., Murphy, G. W., Swisher, S. N.: Hemodynamic studies of the portal circulation in myeloid metaplasia. Amer. J. Med. **41**, 360–368 (1966).

Rothwell-Jackson, R. L., Hunt, A. H.: Proximal gastric resection in the treatment of bleeding gastro-oesophageal varices in patients with portal hypertension due to extrahepatic obstruction. Brit. J. Surg. **57**, 487–494 (1970).

Rottiers, R., Van Egmond, J., Verbruggen, R., Dierick, G., Vermeulen, A., De Groote, J., Standaert, L., Demeulenaere, L.: Cirrhosis, hyperammonemia and lactulose. T. Gastro-ent. **11**, 123–139 (1968).

RUPRECHT, A. L., KINNEY, T. D.: Esophageal varices caused by metastasis of carcinoma to the liver. Amer. J. dig. Dis. 1, 145–154 (1956).

RUZICKA, F. F., JR., ROSSI, P.: Normal vascular anatomy of the abdominal viscera. Radiol. Clin. N. Amer. 8, 3–29 (1970).

SALAM, A. A., WARREN, W. D., LE PAGE, J. R., VIAMONTE, M. R., HUTSON, D., ZEPPA, R.: Hemodynamic contrasts between selective and total portal-systemic decompression. Ann. Surg. 173, 827–844 (1971).

SCHAEFER, J., BRAMSCHREIBER, J., MISTILIS, S., SCHIFF, L.: Gastroesophageal variceal bleeding in the absence of hepatic cirrhosis or portal hypertension. Gastroenterology 46 583–588 (1964).

SCHAEFER, J. W., SCHIFF, L., GALL, E. A., OIKAWA, Y.: Progression of acute hepatitis to postnecrotic cirrhosis. Amer. J. Med. 42, 348–358 (1967).

SCHAFFNER, F.: Principles of management of portal hypertension. In: The therapy of portal hypertension, ed. N. G. MARKOFF, p. 64–68. Stuttgart: Georg Thieme 1968.

SCHAFFNER, F., GADBOYS, H. L., SAFRAN, A. P., BARON, M. G., AUFSES, A. H., JR.: Budd-Chiari syndrome caused by a web in the inferior vena cava. Amer. J. Med. 42, 838–843 (1967).

SCHEINBERG, I. H., GITLIN, D.: Deficiency of ceruloplasmin in patients with hepatolenticular degeneration (Wilson's disease). Science 116, 481–485 (1952).

SCHERL, N. D., KLEIN, R.: Portal thrombosis, bleeding varices and mesenteric infarction in a patient with polycythemia vera. Amer. J. Gastroent. 53, 164–168 (1970).

SCHEUER, P.: Liver biopsy interpretation. London: Baillière, Tindall & Cassell 1968.

SCHEUER, P. J., WILLIAMS, R.: Genetic disorders of the liver. In: Progress in liver diseases, eds. H. POPPER and F. SCHAFFNER, vol. II, p. 272–289. New York: Grune and Stratton Co. 1965.

SCHMID, M.: Zur Leberhistologie der verschiedenen Formen des portalen Hochdruckes. In: The therapy of portal hypertension, ed. N. G. MARKOFF, p. 120. Stuttgart: Georg Thieme 1968.

SCHREIBER, H. W., SCHRIEFERS, K. H., ESSER, G., BARTSCH, W. M.: Spätergebnisse nach 150 direkten porto-cavalen Anastomosen. Dtsch. med. Wschr. 89, 2185–2191 (1964).

SCOBIE, B. A., SCHLEGEL, J. F., CODE, C. F., SUMMERSKILL, W. H. J.: Pressure changes of the esophagus and gastroesophageal junction with cirrhosis and varices. Gastroenterology 49, 67–73 (1965).

SEDACCA, C. M., PERRIN, E., MARTIN, L., SCHIFF, L.: Polycystic liver: unusual cause of bleeding esophageal varices. Gastroenterology 40, 128–136 (1961).

SEDGWICK, C. E., POULANTZAS, J. K., KUNE, G. A.: Management of portal hypertension secondary to bile duct strictures: review of 18 cases with splenorenal shunt. Ann. Surg. 163, 949–953 (1966).

SELMAIR, H., VIDO, I., WILDHIRT, E.: Zur Prognose der chronischen Hepatitis. Dtsch. med. Wschr. 94, 2220–2222 (1969).

SHALDON, S., DOLLE, W., GUEVARA, L., IBER, F. L., SHERLOCK, S.: Effect of pitressin on the splanchnic circulation in man. Circulation 24, 797–807 (1961).

SHALDON, S., SHERLOCK, S.: Portal hypertension in the myeloproliferative syndrome and the reticuloses. Amer. J. Med. 32, 758–764 (1962a).

SHALDON, S., SHERLOCK, S.: Obstruction to the extrahepatic portal system in childhood. Lancet 1962I, 63–68.

SHAPIRO, E., WEINER, H.: The diagnosis of tertiary syphilis of the liver, twenty-five years after McCrae. Amer. J. Med. Sci. 222, 494–499 (1951).

SHARP, H. L., BRIDGES, R. A., KRIVIT, W., FREIER, E. F.: Cirrhosis associated with alpha-1-antitrypsin deficiency: a previously unrecognized inherited disorder. J. Lab. clin. Med. 73, 934–939 (1969).

SHELDON, J. H.: Haemochromatosis. London: Oxford University Press 1935.

SHERLOCK, S.: Haematemesis in portal hypertension. Brit. J. Surg. 51, 746–749 (1964).

SHERLOCK, S.: Hepatic circulatory changes in man. Published by Little, Brown and Company. Reprinted from Gamble and Wilbur [Concepts of clinical gastroenterology 13, 165–189 (1965)].

SHERLOCK, S.: Management of bleeding esophageal varices. Colston Papers, vol. XIX. Proceedings of the nineteenth symposium of the Colston research society, 13, 363–370 (1967).

SHERLOCK, S.: Hepato-lienal fibrosis without cirrhosis: non-cirrhotic intrahepatic portal hypertension. Postgrad. Med. J. 44, 109–111 (1968).

SHERLOCK, S., ALPERT, L.: Bleeding in surgery in relation to liver disease. Proc. roy. Soc. Med. 58, 257–259 (1965).

SHERLOCK, S., FELDMAN, C. A., MORAN, B., SCHEUER, P. J.: Partial nodular transformation of the liver with portal hypertension. Amer. J. Med. 40, 195–203 (1966).

SHUMACKER, H. B., JR., WALDHAUSEN, J. A.: Intrahepatic arteriovenous fistula of hepatic artery and portal vein. Surg. Gynec. Obstet. 112, 497–501 (1961).

SICOT, C., BENHAMOU, J. P.: Portal hypertension and primary biliary cirrhosis. Abstracts 5th E.A.S.L. Meeting, Bern. Digestion 4, 180 (1971).

Sidbury, J. B., Jr., Mason, J., Burns, W. B., Jr., Ruebner, B. H.: Type IV Glycogenosis. Report of a case proven by characterization of glycogen and studied at necropsy. Bull. Johns Hopk. Hosp. **111**, 157–181 (1962).

Silva, I. J., Moffat, R. C., Walt, A. J.: Vasopressin effect on portal and systemic hemo-dynamics. J. Amer. med. Ass. **210**, 1065–1068 (1969).

Simeone, F. A., Hopkins, R. W.: Portarenal shunt for hepatic cirrhosis and portal hyper-tension. Surgery **61**, 153–167 (1967).

Smetana, H. F., Hadley, G. G., Sirsat, S. M.: Infantile cirrhosis. Pediatrics **28**, 107–127 (1961).

Smith, G. W.: Splenectomy and coronary vein ligation for the control of bleeding esophageal varices. Amer. J. Surg. **119**, 122–131 (1970).

Smith, G. W., Edwards, O. E.: Hemorrhage from varices in patients with achlorhydria. Gastroenterology **51**, 1054–1057 (1966).

Smith, J. L., Lineback, M. L.: Hereditary hemorrhagic telangiectasia. 9 Cases in one Negro family, with special reference to hepatic lesions. Amer. J. Med. **17**, 41–49 (1954).

Snodgrass, R. W., Mellinkoff, S. M.: Bleeding varices in the upper esophagus due to obstruction of the superior vena cava. Gastroenterology **41**, 505–508 (1961).

Song, Y. S.: Hepatic lesions in sickle cell anemia. Amer. J. Path. **33**, 331–351 (1957).

Stathers, G. M., Blackburn, C. R. B.: Extrahepatic portal hypertension: the clinical evalua-tion, investigation and results of treatment of 28 patients. Austr. Ann. Med. **17**, 12–19 (1968).

Stelzner, F., Lierse, W.: Die Blutgefäßanordnung vor allem im terminalen Abschnitt der Speiseröhre. Die Venen. Langenbecks Arch. klin. Chir. **321**, 47–64 (1968).

Sternlieb, I., Scheinberg, I. H., Walshe, J. M.: Bleeding oesophageal varices in patients with Wilson's disease. Lancet **1970I**, 638–641.

Sterup, K., Mosbech, J.: Budd-Chiari syndrome after taking oral contraceptives. Brit. med. J. **1967 IV**, 660.

Stolze, T.: Die „atypisch" in den oberen zwei Dritteln des Oesophagus auftretenden Varicen. Radiologe **4**, 232–236 (1964).

Stone, W. D., Islam, N. R. K., Paton, A.: The natural history of cirrhosis. Experience with an unselected group of patients. Quart. J. Med. **37**, 119–132 (1968).

Strohmeyer, G., Dölle, W.: Ösophagusvarizen: Bedeutung, Ursache und Behandlung. Med. Klin. **58**, 1649–1653 (1963).

Sullivan, A., Rheinlander, H., Weintraub, L. R.: Esophageal varices in agnogenic myeloid metaplasia: disappearance after splenectomy. A case report. Gastroenterology **66**, 429–432 (1974).

Sutton, J. P., Yarborough, D. Y., Richards, J. T.: Isolated splenic vein occlusion. Review of literature and report of an additional case. Arch. Surg. **100**, 623–626 (1970).

Sweetham, W. P., Sykes, C. G. W.: Congenital fibrosis of the liver as a familial defect. Lancet **1961I**, 374–376.

Symmers, W. S. C.: Note on the new form of liver cirrhosis due to the presence of the ova of Bilharzia haematobia. J. Path. Bact. **9**, 237–239 (1904).

Tabaqchali, S., Dawson, A. M.: Peptic ulcer and gastric secretion in patients with liver disease. Gut **5**, 417–421 (1964).

Tanner, N. C.: The late results of porto-azygos disconnection in the treatment of bleeding from esophageal varices. Ann. roy. Coll. Surg. Engl. **28**, 153–174 (1961).

Taylor, W. J., Jackson, F. C., Jensen, W. N.: Wilson's disease, portal hypertension and intrahepatic vascular obstruction. New Engl. J. Med. **260**, 1160–1164 (1959).

Teschendorf, W.: Lehrbuch der röntgenologischen Differentialdiagnostik, 4. Aufl., Bd. I, p. 1050–1061. Stuttgart: Georg Thieme 1958.

Thompson, E. N., Sherlock, S.: The aetiology of portal vein thrombosis with particular reference to the role of infection and exchange transfusion. Quart. J. Med. **33**, 465–479 (1964).

Tisdale, W. A., Klatskin, G., Glenn, W. W. L.: Portal hypertension and bleeding esoph-ageal varices. Their occurrence in the absence of both intrahepatic and extrahepatic obstruction of the portal vein. New Engl. J. Med. **261**, 209–218 (1959).

Tsakiris, A., Haemmerli, U. P., Bühlmann, A.: Reduction of portal venous pressure in cirrhotic patients with bleeding from esophageal varices, by administration of a vaso-pressin derivative (phenylalamine²-lysine⁸-vasopressin). Amer. J. Med. **36**, 825–839 (1964).

Tumen, H. J., Cohn, E. M.: Cirrhosis. In: Gastroenterology, ed. H. L. Bockus, vol. III, p. 299–402. Philadelphia-London: W. B. Saunders Co. 1965.

Turner, M. D., Sherlock, S., Steiner, R. E.: Splenic venography and intrasplenic pressure measurement in the clinical investigation of the portal venous system. Amer. J. Med. **23**, 846–859 (1957).

Turrill, F. L., Mikkelsen, W. P.: "Sinistral" (left-sided) extrahepatic portal hypertension. Arch. Surg. **99**, 365–368 (1969).

VARRIALE, P., BONANNO, C. A., GRACE, W. J.: Portal hypertension secondary to pancreatic pseudocysts. Arch. intern. Med. **112**, 191–198 (1963).

VIAMONTE, H., JR., WARREN, W. D., FOMON, J. J.: Liver panangiography in the assessment of portal hypertension in liver cirrhosis. Radiol. Clin. N. Amer. **8**, 147–167 (1970).

VILINSKAS, J., JOYEUSE, R., SERLIN, O.: Hepatic sarcoidosis with portal hypertension. Amer. J. Surg. **120**, 393–396 (1970).

VOORHEES, A. B., JR., HARRIS, R. C., BRITTON, R. C., PRICE, J. B., SANTULLI, T. V.: Portal hypertension in children: 98 cases. Pediat. Surg. **58**, 540–549 (1965).

WAGENKNECHT, T. W., NOBLE, J. F., BARANOFSKY, I. D.: Nature of bleeding in esophageal varices. Surgery **33**, 869–874 (1953).

WALKER, G., WILLIAMS, R., CONDON, R. E., THOMPSON, E. N., SHERLOCK, S.: Gastric cooling in the treatment of bleeding from esophageal varices. Lancet **1964 II**, 328–331.

WALKER, R. M.: Esophageal transection for bleeding varices. Surg. Gynec. Obstet. **118**, 323–329 (1964).

WALSHE, J. M., BRIGGS, J.: Caeruloplasmin in liver disease. Lancet **1962 II**, 263–265.

WANGENSTEEN, S. L., ORANOOD, R. C., VOORHEES, A. B., SMITH, E. B., HEALEY, W. V.: Intragastric cooling in the management of hemorrhage from the upper gastrointestinal tract. Amer. J. Surg. **105**, 401–412 (1963).

WARREN, K. S., REBOUCAS, G.: Blood ammonia during bleeding from esophageal varices in patients with hepatosplenic schistosomiasis. New Engl. J. Med. **271**, 921–926 (1964).

WARREN, W. D., FOMON, J. J., LEITE, C. A.: Critical assessment of the rationale of thoracic duct drainage in the treatment of portal hypertension. Surgery **63**, 7–16 (1968).

WARREN, W. D., FOMON, J. J., VIAMONTE, M., ZEPPA, R.: Preoperative assessment of portal hypertension. Ann. Surg. **165**, 999–1012 (1967).

WARREN, W. D., FOMON, J. J., ZEPPA, R.: Further evaluation of selective decompression of varices by distal splenorenal shunt. Ann. Surg. **169**, 652–660 (1969).

WEINBERG, T.: Observations on the occurrence of varices of the esophagus in routine autopsy material. Amer. J. clin. Path. **19**, 554–557 (1949).

WEINBREN, K.: Diseases of the liver. Recent advances in pathology, ed. C. V. HARRISON, p. 185. London: J. & A. Churchill 1966.

WELCH, C. S.: Portal hypertension. New Engl. J. Med. **243**, 598–610 (1950).

WHITE, J. J., SLAPAK, M., MACLEAN, L. D.: Extracorporeal portosystemic shunt for portal hypertension. Surgery **63**, 17–28 (1968).

WILLIAMS, R., DAWSON, J.: Management of bleeding esophageal varices. Brit. med. J. **1968 I**, 35–37.

WILLIAMS, R., CORDON, R. E., WILLIAMS, H. S., BLENDIS, L. M., KREEL, L.: Splenic blood flow in cirrhosis and portal hypertension. Clin. Sci. **34**, 441–452 (1968).

WILLIAMS, R., PARSONSON, A., SOMERS, K., HAMILTON, P. J. S.: Portal hypertension in idiopathic tropical splenomegaly. Lancet **1966 I**, 329–333.

WODAK, E.: Die konservative Behandlung der Oesophagusvarizen. H.N.O. **13**, 131–133 (1965a).

WODAK, E.: Die Wandsklerosierung der Oesophagusschleimhaut im histologischen Bild. Wien. med. Wschr. **115**, 406 (1965b).

YAMAMOTO, S., REDEKER, A. G., REYNOLDS, T. B.: The effect of thoracic duct drainage on hepatic hemodynamics in cirrhosis. Gastroenterology **46**, 305 (1964).

YOUNG, R. C.: The Budd-Chiari syndrome. Arch. intern. Med. **124**, 754–757 (1969).

ZEEGEN, R., STANSFELD, A. G., DAWSON, A. M., HUNT, A. H.: Bleeding oesophageal varices as the presenting feature in primary biliary cirrhosis. Lancet **1969 II**, 9–12.

ZEEGEN, R., STANSFELD, A. G., DAWSON, A. M., HUNT, A. H.: Prolonged survival after portal decompression of patients with non-cirrhotic intrahepatic portal hypertension. Gut **11**, 610–617 (1970).

ZUIDEMA, G. D., EBERT, P. A.: Mesenteric-caval anastomosis for portal decompression. Johns Hopk. med. J. **120**, 201–209 (1967).

Chapter 11

Hiatus Hernia

E. HAFTER

With 28 Figures

1. Definition and Classification

Hiatus hernia is the usual term to describe the constant or recurrent protrusion of parts of the stomach through the hiatus of the diaphragm into the thorax. Although its most common form, the esophagogastric sliding hernia, is no true hernia, since it does not have a hernial sac, it is classified as such. The classification of ÅKERLUND (1926, 1933), based on anatomical characteristics, distinguishes three forms:

Type 1: hiatus hernia with congenital short esophagus;
Type 2: paraesophageal hiatus hernia;
Type 3: esophagogastric sliding hernia.

The existence of Åkerlund's first type, the congenital short esophagus or thoracic stomach (German: kongenital kurzer Oesophagus; French: brachyœsophage) is a matter of controversy. In most cases a predisposition to the development of hernia in the form of a wide hiatus or an unsuitable fixation of the proximal part of the stomach in the abdomen is probably the congenital factor. It seems, therefore, that the hernia is a primary, the short esophagus only a secondary factor. This view is confirmed by pediatric observations (THOMSEN, 1955). As it is almost impossible to distinguish radiologically Åkerlund's type 1 from his type 3, both types are nowadays designated as "esophagogastric sliding hernia". In Åkerlund's type 2, which is frequently called "rolling hernia", the cardia is in its normal site under the diaphragm. Part of the fundus, surrounded by a peritoneal sac, protrude beside the esophagus into the thorax. The wide hiatus is mostly congenital and there is often a persisting right pneumatoenteric recessus (THOMSEN, 1955).

Åkerlund's third type, the sliding hernia, is by far the most common. The protrusion is often completely or partly reversible and may be brought about by horizontal position or increased intraabdominal pressure.

A number of other classifications have been proposed. ALLISON (1951) distinguishes 5 different types: (1) paraesophageal hernia; (2) paraesophageal sliding hernia; (3) sliding hernia; (4) sliding hernia with paraesophageal sac; (5) congenital short esophagus. BARRETT (1952) describes 3 types: (1) sliding hernia, (2) paraesophageal hernia, and (3) mixed hernia. In infants THOMSEN (1955) distinguishes, besides the paraesophageal hiatus hernia, two types of sliding hernias (a) with an abnormal esophagus and (b) with a normal gullet. This classification is mostly of clinical and therapeutical value.

Most authors agree with a division into two main groups: (1) the common sliding esophagogastric hiatus hernia and (2) the rather rare paraesophageal hernia, along with several mixed types (Fig. 312). The initial stage of a sliding hernia has been called "hiatus insufficiency" (ZAINO et al., 1963). In this condi-

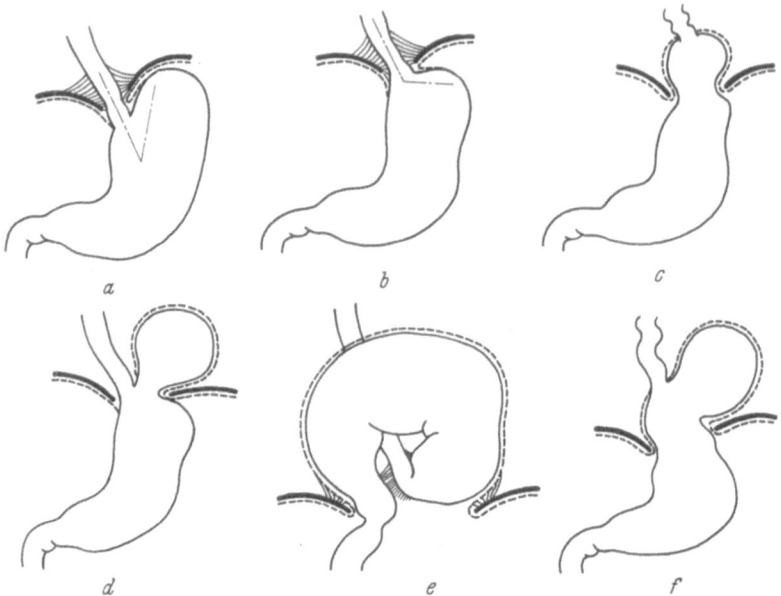

Fig. 312a—f. Types of hiatus hernia (according to HOLLE). a Normal. b Hiatal insufficiency. c Esophagogastric sliding hernia. d Paraesophageal hernia. e Large paraesophageal hernia, "upside-down-stomach". f Mixed type: sliding and paraesophageal hernia. (From HOLLE, 1968, p. 514)

tion only the intraabdominal segment of the esophagus protrudes into the thorax while the stomach itself remains in an intraabdominal position. Hiatus insufficiency corresponds to "hiatal herniation without a sac" (WOLF, 1970). (French: malposition cardiotubérositaire.) This condition is not always easily distinguished from normal.

2. Incidence

In 1926 the incidence of hiatus hernia was reported to be 2 to 3% of the roentgen examinations of the upper gastrointestinal tract (ÅKERLUND, 1926). This figure kept increasing, mainly thanks to improved radiological techniques, until it reached 8 to 15% in 1950. Since then still higher incidences, ranging from 20 to even 100% were reported. These widely divergent figures find their origin not only in different radiological techniques or diverging criteria for diagnosis, but also in the ages of the groups of patients under study. The incidence increases with the age of the patients as well as with the size and hardness of the pillow put under the patient's abdomen during the radiological examination. By (over)interpretation of the X-ray pictures obtained with routine intensive abdominal compression VESTBY and AAKHUS (1966) made a diagnosis of hernia in 100% of their examinations. However, it can be seen from their pictures that phrenic ampullae are designated as hernias while it is accepted by most other authors that these images may be due to a ballooning out of the distal esophagus. Inspiratory protrusions of the vestibulum were taken as "first degree hernias" in the 50% incidence reported by STEIN and FINKEL-STEIN (1960). Protrusions of the stomach, however, were observed in only 24%

Table 31. Incidence of hiatus hernia in 5557 roentgen studies of the stomach in non-hospitalized patients

Age	Males			Females			Total	Data of WOLF et al., 1959		
	Examinations No.	Hiatus hernia		Examinations No.	Hiatus hernia		%	Small hiatus hernia %	Larger hiatus hernia (>3.8 cm) %	Total %
		No.	%		No.	%				
10–19	52	0	0	61	0	0	0	0	0	0
20–29	296	23	7.8	301	10	3.3	5.5	4	0	4
30–39	536	102	19.0	459	41	8.9	14.4	13	3	16
40–49	687	189	27.5	582	112	19.2	23.7	28	4	32
50–59	678	243	35.8	614	179	29.1	32.0	34	10	44
60–69	427	164	38.4	479	173	36.1	37.2	41	18	59
70–79	168	67	40.0	193	48	25.1	31.8	55	21	76
80–89	—	—	—	—	—	—	—	76	22	98
Total	2864	778	27.5	2693	563	20.9	24.3	33.7	11	45

of their cases. Other authors quote similar figures: DEBRAY et al. (1966) 26.4%, HAFTER (1957) 24.3% (Table 31). WOLF et al. (1959) examined 400 patients in the right anterior oblique position using a technique of constant drinking and abdominal compression. They found medium size and big hernias in 11% and small hernias, with a length of less than $1^1/_2$ inches, in 33.7%, totalling 45%. These figures illustrate that reports on incidence depend on where the line is drawn between hernia and norm.

We have classified the results of our examinations according to age and sex. A diagnosis of hernia was made only in those cases in which the gastric mucosa or "middle ring" (see p. 760) was distinctly recognizable above the hiatus. In all cases the esophagogastric junction was examined in both the prone and the supine positions. Additional compression with a pillow under the abdomen was used only in thin patients with symptoms of hiatus hernia, exceptionally, in adipose patients and, in patients without hernia symptoms, when they are over the age of 70. The percentages given in Table 31 are probably below the true incidence, especially in the older age group. Thusfar there is no agreement as to what can be called "still physiological compression".

In most reports the sex distribution of hiatus hernia shows a slight preponderance for females. In our studies male patients seemed somewhat more susceptible. The age of the patient is a very important factor. In old people a small and mostly asymptomatic sliding hernia is next to physiological.

3. Anatomical Basis, Etiology and Pathogenesis

Before debouching into the stomach, the terminal esophagus passes the diaphragm through the esophageal hiatus. This oval or almond-shaped hiatus is located before the aorta in the saddle-shaped subsidence between the 2 diaphragmatic domes, at the level of the 9th and 10th thoracic vertebra, about 12 cm behind the xiphoid processus. Its longitudinal diameter is 3 to 5 cm with a cross diameter of about 1.5 to 2 cm. The opening is formed by a lasso-shaped muscle loop, which originates as the right diaphragmatic crus from the anterior side of the first lumbar vertebra and then swings round the esophagus like a

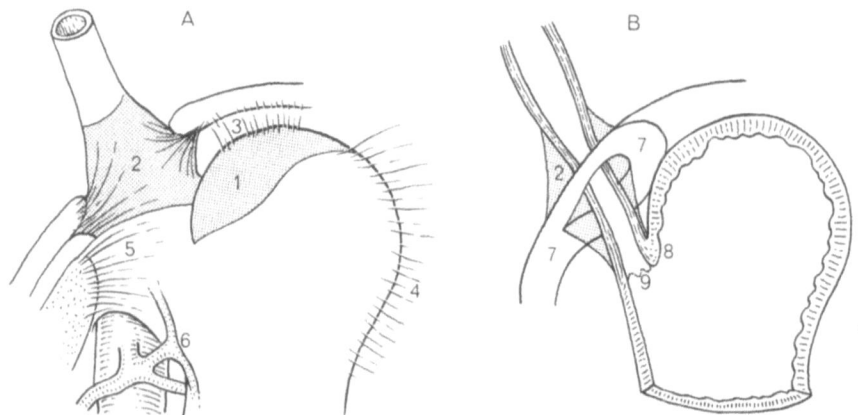

Fig. 313. A Fixation of the gastric fundus in the abdomen. *1* retroperitoneal attachment of the posterior wall of the gastric fundus; *2* esophago-diaphragmatic membrane, surrounding the vestibulum; *3* phrenoesophageal membrane; *4* gastrosplenic ligament; *5* gastrohepatic ligament; *6* left gastric artery; B Structures to which prevention of reflux has been ascribed: *7* lasso-like sling of the right diaphragmatic crus, which constitutes the hiatus; *8* angle of His and Gubaroff's valvule; *9* squamocolumnar mucosal junction

horse-shoe. The musculature of this U-shaped band varies in strength. It often gets atrophic in old age. On deep inspiration it contracts, pulls down the terminal esophagus to the right and compresses its lumen.

The intrahiatal portion of the esophagus has a length of 0.5 to 1.0 cm at its anterior side and of 1.5 to 2.5 cm at its posterior side. The abdominal portion of the gullet lies in the retroperitoneal space and has a length of 3 to 4 cm. This segment is called the vestibulum and is surrounded by the esophagodiaphragmatic membrane, which is attached to the inferior margin of the hiatus. The cardia constitutes the junction of the esophagus and the stomach. On gross anatomy the cardia is located at the transition from the tube (the gullet) into the sac (the stomach). This border is not well identified on the smaller curvature. On the greater curvature it is marked by the incisura cardiaca or the acute angle of His (Fig. 313 B). This angle, formed by the left wall of the abdominal esophagus and the right side of the gastric fundus, is due to the fact that the esophagus does not enter the stomach at the top of the fundus, but more sideward to the right. It is reinforced by traction of the oblique fibers of the stomach, which form a U-shaped band that borders the cardiac incisura and extends downward, one arm located on the anterior and the other on the posterior surface of the stomach. The angle of His may be widened with increasing age and may even be completely obliterated in patients with a hiatus hernia. The only landmark that allows the surgeon to locate the gastroesophageal junction in these cases is the distal insertion of the esophagodiaphragmatic membrane which corresponds roughly to the squamocolumnar epithelial junction. This junction is recognizable on esophagoscopy by the smooth longitudinal folds of the light-red esophageal mucosa, which contrasts with the velvet-like, deep-red surface of the stomach. It zigzags, but becomes more even on dilatation of the lumen.

Under pathological conditions it is often difficult to recognize the squamocolumnar junction, because esophagitis produces hyperemic reddening of the terminal esophageal mucosa, which can be confused with the gastric mucosa.

Daubing with a 1% Lugol solution will color the esophageal epithelium blue and show the esophagogastric mucosal junction clearly.

The submucosa is stronger at the level of the epithelial junction, due to the presence of circular connective tissue fibers. These limit the extensibility of the epithelial junction, as compared with its surroundings, which is important for the formation of a Schatzki ring.

The intraabdominal pressure is about 10 to 20 mm Hg higher than the intrathoracic pressure. This abdominothoracic pressure gradient increases markedly on maximal inspiration. This creates a thoracic vacuum, which would pull the stomach into the thorax, if it were not fastened in the abdomen (Fig. 313 A).

Although respiration and deglutition may move the cardia upward over a short distance, under normal circumstances it remains below the diaphragm. The following fixations retain the gastric fundus in the abdomen (ROSSETTI, 1966).

1. The retroperitoneal fixation of the posterior wall of the junctional segment to the paravertebral tissues at the upper edge of the bursa omentalis. This fixation is broken by surgical exposure of the cardia during vagotomy or Heller's operation.

2. The esophagodiaphragmatic membrane (Laimer-Bertelli membrane). It originates at the inferior surface of the diaphragm around the hiatus and divides into two sheets, which loosely connect hiatus and esophagus. The upper sheet passes the hiatus and penetrates into the esophageal wall 1 to 2 cm higher. The lower, more compact sheet attaches itself to the esophageal wall at the level of the squamocolumnar junction, close to the angle of His. Thus the membrane forms a sheath of about 3 to 4 cm around the vestibule (Fig. 313). It consists of elastic fibers and connective tissue and forms an air-tight partition between abdominal and thoracic cavities. Its elasticity allows the vestibulum some freedom of movement during respiration. In young people it is white, short, thick and strong ligament-like (ZAINO et al., 1963); thus it can resist the higher abdominal pressure and prevent the protrusion of vestibulum and fundus. If some surgeons negate its existence, this is due to variation in development; in old people, due to senile atrophy, it is reduced to a yellow-gray, thin and flabby membrane which yields to intraabdominal pressure. In this stage it has no more significance for the continence of the hiatus and can no longer be used for the fixation of the cardia during surgical repair of the hernia.

3. The ligamentum gastro-phrenicum. This connects the gastric fundus with the inferior surface of the diaphragm and is one of the elements determining the configuration of the esophagogastric angle.

4. The ligamentum gastro-lienale. This forms the direct continuation of (3) along the greater curvature.

5. The ligamentum gastro-hepaticum. This connects the lesser curvature of the stomach with the liver. In its upper part, pars densa, it forms a strong connection, limiting movements of the abdominal portion of the esophagus and the lesser curvature of the stomach.

6. The arteria gastrica sinistra. Called the gastric ancre by MOYNIHAN, it can function as a fixation of the lesser curvature, if it is relatively short.

When these fixations retain the stomach in its infradiaphragmatic position, the thoracic vacuum favors gastroesophageal reflux. Normally this is prevented by a gastroesophageal closing mechanism, discussed on p. 51. Several factors have been said to contribute to this antireflux mechanism: the muscular closing of the diaphragmatic crura on maximal inspiration, a flap valve mechanism by the angle of His, and the compression of the subdiaphragmatic esophagus by the abdominal pressure; however, the most important anti-reflux mechanism is the lower esophageal sphincter.

The formation of a hiatus hernia is possible when the fixations no longer suffice to resist the abdominothoracic pressure gradient and the pull by the longitudinal esophageal musculature. Insufficient fixation can be congenital and causes hiatus hernia in infants. But mostly a hiatus hernia is due to weakness and loss of elasticity of the connective tissue, which increase with age. Surgery also can destroy the fixation of the stomach. Heller's operation and vagotomy disconnect the fixation of the posterior wall of the cardia and fundus, while gastric resection breaks the fixation by the left gastric artery. According to the place of the insufficient fixation an esophagogastric or a paraesophageal hernia will occur.

The gastroesophageal pressure gradient is magnified by an increase in intra-abdominal pressure, due to gain in weight, pregnancy, ascites and intraabdominal tumors. On the other hand the longitudinal tension of the esophagus is increased by sclerosing esophagitis.

Esophagogastric hernia eliminates the compressing effect of the abdominal pressure on the infradiaphragmatic gullet. This leaves only the sphincter to prevent reflux. If the sphincter is sufficiently strong its operation alone will do this. In rare cases the intrasphincteric pressure is increased and causes painful or pressing sensations behind the xiphoid, which may imitate angina pectoris (HEITMANN, 1969); such patients do not suffer from reflux.

4. Pathological Anatomy

Most esophagogastric hiatus hernias are not fixed in the thorax, but are reversible. As a result of post mortem weakening and of the disappearance of the abdominoesophageal pressure gradient, most smaller hernias escape detection on autopsy. Only a large hiatus, having a width of more than 2 fingers, and an atrophic flabby esophagodiaphragmatic membrane can be found. If they are searched for one often finds still other insufficient fixations of the fundus in the abdomen. The surgeon is comfronted with a similar situation. The extension of the angle of His associated with the hernia hampers the detection of the esophagogastric junction; only the insertion of the distal sheet of the esophagodiaphragmatic membrane allows detection. Some indication is given by the width of the hiatus and the strength or overextension of the esophagodiaphragmatic membrane. Under the influence of the traction necessary for the operative repair of the hernia the fundus also assumes a tubular shape. Every surgeon is familiar with the difficulty of measuring this traction in such a way that fundus and vestibulum are in the correct position, and many of the postoperative radiological recurrences are caused by insufficient repositioning.

Because the posterior wall of the gastric fundus does not have a peritoneal covering, no hernial sac is found in esophagogastric hiatus hernia. A covering resembling a hernial sac is formed by the extended esophagodiaphragmatic membrane. In larger hernias only part of the fundus without peritoneal covering protrudes. The paraesophageal hernia, however, has a hernial sac.

The most frequent pathological finding indicating a sliding hernia is a more or less severe esophagitis. This leads to parietal thickening, due to inflammatory infiltration of the submucosa and of the muscular layer. The erosions are mostly patchy, located dorsally in the distal esophagus and subside proximally. In severe cases a peptic ulcer may develop.

5. Clinical Features

5.1. Symptoms

The symptoms of hiatus hernia are caused both by the anatomical condition —the hernia itself—and by the functional disorders—gastroesophageal reflux and motility disorders of the esophagus. It is not always possible to decide which of these factors is responsible for the symptoms (KRAMER, 1970).

The symptomatic triad of local complaints, insufficiency of the cardia (belching, reflux, regurgitation of food, heartburn) and the dependency of these symptoms on the patient's position is characteristic and almost pathognomonic. But the symptoms are in no way obligatory; often only one of them occurs; they may be mild or even absent. PALMER (1968) found symptoms only in half of his 786 cases, diagnosed mostly by esophagoscopy. Personal observations, on the other hand, showed complete lack of symptoms attributable to hiatus hernia in only 5% of 300 cases (HAFTER, 1957). Mild symptoms such as a tendency to belch, heartburn after consumption of acid liquids or after a copious meal, a feeling of pressure coming up in a horizontal position and subsiding on getting up, were mentioned only upon explicit questioning. The selection of the patients may also have played a role, since only patients with epigastric complaints were included in our series. In the 5% of asymptomatic patients other epigastric complaints had motivated the examination.

Local complaints consist of discomfort, a feeling of pressure and fullness, of tightness, cramps, burning or pain of varying intensity. The sensations are localized high in the mid- or left epigastrium and behind the xiphoid. They may radiate behind the sternum, into the neck, on occasion into the jaws and behind the ears. In the neck they are often experienced as strangling. In other instances they radiate straight into the back, mostly into the left paravertebral inter-scapular region, and may often be interpreted as a disease of the spine. Radiations into the heart region, the left shoulder and arm, accompanied by a feeling of anxiety and oppression, respiratory difficulty, tachycardia or extrasystoles are frequent, so that one third of our own patients feared angina pectoris and first visited the cardiologist. The local complaints generally are not caused by physical exertion but occur mostly during rest; they do not show a clear diurnal rhythm or dependency on meals; they have no periodicity but occur episodically. Mostly they depend on the position of the patient, occur at night when going to bed, wake up the patient or begin in the morning on awakening. They are favored by meteorism, constipation, bending down and by every increase in intraabdominal pressure; often they are caused by nervous tension. They can last for seconds or hours and disappear spontaneously or on belching, by flatus, defecation, changing position or intake of antacids. Their occurrence is capricious: they can disappear completely for weeks or months so that the patient forgets about them. The mechanisms of the local complaints are manifold. The protrusion of the stomach through the relatively narrow hiatus slightly strangulates the fundus. It has not yet been established to what extent the complaints are caused by traction on the peritoneum, by compression of the gastric wall or by compression of the vagal nerves. On the other hand, heartburn characteristic of reflux or reflux esophagitis often changes into a dull oppressing or penetrating pain. HEITMANN (1969) has found that 10% of his hernia patients had an abnormally high intrasphincteric pressure, often associated with diffuse esophageal spasm. These patients complained about pressing, cramp-like and often very painful sensations not accompanied by heartburn. The mechanism of local complaints is therefore not recognizable in every single case.

Insufficiency of the cardia manifests itself in belching, in reflux of gastric content and, more rarely, in regurgitation of food. Belching is a frequent and often unrecognized symptom of esophagogastric hiatus hernia. Upon questioning it is revealed in more than 90% of the cases. Air enters the stomach primarly together with food and drink. On the average 2 ml of air are swallowed on every deglutition. The swallowing of larger amounts of air causes a clucking noise. Many types of food contain air, especially new bread and whipped eggs and many soft drinks contain CO_2; a bottle of coca-cola, e.g., produces 500 ml of CO_2. During chewing gum and smoking, especially pipe smoking, air is swallowed. In addition about 1 ml of air enters the stomach on every deep inspiration (MADDOCK et al., 1949). Large quantities of CO_2 develop when gastric acid reacts with predominantly alkaline food. However, CO_2 is absorbed and exhaled fast. The gas in the stomach comes mainly from outside air and contains predominantly nitrogen. When there is an insufficiency of the cardia the air is belched up, particularly after meals or on getting up from a horizontal position.

Gastroesophageal reflux occurs mainly in horizontal position and on leaning forward during sitting or bending down, e.g. on tying one's shoe laces. It is favored by organic or functional hindrance of gastric emptying and can accompany an attack of duodenal ulcer. The gastric content does not always reach the mouth; often it does not pass beyond the lower end of the esophagus. In such a case the patient notices it only when the acid gastric content causes heartburn. However, heartburn can also occur in hiatus hernia when partial resection of the stomach has led to achlorhydria. Then it is due to reflux of bile acids and pancreatic secretions. The individual tolerance for refluxed acid varies within wide limits. It depends on the pH of the gastric content as well as on the sensitivity of the esophageal mucosa. The latter is increased by the inflammatory changes of esophagitis. Opinions about the correlation between heartburn and bioptically established esophagitis vary considerably. ISMAIL-BEIGI et al. (1970) found such a coincidence in 81% of their patients with heartburn; OTTENJANN et al. (1968) found signs of esophagitis in 26% of their patients with, and in 27% of their control patients without heartburn. The cause of this discrepancy may be due not only to diverging criteria of esophagitis but also to the patchy distribution of the lesions. When esophageal erosions occur in patients with reflux of acid gastric contents heartburn is almost predictable.

Heartburn is caused not only by reflux of acid but is often observed after consumption of acid or irritating drinks. The pH values of common drinks are, according to FLICK (1970): lemon 2.2 to 2.5; ginger ale 2.7 to 2.8; orange juice 2.8; coca-cola 2.8 to 2.9; 7-Up 3.0 to 3.1; grape-fruit juice 3.2 to 3.5; grape juice 3.3 to 3.6; pine-apple juice 3.4 to 3.5; coffee 4.9 to 5.1; milk 6.5 to 6.7; tea 6.9 and water 7.6 to 8.2. All drinks whose pH is below 4.0 can cause heartburn.

Heartburn after drinking black coffee, concentrated alcohol or certain spices must be ascribed to factors other than the pH. Heartburn can change into a dull, penetrating, on occasion cramp-like pain, so that sensations other than burning can be a symptom of reflux esophagitis.

Regurgitation of food is rarer than belching or acid reflux. Most frequently it occurs during the night after a copious and late dinner. It can cause aspiration pneumonia so that recurrent bronchopulmonary infections must suggest hiatus hernia.

The third element of the symptomatological triad is the finding that the symptoms depend on the position of the patient. Belching is favored by an upright position and is often elicited by getting up from an horizontal position. Local complaints and reflux, on the other hand, occur mainly when the patient is in a supine position because the esophagus debouches at the right dorsal side of the gastric fundus. Lateral decubitus can provoke or eliminate the complaints. This paradox is explained by the fact that the right lateral decubitus, though favoring reflux into the esophagus, also facilitates gastric emptying through the pylorus; during left lateral decubitus, on the other hand, the gastric content stagnates. The most favorable position to prevent reflux is a fairly upright dorsal decubitus, as most patients experience on their own.

Paraesophageal hernias do not cause reflux but the local complaints are similar to those found in a sliding hernia; in addition breathing difficulties, dyspnoe and coughing occur. Four clinical forms of hiatus hernia must be mentioned explicitly: hiatus hernia in infants, hiatus hernia during pregnancy, postoperative hiatus hernia and traumatic hiatus hernia.

5.2. Hiatus Hernia in Infants

Esophagogastric hernias in infants can mostly be noticed already during the first weeks. ÅKERLUND (1926, 1933) thought that the short esophagus with hernia was congenital. Today the opinion prevails that in most cases neither the hernia nor the short esophagus are congenital, but the insufficient fixation of the gastric fundus in the abdomen is. A wide hiatus is an additional predisposing factor. The resulting hernia leads almost always to severe reflux esophagitis and frequently to ulceration; these are responsible for the shortening of the esophagus (ALLISON, 1948; THOMSEN, 1955).

The rare cases of the Barrett-type of short esophagus (1952), also called "endobrachyesophagus", may be congenital. In these cases the esophagus looks normal on the outside, but in its distal portion a squamous columnar epithelium is found which may reach as high as the cricoid. The lower esophagus lined by columnar epithelium may be combined with hiatus hernia. This entity is discussed in detail on p. 525.

In infants sliding hernias cause vomiting, bleeding and pain. If the esophagitis is not yet too severe early treatment, especially avoidance of horizontal decubitus, can eliminate the complaints. In case of severe esophagitis and stenosis surgery is indicated.

In contrast with esophagogastric hernia, paraesophageal hernia in infants seems to be congenital. It is found in 10% of all hernia cases (THOMSEN, 1955). The hiatus is almost always wide and the hernial sac large. Its symptoms are again vomiting, hematemesis and pain. Surgical treatment is indicated because of the danger of incarceration.

5.3. Hiatus Hernia during Pregnancy

In many women gastroesophageal reflux and heartburn occur during pregnancy. In contrast with pernicious vomiting of pregnancy it does not take place during the first months; usually it starts from the 5th month on and increases in intensity during the further course of pregnancy. The heartburn depends on the position of the patient: it worsens in horizontal decubitus and is ameliorated by getting up. On occasion vomiting occurs. After delivery the complaints all disappear at once, but they can recur during a following pregnancy or under other circumstances. Radiological examinations by HILLEMAND et al. (1953) and MONGES et al. (1956) have shown that a sliding hernia can be demonstrated in most pregnant women with heartburn. MONGES found a hiatus hernia in 28.7% of the examined pregnant women; the incidence given by other authors (MIXSON

and Woloshin, 1956; Sutherland et al., 1956) revolves around 5% for primi-
parae and around 20% for multiparae. The number of hernias increases toward
the end of pregnancy. Part of these hernias remain asymptomatic. The most
important pathogenetic factors are present: an increase in intraabdominal pressure and a loosening and flaccidity of the tissues. The fact that hiatus hernia
is not diagnosed more often during pregnancy is caused by the reluctance to
perform X-ray examinations during pregnancy and by the general experience that
symptoms disappear completely or almost completely in the majority of cases
after childbirth. Radiological follow-up of patients with hiatus hernia during
pregnancy showed this condition in only one third of the patients. These numbers
must be approached cautiously because in the follow-up studies no compression
to increase the intraabdominal pressure was applied, whereas such compression
was automatically present during pregnancy.

5.4. Postoperative Hernias

Postoperative hernias develop after operations during which the region of
the cardia is exposed through loosening of the gastrodiaphragmatic ligament,
of the esophagodiaphragmatic membrane and of the retroperitoneal fixations
of the posterior wall of the fundus. This happens as a rule during subdiaphragmatic
vagotomy, during Heller's operation and during resection of the upper half of
the stomach. Distal gastric resection eliminates the fixation by the left gastric
artery and thus also favors hiatus hernia. Furthermore there is the possibility
of a pre-existing, maybe asymptomatic hernia which is only demonstrated after
the operation. As a rule hernia after partial gastrectomy causes no or only minor
reflux symptoms (Figs. 314, 315).

Often symptoms of an esophagogastric hernia occur after surgical procedures
outside of the stomach, especially following cholecystectomy. These symptoms
are due to pre-existing hernias which were previously asymptomatic, but now
become manifest as a result of esophagitis favored by the long postoperative
bed rest and the use of gastric tubes.

5.5. Traumatic Hiatus Hernias

Often a thoracic or abdominal trauma is held responsible for the pathogenesis of a hiatus hernia. This may be an important medicolegal problem.
Traumatic diaphragmatic hernias protrude through diaphragmatic holes of traumatic origin and not through the hiatus. Unambiguous cases of traumatic hiatus
hernias have not been demonstrated thusfar. But the possibility exists that
a pre-existing asymptomatic hiatus hernia becomes manifest after a trauma,
often followed by a long period of bed rest.

5.6. Signs

Direct examination does not yield findings typical of hiatus hernia. Deep
palpation high in the epigastrium and under the left costal margin occasionally
causes pains similar in character to the spontaneous complaints.

Other signs can at most indicate the presence of factors which are known
to favor the genesis of a hernia: overweight, pregnancy, ascites, abdominal tumors
and organic obstruction of the gastrointestinal tract; belching on getting up
from a horizontal position can also be a sign of hiatus hernia. The most valuable
tools for diagnosis are history taking and X-ray examination.

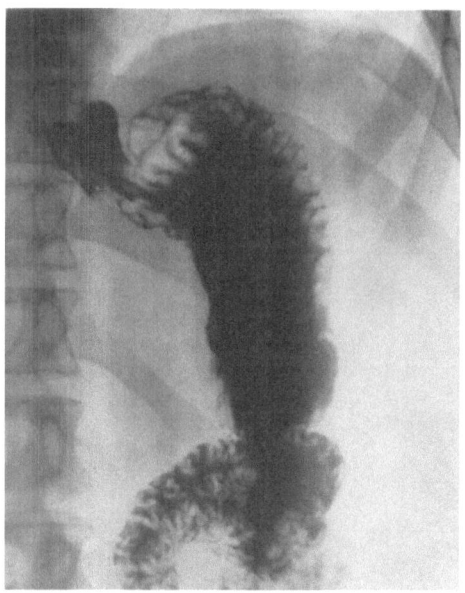 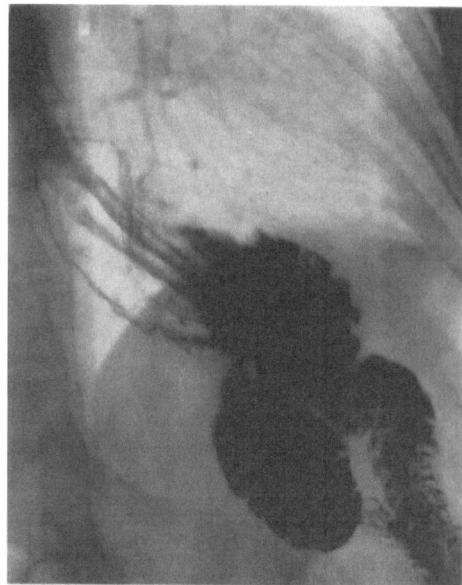

Fig. 314   Fig. 315

Fig. 314. Walnut-sized sliding hernia after hemigastrectomy

Fig. 315. Apple-sized paraesophageal hernia after a three quarter Billroth II gastrectomy

6. Technical Features

6.1. Radiological Examination

6.1.1. Technique of X-ray Examination

On occasion large fixed esophagogastric and paraesophageal hernias are visible on fluoroscopy of the thorax or on chest films even without contrast medium. A medium sized hernia may show up on lateral views as an air shadow behind the heart, often containing a fluid level. Very large hernias can even be recognizable on frontal views, when they project beyond the right heart border. The absence of the subdiaphragmatic gastric air bubble is considered an indirect sign of hiatus hernia. At any rate the diagnosis must be confirmed by examination with contrast material.

The position most favorable to reveal a hernia is determined by fluoroscopy. Modern radiological equipment including image amplifiers and TV monitors greatly facilitate the examination. It is of the utmost importance to take pictures in different positions and with different degrees of filling so that the images can be interpreted with certainty as hernia and can be distinguished from an epiphrenic ampulla.

The demonstration of a hiatus hernia is complemented by standard X-rays of the stomach. As contrast material a thin mixture (barium-water: 1/3 v.v.) is used; for more contrasting pictures a thicker mixture (barium-water: 1/2 v.v.). The mixture will better adhere to the esophageal mucosa if, instead of water, a 1% solution of carboxymethyl cellulose is used. It is best to store carboxymethyl cellulose in a 5% solution and to dilute it with water to 1% just before use.

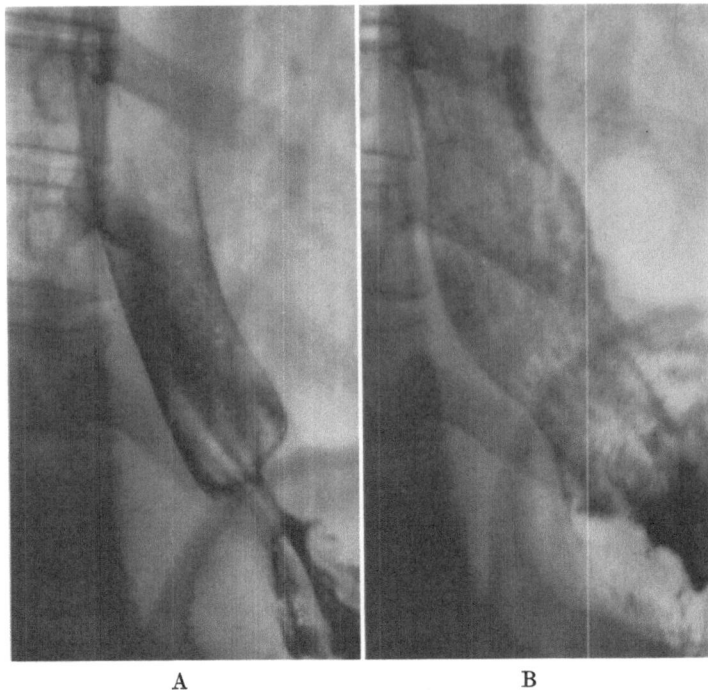

A   B

Fig. 316A and B. Effect of respiration on the normal distal esophagus. On maximal inspiration (A), the barium outflow into the stomach is blocked due to closure of the hiatus and
to compression of the abdominal part of the esophagus by the raised intraabdominal pressure.
On expiration (B), the hiatus opens, allowing barium to pass into the stomach

Exceptionally a thick barium paste is preferred (barium 1% carboxymethyl
cellulose solution: 2/1 or 3/1 v.v.) or one of the commercially available preparations which pass more slowly through the esophagus.

The position of the patient is a decisive factor in demonstrating a hernia.
If he stands up the hernia collapses and can often not be demonstrated. Smaller
hernias are mostly reversible and disappear in the upright position. The only
information yielded by an examination in upright position are the unimpeded
and fast passage of the contrast material through the esophagus and the cardia
and the continence of the hiatus. To test this continence the patient is asked
to inhale deeply immediately after swallowing barium and then to hold his
breath for a while. In normal subjects this maneuver blocks the cardia completely so that the contrast medium is held up in the distal esophagus (Fig. 316).
On expiration the esophageal lumen opens and the contrast medium passes.
Incontinence of the hiatus is associated with passage of the contrast medium even
on maximal inspiration, and is indicative of an abnormally wide hiatus and suggests
hiatus hernia (Fig. 317). However, continence on inspiration does not exclude
hiatus hernia.

A few radiologists recommend that the patient be placed in profile and bend
over maximally with stretched knees, in order to fill the hernia by reflux. This
procedure has not found a wide acceptance. To demonstrate a hiatus hernia
the patient is put in a horizontal position. In dorsal decubitus the contrast

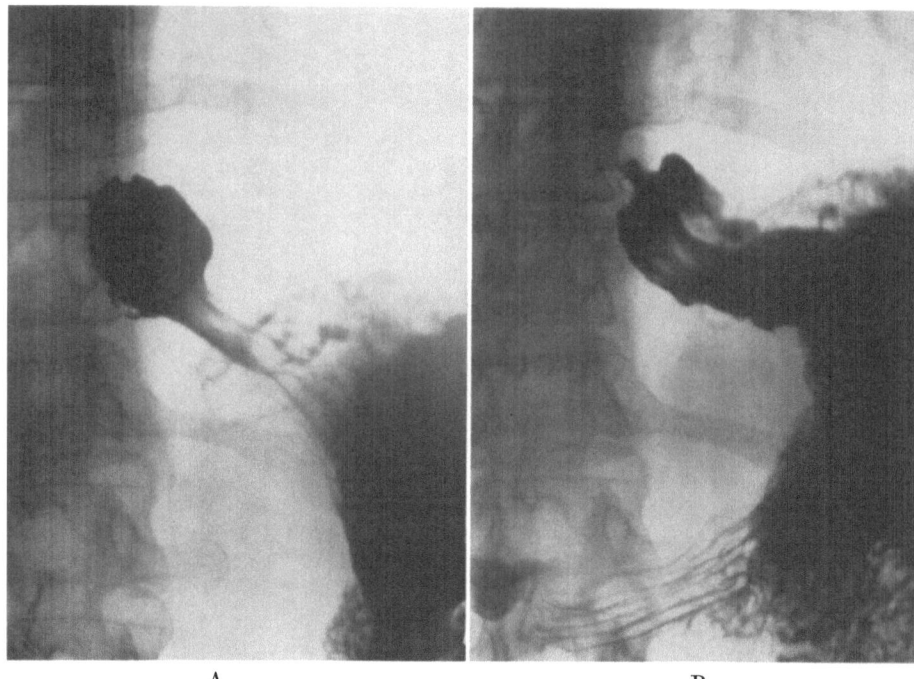

A   B

Fig. 317 A and B. Hiatal insufficiency. A Even on maximal inspiration, the hiatus remains
open. B On expiration the hiatus is wide open and a mandarin-sized hiatal hernia
is recognizable

medium collects in the dorsally located fundus. Large hernias can be well demonstrated in this way, particularly when the hiatus is wide. To demonstrate smaller
and reversible hernias it is recommended to place the patient in a supine left
posterior oblique head-down position and to have him swallow the contrast
material. However, in this position an epiphrenic ampulla is frequently observed,
due to the fact that the vestibulum may slide upward into the thorax, widen and
thus simulate a hernia. Therefore some radiologists do not favor this technique.
But it does allow to reveal the rest of the stomach and the duodenal bulb and
can be recommended as a routine exposure at the beginning of the examination
(Fig. 318). Exposures taken in the prone right anterior oblique position on Bucky
films avoid superposition of the gastroesophageal zone on the spine (Fig. 319).
In this position the cardia is higher than the rest of the stomach, so that the
contrast material flows into the distal part of the stomach and the fundus fills
with air. If the mucosa is still coated with contrast material the fundus and an
eventual hiatus hernia will show up in double contrast. To demonstrate the
terminal esophagus and the gastroesophageal junction the patient is asked to
swallow contrast material in this position. Small reversible hernias may not
protrude in this position and escape detection. A bolster under the right mesogastrium may force it out (Fig. 320), but a negative finding does not exclude
the presence of a hernia. More often a hiatus hernia can be demonstrated in
straight procubitus, after the stomach has been well filled with barium mixture,
if films are taken at the moment when a bolus of contrast material passes the

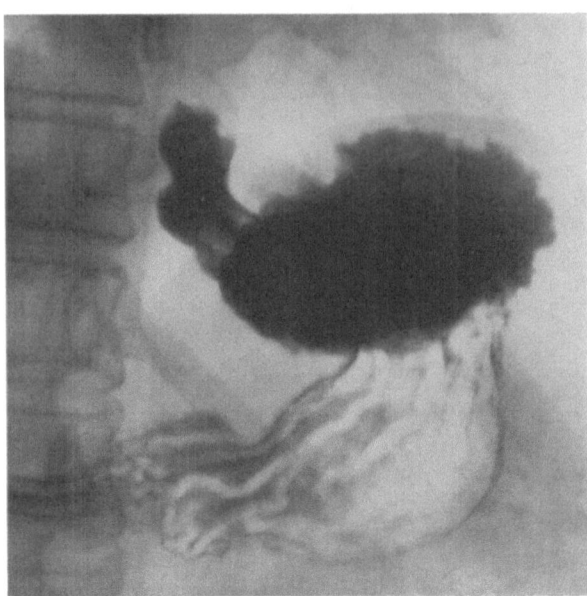

Fig. 318. X-ray taken in supine left-posterior head-down position. Walnut-sized hernia; above it, a hazelnut-sized vestibule

cardia. In obese patients the pressure of the abdomen is sufficient to force out even small reversible hernias (Fig. 321). This is not the case in thin subjects; they need a bolster under the mesogastrium to increase the intraabdominal pressure. The increase in pressure depends on the size and the hardness of the bolster. In our own examinations we use a foam rubber bolster with a diameter of 10 cm; it causes a small increase in pressure, still "within physiological limits". An inflated rubber balloon has the same effect. Some authors use hard bolsters and even sand bags; consequently they will diagnose hernias more often. The degree of pressure which can still be considered "physiological" is not agreed upon. Others prefer a Trendelenburg position of 30 degrees combined with procubitus. The exposures are made preferably during expiration while the hiatus is open. Exposures during inspiration, which creates the epiphrenic ampulla, are recommended in some cases to localize the squamocolumnar epithelial junction.

The hernia may also be demonstrated with the patient in a horizontal position and a horizontal direction of the X-rays (Kinsella-technique). In procubitus the hernia is filled with air, in decubitus with contrast material (LEDOUX-LEBARD et al., 1967). This technique may yield additional information in complicated cases but has not found wide acceptance as a routine method.

6.1.2. Radiological Demonstration of Reflux

On occasion gastroesophageal reflux, the most important clinical symptom of hiatus hernia, can be observed during radiological examination in dorsal decubitus, either spontaneously or after dry swallows. BROMBART and VAN LERBERGHE (1952) placed their patients in profile, had them bend over maximally with stretched

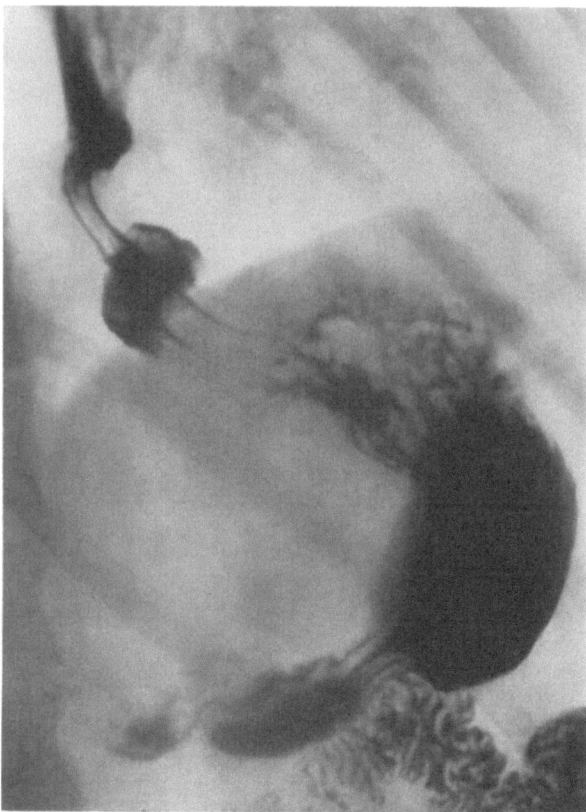

Fig. 319. X-ray taken in prone right-anterior position. Walnut-sized hernia; above it, the contracted vestibule

knees and tried to provoke reflux by asking the patients to contract the abdominal musculature, to strain and cough. To demonstrate reflux other radiologists recommend the water siphonage test described by CARVALHO (1951). The patient's stomach is filled with contrast material and he assumes a supine right posterior oblique position. Through a tube he quickly drinks 250 ml of water. This flushes remnants of the barium mixture from the esophagus into the stomach; at the same time the lower esophageal sphincter opens, allowing reflux. This water siphonage test was used by LINSMAN (1965) in 1000 unselected patients. Positive results were obtained in 78.9% of hiatus hernia patients and in 38.3% of patients with gastrointestinal ulcer. 73.7% of the patients with positive tests had heartburn while the other 26.3% had no complaints. This is to be expected since the lower esophageal sphincter opens for 6 to 8 seconds after most swallows. The clinical significance of an artificially provoked reflux seems minor, but the radiological demonstration of a spontaneous reflux is clinically important (KRAMER, 1969) especially if a significant amount of refluxed material stays in the esophagus and does not elicit propulsive esophageal contractions that return it promptly into the stomach.

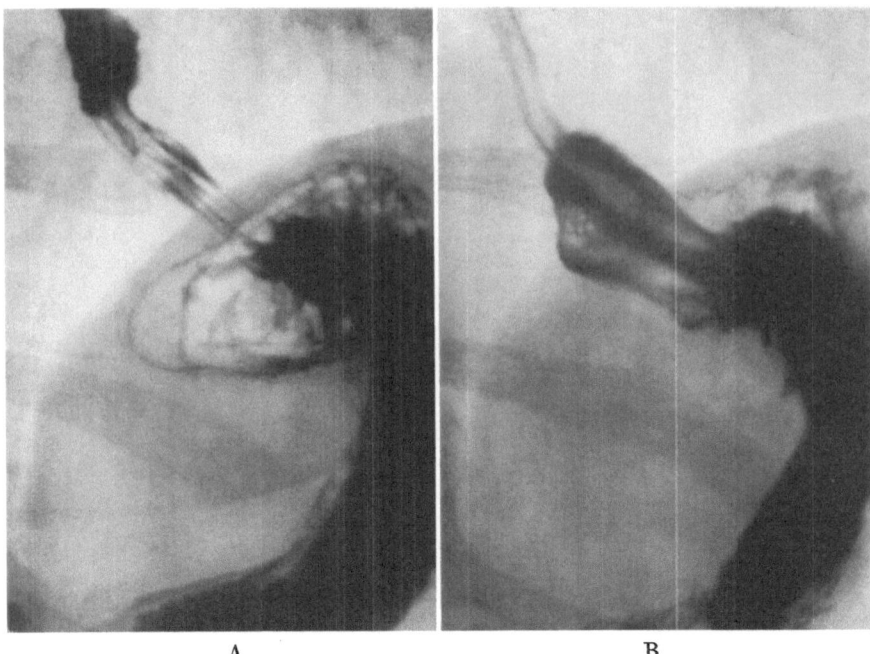

A   B

Fig. 320 A and B. Reversible hiatus hernia. A Contracted vestibular segment above the diaphragm. B When a bolster is placed under the abdomen, a mandarin-sized hernia appears

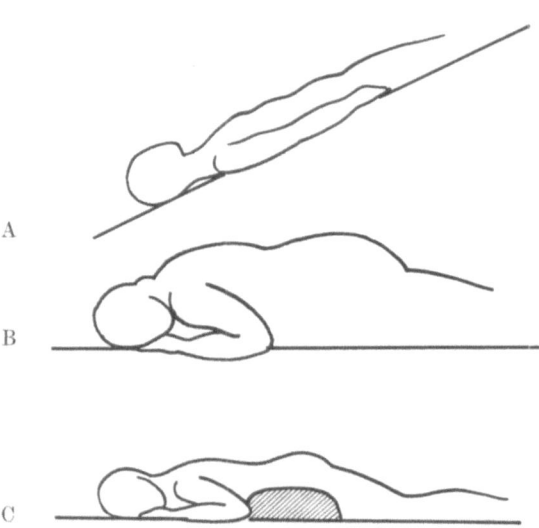

Fig. 321 A—C. Position for demonstrating a hiatal hernia. A Supine left-posterior head-down position. B Prone or prone right-anterior position, Bucky table. In obese patients the prone position is sufficient to bring about a reversible hernia by raising the intra-abdominal pressure. C In thin patients a bolster is used to bring about this effect

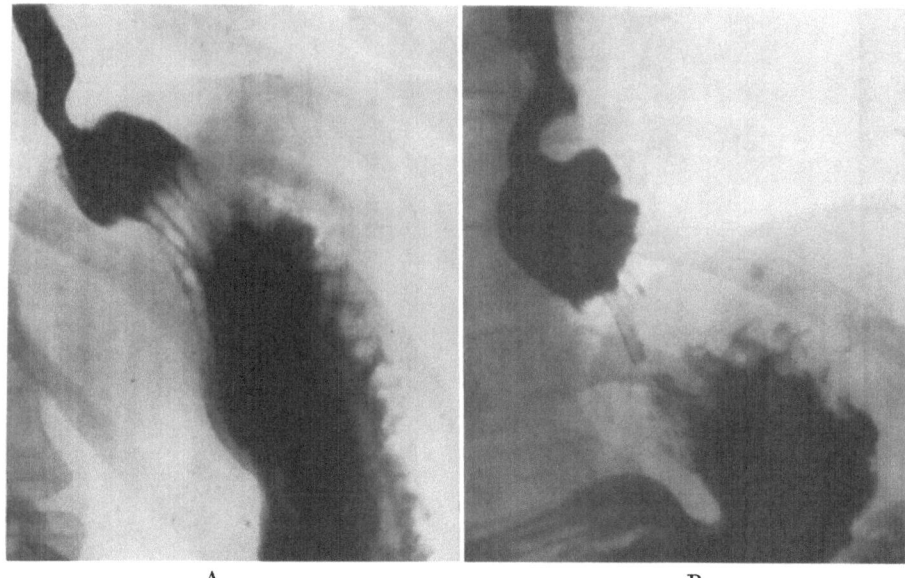

A   B

Fig. 322 A and B. The projection of the hiatus depends on the patient's position. In the prone right-anterior position (A), the hiatus projects below the diaphragmatic dome and in the strict prone position (B), above it

6.1.3. Interpretation of X-ray Findings

The diagnosis of esophagogastric sliding hernia is unambiguous if the pictures taken during expiration reveal a round, oval or bell-shaped accumulation of barium above the diaphragm, the size of a walnut or larger, in which gastric mucosal rugae are discernible or which is connected with the stomach by a segment showing at the level of the hiatus longitudinal mucosal folds of the gastric type (Figs. 317 B, 319, 320 B). When the hernia is small the esophagus usually debouches in the center of the herniated stomach; when it is larger the junction between esophagus and stomach is located at the right upper aspect of the herniated sac. The slightly eccentric pouching of the hernia together with the presence of a clearly visible incisura cardiaca is pathognomic of an esophagogastric sliding hernia. The terminal esophagus immediately above the hernia is narrow over a length of 2 to 3 cm, due to the resting tone of the lower esophageal sphincter (Figs. 319, 337). In a slightly oblique right anterior position and in a slightly oblique left posterior position the hiatus and a diaphragmatic dome project at the same level. A more oblique position will lower the projection of the hiatus below that of the diaphragm (Fig. 322 A). A straight horizontal procubitus shows it a few cms above that of the diaphragm (Fig. 322 B). The width of the hiatus can be estimated during maximal expiration. Normally it has a diameter of 15 to 20 mm and closes completely during maximal inspiration (Fig. 316). In a patient with hiatus hernia the diameter of the barium column is usually more than 20 mm, though not always, and the hiatus closes incompletely during maximal inspiration (Fig. 317).

As a rule gastric mucosal folds in the hernia can be recognized only when some air is still left in the hernia, as is usually the case in right procubitus. At the

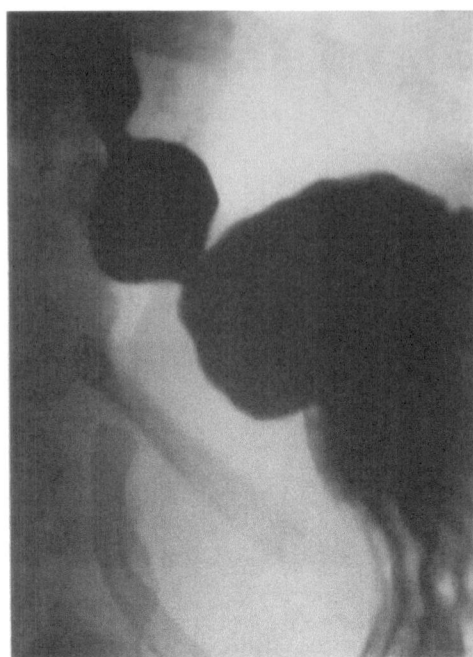

Fig. 323. Supine left-posterior head-down position. Picture taken on maximal inspiration immediately after deglutition. Mandarin-sized, completely filled and spherical image above the hiatus. The differentiation between an epiphrenic ampulla and a small hernia is impossible

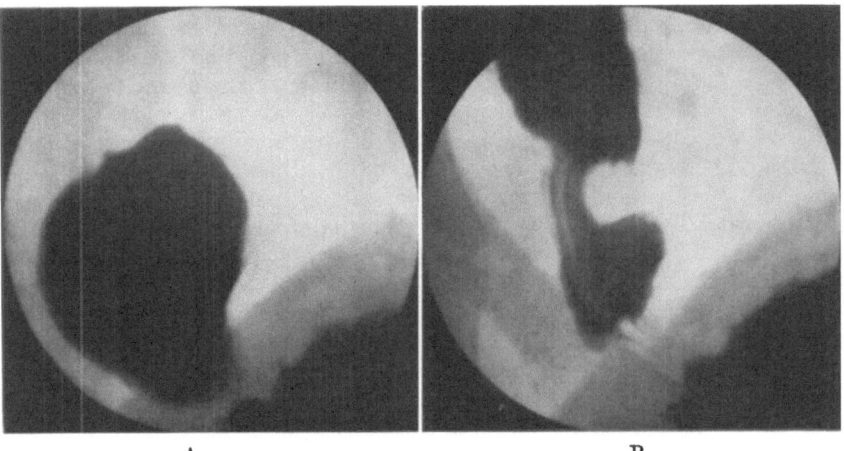

A   B

Fig. 324A and B. Epiphrenic ampulla at different degrees of filling. A few seconds after deglutition, on maximal inspiration, which blocks the barium outflow, the vestibule balloons out to an epiphrenic ampulla. A Pear-shaped epiphrenic ampulla. B If the patient holds his breath, the epiphrenic ampulla empties proximally. The proximal half of the vestibule is contracted. At the transition of vestibule to tubular esophagus, the "upper ring" can be recognized

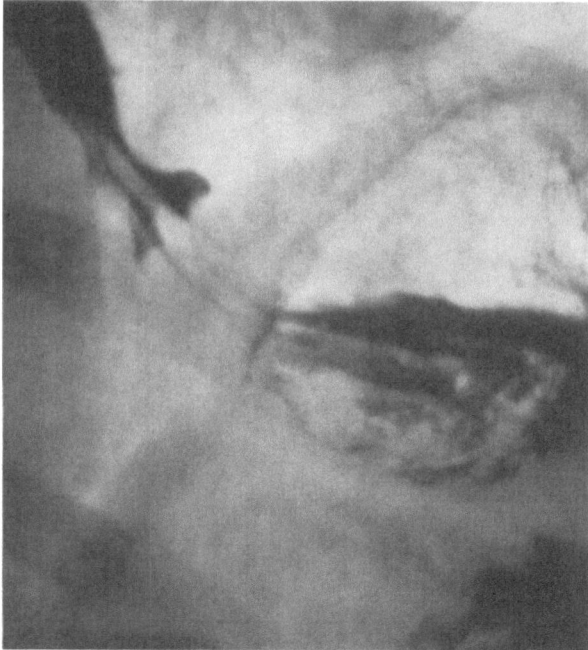

Fig. 325. Z-line (zig-zag line) at the squamocolumnar mucosal junction. Two centimeters above the diaphragmatic dome, a small amount of contrast material is held up on top of the coarse gastric folds and this visualizes the arc-like epithelial junction (incidental finding)

level of the hiatus itself, however, the external compression causes the gastric folds to become visible even when the hernia is full of contrast medium (Figs. 317 B, 318, 320 B, 322 A).

In left posterior oblique position it may be difficult to interpret a round or oval epiphrenic image as a hiatus hernia or an epiphrenic ampulla (Fig. 323). This ampulla is formed by inflation of the terminal few cm of the supradiaphragmatic esophagus. If a patient takes a deep breath after swallowing he blocks the passage of the esophagus into the stomach, thus giving rise to a round or pear-shaped dilatation of the terminal esophagus. This epiphrenic ampulla varies in size, depending upon the level the esophageal contraction has reached at the time of the exposure (Fig. 324 A, B). If he holds his breath for a few more seconds the epiphrenic ampulla empties into the more proximal esophageal segments. It is often hard to distinguish a full epiphrenic ampulla formed only by the terminal esophagus from one formed by both the terminal esophagus and a hiatus hernia (Fig. 323). On incomplete filling of the hernia with barium the epithelial junction can exceptionally be recognized as an arching line (Fig. 325). On complete filling a special technique will reveal a Schatzki ring at the level of the epithelial junction in 50% of patients with a small hernia. To demonstrate it the patient is placed in right anterior oblique position on the Bucky table and drinks the contrast material out of a spouted cup: after 4 to 5 swallows he takes a deep breath and at that moment the pictures are taken. The maximal inspiration blocks the passage into the stomach; the hernia and terminal esophagus are filled and balloon out so that 3 rings appear (Fig. 326). The upper ring is located between the tubular esoph-

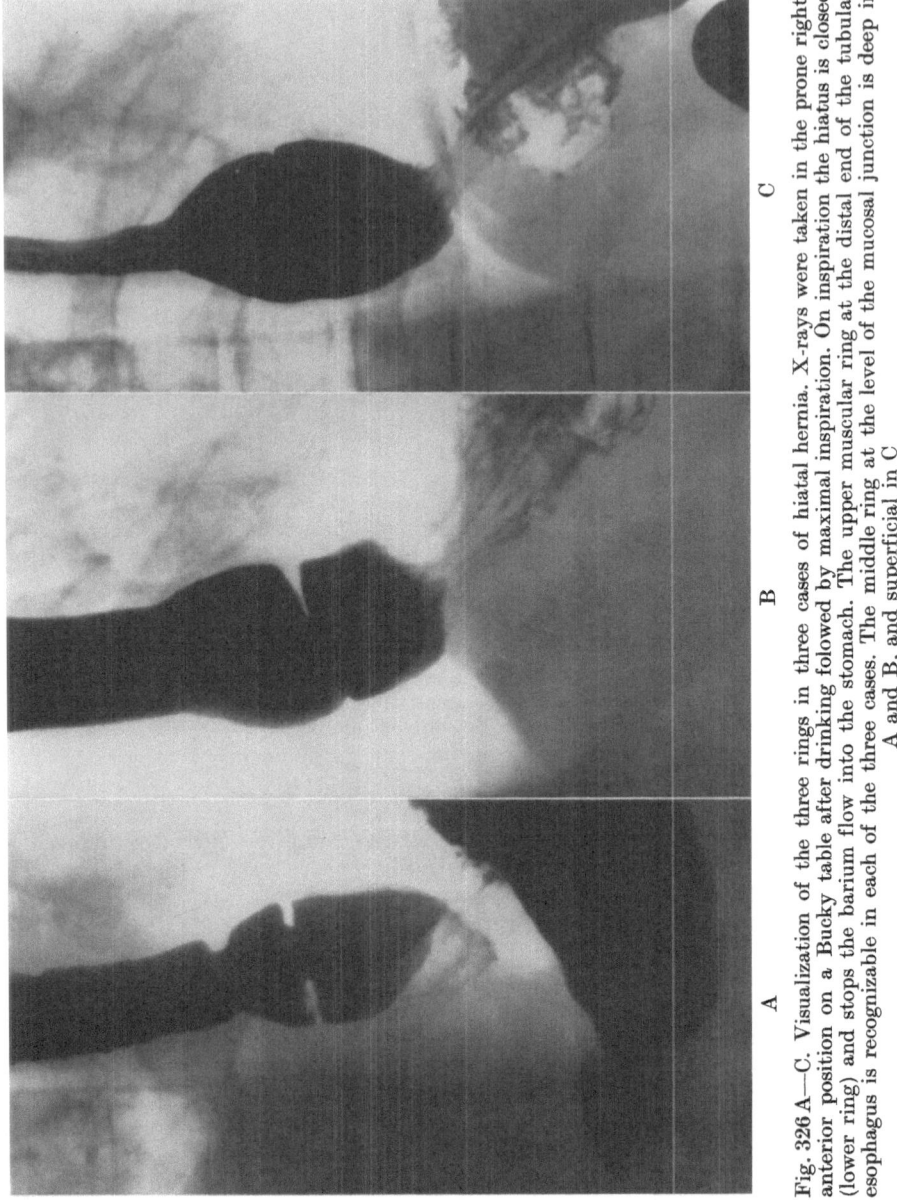

Fig. 326 A—C. Visualization of the three rings in three cases of hiatal hernia. X-rays were taken in the prone right-anterior position on a Bucky table after drinking folowed by maximal inspiration. On inspiration the hiatus is closed (lower ring) and stops the barium flow into the stomach. The upper muscular ring at the distal end of the tubular esophagus is recognizable in each of the three cases. The middle ring at the level of the mucosal junction is deep in A and B, and superficial in C

agus and the vestibulum, is contractile, inconstant and thus of a muscular nature; a lower ring, which separates the hernia from the subdiaphragmatic part of the stomach, is caused by the inspiratory hiatal pinchcock and disappears on expiration. In between both rings, at the level of the squamocolumnar epithelial junction, a middle ring is formed. It may appear as a slight indentation, occasionally visible only on the left, or as a complete ring. It is not contractile and therefore not of muscular nature. This is the "lower esophageal ring" described by SCHATZKI (1956), which is discussed in more detail in Chapter VI.

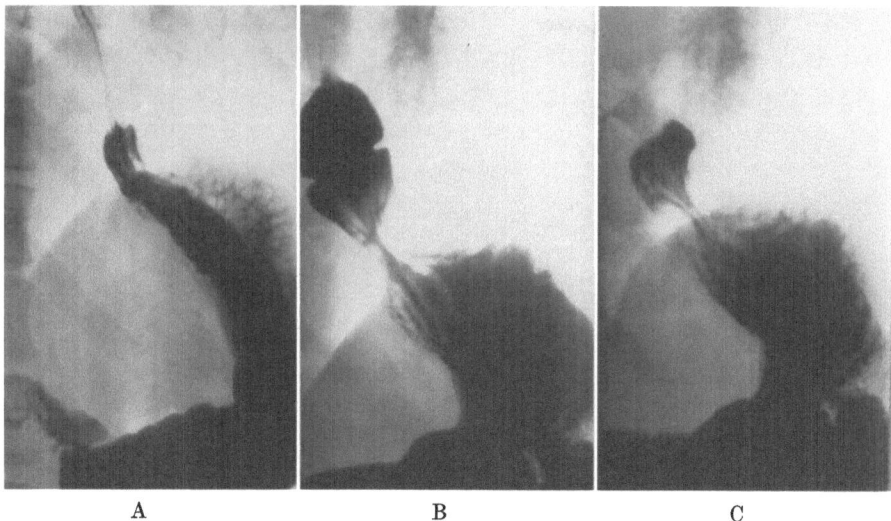

A					B					C

Fig. 327 A—C. Hiatus hernia in different degrees of filling. Prone right-anterior position. Bucky table. A 5 sec after deglutition; expiration. B After drinking, followed by maximal inspiration, visualization of the three rings. C After the next expiration. The vestibule is emptied, the hernia is still filled

The studies of Bauer et al. (1970) indicate that the squamocolumnar junction in patients with a Schatzki ring is situated at the junction of esophageal and gastric mucosa. It is found only in patients with hiatus hernia over 40 years of age, suggesting that it is an acquired condition. The demonstration of a middle ring permits the localization of the transition between the dilated vestibulum and the herniated sac, and therefore the differential diagnosis between a physiological phrenic ampulla and a pathological hiatus hernia. On expiration the inflated vestibulum empties first, while the hernia remains filled for a few more seconds (Fig. 327). Once one is familiar with the morphology of these three rings it is possible to interpret the nature and the localization of rings on X-rays taken with other techniques. Misunderstandings are due to the fact that some radiologists use the term ampulla to designate a transient expansion of the tubular esophagus, immediately above the upper ring, and not to designate the dilated vestibulum. To avoid misunderstandings it seems better to use only the term epiphrenic ampulla.

An indirect symptom of hiatus hernia, often recognizable on pictures of standing patients, is the absence of an air bubble in the gastric fundus. It disappears together with the angle of His when the protrusion of the cardia results in a spindle-shaped fundus.

The width of the hiatus in patients with a hernia is difficult to determine radiologically since the hiatal opening is occupied by a variable amount of soft tissue. The maximal diameter of the barium column traversing the hiatus is of clinical importance. To determine this diameter the lower esophagus should be fully expanded with barium and pictures taken at maximal expiration. If this diameter is large (20 mm or more), it favors gastroesophageal reflux (Fig. 328), if it is small, the patient is likely to have local discomfort rather than symptoms of reflux.

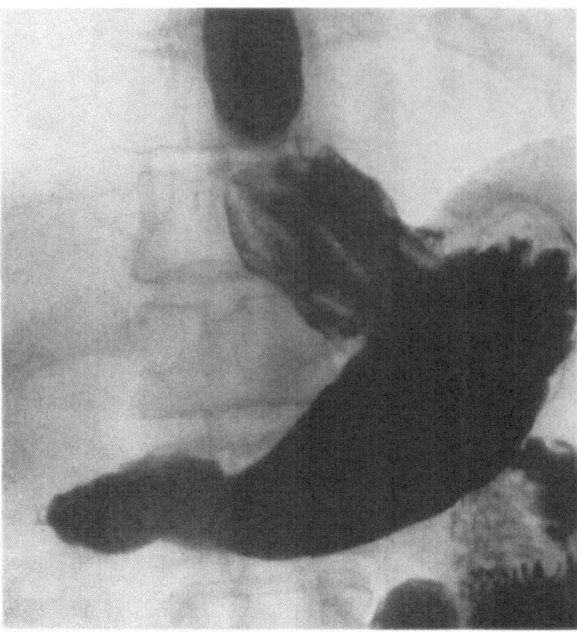

Fig. 328. Apple-sized hiatus hernia with a wide hiatus and major reflux symptoms

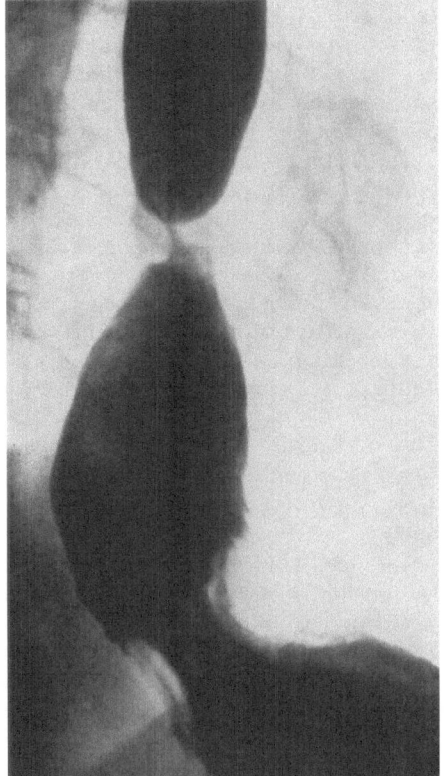

Fig. 329. Short esophagus with stricture and pulled-up hernia

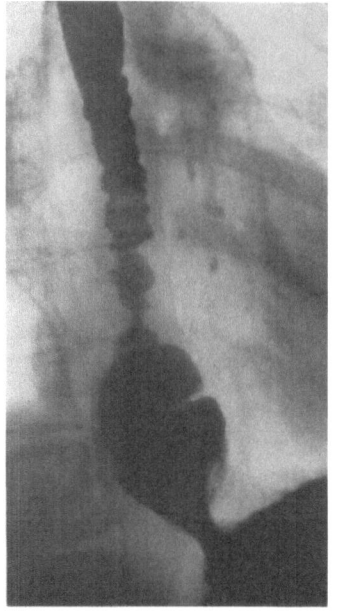 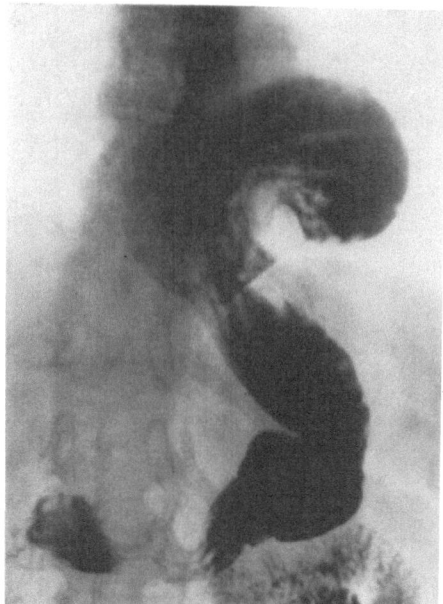

Fig. 330   Fig. 331

Fig. 330. Mandarin-sized sliding hernia with corkscrew esophagus

Fig. 331. Large paraesophageal hernia. The hernia hides the cardiac orifice

In larger sliding hernias the esophagus becomes too long and occasionally tortuous in its distal third. But mostly it is straight and therefore shortened. The shortening may be due to contraction of the longitudinal muscle coat, as the surgeon will notice on severing the esophagus. It is hard to decide radiologically whether a minor shortening is congenital, the result of longitudinal tension or due to sclerosing reflux esophagitis. Major shortenings, particularly when combined with a stricture, are organic lesions (Fig. 329). The differentiation between functional and organic shortening is very important, for it enables the surgeon to opt for an abdominal or a thoracic approach. An especially wide hiatus, a combination of hiatus hernia with other congenital anomalies and a localization of the esophagodiaphragmatic membrane substantially distal from the squamocolumnar epithelial junction indicate a congenitally short esophagus. The esophagoscopic finding of severe extensive circular esophagitis and rigidity of the esophageal wall suggests an organic shortening. The surgeon will then decide on a transthoracic approach. Hiatus hernia can be associated with non-propulsive tertiary contractions of the esophagus (Fig. 330). The ensuing radiological "curling" may be due to the syndrome of painful diffuse spasm of the esophagus, or may not be associated with any clinical symptoms at all (asymptomatic diffuse spasm, KRAMER, 1967).

6.1.4. Paraesophageal Hernia

A large paraesophageal hernia may show up on chest X-rays as an air-filled pouch behind the heart often containing a fluid level. Small paraesophageal hernias can be demonstrated only when the stomach is filled with contrast

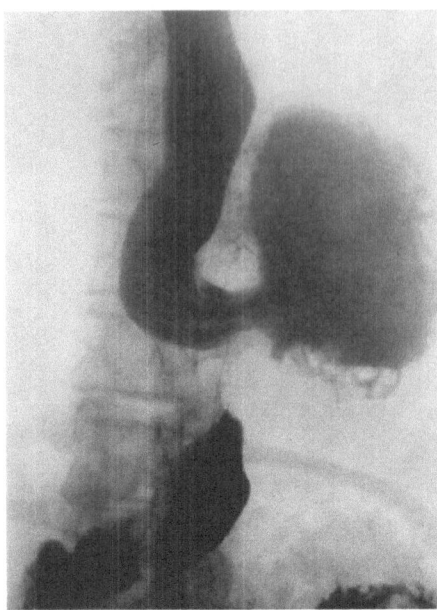

Fig. 332. Large paraesophageal hernia; the cardia occupies its normal subdiaphragmatic position

material. Characteristically the terminal esophagus remains at its normal intra- and subdiaphragmatic position. As a rule the stomach protudes into the thorax at the left of the esophagus through a mostly widened hiatus (Figs. 329, 330). A persisting pneumoenteric recessus is often found (Thomsen, 1955). The herniated stomach can compress the terminal esophagus and thus hinder the passage of food. A filled hernial sac may hide the site of entrance into the stomach so that the hernia seems to be of the esophagogastric type (Fig. 331). By means of the double contrast technique or by rotation of the patient it is possible to determine the location of the cardia (Fig. 332). When in large paraesophageal hernias more than half of the stomach has herniated the greater curvature faces upward. This "upward down stomach" may lead to volvulus. Paraesophageal hernias tend to draw ever increasing portions of the stomach into the thorax and to incarcerate. On the other hand they do not cause reflux.

Sweet (1952) described a special form of paraesophageal hernia, "esophageal hiatus hernia of the diaphragm". This hernia does not protrude through the hiatus, but through an opening so close to it that only a few muscle fibers of the diaphragm separate the hernia from the esophagus.

6.1.5. Mixed Hernias

Small paraesophageal hernias can be combined with a herniation of the cardia (Fig. 333). On the other hand an esophagogastric sliding hernia can be associated with a rising of the fundus above the cardia. In both instances the hernia is of the mixed type. When the hernia is very large the initial type may no longer be recognizable.

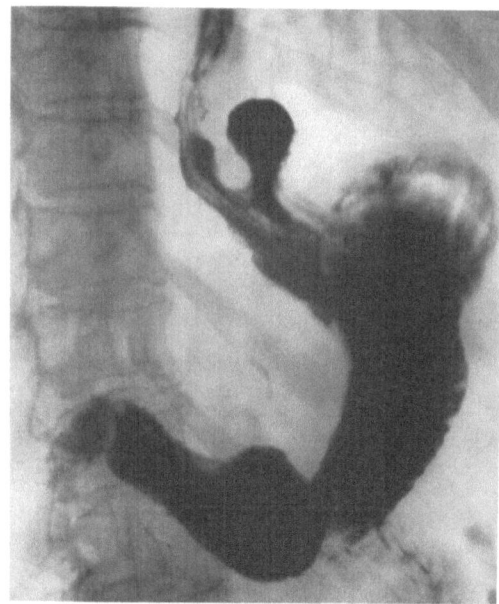

Fig. 333. Mixed hernia

6.1.6. Invagination

Prolapse of the esophageal mucosa into the stomach has been described by
KLINEFELTER (1956), ODEGAARD (1959), DE LORIMIER and WARREN (1960) and
ALDRIDGE (1962). This prolapse manifests itself by a clover-leaf deformity of
the hernia or by a "Saturnus-ring" (Fig. 334). These images may be either the
effect of the projection of the 3 rings or a transient functional phenomenon,
caused by a Valsalva maneuver, and clinically unimportant. The same is true
for the prolapse of the gastric mucosa into the terminal esophagus, described
by FELDMAN (1951), BLUM et al. (1961) and HÄRING (1961).

6.1.7. Note on Terminology

Agreement about radiological findings in the region of the cardia is hampered
by the prevailing anarchy in the nomenclature. This may be due in part to the
great number of synonyms, but mostly to an insufficient distinction between
anatomical, radiological and physiological, especially manometric, notions. Anatomical, radiological and manometrical terms must be kept apart. For instance
"epiphrenic ampulla" is a radiological, "vestibulum" an anatomical and "high
pressure zone" a manometric notion.

6.2. Endoscopy

An esophagogastric hiatus hernia can be diagnosed by means of esophagoscopy, gastroscopy or, in some cases, peritoneoscopy.

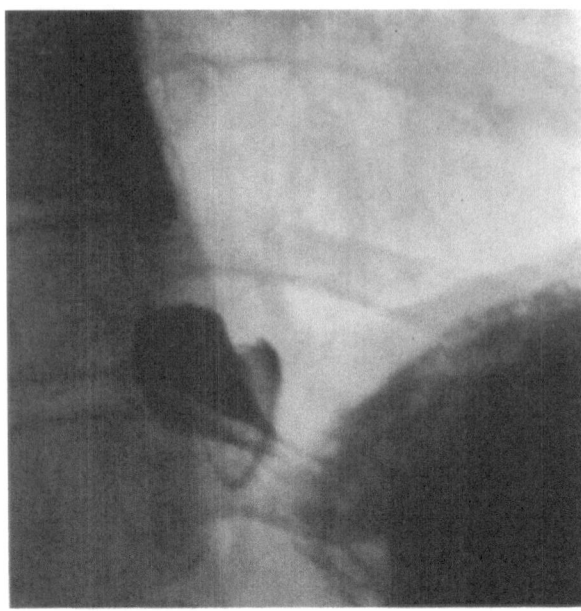

Fig. 334. "Saturnus ring", often interpreted as an esophagogastric invagination, but due to an oblique projection of the middle ring

6.2.1. Esophagoscopy

Esophagoscopy successively reveals (1) the narrowed vestibulum; (2) the squamocolumnar epithelial junction; (3) the hernia with its gastric mucosa; (4) the hiatus; (5) the subdiaphragmatic stomach.

1. The entry into the tonically contracted vestibulum is often recognizable by the circular narrowing of the lumen. It does not resist the passage of the esophagoscope. The opinions and definitions about the distal limit of the vestibulum diverge. Palmer (1968) states that mostly the entire vestibulum is covered with gastric mucosa. Similarly, Savary (1968) finds that in most cases the distal half is covered with gastric mucosa. For Zaino et al. (1965), however, the epithelial junction is the distal limit of the vestibulum. If his definition is accepted Palmer's and Savary's findings correspond to small hiatus hernias. The oblique and spiraling muscle fibers of the terminal esophagus, described by Laimer (1953), et al. Zaino (1963) and Stelzner (1968) can sometimes be recognized on endoscopy as transverse or oblique submucosal fibers. When the vestibulum is in its normal position no respiratory changes of the lumen can be observed in its intrahiatal part. Its subdiaphragmatic part is compressed on inspiration and expanded on expiration. When it is located in the thorax because of hiatus hernia it is compressed on expiration and expanded on inspiration.

2. The squamocolumnar epithelial junction usually looks more or less like a series of arches formed by large gastric folds. The dorsal aspect of the junction seems to be located higher than the ventral aspect. This is due in part to an endoscopic artifact, for the axes of endoscope and hiatus do not run parallel (Savary, 1970). On the other hand reflux esophagitis starts with hyperemic reddening of the dorsal aspect, so that it can easily be confused with gastric mucosa. If the region of the squamocolumnar epithelial junction is inflated

with air the zigzag line stretches and becomes almost straight. On occasion a circular projection becomes visible, corresponding to the Schatzki ring, which is located near or at the level of the squamocolumnar epithelial junction. Often islets of ectopic squamous epithelium are found distally of the demarcation; more rarely islets of ectopic columnar epithelium are found in the terminal esophagus. It may therefore be difficult to determine the exact site of the junction. In the Barrett esophagus the columnar epithelium extends far into the gullet. The mucosa of the normal terminal esophagus is light rose, smooth and slightly transparent. Usually it shows small submucosal blood vessels running parallel to the longitudinal axis. The gastric mucosa is dark red, velvety; its folds are prominent and larger than those of the esophagus. When in doubt the endoscopist can stain the esophageal mucosa blue with a 1% lugol solution.

3. The hiatus hernia with its gastric mucosa extends as a sac from the squamo-columnar epithelial junction to the diaphragmatic pinchcock. In contrast with the intraabdominal stomach the hernia expands on inspiration and collapses on expiration.

4. On esophagoscopy the hiatus can be recognized as a circular narrowing of the distal end of the hernia; on maximal inspiration it becomes tight and moves to the right while on expiration it widens. Its edge can often be felt with the top of the esophagoscope. With the fiber esophagoscope it is quite easy to pass the hiatus and to penetrate into the intraabdominal stomach.

5. The subdiaphragmatic stomach can be differentiated from the hernia by its expiratory dilatation and inspiratory collapse.

Thus all landmarks necessary to diagnose a sliding hiatus hernia can be recognized by esophagoscopy. However, a small reversible sliding hernia can easily be missed on esophagoscopy because no abdominal compression is exerted to elicit the herniation. For this reason the endoscopist often finds reflux esophagitis without hernia. The clinically most important confirmation he can give is not the diagnosis of hiatus hernia, but concerns the state of the mucosa in esophagus and hernia and the presence or absence of complications such as esophagitis, ulcer, stenosis and gastritis. The esophagoscopic signs of reflux esophagitis are described on p. 514.

The incidence of reflux esophagitis in hiatus hernia was found to be 23.9% of 786 cases; the incidence of strictures was 4.3% (PALMER, 1968). In a somewhat differently selected group of 1198 patients with a radiologically demonstrated hiatus hernia or with reflux complaints SAVARY (1966) found signs of esophagitis in 51%. All esophagoscopists agree that severe erosive esophagitis may be completely asymptomatic and that on the other hand patients with endoscopically and bioptically normal mucosa may complain of intensive heartburn. Individual tolerance determines whether reflux of acid gastric secretion will cause heartburn without esophagitis, esophagitis without heartburn or esophagitis with symptoms and maybe complications.

In the opinion of some endoscopists the presence of severe erosive esophagitis, even without symptoms, is an indication for surgery. However, surgical treatment was used by PALMER (1968) for only 3.9% of his 786 patients followed for 20 years, 23.9% of whom had esophagitis and 4.3% strictures. Lesions of the gastric mucosa in the hiatus hernia are less frequent and less pronounced than those due to peptic esophagitis. Superficial gastritis, with or without atrophy, is found with the same frequency as in other comparable age groups. To this histological finding corresponds either a normal endoscopic aspect, or hyperemic reddening of the crests of the folds, associated with dullness and sometimes erosions of the surface. More often the bright red and glossy mucosa is edematous and swollen and bleeds easily on contact with the esophagoscope. Histologically this corresponds to mucosal edema and minor cellular infiltration. This edematous gastritis is remarkably frequent in relatively small hernias with narrow hiatus. The throttling of the blood circulation in the hiatus, lymph stasis and pressure changes in the intrathoracic stomach may play a role in the pathogenesis of this gastritis (SAVARY, 1966). This seems to agree with the fact that no relation can be found between the occurrence and intensity of esophagitis on the one hand and edematous gastritis on the other in hiatus hernia. Esophagoscopy does not yield useful information in cases of paraesophageal hernia.

6.2.2. Gastroscopy

Gastroscopy in hiatus hernia can best be performed with a forward viewing fiber endoscope because the lateral views obtained with other types of gastroscopes only allow the observation of the middle portion of a large hernia. The forward viewing scope reveals most areas of the intraabdominal stomach and, when the inversion technique is used, even the point of entry of the instrument. It is not always possible, however, to distinguish between the point of entry into a hernia and a normal cardia. The gastroscopic inversion technique will reveal an esophagogastric hernia only when the hiatus is so wide that the cardia comes into view behind it. In paraesophageal hernia the entry into the herniated sac can be viewed by means of the inversion technique. In a large paraesophageal hernia it is better to omit an examination with inversion, to avoid damaging the small intraabdominal stomach.

6.2.3. Peritoneoscopy

Peritoneoscopy may show the entry of the stomach into an abnormally wide hiatus. In the literature the presence of a hiatus hernia has often been considered a contraindication for peritoneoscopy. This may be valid for large paraesophageal hernias, which massive insufflation with air may incarcerate. Thusfar no accidents due to peritoneoscopy have been reported in sliding hernias.

6.3. Manometry

Intraluminal pressure measurements have substantially advanced our understanding of the physiology and pathophysiology of the gastroesophageal junctional segment. Contradictory results of manometric studies are mostly caused by the application of different techniques. The original balloon method has become virtually obsolete. Today the most common technique uses small catheters with a lateral opening at the distal end, which are constantly perfused with water during the examination and allow an almost quantitative determination of the closing force and the resistance to stretch of the sphincter (HARRIS et al., 1966; POPE, 1967; WINANS and HARRIS, 1967; HEITMANN, 1969).

In normal subjects the distal 2 to 4 cm of the lower esophagus act as a physiological sphincter, which is closed at rest and opens only in response to certain stimuli. The subdiaphragmatic portion of the sphincter acts as a flutter valve, and is probably an important factor in the antireflux mechanism. When the lower esophageal sphincter has moved into the thorax, it no longer is subject to the intraabdominal pressure. Under these circumstances the sphincter is the only antireflux mechanism left. The intrasphincteric pressure usually drops slightly. This favors gastroesophageal reflux (COHEN and HARRIS, 1970; HADDAD, 1970) (Fig. 328). If in such cases the intragastric pressure is increased by 10 to

15 mm Hg by means of a standardized abdominal compression maneuver, the increased pressure is transferred into the lower esophagus, which demonstrates the lack of an effective closing mechanism (HEITMANN, 1969). If the high pressure is maintained in spite of hernia there is no reflux.

Manometry by means of either perfused catheters or balloon-covered miniature transducers is not a sensitive way of detecting the presence of a hiatal hernia (COHEN, 1970). Several criteria have been used for the manometric diagnosis of hiatus hernia: upward displacement of the sphincteric high pressure zone; the presence of two pressure inversion points (P.I.P. or points where the respiratory pressure swing changes from inspiratory positive to inspiratory negative or vice versa), and two separate peaks of high pressure or an elongation of the high pressure zone. These criteria, used in combination or alone, result in a high incidence of false negative as well as false positive diagnoses. Manometry with a perfused catheter system, however, may give valuable information about the predisposition to reflux. A low resting pressure in the sphincter or the absence of a lower esophageal high pressure zone indicates the presence of an incompetent sphincter. Similarly, when a modest abdominal compression results in an increase of the resting intraesophageal pressure, the closing mechanism at the cardia is considered to be ineffectual or absent. Intraluminal pressure measurements in patients with a hiatal hernia are also important for the evaluation of associated motor disturbances of the esophagus. Vigorous simultaneous and repetitive contractions in the lower esophagus may be associated with pain and dysphagia, suggesting diffuse spasm of the esophagus. HEITMANN (1969) found in 10% of his hiatus hernia patients abnormally high intrasphincteric pressures, i.e. "overcompetent" sphincters. Some of these had diffuse spasm of the esophagus. They did not suffer from reflux complaints but from cramp-like retrosternal pains, often imitating angina pectoris; on occasion they also had dysphagia. On radiological examination the terminal esophagus was found narrowed over about 1 cm, which slowed down the passage through the cardia. The question remains unanswered whether this narrowing is due to primary hypertonicity of the lower esophagus, leading to hernia, or to a consequence of the hiatus hernia, namely, stenosing esophagitis and perhaps unrecognized ulceration.

6.4. pH Measurements

Intraesophageal pH measurements with the aid of a small pH electrode probably constitute the most sensitive test of gastroesophageal reflux (HADDAD, 1970). It is described in detail in Chapter II (pH measurements).

6.5. Acid Infusion Test

Heartburn caused by infusion of acid into the esophagus according to the method of BERNSTEIN (1958) is an objective indication of reflux. Recent evidence indicates that a positive acid infusion test strongly suggests the presence of esophagitis.

7. Diagnosis

The diagnosis of hiatus hernia is based primarily on history and radiology. Interrogation of the patient mostly brings to light one or more symptoms of the triad: local complaints, incontinence of the cardia (belching, reflux, heart-

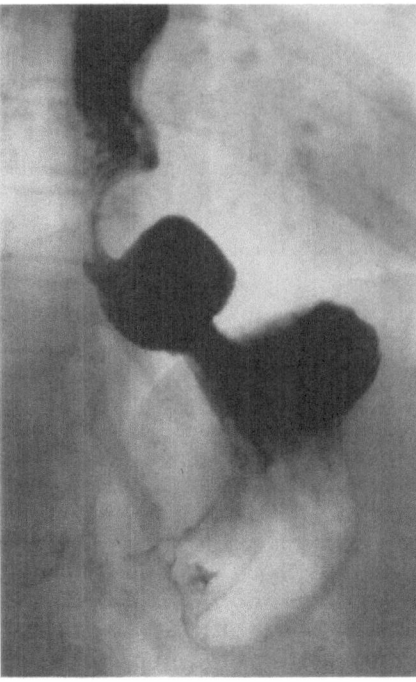

Fig. 335. Mandarin-sized hiatus hernia in a patient presenting with recent reflux complaints
as a first symptom of stenosing carcinoma of the gastric antrum

burn) and dependency of the complaints on the position of the patient. An
appropriate radiological examination will demonstrate all hiatus hernias, even
small ones, and distinguish them from an epiphrenic ampulla. Esophagoscopy
is indicated to diagnose complications (esophagitis, erosions, ulcerations) and to
localize hemorrhages. Intraluminal pressure measurements permit an evaluation
of the competence of the lower esophageal sphincter and pH measurements
may give objective evidence about the presence and duration of gastroesophageal
reflux.

The clinically most important problem, however, is not the presence of a
hiatus hernia, but whether the hernia is responsible for the symptoms. In the
majority of cases this can be determined by history, paying special attention
to the symptomatological triad. If symptoms other than those of the triad are
mentioned, other disorders must be looked for. Frequently a hiatus hernia is
asymptomatic and manifests itself only when other disorders are present such
as bloating, constipation, eating too fast or too much and nervous tension. An
asymptomatic hernia can become symptomatic because of an increase in intraabdominal pressure due to pregnancy, ascites, increase in weight or space-occupying processes; often it may also become symptomatic because of an impediment
of the gastrointestinal passage by carcinoma (Figs. 335, 336). In order not to
miss a much more serious condition it is imperative not to be satisfied with
the impressive radiological finding of a hernia but to search further for the
ultimate cause of the symptoms.

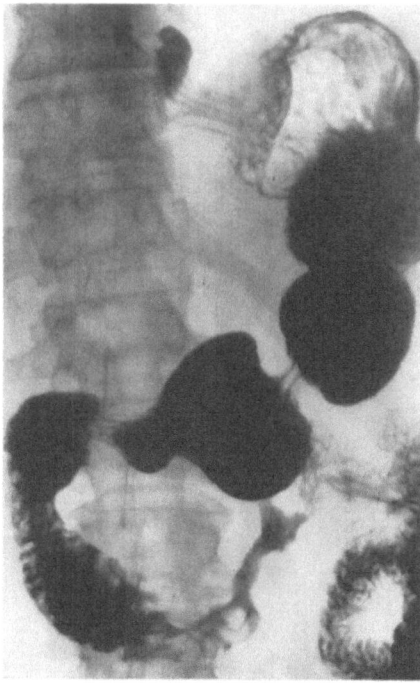

Fig. 336. Small hiatal hernia presenting with reflux symptoms resistant to therapy. Adenocarcinoma of the distal duodenum

8. Complications

The most frequent complication of esophagogastric hiatus hernia is reflux
esophagitis, which in its turn may cause other more serious complications:
acquired brachyesophagus, stenosis and ulcerations. The clinical manifestations
of these complications are heartburn, pain, hemorrhage and dysphagia. Only
the last two will be discussed here.

The hemorrhage can be massive and manifest itself as hematemesis or melena,
or it can be occult and cause iron deficiency anemia. Massive hemorrhage mostly
stems from an ulcer in the stomach or duodenum, more rarely in the hernia
itself. An ulcer in the hernia may be located at the level of the hiatus, mostly
at the right ventral side; there it produces typical ulcer symptoms. More rarely
it is located in the herniated sac; there it is associated with few symptoms.
Its most frequent localization is at the squamocolumnar epithelial junction,
where it simulates an esophageal ulcer. It causes intensive pain on swallowing
(odynophagia), which irradiates into the back or into the upper substernal region.
Pain is also frequently felt when the stomach is empty and the patient lies down.
It is lessened by eating or taking antacids. The ulcer almost always gives rise
to a fibrous stricture, causing dysphagia and stasis. These ulcers do not tend
to heal spontaneously, and can perforate into the pleural cavity, the mediastinum
or, more rarely, into the pericardial sac, the lungs or the peritoneal cavity.

An other cause of massive bleeding in hiatus hernia is the Mallory-Weiss
syndrome. This condition is described on p. 689. Occult bleeding in sliding hernia
mostly stems from erosive esophagitis, demonstrable only by esophagoscopy or

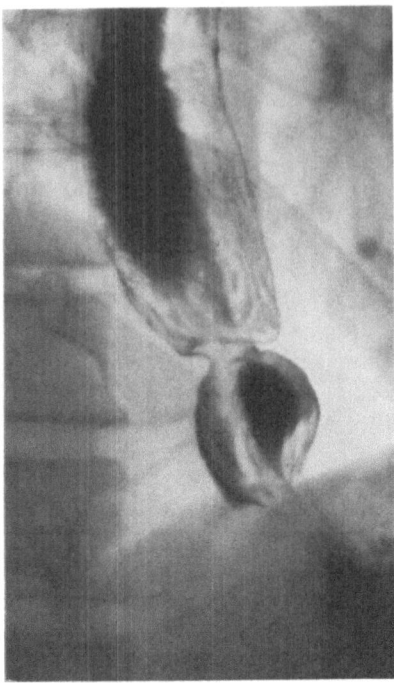

Fig. 337. Hiatus hernia with dysphagia due to a Schatzki ring with a diameter of 11 mm

from edematous gastritis of the hernia. Massive bleeding due to esophagitis is rare. When other symptoms of esophagitis are discrete or lacking, hypochromic anemia may be the only manifestation. This is to be found in large para-esophageal hernias, which bleed from the edematous gastritis of the strangulated part of the stomach.

The incidence of bleeding is differently quoted according to the selection of the cases. It is highest among patients of surgical departments, 24% according to MOUCHET and BARRAYA (1962), 16% according CHAUSSE (1968). Patients of medical departments and outpatients bleed more rarely, but the incidence increases with increasing duration of observation. E. PALMER (1968) found hemorrhages or anemia in 26% of his hernia patients observed for 20 years. In our own studies of 300 outpatients with hiatus hernia (HAFTER, 1957) an anemia of less than 11 g-% Hb was found in only 9.3%, a massive bleeding in no more than 3.7%; 2.7% of them had a gastroduodenal ulcer and only in 1% no source of bleeding could be demonstrated other than the hernia. Therefore other sources of bleeding must be looked for in patients with hiatus hernia who bleed massively. Esophageal varices, ulcers, carcinoma and hemorrhagic gastritis, possibly caused by drugs, bleed more frequently than the hiatus hernia itself.

Dysphagia is mostly due to complications. (1) Stenosing reflux esophagitis is often found in infants (32.7%, THOMSEN, 1955), more rarely in adults with hiatus hernia (4.3%, PALMER, 1968). It may occur in patients with a long history of gastroesophageal reflux, but on occasion, especially during the last weeks of pregnancy, it may progress quickly, without any previous symptoms. The rapid progression, the radiological picture and loss of weight may suggest a carcinoma.

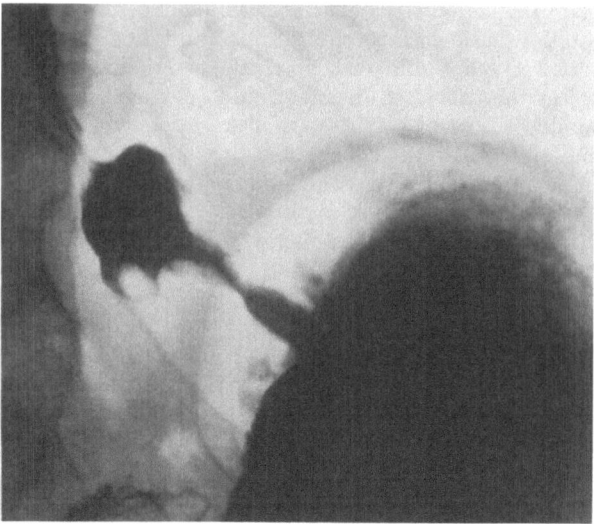

Fig. 338. Carcinoma of the cardia in a walnut-sized hiatal hernia

Esophagoscopy and multiple negative biopsies decide. (2) An ulcer develops mostly at the squamocolumnar epithelial junction and may cause stricture and painful dysphagia. (3) A narrow Schatzki ring with a diameter of less than 20 mm may cause dysphagia. Poorly masticated food can lead to impaction. The ring can be shown radiologically (Fig. 337). (4) Motility disorders of the esophagus and lower esophageal sphincter can also cause dysphagia and substernal pain.

A few authors described a superficial migrating thrombophlebitis. Most authors' observations, including our own, could not confirm this finding. It is probably nothing more than a coincidence in older subjects.

The cooccurrence of carcinoma and hiatus hernia is probably coincidental. A carcinoma of the gastric fundus can develop in the thorax in cases of hiatus hernia (Fig. 338). An asymptomatic hiatus hernia may become manifest because of a partial obstruction of the gastrointestinal tract due to a carcinoma (Figs. 335, 336).

9. Associated Diseases

Not only the complications of hiatus hernia but also the associated diseases are clinically important. They occur frequently in older subjects. Over 50% of our own patients had associated diseases in the abdomen. Gall stones accounted for the greatest number (16.3%). This corresponds fairly well to the incidence of gall stones in outpatients with upper abdominal complaints (18%). No pathogenetic conclusions can be drawn from these figures. Symptoms of hiatus hernia often occur after cholecystectomy. They may be due to the long postoperative bed rest, which, by causing reflux esophagitis, may make an asymptomatic hernia manifest. They may also be the real cause of the complaints, which were originally and wrongly ascribed to the gall stones. The combination of hiatus hernia and gastroduodenal ulcer seems equally coincidental. Stenosing duodenal ulcers slow down the emptying of the stomach and thus contribute to reveal a hiatus hernia.

This may explain the periodicity of the complaints in some cases of hiatus hernia. The combination of hiatus hernia, cholelithiasis and diverticulosis of the sigmoid colon has been called Saint's Triad. Diverticulosis of the sigmoid and hiatus hernia have more or less the same age distribution. A common factor in both is probably the age-induced loss of elasticity and weakness of the connective tissue. The association with gall stones constitutes a pseudo-triad, due to coincidence.

Clinically more important is the connection between hiatus hernia and coronary insufficiency. Their coincidence also is due to age. In the majority of cases symptoms occurring after physical effort point to coronary insufficiency, whereas their occurrence at rest points to hiatus hernia. Yet the symptoms of both diseases can occasionally be so similar that the distinction between them cannot be made on the basis of clinical history. Electrocardiographic signs of ischemia after exercise allow the differential diagnosis. Both diseases seem to be correlated in that they augment each others symptoms. If the acid infusion test (BERNSTEIN and BAKER, 1958) induces pain similar to the "spontaneous" pain of the patient, and if this acid-induced pain is not associated with signs of ischemia on a simultaneously recorded electrocardiogram, the esophagus is likely to be the cause of this pain. The clinical significance of these associated diseases is mainly that their symptoms may be erroneously ascribed to the hiatus hernia. If the symptomatology is uncharacteristic of hiatus hernia other diseases must be tought of and looked for.

10. Evolution and Prognosis

The first symptoms of esophagogastric hiatus hernia in adults occur mostly after the thirtienth year. They are favored by an increase in weight, functional or organic obstruction of the gastrointestinal tract or nervous tension. If no organic lesions are present, apart from the hernia, or if they can be controlled, the complaints can mostly be eliminated or greatly reduced by conservative treatment. Many hernia patients have no symptoms for weeks or months and know what causes and what ameliorates their complaints.

As a rule hiatus hernia increases in size with age. STRAFKA et al. (1954) found in 32% of their hernia patients that small hernias increased in the course of years. In 27% of their 61 patients with large hernias complications developed (esophagitis, strictures and ulcerations). Such a high incidence of complications is found only in very large hernias. Most observers agree that the size of the hernia and the intensity of the symptoms do not correlate, except when the hernia is very big. The hernia symptoms decrease mostly with age and often disappear completely. This is probably due to the decrease in acidity of the gastric secretion, in weight and in tone of the autonomic nervous system; also to the patient's experience in avoiding his symptoms. The decrease of the symptoms with age does not take place in severe reflux esophagitis or in peptic ulcer complicated by stenosis. Apart from these, complications are rare and mortality occurs only in cases of incarceration of a paraesophageal hernia and perforation of an ulcer. Esophagogastric hernia hardly ever leads to deadly complications and mortality is almost always a consequence of surgical treatment (KIESER, 1967).

Paraesophageal hernia, on the other hand, tends to pull an increasingly greater portion of the stomach in the thorax, predisposes to severe hemorrhages and involves the risk of volvulus and incarceration. It is generally agreed that paraesophageal hernia is an absolute indication for surgical treatment.

11. Therapy

11.1. Medical Treatment

Only a small percentage of patients with hiatus hernia need surgical treatment. In most cases conservative measures are sufficient to eliminate the symptoms, or to make them bearable. An asymptomatic and uncomplicated hernia, found incidentally, does not need treatment. One of the most important conservative measures consists of informing the patient about his hiatus hernia, about the mechanism that causes his symptoms, and about its innocence and its good prognosis. Unlike other hernias, a sliding hiatus hernia does not lead to incarceration. This information frees him from his fear of angina pectoris and of esophageal or gastric carcinoma; it spares him the humiliation of having "nothing more than nervous or psychosomatic complaints", a neurosis or even hysteria. It can best be given by means of a sketch or of the X-ray pictures. Additional measures aim at decreasing the intraabdominal pressure, preventing the reflux and treating its consequences (heartburn) with medication.

The intraabdominal pressure can be decreased by weight reduction through dietary measures. The intake of carbohydrates should be reduced and supper must be light and taken early. An increase of a few pounds is often sufficient to provoke complaints and their loss sufficient to eliminate them again. A tight belt or girdle should be avoided.

Gastroesophageal reflux at night can be prevented by keeping the evening meals small and by slanting the bed 15 to 25 cm. The manometric studies of the lower esophageal sphincter have greatly contributed to the medical treatment of gastroesophageal reflux. Smoking, fatty meals, alcohol and anticholinergics result in a decrease of the lower esophageal sphincter pressure and thus favor gastroesophageal reflux. On the other hand gastrin, antacids, which stimulate the secretion of gastrin, protein meals and metoclopramide increase the sphinctric pressure and thus decrease reflux.

The most efficient means to treat heartburn are antacids. They often eliminate not only heartburn but also other oppressing or painful sensations originating from the terminal esophagus or the hiatus hernia. Calcium carbonate is an effective antacid, but recent studies have demonstrated that it is capable of raising the serum gastrin level and markedly increasing gastric secretion of acid, especially in people with peptic ulcer disease (FORDTRAN, 1968; BARRERAS, 1970; REEDER et al., 1972; MORRISSEY and BARRERAS, 1974). Therefore there is a tendency to replace the time-honored mixture (calcium carbonate 80 g, magnesium oxide 20 g, bismuth subnitrate 20 g) by less effective mixtures of magnesium oxide and aluminum hydroxide gels. The proportion of the laxative magnesium should be adjusted to the bowel movements of the patient. It is also recommended to prescribe antacid tablets, which the patient can easily take when needed. If the antacid does not eliminate the symptoms, the addition of a mucosal anesthetic can be tried, e.g. Muthesa®, Tepilta®, Xylocain gel® or a preparation of colloidal-silver 2.0, Procaine 4.0, Mucilage of arabic gum 30.0, water ad 200. This should be taken 10 minutes before meals and whenever symptoms arise. To handle a sudden attack of pain the patient should get up, breath out deeply, raise his arms or drink. Anticholinergics are not indicated in patients with hiatus hernia because they decrease the resting pressure in the lower esophageal sphincter and delay the gastric evacuation, thus favoring gastroesophageal reflux.

Heartburn during or after meals is mostly caused by acid liquids with a pH below 4.0, concentrated alcohol, black coffee or locally irritating spices. The patient will learn to discern which kinds of food and drink are to be avoided.

In the majority of cases these measures do away with these symptoms. If they are persistent or very intensive esophagoscopy is indicated to search for erosive esophagitis or a peptic ulcer. When the patient's symptoms have disappeared the medication is gradually withdrawn, but whenever they recur it should be taken again. Intolerated foods and beverages, and gain of weight must be avoided; a habit of sleeping in a slanting bed should be developed.

Paraesophageal hernia should be treated by surgery.

11.2. Surgical Treatment

In view of the mostly mild complaints, the effectiveness of conservative measures and the often unrewarding results of surgery, the latter is indicated only in cases of paraesophageal and very large esophagogastric hernias and of complications such as acute or chronic bleeding associated with anemia, severe esophagitis with erosions or ulcer, esophageal strictures insufficiently responsive to bougienage, and intensive complaints which do not respond to treatment. In the latter case it is not the radiologist but the patient himself who decides in favor of surgery.

These conditions are fulfilled rather rarely. Surgery was performed in only 3.9% of the 768 hiatus hernia patients followed for 30 years by Palmer (1968). Of our own 5557 cases, observed between 1950 and 1970, only 110 (1.9%) underwent surgery, sometimes without the knowledge of the internist or even against his advice.

The great number of surgical procedures shows that none of them is completely satisfactory or applicable in all cases. Both a thoracic and an abdominal approach can be used. The thoracic approach through the seventh or eighth intercostal space has the advantage of a good exposure of the hiatal region, even in obese patients. It has the disadvantage that the upper abdominal viscera cannot be explored unless a phrenicotomy is done. But even after incision of the diaphragm only minor operations such as a cholecystectomy or a pyloroplasty can be performed. The contention that thoracotomy is less well tolerated than laparotomy is untenable. It is valid only for patients with decreased pulmonary function or previous myocardial infarction. Postoperative thoracic pains do not occur if the intercostal nerves are not injured. The thoracic approach is especially appropriate for patients with a sharp epigastric angle and for the treatment of recurrences (Rudler, 1968). The advantage of the abdominal approach is that it allows the surgical treatment of other abdominal diseases. But in obese patients or in patients of the pycnic type it has the disadvantage that the cardia is barely within reach and that a hernia at the site of the abdominal incision is a frequent complication. The incidence of recurrences is the same for both approaches (Rudler, 1968), so that the choice between them must be made on a case-by-case basis.

In paraesophageal hernias the further herniation and its risk of volvulus and incarceration can be prevented by means of a gastropexy, attaching the lesser curvature to the ventral side of the abdominal wall, either at the left (Nissen and Rossetti, 1959) or at the right side (Boerema and Germs, 1955). A dorsal gastropexy can also be performed by fixing the stomach to the preaortic fascia (Hill, 1967). The results of these procedures are said to be satisactory.

In cases of esophagogastric sliding hernias the surgeon will attempt (1) to replace the cardia and thus the abdominal part of the esophagus in its normal subdiaphragmatic position; (2) to keep them there; (3) to prevent gastroesophageal reflux; and (4) if necessary, to narrow the widened hiatus.

1. Replacement of the cardia poses no problems, except when the esophagus is shortened. Thus the abdominal part of the esophagus is again subjected to the increased abdominal pressure, which many surgeons consider as an important factor in the closing mechanism of the cardia.

2. The fixation of the stomach in the abdomen, on the other hand, poses considerable problems. The tightening of the phrenic or esophageal membrane and its fixation to the hiatus, following ALLISON (1951), is usually insufficient because of the weakness of this membrane; this technique has largely been abandoned. Ventral gastropexy (NISSEN and ROSSETTI, 1959) also is often unsatisfactory in cases of hiatus hernia, and is used nowadays only for the repair of paraesophageal hernias. The results of dorsal gastropexy (HILL, 1967) are said to be better. The technique of BELSEY (SKINNER and BELSEY, 1967) consists of a ventral fundoplication with fixation of the terminal esophagus, 3 to 5 cm above the cardia, and of the stomach to the hiatus, which is narrowed from the dorsal side. The approach is thoracic.

3. The most successful methods seem to be those that prevent reflux by bringing a sufficiently long segment of the esophagus into the abdomen and accentuating the angle of His. Admittedly the "esophagogastropexy" (LORTAT-JACOB, 1957), which sutures the right side of the gastric fundus to the left side of the esophagus, has turned out to be insufficient. Today the best techniques appear to be those that use a fundoplication, such as the Nissen procedure (NISSEN and ROSSETTI, 1959, 1962). It consists of putting an envelope of gastric fundus around the terminal esophagus. A possible consequence of this procedure is inability of the patient to belch. If the envelope of gastric fundus is wrapped too tightly around the terminal esophagus, it may cause dysphagia. But this can be prevented by introducing a wide gastric tube into the esophagus during the operation. Techniques of fundoplication which do not involve the entire esophageal circumference seem to yield equally good results: a posterior hemifundoplication (RUDLER, 1968) or an anterior hemifundoplication according to DOR et al. (1962) or to BELSEY (SKINNER and BELSEY, 1967) can be recommended.

4. The value of narrowing the hiatus is controversial. It is not sufficient by itself, but many surgeons use it in combination with other measures. It should be recommended in cases of an abnormally wide hiatus and when the musculature of the diaphragmatic crus is well developed, which is rather exceptional. Again it is necessary to introduce a large gastric tube into the esophagus and to leave the hiatus wide enough for a finger to pass through, in order to prevent postoperative dysphagia.

In recent years a "balanced operation" consisting of gastropexy, narrowing of the hiatus, vagotomy and pyloroplasty, has been recommended for the treatment of esophagogastric hernia (J. BERMAN and E. BERMAN, 1959; HOLLE, 1968; MEADS and SAWYERS, 1969). This major procedure appears unnecessary in cases of uncomplicated hiatus hernia, but must be recommended if a duodenal ulcer is also present.

If during an abdominal operation cholelithiasis is found, cholecystectomy can be performed; similarly, if an ulcer is found, a gastrectomy or a vagotomy with pyloroplasty can be undertaken. But whether a surgeon should proceed to repair a hiatus hernia diagnosed during cholecystectomy, or not, is a controversial point. If the hernia was asymptomatic before the operation, he should be reluctant because postoperative complaints are not infrequent. The situation is different when the surgeon is faced with esophageal complications such as extensive stenosis due to esophagitis, or a brachyesophagus which cannot be repositioned into the abdomen. Before considering esophageal resection, he should

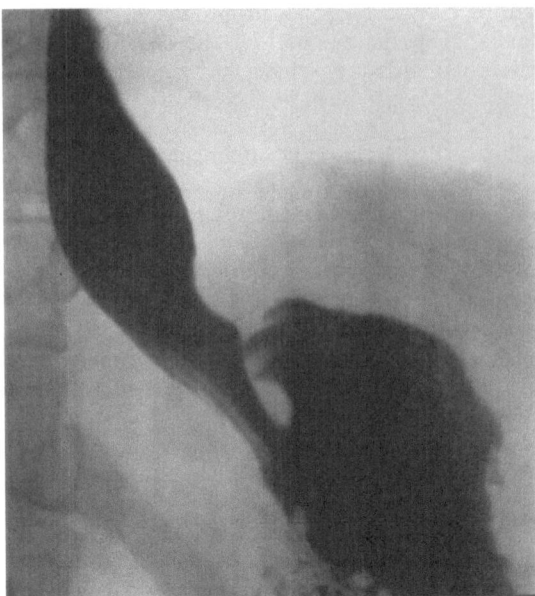

Fig. 339. A too narrow fundoplication causing dysphagia

attempt to treat the stenosis by preoperative bougienage, or digital dilatation during surgery, followed by a procedure to prevent reflux. If the gastro-esophageal junction cannot be brought down within the abdomen, a thoracic fundoplication should be performed. If dilatation of the stricture fails, one can perform the Thal esophagoplasty (Thal et al., 1965) which can be combined with a thoracic fundoplication. The "anastomose continente" according to Lortat-Jacob (Megevand, 1968) and the interposition between esophagus and stomach of a segment of the small intestine or of the colon have also been found valuable techniques.

Opinions vary considerably about the results of surgical treatment. The evaluation of the surgical results is difficult due to the lack of uniformity in the indication for surgery, the presence or absence of preoperative complications, the great number of surgical methods and their variants, the diverging techniques of different surgeons, and especially the necessarily subjective interpretation of the information given by the patient. Objective, i.e. radiologically established-recurrences are mostly observed after fixation of the gastric fundus to the dia-phragm. They can occur days or months after the operation. The majority of postoperative anomalies, however, are not due to real recurrences, but to insuf-ficient repositioning of the hernia and are evident immediately after the operation. The radiological demonstration of recurrences or pseudo-recurrences is less im-portant than the clinical recurrence or persistence of the symptoms of the hernia; therefore, more attention must be paid to the subjective appreciation of the result by the patients who underwent surgery then to the percentage of recur-rences, which can barely be evaluated anyway. The majority of follow-up studies done by surgeons report radiological and clinical improvements in 75 to 90% of the patients. The follow-up studies of internists are less enthusiastic. Debray et al. (1966b) reported unsatisfactory results in 51% of 63 patients. 51 of our own 100 patients were similarly dissatisfied, although the surgical departments in which most of them underwent their treatment reported good results in 92, 84 and 78%. The figures reported by the Geneva University hospital are in between; 63% of its patients were satisfied, 20% improved but still had complaints, and 17% were dissatisfied (CHAUSSE, 1968). Some of the postoperative complaints are identical with the preoperative symptoms (reflux and heartburn), others arise after the operation: dysphagia, stasis in the distal esophagus, a sensation of epigastric pressure or tension, substernal discomfort, attacks of tachycardia, or the painful inability to belch (Fig. 339).

Ultimately the surgeon's experience and skill appear to be more dicisive about success or failure than the method he uses.

References

ÅKERLUND, Å.: Hernia diaphragmatica herniae oesophagei, vom anatomischen und röntgenologischen Gesichtspunkt. Acta radiol. (Stockh.) 6, 3–22 (1926).

ÅKERLUND, Å.: Die anatomischen Grundlagen des Röntgenbildes der sogenannten erworbenen Hiatushernie. Acta radiol. (Stockh.) 14, 523–544 (1933).

ALDRIDGE, N. H.: Transmigration of the lower esophageal mucosa. Radiology 79, 962–968 (1962).

ALLISON, P. R.: Peptic ulcer of oesophagus. Thorax 3, 20–42 (1948).

ALLISON, P. R.: Reflux esophagitis, sliding hiatal hernia, and anatomy of repair. Surg. Gynec. Obstet. 92, 419–431 (1951).

BARRERAS, R. F.: Acid secretion after calcium carbonate in patients with duodenal ulcer. New Engl. J. Med. 282, 1402–1405 (1970).

BARRETT, N. R.: Hiatus hernia. Proc. roy. Soc. Med. 45, 279–286 (1952).

BERMAN, J. K., BERMAN, E. J.: Balanced operations for esophagitis associated with esophageal hiatal hernia. Arch. Surg. 78, 889–893 (1959).

BERNSTEIN, L. M., BAKER, L. A.: A clinical test for esophagitis. Gastroenterology 34, 760–781 (1958).

BLUM, S. D., WEISS, A., WEISELBERG, H. M., SIEGEL, W. B.: Retrograde prolapse of gastric mucosa into the esophagus. Gastroenterology 41, 408–411 (1961).

BOEREMA, I., GERMS, R.: Gastropexia anterior geniculata wegen Hiatusbruch des Zwerchfells. Zbl. Chir. 80, 1585–1592 (1955).

BOEREMA, I., GERMS, R.: Fixation of the lesser curvature of the stomach to the anterior abdominal wall after reposition of the hernia through the oesophageal hiatus. Arch. Chir. Neerl. 7, 351–359 (1955).

BROMBART, M., LERBERGHE, R. VAN: Le reflux gastro-œsophagien. Acta gastro-ent. belg. 15, 66–75 (1952).

CARVALHO, M. DE: Chirurgie du syndrome hiato-œsophagien. Arch. Mal. Appar. dig. 40, 280–293 (1951).

CHAUSSE, J. M.: Statistique de la clinique chirurgicale de Genève 1957/1967. In: RUDLER, J. C.: Hernies hiatales de l'adulte. Genève: Éd. Méd. & Hyg. 1968.

CODE, C. F., SCHLEGEL, J. F.: Motor action of the esophagus and its sphincters. In: Handbook of physiology, sect. 6, vol. 4, pp. 1821–1839. Baltimore: Williams & Wilkins 1968.

COHEN, B. R., WOLF, B. S.: Cineradiographic and intramural pressure correlations in the pharynx and esophagus. In: Handbook of physiology, sect. 4, vol. 4, pp. 1841–1860. Baltimore: Williams & Wilkins 1968.

COHEN, B. S.: Manometry and related techniques in hiatus hernia and its complications. In: Progress in gastroenterology, vol. 2, ed. G. B. JERZY GLASS, pp. 149–161. New York and London: Grune & Stratton 1970.

COHEN, S., HARRIS, L. D.: Lower esophageal sphincter pressure as an index of lower esophageal sphincter strength. Gastroenterology 58, 157–162 (1970).

COLLIS, J. L.: Surgical control of reflux in hiatus hernia. Amer. J. Surg. 115, 465–471 (1968).

DAGRADI, A. E., BRODERICK, J. T., JULER, G., WOLINSKA, S., STEMPIEN, S. J.: The Mallory-Weiss syndrome and lesion. A study of 30 cases. Amer. J. dig. Dis. 11, 710–721 (1966).

DANIELS, B. T.: The phrenoesophageal membrane. Amer. J. Surg. 110, 814–817 (1965).

DAVIS, M. V., FIUZAT, J.: Gastroesophageal reflux and hiatal hernia. Experiences with the Belsey repair. Amer. J. Surg. 118, 883–886 (1969).

DEBRAY, C., CHERIGIE, E., HARDOUIN, J.-P.: Les hernies hiatales. Presse méd. **74**, 607–611 (1966).

DEBRAY, C., LORTAT-JACOB, O.: L'avenir des hernies hiatales opérées. A propos de 63 observations. Le point de vue du médecin. Arch. Mal. Appar. dig. **55**, 853–870 (1966).

DOR, J., HUMBERT, P., DOR, V., FIGARELLA, J.: L'intérêt de la technique de Nissen modifiée dans la prévention du reflux après cardio-myotomie de Heller. Mém. Acad. Chir. **88**, 877–881 (1962).

DAER, N. H., PRIDIE, R. B.: Incidence of hiatus hernia in asymptomatic subjects. Gut **9**, 696–699 (1968).

FELDMAN, M.: Retrograde extrusion or prolapse of the gastric mucosa into the esophagus. Amer. J. med. Sci. **222**, 54–60 (1951).

FLICK, A. L.: Acid content of common beverages. Amer. J. dig. Dis. **15**, 317–320 (1970).

FORDTRAN, J. S.: Acid rebound. New Engl. J. Med. **279**, 900–905 (1968).

GOYAL, R. K., BAUER, J. L., SPIRO, H. M.: The nature and location of lower esophageal ring. New Engl. J. Med. **284**, 1175–1180 (1971).

HADDAD, J. K.: Relation of gastroesophageal reflux to yield sphincter pressures. Gastroenterology **58**, 175–184 (1970).

HÄRING, R.: Magenschleimhautprolaps in den Oesophagus als seltene Ursache einer Dysphagie. Chirurg **32**, 115–119 (1961).

HAFTER, E.: Die Hiatushernie, ihre Häufigkeit und klinische Bedeutung. Dtsch. med. Wschr. **82**, 1709–1712 (1957).

HAFTER, E.: Röntgendiagnose der Hiatushernie. Radiologe **1**, 141–147 (1961).

HAFTER, E.: Der sogenannte untere Ösophagusring. Dtsch. med. Wschr. **89**, 2338–2342 (1964).

HARRINGTON, S. W.: Various types of diaphragmatic hernia treated surgically: report of 430 cases. Surg. Gynec. Obstet. **86**, 735–755 (1948).

HARRIS, L. D., WINANS, C. S., POPE, C. E., II: Determination of yield pressures; a method for measuring anal sphincter competence. Gastroenterology **50**, 754–760 (1966).

HEITMANN, P.: Der gastro-oesophageale Verschlußmechanismus bei Hiatusgleithernien. Internist (Berl.) **10**, 249–258 (1969).

HILL, L. D.: An effective operation for hiatal hernia. An eight year appraisal. Ann. Surg. **166**, 681–692 (1967).

HILLEMAND, P., VIGUIE, R., BERNARD, H., VILLARD, J., DELILLE, R.: Hernie diaphragmatique et grossesse. Ses rapports avec le pyrosis de la femme enceinte. Bull. Mém. Soc. méd. Hôp. Paris **69**, 229–234 (1953).

HOLLE, F.: Spezielle Magenchirurgie. Berlin-Heidelberg-New York: Springer 1968.

IMDAHL, H.: Der terminale Oesophagus. Stuttgart: Schattauer 1963.

ISMAIL-BEIGI, F., HORTON, P. F., POPE, C. E., II: Histological consequences of gastroesophageal reflux in man. Gastroenterology **58**, 163–174 (1970).

JOHNSTON, J. H., JR., GRIFFIN, J. C., JR.: Anatomic location of the lower esophageal ring. Surgery **61**, 528–534 (1967).

KIESER, C.: Untersuchungen über die tödlichen Komplikationen von Hiatushernien. Gastroenterologie **107**, 328–336 (1967).

KLINEFELTER, E. W.: Invagination of the esophagus in hiatus hernia. Radiology **67**, 562–568 (1956).

KRAMER, P.: Does a sliding hiatus hernia constitute a distinct clinical entity? Gastroenterology **57**, 442–448 (1969).

KRAMER, P.: Diffuse esophageal spasm. Mod. Treatm. **7**, 1151–1162 (1970).

KRAMER, P., FLESHLER, B., McNALLY, E.: Oesophageal sensitivity to Mecholyl in symptomatic diffuse spasm. Gut **8**, 120–127 (1967).

LEDOUX-LEBARD, G., HEITZ, F., BEHAR, A.: Les hernies hiatales de l'adulte. Neuchâtel-Paris: Delachaux & Nestlé S.A. 1967.

LERCHE, W.: Esophagus and pharynx in action. Springfield (Ill.): Charles C. Thomas 1950.

LINSMAN, J. F.: Gastroesophageal reflux elicited while drinking water (water siphonage test). Its clinical correlation with pyrosis. Amer. J. Roentgenol. **94**, 325–332 (1965).

LORIMIER, A. A. DE, WARREN, J. P.: Prolapse of the mucosa at the esophagogastric junction. Amer. J. Roentgenol. **84**, 1061–1069 (1960).

LORTAT-JACOB, J. L.: Le traitement chirurgical des maladies du reflux gastro-œsophagien: malpositions cardiotubérositaires, hernies hiatales, brachyœsophages. Presse méd. **65**, 455–456 (1957).

MADDOCK, W. G., BELL, J. L., TREMAINE, M. J.: Gastrointestinal gas. Ann. Surg. **130**, 512–535 (1949).

McNAMARA, J. J., PAULSON, D. L., URSCHEL, H. C.: Hiatal hernia and gastroesophageal reflux in children. Pediatrics **43**, 527–532 (1969).

MEADS, G. E., JR., SAWYERS, J. L.: Reappraisal of the balanced operation for sliding esophageal hiatal hernia. Amer. J. Surg. **117**, 124–129 (1969).

MEGEVAND, R.: Traitement chirurgical. In: RUDLER, J. C.: Hernies hiatales de l'adulte. Genève: Éd. Méd. & Hyg. 1968.

MELCHER, D. H.: Some anatomical considerations in sliding hiatus hernia. Brit. J. Surg. **56**, 904–906 (1969).

MIXSON, W. T., WOLOSHIN, H. J.: Hiatus hernia in pregnancy. Obstet. and Gynec. 8, 249–253 (1956).

MONGES, H., DELMAS, H., MONGES, A.: Hernie hiatale et reflux gastrocœsophagien chez les gastrectomisés subtotaux. Arch. Mal. Appar. dig. **43**, 1075–1082 (1954).

MONGES, H., MONGES, A., GARCIN-NICOLAS, H.: Sur la pyrosis des femmes enceintes: Hernies hiatales et reflux gastro-œsophagien pendant la grossesse. Arch. Mal. Appar. dig. **42**, 1092–1100 (1956).

MORRISSEY, J. F., BARRERAS, R. F.: Antacid therapy. New Engl. J. Med. **290**, 550–554 (1974)

MOUCHET, A., BARRAYA, L.: Les hernies hiatales. 64me Congrès français de Chirurgie 1962.

MULLER-BOTHA, G. S.: The gastro-oesophageal junction. London: Churchill Ltd. 1962.

MUSTARD, R. A.: A survey of techniques and results of hiatus hernia repair. Surg. Gynec. Obstet. **130**, 131–136 (1970).

NISSEN, R., ROSSETTI, M.: Die Behandlung der Hiatushernien und Refluxösophagitis mit Gastropexie und Fundoplicatio. Stuttgart: Thieme 1959.

NISSEN, R., ROSSETTI, M.: Zur Indikation der Fundoplicatio und Gastropexie bei Hiatushernie. Warnung vor einer wahllosen Anwendung. Schweiz. med. Wschr. **92**, 533–534 (1962).

ODEGAARD, H.: Invagination of the esophagus in hiatus hernia. A report of 8 cases. Acta radiol. (Stockh.) **51**, 443–448 (1959).

OTTENJANN, R., LUX, G., STADELMANN, O., ELSTER, K.: Sodbrennen, Perfusionstest und distale Oesophagobiopsie. In: Aktuelle Gastroenterologie, eds. H. BARTELHEIMER and N. HEISIG, p. 303–305. Stuttgart: Thieme 1968.

PALMER, E. D.: The hiatus hernia-esophagitis-esophageal stricture complex. Twenty-year prospective study. Amer. J. Med. **44**, 566–579 (1968).

POPE, E. C., II: A dynamic test of sphincter strength: its application to the lower esophageal sphincter. Gastroenterology **52**, 779–786 (1967).

REEDER, D. D., CONLEE, J. L., THOMPSON, J. C.: Changes in gastric secretion and serum gastrin concentration in duodenal ulcer patients after oral calcium antacid. In: DEMLING, L.: Gastrointestinal hormones, p. 19–22. Stuttgart: Thieme 1972.

RINALDO, J. A., GAHAGAN, T.: The narrow lower esophageal ring: pathogenesis and physiology. Amer. J. dig. Dis. **11**, 257–265 (1966).

ROSSETTI, M.: Die Refluxkrankheit des Oesophagus. Stuttgart: Hippokrates 1966.

RUDLER, J. C.: Hernies hiatales de l'adulte. Genève: Éd. Méd. & Hyg. 1968.

SANDRY, R. J.: The pathology of chronic oesophagitis. Gut **3**, 189–200 (1962).

SAVARY, M.: Aspect endoscopique de la portion gastrique intrathoracique dans la hernie hiatale. Pract. oto-rhino-laryng. (Basel) **28**, 175–189 (1966).

SAVARY, M.: L'aspect endoscopique du vestibule gastro-œsophagien. Pract. oto-rhino-laryng. (Basel) **30**, 134–148 (1968).

SAVARY, M.: La jonction muqueuse gastro-œsophagienne. Rev. méd. Suisse rom. **90**, 25–36 (1970).

SKINNER, D. B., BELSEY, R. H. R.: Surgical management of esophageal reflux and hiatus hernia. Long term results with 1030 patients. J. thorac. cardiovasc. Surg. **53**, 33–54 (1967).

STEIN, G. N., FINKELSTEIN, A.: Hiatal hernia. Roentgen incidence and diagnosis. Amer. J. dig. Dis. **5**, 77–87 (1960).

STELZNER, F.: Der Verschluß der terminalen Speiseröhre. Dtsch. med. Wschr. **93**, 1679–1685 (1968).

STILSON, W. L., SANDERS, I., GARDINER, G. A., GORMAN, H. C., LODGE, D. F.: Hiatal hernia and gastroesophageal reflux. A clinicoradiological analysis of more than 1000 cases. Radiology **93**, 1323–1327 (1969).

SUTHERLAND, C. G., ATKINSON, J.C., BROGDON, B. G., CROW, N. E., BROWN, W. E.: Esophageal hiatus hernia in pregnancy. Obstet. and Gynec. 8, 261–264 (1956).

SWEET, R. H.: Esophageal hiatus hernia of the diaphragm. Ann. Surg. **135**, 1–13 (1952).

TANNER, N. C., HARDY, K. J.: Hiatus hernia. A follow-up of 53 operations. Brit. J. Surg. **57**, 131–134 (1970).

THAL, A. P., HATAFUKU, T., KURTZMAN, R.: New operation for distal esophageal stricture. Arch. Surg. **90**, 464–472 (1965).

THOMSEN, G.: Hiatus hernia in children. Acta radiol. (Stockh.), Suppl. **129**, 1–200 (1955).

VANTRAPPEN, G.: Slokdarmmotiliteit. Brussel: Arscia Uitgaven N.V. 1961.

VESTBY, G. W., AAKHUS, T.: Incidence of sliding hiatus hernia. Invest. Radiol. **1**, 379–385 (1966).

WINANS, C. S., HARRIS, L. D.: Quantitation of lower esophageal sphincter competence. Gastroenterology 52, 773–778 (1967).

WOLF, B. S.: Roentgen features of the normal and herniated esophagogastric region. Clinical correlations. In: Progress in gastroenterology, vol. II, ed. G. B. JERZY GLASS, pp. 288–315. New York and London: Grune & Stratton 1970.

WOLF, B. S., BRAHMS, S. A., KHILNANI, M. T.: The incidence of hiatal hernia in barium meal examination. J. Mt Sinai Hosp. 26, 598–600 (1959).

WOLF, B. S., MARSHAK, R. H., SOM, L. M., GREENBERG, I. I.: The gastro-esophageal vestibule on roentgenexamination. J. Mt Sinai Hosp. 25, 167–200 (1958).

ZAINO, C., POPPEL, M. H., JACOBSON, H. G., LEPOW, H.: The lower esophageal vestibular complex. Springfield: Thomas 1963.

Chapter 12

Resection and Reconstruction of the Esophagus

P. Valembois and G. Vantrappen

With 5 Figures

The partial or total resection of the esophagus and its replacement by stomach or by an interposed segment of intestine has become an accepted procedure in cases of esophageal stricture, atresia, varices and malignancy. Resection has also been recommended for malignant tumors of the esophagus with metastases, because removal of the primary lesion is said to improve the general condition of the patient (Plested et al., 1968). Even when the primary tumor cannot be removed, some surgeons perform a bypass operation (Johnson and Clagett, 1970; Burdette, 1971). They argue that a feeding gastrostomy or jejunostomy is poorly tolerated, does not improve the general condition of the patient and leaves him with his dysphagia and his inability to swallow saliva. A feeding gastrostomy or jejunostomy is performed only as a preterminal or preoperative procedure or in some cases which are treated by radiotherapy. Although the use of tubes placed through the obstructed region and bougienage are simple methods with a reasonable palliation of the dysphagia, they are not without complications. Therefore, a bypass operation without resection may be desirable in some selected cases.

1. Resection of the Esophagus

Theoretically, partial resection of the esophagus should be a satisfactory operation for most benign esophageal lesions. The continuity of the gastrointestinal tract may be restored by an end-to-end anastomosis (Gross, 1948), eventually after the stomach has been brought into the thorax (Wooler, 1952), or by the interposition of an intestinal segment. Partial resections have also been performed in selected cases of malignancy (Parker and Brockington, 1949; Katsura et al., 1958; Kunkel and Kunkel, 1958; Davidson, 1967). Esophagoesophageal anastomoses do not heal easily and are frequently followed by stenoses or leakage. These stenoses can entail dysphagia, or obstruction by bolus impaction.

Due to its intrathoracic localization, the leaking anastomoses will usually have dramatic consequences. In order to avoid an esophago-esophageal anastomosis the esophagus distal to the lesion is completely removed, including the gastroesophageal sphincter. The loss of this sphincter, however, may result in severe reflux esophagitis. After this type of resection the stomach has to be displaced into the thorax for an esophagogastrostomy, or an intestinal segment has to be interposed between the esophagus and the stomach. Many authors are so reluctant to use intrathoracic anastomoses that they do not hesitate to sacrifice the upper part of the gullet in cases of high esophageal lesions (Ong, 1971). Moreover, it is much easier to perform an anastomosis in the neck than to suture high in the thorax; the cervical esophagus is said to heal more easily, due to its richer vascularization; and finally, if complications should occur, this anastomosis is safer and can be better explored. When the esophageal lesion is malignant there is still another reason why a total esophagectomy is frequently carried out. An esophageal carcinoma commonly metastasizes in the submucosa at some distance of the primary lesion. According to Scanlon et al. (1955) such metastases occur in 45% of the cases, and may be located as high as 15 cm above the primary lesion (Parker and Gregorie, 1967). Partial resection would thus entail the risk of leaving behind tumor tissue, even if the site of the anastomosis is free of carcinoma.

1.1. Postoperative Complications

Block dissection of the esophagus in cases of malignant tumors will inevitably result in section of the vagal nerves, if the tumor is situated below the aortic arch. Indeed, from that level on the vagi run close to the esophagus. Complications of this vagotomy are diarrhea and gastric hypomotility with stasis. The frequency with which diarrhea occurs after vagotomy varies, but can be as high as 70% (Harkins et al., 1963). This diarrhea may be long-lasting and severe, but is usually mild and transient so that the incidence of clinically important diarrhea is probably no more than 5%. The pathogenesis of this diarrhea is uncertain, and clinical and experimental data concerning the problem are highly controversial. Esophageal resection is usually supplemented by a gastric drainage procedure in order to avoid delayed gastric emptying and stasis, which, in the absence of the gastroesophageal sphincter, would greatly favor gastroesophageal reflux.

In the neck, both recurrent laryngeal nerves, located in the tracheoesophageal grooves, run close to the esophagus; in the upper mediastinum, only the left one lies close to the gullet. In dissecting the esophagus from the trachea, and in clearing the lymphonodes along it, great care must be exercised, for the nerves can easily be damaged, resulting in vocal cord paralysis. If both nerves are injured serious respiratory difficulties will ensue. For carcinoma of the superior mediastinal esophagus Waddell and Scannell (1957) recommend sacrificing the left recurrent laryngeal nerve, accepting an unilateral vocal cord paralysis.

2. Replacement of the Esophagus

When the entire esophagus has to be replaced or bridged over, the esophageal substitute can be brought into the prethoracic or substernal area or into the posterior mediastinum. The subcutaneous prethoracic route is longer and entails the risk of obstruction because a kink may be formed as the intestine passes the manubrium sterni. Frequently, therefore, the manubrium is partly removed. The subcutaneous route is less esthetic but safer than the other routes, because leakage and infarctions are more easily recognized and treated and remain localized in the subcutaneous area. Another advantage is the possibility of forcing an impacted bolus into the stomach by external pressure. By using the subcutaneous or substernal route a thoracotomy can be avoided in cases when the esophagus is not removed. Blind undermining of the substernal region can be done without undue risk of pneumothorax.

Replacement of the esophagus has been performed by means of skin, stomach, jejunum or colon. Skin reconstruction is the oldest replacement technique, and was first performed by von Mikulicz (1886), in a case of a resected cervical carcinoma. By means of a skin-tube, making use of the chest wall, H. Bircher in 1894 succeeded in connecting a cervical esophagostomy with a gastrostomy (E. Bircher, 1907). This method usually required a long time for completion:

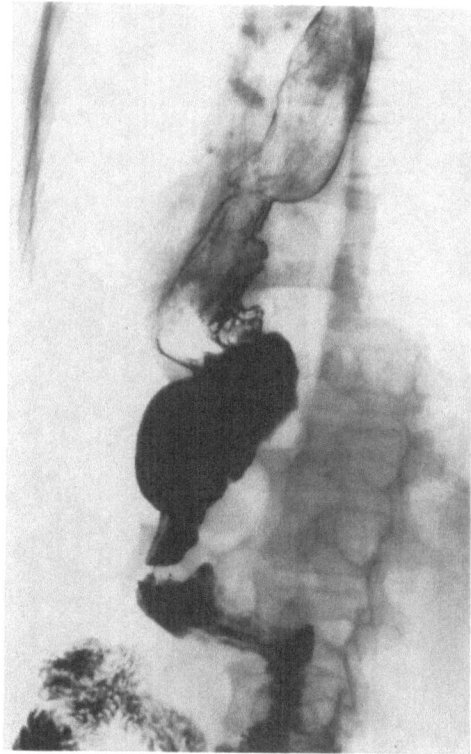

Fig. 340. Intrathoracic end-to-end gastroesophageal anastomosis after resection of a carcinoma in the lower third of the esophagus

sometimes as many as 20 to 30 re-interventions had to be done, usually because of fistulization.] At present, skin reconstruction in various modifications is used only for replacement of the cervical esophagus (LÄMMLI and FISCH, 1971).

The stomach has been used in part or in whole. Tubes made of the greater curvature of the stomach and mounted in a peristaltic or antiperistaltic way have never been widely adopted, although they preserve the normal sequence of esophagus, stomach and small intestine. At present, HEIMLICH (1970) is the main promotor of this technique.

Elevation of the stomach to bridge the defect produced by the esophageal resection has come into general use only after the publications of ADAMS and PHEMISTER (1938), GARLOCK (1944) and SWEET (1945) (Fig. 340). This technique is based on the finding that an adequate blood supply for the stomach remains, if the right gastric and right gastroepiploic vessels with their marginal arcades are left intact. In this way it is possible to bring the gastric fundus up into the neck eventually after mobilization of the duodenum, and to connect it with the pharynx. The esophagogastrostomy is a relatively easy and short procedure, requiring only one intestinal anastomosis and a pyloroplasty. The late results are less satisfactory, because of the frequent occurrence of reflux esophagitis and stenosis.

The use of jejunum or colon as an esophageal substitute has been revived by the experimental work of KIRILUK and MERENDINO (1954), who demonstrated

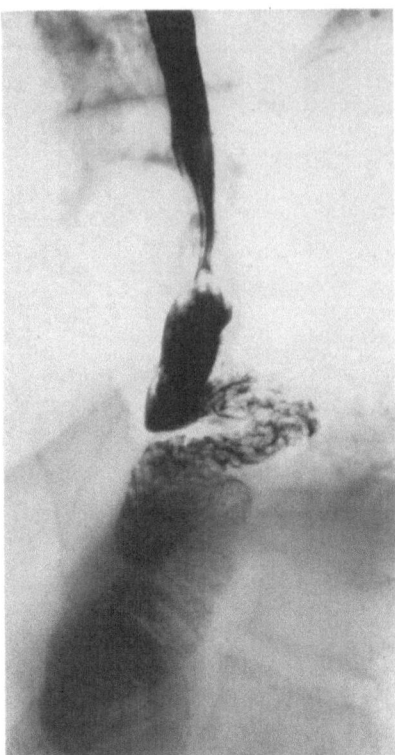

Fig. 341. Intrathoracic esophagojejunal anastomosis after total gastrectomy

that the jejunum and the colon are more resistant to acid peptic digestion than the esophagus, and that in dogs, even when the stomach was stimulated by histamine, ulcerations did not occur in the interposed jejunal segment (Skinner and Merendino, 1955). In addition, the jejunum neutralizes the refluxing acid, thus preventing it from damaging the mucosa of the proximal esophagus. Although the technique of using the jejunum as an esophageal substitute (Fig. 341) was introduced as early as 1904 by L. Wullstein it has never been widely adopted, in spite of the fact that both organs have about the same diameter. The disposition of the vessels in the mesentery is frequently so unfavorable that the available intestinal segment is too short to bridge the whole length of the esophagus. Attempts have been made to solve this problem by anastomosing a proximal mesenteric artery to the internal mammary artery (Longmire, 1947). As the small bowel substitute retains its direction of propulsion (Hanna et al., 1967b) it must be mounted in an isoperistaltic way. A heteroperistaltic substitution almost always gives rise to complications (Portes et al., 1962), particularly if the interposed segment is longer than 10 cm. As a result of its inherent peristaltic pattern the isoperistaltic segment will prevent reflux of gastric contents into the proximal esophagus. The fluoroscopic observations of Moylan et al. (1970) indicate that the backward flow of barium extends over a distance of not more than 8 cm. Therefore these authors recommend that the interposed jejunal segment should have a length of at least 15 cm.

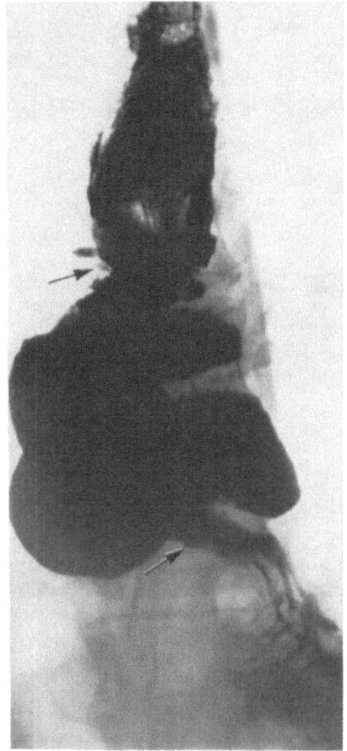

Fig. 342. Colon transplant (between arrows) for stenosing caustic esophagitis

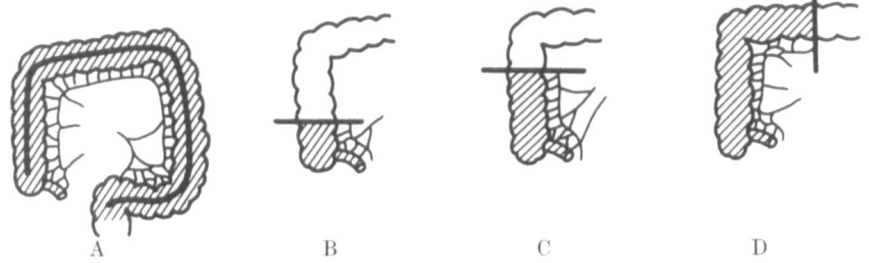

Fig. 343A—D. Variation in venous drainage of the right colon in 25 specimens. A Continuity coecum to sigmoid: 20 specimens. B, C, D Lack of marginal anastomosis between ileocolic and right colic vein (2 specimens), right colic and middle colic vein (2 specimens), two independent branches of the middle colic vein (1 specimen). [From NICKS, R.: Brit. J. Surg. 54, 124 (1967)]

In spite of the good results reported by these authors most surgeons prefer the colon as an esophageal substitute. Due to the favorable disposition of its blood vessels, the colon can be used to bridge the whole length of the esophagus. Esophagocoloplasty was originally proposed by KELLING (1911). The ascending colon, with or without the terminal ileum can be utilized as well as the transverse or the descending colon (Fig. 342). Unlike the small bowel the colon has a marginal artery which runs close to its wall. The blood vessel pattern to the right side of

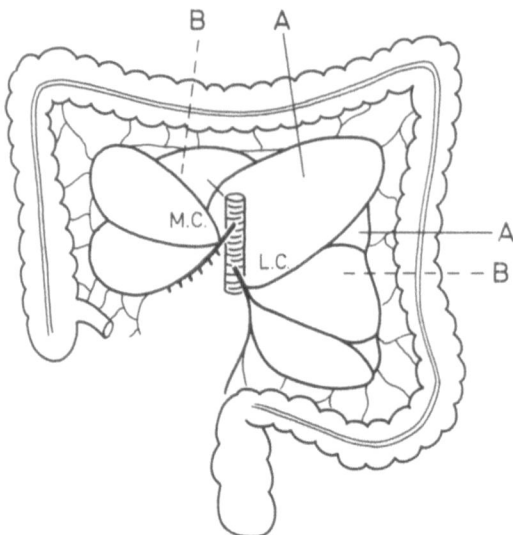

Fig. 344. Blood supply to the colon showing points of division for short (A–A) and long (B–B) colon transplants. [From BELSEY, R.: J. thorac. cardiovasc. Surg. 49, 33 (1965)]

the colon, however, is more variable than the vascularization of the left colon (BECK and BARONOFSKY, 1960). Very few studies are available concerning the venous drainage of the large bowel. If the venous return is compromised the viability of the transplant will equally be jeopardized. R. NICKS (1967) found a lack of adequate marginal venous anastomosis between the major veins of the right colon in 5 of 25 specimens (Fig. 343). On the left side an excellent marginal vein continued into the left colic vein in all specimens he examined. It may be assumed that in the past an inadequate arterial supply and/or venous congestion have been important causes of leakage, fistula formation, stricture and infarction after colonic replacement of the esophagus. For this reason several surgeons who had been using the right colon as an esophageal substitute have now turned to the left half of the colon. When the arterial blood supply is derived from the middle colic artery, the ascending colon can easily be mounted as an isoperistaltic segment. If, however, this artery is used for a left colon interposition a hetero-peristaltic disposition is inevitable, unless the interposed segment is short. CHRY-SOSPATHIS and GOLEMATIS (1962) and BELSEY (1965), who published a series of 105 cases, have demonstrated that transposition in an isoperistaltic manner of the left half of the colon with its blood supply maintained from the left colic artery is quite feasible (Fig. 344). According to these authors the isoperistaltic inter-position gives less postoperative complications and better functional results than the heteroperistaltic colon substitute. It is apparent that a careful examination of the arterial supply will determine the portion of the intestine best utilized for the procedure in each individual case. A preoperative selective arteriography may give valuable information.

2.1. Mortality and Morbidity of the Esophageal Substitution

Resection of the esophagus for benign lesions usually carries with it a lower mortality than resection carried out for malignancy. Patients with malignant lesions are usually older and in a poor general condition, and the dissection has to be more extensive. Recent reports indicate that the mortality after esophageal resection and reconstruction for malignant lesions amounts to 20% versus 7% for benign lesions (MULLEN et al., 1970). It is generally agreed that, except in selected cases, colon interposition should not be used following resection of malignant lesions, if reconstruction can be effected by a simpler and easier technique, such as esophagogastrostomy. High esophagogastrostomies yield better results than lower anastomoses. Not only are postoperative complications less frequent (GRIMES and STEPHENS, 1960), but the mortality of this procedure is also lower, i.e. 6% versus 12% (BELSEY, 1972). Respiratory failure is one of the most important causes of death after esophageal substitution. In addition to the pulmonary complications that may follow any laparotomy or thoracotomy, many patients who are considered for esophagoplasty already have bronchopulmonary infections as a result of their esophageal obstruction. As patients in the immediate postoperative period spend more time in a reclining position, the regurgitation will contribute to the pneumonitis usually associated with the terminal period. Therefore, good preoperative care and treatment, including antibiotics, respiratory exercises, and a semi-sitting position are of the utmost importance.

2.1.1. Necrosis of the Esophageal Substitute

Necrosis of the esophageal substitute is a rare complication if the entire stomach is used to bridge the esophageal defect, but is more frequent with jejunal or colonic transplants. MULLEN et al. (1970) reviewed the recent literature and found a mean incidence of necrosis in 8% of colon substitutes. As the blood supply of the jejunum is more vulnerable the incidence of necrosis is higher and may reach 50% when jejunal segments are interposed (HUGUIER et al., 1970). The mortality of this complication is very high, even if necrosis is not complete.

The persistence of old blood-stained fluid in the aspirate of an esophageal indwelling catheter 48 hours after the operation is an indication of serious trouble with the blood supply (BRAIN, 1967). The presence of brown blood-stained fluid draining from the cervical incision has the same significance. Daily X-ray control of the chest also gives important information. Should there be fluid levels with distension of the intestinal loop, or pleural effusion with a tendency to increase, surgical exploration is indicated. As gangrene develops, pulse rate and fever begin to rise and the patient becomes more and more toxic, but pain may not occur. Immediate removal of the transposed substitute is then compulsory. If the proximal anastomosis is postponed and the proximal end of the intestinal segment is fixed to the skin in the neck, the color of the stomy will give a good idea of the nutritional state of the transplant. REYNOLDS et al. (1961), who perform the proximal anastomosis as a primary procedure, wait for 24 hours before closing the cervical incision in order to check the color of the anastomosed segment.

A meticulous technique during the substitution procedure is essential to prevent this complication. The blood vessels of the intestinal segment should be handled carefully and should not be subjected to traction. The veins are more easily traumatized than the arteries. Venous congestion and thrombosis is the most frequent cause of partial or total necrosis of the transplant.

Impairment of the blood supply may also have less acute consequences. HONG et al. (1964) reported 4 cases with dysphagia gradually developing several months after esophageal substitution with colon. Re-exploration showed the bowel segment to have narrowed to a fibrous cord.

2.1.2. Leakage at the Anastomosis

Leakage at the anastomosis is the most common complication, occurring in 23.5% of 289 procedures collected from the literature since 1962 (Mullen et al., 1970). The nature of the underlying disease, benign or malignant, does not seem to influence the incidence of this complication. The least favorable anastomotic site is the middle third of the esophagus (Maillard et al., 1969). Antiperistaltic substitutes give rise to leakage more frequently than isoperistaltic transplants. Huguier et al. (1970) reported 3 leakages in 6 antiperistaltic left colon transplants, and only 2 in 12 isoperistaltic substitutes. Belsey (1965) also reported a low incidence with isoperistaltic left colon substitution (2 leakages in 92 procedures).

It is generally agreed that the esophageal suture does not heal easily. This is due, among other factors, to the absence of a sealing serosa and to the fact that the esophageal mucosa is not sterile. An impaired blood supply and traction on the anastomosis will also favor leakage. The anastomosis has to be made with the greatest care. Accurate apposition of the divided segment of the esophagus and the stomach, colon or jejunum is an absolute necessity. A continuous suture should not be used, because it may compromise the blood supply. A one layer through-and-through suture is used by some surgeons (Belsey, 1965; Ong, 1971). The suture can be invaginated in the stomach or in the colon; it may also be covered by a pleural flap. The esophageal substitute should have sufficient length to avoid traction on the anastomosis, but if it is too long the evacuation may be hampered as a result of tortuosity and kinking. Traction on the anastomosis during the postoperative period may be avoided by anchoring the transplant to the prevertebral fascia.

The absence of the lower esophageal sphincter may also be an important cause of leakage at the anastomosis. In patients with a fistula at the proximal anastomosis the gastrostomy feeding may be expelled through the fistula tract on coughing. Nicks (1967) observed fluoroscopically that barium passed directly into the thoracic colon, in preference to the duodenum. This was most marked on coughing, on deep breathing and with changes in posture. When the gastroesophageal sphincter has been removed, coughing results in an expulsion of the gastric contents into the esophagus. As the upper esophageal sphincter is closed at that time the intraesophageal pressure will rise sharply. The high intraluminal pressure at the level of the anastomosis in the neck will favor the disruption of the suture, particularly because there is no extraluminal counterpressure in the neck during coughing.

It has not yet been determined which site of the stomach is best suited for a jejuno- or cologastrostomy. Belsey (1965) prefers the back of the stomach, a third of its length from the cardia. Most other surgeons use either the anterior aspect of the stomach, immediately proximal to the antrum, the fundus, or the site of the transection of the stomach. When the esophageal substitute is placed in the subcutaneous or substernal area the easiest site of anastomosis is the anterior aspect of the stomach.

The esophageal substitute and the stomach should be decompressed during the postoperative period. Decompression of the stomach is usually achieved by a gastrostomy, which may also serve as a temporary feeding stomy. A pyloroplasty is also carried out because of the vagotomy which is necessarily associated with the esophageal resection. Intubation of the transplant is also a necessity to insure its decompression, although an indwelling tube may compromise healing of the anastomosis if left in the esophagus for a long time (Borgström and Lundh, 1959). If the proximal anastomosis or the esophagogastrostomy is located in the neck, wound drainage of this region will indicate the presence of a leak. If an intrathoracic anastomosis has been performed, leakage results in mediastinitis, a serious complication which is responsible for 50% of the postoperative deaths (LORTAT-JACOB et al., 1970; INBERG et al., 1971). The symptoms and treatment are similar to those of an esophageal perforation. Sometimes the leak becomes encapsulated; secondary perforation may then result in an esophagopleural or esophagobronchial fistula. Fistulas in the neck usually heal spontaneously after a few days or weeks, if there is no distal stenosis. A kink of the antethoracic interposed viscus at the level of the manubrium sterni, or of the retrosternal transplant around the trachea may also be the cause of a persisting neck fistula. If the fistula does not heal spontaneously, a re-intervention with a new anastomosis is necessary.

When the anastomosis heals with difficulty, particularly when there has been leakage at the anastomosis, a stricture is likely to develop (HONG et al., 1964). Benign stenoses are best treated by progressive dilatations. In case of malignancy however, one should always consider the possibility that the stricture formation is due to recurrence of the growth.

2.1.3. Other Complications

MALCOLM (1968) reviewed 11 published cases of peptic ulcer in colon used for esophageal replacement. In none of these 11 patients a gastric drainage procedure had been performed. This rare complication can entail others, such as perforation and hemorrhage. Compression of the gastric outflow tract by the blood vessels of the substitute may lead to gastric obstruction. This complication may occur even if these blood vessels pass behind the stomach (MENGUY, 1965).

2. 2. Functional Results

The functional results of visceral esophageal substitutes have not been studied extensively. According to BELSEY (1965) only 44% of the patients are free of symptoms after esophagogastrostomy. The patients frequently complain of varying degrees of regurgitation, substernal burning and pain, dysphagia or fullness, nausea and weakness after meals, or diarrhea. Dumping-like symptoms occur more frequently in patients in whom a gastric drainage procedure has been performed (HANNA et al., 1967a). 27% of the patients with an esophagogastrostomy develop reflux esophagitis, which may lead to stricture at or proximal to the anastomosis. To avoid this complication GRIMES and STEPHENS (1960) recommend performing a high esophagogastrostomy and bringing the entire stomach into the thorax. As there is no longer an intraabdominal portion of the stomach, inspiration will not result in an aspiration of the gastric contents into the thorax.

At present the esophagogastrostomy is carried out only after resection of malignant tumors of the esophagus or of the cardia or as a palliative bypass procedure for inoperable carcinomas of the esophagogastric junction (JOHNSON and CLAGETT, 1970). This procedure is simple and well tolerated and carries with it a lesser risk of complications in the immediate postoperative period, compared with the other substitution procedures. Because of short survival, reflux probably will not become a significant problem, and this operation provides a very effective palliation of the dysphagia. Jejunal replacement of the esophagus does not constitute a generally accepted procedure. However, when this operation succeeds, the functional results are very good. BRAIN (1967) and HANNA et al. (1967a) report complete relief of all symptoms in 73 and 70% of their patients. Dumping symptoms are rare. Fluoroscopic observations indicate that the evacuation of the jejunal segment takes from 10 seconds to 1 hour, whereas the emptying of colon substitutes may atke several hours (HANNA et al., 1967b). Another advantage of

the succesfull jejunal interposition is that the propulsive activity of the interposed segment, if it measures at least 15 cm, prevents the refluxing gastric contents from reaching the esophagus and the pharynx (Moylan et al., 1970). The
procedure most frequently used for the treatment of benign lesions is the colon
interposition. The function of the interposed colon segment has usually been
considered to be that of an inert tube, conducting food passively into the stomach.
Recently, however, Jones et al. (1971) presented experimental and clinical
evidence that the transposed colon exhibits peristaltic activity and a rapid acid-
clearing capacity (Jones et al., 1973). Peristaltic activity is rarely seen at roentgen
examination of colonic transplants, but regurgitation into the pharynx is common
when the colon is interposed in an antiperistaltic manner.

Hanna et al. (1967a) report 50% good to excellent results after right colon
interposition in an isoperistaltic manner as well as after antiperistaltic left colon
interposition. As the arterial blood supply and venous return are richer and more
constant in the left than in the right colon, isoperistaltic substitution with the
left colon is presently the safest procedure. Belsey (1965) used this operation
with good results, 81% of his 88 patients being asymptomatic.

References

Adams, W. E., Phemister, D. B.: Carcinoma of the lower thoracic esophagus. Report of
succesful resection and esophagogastrostomy. J. thorac. Surg. 7, 621–632 (1938).
Beck, A. R., Baronofsky, I. D.: A study of the left colon as a replacement for the resected
esophagus. Surgery 48, 499–509 (1960).
Belsey, R.: Reconstruction of the esophagus with left colon. J. thorac. cardiovasc. Surg. 49,
33–55 (1965).
Belsey, R.: Recent progress in oesophageal surgery. Acta chir. Belg. 4, 230–238 (1972).
Bircher, E.: Ein Beitrag zur plastischen Bildung eines neuen Oesophagus. Zbl. Chir. 34,
1479–1482 (1907).
Borgström, S., Lundh, B.: Healing of esophageal anastomosis. Ann. Surg. 150, 142–148
(1959).
Brain, R. H. F.: The place for jejunal transplantation in the treatment of simple strictures
of the esophagus. Ann. roy. Coll. Surg. Engl. 40, 100–118 (1967).
Burdette, W. J.: Palliative operation for carcinoma of cervical and thoracic esophagus.
Ann. Surg. 173, 714–732 (1971).
Chrysospathis, P. J., Golematis, B.: The use of the colon as a substitute for the esophagus.
Gut 3, 162–166 (1962).
Davidson, J. S.: Resection of squamous-cell carcinoma of the oesophagus with end-to-end
oesophageal anastomosis. Brit. J. Surg. 54, 63–70 (1967).
Garlock, J. H.: The reestablishment of esophagogastric continuity following resection of the
esophagus for cancer of the middle third. Surg. Gynec. Obstet. 78, 23–28 (1944).
Grimes, O. F., Stephens, H. B.: Surgical management of acquired short esophagus. Ann.
Surg. 152, 743–766 (1960).
Gross, R. E.: Treatment of short stricture of the esophagus by partial esophagectomy and
end-to-end esophageal reconstruction. Surgery 23, 735–744 (1948).
Hanna, E. A., Harrison, A. W., Derrick, J. R.: Long-term results of visceral esophageal
substitutes. Ann. thorac. Surg. 3, 111–118 (1967a).
Hanna, E. A., Harrison, A. W., Derrick, J. R.: Comparative function of visceral esophageal
substitutes by cinefluoroscopy. Ann. thorac. Surg. 3, 173–176 (1967b).
Harkins, H. N., Stavney, S., Griffith, C. A., Savage, L. E., Kato, T. Y., Nyhus, L. M.:
Selective gastric vagotomy. Ann. Surg. 158, 448–460 (1963).
Heimlich, H. J.: Carcinoma of the cervical esophagus. J. thorac. cardiovasc. Surg. 59, 309–
318 (1970).
Hong, P. W., Seel, D. J., Dietrick, R. B.: The use of the colon in the surgical treatment of
benign stricture of the esophagus. Ann. Surg. 160, 202–209 (1964).
Huguier, M., Gordin, F., Maillard, J. N., Lortat-Jacob, J. L.: Results of 117 esophageal
replacements. Surg. Gynec. Obstet. 130, 1054–1058 (1970).
Inberg, M. V., Linna, M. I., Scheinin, T. H., Vänttinen, E.: Anastomotic leakage after
excision of esophageal and high gastric carcinoma. Amer. J. Surg. 122, 540–544 (1971).

JOHNSON, C. L., CLAGETT, O. T.: Palliative esophagogastrostomy for inoperable carcinoma of the esophagogastric junction. J. thorac. cardiovasc. Surg. 60, 269–274 (1970).

JONES, E. L., BOOTH, D. J., CAMERON, J. L., ZUIDEMA, G. D., SKINNER, D. B.: Functional evaluation of esophageal reconstructions. Ann. thorac. Surg. 12, 331–346 (1971).

JONES, E. L., SKINNER, D. B., DEMEESTER, T. R., ELKINS, R. C., ZUIDEMA, G. D.: Response of the interposed human colonic segment to an acid challenge. Ann. Surg. 177, 75–78 (1973).

KATSURA, S., YOSHINOBU, I., OKAYAMA, G.: Transplantation of the partially resected middle esophagus with a jejunal graft. Ann. Surg. 147, 146–156 (1958).

KELLING, G.: Oesophagoplastik mit Hilfe des Querkolon. Zbl. Chir. 38, 1209–1212 (1911).

KIRILUK, L. B., MERENDINO, K. A.: An experimental study of the buffering capacity of the contents of the upper small bowel. Surgery 35, 532–537 (1954).

KIRILUK, L. B., MERENDINO, K. A.: The comparative sensitivity of the mucosa of the various segments of the alimentary tract in the dog to acid-peptic action. Surgery 35, 547–556 (1954).

KUNKEL, W. M., KUNKEL, P. A.: Resection of carcinoma of the mid-esophagus with primary anastomosis. J. thorac. Surg. 36, 49–52 (1958).

LÄMMLI, K., FISCH, U.: Die Reconstruction des Oesophagus mit deltopektoralen Hautlappen. Pract. oto-rhino-laryng. (Basel) 33, 11–17 (1971).

LONGMIRE, W. P., JR.: A modification of the Roux technique for antethoracic esophageal reconstruction. Anastomosis of the mesenteric and internal mammary blood vessels. Surgery 22, 94–100 (1947).

LORTAT-JACOB, J. L., MAILLARD, J. N., RICHARD, C. A., FÉKÉTÉ, F., LAUNOIS, B.: Surgical treatment of cancer of the esophagus. Brit. J. clin. Pract. 24 (1), 13–16 (1970).

MAILLARD, J. N., LAUNOIS, B., LAGAUSIE, P. DE, LELLOUCH, J., LORTAT-JACOB, J. L.: Cause of leakage at the site of anastomosis after esophagogastric resection for carcinoma. Surg. Gynec. Obstet. 129, 1014–1018 (1969).

MALCOLM, J. A.: Occurence of peptic ulcer in colon used for esophageal replacement. J. thorac. cardiovasc. Surg. 55, 763–772 (1968).

MENGUY, R.: Intrathoracic perforation of the colon: An unusual complication of colonic interposition for esophageal stricture. Amer. J. Surg. 31, 328–332 (1965).

MIKULICZ, J. VON: Ein Fall von Resection des carcinomatösen Oesophagus mit plastischem Ersatz des excidierten Stückes. Prag. med. Wschr. 11, 93 (1886).

MOYLAN, J. P., BELL, J. W., CANTRELL, J. R., MERENDINO, K. A.: The jejunal interposition operation: a follow-up on seventeen patients followed 10 to 17 years. Ann. Surg. 172, 205–211 (1970).

MULLEN, D. C., POSTLETHWAIT, R. W., DILLON, M. L.: Complications of substernal colon interposition. Amer. Surg. 36 (2), 80–84 (1970).

NICKS, R.: Colonic replacement of the esophagus. Some observations on infarction and wound leakage. Brit. J. Surg. 54, 124–129 (1967).

ONG, G. B.: Resection and reconstruction of the esophagus. Current problems in surgery. Chicago: Year Book Medical Publishers, September 1971.

PARKER, E. F., BROCKINGTON, W. S.: Esophageal resection with end-to-end anastomosis. Experimental and clinical observations. Ann. Surg. 129, 588–605 (1949).

PARKER, E. F., GREGORIE, H. B.: Carcinoma of the esophagus. Current problems in surgery. Chicago: Year Book Medical Publishers, April 1967.

PLESTED, W. G., TILDON, T. T., HUGHES, R. K.: A philosophy of treatment of esophageal carcinoma. Amer. Surg. 35, 650–656 (1968).

PORIES, W. J., GERLE, R. D., SHERMAN, C. D., HINSHAW, J. R.: The danger of esophageal replacement with antiperistaltic loops of small bowel. Ann. Surg. 156, 68–73 (1962).

REYNOLDS, J. T., GUYNN, V. L., GROVE, W. J., JAVID, H.: Experience with the use of the right colon to replace the esophagus. Amer. J. Surg. 101, 39–43 (1961).

SCANLON, E. F., MORTON, D. R., WALKER, J. M., WATSON, W. L.: The case against segmental resection for esophageal carcinoma. Surg. Gynec. Obstet. 101, 290–296 (1955).

SKINNER, H. H., MERENDINO, K. A.: Experimental evaluation of an interposed jejunal segment between the esophagus and the stomach combined with upper gastrectomy in the prevention of esophagitis and jejunitis. Ann. Surg. 141, 201–207 (1955).

SWEET, R. H.: Surgical management of carcinoma of the mid-thoracic esophagus. Preliminary report. New Engl. J. Med. 233, 1–7 (1945).

WADDELL, W. R., SCANNELL, J. G.: Anterior approach to carcinoma of the superior mediastinal and cervical segments of the esophagus. J. thorac. Surg. 33, 663–669 (1957).

WOOLER, G. H.: Discussion on head and neck cancer. Proc. roy. Soc. Med. 45, 264 (1952).

WULLSTEIN, L.: Über antethorakale Oesophago-jejunostomie und Operationen nach gleichem Prinzip. Dtsch. med. Wschr. 30, 734–736 (1904).

Chapter 13

Etiology and Non-Surgical Treatment of Organic Esophageal Stenosis

G. Vantrappen, J. Hellemans and K. Geboes

With 7 Figures

Esophageal stenosis is a not uncommon condition and has a varied etiology. It can occur in all age groups and in varying segments of the esophagus. The most characteristic symptom of an organic narrowing without complete obstruction is dysphagia for solids whereas drinking remains relatively easy. When the stenosis narrows further, drinking may become more and more difficult if not impossible. A prolonged swallowing time, impaction pain and regurgitation are common symptoms. X-ray examination does not always differentiate an organic stenosis from spasm and often leaves some doubt about the underlying pathology. Endoscopic examination with biopsy is nearly always indicated. The simplest method to rule out organic stenosis as the cause of dysphagia is to pass a large metal olive into the stomach.

1. Etiology

Especially in the elderly, esophageal stenosis should always arouse suspicion of malignancy. Most benign strictures are caused by acid or bile reflux, which is responsible for the chronic inflammatory process that results in stenosis. Such strictures are located at the distal end of the esophagus, unless the lower segment of the gullet is lined by columnar epithelium. Indwelling nasogastric tubes, especially with the patient in the supine position (Bingam, 1958; Nagler and Spiro, 1965), persistent vomiting (Smith and Nelson, 1965) and surgical destruction of the antireflux mechanism (Rider et al., 1969) have been implicated as predisposing toward esophagitis and stricture formation. Esophagitis occurs in 10 to 24% of the hernia patients, and scarring with subsequent stricture formation has been noted in 2 to 4% (Koch, 1960; Palmer, 1968; Johnson and Lukash, 1970). Reflux esophagitis without hiatus hernia is less frequent, but stricture formation has been found in 5% of these cases (Palmer, 1968). The annual incidence of severe esophagitis with chronic ulceration or stricture formation is about 4.5 per 100000 in North-East Scotland. The incidence of severe peptic esophagitis increases sharply after the age of 50 (Brunnen et al., 1969). However, tight peptic stricture of the lower esophagus may occur at any age and has been described in a 17-day old infant (Kundert and Morger, 1970; Belsey and Skinner, 1972). Peptic stenosis should be suspected when a long history of heartburn and recumbency regurgitation is complicated by dysphagia. Heartburn often disappears when dysphagia develops. Some patients present with a peptic stenosis without prior heartburn.

Ingestion of caustic agents, either accidentally or as suicidal attempt, is frequently complicated by stricture formation (Fig. 345A). In untreated cases stenosis can be expected in 56% of the patients (Hardin, 1956; Johnson and

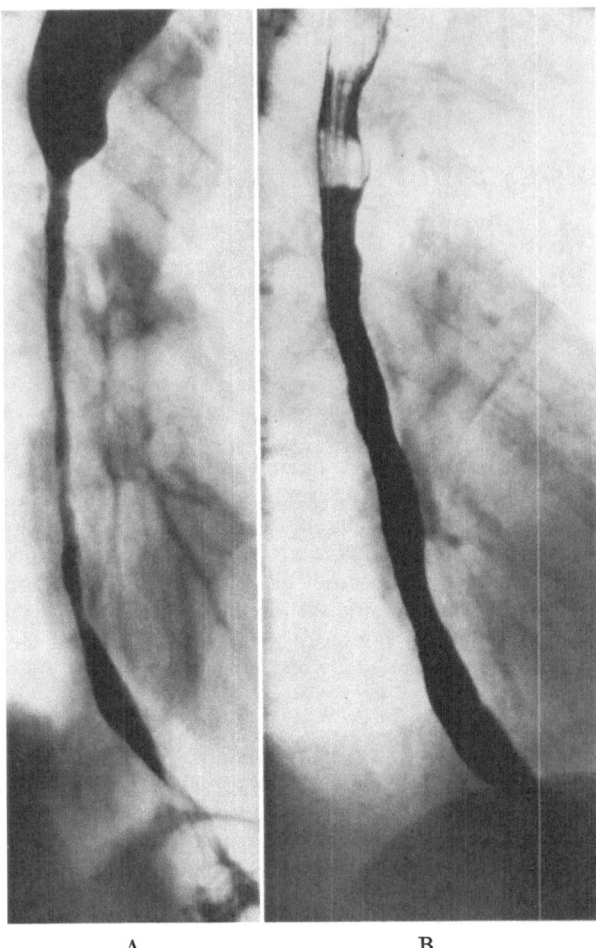

Fig. 345A and B. Extensive narrowing due to caustic esophagitis. Before (A) and after (B) dilatation

LUKASH, 1970). The overall incidence of stricture formation has been lowered by modern therapy with antibiotics and steroids, but still remains considerable (see Caustic Lesions of the Esophagus).

Esophageal transit may be hindered after surgical interventions. A faulty suture technique may excessively narrow the esophageal lumen, anti-reflux mechanisms may be destroyed (which can result in peptic esophagitis), or an anastomosis may give rise to stricture formation (Fig. 346A). Stenosis following surgical repair of the esophagus for congenital atresia with or without fistula is not infrequent. Operation techniques such as HAIGHT's end-to-end repair (HAIGHT and TOWSLEY, 1943) and GROSS's (1953) side-to-side anastomosis are complicated by stricture formation at the level of the anastomosis in 32 to 77% of the survivors (SHAW et al., 1955; KOCH, 1960; BURGESS et al., 1968; HOLDEN and WOOLER, 1970; BUKER et al., 1972).

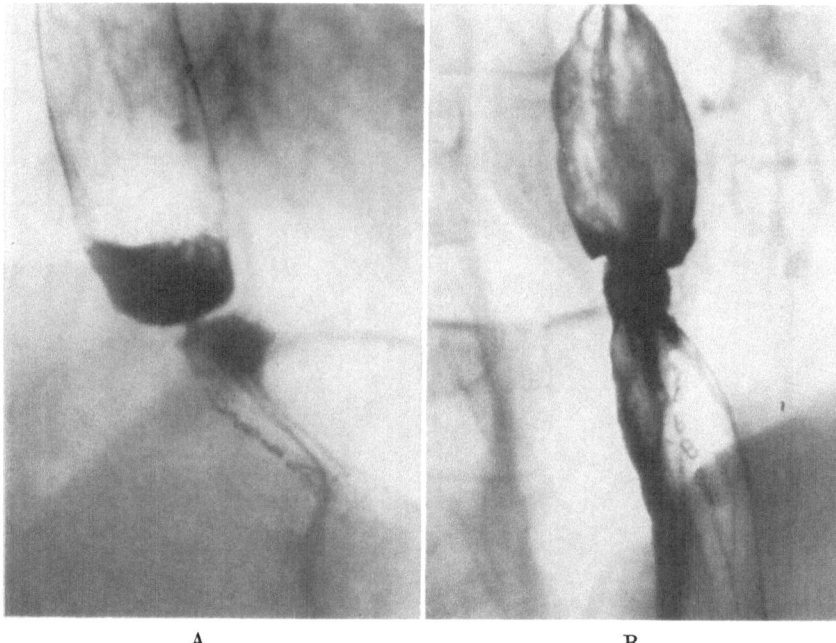

A   B

Fig. 346 A and B. Stenosis at the level of an esophagogastric anastomosis following a large
polar gastrectomy before (A) and after (B) dilatation

Acquired esophageal strictures can occur after resection of a Zenker diverticulum or after resection of the cardia with esophagogastrostomy. Small intestine and colon interposition may be complicated by swallowing difficulties due to motility disturbances or to an incompetent anti-reflux mechanism and stricture formation (HOOVER, 1955; KNUDSEN and OBERHELMAN, 1970).

Heterotopic gastric epithelium (MOSSBERG, 1966), radiation therapy, congenital strictures (Fig. 347 A), external trauma, traumata caused by instrumentation or ingested foreign bodies, and esophageal webs and rings are among the less common causes of esophageal stenosis. Webs and rings are easily missed on roentgenograms so that their incidence can be underestimated. When carefully sought, a lower esophageal ring will be found quite often (CAUTHORNE, 1970) and it is a common cause of benign stricture in middle-aged and older people (Fig. 348 A). Rare causes of stricture formation are pemphigus, benign mucous membrane pemphigoid, and recessive dystrophic epidermolysis bullosa (see The Esophagus in Cutaneous Diseases).

2. Techniques of Dilatation

Treatment of strictures by means of dilatation was suggested as early as 1821 by HILDRETH (BOLSTAD, 1966). At the first reported attempt at dilatation it seemed to be more difficult to withdraw the dilating "common probang" than to pass it into the stomach (PURTON, 1821).

Dilatation can be performed in four ways: by blind bougienage, by peroral endoscopic bougienage, by peroral bougienage using a guide previously passed through the stenosis, and by anterograde or retrograde bougienage through a

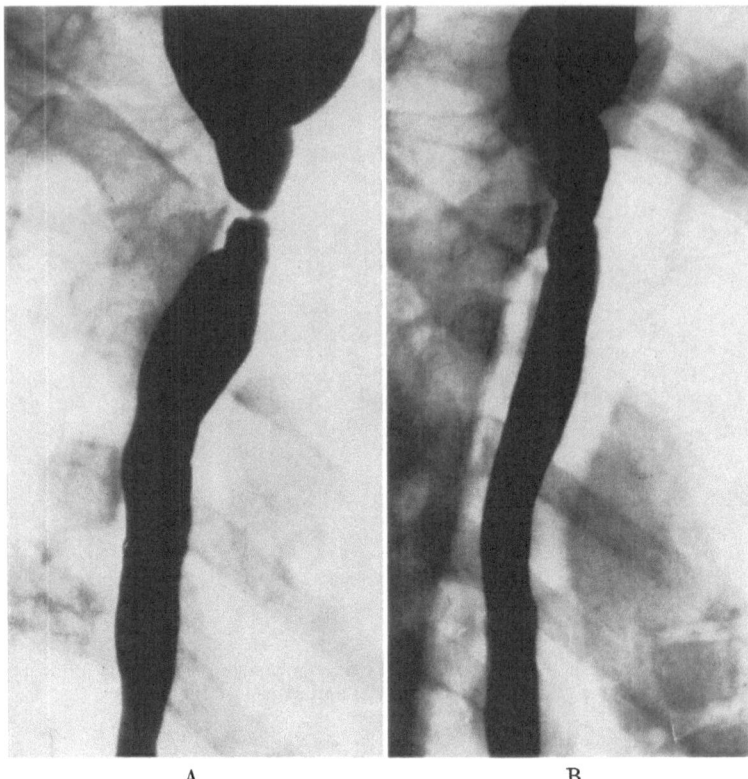

A   B

Fig. 347A and B. Congenital ring in the cervical esophagus, before (A) and after (B) dilatation

gastrostomy opening. In all these methods dilators of progressively increasing
diameter are passed through the stenosis. The risk of perforation is highest with
blind or endoscopic peroral bougienage. Because of this danger, blind bougienage
should be avoided.

Several types of dilators have been proposed for the treatment of esophageal
strictures. Conventional bougies have been made out of wax-impregnated woven
silk, gum, rubber, plastic, and recently, teflon. The latter material becomes
slippery in the presence of mucus so that the application of lubricant jellies is not
necessary (Emerson, 1965, 1966). Bougies have a conic or blunt tip (Fig. 349).
They are usually graduated in French (1 French = 1 mm of circumference). Boring
a channel through the olive tip of a teflon dilator makes it possible to pass the
dilator over a string which is a much safer procedure. Flexible mercury-filled
rubber bougies are still frequently used. The most important ones are the Maloney
tapered dilators, graduated in size from 12 to 60 French and the Hurst dilators
with blunt endings. The Sippy dilating metal olives, size 10 (for children) or 18 (for
adults) (Fig. 350) to 51 French, the conically shaped Plummer olives, size 15 to
45 French, and the Eder-Puestow olives, size 21 to 45 French (Fig. 351) have
several advantages. They can be used even when the stricture is old, hard or
rigid; they allow a brief procedure in contrast to some bougies which are left in
place for hours; and their use is safer than blind or endoscopic methods. Generally

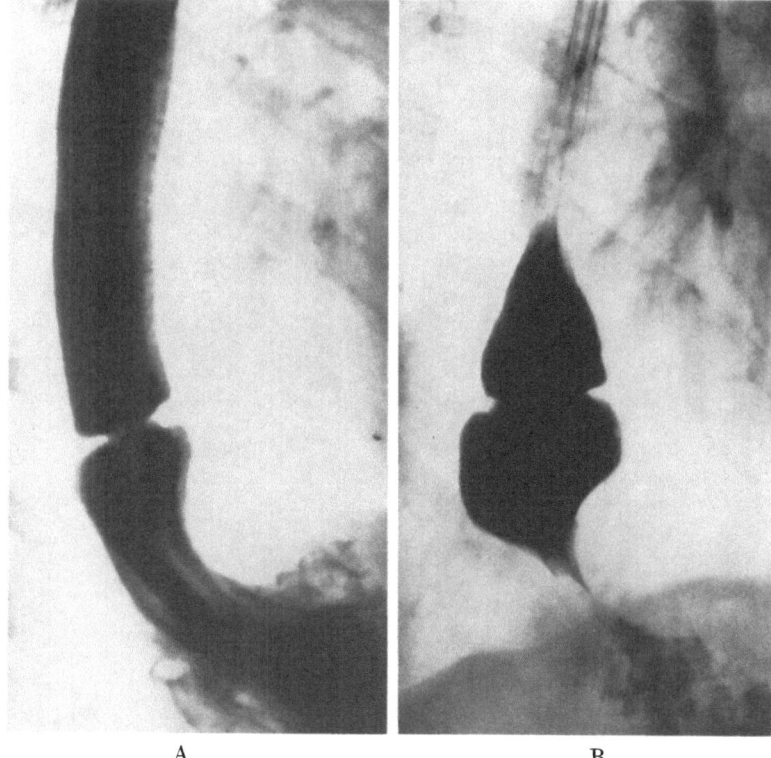

A   B

Fig. 348 A and B. Schatzki ring. Before (A) and after (B) pneumatic dilatation

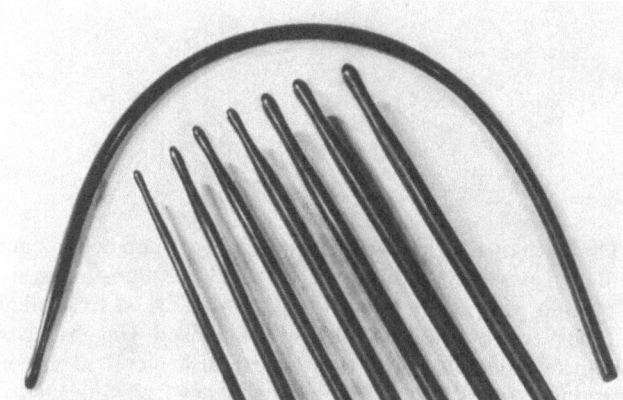

Fig. 349. Conically tipped bougies for blind or endoscopic use

a dilation is performed without analgesic premedication except when the stenosis is tight or the procedure very painful. Sedation is useful in anxious patients. Local anesthesia of the throat is appreciated by some but refused by others. The danger of spill-over into the trachea is increased considerably when local anesthetics

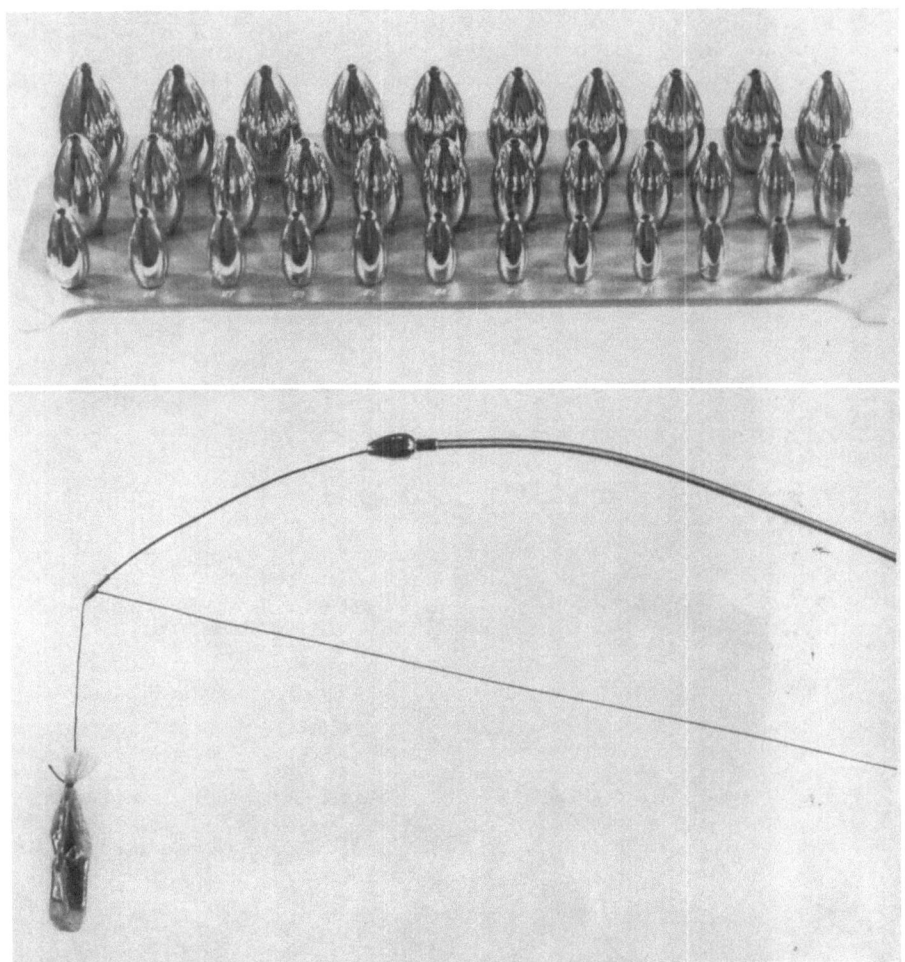

are applied. The patient is asked to sit upright in a chair with a support for his head. As a rule we use the Sippy olives or the Eder-Puestow system. The day before the dilatation with Sippy olives the patient is asked to swallow a mercury-weighted latex bag, to which a nylon thread is attached. Once the bag is anchored in the intestine the nylon thread is tightened and a metal wire, with an eye on its end, is introduced over it to a distance of 50 cm from the incisors. This wire serves as a solid guide for a coiled steel spring wire with the metal olive screwed to its end. The latter is inserted into the stomach over the metal wire, which is retained by a helper. The olive and the spring wire are withdrawn but the wire guide is left in place throughout the procedure. Progressively larger olives are pushed past the stenosis. The decision whether or to what extent to increase the size of the olive during one session depends on the resistance met at the level of the stenosis, the nature of the stenosis, and the reactions of the patient. In one session a progress of 1 to 10 units French may be made. As a routine safety measure

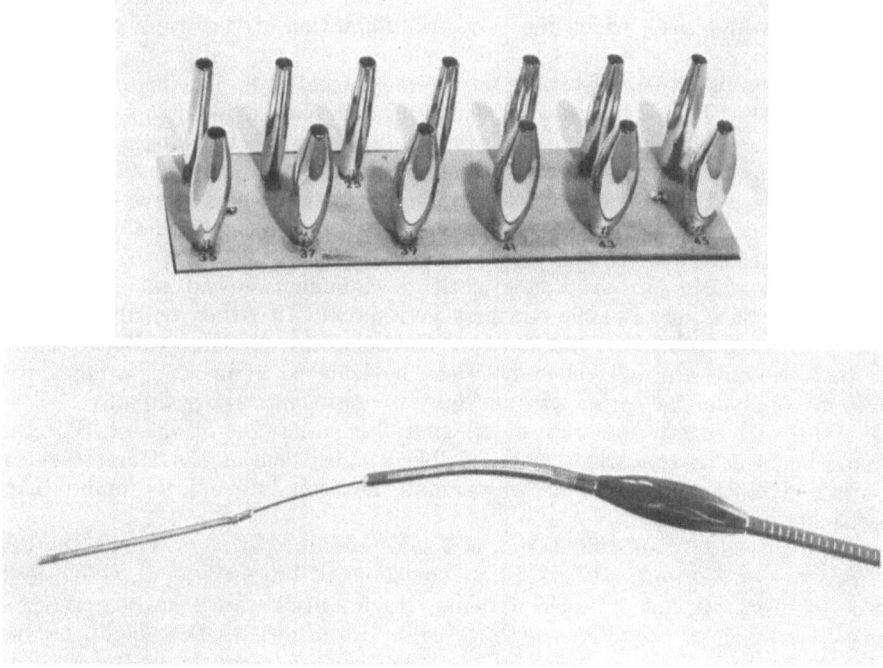

Fig. 351. Eder-Puestow dilator

the patient is requested not to eat or drink for the first two hours after the dilatation. The procedure may be repeated the next day. In cases of benign stenosis drinking markedly improves when a 30 F olive can be passed. Some patients are able to take solids after they have been dilated with a 38 F dilator; however, dysphagia for most solids generally disappears only after a 41 to 45 F dilator has been passed. Most patients are able to eat almost normally, if they chew sufficiently, once they have been treated with a 45 F dilator. Generally we do not attempt to exceed this diameter. At this stage an esophagoscope can be passed through the stenosis (Figs. 345 to 348 B).

Narrow stenoses often prevent the passing of the mercury-filled bag. In that case an attempt can be made to pass a silk wire to which a small lead shot is attached, or to pass a bougie under esophagoscopic control. In most cases, however, it is possible to pass the piano wire of the Eder-Puestow system through the stenosis, either blindly, or under fluoroscopic control. As this wire has a blunt and flexible finger tip at its end, there is virtually no risk of perforation. If that fails, the coiled steel spring wire of the Sippy system with a 18 F olive attached to it, is introduced until just above the stenosis. Through the lumen of the spring wire a Seldinger wire of the type used for catheterization of blood vessels is inserted. Under fluoroscopic control the Seldinger wire is passed gently beyond the first dilatation, or as a guide to insert the more rigid metal piano wire into the stomach. With these techniques we have thusfar been able to dilate all patients for whom dilatation was indicated.

The Eder-Puestow system has certain advantages. Swallowing a nylon thread with a mercury-filled latex bag the day before the dilatation is superfluous. The system is more rigid than the Sippy or the Plummer system and the olives are long and symmetrical, which facilitates the dilatation of very tight stenoses. In order to dilate a tight stenosis, a rigid system is necessary; otherwise part of the exerted force is directed laterally on the esophageal wall. The olive is preceded by a conical and flexible finger which has already passed the stenosis when the olive must be pushed through it. This flexible finger lessens the danger of perforating the esophageal wall. In gastrectomized patients, however, this finger may be cumbersome, as it pushes against the gastric or intestinal wall. The relative rigidity of the system, however, makes for a more uncomfortable passage through the patient's throat.

In some patients, for example in patients who underwent a total gastrectomy, a system with a very flexible end may be required. It is then possible to insert the coiled steel spring wire directly over the nylon thread. The rigidity necessary to push the olive through the stenosis can be achieved by inserting a metal wire into the lumen of the spring wire until a few centimeters above the olive.

Self-bougienage to maintain an adequate lumen has been proposed (PALMER, 1961) and can be safe when more flexible bougies such as the Hurst type are entrusted to the patient. Not all patients, however, are able to maintain an adequate lumen.

In experienced hands dilatation is a safe procedure, as is proved by the vast experience of BENEDICT (1966a, b). In the series of BRUNNEN et al. (1969), only 1 perforation was noted in 129 patients. No fatalities were seen in a series of 220 cases of OLSEN and HARRINGTON (1948). In our own series of 90 dilated patients one perforation occurred in a patient with a recurrence after subtotal gastrectomy for carcinoma. Moderate bleeding may occur in peptic esophagitis or cancer patients. Intestinal retention of a silk thread or of a mercury bag causing small bowel obstruction is an unusual complication (WHITE, 1967). Of a total of 2400 self-dilatations in 16 patients one perforation occurred as the only complication (PALMER, 1961).

Most patients have to be dilated regularly, because of recurrent stenosis. It is our policy to dilate the patients at regular intervals without waiting for severe complaints to develop again. The intervals are determined in such a way that the patient can take a normal diet between the dilatations, that he can be treated up to a 45 to 46 F dilator in one session as an out-patient and that the stenosis is sufficiently narrow to be felt on passing a 37 to 40 F dilator. After one year of treatment according to these criteria, the frequency of the sessions tends to decrease markedly in the case of benign stenosis.

Infants are often treated with retrograde dilatation, if necessary under general anesthesia (KUNDERT and MORGER, 1970). Retrograde dilatation was first suggested by SCHEDE (1883), and the first successful case was treated by TRENDELENBURG (BOLSTAD, 1966). It has been advocated for caustic burns because of the fact that the stricture is often eccentric and the esophageal wall beneath the lesion is usually in better condition. The direct method is effected using a fine caliber esophagoscope or a cystoscope introduced through a gastrostomy opening. Initial dilatations are done to 12 or 14 French. Then the gastrostomy is allowed to close and further treatment is performed perorally. The indirect method, the method of the endless string, was developed by DUNHAM in 1903. A silk thread about 1 m long with 3 or 4 lead shots at intervals of 10 cm is swallowed by the patient. The upper end is fixed at the cheek of the patient. The lower end is washed down, picked up through the gastrostomy opening with a forceps or a filiform (PUTNAM, 1967) and fixed at the abdominal wall. Dilatations are best performed from below, using gum or rubber bougies, for instance the Tucker

Soulas or the longer Aubin bougies. The procedure is started by pulling a bougie of small caliber, firmly attached to the string, through the area of stricture. The bougie is left in place for a while and followed by another with increased size. In each session about three bougies are used. The thread is left in place during the intervals.

Almost complete obliteration of the lumen can be treated with the aid of filiforms introduced by endoscopic way. A wire is tied onto the bougie, and left in place. Additional dilatations are performed using the attached thread as a guide.

A special and complicated technique for the treatment of severe stenosis has been described. It consists of inserting two esophagoscopes, one through the mouth, the other through a gastrostomy. Thoracotomy is performed and under direct vision a long needle bearing a thread is introduced through a cannula in the esophageal lumen and pushed through the atretic portion. The thread is later used to carry dilators. This technique is called the Barreto technique (BARBOSA et al., 1953; HARDIN, 1956).

3. Indications for Dilatations
3.1. Benign Strictures

If possible, stricture formation should be prevented. Medical treatment of esophageal reflux is effective in most cases. When a strictly applied medical regime fails, a surgical antireflux procedure should be considered before stenosis has developed. Old age or a poor general condition, however, may make surgery hazardous. Surgery is also indicated in the presence of severe bleeding or perforation.

In patients with caustic lesions of the esophagus, early dilatations, namely the Salzer technique performed within the first 24 to 48 hours after the accident by means of Maloney or Hurst dilators, have been advocated in order to prevent stricture formation (HOLINGER et al., 1953; APPELBERG, 1960; JOHNSON and LUKASH, 1970). The procedure is performed daily for about 2 to 4 weeks using bougies of progressively increasing size. Healing with good functional result was obtained in 82% of the patients treated by prophylactic bougienage (DALY and CARDONA, 1961). This method, however, seems rather hazardous. As it is effectuated during the inflammatory and necrotic phase of the burn, it may increase tissue damage, introduce infection, and delay the reparation phase; it is often unnecessary (BURFORD et al., 1953; HARDIN, 1956; HALLER and ANDREWS, 1970).

The early use of steroids and antibiotics reduces the rate of stricture formation considerably. It has been suggested that steroids should be combined with early dilatation. Whether this method further reduces the incidence of stricture formation is not yet clear. In cats HALLER and BACHMAN (1964) could not decrease the incidence of stricture formation by adding early dilatation to steroid treatment. In dogs treated medically and with bougienage started at the 7th to 10th day after the burn, stricture formation after the caustic burn was less frequent than in animals treated by either methode alone (KNOX et al., 1967). Out of 61 patients with caustic esophagitis treated with steroids, antibiotics and feeding tube, 55 healed without stricture, and only 4 required dilatations later on (DALY and CARDONA, 1961). In spite of the good results obtained with this treatment, the lumen should be kept patent by insertion of a nasogastric feeding tube or of a thread in order to maintain a pathway for further dilatations (OLSEN, 1969).

Instrumental dilatation almost always succeeds in relieving dysphagia caused by a benign stricture. However, lower esophageal rings are better managed by means of pneumatic dilatations. In patients who are not adequately relieved additional disturbances are often found. Incomplete relief by dilatation is to be expected, for instance, in scleroderma patients with aperistalsis, in achalatic patients who developed a stricture after a cardiomyotomy, in patients with aperistalsis of the lower segment caused by caustic lesions, in patients with total gastrectomy, and in patients with severe reflux esophagitis. BENEDICT (1966a) analyzed 233 cases of peptic stenosis; 133 of them were treated with bougienage alone; results were excellent in 55.6%, good in 14.3%, fair in 15% and unsatisfactory or failures in 15.1%. This compared well with the results in the 48 cases treated by surgery alone; 62.6% of these were symptom free, 4.2% still had some occasional trouble, fair results were obtained in 12.5%, 4.2% had daily trouble and 16.6% died in the hospital. Another 43 patients had been treated by surgery and required bougienage after the procedure. Still another 9 patients had been treated by bougienage before surgery and after surgery as well.

BRUNNEN et al. (1969) reported comparable results in a series of 182 patients with peptic stenosis; 149 were treated initially with medical regime and bougienage. 77 were much improved and 20 were later referred to surgery. Good results were obtained in 39 cooperative patients out of 45, treated with progressive bougienage by PALMER (1968). Some surgeons were less successful and could manage only 9% of their 270 patients by dilatation alone (BELSEY and SKINNER, 1972).

In a series of 342 corrosive burns reported by APPELBERG (1960), bougienage was required in 132 patients. Results were good in 86.8% and poor in 1.5%; 14 perforations were noted. 22 patients needed retrograde dilatations. Radical surgery has been proposed in advanced cases responding unsatisfactorily to conservative treatment, especially because of the risk of malignant degeneration which amounted to 15.1% in one series (GIULI et al., 1972). Morbidity and mortality of surgical procedures is relatively high, however (ZEPPA, 1970).

Dilatation following repair for esophageal atresia is started approximately two weeks after the operation, or even later. A nasogastric string may be introduced during the operation (KOCH, 1960) or one or two days after the procedure, providing a pathway for the dilatation. Silicone rubber tubing may be used instead of the thread because it is not as irritating for the nasal mucosa (MORGAN and HARKINS, 1972). Retrograde dilatation with Tucker bougies has proved to be a safe and satisfactory procedure. Afterwards bougienage can be continued perorally with Salzer shot-filled dilators or Hurst dilators, while the nasogastric string is still in place (KUNDERT and MORGER, 1970). In a series of 109 infants with esophageal atresia treated by end-to-end anastomosis, 70% needed less than 12 dilatations during the first few months of life; 24% required dilatations for approximately one year (the lumen was well established and increased as the child grew up); 6% had prolonged trouble and needed long-term treatment of the postoperative stricture (MORRISON, 1959).

In adults, dilatation of postoperative strictures is nearly always easy. After dilatation of gastrectomized patients, dumping symptoms may manifest themselves for the first time. If the gastrointestinal tract beyond the stenosis is tortuous a special technique can be used (see 2). To treat similar cases KNUDSEN and OBERHELMAN (1970) used a leading filiform catheter welded on the spring-tip of a Plummer-Vinson dilator.

3.2. Malignant Stenoses

Dilatation of malignant esophageal stenoses can be useful in some cases. It may permit diagnostic procedures such as endoscopy beyond the stenosis, or biopsy taking at different levels of the lesion. It may also improve the quality and interpretation of the X-ray pictures as a result of a more complete filling of the segment distal from the stenosis. Secondly, it may permit oral feedings to be resumed in patients who are to undergo surgery or radiation treatment. This may considerably improve the general condition of the patient. Thirdly, dilatation may play its role in the symptomatic treatment of malignant stenosis. A palliative surgical reconstruction is a major procedure with a non-negligible mortality. Bougienage is an alternative form of therapy, often to be preferred over intubation with Mousseau-Barbin, Celestin or Souttar tubes.

The Eder-Puestow metal olives are the most apropriate dilators to treat these tight stenoses. The symptomatic improvement in these patients, however, is markedly less than that of a patient treated for benign stenosis.

References

APPELBERG, H. R.: Corrosive burns of the esophagus and their treatment. Acta oto-laryng. (Stockh.) Suppl. **158**, 138–143 (1960).

BARBOSA, J. DE CASTRO, DA ROCHA, R. M., DA CUNHA, F. C.: Impenetrable cicatricial obliteration of the thoracic esophagus. Treatment by combined thoracotomy and endoscopy, with report of two cases. J. Amer. med. Ass. **152**, 1103–1105 (1953).

BELSEY, R. H. R., SKINNER, D. B.: Management of esophageal strictures. In: Gastroesophageal reflux and hiatal hernia, p. 173–196, ed. by D. B. SKINNER, R. H. R. BELSEY, T. R. HENDRIX and G. D. ZUIDEMA. Boston: Little, Brown & Co. 1972.

BENEDICT, E. B.: Peptic stenosis of the esophagus. A study of 233 patients treated with bougienage, surgery, or both. Amer. J. dig. Dis. **11**, 761–770 (1966a).

BENEDICT, E. B.: Esophageal stenosis caused by peptic esophagitis or ulceration. Surg. Gynec. Obstet. **122**, 613–620 (1966b).

BINGHAM, J. A. W.: Oesophageal strictures after gastric surgery and nasogastric intubation. Brit. med. J. **1958 II**, 817–819.

BOLSTAD, D. S.: The management of strictures of the esophagus. Ann. Otol. (St. Louis) **75**, 1019–1028 (1966).

BORJA, A. R., RANSDELL, H. T., JR., THOMAS, T. V., JOHNSON, W.: Lye injuries of the esophagus. J. thorac. cardiovasc. Surg. **57**, 533–538 (1969).

BRUNNEN, P. L., KARMODY, A. M., NEEDHAM, C. D.: Severe peptic oesophagitis. Gut **10**, 831–837 (1969).

BUKER, R. H., COX, W. A., PAULING, F. W., SEITTER, G.: Complications of congenital tracheoesophageal fistula. Amer. J. Surg. **124**, 705–710 (1972).

BURFORD, T. H., WEBB, W. R., ACKERMAN, L.: Caustic burns of the esophagus and their surgical management: a clinicoexperimental correlation. Ann. Surg. **138**, 453–460 (1953).

BURGESS, J. N., CARLSON, H. C., ELLIS, F. H., JR.: Esophageal function after successful repair of esophageal atresia and tracheoesophageal fistula. J. thorac. cardiovasc. Surg. **56**, 667–673 (1968).

CAUTHORNE, R. T.: Management of a lower esophageal ring. Mod. Treat. **7**, 1163–1168 (1970).

DALY, J. F., CARDONA, J. C.: Acute corrosive esophagitis. Arch. Otolaryng. **74**, 629–634 (1961).

DUNHAM, T.: New instruments for the treatment of oesophageal stricture. Ann. Surg. **38**, 350 (1903).

EMERSON, E. B., JR.: Teflon esophageal dilators. Arch. Otolaryng. **81**, 213–214 (1965).

EMERSON, E. B., JR.: Teflon esophageal dilators for children. J. thorac. cardiovasc. Surg. **52**, 579–580 (1966).

GIULI, R., CLOT, P., ESTENNE, B., RICHARD, C.-A.. LORTAT-JACOB, J. L.: Valeur de l'œsophagoplastie dans le traitement des sténoses caustiques de l'œsophage. Etude de 63 cas. Ann. Chir. **26**, C1279–C1282 (1972).

GROSS, R. E.: The surgery of infancy and childhood. Philadelphia-London: W. B. Saunders Co. 1953.

HAIGHT, C., TOWSLEY, H. A.: Congenital atresia of the esophagus with tracheoesophageal fistula. Extrapleural ligation of fistula and end-to-end anastomosis of esophageal segments. Surg. Gynec. Obstet. **76**, 672–688 (1943).

HALLER, J. A., JR., ANDREWS, H. G.: Pathophysiology and management of acute corrosive burns of the esophagus. Mod. Treatm. **7**, 1182–1189 (1970).

HALLER, J. A., JR., BACHMAN, K.: The comparative effect of current therapy on experimental caustic burns of the esophagus. Pediatrics **34**, 236–245 (1964).

Hardin, J. C., Jr.: Caustic burns of the esophagus. A ten year analysis. Amer. J. Surg. 91, 742–748 (1956).

Holden, M. P., Wooler, G. H.: Tracheo-oesophageal fistula and oesophageal atresia: results of 30 years' experience. Thorax 25, 406–412 (1970).

Holinger, P. H., Tamari, M. J., Bear, S. H.: Corrosive esophagitis due to nitric acid. Laryngoscope (St. Louis) 63, 789–807 (1953).

Hoover, W. B.: Pharynx and esophagus: esophagologic consultation as aid to surgeon in diagnosis and treatment. Surg. Clin. N. Amer. 35, 629–646 (1955).

Johnson, R. B., Lukash, W. M.: Dilatation of esophageal strictures. Mod. Treatm. 7, 1190–1203 (1970).

Knox, W. G., Scott, J. R., Zintel, H. A., Guthrie, R., McCabe, R. E.: Bouginage and steroids used singly or in combination in experimental corrosive esophagitis. Ann. Surg. 166, 930–941 (1967).

Knudsen, D. F., Oberhelman, H. A., Jr.: A new bougie. Amer. J. Surg. 120, 420–421 (1970).

Koch, H. J.: Acquired oesophageal strictures. Acta oto-laryng. (Stockh.) Suppl. 158, 113–121 (1960).

Kundert, J. G., Morger, R.: Zur Behandlung der erworbenen Ösophagusstenosen im Säuglings- und Kindesalter. Schweiz. med. Wschr. 100, 273–280 (1970).

Morgan, W. W., Jr., Harkins, G. A.: Silicone rubber tubing as a guide in dilating chronic esophageal stricture in children. J. pediat. Surg. 7, 412–413 (1972).

Morrison, L. E.: Experiences with dilatation of the esophagus following surgery for esophageal atresia. Ann. Otol. (St. Louis) 68, 580–595 (1959).

Mossberg, S. M.: The columnar-lined esophagus (Barrett syndrome)—an acquired condition? Gastroenterology 50, 671–676 (1966).

Nagler, R., Spiro, H. M.: Persistent gastroesophageal reflux during prolonged gastric intubation. New Engl. J. Med. 269, 495–500 (1965).

Olsen, A. M.: Dysphagia and esophageal obstruction. In: Current therapy, section 5: The digestive system, p. 308–312. Philadelphia-London-Toronto: W. B. Saunders Comp. 1969.

Olsen, A. M., Harrington, S. W. J.: Esophageal hiatal hernias of the short esophagus type; etiologic and therapeutic considerations. J. thorac. Surg. 17, 189–209 (1948).

Palmer, E. D.: Management of esophageal stricture in the elderly patient. Arch. Otolaryng. 74, 703–706 (1961).

Palmer, E. D.: The hiatus hernia-esophagitis-esophageal stricture complex: twenty year prospective study. Amer. J. Med. 44, 566–579 (1968).

Purton, T.: An extraordinary case of distension of the oesophagus, forming a sac, extending from two inches below the pharynx to the cardia orifice of the stomach. London Med. Phys. J. 46, 540–542 (1821).

Putnam, T. C.: Placement of an esophageal string for retrograde dilatation. Surg. Gynec. Obstet. 124, 840–841 (1967).

Rider, J. A., Moeller, H. C., Puletti, E. J., Desai, D. C.: Treatment of post-operative esophageal stricture by dilatation with metal olive bougies. Gastrointest. Endoscopy 15, 151–155 (1969).

Shaw, R. R., Paulson, D. L., Siebel, E. K.: Congenital atresia of the esophagus with tracheo-esophageal fistula. Treatment of surgical complications. Ann. Surg. 142, 204–213 (1955).

Smith, R. A., Nelson, C. S.: Oesophageal obstruction following hyperemesis gravidarum. Thorax 20, 528–531 (1965).

White, J. F.: An unusual complication of esophageal dilatation. Arch. Otolaryng. 85, 416–417 (1967).

Zeppa, R.: Surgical therapy of esophageal strictures. Mod. Treatm. 7, 1204–1216 (1970).

Chapter 14

Acquired Esophageal Fistula

K. Geboes and P. Valembois

With 3 Figures

1. Esophagorespiratory Fistula

1.1. Etiology

The vast majority of acquired abnormal esophageal communications are esophagorespiratory fistulas. 50 to 90% of them are due to intrathoracic malignant disease (Monserrat, 1941; Moersch and Tinnea, 1944; Coleman, 1957; J. Dor and V. Dor, 1964; Sebastian et al., 1969).

1.1.1. Malignant Esophageal Fistula

In a series of 111 malignant respiratory fistulas esophageal carcinoma was found in 96 patients, lung carcinoma in 9 and tracheal malignancy in 6 (Martini et al., 1970). Rarely malignant disease of the thyroid or of mediastinal lymph nodes [such as Hodgkin's disease (Fig. 352) or lymphosarcoma] can be complicated by an esophagorespiratory fistula (Bories-Azeau and Dayan, 1972). According to Martini et al. (1970) 15% of tracheal cancers, 5% of esophageal cancers and 0.16% of lung cancers develop an esophagorespiratory fistula. The incidence of fistula formation increases after external radiation therapy (Fig. 353).

1.1.2. Esophagorespiratory Fistula of Benign Origin

Benign esophagorespiratory fistulas are rare (Sacks et al., 1967). Only 300 cases were published up to 1971 (Bories-Azeau and Dayan, 1972). On the basis of etiology the following classification can be proposed: (1) Fistulas caused by mechanical or chemical trauma (foreign bodies, caustic agents, instrumentation or thoracic wounds). (2) Fistulas secondary to esophageal diverticula and (3) Fistulas complicating infectious diseases such as tuberculosis, syphilis, fungal infection or non-specific bacterial agents.

1.1.2.1. Traumatic Fistula

Traumatic fistulas constitute about 20 to 25% of all benign esophagorespiratory communications (Mathey et al., 1960; J. Dor and V. Dor, 1964). External penetrating wounds rarely have been described as a cause of fistula because the accompanying lesions of major blood vessels are usually fatal (Coleman, 1957). Esophagorespiratory fistulas secondary to thoracic trauma occur now more frequently as a by-product of high-speed automobile travel; 9 cases were collected by Deaton and Coggeshall (1962) and 17 by Killen and Collins (1965). Steering-wheel injuries and other indirect traumas, which cause a sudden violent compression of the chest, may produce a tracheoesophageal fistula by direct compression of the trachea and esophagus between sternum and dorsal

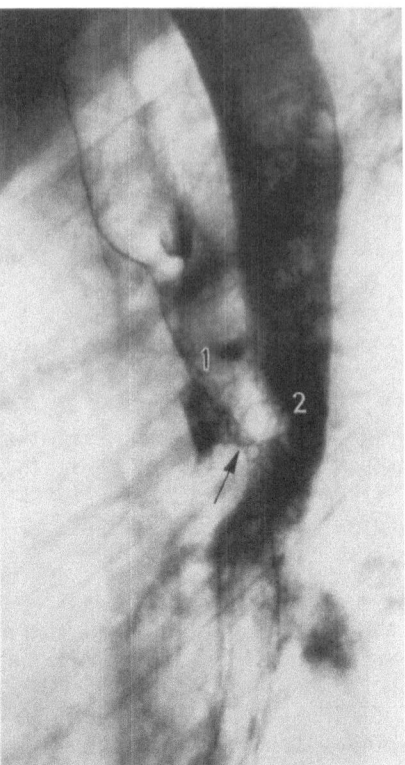

Fig. 352. Fistulous tract (arrow) between the esophagus (2) and the left main bronchus (1) in a patient with recurrent Hodgkin's disease. Biopsy of the bronchial end of the fistula showed lymphogranulomatous involvement

vertebrae or by partial rupture of the esophagus followed by infection and fistulization (Gelissen and Persijn, 1968). Esophagorespiratory fistulas following blunt trauma are usually seen in young persons with a pliable compressible thorax (Kronberger, 1962; Bories-Azeau and Dayan, 1972). They are not necessarily associated with rib fractures. Pre-existing esophageal diverticula may play an important etiologic role (Holmes and Netterville, 1956; Coleman, 1957). These fistulas usually develop just above the carina (Deaton and Coggeshall, 1962; Killen and Collins, 1965).

Operative trauma of the esophagus and trachea following tracheotomy, thyroidectomy, surgical repair of an esophageal diverticulum, Heller's operation, and other surgical interventions on the esophagus may rarely be complicated by fistula formation (Mathey et al., 1960). Ingestion of lye and other caustic agents in an attempted suicide rather frequently causes perforation of the esophagus into the trachea or mediastinum. A fistulous tract can be formed early after ingestion of lye, or secondary to stricture formation, esophageal dilatation and ulceration (Waller and Rumler, 1963). All types of esophageal dilatation can produce fistulization, especially when the esophageal wall is abnormally weak (Mathey et al., 1960). Ingestion of foreign bodies may cause no harm to the patient when they are small and smooth so that they can pass easily along the alimentary tract. Large and sharp objects and occasionally even smooth foreign bodies can produce

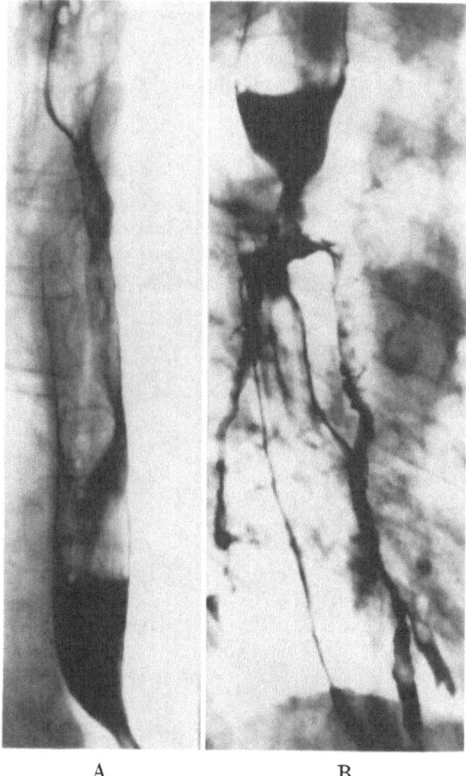

Fig. 353. A Bronchus carcinoma, causing an extrinsic impression on the right lateral border of the esophagus in its middle third. B Two months after radiation therapy, the patient developed an esophagobronchial fistula

a variety of complications but an esophagorespiratory fistula was observed in only 1 out of 200 cases (EL BARBARY et al., 1969). The development of a fistulous tract may be secondary to direct penetration of the esophagus by the swallowed object, occuring during the first days after ingestion, or to mediastinal infection. Endoscopic manipulation of the foreign body is another rare cause. Prolonged intubation for assisted ventilation may also produce ulceration and esophago-tracheal communication.

1.1.2.2. Fistula Secondary to Esophageal Diverticulum

A traction diverticulum of the esophagus, usually due to pre-existing peri-esophageal infection with subsequent contraction of scar tissue, may lead to a fistulous communication with the respiratory tree by continued activity of the initial infection, by superimposed secondary infection with ulceration or by erosion, for instance by calcified lymph nodes (COLEMAN, 1957; SAEGESSER et al., 1968). Some authors feel that these fistulas have a congenital origin (J. DOR and V. DOR, 1964).

1.1.2.3. Infectious Fistula

Infection is responsible for the majority of the benign acquired esophago-respiratory fistulas. The most common specific etiological factors are tuberculosis

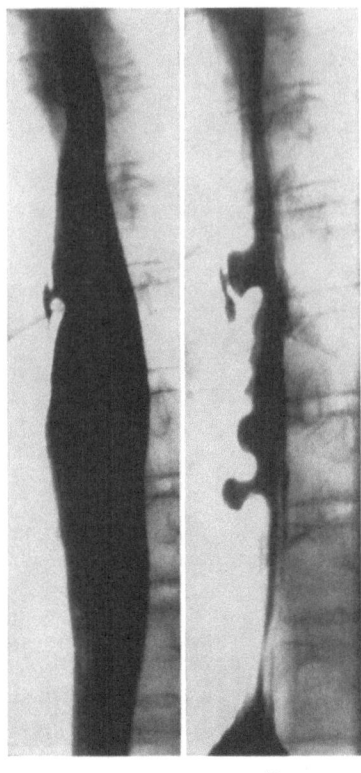

A   B

Fig. 354 A and B. Blind fistula originating in the middle third of the esophagus after mediastinal surgery for abscess formation in tuberculous lymphnodes. A Esophagogram during
filling: the sinus tract begins at the right border of the esophagus. B Esophagogram during
emptying: the fistula originates at the top of a traction diverticulum

(about 30%) (Fig. 354) and syphilis (about 25%) (COLEMAN, 1957; J. DOR and
V. DOR, 1964; WYCHULIS et al., 1966; SAEGESSER et al., 1968). More rare causes
include mycotic infections such as actinomycosis, histoplasmosis and coccidioidomycosis, Rickettsiae, common bacterial agents, thyroid abscesses and collagenous
diseases such as WEGENER's granulomatosis (KULIS and NEQUIN, 1965). Infectious
fistula formation almost always results from inflammatory processes in and around
the mediastinal lymph nodes. Primary infections of the esophagus or the trachea
seldom cause a fistulous tract. Broncholithiasis, calcified lymph nodes eroding the
trachea or the bronchi, peptic ulceration of an esophageal diverticulum and
necrosis of a syphilitic gumma or erosion by syphilitic aneurysm may all play an
etiologic role.

1.1.2.4. Esophageal Fistula and Bronchopulmonary Sequestration

The association of esophagobronchial fistula formation with pulmonary sequestration has been reported (HALASZ et al., 1962; WESTERHEIDE, 1964).

1.2. Location of the Fistula

The esophagus lies in immediate contact with the membraneous portion of the trachea and the left bronchus. This predisposes to the formation of a fistulous tract between these structures. Most esophagorespiratory fistulas are single; double or more complicated trajects have been recorded in cancer (MARTINI et al., 1970) and after ingestion of lye (WALLER and RUMLER, 1963). The fistulous opening is located in the middle third of the esophagus in 50 to 60% of the cases (MARTINI et al., 1970; BORIES-AZEAU and DAYAN, 1972) and in the upper third in 25%; the remainder is located in the lower third or the cervical esophagus. Usually the esophageal opening is found on the anterior or the right anterolateral wall. Esophagorespiratory fistulas caused by trauma, foreign bodies or cancer, most commonly end in the trachea, seldom in the bronchi (COLEMAN, 1957; J. DOR and V. DOR, 1964; SAEGESSER et al., 1968). 61 of the 117 fistulas reported by MARTINI et al. (1970) were esophagotracheal. Infectious fistulas end in the bronchi more often.

1.3. Symptoms

Though the primary lesion is frequently located in the esophagus, most complaints are of pulmonary nature. Clinical manifestations among individuals with esophagorespiratory fistula vary considerably as to degree and duration. A pathognomic triad has been proposed (SAEGESSER et al., 1968): paroxysmal cough after ingestion of liquids, episodical abdominal distension and recurrent bronchopulmonary infections.

Undoubtedly the most frequent symptom is a paroxysmal cough following the ingestion of liquids. It may be initiated when the patient is lying in a certain position, usually lateral decubitus, which makes the fistulous tract accessible to swallowed fluids. Relief may be obtained by change of position or by taking liquids in a position placing the tract out of access. Irritating food or liquids and gazeous liquids more often produce episodes of cough. The symptom is inconstant. Usually coughing starts immediately after the pharyngeal swallowing movement. In the early stages of a fistulous track, however, it may take a few seconds before the swallowed liquid reaches the sensitive tracheobronchial mucosa and elicits coughing. When the fistula is of benign origin, paroxysmal cough may be inconsequential and supported well by the patient for years. Small fistulas may be temporarily plugged by solid food, which accounts for the periodic disappearance of symptoms. In large fistulas the clinical course following ingestion of food may be dramatic with severe dyspnea and cough. Ingestion of solid food is usually easy, unless the fistula is very large. Expectoration of liquids or food particles is a common complaint (MATHEY et al., 1960). Hemoptysis and dyspnea occur frequently, probably because of associated tracheobronchitis caused by aspiration of liquid and food particles.

Passage of air into the gastrointestinal tract may produce no symptoms, although megaesophagus and/or abdominal distension due to the presence of large volumes of air have been reported.

Recurrent bronchopulmonary infections, which are frequently observed, may often masquerade the presence of a fistulous traject. Pneumonia without a history of cough may even be the presenting complaint. Bronchiectases or lung abscesses are occasionally found, and it may be difficult to ascertain whether or not these are the result or the cause of the fistula. Dysphagia, nausea and hematemesis have been noticed. Severe weight loss and debilitation usually occur when the fistula is very large or of cancerous origin. Most patients with benign esophagorespiratory fistula, however, maintain a satisfactory nutritional state. When cancer, ingestion of foreign bodies or caustic agents, or trauma are responsible for the fistula, associated symptoms are possibly more important and may mask the existence of the fistulous tract; the presence in such patients of rapidly accumulating mediastinal emphysema or tension pneumothorax, however, should arouse suspicion. If the fistula is caused by non-penetrating trauma, usually two days to several weeks pass before symptoms become manifest. An early pneumothorax, mediastinal emphysema, broadening of the mediastinal shadow, inability to allay a rapidly accumulating pneumothorax by closed intercostal tube drainage may all be indications of a fistula. Pulmonary hemorrhage is not an unusual symptom and may occasionally terminate in death.

1.4. Diagnosis

A proper interpretation of the history and complaints of the patient is often the clue to the diagnosis. On the basis of clinical symptoms alone, Martini et al. (1970) established the diagnosis in 29 of his 111 cases.

Physical examination may reveal associated abnormalities such as chest trauma, respiratory infections or granulomatous disease. Basilar rales, malodorous breath and a chronically ill appearance of the patient may be observed. Occasionally abdominal distension and tympanism are present. Patients with a positive history who can cooperate may be given a swallow of water to observe the typical coughing spell. It the swallow-cough sequence is evoked by this maneuver, the diagnosis of esophagorespiratory fistula is likely (Anderson and Sabiston, 1965). Rales may be found to appear following the coughing spell (Ono's sign). Routine chest roentgenograms with or without tomograms may demonstrate the presence of pleuropulmonary lesions, of air in the esophagus and of various associated anomalies.

The radiological examination of the esophagus by means of barium or aqueous medium is diagnostic in most cases. As the fistulous tract may vary in size and patency, repeated examinations in various positions may be necessary. With a small fistula, little of the contrast medium enters the trachea or bronchi and a vigorous cough clears the material almost immediately. Hence precise localization may be difficult especially when barium, which irritates the bronchi, is used. Cineroentgenography has been of considerable value to localize the fistula and exclude other causes of aspiration of contrast medium. If possible the patient should be placed in the position in which his symptoms are most marked; otherwise the tract may be missed. The contrast agent may be given by mouth or by tube.

Bronchography is of less value to visualize the fistulous tract but it is mandatory to deliniate damaged lung tissue and to orient surgeons at the time of closure of the fistulous connection.

Whereas bronchography is of less value than esophagography, bronchoscopy will more often permit direct observation of the fistula, because mucosal folds may hide the lesion during esophagoscopy. As both these endoscopic examinations are often negative, they are mainly indicated to obtain material for histologic, cytologic and bacteriologic studies, and to show the underlying disease. Bronchoscopic examination usually reveals hyperemia, inflammation and the presence of mucopurulent secretions. The fistulous opening may be seen as an ulcerated or a proliferating lesion. Esophagoscopy in benign fistula often shows inflammation. During periods of cough, air and pus may be seen passing into the lumen. To identify and localize a fistulous tract it may be useful to instill methylene blue into the esophagus and to try and observe its entrance into the bronchial tree

(COLEMAN and BUNCH, 1950). Another diagnostic test was described by J. DOR and V. DOR (1964). It consists of inflating a balloon at different levels of the trachea, in order to produce esophageal eructation and to localize the fistula.

Laryngoscopy may be of particular value in excluding the presence of a pharyngeal or laryngeal lesion. Mediastinoscopy may be useful to identify mediastinal granulomatous disease. Occasionally the fistula may be seen through a tracheostomy opening (in 6 cases—MARTINI et al., 1970).

Skin tests, serologic studies and cultures may be of value to obtain a precise diagnosis when infection is suspected as an etiologic factor.

1.5. Treatment

Spontaneous closure of the fistula cannot be expected in view of the recurrent infections due to the passage of food and saliva into the respiratory tract. In some cases no treatment is necessary because the patient's complaints are minor and because he has learned to take food in an appropriate position. Non-surgical methods such as electrical cauterization or application of silver nitrate or sodium hydroxide by endoscopic way have been tried. Results are most often unsatisfactory, although small fistulas (3 mm or less in diameter) can be closed by this method (COLEMAN, 1957). COLEMAN reported the outcome in 27 patients treated without surgery: 16 died, 6 showed no improvement, and 5 were cured. The results of radiotherapy were also discouraging.

The proper therapy is surgical and comprises division of the fistulous tract and resection of irreversibly damaged lung tissue. Patients in good general condition may undergo the surgical intervention immediately. Preoperative treatment is necessary in debilitated patients with or without associated pneumonia. Broad spectrum antibiotics, postural drainage, pleural drainage and respiratory exercises are often necessary. Prevention of pulmonary infection from the fistulous tract by parenteral feeding is helpful. When the fistula is small, nasogastric tube feeding can be used. Active syphilis, tuberculosis and fungal infections should receive proper treatment. Associated traumas should be managed.

The choice of surgical approach depends upon the location and extent of the communication. A high esophageal fistula can be approached via a lateral cervicotomy in front of the M. cleidomastoideus. If necessary, the incision can be extended by section of this muscle and resection of the inner third of the clavicle and the anterior portion of the upper ribs. Thoracic fistulas are approached via a thoracotomy. A right posterolateral approach is advocated, unless major pulmonary disease exists on the left (HUTCHIN and LINDSKOG, 1964; ANDERSON and SABISTON, 1965). Simple ligation of the fistulous tract is not recommended because of the possibility of recurrence. Resection of the tract, closure of the defect and inversion with interrupted sutures are necessary.

Treatment of esophagorespiratory fistulas of malignant origin raises difficult problems, especially when healing is compromised by prior irradiation. The majority of patients die from aspiration pneumonia unless palliative treatment is undertaken. Curative surgery has been proposed, consisting of esophagectomy and bypass with repair of the tracheobronchial tree (ONG and KWONG, 1970). Many of these patients, however, are very debilitated and major surgery is not possible. Usually only palliative treatment is indicated. If the fistula is small, aspiration pneumonia can usually be prevented by stopping all peroral food and drink and feeding the patient after a jejunostomy. A gastrostomy is not advocated because of the danger of gastroesophagobronchial reflux. Large fistulas are treated by jejunostomy and cervical esophagostomy (with transection of the cervical esophagus and closure of its distal end). Palliative intubation of malignant fistulas by means of Souttar, Célestin, Mousseau-Barbin or other tubes has been succesful in the hands of some (Heimlich, 1962; Kovarik, 1963; Provan, 1969) but this procedure has not been generally accepted.

2. Aortoesophageal Fistula

Acquired communications between esophagus and blood vessels are rare, and have a very poor prognosis due to the massive hemorrhage they produce. Aorto-esophageal fistulas can be divided into two categories, benign and malignant.

2.1. Benign Aortoesophageal Fistula

Apparently Dubreuil, a French naval doctor, was the first to report a case of benign aortoesophageal fistula in 1818. His patient was a 28 year old soldier who swallowed a 3.3 cm fragment of beef rib. Most cases of benign aortoesophageal communications have been associated with the ingestion of foreign bodies, especially bones (50 out of the 81 cases collected by Sloop and Thompson, 1967). More recently metal objects such as dental prostheses, coins, safety pins, coil springs and nails have been reported to cause fistulas. The next most common cause is a fistula developing between the esophagus and an aneurysm of the aorta, either arteriosclerotic, syphilitic or traumatic (Gittleman and Leichtling, 1952; Calenda and Uricchio, 1953; Salmons, 1954; Pewters, 1955). Erosion of the aorta by an esophageal peptic ulcer, esophageal instrumentation, an ulcer developing in an achalatic megaesophagus, a mediastinal abscess or a Hufnagel aortic valve are other rare causes (Smith and Brodman, 1953; Powell, 1957; Couves et al., 1958; Kittle, 1958; MacPherson and Thompson, 1958; Ullmann et al., 1961; Waller and Rumler, 1963).

Some 90 cases of aortoesophageal fistula as a result of injury arising from swallowed foreign bodies have been reported (Sloop and Thompson, 1967; El Barbary et al., 1969; Bories-Azeau and Dayan, 1972). Surgical treatment was attempted in only a few cases and survival is exceptional. The first case of perforation of the aorta by a foreign body with a successful outcome was presented by Taniewski in 1961 (cited by Valtonen and Koivuniemi, 1967). Only rarely does an ingested foreign body immediately penetrate into the aorta, producing massive hemorrhage (the so-called primary perforation, Poulet, 1880). In most cases there is a latent period not exceeding 5 days. The clinical course is characterized by the occurence of a "signal hemorrhage" usually followed in hours to days by an exsanguinating bleeding. In 50 of the 81 cases collected by Sloop and Thompson (1967), massive hemorrhage did not occur until more than 6 hours after the first bleeding. The signal hemorrhage may be followed by recurrent more severe episodes of blood loss or numerous small hemorrhages. The blood is bright red which is a diagnostic clue of the arterial origin of the bleeding. In most cases of fistulas caused by foreign bodies, the aortic opening is located 1 to 5 cm from the origin of the left subclavian artery. Less commonly perforation occurs at the upper edge of the aortic arch and the lower thoracic aorta. Perforation is probably caused by gradual erosion associated with infection.

2.2. Malignant Aortoesophageal Fistula

Fatal hemorrhage as a result of an aortoesophageal fistula, complicating carcinoma of the esophagus or esophageal metastases from other tumors, is uncommon. The first case seems to have been reported by Van Doevereen in 1789.

In 1896, 50 cases of perforation of large vessels as a complication of esophageal cancer were collected by KNAUT. Among these were 34 cases of abnormal aorto-esophageal communications. At last 72 more cases were reported between 1896 and 1946 (POSTOLOFF and CANNON, 1946; VALTONEN and KOIVUNIEMI, 1967). Although upper gastrointestinal bleeding is not uncommon in esophageal carcinoma, it is rarely due to communication with the aorta. Only one case was noted in a series of 1859 patients with esophageal cancer (GHOSH et al., 1972). As in aortoesophageal fistula caused by foreign bodies, massive exsanguinating hemorrhage usually seems to occur after several hours of more or less intensive bleeding. The bleeding may also start slowly and progress steadily until sudden exsanguination (BOTTIGLIERI et al., 1963). Penetration of the aorta is due to bacterial invasion of the carcinoma or necrosis of the aortic wall (POSTOLOFF and CANNON, 1946). Direct invasion of the whole aortic wall by tumorous tissue has not been reported, the invasion being limited to adventitia.

Esophageal cancer can be complicated by other abnormal communications with large vessels such as the left common carotid artery, the left subclavian artery, the first, second, third, or fourth intercostal arteries, the right subclavian artery, the left internal carotid and esophageal arteries (KNAUT, reported by GHOSH et al., 1972).

2.3. Other Fistulas between the Esophagus and the Cardiovascular System

2.3.1. Fistula between the Esophagus and the Pericardial Cavity

Fistulous communications between the esophagus and the pericardial cavity are rare. 17 cases were collected in 1957 by McDANIEL and KNEPPER; 4 of these were caused by a benign, apparently idiopathic ulcer of the esophagus; in 5 cases there was a history of a swallowed foreign body; 5 cases were associated with esophageal carcinoma, 1 was due to ulceration of a necrotic lymph node and 1 occurred after ulceration of a congenital tracheoesophageal diverticulum. 22 cases were reviewed by PROLLA et al. (1967). The fistula formation is usually followed by a rapid decline of the patient's condition. Penetration into the pericardium leads to a pyopneumopericardium. The clinical course is usually characterized by a sudden onset of precordial or upper epigastric pain. Dyspnea, cyanosis, shock and fever may occur. Clinical findings include augmented heart dullness on percussion, precordial gaseous tympanism, and splashing metallic sounds (water-wheel murmur), synchronous with the heartbeat and often heard at a distance from the patient. The chest X-ray shows an enlarged heart shadow with an air-fluid level. The diagnosis can be made by an esophagogram, which in some cases will demonstrate the abnormal communication. Microscopic examination of pericardial fluid may be useful (DONS et al., 1964). Although the condition carries a poor prognosis, surgical intervention may be lifesaving.

2.3.2. Kommerell's Diverticulum

Kommerell's diverticulum is caused by the persistence of the distal end of the fifth aortic arch. Eventually the right subclavian artery may take its origin from this aneurysmal dilatation and cause extrinsic compression of the esophagus with dysphagia. Rupture of the aneurysm into the thoracic esophagus will result in massive upper gastrointestinal hemorrhage (LYNN, 1969).

2.3.3. Esophagocardiac Fistula

Esophagocardiac fistulas have also been reported. Of 22 esophagopericardiac fistulas, presented by Prolla et al., 1967), 7 penetrated the heart. Another case was reported by Laubscher (1970). This patient had minimal prodromic symptoms and was found dead in bed. Perforation can be caused by foreign bodies, carcinoma, or ulcers penetrating into the left atrium (Prolla et al., 1967).

2.3.4. Fistula between Larger Veins and Esophagus

Development of a fistulous connection between larger veins and the esophagus is uncommon. It may occur as a complication of esophageal cancer. In the review of Knaut (1896, cited by Ghosh, 1972) two cases are mentioned. Esophageal tuberculosis is another cause of an abnormal communication between the esophagus and a larger vein (Grasso, 1951). Although most diverticula of the midesophagus remain asymptomatic, abnormal esophagovenous communication is one of the rare complications (Cheitlin et al., 1961; Renfer, 1951). The clinical picture may be misleading. The fistula formation may present itself as septic fever, progressive pulmonary infiltration and septicemia, eventually resulting in exsanguinating esophageal hemorrhage.

3. Esophagocavitary Fistulas

Esophagocavitary fistulas are abnormal connections between the esophagus on the one hand and the pleural cavity, an extrapleural cavity, or an extramusculoperiostal cavity on the other.

3.1. Etiology and Pathogenesis

The fistula formation may be secondary to malignant tumor of the esophagus, surgical interventions, trauma or spontaneous panmural rupture of the esophagus (Gaubert et al., 1961). Most common are the postoperative fistulas, particularly those occurring after lung resections, surgical procedures, for esophageal carcinoma, after hiatus hernia repair, Heller's operation, or interventions for diverticulum (Takaro et al., 1960; Eriksen, 1964; Bories-Azeau and Dayan, 1972). They are due to leakage of the esophagointestinal anastomosis or to necrosis of the esophageal wall caused by devascularization. Fistulas following esophageal surgery are most likely to develop when the lesion for which the resection is carried out is a carcinoma, a caustic stenosis or an ulcer, when the anastomosis is made in the thoracic esophagus and when the vascularization of the distal segment is compromised. Other factors are the duration of the procedure (Maillard et al., 1969) and the surgical technique (a terminolateral anastomosis tends to give fewer complications).

Thoracic interventions not directly related to the esophagus can also be complicated by fistula formation. 33 such cases were collected by Takaro et al. (1960); of these, 29 were secondary to surgery of the lung, one was due to thoracic aneurysm resection, another to removal of a bronchogenic cyst, and still another to lysis of adhesions during intrapleural artificial pneumothorax. Operations for gastric, pleural or mediastinal tumors are also on rare occasions complicated by fistula formation.

Endoscopic examinations and dilatations may also produce perforation and fistulization.

Based on the pathogenesis and the localization of the fistulas, several types can be distinguished (TAKARO et al., 1960). Type I is the esophagopleural fistula, often secondary to pneumonectomy for tuberculosis or cancer (MATHEY et al., 1960). These fistulas can be diagnosed early (within 3 months) or late after the operation. Surgical trauma often contributes directly to the early development of a fistula. Fibrous retractions of the esophagus, esophageal diverticula and lymph-adenopathies of the mediastinum favor surgical esophageal perforations. Pre-operative radiological examination of the esophagus is indicated to prevent such complications. The late development of a fistula is favored by mechanical traction on the esophagus and possibly by a pre-existing chronic infection (DUMONT and DE GRAEF, 1961). The incidence of esophagopleural fistulas after pulmonary resections is about 0.4% (TAKARO et al., 1960; SANBE, 1965). Type II, esophagoextra-pleural fistulas, develop after extrapleural surgery (thoracoplasty or extrapleural pneumolysis). This condition is rare and was observed mainly at the time when tuberculosis was still treated by extrapleural pneumothorax (JACOTTET, 1954, 8 out of 1500 cases; LE BRIGAND, 1960, 3 out of 2550 cases). LE BRIGAND (1960) collected 32 cases from the literature. The fistula developed early in only 2 cases, probably as a direct consequence of esophageal trauma. The other cases were probably due to juxtaesophageal adenitis, peripleuritis of the mediastinal pleura, or devascularization of the esophagus during the intervention. Type III are the esophagopleural fistulas which develop without previous surgical intervention, mostly as a complication of a pre-existing, intrapleural empyema. Chronic pleural, extrapleural or mediastinal empyemas, if drained inadequately, may perforate into the esophagus. Pleuropulmonary lesions and suppurating or caseating lymph-nodes may connect the esophagus with the pleural cavity. 35 cases have been collected by TAKARO et al. (1960), most of which were described before the intro-duction of antibiotics.

3.2. Localization

Esophagopleural and esophagoextrapleural fistulas are mostly located on the right because of the close anatomic relation between esophagus and mediastinal pleura on that side (LE BRIGAND, 1960; TAKARO et al., 1960). The localization of the orifice depends on type and cause of the fistula. After pneumothorax the fistulous tract is mostly located in the upper third of the esophagus, after pneumonectomy or chronic empyema in the middle third. A fistula opening in the lower third is rare, but may occur, for instance after hiatus hernia repair. Generally the orifice is quite wide, 5 to 15 mm after pneumothorax, 3 cm after pneumonectomy and even more after leakage of an anastomosis.

3.3. Symptoms

Esophagopleural fistulas do not conform to a characteristic clinical pattern. The symptoms can begin suddenly and dramatically or develop more insiduously. Early fistulas are characterized by the abrupt onset of pain high in the thorax, rarely in the abdomen and by sudden fever and dyspnea. Shock, agitation and delirium may mask the clinical picture. In rare instances the patient also com-plains about dysphagia. Late fistulas are associated with fever and vague thoracic pain and ofter suggest a bronchopleural fistula or an empyema. An extrapleural fistula also gives rise to atypical symptoms and should be suspected when a severe extrapleural pyothorax does not respond to good medical treatment.

3.4. Diagnosis

The clinical examination generally suggests a pleural effusion. In some acute cases there is cutaneous emphysema, in others recurrent nerve paralysis (Bories-Azeau and Dayan, 1972). Chest X-rays confirm the existence of a pleural effusion, sometimes with a fluid level and can reveal a pneumomediastinum, pneumoperi-cardium, broadening of the mediastinum or paresis of the diaphragm. The radio-logical examination of the esophagus is best performed with lipidol or dionosyl (see Radiological Examination 2.1.2.). The passage of contrast medium into the pleural cavity confirms the diagnosis (Le Brigand, 1960). The existence of a small outpouching of the esophagus, especially at the upper pole of a pneumo-thorax should arouse suspicion. Not infrequently the radiological examination of the esophagus is normal. Esophagoscopy may reveal the existence of an abnormal opening, as well as the presence of esophageal lesions. The fluid obtained by puncture of the pleural cavity may have a sour smell, if food particles are present in it. Examination of this fluid may be conclusive (Dumont and De Graef, 1961). Sometimes the patient notices that the closure of a pleural drainage results in malodorous belching, or he may feel air escaping through an external fistula opening on swallowing. The pleural exudate may be tested for hydrochloric acid. In dubious cases the presence of squamous epithelial cells and microorganisms usually found in saliva may be helpful (Eriksen, 1964). The diagnosis can also be confirmed by the passage of methylene blue into the pleural cavity a few minutes after its ingestion. Another test consists of injecting a substance with a characteristic smell or odor into the pleural or extrapleural cavity.

3.5. Treatment

Treatment depends on the size and the cause of the fistula. Complete healing is possible but the overall mortality is high (49% mortality versus 21% complete healing after surgical correction) (Takaro et al., 1960). It is important to maintain or to restore the general condition of the patient by means of adequate feeding. This can be achieved by administering a protein-rich diet via a jejunostomy, or by parenteral hyperalimentation (Dudrick and Ruberg, 1971). Effective drainage and administration of antibiotics into the pleural or extrapleural cavity are the first steps in the surgical treatment of these fistulas, but even if associated with a gastrostomy of jejunostomy, they will result in complete healing only rarely. Ex-tensive procedures on the thoracic wall to reduce the residual cavity may influence the morbidity favorably but are not curative (Dumont and De Graef, 1961). To obtain a complete healing, drainage and lavage of the empyema must usually be followed by closure of the esophageal fistula which should be covered with a pleural flap. In cases of malignancy drainage of the empyema will usually be the only therapeutic measure.

4. External Esophageal Fistula

External fistulas almost always occur as a complication of thoracic, diaphrag-matic or esophageal surgery. They are due to local necrosis and break-down of the esophageal wall, or to anastomotic leakage. (Resection and reconstruction of the esophagus 2.1.2.)

References

ANDERSON, R. P., SABISTON, D. C., JR.: Acquired bronchoesophageal fistula of benign origin. Surg. Gynec. Obstet. **121**, 261–266 (1965).

BORIES-AZEAU, A., DAYAN, L.: Les fistules non congénitales de l'œsophage. Encycl. Médico-Chirurgicale (Paris) **920 A¹⁰**, 1–14 (1972).

BOTTIGLIERI, N. G., PALMER, E. D., BRIGGS, G. W., CONANT, C. N.: Aortoesophageal fistula complicating carcinoma involving the esophagus, report of 3 cases. Amer. J. dig. Dis. **8**, 837–844 (1963).

BOWLIN, J. W., HARDY, J. D., CONN, J. H.: External alimentary fistulas. Analysis of seventy-nine cases, with notes on management. Amer. J. Surg. **103**, 6–14 (1962).

CALENDA, D. G., URICCHIO, J. F.: Gastrointestinal hemorrhage due to rupture of aortic aneurysm into the esophagus. J. Amer. med. Ass. **153**, 548–549 (1953).

CHEITLIN, M. D., KAMIN, E. J., WILKES, D. J.: Midesophageal diverticulum. Report of a case with fistulous connection with the superior vena cava. Arch. intern. Med. **107**, 252–259 (1961).

COLEMAN, F. P.: Acquired non-malignant esophagorespiratory fistula. Amer. J. Surg. **93**, 321–328 (1957).

COLEMAN, F. P., BUNCH, G. H.: Acquired nonmalignant esophago-tracheobronchial fistula. J. thorac. Surg. **19**, 542–558 (1950).

COUVES, C. M., HOWARD, J. M., AMERSON, J. R.: Fatal perforation of the thoracic aorta by a gastric ulcer. A late complication of esophageal resection. Amer. J. Surg. **95**, 878–881 (1958).

DEATON, W. R., JR., COGGESHALL, A. B.: Acquired tracheoesophageal fistula following compression injury to the chest. J. thorac. cardiovasc. Surg. **44**, 84–89 (1962).

DONS, N., ERIKSEN, K. R., RYSSING, E., THERKELSEN, F.: Pyopneumopericardium with oesophagopericardial fistula. Report of a case with recovery. Acta chir. scand. **128**, 766–770 (1964).

DOR, J., DOR, V.: Les fistules œso-aériennes bénignes. J. franç. Méd. Chir. thor. **18**, 377–423 (1964).

DUBREUIL: Observation sur la perforation de l'œsophage et de l'aorte thoracique par une portion d'os avalé; avec des réflexions. J. Univ. Sci. Méd. **9**, 357–363 (1818).

DUDRICK, S. J., RUBERG, R. L.: Principles and practice of parenteral nutrition. Gastroenterology **61**, 901–909 (1971).

DUMONT, A., GRAEF, J. DE: La fistule œsophago-pleurale, complication tardive de la pneumonectomie. Lyon chir. **57**, 481–488 (1961).

EL BARBARA, A. S., FOAD, H., FATHI, A.: Oesophageal fistulae caused by swallowed foreign bodies. J. Laryng. **83**, 251–259 (1969).

ERIKSEN, K. R.: Oesophagopleural fistula diagnosed by microscopic examination of pleural fluid. Acta chir. scand. **128**, 771–777 (1964).

GAUBERT, J., MATHÉ, J., LARENG, L., GAUBERT, Mme J.: Une fistule œso-pleurale après plaie de l'œsophage chez un enfant. Poumon **17**, 257–265 (1961).

GELISSEN, H. J., PERSIJN, N.: Fistules œsophago-trachéobronchiques. Bronches **18**, 180–195 (1968).

GHOSH, B. C., CHOUDHRY, K. U., BEATTIE, E. J., JR.: Massive bleeding from esophageal cancer. J. thorac. cardiovasc. Surg. **63**, 977–979 (1972).

GITTLEMAN, S. E., LEICHTLING, M.: Dissecting aneurysm of the aorta with perforation into the esophagus. N.Y. St. J. Med. **52**, 2517–2519 (1952).

GRASSO, M.: Case of tuberculous fistula of the esophagus and superior vena cava. Arch. ital. Anat. Istol. pat. **24**, 530 (1951).

HALASZ, N. A., LINDSKOG, G. E., LIEBOW, A. A.: Esophagobronchial fistula and bronchopulmonary sequestration. Report of a case and review of the literature. Ann. Surg. **155**, 215–220 (1962).

HEIMLICH, H. J.: Two palliative operations for cancer of the esophagus using plastic procedures. Amer. J. Surg. **103**, 376–382 (1962).

HOLMES, T. W., JR., NETTERVILLE, R. E.: Complications of first rib fracture, including one case each of tracheoesophageal fistula and aortic arch aneurysm. J. thorac. Surg. **32**, 74–91 (1956).

HUTCHIN, P., LINDSKOG, G. E.: Acquired esophagobronchial fistula of infectious origin. J. thorac. cardiovasc. Surg. **48**, 1–12 (1964).

JACCOTTET, H.: Les fistules œsophagiennes du pneumothorax extra-pleural. Thèse, Lausanne 1954.

KILLEN, D. A., COLLINS, H. A.: Tracheoesophageal fistula resulting from nonpenetrating trauma to the chest. J. thorac. cardiovasc. Surg. **50**, 104–110 (1965).

Kittle, C. F.: Aorto-esophageal fistula: A late complication following insertion of a Hufnagel valve. J. thorac. cardiovasc. Surg. **36**, 44–48 (1958).

Knaut, B.: Über die durch Speiseröhrenkrebs bedingte Perforation der benachbarten Blutbahnen, nebst einer Beobachtung von primärer Oesophagus-Dilatation und von Leukoplakia Esophagi. Berlin 1896, reported by B. C. Ghosh, K. V. Choudhry and E. J. Beattie.

Kovarik, J. L.: Palliative treatment of a broncho-esophageal fistula. J. thorac. cardiovasc. Surg. **46**, 252–255 (1963).

Kronberger, L.: Zum Entstehungsmechanismus der traumatischen Ösophagotrachealfisteln. Klin. Med. **17**, 228–292 (1962).

Kulis, J. C., Nequin, N. D.: Tracheo-esophageal fistula due to Wegener's granulomatosis. J. Amer. med. Ass. **191**, 54–55 (1965).

Laubscher, F. A.: Esophagocardiac fistula, report of a case. New Engl. J. Med. **282**, 794–795 (1970).

Le Brigand, H.: Les fistules œsophagiennes du pneumothorax extra-pleural. Ann. Chir. **14**, 653–660 (1960).

Lynn, R. B.: Kommerell's diverticulum with esophago-arterial fistula. Canad. J. Surg. **12**, 331–353 (1969).

MacPherson, D. J., Thompson, W. R.: Aortic esophageal fistula secondary to achalasia accompanied by megaesophagus and esophageal ulceration. New Engl. J. Med. **259**, 1027 (1958).

Maillard, J. N., Launois, B., Lagausie, P. H., de, Lellouch, J., Lortat-Jacob, J. L.: Cause of leakage at the site of anastomosis after esophagogastric resection for carcinoma. Surg. Gynec. Obstet. **129**, 1014–1018 (1969).

Martini, N., Goodner, J. T., D'Angio, G. J., Beattie, E. J., Jr.: Tracheoesophageal fistula due to cancer. J. thorac. cardiovasc. Surg. **59**, 319–324 (1970).

Mathey, J., Fékété, F., Lortat-Jacob, J. L., Maillard, J. N.: Traitement des fistules œsophago-thoraciques. (Fistules après résections œsophagiennes, fistules néoplasiques et malformations néo-natales exceptées.) J. Chir. (Paris) **79**, 377–397 (1960).

McDaniel, J. R., Knepper, P. A.: Esophagopericardial fistula: report of a case and review of the literature. J. thorac. Surg. **34**, 173–176 (1957).

Moersch, H. J., Tinney, W. S.: Fistula between the esophagus and the tracheobronchial tree. Med. Clin. N. Amer. **28**, 1001–1007 (1944).

Monserrat, J. L.: Fistulas tuberculosas esófago-tráqueobrónquicas. Rev. Asoc. méd. argent. **55**, 438–441 (1941).

Ong, G. B., Kwong, K. H.: Management of malignant esophagobronchial fistula. Surgery **67**, 293–301 (1970).

Pewters, J. T.: Rupture of aortic aneurysm into esophagus. J. Amer. med. Ass. **158**, 587 (1955).

Postoloff, A. V., Cannon, W. M.: Genesis of aortic perforation secondary to carcinoma of the esophagus. Report of observations in two cases. Arch. Path. **41**, 533–539 (1946).

Poulet, A.: A treatise on foreign bodies in surgical practice, vol. 1. New York: William Wood & Co. 1880.

Powell, M. E. A.: A case of aortic-esophageal fistula. Brit. J. Surg. **45**, 55–57 (1957).

Prolla, J. C., Taebel, D. W., Kirsner, J. B.: Perforation of an esophagogastric anastomotic ulcer into the left atrium. Case report and review of the literature. Gastroenterology **52**, 871–874 (1967).

Provan, J. L.: Use of celestin tube for palliation of malignant oesophageal obstruction. Thorax **24**, 599–602 (1969).

Renfer, H. R.: Trombophlebitis der Vv. anonyma und subclavia sin. als Komplikation eines Oesophagusdivertikels. Schweiz. med. Wschr. **81**, 750–751 (1951).

Sacks, R. P., Dubois, J. J., Geiger, J. P., Severance, R. C.: The esophagobronchial fistula. Case report and review of the literature. Amer. J. Roentgenol. **99**, 204–209 (1967).

Saegesser, F., Waridel, D., Aguet, F.: Les fistules œsoaériennes bénignes acquises non traumatiques. Helv. chir. Acta **1**, 1–20 (1968).

Salmon, J. A.: Gastrointestinal hemorrhage due to rupture of aortic aneurysm into the esophagus. Gastroenterology **27**, 474–477 (1954).

Sanbe, Y., Tongu, S.: Three cases of coincidence of esophageal fistula by pyothorax and bronchopleural fistula after pulmonary resection against pulmonary tuberculosis. Jap. J. thorac. Surg. **18**, 913–916 (1965).

Sebastian, S., Parker, J. O., Lynn, R. B.: Acquired esophagobronchial fistulas in adults. Canad. med. Ass. J. **101**, 517–519 (1969).

Sloop, R. D., Thompson, J. C.: Aorto-esophageal fistula: report of a case and review of the literature. Gastroenterology **53**, 768–777 (1967).

Smith, J., Brodman, H. R.: Esophageal fistula complicated by mycotic empyema and esophago-aortic perforation. Dis. Chest **24**, 66–71 (1953).

Takaro, T., Walkup, H. E., Okano, T.: Esophagopleural fistula as a complication of thoracic surgery. A collective review. J. thorac. cardiovasc. Surg. **40**, 179–193 (1960).

Ullmann, A. S., Shier, K. J., Horn, R. C., Jr.: Aorto-esophageal fistula: an unusual complication of esophago-gastrostomy following resection for carcinoma of the esophagus. Canad. med. Ass. J. **85**, 27–31 (1961).

Valtonen, E. J., Koivuniemi, A.: Aortoesophageal fistula complicating carcinoma of the esophagus. Report of observations in two cases. J. thorac. cardiovasc. Surg. **53**, 448–452 (1967).

Waller, H., Rumler, W.: Über den ungewöhnlichen Ausgang einer Laugenverätzung. Med. Klin. **58**, 1719–1721 (1963).

Westerheide, R. L.: An unusual complication of a bronchogenic cyst. J. thorac. cardiovasc. Surg. **47**, 389–393 (1964).

Wychulis, A. R., Ellis, F. H., Jr., Andersen, H. A.: Acquired non-malignant esophago-tracheo-bronchial fistula. J. Amer. med. Ass. **196**, 103–108 (1966).

Chapter 15

The Esophagus in Cutaneous Diseases

K. Geboes and J. Janssens

With 2 Figures

1. Bullous Dermatoses
1.1. Pemphigus

Pemphigus vulgaris is a bullous dermatosis characterized by the formation of intraepithelial bullae. Acantholysis, the separation of intercellular contacts between malphigian cells, is the basic lesion. It means that epidermal cells have lost their ability to establish intercellular contact points. The basal cell layer remains intact. Rupture of the bullae usually leaves large erosions, which heal rather slowly without scarring if they are not infected. The prognosis of this disease was very poor before the use of steroids.

Esophageal involvement is rare (WIENER, 1955). A typical case of esophageal involvement in a patient with proven lesions of oral pemphigus was described by RAQUE et al. (1970). The patient complained about progressively increasing dysphagia and painful recurring oral lesions. Typical intraepithelial bullae and acantholytic cells were found in a biopsy of the mucosa of the cervical esophagus. On radiological and endoscopic examination a stenosis of the esophagus was found at the level of the first thoracic vertebra, 2 to 3 cm below the cricopharyngeal muscle. Direct examination of the proximal esophagus revealed narrowing of the lumen and an irregular superficial erosion of the mucosa with surrounding erythema. Introduction of the esophagoscope produced some bleeding of the inflamed mucosa. The response to steroid therapy was favorable.

Pemphigus may lead to severe stenosis of the esophagus (TRIGLIANOS, 1970). In such cases dilatations are indicated. The diagnosis is established on the basis of the clinical evolution, the appearance of the lesions and the histological changes.

The sera of virtually all patients with active pemphigus contain autoantibodies to an intercellular substance of stratified squamous epithelium, demonstrable by indirect immunofluorescence (ABLIN and BEUTNER, 1968). The reactive antigen is obtained by extraction from stratified squamous epithelium, and from the mucosa of human, monkey and bovine esophagus.

1.2. Bullous Pemphigoid (Parapemphigus)

A clear differentiation between pemphigus and pemphigoid was first made by LEVER in 1953. He pointed out that the lesions of pemphigoid are characterized pathologically by the subepithelial location of the bullae, as in epidermolysis bullosa, and by the complete absence of acantholysis, whereas the lesions of pemphigus vulgaris are characterized by intraepithelial bullae. The disease is not hereditary and usually affects the elderly. Its course is more benign and the regeneration of epithelium and epidermis is adequate. Basement membrane autoantibodies can be found by indirect immunofluorescence in the sera of these patients (PECK et al., 1968).

Bullous pemphigoid may involve the esophagus. Foroozan et al. (1967) described a case of esophageal involvement resulting in the expulsion of an "epithelial cast". Shortly after the development of bullae on several parts of the body the patient began to complain about dysphagia. During the hospitalization he regurgitated a long thin, membranous cast which remained adherent to the posterior pharynx at its proximal end. This cast did not break off with moderate traction and was therefore cut from its attached end with a pair of scissors. Immediately after expelling this tissue the patient vomited his breakfast. There was no evidence of blood in the vomitus. The membranous cast consisted histologically of squamous epithelium which was intact throughout its circumference. The peripheral layer was composed of basal squamous epithelial cells with large dense nuclei, whereas the luminal layers consisted of partially keratinized epithelium with degenerating, paler-appearing nuclei. Esophageal biopsies were obtained 48 hours after the patient had expelled the cast. The luminal surface of the biopsy was devoid of squamous epithelium. There was evidence of acute inflammation of the submucosal connective tissue. After 4 weeks a partial regeneration of the epithelium had occurred; after 8 months the epithelium was still clearly thinner than in normal subjects. The radiological examination of the esophagus remained normal throughout. Esophageal motility was severely disturbed in the beginning of the disease but after two months it had become normal again. No stricture formation was noted.

1.3. Benign Mucosal Pemphigoid (Cicatricial Pemphigoid)

Benign mucosal pemphigoid is a chronic disease with subepithelial vesicle and bulla formation, erosions, inflammation and scarring with loss of continuity between dermis and epidermis. It may affect the mucous membranes of the eyes, mouth, pharynx, esophagus, larynx, nose, vagina and penis (Braun-Falco, 1969). The skin is involved in one third of the cases (Bean et al., 1972). Both dermis and epithelium are affected and show an increased cellular activity. Scarring is the most specific feature of this disease (Lindemayr and Lofferer, 1969).

The disease occurs mainly in older subjects. As a consequence of the scarring esophageal strictures may occur, which may be treated with dilatation or surgically (Parker Cross, 1968; Brauner and Jimbow, 1972). Tissue-fixed, basement membrane zone antibodies have been demonstrated by direct immunofluorescent staining of specimens from the buccal mucosa and skin (Bean et al., 1972).

1.4. Epidermolysis Bullosa Dystrophica

Epidermolysis bullosa is a hereditary disease of the skin characterized by subepidermal serous or serohemorrhagic bullae. Traumata, however, slight and superficial, tear the epiderm from the underlying derm and cause bullae. In some types the mucous membranes may be involved. Esophageal involvement occurs in epidermolysis bullosa dystrophica polydysplastica, a type characterized by autosomal recessive transmission (Wey and Schnyder, 1963; Bergenholtz et al., 1963; Bergenholtz et al., 1965; Nix and Christianson, 1965). The symptoms, already present at birth, consist of a diffuse involvement of skin and mucous membranes of mouth and pharynx. The larger airways, the anus and the esophagus may but need not be involved. Another type in which the mucous membranes may be involved is the epidermolysis bullosa lethalis (Herlitzch' disease), which is usually fatal in the first years of life.

Schuman and Arciniegas (1972) collected 50 cases of epidermolysis bullosa dystrophica dysplastica involving the esophagus. The lesion of the esophageal

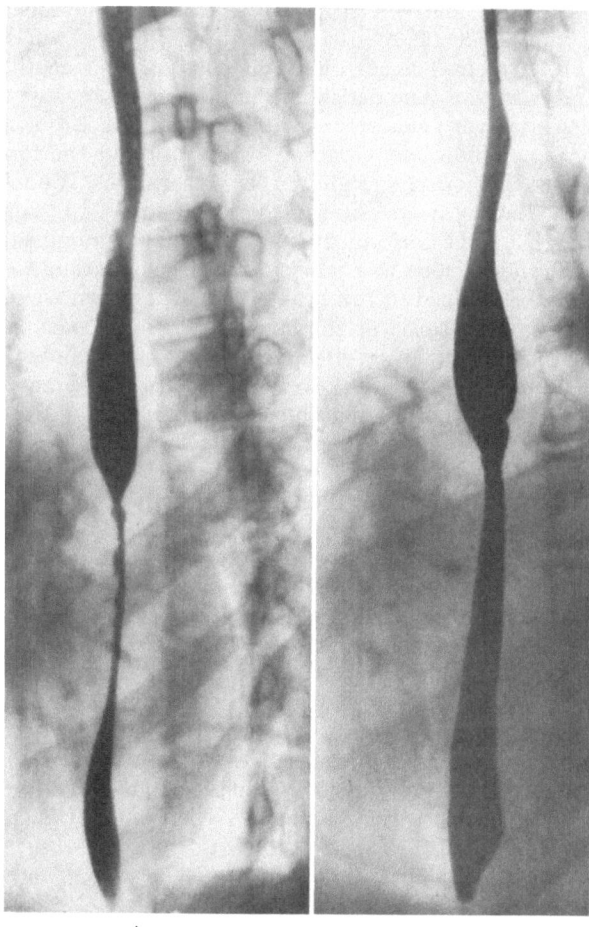

A   B

Fig. 355 A and B. Epidermolysis bullosa in a 12-year old child. Tapered esophageal stenosis before (A) and after (B) treatment by dilatation

mucosa is basically the same as that of the skin. The subepithelial bullae are thought to be caused by the intake of rough or hot food, by reflux of acid gastric contents, or by pressure and pulsations from heart and aorta. Diffuse esophageal lesions are rare. Mostly the esophagus is affected at the level of its normal narrowings. When the esophagus becomes involved dysphagia is the most important symptom, and usually begins already at an early age, rarely in the second or third decade. Involvement of the esophagus beginning at a later age is exceptional unless after a specific trauma. The disease occurs more commonly in men than in women (KATZ et al., 1967; SCHUMAN and ARCINIEGAS, 1972). At first the dysphagia is mostly intermittent and caused by active lesions. Later it becomes continuous and progressive as a result of cicatricial stenosis (Fig. 355). Half of the strictures occur in the proximal third, one fourth in the distal third of the esophagus (KATZ et al., 1967). Proximal lesions may lead to severe complications such as food impaction, malnutrition and aspiration pneumonia. During the active phase spontaneous strictures of the esophagus may occur. The diagnosis is based mainly on the clinical appearance and histology of associated skin lesions. Radiological examination of the esophagus reveals a narrowing which is usually limited to a short segment of 2 to 6 cm. The narrowed zone may have a smooth outline or may be ulcerated and irregular. The peristalsis may be normal (Dupree et al., 1969) or disturbed. Pseudodiverticula or prestenotic dilatations are sometimes noted. Esophagoscopy is not indicated because it may result in the formation of new bullae, ulcerations, hemorrhages, and even perforations. Endoscopy may be difficult anyhow because of an associated microstomia. If in spite of these inherent dangers it has to be performed, steroids should be administered (Wey and Schnyder, 1963) and as soon as friability and desquamation are observed, the examination must be stopped (Katz et al., 1967). The prognosis of epidermolysis bullosa is fair to poor because of the generalized involvement and of feeding difficulties. Treatment is not very effective and consists mainly of prescribing a fluid or semi-fluid diet in order to prevent local mechanical trauma as much as possible, of local anesthesia of the mouth and of antibiotics, in the case of secondary infection.

Slow acting heparine and vitamines A and C have been tried without appreciable result (Wey and Schnyder, 1963). Vitamine E seems to give good results (Sehgal and Sanyal, 1972). Steroid treatment has improved the prognosis but the outcome is variable and hard to predict. It is generally accepted that high doses are required (20 to 40 mg of prednisone a day for children under 5 years, 80 mg for older children and adults) (Katz et al., 1967). The dosis must be tempered down slowly to avoid recurrence. Prolonged treatment is dangerous, not only because of the well known side effects of steroids but mainly because they seem to interfere with the development of a natural resistance against bulla formation. Indeed, as the child grows up the skin fragility decreases and the dystrophic changes increase. Organic strictures can be treated with bougie dilatations though these risk to produce new lesions. Surgical treatment consists of gastrostomy or a bypass operation. Transplantation of the right colon has been found useful (Absolon, 1970).

There are reports of esophageal carcinoma developing in patients with epidermolysis bullosa (Wetteland and Hovding, 1956).

1.5. Toxic Epidermal Necrolysis (Lyell's Disease, Ritter's Disease)

Toxic epidermal necrolysis is a syndrome characterized by a diffuse involvement of the skin which becomes erythematous. The inflamed and necrotic epidermis strips off, usually after a phase of subepidermal blister formation. The etiology of this disease is not precisely known. Multiple factors have been suggested, the most common being drugs, particularly phenylbutazone, barbiturates and sulfonamides, and staphylococcal infection (phage type 71).

In some patients, mainly middle-aged women, however, there is little evidence of such causes.

Both infants and adults can be affected by the disease. The diagnosis is established on the basis of the clinical picture and the histological appearance of the lesions. Ulceration of the mucous membrane of the oral cavity, pharynx and esophagus has been noted (Koblenzer, 1967). Cases previously reported as acquired epidermolysis bullosa may in fact be manifestations of toxic epidermal necrolysis (Rook et al., 1972).

Johnson (1967) described a 59 year old patient with "epidermolysis bullosa acquisita" who expelled 4 "esophageal casts" and later developed organic strictures.

1.6. The Stevens-Johnson Syndrome

The Stevens-Johnson syndrome is a severe form of erythema multiforma, characterized by fever and extensive bullae formation of the oral mucosa, followed by erosions, variable skin lesions and the involvement of numerous organs. The etiology is unknown. The disease may occur at all ages but is more often seen in the first three decades. A recurrence rate of 25% has been reported. During the acute stages of oral involvement swallowing is usually very painful and excessive salivation occurs. The mucous membrane involvement may extend to the esophagus, causing a necrotizing esophagitis (CALCATERRA and STRAHAN, 1971). The differential diagnosis with Lyell's syndrome may be difficult.

1.7. Recurrent Aphtae

Recurrent aphtae is a common disease characterized by recurrent ulcerations of the mucous membranes. The cause of this disorder is not known. The herpes simplex virus is not responsible for it. Various types have been described which may all be manifestations of a same disease process: "la grande aphtose de Touraine".

Involvement of the esophagus is rare. During the active phase the patient may complain about burning and epigastric pain, increasing after the ingestion of food or in the recumbent position. The pain is alleviated only slightly by antacids; COLLINS and WELLS (1971) described a case in which esophagoscopy revealed three irregular ulcerations in the middle third of the gullet and a diffusely inflamed and friable mucosa in the lower third. Several bullous eruptions were noted on the left posterolateral aspect of the esophagogastric junction. Radiologically the esophagus appeared normal. The patient, a 32 year old woman, responded well to conservative therapy. Recurrent aphtae can lead to stenosis which may require dilatations (GAILLARD, 1970).

1.8. Esophagitis Superficialis Dissecans.
Benign or Idiopathic Esophageal Casts

Expulsion of the complete or almost complete esophageal mucosa as a "cast", without associated skin lesions, is rare though several cases have been reported (WILLCOX, 1949; BAIRD and COHEN, 1953; DONALD and PATERSON, 1967). Usually the patients experience a vague epigastric discomfort a few weeks before the expulsion of the mucosa. Sometimes there is slight dysphagia or frequent belching. Hematemesis is rare. The esophageal mucosa of the cast is generally well preserved and shows no histological signs of necrosis. The regeneration is almost always complete without scarring. In a few cases lesions of the basal cell-layer were found, i.e. hydropic vacuolization of the cytoplasm and pyknosis of the nuclei. Epithelial bulla-formation due to abnormalities of the basal cell-layer is thought to be the cause of the loss of cohesion between the epithelium and the underlying tissue (DONALD and PATERSON, 1967). BADHAM (1967) described an association of blood blisters in the oral mucosa with esophagitis dissecans. He suggested that both lesions are basically the same and proposed the name angina bullosa hemorrhagica. Usually only one esophageal cast is expelled. The low incidence of recurrences might be explained by the fact that the formation of groups of cells with weak desmosomes is rare. The intramural dissection of the esophagus can cause typical radiological pictures (Fig. 356). LOWMAN et al. (1969) described the "mucosal stripe sign" characterized by two lumens in the esophagus separated by a fine radiolucent stripe. Swallowing water did not remove the barium from the outer lumen. There was no extraluminal effusion.

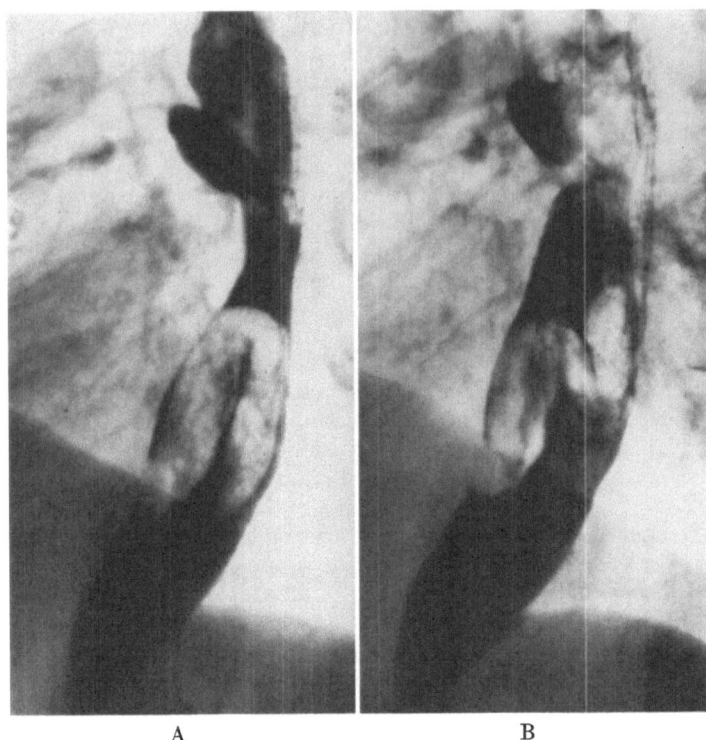

Fig. 356. Intraluminal defect due to membranous cast in a 42-year old patient with chronic renal failure treated by chronic hemodialysis. A and B show the variable position of the loose end and the site of attachment to the anterior esophageal wall

2. Disorders of Keratinization
2.1. Keratosis Follicularis, Darier's Disease

This dominant autosomally transmitted disease is characterized by a widespread eruption, consisting of confluent areas of erythema with follicular hyperkeratotic papules. The small papules tend to enlarge and coalesce to produce more or less circumscribed patches or regions of diffuse involvement. The earliest lesion consists of the formation of cleft-like intraepidermal lacunae, suprabasilar in location. Later they extend irregularly throughout the Malpighian layer.

Small groups of cells around the lacunae become separated, and form two variants of dyskeratotic cells: "Corps ronds" which are cells with homogenous eosinophilic material surrounding a basophilic pyknotic nucleus and intensily basophylic-staining small elongated "grains". Hyperkeratosis, acanthosis and dyskeratosis are present in variable degrees. Acantholysis affects single cells. DARIER (1889) was the first who described the disease, which he called "psorospermosis". Other synonyms are: dyskeratosis follicularis vegetans and keratosis follicularis. Besides oral and rectal involvement this disease may also, in extremely rare instances, affect the esophagus. The whole length of the esophageal mucosa is covered by multiple, pinhead-sized, round, wide papules which occasionally may coalesce to patches (HALTER, 1949).

Radiologically the outline of the esophagus is irregularly indented (STEIN, 1962). Usually the disease remains asymptomatic.

2.2. Keratoderma

Keratoderma (tylosis palmaris et plantaris) is a hereditary skin disease characterized by dyskeratosis often associated with hyperhydrosis and sometimes with hypohydrosis. Usually it appears as a hyperkeratosis of the soles of the feet and palms of the hands, manifested clinically by a thickening and sometimes a fissuration of the affected skin. The histological findings are acanthosis, thickening of the epiderm due to an increase in the number of non-keratinized epithelial cells and hypertrophy of the sweat glands and ducts. The disease is rare although the precise incidence is unknown because usually it is asymptomatic. The prevalence of keratoderma in the population of Northern Ireland has been calculated at 1 in 40000 (SWAN, 1956). Both sexes are affected and there is no racial preference. Tylosis is transmitted in an autosomal dominant way. In its variant, sclerotylosis, the hyperkeratosis of hands and feet is associated with atrophic changes of the rest of the skin and of the nails (HURIEZ et al., 1968). Sclerotylosis shows extremely close linkage with the MNS blood group system.

HOWEL EVANS (1958) recognized the association of keratoderma and esophageal carcinoma. He described two families from the Liverpool area; esophageal carcinoma was found in 18 of the 48 members with keratoderma and in 1 of the 87 without it. At first it was thought that the association was very frequent and that the risk of carcinomatous degeneration of the esophageal mucosa was as high as 91% at the age of 60 and 95% at the age of 65. Further follow-up of these two families and the study of other families indicated that the risk had been overestimated, but the association itself between esophageal carcinoma and tylosis cannot be doubted (HARPER et al., 1970). Besides esophageal carcinoma, patients with tylosis may also develop carcinoma of bronchus, larynx or stomach (DE ANGELIS PARNELL and JOHNSON, 1969; SCHWINDT et al., 1970). Carcinomatous degeneration of the skin occurs in association with sclerotylosis. SHINE and ALLISON (1966) described a family in which two and perhaps three generations were affected with a late onset type of keratoderma associated with congenital hernia and a lower esophagus lined by columnar epithelium. Keratoderma may also be acquired. An association of this acquired form with internal cancer has been suggested (DOBSON et al., 1965) but is not generally accepted (BEAN et al., 1968).

2.3. Acanthosis Nigricans

Two forms of acanthosis nigricans occur; a malignant and a benign form. The malignant form is usually seen in adults in association with a neoplastic process. Cutaneous involvement is characteristically symmetrical, with development of hyperpigmentation and exaggerated skin markings. Epidermal changes are typical and include hyperkeratosis, areas of atrophy and acanthosis, and hyperpigmentation of the basal layer. Acanthosis nigricans maligna can be the first manifestation of an esophageal carcinoma (JANSEN, 1965; ANSCOMBE et al., 1967); usually however, the associated tumor is located in the abdomen. Another possibility is the development of acanthosis nigricans in the esophageal mucosa, associated with a tumor localized elsewhere. This was first described by SSUTJEV and TALAJEV in 1926. In a patient with metastasis from a visceral carcinoma KREBS (1962) found a smooth and pale-looking esophageal mucosa dotted with numerous flesh-colored nodules with a diameter of 5.5 mm and a slightly granulating surface. On microscopic examination he found marked papillary changes, local parakeratotic lesions of the epithelium, a diffuse infiltration of the corium by lymphocytes, rare plasma cells and neutrophilic leukocytes. The involvement of the mucous membranes is not associated with hyperpigmentation.

3. Hypertrophic Osteoarthropathy

The symptoms of this disease, described for the first time by Marie in 1890, are clubbing of the fingers and toes, soft tissue swelling of the distal portions of the limbs, in particular around the large distal joints, which may exhibit painful effusions, a coarsening and overgrowth of the facial features and the deposition of subperiostal new bone (Hollis, 1967). In about 90% of the cases it is combined with primary malignant tumors of lungs or pleura. Maurice-Williams and Wilson (1969) collected 8 cases of hypertrophic osteoarthropathy associated with esophageal disease. 5 of these patients had esophageal carcinoma, 2 had benign esophageal polyps and 1 patient suffered from achalasia. These authors described a patient with a squamous cell carcinoma in the esophagus.

4. Dermatomyositis

Dermatomyositis is a disorder of skin, muscle and blood vessels, characterized by erythematous and edematous changes in the skin and a non-suppurative, non-hemorrhagic inflammation of the muscles. The cause is not known. It occurs twice as frequently in females as in males and may begin in childhood, or between the ages of 40 and 60.

There is some relation to malignancy. The incidence of cancer associated with dermatomyositis varies widely from 15.3% to 52.2% (Williams, 1959; Arundell et al., 1960). Most commonly involved in these are cancers of the stomach, breast, lung, ovary and lymph nodes, in that order of frequency (Bhattachary and Sealy, 1972). Dysphagia can occur in most of the so-called collagen diseases, but especially in dermatomyositis. Generally the swallowing difficulties are a consequence of the involvement of the pharynx. The incidence of dysphagia was 60% in the series of Christianson (1956; 270 cases) and 84% in that of Donoghue et al. (1960; 38 cases). The symptoms may begin in an early stage of the inflammation, and are generally more pronounced for solid food; steroid treatment is effective. Disturbances in the peristaltic movements can sometimes be discovered radiologically. Esophagoscopy may reveal a generalized mucosal atrophy. Unlike systemic sclerosis, dermatomyositis is rarely associated with traces of esophagitis.

5. Leukoplakia and Other Yellow-White Spots on the Esophageal Mucosa

Leukoplakia or leukokeratosis is due to hyperkeratinization of the superficial layers of the epithelium, associated with a variable degree of dyskeratosis and an inflammation of the underlying connective tissue. The lesions can be found on the mucosa of tongue, cheeks, lips and palate as yellow-white patches. They are mostly painless unless fissuration occurs. Generally leukoplakia is considered precancerous. It is thought to be caused by local traumata, smoking, or systemic conditions such as food deficiences and syphilis. The lesions may also be found in the esophagus. Leukoplakia is thought to occur more frequently in cirrhosis patients (Etienne et al., 1969).

Oral submucous fibrosis is a disease mainly observed in India, characterized by blanching and stiffness of the oral mucosa, difficulty in opening the mouth and inability to tolerate spicy foods. Dysphagia has been reported as one of the symptoms. Esophagoscopy reveals evidence of submucous fibrosis involving the esophageal mucosa at varying degrees of intensity in several cases.

Examination shows complete or local blanching, leukoplakia or normal appearance. Histologically there may be atrophy of the epithelium, normal thickness, or atrophy and hyperplasia side by side. Spongiosis, inter- and intracellular edema causing a disruption of intercellular contact may occur. Oral submucous fibrosis is considered a precancerous condition by some investigators (MATHEW et al., 1967). Not all grey-white or yellow-white, slightly raised spots must a priori be diagnosed as leukoplakia.

Hereditary leukokeratosis or white spongy naevus is an autosomal dominant hereditary disease whose symptoms may be present at birth or appear during the first years of life. They are yellow-white, soft lesions which have an irregular surface of hyperkeratosis, and may be found on the mucosal surfaces of cheeks, floor of mouth, tongue, lips, and peritonsillar and hypopharyngeal areas. No malignancy has been reported. These lesions may also affect the esophagus (HAYE and WHITEHEAD, 1968), and cause intermittent dysphagia. On endoscopy diffuse hyperkeratosis is found almost throughout the esophagus. The pathological signs of the disease are acanthosis, extensive intra- and intercellular edema of the prickle cell layer, and a diffuse, not very intensive infiltration of the corium by chronic inflammatory cell infiltration. The histologic appearance is not pathognomic since similar changes can occur in Vitamine A deficiency.

Glycogenic acanthosis is another benign lesion of the esophagus, which appears as a grey-white, slightly elevated discrete or confluent mucosal plaque (RYWLIN and ORTEGA, 1970; BENDER et al., 1973).

References

ABLIN, R. J., BEUTNER, E. H.: Absorption studies on antigen(s) of the esophageal mucosa reactive with autoantibodies of pemphigus. Int. Arch. Allergy 33, 227–238 (1968).

ABSOLON, K. B.: Surgical considerations of epidermolysis bullosa. Bull. Soc. int. Chir. 29 134–138 (1970).

ANSCOMBE, A. R., Fox, H., GUNN, A. D. G.: Acanthosis Nigricans. Brit. J. Surg. 54, 525–529 (1967).

ARUNDELL, F. D., WILKINSON, R. D., HASERICK, J. R.: Dermatomyositis and malignant neoplasms in adults. A survey of 20 years' experience. Arch. Derm. 82, 772–775 (1960).

BADHAM, N. J.: Blood blisters and the oesophageal cast. J. Laryng. 81, 791–803 (1967).

BAIRD, I. M., COHEN, H.: Simple oesophageal cast. Lancet 1953 II, 1187–1189.

BEAN, S. F., FOXLEY, E. G., FUSARO, R. M.: Palmar keratoses and internal malignancy. A negative study. Arch. Derm. 97, 528–532 (1968).

BEAN, S. F., WAISMAN, M., MICHEL, B., THOMAS, C. I., KNOX, J. M., LEVINE, M.: Cicatricial pemphigoid immunofluorescent studies. Arch. Derm. 106, 195–199 (1972).

BENDER, M. D., ALLISON, J., CUARTAS, F., MONTGOMERY, C.: Glycogenic acanthosis of the esophagus: a form of benign epithelial hyperplasia. Gastroenterology 65, 373–380 (1973).

BERGENHOLTZ, A., OLSSON, O., ARWILL, T., LUNDSTRÖM, N. R.: Die Epidermolysis bullosa hereditaria dystrophica mit Oesophagusveränderungen. Arch. klin. exp. Derm. 217, 518–533 (1963).

BERGENHOLTZ, A., OLSSON, O., ARWILL, T., LUNDSTRÖM, N. R.: Epidermolysis bullosa hereditaria. II. Oesophageal changes in epidermolysis bullosa hereditaria dystrophica. Pract. oto-rhino-laryng. (Basel) 27, 219–232 (1965).

BHATTACHARYA, S. K., SEALY, W. C.: Paraneoplastic syndromes. Curr. Probl. Surg. 1–49 (May) (1972).

BRAUN-FALCO, O.: The pathology of blister formation. Year Book Dermatol.; eds. A. W. KOPF and R. ANDRADE, p. 6–37. Chicago: Year Book Med. Publ. 1969.

BRAUNER, G. J., JIMBOW, K.: Benign mucous membrane pemphigoid. An unusual case with electron microscopic findings. Arch. Derm. 106, 535–540 (1972).

CALCATERRA, T. C., STRAHAN, R. W.: Stevens-Johnson syndrome. Oropharyngeal manifestations. Arch. Otolaryng. 93, 37–41 (1971).

CHRISTIANSON, H. B.: Dermatomyositis: unusual features, complications and treatment. Arch. Derm. Syph. (Chic.) 74, 581–589 (1956).

Collins, W. J., Wells, R. F.: Aphtous esophagitis. Gastrointest. Endoscopy 17, 115–116 (1971).

Darier, J.: De la psoropermose folliculaire végétante. Ann. Derm. Syph. (Paris) 10, 597–612 (1889).

De Angelis Parnell, D., Johnson, S. A. M.: Tylosis palmaris et plantaris. Its occurrence with internal malignancy. Arch. Derm. 100, 7–9 (1969).

Dobson, R. L., Young, M. R., Pinto, J. S.: Palmar keratoses and cancer. Arch. Derm. Syph. (Chic.) 92, 553–556 (1965).

Donald, K. J., Paterson, R. A.: Idiopathic oesophageal epithelial cast. Aust. Ann. Med. 16, 255–257 (1967).

Donoghue, F. E., Winkelmann, R. K., Moersch, H. J.: Esophageal defects in dermatomyositis. Ann. Otol. (St. Louis) 69, 1139–1145 (1960).

Dupree, E., Hodges, F., Jr., Simon, J. L.: Epidermolysis bullosa of the esophagus. Amer. J. Dis. Child. 117, 349–351 (1969).

Etienne, J.-P., Delavierre, P., Petite, J.-P., Sauleau, P.: Les leucoplasies œsophagiennes au cours des cirrhoses. Sem. Hôp. Paris 45, 1589–1596 (1969).

Foroozan, P., Enta, T., Winship, D. H., Trier, J. S.: Loss and regeneration of the esophageal mucosa in pemphigoid. Gastroenterology 52, 548–558 (1967).

Gaillard, J.: Un nouveau cas d'apthose sténosante de l'œsophage. J. franç. Oto-rhino-laryng. 19, 744–745 (1970).

Halter, K.: Röntgenologisch und endoskopisch erfaßbare Speiseröhrenveränderungen beim Morbus Darier und Morbus Pringle. Arch. Derm. Syph. (Berl.) 189, 401–403 (1949).

Harper, P. S., Harper, R. M. J., Howel-Evans, A. W.: Carcinoma of the oesophagus with tylosis. Quart. J. Med. 49, 317–333 (1970).

Haye, K. R., Whitehead, F. I. H.: Hereditary leukokeratosis of the mucous membrane. Brit. J. Derm. 80, 529–533 (1968).

Hollis, W. C.: Hypertrophic osteoarthropathy secondary to upper-gastrointestinal-tract neoplasm. Ann. intern. Med. 66, 125–130 (1967).

Howel Evans, W.: Thesis for degree for M.D., University of Liverpool 1958.

Huriez, C., Deminatti, M., Agache, P., Mennecier, M.: Une génodysplasie non encore individualisée: la génodermatose scléro-atrophiante et kératodermique des extrémités fréquemment dégénérative. Sem. Hôp. Paris 44, 481–488 (1968).

Jansen, L. H.: Huidafwijkingen bij interne maligne processen, in het bijzonder acanthosis nigricans. Ned. T. Geneesk. 109, 1641–1647 (1965).

Johnson, M. L.: Epidermolysis bullosa acquisita with esophageal casts. Proc. roy. Soc. Med. 60, 1272 (1967).

Katz, J., Gryboski, J. D., Rosenbaum, H. M., Spiro, H. M.: Dysphagia in children with epidermolysis bullosa. Gastroenterology 52, 259–262 (1967).

Koblenzer, P. J.: Acute epidermal necrolysis. (Ritter von Rittershain-Lyell.) A clinicopathologic study. Arch. Derm. Syph. (Chic.) 95, 608–617 (1967).

Krebs, A.: Acanthosis nigricans mit Befall des Oesophagus und Mangel an Vitamin A. Schweiz. med. Wschr. 92, 545–552 (1962).

Lever, W. F.: Pemphigus. Medicine (Baltimore) 32, 1–123 (1953).

Lindemayr, H. W., Lofferer, O.: So called benign mucous membrane pemphigoid. Wien. klin. Wschr. 77, 909–912 (1965).

Lowman, R. M., Goldman, R., Stern, H.: The roentgen aspects of intramural dissection of the esophagus. The mucosal stripe sign. Radiology 96, 1329–1331 (1969).

Marie, P.: De l'ostéo-arthropathie hypertrophiante pneumique. Rev. Méd. (Paris) 10, 1–36 (1890).

Mathew, B., Warrier, P. K. R., Zachariah, J., Ramchandran, P.: Oesophageal changes in oral submucous fibrosis. Indian J. Path. Bact. 10, 350–353 (1967).

Maurice-Williams, R. S., Wilson, R. J.: Hypertrophic osteoarthropathy associated with carcinoma of the oesophagus. Postgrad. med. J. 45, 743–744 (1969).

Nix, T. E., Christianson, H. B.: Epidermolysis bullosa of the esophagus. Report of two cases and review of the literature. Sth. med. J. (Bgham., Ala.) 58, 612–620 (1965).

Parker Cross, J., Jr.: Benign mucous membrane pemphigoid. Virginia med. Mth. 95, 337–339 (1968).

Peck, S. M., Osserman, K. E., Weiner, L. B., Lefkovits, A., Osserman, R. S.: Studies in bullous diseases. Immunofluorescent serologic tests. New Engl. J. Med. 279, 951–958 (1968).

Raque, C. J., Stein, K. M., Samitz, M. H.: Pemphigus vulgaris involving the esophagus. Arch. Derm. Syph. 102, 371–373 (1970).

Rook, A., Wilkinson, D. S., Ebling, F. J. G.: Textbook of dermatology, second edition. Oxford: Blackwell scientific Publications 1972.

RYWLIN, A. M., ORTEGA, R.: Glycogenic acanthosis of the esophagus. Arch. Path. **90**, 439–443 (1970).

SCHUMAN, B. M., ARCINIEGAS, E.: The management of esophageal complications of epidermolysis bullosa. Dig. Dis. **17**, 875–880 (1972).

SCHWINDT, W. D., BERNHARDT, L. C., JOHNSON, S. A. M.: Tylosis and intrathoracic neoplasms. Chest **57**, 590–591 (1970).

SEHGAL, V. N., SANYAL, R. K.: Vitamin E therapy in dystrophic epidermolysis bullosa. Arch. Derm. **105**, 460 (1972).

SHINE, I., ALLISON, P. R.: Carcinoma of the oesophagus with tylosis (keratosis palmaris et plantaris). Lancet **1966I**, 951–953.

STEIN, G.: Röntgenologisch erfaßbare Veränderungen am Oesophagus bei der Darierschen Krankheit. Radiol. diagn. (Berl.) **3**, 483–485 (1962).

SSUTJEV, G., TALAJEV, W.: Russkij vestnik derm. **3**, 670 (1925), cited in Zbl. Haut- u. Geschl.-Kr. **19**, 128 (1926).

SWAN, H. P.: Inheritance of tylosis palmaris et plantaris in 2 families of Northern Ireland. Ulster med. J. **25**, 27–30 (1956).

TRIGLIANOS, A.: Pemphigus et sténose de l'œsophage. Ann. Oto-laryng. (Paris) **87**, 663–668 (1970).

WETTELAND, P., HÖVDING, G.: Squamous-cell carcinoma in epidermolysis bullosa. Acta derm.-venereol. (Stockh.) **36**, 27–36 (1956).

WEY, W., SCHNYDER, U. W.: Über Ösophagusstenosen bei Epidermolysis bullosa hereditaria und ihre Behandlung. Schweiz. Ges. Derm. Vener. Colloquium, Luzern. Dermatologica (Basel) **128**, 173–183 (1964).

WIENER, K.: Systemic association and treatment of skin diseases, p. 280. St. Louis: C. V Mossby Co. 1955.

WILLCOX, J. M.: Simple oesophageal cast. Lancet **1949II**, 417.

WILLIAMS, R. C.: Dermatomyositis and malignancy. A review of the literature. Ann. intern. Med. **50**, 1174–1181 (1959).

Miscellaneous and Rare Diseases

K. Geboes and W. Pelemans

With 2 Figures

1. Idiopathic Retroperitoneal Fibrosis

Idiopathic retroperitoneal fibrosis was first described by Ormond (1948). Its cause is still unknown. Five cases of esophageal involvement have been collected by Mitchell (1971). In three of these patients it led to obstruction of the azygos and hemiazygos veins, resulting in a venous return via the esophagus and esophageal varices. In two cases the esophagus itself was involved. Obstruction of the distal segment of the esophagus by retroperitoneal fibrosis can mimic the radiological picture of achalasia (Nelson et al., 1968).

2. Amyloidosis

Amyloidosis is characterized by the intercellular, sometimes intracellular accumulation of hyaline material with typical staining characteristics in various tissues of the body. This material has a fibrous structure and probably consists of proteins synthesized by the reticuloendothelial system. Histologically two patterns of distribution are found in the gastrointestinal tract, corresponding to the classification of amyloid in the perireticulin and pericollagen type (Gilat et al., 1969).

A distinction is made between primary amyloidosis, secondary amyloidosis associated with chronic inflammatory diseases, amyloidosis secondary to multiple myeloma and heriditary amyloidosis frequently associated with neurological symptoms. The amyloidosis can be diffused or localized and pseudo-tumorous. Primary amyloidosis mainly affects heart, tongue and gastrointestinal tract. Stomach, small intestine and colon are involved in 30 to 90% of the cases (Gilat et al., 1969; Chernenkoff et al., 1972). Esophageal involvement occurs in 20% of the cases (Mathews, 1954) and frequently leads to dysphagia (Korelitz and Spindell, 1956). Although gastrointestinal bleeding is a frequent complication of primary amyloidosis, it rarely originates in the esophagus (Pocock and Dickens, 1953). Radiological examination of the esophagus may reveal only minimal abnormalities such as an abnormal barium retention in the valleculae and the pyriform sinusses. In other cases it produces localized stenosis, due to a pseudo-tumorous mass (Heitzman et al., 1962; Solanke et al., 1967), rigidity suggestive of diffuse infiltration (Brown, 1964) or a large atonic esophagus suggesting achalasia (Fig. 357) (Miller, 1969). In the case of localized obstructions surgery can be attempted (Solanke et al., 1967).

3. Lupus Erythematosus Disseminatus

The gastrointestinal tract is rarely involved in this disease. Esophageal lesions were found in 7 of the 138 cases collected by Harvey et al. (1954) and consisted of diphteroid esophagitis in 3 patients and ulcerations in 4. Six percent of the

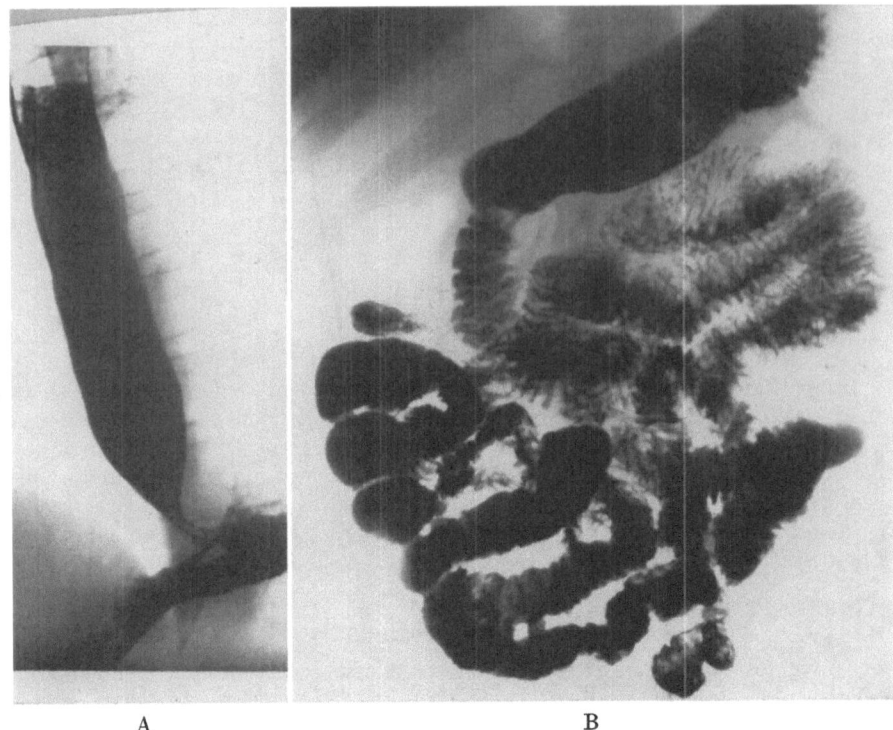

Fig. 357 A and B. Esophageal involvement in a 17-year old patient with amyloidosis secondary to juvenile chronic polyarthritis. A Achalasia-like aspect of the esophagus. B Diffusely abnormal pattern of the small bowel

patients complained about dysphagia. In another series of 87 cases no esophageal lesions were mentioned (Brown et al., 1956). Abnormal peristalsis and an atonic dilated esophagus have also been reported (Gould and Daves, 1958; Stevens et al., 1964).

4. Intramural Diverticulosis

This condition was described for the first time as a separate entity in 1960 (Mendl et al., 1960). The intramural diverticula consist of small hernia-like protrusions of the mucosa (Creely and Trail, 1970). The condition may be present from birth on (Culver and Chaudhari, 1967); it may also affect old people, but occurs mainly in middle-aged subjects. The cause of the disease is unknown. Candida albicans infection sometimes produces a radiological picture resembling intramural diverticulosis. In several cases candida have been found and lesions have been described disappearing after the administration of fungistatics (Smulewicz and Dorfman, 1971).

The main symptom is slowly progressive dysphagia, with a sensation of food sticking retrosternally. Some patients complain about pain in the upper third of the thorax after swallowing. There seems to be no racial or sexual preference (Creely and Trail, 1970). Radiologically multiple "flask-shaped" diverticula, 1 to 3 mm in size with narrow necks communicating with the esophageal lumen

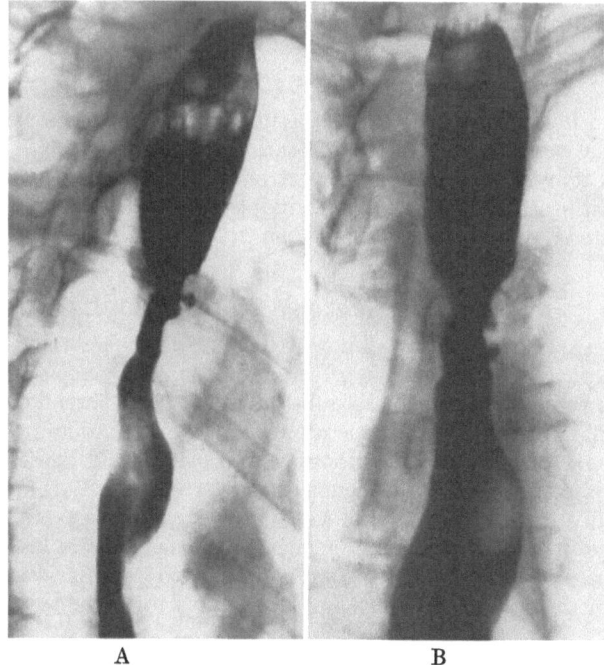

A   B

Fig. 358. Intramural diverticula in a 46-year old woman with severe dysphagia

are found, usually over the entire length of the esophagus. These are frequently accompanied by organic strictures in the upper third of the gullet (Fig. 358). Esophageal peristalsis may also be disordered. Esophagoscopy may show not only the mouths of the diverticula, but also hyperemia, edema and white spots, as well as an organic stricture which can be treated with dilatations. The pathological examination of biopsy specimens usually shows nothing but chronic inflammation. The differential diagnosis must be made with moniliasis, hyperdeveloped esophageal glands filled with contrast medium, tuberculous esophagitis and the "collar-button" abscesses found with ulcerative colitis.

5. Pneumatosis Cystoides

This condition is characterized by multiple submucosal or subserosal air-filled cysts found mainly in small intestine and colon. It may be primary or secondary to other gastrointestinal conditions such as pyloric stenosis, diaphragmatic hernia, Crohn's disease and ulcerative colitis. A case of esophageal involvement has been described by VANASIN et al. (1971). This 62-year old patient had a history of dysphagia due to a stricture in the distal segment of the esophagus. At autopsy multiple submucosal air-containing cysts were found which filled the lumen of the middle part of the esophagus. The cysts had dissected deeply into the muscle layers as far distally as the fibrous stricture. Air-filled cysts were also evident in the loose areolar submucosal tissue overlying the stricture.

6. Eosinophilic Granuloma

Eosinophilic granulomas have been described mainly in the stomach. Their etiology is unknown. A case of eosinophilic granuloma at the esophagogastric junction was reported by Schreiber (1962). This patient complained about epigastric and low retrosternal pain. On endoscopic examination a pedunculated polypoid lesion was found, without ulceration and slightly lobulated. On pathologic examination an edematous fibrous stroma with fibroblasts and lymphocytes was found, diffusely infiltrated with eosinophylic leucocytes. The mucosa of the polyp consisted partially of columnar epithelium and partially of squamous epithelium.

7. Extensive Necrosis of the Esophagus

Although vascular lesions are known to cause necrosis in the gastrointestinal tract, the esophagus is only rarely affected. Extensive necrosis of the esophagus is mostly due to ingestion of caustic substances or to the spread of mediastinal or gastrointestinal infection. In some cases, however, it occurs without a pre-existing esophageal disease and without a well established cause. In these cases the necrosis is perhaps due to ischemia (Brennan, 1967; Etienne et al., 1969). Macroscopically large zones of homogenously black mucosa are found, sharply bounded by still normal mucosa. Sometimes the necrosis is less extensive and appears as patchy lesions. Microscopic examination reveals necrosis of mucosa and of part of the submucosa as well as underlying inflammatory reactions.

8. Esophagogastric Invagination. Transmigration of the Esophageal Mucosa

Although esophagogastric invagination has been described as a separate entity (Aldridge, 1962; Bielecki, 1964), it is of limited clinical significance and its existence as a clinical syndrome is not generally accepted (Stiennon, 1967). The retrograde or descending prolaps of esophageal mucosa into the stomach is said to be the most frequent form, but ascending or prograde invagination of the gastric mucosa also occurs. The condition is due to intrinsic mobility of the mucosa at the level of the cardia and the distal esophagus.

The symptoms are atypical. Dysphagia is reported as the most common complaint, occuring in 50% of the patients. The radiological images produced by the invagination have been described under various names such as "the Saturnus ring" (Jutras et al., 1949); "a jack in the pulpit" (Klinefelter, 1956); "an arum lily" (Aldridge, 1962) or "a candle flame" (l'image en chandelle flamboyante) (Bielecki, 1964). Mostly these images are temporary and occur during a Valsalva maneuver or with the patient in the head-down position.

At operation a case of prograde invagination was found to be associated with fatty hypertrophy of the submucosa at the level of the cardia (Van de Vijver, 1969a, b). In analogy with lipomatosis of the ileocoecal sphincter the term lipomatosis of the cardia was proposed.

9. Cervical Osteophytes
External Compression

Large osteophytes of the cervical spine can cause extrinsic compression of the esophagus (Hilding and Tachjian, 1960; Hargrove, 1966). The dysphagia and the radiological and endoscopical signs they produce may even suggest a tumor (El Sallab and Laws, 1965).

10. Ulcerative Colitis

Ulcerative colitis is only rarely associated with ulcerations of the esophagus. Two patients with ulcerative colitis, esophagitis and esophageal strictures were reported by BENEDICT and SWEET in 1948. ACHENBACH et al. (1956) described a case of ulcerative esophagitis associated with perianal abscesses, arthritis, erythema nodosum, pyoderma gangrenosum and intermittent jaundice. This patient, however, did not have the typical lesions of ulcerative colitis. Cases of diffuse ulcerative esophagitis accompanying colitis have been reported by KNUDSEN and SPARBERG (1967), ROSENDORF and GRIEVE (1967) and by ALEA (1969). An autopsy study of patients who died from ulcerative colitis showed that ulcerative lesions of the esophagus were more frequent in these patients than in a control series of patients who died from other severe chronic diseases. It seems possible therefore that well developed chronic ulcerative esophagitis constitutes an additional expression of the widening pathologic spectrum of ulcerative colitis (CHRISTOPHER et al., 1969).

11. Pancreatitis

The peritoneal exudate of acute pancreatitis may migrate into the mediastinum and cause cicatricial fibrosis, leading to a smooth and progressive narrowing of the lower third of the esophagus (GOUIN et al., 1972). Acute pancreatitis may even cause esophageal perforation (HOOPER and STOKER, 1970). Chronic pancreatitis has also been reported to produce dysphagia, due to the formation of mediastinal pseudocysts (LÉGER et al., 1970).

12. Amebic Abscess

BAKER and MURRAY (1969) described a patient with an amebic abscess of the left hepatic lobe which caused compression and obstruction of the distal end of the esophagus. Both the dysphagia and the external compression disappeared after the aspiration of the abscess.

13. Worms
13.1. Hydatid Cyst

A hydatid cyst may involve the esophagus and even perforate into the lumen (TRENTA and BIRARELLI, 1960). On radiological and endoscopical examination it resembles a benign tumor.

13.2. Spirocerca Lupus

The esophagus can also play a role in the "life cycle" of worms. Spirocerca lupus, a nematode usually found in dogs and in wild Canidae, lives in its adult stage in submucosal nodules of the terminal segment of the esophagus. Its eggs are laid in the esophageal lumen (MURRAY, 1968).

14. Ectopic Tissues
14.1. Primary Melanosis of the Esophagus

Typical melanoblasts with melanin granules and dendrites have been found in the esophageal mucosa. In a systematic study of the esophagus by means of the Swiss Roll technique, melanoblasts were found in 4 out of 100 non-selected autopsies (DE LA PAVA et al., 1963). The pigment was localized in the basal layer of the mucosa in areas 1 to 3 cm long. In two cases these areas were found in the upper third of the esophagus, in two others in the lower third. On macroscopic examination the esophagus appeared normal. The presence of melanoblasts in the esophageal mucosa suggests that this is indeed possible. The question has been raised whether or not malignant melanomas ever originate in the esophagus.

14.2. Sebaceous Glands

A similar systematic study of the esophagus revealed sebaceous glands at different levels of the gullet in 2% of the cases (De la Pava and Pickren, 1962). The presence of these glands in the mucosae of mouth, salivary glands, lips, prepuce and vulva has been described before and is known as Fordyce's syndrome.

14.3. Liver Tissue

Jimenez and Hayward (1971) reported the presence of ectopic liver tissue in the esophageal wall. They described a 70 year old patient with progressive dysphagia of three years duration. On radiological examination the distal third of the esophagus was found to be almost completely obstructed by a tumor, which on operation was found to consist of liver tissue.

14.4. Pancreatic Tissue

The presence of aberrant pancreatic tissue in the thorax is exceedingly rare. Massive upper-gastrointestinal bleeding caused by ectopic pancreatic tissue of the esophagus has been reported by Razi (1966). Baar and d'Abreu (1949) have reported on a 6 year old girl with recurrent pneumonia who had an epiphrenic esophageal diverticulum containing pancreatic tissue. Tilson and Touloukian (1972) collected 5 cases from the literature and added another of a two year old girl with multiple congenital anomalies. Barium swallow revealed a mediastinal mass connected by a fistulous tract to the esophagus. Exploration of the mediastinum showed that the mass was 8 cm in diameter and formed the anterior wall of the esophagus and proximal stomach. On microscopic examination it was found to consist of ectopic pancreatic tissue.

14.5. Heterotopic Gastric Mucosa

Gastric mucosa has been found in the esophagus mainly in the lower third, but it may also be present in other locations. Besides the heterotopic gastric mucosa which can be found in the condition called "the lower esophagus lined by columnar epithelium", there are also instances of ectopic islets of gastric mucosa at different levels of the gullet (Emery and Haddadin, 1971). There has been a case report of a 23 day old child who died suddenly as a result of aspiration of large quantities of mucus secreted by gastric glands high in the gullet (Libcke, 1969). According to Foxen (1957) the secretions of aberrant gastric mucosa may lead to spasm of the cricopharyngeal muscle and dysphagia. Another child was described with a complete obstruction of the esophagus due to the presence of a congenital membrane consisting of gastric glands and smooth muscle tissue (Schwartz, 1961).

14.6. Tracheobronchial Remnants

Kumar (1962) reported on a 10 month old child with a congenital stenosis of the esophagus caused by a cartilaginous ring, resembling a trachea ring, in the distal third of the esophagus. The radiological picture mimicked that of achalasia. Two other cases were reported by PAULINO et al. (1963). A constricting band containing tracheobronchial remnants (respiratory glands and epithelium) was the cause of dysphagia in another, one year old girl (FONKALSRUD, 1972).

14.7. Aberrant Origin of Right Main Bronchus

Exceptionally the right main bronchus may originate from the gullet. NIKAIDO and SWENSON (1971) collected from the literature 5 cases and added one of their own. Respiratory difficulties, feeding problems, decreased breath sounds on the right side of the chest and a shift of the heart to the right side of the thorax were the main symptoms.

14.8. Thyroid Tissue

In a patient who was admitted to the hospital because of acute dysphagia, endoscopic examination revealed a hard bleeding tumor which completely obstructed the esophagus and consisted of thyroid tissue. The tumor originated on the mucosal side of the esophagus (ORSO, 1970).

References

ACHENBACH, H., LYNCH, J. P., DWIGHT, R. W.: Idiopathic ulcerative esophagitis. Report of a case. New Engl. J. Med. **255**, 456–459 (1956).

ALDRIDGE, N. H.: Transmigration of the lower esophageal mucosa. Radiology **79**, 962–968 (1962).

ALEA, J. A.: Dysphagia and ulcerative colitis. Gastrointest. Endoscopy **16**, 111–113 (1969).

ANDRESS, M.: Submucosal haematoma of the oesophagus due to anticoagulant therapy. Report of a case. Acta radiol. Diagn. **11**, 216–219 (1971).

BAAR, H. S., D'ABREU, A. L.: Duplications of foregut; superior accessory lung (2 cases); epiphrenic oesophageal diverticulum; intrapericardial teratoid tumour, and oesophageal cyst. Brit. J. Surg. **37**, 220–230 (1949).

BAKER, N. M., MURRAY, J. A.: Oesophageal obstruction due to an amoebic liver abscess. Cent. Afr. J. Med. **15**, 129–131 (1969).

BENEDICT, E., SWEET, R.: Benign stricture of the esophagus with special reference to esophagitis, hiatus hernia, esophageal ulcer and duodenal ulcer. Gastroenterology **11**, 618–628 (1948).

BIELECKI, M.: Les invaginations œsophago-gastriques. Aspects radiologiques et discussion pathogénique. Ann. Radiol. **7**, 39–56 (1964).

BRENNAN, J. L.: Case of extensive necrosis of the oesophageal mucosa following hypothermia. J. clin. Path. **20**, 581–584 (1967).

BROWN, C. H., SHIREY, E. K., HASERICK, J. R.: Gastrointestinal manifestations of systemic lupus erythematosus. Gastroenterology **31**, 649–664 (1956).

BROWN, J.: Primary amyloidosis. Clin. Radiol. **15**, 358–367 (1964).

CHEN, P.: Spontaneous hematoma of the esophagus. A complication of uremia. Radiology **100**, 281–282 (1971).

CHERNENKOFF, R. M., COSTOPOULOS, L. B., BAIN, G. O.: Gastrointestinal manifestations of primary amyloidosis. Canad. med. Ass. J. **106**, 567–569 (1972).

CHRISTOPHER, N. L., WATSON, D. W., FARBER, E. R.: Relationship of chronic ulcerative esophagitis to ulcerative colitis. Ann. intern. Med. **70**, 971–976 (1969).

CREELY, J. J., TRAIL, M. L.: Intramural diverticulosis of the esophagus. Sth. med. J. (Bgham, Ala.) **63**, 1257–1260 (1970).

CULVER, G. J., CHAUDHARI, K. R.: Intramural esophageal diverticulosis. Amer. J. Roentgenol. **99**, 210–211 (1967).

DE LA PAVA, S., NIGOGOSYAN, G., PICKREN, J. W., CABRERA, A.: Melanosis of the esophagus. Cancer (Philad.) **16**, 48–50 (1963).

DE LA PAVA, S., PICKREN, J. W.: Ectopic sebaceous glands in the esophagus. Arch. Path. **73**, 397–399 (1962).

DINES, D. E., ANDERSON, M. W.: Giant left atrium as a cause of dysphagia. Ann. intern. Med. **65**, 758–761 (1966).

El-Sallab, R. A., Laws, J. W.: Oesophageal and tracheal pseudo-tumours due to anterior cervical osteophytes. Brit. J. Radiol. **38**, 682–684 (1965).

Emery, J. L., Haddadin, A. J.: Gastric-type epithelium in the upper esophageal pouch in children with tracheoesophageal fistula. J. pediat. Surg. **6**, 449–453 (1971).

Etienne, J.-P., Roge, J., Delavierre, P., Veassier, P.: Nécroses de l'œsophage d'origine vasculaire. Sem. Hôp. Paris **45**, 1599–1606 (1969).

Fonkalsrud, E. W.: Esophageal stenosis due to tracheobronchial remnants. Amer. J. Surg. **124**, 101–103 (1972).

Forrester, R. M., Cohen, S. J.: Esophageal atresia associated with an anorectal anomaly and probable laryngeal fissure in three siblings. J. pediat. Surg. **5**, 674–675 (1970).

Foxen, E. H. M.: Ectopic gastric mucosa in the cervical esophagus, a possible cause of dysphagia. J. Laryng. **71**, 419–424 (1957).

Gilat, T., Revach, M., Sohar, E.: Deposition of amyloid in the gastrointestinal tract. Gut **10**, 98–104 (1969).

Gouin, B., Gosset, F., Hardouin, J. P.: Dysphagie et pancréatite chronique. Nouv. Presse Méd. **1**, 2550 (1972).

Gould, D. M., Daves, M. L.: Review of roentgen findings in systemic lupus erythematosus. Amer. J. med. Sci. **235**, 596–610 (1958).

Hargrove, M. D.: Dysphagia associated with inflammatory reaction within the esophagus at the level of a vertebral spur. Gastrointest. Endoscopy **13**, 28–39 (1966).

Harvey (McGehee), A., Shulman, L. E., Tumulty, P. A., Conley, E. L., Schoenrich, E. H.: Systemic lupus erythematosus: review of the literature and clinical analysis of 138 cases. Medicine (Baltimore) **33**, 291–437 (1954).

Heitzman, E. J., Heitzman, G. C., Elliott, C. F.: Primary esophageal amyloidosis. Arch. intern. Med. **109**, 595–600 (1962).

Hilding, D. A., Tachdjian, M. O.: Dysphagia and hypertrophic spurring of the cervical spine. New Engl. J. Med. **263**, 11–14 (1960).

Hooper, J. C., Stoker, T. A. M.: Rupture of the oesophagus associated with acute pancreatitis. Brit. J. clin. Pract. **24**, 481–484 (1970).

Jimenez, A. R., Hayward, R. H.: Ectopic liver. A cause of esophageal obstruction. Ann. thorac. Surg. **12**, 300–304 (1971).

Jutras, A., Levrier, P., Longtin, M.: Étude radiologique de l'œsophage para-diaphragmatique et du cardia. J. Radiol. Électrol. **30**, 373–416 (1949).

Klinefelter, E. W.: Invagination of the esophagus in hiatus hernia. Radiology **67**, 562–568 (1956).

Knudsen, K. B., Sparberg, M.: Ulcerative esophagitis and ulcerative colitis. J. Amer. med. Ass. **201**, 154 (1967).

Korelitz, B. I., Spindell, L. N.: Gastrointestinal amyloidosis. J. Mt Sinai Hosp. **23**, 683–695 (1956).

Kumar, R.: A case of congenital oesophageal stricture due to a cartilaginous ring. Brit. J. Surg. **49**, 533–534 (1962).

Léger, L., Pagniez, G., Lenriot, J.-P.: Dysphagie révélatrice d'une pancréatite chronique. A propos de 2 observations de faux kystes médiastinaux. J. Chir. (Paris) **99**, 217–234 (1970).

Libcke, J. H.: Heterotopic gastric mucosa in the cervical esophagus, a possible cause of fatal aspiration. Pediatrics **44**, 447–448 (1969).

Longley, E. O.: Oesophageal compression due to silicotic mediastinal lymph glands. Trans. Soc. Occup. Med. **20**, 69 (1970).

Mathews, W. H.: Primary systemic amyloidosis. Amer. J. med. Sci. **228**, 317–333 (1954).

Mendl, R., McKay, J. M., Tanner, C. M.: Intramural diverticulosis of the oesophagus and Rokitansky-Aschoff sinuses in the gall-bladder. Brit. J. Radiol. **33**, 496–501 (1960).

Miller, R. H.: Amyloid disease. An unusual cause of megalo-oesophagus. S. Afr. med. J. **43**, 1202–1203 (1969).

Mitchell, R. J.: Alimentary complications of non-malignant retroperitoneal fibrosis. Brit. J. Surg. **58**, 254–256 (1971).

Murray, M.: Incidence and pathology of Spirocerca Lupi in Kenya. J. comp. Path. **78**, 401–405 (1968).

Nelson, R. M., Jenson, C. B., Horsley, B. L., Ershler, I.: Idiopathic retroperitoneal fibrosis producing distal esophageal obstruction. J. thorac. cardiovasc. Surg. **55**, 216–224 (1968).

Nikaido, H., Swenson, O.: The ectopic origin of the right main bronchus from the esophagus. A case of pneumonectomy in a neonate. J. thorac. cardiovasc. Surg. **62**, 151–160 (1971).

Nye, S. W., Chittayasothorn, K.: Ceroid in the gastrointestinal smooth muscle of the Thai-Lao ethnic group. Amer. J. Path. **51**, 287–299 (1967).

Ormond, J. K.: Bilateral ureteral obstruction due to envelopment and compression by inflammatory retroperitoneal process. J. Urol. (Baltimore) **59**, 1072–1079 (1948).

ORSO, L.: Speiseröhrenverschluß verursachende Schilddrüsenwucherung. HNO (Berl.) 18, 53–55 (1970).

PAULINO, F., ROSELLI, A., APRIGLIANO, F.: Congenital esophageal stricture due to tracheo-bronchial remnants. Surgery 53, 547–550 (1963).

POCOCK, D. S., DICKENS, J.: Paramyloidosis with diabetes mellitus and gastrointestinal hemorrhage. New Engl. J. Med. 248, 359–363 (1953).

RAZI, M. D.: Ectopic pancreatic tissue of esophagus with massive upper gastrointestinal bleeding. Arch. Surg. 92, 101–104 (1966).

ROSENDORFF, C., GRIEVE, W.: Ulcerative oesophagitis with ulcerative colitis. Gut 8, 344–347 (1967).

SCHREIBER, M. H.: Granuloma of the esophagogastric junction with eosinophilic infiltration. Gastroenterology 43, 206–211 (1962).

SCHWARTZ, S. I.: Congenital membranous obstruction of esophagus. Arch. Surg. 85, 480–482 (1962).

SMULEWICZ, J. J., DORFMAN, J.: Esophageal intramural diverticulosis: A re-evaluation. Radiology 101, 527–529 (1971).

SOLANKE, T. F., OLURIN, E. O., NWAKONOBI, F., UDEOZO, I. O. K.: Primary amyloid tumour of the oesophagus treated by colon transplant. Brit. J. Surg. 54, 943–946 (1967).

STEVENS, M. B., HOOKMAN, P., SIEGEL, C. I., ESTERLY, J. R., SHULMAN, L. E., HENDRIX, T. R.: Aperistalsis of the esophagus in patients with connective-tissue disorders and Raynaud's phenomenon. New Engl. J. Med. 270, 1218–1222 (1964).

STIENNON, O. A.: The "Captive bolus" test and the pinchcock at the diaphragm. An esophageal pump and some non-diseases of the esophagus. Amer. J. Roentgenol. 99, 223–232 (1967).

TILSON, M. D., TOULOUKIAN, R. J.: Mediastinal enteric sequestration with aberrant pancreas: A formes frustes of the intralobar sequestration. Ann. Surg. 176, 669–671 (1972).

TRENTA, A., BIRARELLI, B.: On a case of perforated echinococeal cysts in the esophagus with successive appearance of a tumor in the same portion of the esophagus. Radiol. med. (Torino) 46, 380–384 (1960).

VANASIN, B., WRIGHT, J. R., SCHUSTER, M. M.: Pneumatosis cystoides esophagi. Case report supporting theory of submucosal spread. J. Amer. med. Ass. 217, 76–77 (1971).

VIJVER, W. VAN DE: Hypertrophie des lèvres du cardia et prolapsus muqueux de l'œsophage. Acta gastro-ent. belg. 32, 662–669 (1969a).

VIJVER, W. VAN DE: Hypertrophie graisseuse et prolapsus des lèvres du cardia. J. belge Radiol. 52, fasc. 3 (1969b).

ZATZKIN, H. R., GREEN, S., LAVINE, J. J.: Esophageal intramural diverticulosis. Radiology 90, 1193–1194 (1968).

Subject Index

Abdominal esophagus
   importance in gastroesophageal sphincter
      competence   51, 423, 424, 425
   in neonatal infants   380, 494
Abdominal pressure, effect on gastroesophageal sphincter   56
Abrasive techniques for cytology   219
Abscess
   intraluminal   694
   intramural, caused by foreign body   666,
   672
   submucosal   551
Acanthosis   444
Acanthosis nigricans
   and carcinoma   830
   distinction between benign and malignant
      type   830
Acetyl-beta-methylcholine, see Mecholyl
Acetylcholinesterase
   in achalasia   292
   decreased activity in achalasia   266
   in ganglion cells   292
Achalasia   287–354
   acetylcholinesterase in ganglion cells
      292
   achalasia-like syndrome produced by
      lesions of motor nuclei   82
   in animals   289
   association with esophageal carcinoma
      444
   atypical cases   314–316
   Chagas' disease   309–312
   complications   317–319
   cricopharyngeal   595
   cytological diagnosis of cancer in — 225
   diameter of esophagus   304
      after treatment with pneumatic
         dilatation   328
   differential diagnosis   309–317
   endoscopic examination   308
   and epiphrenic diverticula   607
   and esophageal carcinoma   460
   experimental production of — 292
   gastrin in — 53
   and hiatal hernia   320, 516
   hypersensitivity to cholinergic drugs   266
      of gastroesophageal sphincter   292,
      293
   hypersensitivity of gastroesophageal
      sphincter to gastrin   292, 305
   incidence   288
   in infants and children
      differential diagnosis   316
      incidence   288
      symptoms   294
      treatment   341

inheritance in animals   289
inheritance and familial incidence   289
intramural ganglion cells in animals   289
intramural ganglion cells in patients   291
lesions of vagal nuclei and nerves in — 290
life expectancy   321
manometry   304–307
Mecholyl test   308
and mycosis of esophagus   559
natural history   295
pain, characteristics   108, 294
pharmacological studies   292
radiological distinction from amyloidosis
   835
radiological distinction from malignant
   narrowing   179, 194, 460
radiology   297–304
retroperitoneal fibrosis, distinction from
   — 835
smooth muscle changes   291
stages
   clinical   295
   radiological   300–304
symptoms   293–295
synonyms   287
treatment   321–341
   dilatations   321–330, 332, 339–341
   myotomy versus forceful dilatations
      339–341
   surgical   331–341
ulcer-like picture in narrow segment   304
vigorous — 296
Achalasia-like syndrome, see Obstruction
   syndrome
Achlorhydria, in upper esophageal web   575
Acid barium, see Contrast materials
Acid, causing corrosive esophagitis   539
Acid clearing test   250, 501
Acid infusion test   262–269
   anginal pain during test   263
   criteria for positive test   262
   in differential diagnosis of reflux eso-
      phagitis and diffuse spasm   363
   evaluation   264, 501
   "false positive" and "false negative" test
      265
   hasards   263
   mechanism of acid induced pain   263
   procedure   262
Acidification of antrum and gastroesophageal
   sphincteric pressure   53
Acrosclerosis   383
Actinomycosis,   565
   causing esophagorespiratory fistula   810
Adenocarcinoma, see Carcinoma
Adenoid cystic tumor   456

Adenoma   431, 444
Adrenergic drugs, in treatment of achalasia
   321
Adrenergic fibers in motor innervation of
   smooth muscle esophagus   85
Adventitia   37
Aerophagia, causing eructation   414
Age, see Presbyesophagus; Neonatal infants
Aime's apparatus for immobilisation of children during radiological examination
   195
Air bubble in gastric fundus
   and belching   414
   in achalasia   300
Air esophagogram   157–159
   causes   157
   in esophageal atresia   623
   in esophageal carcinoma   462
   in esophageal belching   412
   in isolated tracheoesophageal fistula
      640
   in polymyositis   380
   in progressive systemic sclerosis   387
Air fluid level
   in achalasia   297, 302
   causes   160
Alcohol
   effect on esophageal motility   408
   harmfull effects in reflux esophagitis
      517
Alcoholic neuropathy, causing esophageal
   motility disorders   408
Alcoholism, predisposing to esophageal
   carcinoma   444
Alfa-1-antitrypsine deficiency, causing
   varices   707
Alfa-spikes   277
Alkali, causing corrosive esophagitis   539
Alkalinization of antrum and gastroesophageal sphincteric pressure   53
Alkylating agents in esophageal carcinoma
   482
Allison operation, in treatment of hiatus
   hernia   777
Ammonia tolerance test   718
Ammonium, causing corrosive esophagitis
   539
Amebic abscess, compressing distal esophagus
   839
Amphotericin B, in treatment of esophageal
   mycosis   564
Ampulla epiphrenica, distinction from hiatus
   hernia   759
Amyenteric achalasia   297
Amyl nitrite
   effect on narrow segment in achalasia   304
   in pharmacoradiology   194
Amyloidosis
   causing esophageal dilatation   313
   involving esophagus   835
Amyotrophic lateral sclerosis, causing
   swallowing difficulties   403
Anastomosis of the esophagus   783
   in atresia, transpleural vs extrapleural
      approach   628

intrathoracic vs cervical   784
leakage on the suture line   629, 790
types of sutures, advantages and complications   627, 630
Anatomy   1–13
   of hiatus diaphragmaticus   743–745
   of hypopharyngeal musculature in relation
      to diverticula   594
   of neonates   1
Andersen's disease, causing varices   707
Anesthetic agents, in pharmacoradiology
   194
Anesthetics, local
   in treatment of heartburn   775
   in treatment of post-vagotomy dysphagia
      370
Angina bullosa hemorrhagica   897
Angina pectoris and diffuse spasm   356, 364
Angio-architecture   35
Antacids
   in treatment of recurrent aphtae   827
   in treatment of reflux esophagitis   517
   in treatment of sphincter incompetence
      775
Antibiotics
   in treatment of atresia   627
   in treatment of corrosive esophagitis
      546, 547, 548, 803
Anticholinergics
   and first positive wave of deglutitition
      complex   72
   and competence of gastroesophageal
      sphincter   58, 423
   and reflex response of esophagus   88
   and relaxation of gastroesophageal sphinc-
      ter   91
   harmful effects in reflux esophagitis   517,
      775
   in pharmacoradiology   194
   producing disconnection between striated
      and smooth muscle contraction in
      transitional zone   276, 284
   in radiological detection of varices   713
   in treatment of diffuse spasm   364
Anticholinesterases
   in myasthenia gravis   398
   in treatment of familial dysautonomia
      404
Antispasmodics
   in treatment of achalasia   321
   in treatment of diffuse spasm   364
   in treatment of post-vagotomy dysphagia
      370
Aorta, descending, producing impression on
   thoracic esophagus   150, 151, 154, 175
Aortic aneurysm, causing downhill varices
   709
Aortic arch
   cervical   657
   double   653–655
   left-sided with right-sided descending
      aorta   657
   right-sided   655–657
Apathic hyperthyroidism and muscle wasting
   399

Aperistalsis, causes 313
  see also Achalasia
Aphtae, recurrent, involving esophagus 827
Apical cap 69
Arfonad in treatment of bleeding esophageal
  varices 721
Argyrophil neurons 85
  intramural, in achalasia 291
Argyrophobe neurons 85
  intramural, in achalasia 291
A-ring of Wolf, *see* Wolf
Arteria lusoria 650–653
Arterial blood supply 9
Arteriography
  in diagnosis of Mallory-Weiss syndrome
    691
  in diagnosis of vascular rings 650
  selective
    in patients with esophageal varices
      717
Arteriovenous shunts in portal system, causing varices 701
Artery
  aberrant left pulmonary 658
  left gastric 9
  left lower phrenic 9
  left subclavian, role in right-sided aortic
    arch syndrome 656
  lower thyroid 9
  posterior inferior cerebellar, and swallow-
    ing disturbances 402
  right subclavian 650–653
    compression during endoscopy 652
Ascites and gastroesophageal reflux 426
Aspiration of air into the esophagus in esophageal belching 410, 411, 412
Aspiration into airways, *see* Spill-over into airways; Bronchopulmonary complications
Ataxia heriditary and ocular myopathy 397
Atresia 615–638
  association with other conditions 619
  distinction from intramural rupture
    695
  early diagnosis 622
  embryology 616
  incidence 615
  nasogastric intubation for diagnosis 622
  proximal and distal segments 617–619
  radiology 623–625
  risk factors 633
  technique of bougienage 804
  technique of radiological examination
    197
  treatment 625–629
  types 617
Atrial fibrillation after esophagogastrectomy
  480
Atrium, left, producing impression on thoracic esophagus 154, 175
Atropine, *see* Anticholinergics
Atrophic gastritis
  predisposing to Mallory-Weiss syndrome
    690
Aubin bougies 803
Auerbach's plexus, *see* Myenteric plexus

Balanced operation in hiatus hernia associ-
  ated with ulcer diseases 777
Balloon kymography 235
Balloon tamponade, in treatment of bleeding
  esophageal varices 721
Banti-syndrome, causing varices 699–701
Barium pill, *see also* Contrast materials
  in diagnosis of foreign body 670
  in diagnosis of peptic stricture 134, 505
Barium sulfate, *see* contrast materials
Barrett
  triade of — 677
  ulcer of — 525
    vs squamocolumnar marginal ulcer 498
Barreto technique, for treatment of severe
  stenosis 803
Basal lamina of squamous epithelium 21
Basal layer of squamous epithelium 18
Basic electrical rhythm, *see* Electrical activity
Belching 414
  in hiatus hernia 747
  mechanism 93
Belching (esophageal—) 410–413
  radiological analysis 412
Belsey procedure (Mark IV)
  influence on sphincteric pressure 52, 424
  in treatment of hiatus hernia 777
Benign tumors and cysts, *see also* Leiomyoma
  431–446
  classification 431
  incidence 431–433
  intraluminal 443
  intramural 433–443
    causing midesophageal diverticula 605
  radiological aspects 171, 173
Betanechol 308, *see also* Mecholyl
Beta-spikes 277
Bicarotid truncus, role in lusoria syndrome
  651
Biphasic waves in diffuse spasm 358
Blastomycosis 565
Bleeding, *see* Hemorrhage
Bleomycin, in treatment of esophageal carcinoma 482
Boerhaave-syndrome 164
Bolus
  effect on amplitude of primary peristaltic
    wave 74
  effect on peristalsis 82–84
  necessity for swallowing act 76, 80
  transport 59–85, *see also* Transport
Bone anomalies in esophageal atresia 622
Bougienage
  causing iatrogenic perforation 685
  to elongate the pouches in atresia 628
  to enable endoscopy
    in peptic stricture 514
  in stenosing carcinoma 463, 804
    in stricture due to columnar epithelium
      lined esophagus 533
  in esophageal stenosis
    caused by benign mucosal pemphigoid
      824
    caused by epidermolysis bullosa dys-
      trophica 826

Bougienage — *cont.*
　caused by esophageal pemphigus　823
　　caused by intramural diverticulosis
　　　837
　　caused by radiation therapy　476
　　caused by recurrent aphtae　827
　　caused by surgical repair of atresia
　　　631
　preventive, in corrosive esophagitis　546,
　　547, 548, 803
　retrograde　802–803
　self-bougienage　802
　techniques　797–803
Brachyesophagus, in reflux esophagitis　498,
　763
Brainstem lesions, causing pharyngoesoph-
　ageal disorders　402
B-ring of Wolf, *see* Wolf
Bronchography, in diagnosis of esophagorespi-
　ratory fistula　812
Bronchopulmonary complications, *see also*
　Spill-over into airways
　in achalasia　319
　in atresia　620
　in carcinoma of esophagus　459
　in congenital bronchoesophageal fistula
　　644
　in corrosive esophagitis　542
　after esophageal substitution　789
　after esophagogastrectomy with espha-
　　geal substitution　480
　in isolated tracheoesophageal fistula　639
　in laryngotracheoesophageal cleft　647
　in leiomyoma　411
　in mycoses of esophagus　563
　in reflux esophagitis　504
　in tracheoesophageal compression by vas-
　　cular rings　649
Bronchopulmonary sequestration
　and esophageal fistula　810
Bronchoscopy
　in diagnosis of esophagorespiratory fistula
　　812
　indication for bronchoscopy in esophageal
　　carcinoma　462
Bronchus
　left main, producing impression on thora-
　　cic esophagus　150, 151, 154
　right main, originating in esophagus
　　841
Browne-Mc Hardy bag for dilatations　323
Budd-Chiari syndrome, causing varices
　708
Bulbar paralysis, causing esophageal dilata-
　tion　313
Bullous dermatoses, involving esophagus
　823–827

Caerulein, effect on gastroesophageal sphinc-
　ter　55
Calcifications
　in leiomyoma　434, 437
　in mediastinum　161, 177
Calcitonin, effect on gastroesophageal sphinc-
　ter　56

Candida involving esophagus　558–564
Cannon, law of denervation　266
Carbon dioxyde snow, causing achalasia-like
　disturbances　292
Carcinoid tumor　486
Carcinoma　447–484
　adenocarcinoma
　　disappointing results of radiation ther-
　　　apy　477
　　originating in heterotopic columnar
　　　epithelium　456
　　originating in lower esophagus lined by
　　　columnar epithelium　456
　　pathology　456
　associated with
　　acanthosis nigricans　830
　　achalasia　317–319, 460
　　hiatal hernia　460
　　hypertrophic osteoarthropathy　830
　　keratoderma　829
　　leiomyoma　436
　　lye stricture　460, 549
　bronchoscopy, indication for — 462
　bougienage of stenotic esophagus to enable
　　endoscopy　463, 804
　causing achalasia-like syndrome　311
　causing aortoesophageal fistula　814
　causing diffuse spasm syndrome　362
　causing esophagocavitary fistula　816
　causing esophagovenous fistula　815
　causing hypertensive sphincter syndrome
　　362
　causing tracheoesophageal fistula　459, 807
　cervical lymph node biopsy　463
　classification into "high and low" tumors
　　in pre-operative assessment　470
　clinical differences between squamous cell
　　carcinoma and adeno-carcinoma　459
　clinical signs　549
　complications of esophagogastrectomy
　　479, 789
　cytology, *see* Cytology
　diagnosis of liver metastases　464
　distinction between carcinoma and benign
　　extramucosal tumor　439, 441
　distinction from lower esophageal ring
　　587
　distinction from midesophageal ring　579
　distinction from reflux esophagitis　516
　dysphagia due to radiation therapy　468
　endoscopy　462
　esophagorespiratory fistula　459, 807
　etiology　448
　of gastroesophageal region, causing varices
　　709
　incidence　447
　　of primary esophageal adenocarcinoma
　　　449, 456
　location in esophagus, influence on results
　　of treatment　465, 477, 484
　manometry in differential diagnosis with
　　achalasia　464
　Mecholyl test　308
　mixed squamous and adenocarcinoma
　　458

pathology 448
P.D. measurements 259
pleomorphic carcinoma, distinction from carcinosarcoma 485
pneumomediastinography 463
postcricoid carcinoma, and upper esophageal webs 576
prognosis 464–466
    influence of location of tumor 465, 477, 484
    influence of sex 465
    in relation to histological type of tumor 466
radioactive phosphorus and miniature Geiger-counter in diagnosis 464
radiological aspects 166–171, 173, 178, 460–462
    air esophagogram 462
    distinction from achalasia 179, 194, 460
    distinction from peptic stricture 178, 460
    early radiological signs 460
    impression or invasion by extraesophageal tumor 169, 173, 176
    metastases in esophagus 169
    smooth stenosis caused by submucosal growth 460
    transmural extension 169
    widening of esophageal lumen 462
squamous cell carcinoma 449–456
    blood-borne metastases 455
    cytological criteria of malignancy 222
    direct spread 451–453
    extent of submucosal spread 452
    lymphatic metastases 454
    pathology 449–456
    relative resistence of stomach to invasion 456
    site and size 449
subjective localization of obstruction 459
submucosal nodules as local metastases 452, 463
survival without treatment 459
symptoms 458–460
tracheoesophageal fistula 482
treatment 466–484
    advantages of radiation therapy 472–476
    bougienage 804
    chemotherapy 481
    colon or stomach as esophageal substitute after resection 479, 784
    comparison of surgery and radiotherapy 467–470
    complications of radiotherapy 471
    drawbacks of radiation therapy 476
    influence of level of tumor on results of treatment 465, 477, 484
    intubation 468, 481
    operative mortality of esophagogastrectomy 483, 789
    preoperative and postoperative irradiation 480
    pretreatment assessment of the patient 464, 470
    radiation therapy 468, 470, 470–477
    radium bougie or implantation techques 472
    results of irradiation 484
    results of surgery 483
    sequels of radiation therapy 476
    surgical procedures 478, 783, 784
    5-year survival rate after irradiation 484
    5-year survival rate after surgical treatment 483
    verrucous squamous cell carcinoma 487
Carcinosarcoma 485
    distinction from pleomorphic carcinoma 485
    radiological aspects 172
Cardiac, see Sphincter, gastroesophageal
Cardiac glands, origin of — 24
Cardiac incisura 6
    see also His
Cardiac orifice 68, 69
Cardiac rhythm
    disturbance in achalasia 320
    disturbance in diffuse spasm 356
Cardiaparalysis, see Achalasia
Cardiomyotomy, see Myotomy (Heller)
Cardioplasty in treatment of achalasia 332
Cardiospasm, see Achalasia
Cardiospasme réactionnel 305
Cardiovascular anomalies associated with esophageal atresia 621
Cardiovascular pulsations 45
Carminatives, effect on gastroesophageal sphincter 56, 423
Caroid, to remove impacted meat 673
Cast epithelial
    benign or ideopathic, in esophagitis superficialis dissecans 827
    in bullous pemphigoid 824
    in toxic epidermal neurolysis 826
Caustic lesions 539–550,
    causing esophagorespiratory fistula 808
    clinical features 541
    diagnostic significance of oral lesions 542
    esophagoscopy 544
    etiologic agents 539
    successive phases of pathologic lesions 541
    treatment 546–549
Celestin's tube 481, 805
Central afferent system, see Innervation, Afferent pathway
Central nervous system disorders, causing pharyngoesophageal disorders 402–406
Cerebrovascular accidents, causing pharyngoesophageal disorders 402
Cervical esophagus, motor innervation by vagal nerve 81, 84
Chagas' disease 309–312
    Mecholyl test in — 266, 308
Chalasia
    in adults 495
    in infants 380, 494

Cheilosis, in upper esophageal web 574
Chemoreceptors in heartburn 503
Chemotherapy of esophageal carcinoma 481
Chewing center, interference with deglutition
    center 80
Chlorambucil (Leuceran)
    in treatment of progressive systemic scle-
        rosis 385, 389
Choking
    causes 112
    definition 105
Choking impression in globus hystericus
    409
Cholecystectomy, followed by symptoms of
    hiatus hernia 773
Cholecystokinin, effect on gastroesophageal
    sphincter 55, 423
Cholinergic drugs, see also Mecholyl
    effect on gastroesophageal sphincter 85,
        423
    effects in achalasia 292, 293
    hypersensitivity in achalasia 266
    in treatment of reflux esophagitis 517
    use in pharmacological tests 266–268
Cholinergic excitatory fibers in motor inner-
    vation of smooth muscle esophagus
    85
Cholinesterase (see Acetylcholinesterase)
Chorea
    causing swallowing difficulties 404
Chylothorax, after esophagogastrectomy
    480
Ciliated epithelium
    during embryonic development 15
    persistence in post-embryonic life 24
Cinefluorography 128–131
    of swallowing act 187
Cinelix 122
Cirrhosis of liver, causing varices 704–708
Claude-Bernard-Horner syndrome
    in hypopharyngeal diverticula 598
Cleaners, causing corrosive esophagitis 539
Cleft larynx 646–648
Clinitest tablets, causing corrosive eso-
    phagitis 539
Clorox, causing corrosive esophagitis 539
Clotrimazole, in treatment of monilial eso-
    phagitis 564
Cobblestone appearance, in progressive sys-
    temic sclerosis 387
Coccidioidomycosis, causing esophagorespir-
    atory fistula 810
Collagen diseases
    causing esophagorespiratory fistula 810
    causing disorders 383–393
    see also Lupus erythematosus; Polymyo-
        sitis; Progressive systemic sclerosis;
        Raynaud's phenomenon; Sjøgren's
        syndrome
Colon
    as esophageal substitute 787
        functional results 792
    involvement in Chagas' disease 310
    involvement in progressive systemic scle-
        rosis 384

Columnar epithelium 25
    electromicroscopy 27
    histology 24–26
    lower esophagus lined with 525–538
        see also Lower esophagus
Common cavity test 500, 515
Concentric type of hiatal hernia 494
Congenital lesions
    atresia 615–638
    bronchoesophageal fistula 643–645
    cleft larynx 646–648
    hepatic fibrosis causing varices 703
    laryngotracheoesophageal cleft 646–648
    lateral pharyngeal diverticula 593
    persistent esophagotrachea 646–648
    vascular rings 649–660
Congestive heart failure, causing varices
    706, 709
Constrictor cardiae 7
Contrast materials
    acid barium meal 134, 501
    barium sulfate 133–135
        aspiration into airways 135
        contra-indications 135
        different types of barium preparations
            134
    for demonstration of hiatus hernia 751
    for demonstration of varices 192–194
    iodinated products 135–137
        aspiration into airways 136
        complications 136
    for radiological examination of children
        196
    for radiological examination of infants
        with esophageal atresia 624
    Tantalum powder 137
Corckscrew esophagus 355
Coronary insufficiency and hiatus hernia
    774
"Corps ronds" 828
Corrosive esophagitis 539–550
    and esophageal mycosis 559
Corticofugal fibers to deglutition center 78
Corticosteroids
    in treatment of dysphagia due to poly-
        myositis 390
    in treatment of progressive systemic scle-
        rosis 385, 389
    injection into strictures 631
Crater-like images
    causes 180–184
    radiological aspects 180–184
Cricoid cartilage 1
Cricopharyngeal indentation, normal and ab-
    normal radiological pictures 190
Cricopharyngeal muscle, see also Musculature,
    pharyngeal; Sphincter pharyngoesopha-
    geal
    identity with pharyngoesophageal sphinc-
        ter 41, 42
    innervation 12, 40
Crohn's disease of the esophagus 568
Crura, see Diaphragm
Curling, see also Tertiary contractions
    in diffuse spasm 356

Cutaneous disease, involving esophagus 823
    –833
Cylindroma 456
    bronchogenic 441
    enterogenous 441
    radiological aspect 173
    retention cysts 443
Cystic fibrosis of pancreas, causing varices
    707
Cytology
    appraisal of different sampling techniques
        221
    causes of false positive results 226, 229
    correlation with histological features 225
    criteria for malignancy 221–225
    for diagnosis of cancer in achalasia 225
    for diagnosis of cancer in Plummer-Vinson
        syndrome 225
    distinction between cells of esophageal
        and oral origin 221
    distinction between malignant and
        "chronic esophagitis" cells 226
    distinction between squamous cell car-
        cinoma and esophageal adenocar-
        cinoma 222
    and early diagnosis of esophageal cancer
        231
    effect of roentgen therapy on esophageal
        cells 230
    in esophageal adenocarcinoma 222–224
    in esophageal lymfoma 224
    false diagnosis of cancer in vitamine B_{12}
        or folic acid deficiency 227–229
    fluorescent techniques 228
    as an index of roentgen sensitivity 231
    indications 225
    normal esophageal smears 221
    preparation of slides 220
    results of cytology in diagnosis of eso-
        phageal carcinoma 225
    specific characteristics of malignant squa-
        mous cells 222
    techniques of sampling 218–221
Cytometry
    of carcinomatous squamous cells 225
    of normal esophageal cells 221
"Cyto-rape" for cytology 219

Darier's disease, see Keratosis follicularis
Deglutitition act, see Swallowing act
Deglutitition center, see Innervation
Deglutitition complex
    in esophagus proper 71–74
    in gastroesophageal sphincter 74
    in pharynx 69–71
    in pharyngoesophageal sphincter 69–71
Delcalix 122, 124, 126
Denervation law 266
Denervation potential 270, 283
Dentate line, see Squamocolumnar junction
Dermatosis, see Cutaneous disease
Dermatomyositis, see Polymyositis 389, 830
Desmosomes 21, 23, 27
Detergents, causing corrosive esophagitis
    539

Dextran infusion, in radiological detection of
    varices 713
Diabetes, causing esophageal motility dis-
    orders 407
Diaphragm
    crura 7, 743
    hiatus and pressure inversion point 46,
        47–48, see also Hiatus
    importance in gastroesophageal compe-
        tence 50, 424, 496
Diazepam (valium)
    in treatment of diffuse spasm 364
    in treatment of stiff-man syndrome 404
Diet, in treatment of esophagitis 517
Diffuse spasm 355–366
    asymptomatic 355
    distinction from achalasia 316, 363
    distinction from vigorous achalasia 296
    and epiphrenic diverticulum 607
    and hypertensive, hyperreactive, hyper-
        contracting gastroesophageal sphincter
        362
    and idiopathic muscular hypertrophy of
        lower esophagus 361
    incidence 355
    manometry 358–361
        after succesful treatment 364
    Mecholyl test 266–268, 308
    pain
        caracteristics 108
        and esophageal contractions 360
        and hypertensive gastroesophageal
            sphincter 362
    pathology 356
    radiology 357
    secondary — 362
    smooth muscle changes in — 356
    symptoms 356
    transition to achalasia 314, 363
    treatment 364
Di-isopropylfluorophosphate (D.F.P.), caus-
    ing achalasia-like disturbances 292
Dilatatio fusiformis, ingluviformis, see
    Achalasia, synonyms
Dilatations (forceful), see also Bougienage
    as a cause of iatrogenic perforation
        685
    in treatment of achalasia 321–331
    in treatment of diffuse spasm 364
    in treatment of hypopharyngeal diverti-
        cula 601
    in treatment of lower esophageal ring
        587
    in treatment of post-vagotomy dysphagia
        370
Dilatation of the esophagus
    causes 309–313
    causing esophagorespiratory fistula 808
    diagnosis on plain X-ray films 159
    in myotonic dystrophy 396
    in neonatal infants 380
    in old age 372
    in progressive systemic sclerosis 387
    after surgical treatment of atresia 630
Dionosil, see Contrast materials

Diphenylhydantoin, in treatment of myotonic
    dystrophy 394
Diphteria, causing esophagitis 552
Dissection, intramural 694
Distension of esophagus
    by obstructing bolus 87
    transient distension 86, 87
Diverticulum 591–613
    association with achalasia 320
    association with leiomyoma 436
    complicated by esophagovenous fistula
        815
    congenital and acquired diverticula 591
    consequence of corrosive esophagitis 545
    in diffuse spasm 356
    distinction from pseudodiverticula 591
    epiphrenic 606–610
        association with achalasia 607
        association with diffuse spasm 607
        association with hiatus hernia 607
        association with leiomyoma 610
        association with peptic esophagitis
            607
        complications 609
        diagnosis of associated lower esopha-
            geal lesions in pretreatment as-
            sessment 610
        endoscopy 609
        etiology 607
        incidence 606
        motility disorders 607
        pathology 607
        on plain chest X-ray 608
        radiological distinction from penetrat-
            ing peptic ulcer 608
        radiological features 608
        relation to motility disorders of distal
            esophagus 607
        symptoms 608
        treatment 610
    hypopharyngeal 593–603
        cineradiographic studies of pharyngo-
            esophageal region 596
        complications 598–601
        complications of surgical treatment
            601–602
        compression of esophagus by — 597
        discriminative symptoms 113
        and dysfunction of pharyngoesopha-
            geal region 595
        endoscopic treatment 603
        endoscopy 598
        incidence 593
        location 594
        manometric data 595
        myotomy of cricopharyngeal muscle in
            treatment of — 602
        natural history 601
        pathogenesis 594–596
        pathology 596
        recurrence after surgery 602
        stages of development 596, 597
        surgical procedures in treatment of
            —601
        symptoms 596

        treatment 601–603
        treatment by dilatations 601
        weak spots, in muscular wall of hypo-
            pharynx 594
    intramural diverticulosis 836
        and esophageal mycosis 563
    Kommerell's diverticulum 815
    lateral pharyngeal 591–593
        characteristics of congenital 593
        distinction from lateral pharyngeal
            pouch 591
        location 591
        radiological appearances 593
    midesophageal 605
        causing esophagorespiratory fistula
            809
    pseudo-diverticula
        in diffuse spasm 357
        lateral pharyngeal 147
    pulsion and traction diverticula 591
    retrocricoid 593
    subphrenic 610
    true and false diverticula 591
Diverticulum (traction), caused by esophagitis
    553
Diverticulopexy, in treatment of hypopha-
    ryngeal diverticula 602
Diverticulosis
    intramural 836
        and esophageal moniliasis 563
    spastic pseudo 355, 356
Dolichoesophagus, see Achalasia, synonyms
Double aortic arch 653–655
Double barrelled esophagus, in intramural
    esophageal rupture 695
Double contrast method of examination, see
    Radiology
Downhill varices 709
Ductus arteriosus (ligamentum), role in vas-
    cular ring syndrome 650, 653, 655, 657
Duhamel's end-to-side anasotmosis 628
Duodenal ulcer
    and hiatus hernia 773
Duplications of esophagus, radiological dist-
    inction from intramural rupture 695
Duration response 89
Dysarthria, associated with "spill-over"
    109
Dysautonomia (familial)
    causing esophageal dilatation 313
    causing swallowing difficulaties 404
Dysachalasia 314, 315
Dyskeratosis follicularis vegetans 828
Dysphagia, see also History and Symptoms
    of Esophageal Disease 103–118
    in achalasia 293
    in amyloidosis 835
    in bullous pemphigoid 824
    in corrosive esophagitis 541
    definition 104
    in diffuse spasm 356
    in epidermolysis bullosa dystrophica 825
    in epiphrenic diverticula 608
    in esophageal carcinoma 449, 458
    in esophageal mycosis 560

in esophagitis superficialis dissecans (idiopathic esophageal casts)   827
in esophagocavitary fistula   817
in esophagorespiratory fistula   811
in familial dysautonomia   404, 405
in fibrovascular polyp   443
and foreign body   667
"functional" or psychogenic   111
in heriditary leukokeratosis   83
and heterotopic gastric mucosa   840
in hiatus hernia   504, 772
in Hodgkin's disease   486
in hypopharyngeal diverticula   596
in iatrogenic perforation   685
inability to swallow   112
in intramural diverticulosis   836
in intramural rupture and bleeding   694
in leiomyoma   436
and lesions of nucleus ambiguus   81
in lower esophageal ring   584
in lower esophagus lined with columnar
   epithelium   531
in lupus erythematosis disseminatus   835
in midesophageal diverticula   605
in midesophageal web   578
in myasthenia gravis   398
in myotonic dystrophy   395
in ocular myopathy and oculopharyngeal
   dystrophy   397
in oral submucous fibrosis   830
in organic stenosis   795
in pemphigus   823
in polymyositis   390
postoperative, after treatment of hypopharyngeal diverticulum   602
post-vagotomy   367–371
   differential diagnosis with achalasia
      316, 368, 370
   pathogenesis   367–370
in progressive systemic sclerosis   386
pseudo dysphagia   104
after radiation therapy   468
in reflux esophagitis   516
in spontaneous rupture of esophagus   677
in Stiff-man syndrome   404
subjective localization of site of obstruction   104, 111
in suppurative esophagitis   551
   in upper esophageal web   574
by vascular rings   650
Dysphagia paradoxa, see Achalasia, synonyms
Dysplastic (dyskariotic) cells, distinction from
   malignant cells   226
Dystonia, esophageal, see Achalasia, synonyms

Eccentric type of hiatal hernia   494
Ectasia of the esophagus   288
Ectopic mucosa   24, 25, 526
   origin of esophageal adenocarcinoma   456
Ectopic tissues in esophagus   839–841
Edentula, in upper esophageal web   574
Eder-Hufford esophagoscope   206
Eder-Puestow dilating metal olives   798, 801
Edrophonium (Tensilon), see
   Anticholinesterases

Elastic muscular system   37
Electrical activity, see Electromyography
Electrodes
   for PD measurements   256
   for pH measurements   246
Electromyography   270–285
   deglutitive electrical activity in animals
      270, 271
   deglutitive electrical inhibition   270,
      280–282
      in human pharyngoesophageal
         sphincter   274
   in esophageal diseases   282–284
   of esophageal muscle strips   270
   of human esophagus   271
      correlation between electrical and
         mechanical activity   274, 275,
         278, 280
   of human gastroesophageal sphincter
      273, 279, 423
   of human pharyngoesophageal sphincter
      273
   of human smooth muscle esophagus
      276–278
   of human striated muscle esophagus
      274
   in myasthenia gravis   398
   in myotonic dystrophy   394
   in ocular myopathy and oculopharyngeal
      myopathy   397
   of pharyngoesophageal sphincter   43, 44
   phasic resting activity in gastroesophageal
      sphincter of dogs   270, 279, 423
   registration methods in animals   270
   registration methods in humans   272
   slow waves   67
   in stiff-man syndrome   404
   of swallowing act   63–65
   technical requirements of registration
      apparatus   272
   after vagotomy   67, 84, 230, 271, 282
Embryogenesis
   of bronchoesophageal fistula   643
   of cysts (bronchogenic, enterogenous)
   of esophageal atresia   616
   of esophageal diverticula   604
   of isolated tracheoesophageal fistula   639
   of laryngotracheoesophageal cleft   646
Embryology   13–15, 616
Emotional disorders of the esophagus
   409–421
Emphysema, cervical
   in esophagocavitary fistula   818
   in esophagorespiratory fistula   812
   in iatrogenic perforation   686
   in perforation by foreign body   670
   in spontaneous rupture of esophagus   677
Encephalopathy
   preventive measures during variceal
      bleeding   720
   after shunt operations   727
Endless string method for bougienage   802
Endobrachyesophagus, see Lower esophagus
   lined with columnar epithelium   526
Endocrine disorders of muscle   399

Enzymes of squamous epithelium   19–21
Eosinophilic granuloma   838
Epidermoid carcinoma, see Carcinoma,
   squamous cell carcinoma
Epidermolysis bullosa dystrophica 824–826
   treatment   826
Epithelial occlusion theory as a cause of
   atresia   616
Epithelium lining congenital bronchoesophageal fistula   643
Eructation, see Belching
Eructation (esophageal), see Belching,
   esophageal
Esophageal speech   80
Esophagitis
   in achalasia   308, 319
   acute, predisposing to spontaneous
      rupture   676
   in bleeding esophageal varices   711
   causing diffuse spasm syndrome   363
   candidosa, see Esophagitis, monilial
   characteristics of pain in — 107
   chronic superficial   497, 498
   corrosive   539–550
   cytological differentiation from
      malignancy   226
   granulomatous   568–570
   in infectious diseases   551
   ischemic   503
   in lower esophagus lined with columnar
      epithelium   531
   monilial   558–564
      distinction from reflux esophagitis 517
   pathological changes   497–499
   PD measurement   259
   peptic, see Esophagitis, reflux
   suppurative   551
   syphilic   556
   tuberculosus   553–555
   viral   551
   reflux — 493–524
      acid infusion test   664
      in children   519
      clinical classification   498
      differential diagnosis   515–517
      distinction from carcinoma   178, 516
      distinction from moniliasis   517
      endoscopy   514
      and epiphrenic diverticulum   607
      after gastrectomy   426
      in hiatus hernia   746
      and lower esophageal ring   583
      manometry   515
      pathological types   497
      predisposing to intramural rupture
         694
      predisposing to spontaneous rupture
         676
      in polymyositis   390
      in post vagotomy dysphagia   368, 369
      in progressive systemic sclerosis
         386, 387
      radiology   505–514
      stricture formation   497, 499
      therapy   517–519

Esophagitis superficialis dissecans,
   (idiopathic esophageal cast)   827
Esophago-esophageal anastomosis
   complications   629–633, 783
   in treatment of esophageal atresia   627
Esophagogastrectomy
   complications   479, 519
   in treatment of stricture in reflux
      esophagitis   518
Esophagogastrostomy
   functional results   791
   predisposing to stricture formation   797
   in reconstruction procedures   785
Esophagomyotomy, see Myotomy, esophageal
Esophagoscopy
   accidental perforation   216
   in achalasia   308–309
   biopsy taking   214
   in caustic esophagitis   544
   cinematography   214
   cytological sampling   214, 218
   equipment   204–209
   fiber esophagoscopy, advantages and
      drawbacks   214–215
   general anesthesia   209
   general rules of examination   204
   hemorrhage caused by — 216
      significance of slight bleeding   217
   in hiatal hernia   213, 514, 766–768
   indications and contraindications   215
   in isolated tracheoesophageal fistula
      640
   local anesthesia   209
   in lower esophagus lined with columnar
      epithelium   532–533
   in moniliasis   563
   normal appearances   213
   pain as an alarm signal   217
   premedication   209
   in reflux esophagitis   514
   and respiratory spasm   217
   rigid esophagoscopes, limitations   206
   squamocolumnar mucosal junction   213
   still photography   213
   in syphilis   556
   technique of fiber esophagoscopy
      209–215
   technique of passing pharyngoesophageal
      sphincter   216
   techniques of rigid esophagoscopy   205
   in tuberculosis   554
   urgent examination   209
Esophagotrachea   646–648
Esophagus proper
   cervical
      radiological landmarks   139
   electromyographic studies, see Electrom-
      myography
   radiological appearance of mucosal folds
      154
   thoracic
      normal radiological appearance
         147–154
      radiological landmarks   147
      thickness of wall   153

Evoked potentials, in myasthenia gravis 398
e-Wave 71
Exanthematous infectious diseases, causing
    esophagitis 551
Extrapyramidal disturbances, causing
    swallowing difficulties 404
Extrinsic compression
    esophageal symptoms 107
    radiological appearances 166, 175–178,
        185, 190
    by vascular rings 649–660

Facilitation in deglutition center 77, 78
Fasciculus solitarius (tractus and nucleus)
    78
Fat ingestion, effect on gastroesophageal
    sphincter 55
Fatty liver, causing varices 704
Feeding disturbances in infants, due to
    merycism 416
Fiber cells as cytological sign of
    malignancy 222
Fibroangioadenomatosis causing varices 703
Fibrocongestive sphenomegaly causing
    varices 701
Fibrolipoma 431, 443
Fibroma 431, 443
Fibromyoma 431
Fibrosarcoma 484
Fibrovascular polyp 431, 443
Filling defects
    causes 166–173
    distinction between intramural extra-
        mucosal and attached extrinsic
        growth 439
    distinction between intramural extra-
        mucosal and benign sessile polypoid
        growth 439
    in esophageal carcinoma 460
    intraluminal defect 171–173
    intramural extramucosal defects 173
    in leiomyoma 437
    radiological aspects 166–173
    radiological distinction between intrinsic
        and extrinsic masses 166
    varices 712
Final positive wave of esophageal
    deglutition complex 73
First positive wave of esophageal deglutition
    complex 72
Fistula
    acquired 807–821
    anastomotic leak 629, 791
    aortoesophageal 814
    and bronchopulmonary sequestration 810
    congenital
        bronchoesophageal 643–645
        tracheoesophageal
            in association with atresia 617,
                619
            embryogenesis 617
            isolated (H-type) 617, 639–642
            operative management of — 627,
                628, 640
            reccurence after treatment 631

in esophageal diverticula 606, 609
in esophageal mycosis 563, 565
esophagocardiac 816
esophagocavitary 816–818
esophago-esophageal, in achalasia 319
esophagopericardial 815
esophagopleural, see also Fistula,
    esophago-cavitary
    secondary to anastomotic leak 629,
        791
esophagorespiratory 807–814
    causes 807–810
    clinical features 811
    diagnosis 812
    secondary to suppurative
        esophagitis 551
    secondary to syphilis 556, 557
    secondary to traumatic lesions
        807–809
    secondary to tuberculosis 553
esophagovenous 815
external esophageal 818
and foreign body 666, 672, 807
tracheoesophageal, see also Fistula,
    congenital
    and esophageal carcinoma 459
        intubation treatment of cancerous
            fistula 482
    and foreign body 672
    traumatic 661, 807
Fluorescence, formaldehyde—induced 36
Fluorescent techniques in esophageal
    cytology 228
5-Fluorocytosine, in treatment of monilial
    esophagitis 564
5-Fluorouracil, in treatment of esophageal
    carcinoma 482
Flutter valve mechanism, importance in
    gastroesophageal sphincteric
    competence 51
Foley catheter, for removal of foreign
    body 672
Folic acid deficiency, false positive cyto-
    logical diagnosis of cancer 227, 229
Force tranducers, in evaluation of eso-
    phageal contraction 241
Fordyce's syndrome 840
Foregut, see also Embryogenesis of congenital
    anomalies 13, 843
Foreign bodies 665–674
    atypical symptoms in children 668
    complications 672
    dangerous "urgent measures" 670
    diagnostic approach 669
    esophagoscopy, indications and
        contraindications 670
    fistula formation 666, 672, 807, 808, 814
    meat impaction 672
        enzymatical removal 673
    pathology 665
    plain films in diagnosis of — 669
    prevertebral space enlargement 185
    site of pain sensation in relation to
        location of obstruction 667
    suppurative esophagitis 551

Foreign bodies — *cont.*
  symptoms and signs 667
  tabulated data of Jackson's collection
    671
  treatment 670–672
  usual location in esophagus 665
Formaldehyde causing corrosive esophagitis
  539
f-phase of pharyngeal deglutition complex
  71
French gradation of bougies 798
Fructose intolerance, causing varices 707
Fundic-like heterotopic mucosa 526
Fundoplication
  influence on sphincteric pressure 52, 424
  in treatment of hiatus hernia 777
Fungal infections 558–567

Gagging 77
Galactosuria, causing varices 707
Gastrectomy and gastroesophageal reflux
  54, 426
"Gastric brush" for cytology 219
Gastric cooling, in treatment of bleeding
  esophageal varices 721
Gastric distension
  in atresia with fistula 620
  in belching 411, 413, 414
  in isolated tracheoesophageal fistula 639
Gastric mucosa in esophagus
  ectopic 24, 25, 526
  heterotopic 840
Gastric pressure, effect of increased pressure
  on gastroesophageal sphincter 57
Gastric rupture, in atresia with fistula 620
Gastric surgery, predisposing to esophageal
  carcinoma 444
Gastrin
  in achalasia patients 53, 292, 305
  dose-response curve of gastroesophageal
    sphincter 53
  effect on gastroesophageal sphincter
    53–55, 56, 423
    in progressive systemic sclerosis 387
  mechanism of action on smooth muscle
    56
Gastrin antiserum 53
Gastroesophageal anomalies
  in esophageal atresia 622
Gastroesophageal region, *see* Vestibule;
  Sphincter, gastroesophageal
  normal radiological appearance 154–156
  radiological landmarks 154–156
Gastroesophageal sphincter, *see* Sphincter,
  gastroesophageal
Gastroesophagostomy, in treatment of
  achalasia 332, 338
Gastrographin, *see* Contrast materials
Gastropexy, posterior, effect on sphincteric
  pressure 52, 424
Gastrostomy
  after interposition procedures 790
  in the management of atresia 627, 628
  in the management of esophageal tumor
    783

Gaucher's disease, causing varices 707–708
Germinative layer of squamous epithelium
  18
Glands in esophagus
  cardiac, origin of — 24
  deep esophageal, in high esophageal
    stricture 525
  sebaceous 840
Globus hystericus 409
Glomus tumor 431
Glossopharyngeal respiration 80
Glucagon, effect on gastroesophageal
  sphincter 56, 423
Glycogenic acanthosis 19
  involving esophagus 831
Glycogenosis type IV, causing varices 707
Goiter, intrathoracic compressing esophagus
  176
Gradient of contraction in esophagus 89
"Grains", in keratosis follicularis 828
Granular cell myoblastoma 431, 487
Granules
  in cells of stratum spinosum 24
  in columnar epithelium cells 27
Granulomatous diseases, causing varices
  703
Granulomatous esophagitis 568–570
Granulomatous proliferation, distinction
  from papilloma 444
Gross' side-to-side anastomosis
  predisposing to stricture formation 796

Haight's end-to-end repair, predisposing to
  stricture formation 796
Haight's telescopic end-to-end anastomosis
  628, 630
Halogens, causing corrosive esophagitis
  539
Hamartoma 443
Hamman sound 677
Heart, hypertrophy, associated with esophageal muscular hypertrophy 362
Heartburn, *see also* Reflux, gastroesophageal
  and acid infusion test
  in hiatal hernia 747–749
  in lower esophagus lined with columnar
    epithelium 532
  pathophysiological basis and conditions
    associated with gastroesophageal
    reflux 424–426
  in pregnancy 426
  in reflux esophagitis 501, 504
  in systemic sclerosis 386, 425
Heidelberg capsule for pH measurements
  247
Heller's myotomy, *see* Myotomy
Hemangioma 431, 444
Hematemesis, *see* Hemorrhage
Hematoma
  intramural 694–696
    mimicking achalasia 695
  postoperative, causing dysphagia 368,
    370
Hemidesmosomes in germinative layer 21
Hemochromatosis, causing varices 706

Hemorrhage
  in achalasia 294
  from aortic erosion, complicating eso-
    phagogastrectomy 479
  in aortoesophageal fistula 814
  from Barrett ulcer 532
  in carcinoma 459
  from colon used for esophageal replace-
    ment 791
  diagnostic approach when bleeding from
    varices is suspected 71
  distinction between variceal bleeding and
    hemorrhage from other source
    719–720
  from diverticulum 606, 608
  from ectopic pancreatic tissue 840
  in hiatal hernia 771
  in intramural rupture and bleeding 694
  in Mallory-Weiss syndrome 691
  in mycosis of esophagus 560, 563
  in reflux esophagitis 505
  "signal hemorrhage", in aorto-
    esophageal fistula 814
Hemoptysis, due to esophagorespiratory
  fistula 811
Hepatitis, acute, causing varices 704
Hernia, see Hiatus hernia
Herlitzch disease 824
Herpetic esophagitis 551
Heterotopic columnar epithelium, see Lower
  esophagus lined with columnar
  epithelium
  and esophageal adenocarcinoma 528
Hexamethonium in treatment of achalasia
  321
Heyrowsky's esophagofundostomy, see
  Gastroesophagostomy
Hiatal continence, maneuver for radiological
  evaluation 752–754
Hiatal herniation without a sac 502, 742
Hiatus, diaphragmatic
  anatomy 7, 743
  radiological evaluation of hiatal width
    761
  radiological localization 154
Hiatus esophagismus, see Achalasia, synonyms
Hiatus hernia 741–782
  and achalasia 320, 516
  acid infusion test, see Acid infusion test
  associated diseases 773
  classification 741
  complication 771–773
  concentric type 494
  and congenital short esophagus 741
  and coronary insufficiency 774
  dependency of symptoms on position
    748
  diagnostic approach 769
  and diffuse spasm 356
    effect on sphincteric pressures 359
    associated with hypertensive sphincter
      362
  causes of dysphagia 772
  eccentric type 494
  and epiphrenic diverticula 607

and eructation 414
and esophageal carcinoma 460
esophageal rings in diagnosis of small
  hernia 761
esophageal shortening as a factor in
  determining the surgical approach
  763
esophagoscopic localization of diaphragmatic hiatus 767
esophagoscopy 213, 766
findings at operation and autopsy 746
and gastric carcinoma 773
and gastroesophageal reflux 51, 423, 424
and gastroesophageal sphincter pressure
  50, 423, 424
gastroscopy 768
hiatal herniation without a sac 742
hiatus insufficiency 742
and hypertensive gastroesophageal
  sphincter 362, 423, 747, 764
hypochromic anemia, due to chronic
  blood loss 771
incidence 424, 504, 742
indirect radiological signs 761
in infants 749
influence of age on incidence 742, 743
influence of repair on sphincteric pressure
  52, 424
and keratoderma 829
and leiomyoma 436
local complaints 747
and lower esophageal ring 587
and lower esophagus lined with columnar
  epithelium 529, 532
  mucosal lesions in hernia sac 767
manometric data 496, 768
manometric evaluation of sphincter
  competence
medical treatment 775
mixed type 764
and associated motor disturbances of
  esophagus 769
natural history 774
paraesophageal 494, 741, 763
  causing hypochromic anemia 772
  in infants 749
  symptoms 749
pathogenesis 502, 503
pathology 746
PD-profile in gastroesophageal region
  257
peritoneoscopy 768
pH measurements, see pH measurements
and phrenic ampulla 742, 754
plain chest X-rays 751
and pneumatosis cystoides 837
and polymyositis 390
positions used for radiological demonstration 752–754
postoperative 750
predisposing to Mallory-Weiss syndrome
  690
during pregnancy 749
prognosis 774
and progressive systemic sclerosis 387

Hiatus hernia — cont.
    radiological signs 496, 497, 757–763
    recurrence after surgical treatment 778
    and reflux esophagitis 767
    rolling type 494
    and short esophagus 763
    signs 750
    sliding type 494, 741
    surgical treatment 776–779
        in case of brachyesophagus 777
        different techniques 777
        indications 776
        results 778
        thoracic vs abdominal approach 776
    symptoms 747–749
    symptoms mimicking angina pectoris
        747
    technique of radiological examination
        751
    temporary — in merycism 418, 502
    traumatic 750
    treatment, if found incidentally during
        operation 777
Hiatus insufficiency 742
Hiccup, associated with esophageal carci-
    noma 459
High pressure zone, see Sphincter
Hill repair
    influence on sphincteric pressure 52, 424
    in treatment of hiatal hernia 777
His
    angle of — 744
    in belching 414
    importance in gastroesophageal sphinc-
        teric competence 51
Histoplasmosis 565
History taking, sequence of questionning
    in diagnostic approach 112–118
Histoplasmosis, causing esophagorespiratory
    fistula 810
Hoarseness in esophageal carcinoma 459
Hodgkin's disease 485, 486
    causing varices 703
Honeywell motility probe 241–243
Hormones, influence on gastro-esophageal
    sphincter 53–56
Hurst dilator 798
Hydatid cysts
    causing varices 703
    involving esophagus 839
Hydramnios, incidence in esophageal atresia
    619
Hyoid bone, during swallowing in
        myotonic dystrophy 396
    in treatment of achalasia 321
    in treatment of post-vagotomy dysphagia
        370
Hypaque, see Contrast materials
Hyperkeratosis 444
Hypermethioninemia, causing varices 707
Hyperplasia, epithelial 444
Hypersplenism in Banti syndrome 701
Hypertensive, hyperreactive, hypercontract-
    ing gastroesophageal sphincter 362
    in hiatal hernia 423, 747, 749

Hyperthyroidism and muscle wasting 399
Hypertrophic osteoarthropathy associated
    with esophageal disease 830
Hypnosis
    in treatment of achalasia 321
Hypoglycemia, effect on gastroesophageal
    sphincter 55
Hypothyroidism 399
Hyterical globe 409
Hysterical spasm 355
Hytrast, see Contrast materials

Iatrogenic perforation of esophagus
    683–688
    causing esophagocavitary fistula 816
    complication of endoscopy 216, 684
    complication of myotomy 336
    complication of pneumatic dilatations
        325–327
    complication of surgery 685
    etiology and pathogenesis 684
    incidence 683
    pain after endoscopy as indication of
        perforation 685
    radiological distinction from intramural
        rupture 695
    symptoms and signs 685
    treatment 686
Idiopathic muscular hypertrophy of the
    lower esophagus 361
Idiopathic splenomegaly, causing varices
    701
Image intensifier 122–124
Impaction, see Obstruction syndrome;
    Stricture syndrome
    in carcinoma of the esophagus 105, 118,
        459
    in diffuse spasm 356
    in epidermolysis bullosa dystrophica 825
    in esophageal webs 574, 577, 579
    by foreign body 667
        see also, Foreign bodies
    in lower esophageal ring 584
    in lower esophagus lined with columnar
        epithelium 532
    meat impaction 672
    in peptic stenosis 504
    in post-vagotomy dysphagia 367
    site of pain sensation in relation to
        location of obstruction 667
Impression
    by anomalous vessels 651, 653, 656
    causes of pathological impression
        175–177, 190
    by normal structures 144, 150, 154
    by pathological conditions 152
    radiological aspects of pathological
        impression 175–177, 190
    radiological distinction between intrinsic
        and extrinsic masses 166
Incisura cardiaca 744
Incarceration, complication of para-
    esophageal hernia 764
Incompetent gastroesophageal sphincter,
    see Reflux, gastroesophageal

Infants, *see* Neonates and children
Influenza, involving the esophagus 551
Inhibition
  deglutitive inhibition 89–91
    in different animal species 89
    electromyographic studies 230, 270, 273, 274, 280–282
    of esophageal propulsive force 87
    of oropharyngeal phase of swallowing 64
    of peristalsis 82
    by distension 91
  interference between deglutition- and other centers 80
Inhibitory fibers, in motor innervation of smooth muscle esophagus 85
Initial negative deflexion of esophageal deglutition complex 72
Innervation 75–85
  adrenergic
    and gastroesophageal sphincter relaxation 91, 423
      deficit in achalasia 293
    histochemical studies and functional correlations 36
    and motor innervation of smooth muscle esophagus 85
  afferent pathways
    central afferent system 78
    influence of afferent impulses on pattern of vagal discharge 82
    influence of afferent impulses on peristalsis 82
    of esophageal peristalsis 82–84
    peripheral afferent nerves of esophageal phase of swallowing 76
    receptors for initiation of swallowing 76, 80
    receptors in smooth muscle part of esophagus 82
    receptors in swallowing muscles 75
  anatomy 12
  cholinergic
    histochemical studies and functional correlations 37
    and motor innervation of smooth muscle esophagus 85
  cortical control of chewing 78
  cortical control of deglutition center 78–80
  deglutition center 75
    excitation of — 75
    functional connection between half centers 75
    interference with other centers 80
    localization 75
  efferent pathways
    of esophageal peristalsis 84
    of pharyngeal constrictors 75
    of striated esophageal muscle 81
    of swallowing act 81
  elementary reflexes 77, 78
  of esophageal phase of swallowing 82–85
  fasciculus solitarius (tractus and nucleus) 78

  of gastroesophageal sphincter 57, 423
  intrinsic, *see* Myenteric plexus; Submucosal plexus
  motoneurons activated during swallowing act 81
  motor nerve fibers of smooth muscle esophagus 85
  motor nuclei of vagus 82
  of oropharyngeal phase of swallowing 75–81
  of pharyngoesophageal sphincter 81
  of pharynx, *see* Pharynx, innervation
  reflex responses of esophagus 86–89
  sensory 36, *see also* Innervation, afferent pathways
  sympathetic, *see also* Nerve
    role in esophageal peristalsis 84
Interferential tracing (electromyographic) 274
Intermediary tracing (electromyographic) 274
Interposition procedure 783, *see also* Reconstruction
  in achalasia 333
  gastric sites for implantation of esophageal substitute 790
  in treatment of stricture in progressive systemic sclerosis 389
  in treatment of stricture in reflux esophagitis 518
Intestinal cells in esophageal mucosa 25
Intraarterial infusion of vasoactive drugs, in treatment of bleeding esophageal varices 721
Intraluminal pressure measurement, *see* Manometry
Intramural bleeding, *see* Rupture, intramural
Intramural diverticulosis 836, *see also* Diverticula, intramural
Intramural nervous system, *see* Myenteric plexus
Intubation, gastric, inducing reflux esophagitis 426, 519, 750, 795
Invagination
  esophagogastric 838
  in treatment of hypopharyngeal diverticula 602
Iron deficiency and upper esophageal web 573, 574, 575
Irradiation, causing achalasia-like disturbances 292
Ischemia
  causing achalasia-like disturbances 292
  causing extensive necrosis of esophagus 838
  in the pathogenesis of reflux esophagitis 520
Ischemic esophagitis 503

Jejunostomy
  in the management of esophageal tumor 783
Jejunum, as an esophageal substitute 785
  functional results 791–792
Junction line, posterior, *see* Line

Kelly-Paterson syndrome, *see* Paterson-
  Kelly syndrome
Keratoderma
  and carcinoma 829
  involving esophagus 829
Keratosis follicularis
  involving esophagus 828
Killian's triangle 594
Kinsella-technique for radiological demon-
  stration of hiatus hernia 755
Koilonychia in upper esophageal web 571
Kommerell's diverticulum 651, 815
Kupffer cell hypertrophy, causing varices 704

Lactulose in treatment of bleeding eso-
  phageal varices 720
Ladder spasm 355
Laimer's triangle 4, 32, 594
Laimer-Bertelli's membrane, *see*
  Phrenoesophageal membrane
Laryngectomy
  and esophageal speech 42, 80
  and pharyngeal transport 62
Laryngopharyngography with contrast
  material 187–190
Laryngo-tracheo-esophageal cleft 646–648
Lavage technique for cytology 220
L-dopa in treatment of dysphagia in
  Parkinsonism 404
Leading complex 63
Leakage of anastomosis after esophagogastrectomy 479, 790
Leiomyoma 431, 433–441, *see also* Benign
  tumors and cysts
  age and sex incidence 433
  association with esophageal carcinoma
    436
  association with esophageal diverticula
    436, 610
  association with hiatal hernia 436
  calcification 434
  complications 441
  degeneration 441
  diagnosis 439–441
    distinction between benign extra-
      mucosal tumor
      and carcinoma 439, 441
    distinction from contraction of crico-
      pharyngeal muscle 439
    distinction between intramural
      extramucosal and benign sessile
      polypoid growth 439
    distinction between intramural extra-
      mucosal and extrinsic growth 439
  esophagoscopy 438
  indication for bronchoscopy 439, 441
  multiple tumors 433
  pathology 433–436
  radiographic signs 436–438
    barium swallow examination 173,
      179, 437
    plain chest film 436
  size and shape of the tumor 433
  symptoms 436
  treatment 441

Leiomyomatosis 433
Leiomyosarcoma 484
Leishmania, pseudocyste in Chagas' disease
  309
Lerche's lower esophageal sphincter 7, 68
Leukemia, causing varices 703
Leukokeratosis, *see also* Leukoplakia
  heriditary, involving esophagus 831
Leukoplakia 444, 487
  involving esophagus 830
  in progressive systemic sclerosis 386,
    387
  in syphilis 557
Ligamentum
  gastrohepaticum 745
  gastrolienale 745
  gastrophrenicum 745
Line
  paraesophageal, right and left
    normal 150, 152
    displaced by mediastinal or eso-
      phageal widening 159, 160, 172
  posterior mediastinal (posterior junction)
    normal 153
    obscured by mediastinal or esophageal
      widening 160
Lipiodol, *see* Contrast materials
Lipoma 431, 443
Lipomatosis of cardia 838
Lipomyoma 431
Liver tissue in esophagus 840
Localized esophageal spasm 355
Lortat-Jacob's esophagogastropexy, in
  treatment of hiatus hernia 777
Low's muscle 8
Lower esophageal sphincter (L.E.S.), *see*
  Sphincter, gastroesophageal
Lower esophageal sphincter of Lerche,
  see Lerche
Lower esophagus lined with columnar epithe-
  lium 525–538
  acquired vs congenital origin 529–531
  associated with keratoderma 829
  and esophageal adenocarcinoma 456
  in infants 749
  local production of gastric juice 531
  origin 25, 26
  and peptic stricture 528
  PD measurements 258
  structure of epithelium 526
Lump
  sensation of — in the throat 409
Lupus erythomatosus involving esophagus
  389, 835
  and monilial esophagitis 559
Lye, causing corrosive esophagitis 539
Lyell's disease, see Toxic epidermal neurolysis
Lymphatic drainage 11
  direction of flow 11
  thoracic duct 3
  lymphatico venous anastomoses 11
Lymph nodes
  anatomy 11
  cervical lymph node biopsy in esophageal
    carcinoma 463

compressing the esophagus 177
malignant mediastinal, causing eso-
    phagorespiratory fistula 807
metastases of esophageal carcinoma
    454
Lymphoma, malignant 484
Lymphosarcoma 485
Lysol, causing corrosive esophagitis 539

Machado-Guerreiro's complement fixation
    test in Chagas' disease 309, 311
Malabsorption syndrome, predisposing to
    esophageal carcinoma 444
Malignant tumors 447–492
    see also Carcinoma; Carcinosarcoma;
        Sarcoma
Mallory-Weiss syndrome 689–693
    arteriography of celiac artery 691
    clinical distinction from intramural rup-
        ture and bleeding 695
    endoscopy 691
    incidence 689
    intraluminal pressures required for 690
    pathogenesis 690
    pathology 692
    radiological features 692
    and spontaneous rupture 690
    symptoms and signs 691
    treatment 692
Malocclusion of teeth associated with infantile
    pattern of swallowing 65
Maloney dilator 798
Malposition cardiotubérositaire 742
Manometry
    in achalasia 304–307
    in atresia 631
    in belching 414
    in brainstem lesions 402
    in diabetic motility disorders 407
    in diffuse spasm 358–361
        after succesful treatment 364
    in esophageal belching 413
    in esophageal carcinoma 464
    in esophageal involvement by bullous
        pemphigoid 824
    in esophagus proper, see Resting pressure;
        Deglutition complex
    in gastroesophageal sphincter, see Sphinc-
        ter, gastroesophageal
    in hiatus hernia 496, 497
    in hypopharyngeal diverticula 595
    in lower esophageal ring 586
    in lower esophagus lined with columnar
        epithelium 529, 533
    in lupus erythematosus disseminatus 836
    manometric technique 235–245
        balloon-kymography 235
        disadvantages of open-tip catheter
            238
        factors responsible for variability of
            results 239
        influence of spatial orientation of
            sensors 239
        intraluminal pressure measurements
            236–238

measurement of squeeze of contrac-
    tion 240
method of analyzing motility records
    243
method of performing motility studies
    in humans 243
miniature balloons 235, 238
perfused catheter system 238–241
pull-through technique of examination
    238
in myasthenia gravis 398
in myotonic dystrophy 396
in myxedema 399
in neonatal infants 379–381
in ocular myopathy and oculopharyngeal
    myopathy 397
in old age 372–376
in pharynx, see Pharynx
in pharyngoesophageal sphincter, see
    Sphincter, pharyngoesophageal
in poliomyelitis 403
in polymyositis 390
in post-vagotomy dysphagia 368
in progressive systemic sclerosis 387
in reflux esophagitis 515
in scleroderma 313
and simultaneous radiological studies
    in diffuse spasm 360
    of esophageal peristalsis 66
    in pharynx and pharyngoesophageal
        sphincter 42, 69–71
Marginal ulcer, see Ulcer
Measles, causing esophagitis 551
Mecholyl
    in achalasia 293, 308
Mecholyl test
    in achalasia 308
    in Chagas' diasease 308, 311, 312
    in distal esophageal obstruction 267
    in familial dysautonomia 405
    in motility disorders 266–268
    in myotonic dystrophy 397
    in old age 377
    in presbyesophagus 267
    in progressive systemic sclerosis 267,
        387
    in symptomatic diffuse spasm 308,
        359
Mediastinal abscess, complication of
    esophagogastrectomy 479, 791
Mediastinal cysts, radiological signs of
    esophageal impression 176
Mediastinal emphysema 163
Mediastinal fibrosis, causing downhill varices
    709
Mediastinal line, see Line
Mediastinal widening
    on chest X-rays 436
    in esophageal carcinoma 462
    in esophageal diseases 159–161
Mediastinitis
    caused by iatrogenic perforations 686
    in spontaneous rupture of esophagus 677
Mediastinoscopy, in esophageal carcinoma
    463

Megacolon
  in Chagas' disease 310
  in familial dysautonomia 405
Megaesophagus idiopathic 287
Meissner plexus, see Submucosal plexus
Melanoma, malignant 486
Melanosis of esophagus 486, 839
Membrane, esophagodiaphragmatic 725, 744
  see also Phrenoesophageal membrane
Meniscus sign, in esophageal carcinoma
  167, 460
Mercuric chloride, causing achalasia-like
  disturbances 292
Merycism 415–421
  in adults 417–421
  in infants 415–417
    neuropsychiatric aspects 416
  mechanism 416, 418, 502
Metastases, see also Carcinoma
  diagnosis of liver metastases from esopha-
    geal carcinoma 464
  in esophagus 169, 486
  in liver, causing varices 703
Metaplastic squamous cells, distinction from
  malignant cells 226
Methotrexate in esophageal carcinoma 482
Methylene blue
  in diagnosis of congenital bronchoesopha-
    geal fistula 644
  in diagnosis of esophagocavitary fistula
    818
  in diagnosis of esophagopleural fistula
    679
  in diagnosis of esophagorespiratory
    fistula 812
  in diagnosis of isolated tracheoesophageal
    fistula 640
Metoclopramide
  effect on gastroesophageal sphincter
    423
  in treatment of sphincter incompetence
    775
Migration time of epithelial cells 19
Millhon-Crites motility probe 241
Miniature balloons in esophageal manometry
  235, 238
Modulation transfer function 124
Monilial esophagitis 558–564
  characteristics of pain 107
  and intramural diverticulosis 836
Morphine, causing esophageal dilatation 313
Mosher bag for dilatations 324
Motility disorders, 287–421
  see also Manometry; Reflux, gastroeso-
    phageal; Sphincter, gastroesophageal;
    Sphincter, pharyngoesophageal
  in esophageal atresia 631
  in esophageal carcinoma 464
  in epiphrenic diverticula 607
  in hiatal hernia 768
  in hypopharyngeal diverticula 595
  in lower esophagus lined with columnar
    epithelium 529
Motor endplates in striated esophageal muscle
  67, 84

Motor nerve fibers of smooth muscle esophagus
  adrenergic fibers 85
  cholinergic excitatory fibers 85
  non-cholinergic excitatory fibers 85
  non-cholinergic, non-adrenergic inhibitory
    fibers 85
Motor neurons, see Innervation
Motor neuron disease, causing swallowing difficulties 403
Motor nuclei for swallowing act 81
Mould effect 438
Mousseau's tube 481, 805
Mucormycosis 565
Mucosal folds
  distinction from esophageal varices at eso-
    phagoscopy 714, 715
  gastric folds above diaphragm as a sign of
    hiatus hernia 757
  transmucosal fold in lower esophagus; dis-
    tinction from lower esophageal ring
    583
Mucosal pattern
  abnormal radiological images 180–184
  normal radiological appearance 154
Mucosal seal, in gastroesophageal sphincter
  competence 51
Mucosal stripe sign
  in esophagitis superficialis dissecans (ideo-
    pathic esophageal casts) 827
  in intramural rupture 695
Mucosal tears at cardia, see Mallory-Weiss
  syndrome
Mucoviscidosis, causing varices 707
Mueller maneuver, and pH measurements
  249
Multiple sclerosis, causing swallowing difficulties 402
Muscle contraction in lower esophagus, distinction from lower esophageal ring 586
  distinction from midesophageal ring 579
  radiological distinction between muscle
    contraction and webs and rings 571
Muscle, see also Musculature
  bronchoesophageal 4
  cricopharyngeal 4, 6
  pleuroesophageal 4
  pharyngeal constrictors 6
    electromyography of — 64
  oropharyngeal, in myotonic dystrophy
    394
  thyropharyngeus 42
  tracheoesophageal 1
Muscle disorders, involving esophagus 394–
  401
  see also Myotonic dystrophy; Ocular myo-
    pathy; Myasthenia gravis; Hyperthy-
    roidism; Myxedema
Muscular hypertrophy of the esophagus 355
Muscularis mucosae, histology 29
Musculature
  anatomy 4
  arrangement of circular bundles at eso-
    phageal entrance 32
  arrangement of muscle layers 4, 30–34

arrangement of muscle layers at lower
    sphincter   32, 422
circular muscle layer,
    anatomy   6
    deglutitive electrical activity   277
    pharmacology   67
coordination of longitudinal and circular
    muscle layer
during peristalsis   65
    electromyographic data on sequence
        of contraction   275
    histology   30–34
longitudinal muscle layer
    anatomy   6
    deglutitive electrical activity of — 277
oblique fibers of stomach   744
pharyngeal constrictors   6
    electromyography   64
smooth
    changes in achalasia   291
    changes in diffuse spasm   356
    changes in myotonic dystrophy   394
    changes in myasthenia gravis   398
    changes in progressive systemic scle-
        rosis   386
        correlation with motility disturb-
            ances   386
    distribution   4, 33, 67
    dysfunction in myotonic dystrophy
        395, 397
    electrical and mechanical properties
        67
    idiopathic muscular hypertrophy of
        lower esophagus   361
striated
    changes in myotonic dystrophy   394,
        395, 396, 397
    changes in myasthenia gravis   398
    distribution   4, 32, 67
    electrical and mechanical properties
        67
thickness of muscle layers   31
    in achalasia   291
    in diffuse spasm   356
    in idiopathic muscular hypertrophy
        361
transitional zone of striated and smooth
    muscle
    location   4
    progression of peristalsis   73
Myasthenia gravis   398
Mycelial form of monilia   560, 563
Mycoses   558–567
    causing esophagorespiratory fistula   810
Myenteric plexus (Auerbach's plexus)
    in animal achalasia   289
    argyrophile and argyrophobe ganglion
        cells in achalasia   291
    in diabetic neuropathy   407
    and efferent innervation of smooth eso-
        phageal muscle   84, 85
    and efferent innervation of striated eso-
        phageal muscle   81
    embryonic development   15, 379
    in familial dysautonomia   404

in idiopathic muscular hypertrophy   362
importance for peristaltic esophageal con-
    traction in smooth muscle esophagus
    85
histology   36
motor neurons   85
in myasthenia gravis   398
in myotonic dystrophy   394, 397
in old age   377
in patients with achalasia   291
in patients with Chagas' disease   309, 310
    311
in patients with diffuse spasm   356
in progressive systemic sclerosis   387
Myoma   431
Myopathy, see Muscle disorders
Myotomy
    cricopharyngeal, in treatment of hypo-
        pharyngeal diverticula   602
    esophageal
        in treatment of diffuse spasm   364
        in treatment of epiphrenic diverticula
            610
        in treatment of familial dysautonomia
            404
        in treatment of post-vagotomy dys-
            phagia   370
    Heller
        in treatment of achalasia   334, 338
        causes of failure   336
        complications   336
        technique   332
        vs forceful dilatation   339–341
Myotonic dystrophy, involving esophagus
    394–397
Myxedema, involving esophagus
Myxofibroma   431, 443
Myxoma   431, 443

Nacleiro's V-sign in rupture of esophagus
    164, 678
Naevus, white spongy, see Leukokeratosis,
    hereditary
Narrowings, see also Stenosis
    esophageal, causes of — 178–180
    hypopharyngeal, causes of — 190
Narrowings of normal esophagus
    anatomy   3
    importance for caustic lesions   541
Nasogastric tube, in treatment of corrosive
    esophagitis   546, 803
Necrosis of esophagus, due to ischemia   838
Negus' hydrostatic dilator   322
Neomycine
    in treatment of bleeding esophageal
        varices   720
Neonates and children
    anatomy   1
    development of gastroesophageal sphinc-
        ter   380, 425
    esophageal motility   379–382
    radiological examination   194–198
        prevertebral layer bulging into the pha
            rynx   140
    webs and rings   575, 578

Neostigmine in achalasia, *see* Mecholyl   308
Nerve, *see also* Innervation
  lesions (peripheral), causing esophageal
    motility disorders   407
  recurrent   1, 2, 3, 81
    compression in hypopharyngeal diver-
      ticula   596, 598
    damage in upper esophageal resection
      784
    innervation of esophagus   12
    invasion by metastases   459
    paralysis in tuberculosis   554
  superior laryngeal
    elementary reflexes   77
    faradization   78
    initiation of swallowing by stimulation
      of —   75, 77
  vagal   2, 3
    anatomy   12
    conduction velocity in efferent fibers
      84
    degenerative lesions in achalasia
      290
    degenerative lesions in diffuse spasm
      356
    dysfunction in achalasia patients
      291
    electrical stimulation   82, 84
    motor innervation of cervical eso-
      phagus   81, 84
    motor innervation of thoracic eso-
      phagus   84
    sympathetic and parasympathetic fi-
      bers   12, 13, 36
Nervous plexus
  esophageal   2, 3, 12, 35–37
  pharyngeal   13, 81
Neurofibroma   431
Neuromuscular disorders, *see* Motility disorders
Neuromuscular incoordination at the cardia
  of the newborn   317
Neuropathy (peripheral), causing esophageal
  motility disorders   407
Nissen's
  fundoplication in treatment of hiatus
    hernia   777
  ventral gastropexy in treatment of hiatus
    hernia   777
Nitrites
  in treatment of achalasia   321
  in treatment of diffuse spasm   364
  in treatment of post-vagotomy syndrome
    370
Nodose ganglion, and detection of afferent
  esophageal impulses   82
Non-cholinergic excitatory fibers in motor
  innervation of smooth esophageal muscle
  85
Non-cholinergic excitatory nerve in "off"
  response   89
Nucleus, *see also* Motor nuclei
  ambiguus   81, 82
    in achalasia patients   290
    in animal achalasia   289

dorsalis nervi vagi   82
  in achalasia patients   290
  in Chagas' disease   309
tracti solitarii   78
Nystatin, in treatment of esophageal mycoses
  564

Obstruction syndrome   109–111, *see also* Impaction; Stricture syndrome
  of achalasia type   110, 115
    distinction from carcinoma   110, 115–
      118
  of advanced cancer type   115
  of stricture type
    characteristics   115
    characteristics of benign stricture   110
    characteristics of malignant stricture
      110
    characteristics of peptic stricture
      110
    distinction between benign and malig-
      nant lesions   110, 118
    distinction between esophageal and
      fundal carcinoma   110, 118
    distinction between peptic strictures
      and carcinoma   110
Obstruction of vena cava superior, causing
  varices   709
Ocular myopathy   397
Oculopharyngeal myopathy   397
Odynophagia
  and esophageal ulcer   771
  and foreign body   667
  and monilial esophagitis   107, 560
Off-response   88
Ono's sign   812
On-response   87
Open-tip catheter, in intraluminal pressure
  measurements   236–238
Oral submucous fibrosis, involving esophagus
  830
Organelles
  of columnar epitheliumcells   27
  of germinative cells   21–23
  of stratum spinosum cells   23
Osteochondrome   431
Osteophytes
  predisposing to iatrogenic perforation
    684
  producing impression on posterior wall
    142, 185, 190, 838

Paget's disease   486
Pain of esophageal origin   107
  in achalasia   294
  acid induced pain and acid barium meal
    134, 501
  in carcinoma of esophagus   459
  in corrosive esophagitis   541
  diagnostic significance of character of —
    107
  diagnostic significance of distribution of—
    107
  diagnostic significance of posture in which
    it occurs   108

diagnostic significance of timing of — 107
in diffuse spasm 356
    pathophysiological basis 360
and foreign body 667
from gastroesophageal reflux 108
in hypertensive sphincter syndrome 362
in intramural diverticulosis 836
and "irritating" drinks 108, 112
in leiomyoma 436
in lower esophagus lined with columnar epithelium 532
in monilial esophagitis 107, 560
in motility disturbances 108
in post-vagotomy dysphagia 367
in reflux esophagitis 107, 505
in stricture of esophagus 107
in suppurative esophagitis 551
in ulcer esophagus 107
Palsy of pharynx 191, see also Central nervous system disorders
Pancreatitis, causing esophageal stenosis 839
Pancreatic tissue in esophagus 840
Papillae of squamous epithelium 17
in esophagitis 497
Papilloma 431, 444
treatment 444
Paraesophageal line, see Line, paraesophageal
Paraesophageal type of hiatal hernia 494
Parapemphigus, see Pemphigoid, bullous
Parasympathetic, see Innervation
Parathyroid masses, producing impression on pharyngoesophageal region 190
Parietal cells in esophageal mucosa 25
Parkinson's disease, causing swallowing difficulties 404
Partial nodular transformation of liver, causing varices 708
Passevant's ridge 62, 71
Paterson-Kelly syndrome, (Plummer-Vinson syndrome) see also Webs, upper esophageal
cytological diagnosis of cancer 225
predisposing to esophageal carcinoma 448, 460
PD measurements 253–261
comparison of pH- and PD recording techniques 255
electrodes 256
in esophageal carcinoma 259
in esophageal ulceration 258
in esophagitis 259
location of reference electrode 256
location of squamocolumnar junction 257
in lower esophagus lined with columnar epithelium 258
origin of PD 253–255
and presence of parietal cells 258
PD profile in gastroesophageal region 257
PD profile in pharyngoesophageal region 259
role of active Na+ absorption in origin of PD 254

role of Cl⁻ secretion in origin of PD 254
technique of PD measurements 255–257
Pemphigoid
benign mucosal, involving esophagus 824
bullous, involving esophagus 823
cicatricial 824
Pemphigus vulgaris, involving esophagus
antigenicity of esophageal mucosa 823
pathology 823
Pentagastrin, see gastrin
Peptic stricture, see Stenosis; Stricture; Obstruction syndrome
Perforation
in colon used for esophageal replacement 791
distinction between perforation and rupture 675
in esophageal mycosis 563
iatrogenic, see Iatrogenic perforation
radiological signs on plain chest films 163–165
Perfused catheter system in manometry 238–241
rate of perfusion for yield pressure 239
rate of perfusion for squeeze pressure 240
Periesophageal edema or granulomatous reaction, postoperative, causing dysphagia 368, 370
Peptic esophagitis, see Esophagitis, reflux
Peptic ulcer in hiatus hernia 771
Peristaltic esophageal contraction
in achalasia 307
afferent pathway for esophageal phase 82–84
in atresia 631
in carcinoma (vs. achalasia) 313
and central nervous system 82, 85
coordination of longitudinal and circular muscle coats 65
in diabetic motility disorders 407
in diffuse spasm
    manometry 359
    radiology 356
effect of vagotomy 82, 84
efferent pathway for esophageal phase 84
and electrical stimulation of efferent vagal fibers 82
electromyographic studies, see Electromyography
gradient of contraction in esophagus 89
in infants 381
influence of afferent impulses 82
influence of age 65
influence of bolus on speed of — 82
influence of esophageal distension on progression of — 82
in motor neuron disease 403
in myasthenia gravis 398
in myotonic dystrophy 396, 397
in ocular myopathy and oculopharyngeal myopathy 397, 398

Peristaltic esophageal contraction — *cont.*
  in old age 372–375
  in polymyositis 390
  in post-vagotomy dysphagia 368, 369
  primary 59–85
    influence of preceding peristalsis on
      amplitude and progression 89
      young vs. old subjects 375
    length of contracting segment 65
    pressure changes 73
    speed 65, 67, 73
      in myxedema 399
      young vs. old subjects 374
    manometry 387
  propagating mechanisms of primary and
    secondary peristalsis 86
  in progressive systemic sclerosis 387
  radiological appearance 148
  secondary 86
    after transection of striated muscle
      esophagus 86
    speed 86
    stimuli for initiation 86
    threshold for initiation 86
  and sympathetic innervation 84
  after transection of striated muscle eso-
    phagus 85
  and vagal innervation 84
Pernicious anemia and gastroesophageal
  sphincter 54
Pharmacological agents in radiological examination 194
Pharmacological tests 266–269
Pharmacoradiography 194
Pharyngeal dimple 594
Pharyngeal nervous plexus 12
Pharyngocoele 591, 593
Pharyngoesophageal junction
  anatomy 6
  innervation 12
  special procedures for radiological examin-
    ation 184–192
Pharyngoesophageal sphincter, *see* Sphincter,
  pharyngoesophageal
Pharynx
  in brainstem lesions 402
  deglutition complex 69–71
  dilatation due to bilateral pharyngeal
    palsy 191
  hypopharynx
    radiological landmarks 138–140
  innervation 75–81
    afferent nerve supply 76
    central afferent system 78
    efferent pathway for pharyngeal con-
      strictors 75
    motor neurons 81
    motor nuclei 81
    plexus pharyngeus 81
    receptors for initiation of swallowing
      76
  motility disorders 191
    discriminative symptoms 114
  in motor neuron disease 403
  in myasthenia gravis 398
  in myotonic dystrophy 394, 396
  in neonatal infants 379
  normal radiological appearance 138–147
  in ocular myopathy and oculopharyngeal
    dystrophy 397
  in old people 147, 191, 372, 593
  pharyngeal constrictors
    anatomy 6
    electromyography 64
  in poliomyelitis 390, 402
  radiological landmarks of hypopharynx
    138–140
  special procedures for radiological exami-
    nation 184–192
  stricture, discriminative symptoms
  stricture, discriminative symptoms 114
  web, discriminative symptoms 114
Phenol
  causing achalasia-like disturbances 292
  causing corrosive esophagitis 539
Phlegmon of esophagus 551, 694
pH measurements 246–252
  acid clearing test 250
  clinical significance of duration of pH drop
    242, 250
  comparision of PD and pH recording
    techniques 255
  comparision with other techniques for
    evaluation of reflux 250
  electrodes 246
  interpretation of reflux 249
  location of reference electrode 246
  maneuvers to induce gastroesophageal
    reflux 248
  methods for performing pH studies in
    human esophagus
    pull-through techniques 247
    technique of fixed location of pH
      electrode 248, 500
  occasional reflux in normal persons 250,
    251
  pH profile in gastroesophageal region
    247
  protracted pH measurements 251
  technique of in vivo recording 246
Photofluorography of swallowing act 127,
  187
Phrenic ampulla 69, 156
  and hiatus hernia 742
Phrenoesophageal membrane 7
  importance in gastroesophageal sphincter
    competence 51, 502
Phrenospasm, *see* Achalasia, synonyms
Physiology 40–102
Pinchcock mechanism of diaphragmatic hiatus 51
Pleuroesophageal stripe, *see* Line, paraesophageal
Pleural complications after esophagogastrec-
  tomy 480
Plummer's
  dilating metal olives 798
  hydrostatic dilator 322
Plummer-Vinson syndrome, *see* Paterson-
  Kelly syndrome; Web, upper esophageal

Pneumatosis cystoides, involving esophagus 837
Pneumo (hydro) thorax
  as early sign of anastomotic leak 479, 629
  in esophageal perforation by foreign bodies 670
  after esophagogastrectomy 480
  and esophagorespiratory fistula 812
  in iatrogenic esophageal perforation 686
  in spontaneous rupture of esophagus 677
Pneumomediastinography, in esophageal carcinoma 463
Pneumomediastinum, as diagnostic aid in leiomyoma 437
Pneumonia, complicating esophageal atresia 620
Poliomyelitis
  and swallowing disorders 75, 402
  and glossopharyngeal respiration 80
Polishers, causing corrosive esophagitis 539
Polycystic liver disease, causing varices 703
Polymyositis 389
Polypoid lesions 431
  eosinophilic granuloma 838
  fibrovascular polyp 443
  pedunculated carcinosarcoma 485
  pedunculated cyst 443
  pedunculated esophageal carcinoma 449
  pedunculated leiomyoma 439
  pedunculated mucosal growth 439
  pedunculated pseudosarcoma 485
  pedunculated sarcoma 485
  radiological aspects 171–173
Polyposis coli, associated with esophageal carcinoma 444
Porphyria hepatica, causing varices 708
Portal hypertension 699–709
Portal venous thrombosis and compression, causing esophageal varices 701
Portocaval anastomosis, as emergency procedure for bleeding varices 722
Postcricoid impression, see Venous impression postcricoid
Post-vagotomy diarrhea, after resection of the esophagus 784
Post-vagotomy dysphagia 367–371
  see also Dysphagia
Post-vagotomy syndrome due to intramural hematoma 695
Potassium permanganate, causing corrosive esophagitis 539
Pouch, see Diverticulum
Pregnancy
  and achalasia 320
  and esophagitis 502
  and heartburn 426, 521
  and hiatus hernia 749
Prematurity
  and esophageal atresia 619
Presbyesophagus 372–378
  mecholyl test 267
  radiology
    air esophagogram 158

asymmetric swallowing 191
hypopharynx 147, 593
indentation due to tortuosity of the descending aorta 175
retention of contrast material in the esophagus 165
thoracic esophagus, deviating to the left 151
Pressure gradient
  in esophagus proper at rest 45
  gastroesophageal
    and Mallory-Weiss syndrome 690
    and rupture of the esophagus 676
Pressure inversion point (P.I.P.)
  in gastroesophageal sphincter 46–48
  in pharyngoesophageal sphincter 43
  in relation to diaphragmatic hiatus 46, 47
Pressure measurements, see Manometry
Pressure profile
  of gastroesophageal sphincter 46–48
  of pharyngoesophageal sphincter 41
Pressure waves
  of esophageal deglutition complex
    final positive wave 73
    first positive wave 72
      electrical equivalent 278
    initial negative deflection 72
      in old age 373
    second positive wave 73
      in old age 373
  giant, in diffuse spasm 358, 359, 363, 364
  inspiratory positive pressure wave in pharyngoesophageal sphincter 240
  peristaltic contraction in esophagus proper 73
  of pharyngeal deglutition complex
    e-wave 71
    f-phase 71
    p-wave 71
    t-wave 71
  tertiary contraction, see Tertiary contraction
Prevertebral space
  causes of enlargement 184
  false enlargement in children 184
  normal radiological appearance 139
  widening by foreign body 669, 670
Primary lateral sclerosis, causing swallowing difficulties 403
Procainamide, in treatment of myotonic dystrophy 394
Progressive bulbar palsy, causing swallowing difficulties 403
Progressive muscular atrophy, causing swallowing difficulties 403
Progressive systemic sclerosis 383–389
  differential diagnosis with achalasia 313
  esophageal involvement 425
  gastrointestinal involvement 384, 385–389
  general data 383–385
  mecholyl test 267
  treatment 385

Prolaps
  of esophageal mucosa into stomach 765
  of gastric mucosa into esophagus 765
Propulsive force of esophagus 87
Prostaglandins, effect on gastroesophageal
  sphincter 55
Prostigmine, see Anticholinesterases 398
Proteinase A, in treatment of meat impac-
  tion 672
Protein ingestion, effect on gastroesophageal
  sphincter 55
Proventriculosis, see Achalasia, synonyms
Pseudobulbar palsy, causing swallowing diffi-
  culties 402
Pseudocysts, mediastinal 839
Pseudodiverticula, see also Diverticula
  distinction from diverticula 591
  in epidermolysis bullosa dystrophica 826
Pseudosarcoma 172, 485
Psorospermosis 828
Pull-through technique
  in pressure measurements 238, 243
  in PD measurements 257
  in pH measurements 247
Pulmonary sequestration causing bronchoesophageal fistula 843
Pyloric competence and esophagitis 502
Pylorospasm in familial dysautonomia 405
Pylorus hypertrophy
  and esohageal atresia 622
  and esophageal muscular hypertrophy
    362
Pyriform sinuses 138
  iatrogenic perforation 684
  location 138
  radiological aspect
    in contrast laryngo-pharyngography
      188
    during modified Valsalva maneuver
      147
    in motility disorders causing stasis of
      contrast material 191
    in pharyngeal palsy 191
    during swallowing 144
    after swallowing 146

Quinidine, in treatment of myotonic dystrophy 394

Radiation predisposing to esophageal carcinoma 444
Radiologic-manometric correlations, see
  Manometry
Radiological examination
  in aberrant right subclavian artery 651
  in achalasia 297–304
  in atresia 623–625
  in belching 414
  in brainstem lesions 402
  in children 194–198
  in congenital fistulas 638–648
  in corrosive esophagitis 545
  in diabetic motility disorders 407
  in diffuse spasm 357
  in double aortic arch 653

  double contrast method of examination
    166, 194
  in esophageal belching 412
  equipment 119–127
    cinefluorography 128–131
    image intensifier 122–124
    spot filming 126
    spot film device 120
    television fluoroscopy 125
  in hiatus hernia 494, 496, 751–765
  in lower esophagus lined with columnar
    epithelium 532
  in merycism 418
  in myasthenia gravis 398
  in mycosis of esophagus 561–563
  in myotonic dystrophy 395
  of normal esophagus 138–156
  in ocular myopathy and oculopharyngeal
    myopathy 397
  in old age 372, see also Presbyesophagus
  pharmacoradiography 194
  in poliomyelitis 403
  in polymyositis 390
  in progressive systemic sclerosis 387
  procedures
    basic 165
    special, for examination of pharyngo-
      esophageal region 184–192
    special, for examination of distal
      pouch in atresia 624
  recording techniques
    cinefluorography 131
    contrast laryngopharyngography
      187–190
    photofluorography 127
    videorecording 131–133
  in reflux esophagitis 505–514
  röntgenographic positions
    for visualization of esophagogastric
      junction 120
    for visualization of varices 192–194
  semiology 166–194
    abnormal images on barium swallow
      of esophagus 166–184
      of pharynx 190–192
    abnormal images on plain films of
      neck 184–186
    abnormal images on plain films of
      chest 157–165
  in tuberculosis 554
Raynaud's phenomen
  and esophageal motility disorders 390
  in myotonic dystrophy 394
  in progressive systemic sclerosis 383,
    386
Receptive relaxation of stomach 91
Receptors, see Innervation, afferent pathways
Reconstruction of esophagus 784–792
  by means of colon 787
    right vs left colon 788
  functional results 791
  by means of jejunum 785
  leakage at the anastomosis 790
  mortality and morbidity 788

necrosis of esophageal substitute 788, 789
by means of skin-tube 784
by means of stomach 785
subcutaneous prethoracic route 784
substernal route 784
in treatment of atresia 628
Reflex, *see* Innervation
Reflux, *see* also Sphincter, gastroesophageal, competence and incompetence; Pain of esophageal origin
of air without belching 93
gastroesophageal
and ascites 426
in atresia 620
in bronchoesophageal fistula 644
characteristics of pain 108
comparison different detection techniques 250, 500
and lower esophageal ring treated by dilatation 587
distinction from regurgitation 105
after esophagogastrectomy 791
in experimental hiatal hernia 51, 423
free reflux and long duration reflux 248
after gastrectomy 54, 426
and gastric intubation 426, 502, 519
after Heller's myotomy 337, 340, 425
in hiatus hernia 51, 424, 747, 748
without hiatus hernia 425, 495, 502
see also Hiatal herniation without a sac
after interposition, producing leakage at the anastomosis 790
maneuvers to induce reflux 248, 500
occasional reflux in normal persons 250, 251, 424, 499
pathophysiological basis 422–430
pH-measurements (technique of fixed location of electrodes) 248
pH-profile in gastroesophageal region 247
predisposing to spontaneous rupture of esophagus 676
in pregnancy 426, 502, 521
in progressive systemic sclerosis 386
radiological demonstration 754
and reflex contraction of gastroesophageal sphincter 57
and sphincter tone 50, 422, 424, 425
after vagotomy 426
intestinoesophageal 426, 502, 519
in merycism 416, 418, 502
Reflux esophagitis, *see* Esophagitis, reflux 493–524
Regeneration potentials 270, 283
Regurgitation
abnormal regurgitation in children, techniques of radiological evaluation 198
in achalasia 294
in atresia 620
in carcinoma of esophagus 459
definition 105

diagnostic significance of various characteristics of — 105
distinction from reflux 105
distinction from vomiting 105
in diffuse spasm 356
in epiphrenic diverticulum 608
in fibrovascular polyps 443
in hiatus hernia 747, 748
in hypopharyngeal diverticulum 597
in mycosis of esophagus 560
in neonates and children 380
in post-vagotomy dysphagia 367
Regurgitation (nasal)
in brainstem lesions 402
in myotonic dystrophy 396
in ocular myopathy and oculopharyngeal dystrophy 397
Relaxation, *see* also Sphincter
of gastroesophageal sphincter 66, 68, 69, 74
of pharyngoesophageal sphincter 43, 69
Repetitive waves
in achalasia 307
in diffuse spasm 358, 359, 363
in heartburn 503
in old age 372, 373
Replacement of esophagus, *see* Reconstruction 784–792
Resection and reconstruction 783–793
Reserpin, in treatment of progressive systemic sclerosis 385, 389
Respiration, influence on location of gastroesophageal high pressure zone 47
Respiratory center, interference with deglutitive center 80
Respiratory pressure variations 45
in esophagus proper 45
in gastroesophageal sphincter 46
in pharyngoesophageal sphincter 43
Respiratory spasm provoked by esophagoscopy 217
Resting pressure
in esophagus proper
in achalasia 305
in neonatal infants 380
in normal subjects 45
in gastroesophageal sphincter
in achalasia 304
correlation with gastroesophageal reflux 50, 442–424, 500
in diffuse spasm 359
in hypertensive sphincter 362, 747, 769
in neonatal infants 380
in normal subjects 48–50
in progressive systemic sclerosis 387
respiratory influence on location 47
and spatial orientation of sensors 47, 239
in pharyngoesophageal sphincter 42
in neonatal infants 379
in normal subjects 42
Retching, mechanism of — 92
Reticular formation, and deglutition center 75, 78

Reticulum cell sarcoma 485
Retroperitoneal fibrosis
    involving esophagus 835
    mimicking achalasia 835
Retropharyngeal abscess, producing enlarge-
    ment of prevertebral space 184, 190
Rhabdomyosarcoma 484
Rhizopus, in myotic esophagitis 565
Riboflavin deficiency in upper esophageal web
    573
Ridges of squamous epithelium 17
Riley-Day syndrome 313, 404
Ring 581–588
    A-ring of Wolf 68
    in achalasia 304
    B-ring of Wolf 68
    definition 572
    distinction between ring and web 571
    lower esophageal 581, 588
        association with hiatal hernia 587,
            759, 761
        distinction from carcinoma 587
        distinction from lower esophageal web
            572, 579, 580, 581
        distinction from muscular contraction
            586
        distinction from peptic stenosis 586
        distinction from transmucosal fold
            586
        dysphagia in relation to diameter of
            ring 584
        endoscopic appearance 586
        etiology and pathogenesis 583
        incidence 581–583
        location in relation to gastroesopha-
            geal sphincter 585, 586
        location in relation to vestibule 69,
            585
        manometric data 586
        pathology 584
        radiological appearance 584–586
        radiological technique for visualization
            584
        symptoms and signs 584
        treatment 587
    radiological appearance 180
    radiological distinction between ring,
        stenosis and muscle contraction
        571
    radiological technique of visualization
        571
    Schatzki, see Ring, lower esophageal
    squamocolumnar, see Ring, lower esopha-
        geal
Ring sign in benign esophageal tumor 437
Ritter's disease, see toxic epidermal neurolysis
Rolling type of hiatal hernia 494, 741
Rosary bead esophagus 355
Rubber bougies 798
Ruffini's sensory corpuscles 36
Rumination in cud-chewers 92, see also
    Merycism
Rupture
    intramural 694–696
        distinction from duplication 695

    distinction from esophageal atresia
        695
    distinction from esophageal perfora-
        tion 695
    distinction from Mallory-Weiss syn-
        drome 695
    etiology and pathogenesis 694
    radiological appearance 695
    symptoms and signs 694
    treatment 695
spontaneous 675–682
    in achalasia 319
    causing esophago cavitary fistula 816
    differential diagnosis 679
    distinction from intramural rupture
        695
    distinction between perforation and
        rupture 675
    intraluminal pressures required for —
        676
    location of tear 676
    and Mallory-Weiss syndrome 680
    occurence in childhood 680
    pathogenesis 675
    pathology 676
    radiological localization of site of per-
        foration 678
    radiological signs on plain chest films
        163–165, 678
    symptoms and signs 677
    and syphilis of esophagus 557
    treatment 680

Saint's triad of — 774
Saltzer shot-filled dilator 804
Saltzer technique of preventive bougienage
    546, 803
Sarcoidosis of esophagus 569
    causing varices 763
Sarcoma 484
Saturnus-ring 765
Scaffer and Rüdinger, glands of — 24
Scarlet fever, causing esophagitis 551
Schatzki ring, see Ring, lower esophageal
Schatzki-like ring
    in lower esophagus lined with columnar
        epithelium 532
Schistosomiasis, causing varices 702
Schluckatmung 72, 80
Scleroderma, see Progressive systemic
    sclerosis
Sclerotylosis 829
Screw arrangement of esophageal muscle
    layers 31
Sebaceous glands in esophagus 840
Second positive wave of deglutition com-
    plex 73
    see also Pressure waves
Secondary parasympathetic ganglion cells
    85
Secretin, effect on gastroesophageal sphincter
    55, 423
Sedatives
    in treatment of belching 415
    in treatment of esophageal belching 413

Segal and Dubois de Montreynaud's esophagoscope   205
Segmental esophagitis   568
Segmental spasm   355
Seidlitz powder
in differential diagnosis of achalasia and
carcinoma   313
effect on narrow segment in achalasia
304
Sengstaken-Blakemore tube
cause of iatrogenic perforation   685
in treatment of bleeding esophageal varices   721
in treatment of Mallory-Weiss syndrome
692
Short esophagus
congenital   741
secondary to esophagitis   494, 763, 778
Sickle-cell disease, causing varices   708
Silvernitrate cauterization in congenital bron-
choesophageal fistula   644
Single tracing (electromyographic)   274
Siphonage test, to demonstrate gastroesophageal reflux   755
Sippy's bag for dilatations   324
Sippy's dilating metal olives   798, 800
Sjögren's syndrome, involving esophagus
390
Skin as esophageal substitute   784
Sliding hernia, see Hiatus hernia
Slow waves, see Electrical activity
Small intestine, involvement in progressive
systemic sclerosis   384
Smallpox, involving the esophagus   552
"Smear effect"   438
Smoking
effect on gastroesophageal sphincter   58,
423
predisposing to esophageal carcinoma
444
Sodium hypochlorite (clorox), causing corrosive esophagitis   539
Souttar tube   481, 805
Speed of peristaltic esophageal contraction,
see Peristaltic esophageal contraction
Sphincter
gastroesophageal
in achalasia
deglutitive pressures   305, 306
hypersensitivity to gastrin   305
pressure after successful treatment
338
relaxation   306
resting pressure   304
yield pressure   305
afferent vagal impulses   51
anatomy   6, 422
in atresia   631
in belching and eructation   414
competence and incompetence, see also
Reflux, gastroesophageal
evaluation by pH measurements
249
hormonal control of sphincter
strength   53–56

incompetence and endogenous
gastrin   53
incompetence and eructations
414
incompetence in progressive systemic sclerosis   387
mechanism of competence   51,
422–424
nervous control of sphincter
strength   57, 423
yield pressure, correlation with
gastroesophageal reflux   50,
239, 422, 424, 500, 515
yield pressure as a measure of
sphincter strength   50
correlation of anatomical and radiological data   68
deglutition complex   74
in diabetic motility disorders   407
in diffuse spasm
deglutitive pressures   360
pressures after successful treatment   364
relaxation   359
resting and yield pressures   359
effect of atropine on competence   58,
423
effect of increased gastric and abdominal pressure   56, 57, 423
effect of sympathectomy   57, 58
effect of vagotomy
on relaxation   58, 84, 368, 369
on sphincteric pressures   57, 425
electromyography, see Electromyography
evaluation of competence by pH
measurements   249
in hiatal hernia   496, 747, 769
hormonal control   53–56, 423
hypertensive, hyperreactive, hypercontracting   355, 362, 423, 747,
769
hypersentivity to gastrin in achalasia
305
hypersensitivity to gastrin in progressive systemic sclerosis   387
in isolated preparations   51
location in relation to squamo-columnar junction   46
location in relation to lower esophageal ring   585, 586
in lower esophagus lined by columnar
epithelium   529, 532
manometric localization in relation to
pressure inversion point   380
in merycism   418
in myotonic dystrophy   397
in neonatal infants
manometry   380, 381, 425
radiology   380, 494
nervous control   57, 423
in ocular myopathy and oculopharyngeal myopathy   398
in old people   375
PD profile   257

Sphincter
  gastroesophagial — *cont.*
    in pernicious anemia   54
    pH profile   247
    in polymyositis   390
    in post-vagotomy dysphagia   368
    pressure inversion point   46–48
    pressure profile   46–48
    in progressive systemic sclerosis   387
    in pseudobulbar palsy   402
    relaxation   74
      in achalasia   305
      in atypical achalasia   314
      in difuse spasm   359
      after destruction of superficial
        receptors   82
      effect of vagotomy   58, 84
      in isolated preparations   91
      manometric characteristics   74
      mechanism   91
      in neonates   381
      in old age   373, 375
      in post-vagotomy dysphagia   368,
        369
      role of adrenergic innervation   91
      after sympathectomy   58
    respiratory pressure variations   46
    rhythmic electrical activity of —   51
    yield pressure   50, *see also* Yield
      pressure
    in Zollinger-Ellison syndrome   54
  pharyngoesophageal (upper esophageal)
    anatomy   6, 40
    in brainstem lesions   402
    deglutition complex   69–71
    electromyographic studies, *see* Electro-
      myography
    in familial dysautonomia   404
    and gastroesophageal reflux   42
    identity with cricopharyngeal muscle
      41, 42
    innervation   81
    location   40
    manometry   396
    mechanism of relaxation   43, 70
    mechanism of tonus   43
    motility disorders
      causes   191
      radiological signs   191
    in neonatal infants   379, 381
    normal radiological appearance   142
    in myasthenia gravis   398
    in ocular myopathy and oculopharyn-
      geal dystrophy   397
    and pathogenesis of hypopharyngeal
      diverticulum   595
    PD profile   259
    in poliomyelitis   403
    in polymyositis   390
    pressure profile   41
    radiological characteristics of cricopha-
      ryngeal indentation   190
    reflex responses   42, 86
    relaxation   300
    respiratory pressure variations   43
      resting pressure   42
      in stiff-man syndrome   404
      voluntary control   42–80
      yield pressure   42
      and Zenker's diverticulum   42
    post-cricoid   41
Spill-over into airways, *see also* Bronchopulmonary complications
    in atresia   620
    causes   108
    diagnostic significance of delay between
      swallow and cough   108
    and dysarthria   109
    and dysphonia   109
    in epidermolysis bullosa dystrophica   825
    in epiphrenic diverticulum   608
    in familial dysautonomia   404
    and foreign body   667
    in hypopharyngeal diverticulum   597
    in myotonic dystrophy   396
    in ocular myopathy and oculopharyngeal
      myopathy   397
    in poliomyelitis   403
    in poliomyositis   390
Spirocerca lupus, involving the esophagus
  839
Splenic vein thrombosis, causing varices
  702
Splenoportography, in patients with esophageal varices   715–717
Spontaneous activity
  in achalasia   307
  in diffuse spasm   358, 364
  in old age   372
Spondylarthrosis, see Osteophytes
Spot film device   120
Spot filming   126
Squamo columnar junction   25, 744
  endoscopic appearance
    in hiatus hernia   766
    in normal subjects   213
  location
    in relation to gastroesophageal sphinc-
      ter   46
    in relation to lower esophageal ring
      584
    in relation to vestibule   766
  localization by PD measurements   257
Squamous-cell carcinoma, *see* Carcinoma
Squamous epithelium
  cell kinetics of —   19
  electron microscopy   21–24
  histochemistry   19–21
  histology   17–19
Squeeze of contraction, technique of measurement   240
Starck dilator   322
Stasis
  in esophagus, *see* Transport, esophageal
  in hypopharynx
    in brainstem lesions   402
    in myasthenia gravis   398
    in myotonic dystrophy   396
    in ocular myopathy and oculopharyn-
      geal myopathy   397

in poliomyelitis 403
in polymyositis 390
Steering-wheel injuries, causing esophagorespiratory fistula 661, 807
Steinert's disease, see Myotonic dystrophy
394–397
Stenosis, benign, see also Obstruction syndrome; Stricture; Stricture syndrome
in achalasia 320
in amyloidosis 835
in benign mucosal pemphigoid 824
distinction between conventional stenosis
and stenosis in lower esophagus lined
with columnar epithelium 535
distinction from esophageal webs and
rings 571, 576, 579, 586
in epidermolysis bullosa dystrophica 825
etiology 795–797
in hypertrophic tuberculosis 553
in intramural diverticulosis 837
and intramural rupture 695
and lower esophageal ring 583, 586, 571
of lower esophageal segment, importance
for the outcome of atresia 622
and Mecholyltest 267
in pancreatitis 839
in pemphigus 823
predisposing to spontaneous rupture
676
after radiation therapy 476
radiological aspects 179
radiological demonstration 134, 137 166
180, 505
radiological distinction between benign
and malignant stenosis 169, 460
in reflux esophagitis 497, 499, 517, 771,
772, 777, 795, 805
in recurrent aphtosis of the esophagus
827
after surgical interventions 796
and syphilis 556, 557
in toxic epidermal neurolysis 826
treatment non-surgical 797–805
"Step effect" 437
Steroids, treatment of corrosive esophagitis
547, 548, 803
Stevens-Johnson syndrome, involving esophagus 827
Stiff-man syndrome, causing dysphagia 404
Stomach as esophageal substitute 785
functional results 791
Stratum spinosum of squamous epithelium,
electronmicroscopy 23
Stricture, see also Obstruction syndrome;
Stenosis; Stricture syndrome
characteristics of pain 107
corrosive 541–549, 795
and esophageal carcinoma 444, 460,
549
incidence 546, 547, 795
predisposing to esophageal carcinoma
444, 549
preventive measures 546, 547
time of onset 542
after esophageal anastomosis 630, 796

in lower esophagus lined with columnar
epithelium 528, 531, 532
vs conventional peptic stenosis 535
in mycosis of esophagus 563
pharyngeal
discriminative symptoms 113
in progressive systemic sclerosis 386
radiological appearance 512
in reflux esophagitis 497, 499, 795
Stricture syndrome, see also Obstruction
syndrome
definition 109
discriminative symptoms 113–118
Stripe, pleuroesophageal, see Line, paraesophageal
Struma, causing down-hill varices 709
Submerged segment 68, 69, 154
see also Abdominal esophagus
Submucosal abscess 551
Submucosal glands 29
Submucosal plexus 36
embryonic development 379
in diffuse spasm 356
Sucking in prematures and infants 379
Swallow, dry,
resulting in globus sensation 410
Swallow-cough, see also Spill-over into airways
in esophagorespiratory fistula 811, 812
in tracheoesophageal fistula 109, 662
Swallowing act
ancillary muscle contractions 65
asymmetric, in brainstem lesions 402
asymmetric passage of bolus through
pharynx 141, 191
in brainstem lesions 402
in bulbar poliomyelitis 402
electromyographic studies 63–65
elicitation of swallowing 76
in familial dysautonomia 404
in fetuses and neonates 379
infantile pattern 65
in motor neuron disease 403
muscles involved in — 63
in myasthenia gravis 398
in myotonic dystrophy 395
normal radiological appearance 141
nervous regulation 75–81
in ocular myopathy and oculopharyngeal
myopathy 397
oral phase 59 62
in Parkinsonism 404
peripheral receptors for initiation of swallowing 76
pharyngeal phase 62
radiological examination 186 192
in thyrotoxicosis 399
timing of deglutitive movements 63
variants
in beer guzzling 63
with viscous material 63
Swallowing incidence 59
Sympathectomy
effect on gastroesophageal sphincter 57, 58
in treatment of achalasia 331, 333

Sympathetic, see Innervation
Syphilis, causing esophagorespiratory fistula
    810
    involving the esophagus 556
Systemic sclerosis, see Progressive systemic
    sclerosis

Tabes, causing swallowing difficulties 402
Tadpole cells as cytological sign of malig-
    nancy 222
Taste buds in upper esophagus 24
Telangiectasia, familial hereditary, causing
    esophageal varices 701
Television fluoroscopy 125
Tender esophagus 112
Tensilon (edrophonium), see Anticholinester-
    ases 398
Tertiary contractions
    in achalasia 300, 307
    in alcoholic neuropathy 408
    causes 362
    definition 59
    in diabetic motility disorders 407
    in diffuse spasm
        manometric examination 358, 359, 364
        radiological examination 356
    in motor neuron disease 403
    in myasthenia gravis 398
    in myotonic dystrophy 396
    in myxedema 399
    in neonates 381
    in ocular myopathy and oculopharyngeal
        myopathy 397, 398
    in old age 372, 373
    in polymyositis 390
    in progressive systemic sclerosis
        manometric examination 387
        radiological examination 387
    in pseudobulbar palsy 403
    radiological appearance 149
Tertiary peristaltic contractions 84
Tetrodotoxin, abolishing peristalsis in isolated
    opossum esophagus 82–85
Thal operation for esophageal stricture 778
    in achalasia 332, 338
    in hiatus hernia
    in post-vagotomy dysphagia 370
    in progressive systemic sclerosis 389
    in reflux esophagitis 518
Third type cells, cytological sign of malign-
    ancy 222
Thoracic esophagus
    motor innervation by vagal nerve 84
Thrush of the esophagus, see Monilial eso-
    phagitis
Thymectomy in myasthenia gravis 398
Thymoma in achalasia 320
Thyroid enlargement, producing enlargement
    of prevertebral space 185, 190
Thyroid tissue in esophagus 841
Thyrotoxicosis and muscle wasting 399
Tonus of pharyngoesophageal sphincter 43
Torulopsis glabrata 559
Toxic epidermal neurolysis, involving eso-
    phagus 826

Trachea
    compression and deviation
        by carcinoma 460
        by fibrovascular polyp 443
        by leiomyoma 436
    invasion by esophageal carcinoma 459
    producing impression on esophagus at
        thoracic inlet 144
Tracheobronchial remnants in esophagus
    840
Tracheoesophageal septum
    in atresia 616
    in laryngotracheoesophageal cleft 646
    in tracheoesophageal fistula 616
Tracheoscopy
    for diagnosis of isolated tracheoesophageal
        fistula 640
Transection of esophagus
    effect on esophageal peristalsis 85
    effect on gastroesophageal sphincter 58
Transitional zone between striated and
    smooth muscle
    deglutitive electrical activity 271
    location 4
    progression of peristalsis in — 73
    young vs old subjects 375
Transmigration of esophageal mucosa, see
    Invagination, esophagogastric
Transmucosal fold
    distinction from lower esophageal ring
        586
Transport
    esophageal 65–67
        in diabetic motility disorders 407
        in diffuse spasm 356, 360
        in familial dysautonomia 404
        in myasthenia gravis 398
        in myotonic dystrophy 396
        in myxedema 399
        in old age 165, 372
        in progressive systemic sclerosis 387
    oral 59–62
    pharyngeal 62
    retrograde 92–93
        see also Belching; Belching (esopha-
            geal); Merycism
    through gastroesophageal sphincter 68
Traumata of the esophagus 661–664
    producing esophagorespiratory fistula
        807–809
Trinitrine, see Nitrites
Tropical splenomegaly, causing varices 701
Trypanosoma 309
Trypsin, in treatment of meat impaction
    672
Tuberculosis 553–555
    causing esophagorespiratory fistula 809,
        815
    causing midesophageal diverticulum 605
Tucker bag for dilatations 323
Tucker-Soulas bougies 802, 804
Tunica adventitia, see Adventitia
Tunica muscularis 30–34
Tuttle test, to detect gastroesophageal reflux
    500

t-Wave of pharyngeal deglutition complex 71
Tylosis palmaris et plantaris, see Keratoderma
Tylosis, predisposing to esophageal carcinoma 444
Typhoid fever, involving the esophagus 352
Tyrosinosis, causing varices 707

Ulcer
    in Crohn's disease 184
    in lower esophagus lined with columnar epithelium (Barrett ulcer) 180, 525, 528, 531, 532, 533
    in midesophageal diverticula 606
    in monilial esophagitis 558
    PD measurements 258
    peptic, in colon used for esophageal replacement 791
    peptic, at squamocolumnar junction (marginal ulcer) 180, 498, 499, 505, 513
    after radiation therapy 476
    radiological aspects 180–184
    radiological distinction from epiphrenic diverticula 608
    syphilitic 556
    tuberculous 553
Ulcerative colitis, involving esophagus 568, 839
Ulcer of duodenum, in pathogenesis of reflux esophagitis 519
Umbilical vein portography, in patients with esophageal varices 717
Upper esophageal sphincter, see Sphincter, pharyngoesophageal
Upside-down stomach 494, 764
Urecholine, in progressive systemic sclerosis 389
Urogenital anomalies in esophageal atresia 620

Vagal nerve, see Nerve
Vagotomy
    effect on esophageal peristalsis 82, 84
    effect on gastroesophageal sphincter 57, 58, 84, 91, 425
    electrical activity after — 67, 84, 270, 271, 282
    post-vagotomy diarrhea after resection of the esophagus 784
    post-vagotomy dysphagia 367–371
    and secondary peristalsis 86
    in treatment of achalasia 331, 333, 338
    in treatment of esophagitis 502
Valleculae 139–146
    stasis of contrast material 191
Valsalva maneuver
    for localization of cricopharyngeal muscle 146
    modified
        for examination of hypopharynx 139, 147, 184, 187
        and lateral pharyngeal diverticulum 591
        during pH measurements 249

Valve mechanism, in gastroesophageal sphincter competence 51
Varices 697–739
    ammonia tolerance test 718
    bleeding 711
        distinction between variceal and other origin 719
        emergency endoscopy 720
        emergency surgical treatment 722, 723, 726
        incidence 711
        influence of variceal size and portal pressure on severity 712
        localization of bleeding site 719
        medical management 720–722
        mortality 711, 712
        pathogenesis 711
        prevention of hepatic encephalopathy 720
        results of different types of therapy 723–725
        from solitary point in lower esophagus 699, 711
        symptoms 712
        treatment by balloon tamponade 721
        treatment by ganglionic blocking agents 721
        treatment by gastric cooling 721
        treatment by intraarterial infusion of vasoactive drugs 721
        treatment by vasopressive agents 720
    causes
        acute hepatitis 704
        arteriovenous shunt in portal system 701
        Budd-Chiari syndrome 708
        Banti syndrome 699–701
        carcinoma of gastroesophageal region 709
        cirrhosis of liver 705–708
        congenital hepatic fibrosis 703
        congestive heart failure 706, 709
        fatty liver 704
        granulomatous diseases 703
        hepatic schistosomiasis 702
        hydatid cysts 703
        Kupffer cell hypertrophy 704
        liver metastasis 703
        myeloproliferative diseases 703
        obstruction of vena cava superior 709
        occurring without portal hypertension 709
        partial nodular transformation 708
        polycystic liver disease 703
        portal vein thrombosis and compression 701
        primary biliary cirrhosis 704
        retroperitoneal fibrosis 835
        splenic vein thrombosis 702
        tropical splenomegaly 701
        veno-occlusive disease 708
        Wilson's disease 704–707
    in childhood 701, 703, 706

Varices — *cont.*
   cineradiography in diagnosis   713
   detection rates by different diagnostic
      techniques   719
   diagnostic approach when bleeding from
      varices is suspected   719
   esophagoscopy
      appearance   714
      in diagnosis of bleeding point   715
      distinction from mucosal folds   714,
         715
      grading   714
   etiology and pathogenesis   699–711
   incidence   699
   intrahepatic or extrahepatic causes   699
   presinusoidal or postsinusoidal causes
      699
   radiological aspects   173
   radiological diagnosis   712, 715
      influence of esophageal contraction on
         visualization   713
      influence of posture on visualization
         713
      measures to improve visualization
         713
      special procedures   192–194
   sclerosing injection for esophageal varices
      728
   splenoportography   715–717
   subepithelial localization in distal eso-
      phagus   697
   surgical treatment   722–728
      elective treatment   724, 727
      emergency procedures   722, 723, 726
      prophylactic operations   727
      thoracic duct drainage   728
      transumbilical portal decompression
         728
   therapy   720–728
   umbilical vein portography   717
   venous drainage of esophagus   697–699
Vascular anomalies
   and esophageal atresia   616, 621–623
   producing impression on thoracic eso-
      phagus   175
Vascular rings
   causing tracheoesophageal compression
      649–660
Vasomotor center, interference with deglutitive center   80
Vasopressine, in treatment of bleeding esophageal varices   720, 721
Venae comitantes nervi vagi   10
Venoocclusive disease, causing varices   708
Venous drainage, after colonic interposition
   9–11, 697–699, 788, 789
Venous impression
   postcricoid   139, 142
      distinction from upper esophageal web
         143, 576
Venous plexuses   10, 697–699
   at gastroesophageal junction   10, 35
Verrucous squamous cell carcinoma   487
Vestibule
   anatomy   7

endoscopic appearance in hiatus hernia
   766
location in relation to lower esophageal
   web and ring   581, 585
radiological appearance   148, 154
   in hiatal hernia   496, 497
relation to manometrical and radiological
   points of reference   68, 69
subepithelial venous drainage   10–35
Video recording   131–133
Vignetting   124, 126
Vigorous achalasia   296, 307
Viral involvement of the esophagus   551
Vitamine B_{12} deficiency,
   false positive cytological diagnosis of
      cancer   224, 227
Volvulus, complicating paraesophageal hernia
   764
Vomiting
   mechanism   92
   and Mallory-Weiss syndrome   690
   vs merycism   416
   and reflux esophagitis   521
   and spontaneous rupture   675
   and stricture formation   795
V-shaped defect in posterior esophageal wall
   4
V-sign, of Nacleiro, in rupture of esophagus
   678

Wallenberg's syndrome, causing pharyngoesophageal disorders   402
Wallerian degeneration of vagal nerve
   in achalasia   290
   in diffuse spasm   356
War gass, causing esophageal dilatation
   313
Washing products, causing corrosive esophagitis   539
Water-wheel murmer in esophagopericardial
   fistula   815
Webs and rings   571–589, see also Patter-
   son-Kelly syndrome
   in achalasia   320
   definition   572
   distinction between web and ring   571
   division of esophagus into 3 segments in
      relation to webs and rings   572
   middle esophagus   577–579
      in infancy   578
      symptoms and signs   578
      treatment   579
   lower esophageal   579–581
      distinction from lower esophageal ring
         572, 579, 580, 581
      distinction from middle esophageal
         web   580
      location in relation to vestibule
         581
   pharyngeal
      discriminative symptoms   114
      radiological distinction between web,
         stenosis and small contraction   571
      technique of radiological examination
         187, 571

upper esophageal (postcricoid)
    clinical features   574
    definition   572
    distinction from postcricoid venous
        impression   143
    endoscopic appearance   576
    etiology and pathogenesis   573
    geographical distribution   573
    incidence   573
    in infancy   575
    and iron deficiency   573, 574
    pathology   574
    radiological examination   575
    and riboflavin deficiency   573
    and Sjögren's syndrome
    treatment   577
Wegener's syndrome   810
Whisky, effect on esophageal motility
    408
White clay-pipestem fibrosis   702
Wilson's disease, causing varices   704–707
Willis' loop, importance in gastroesophageal
    sphincteric competence   51

Wolf
    A-ring   7, 64, 68, 154, 585
        in achalasia   304
        in hiatus hernia   496, 497
        radiological aspect   180
    B-ring   68, 69, 154
        radiological aspect   180

Xenodiagnosis of Chagas' disease   309

Yield pressure   238, 239
    in gastroesophageal sphincter   50
        correlation with gastroesophageal re-
            flux   50, 239, 422, 424, 500, 515
    in paryngoesophageal sphincter   42
Yperite, causing esophageal dilatation   313

"Zelltupfsonde" for cytology   219
Zenker's diverticulum, see Diverticulum,
    hypopharyngeal
Z-line, see Squamocolumnar junction
Zollinger-Ellison syndrome
    and gastroesophageal sphincter   54